Lecture Notes in Computer S

Commenced Publication in 1973
Founding and Former Series Editors:
Gerhard Goos, Juris Hartmanis, and Jan van Leeuwen

WITHDRAWN
WRIGHT STATE UNIVERSITY LIBRARIES

Editorial Board

David Hutchison
Lancaster University, UK

Takeo Kanade
Carnegie Mellon University, Pittsburgh, PA, USA

Josef Kittler
University of Surrey, Guildford, UK

Jon M. Kleinberg
Cornell University, Ithaca, NY, USA

Friedemann Mattern
ETH Zurich, Switzerland

John C. Mitchell
Stanford University, CA, USA

Moni Naor
Weizmann Institute of Science, Rehovot, Israel

Oscar Nierstrasz
University of Bern, Switzerland

C. Pandu Rangan
Indian Institute of Technology, Madras, India

Bernhard Steffen
University of Dortmund, Germany

Madhu Sudan
Massachusetts Institute of Technology, MA, USA

Demetri Terzopoulos
University of California, Los Angeles, CA, USA

Doug Tygar
University of California, Berkeley, CA, USA

Moshe Y. Vardi
Rice University, Houston, TX, USA

Gerhard Weikum
Max-Planck Institute of Computer Science, Saarbruecken, Germany

WITHDRAWN
WRIGHT STATE UNIVERSITY LIBRARIES

Nicholas Ayache   Sébastien Ourselin
Anthony Maeder (Eds.)

Medical Image Computing and Computer-Assisted Intervention – MICCAI 2007

10th International Conference
Brisbane, Australia, October 29 – November 2, 2007
Proceedings, Part I

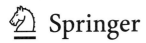 Springer

Volume Editors

Nicholas Ayache
INRIA, Asclepios Project-Team
2004 Route des Lucioles, 06902 Sophia-Antipolis, France
E-mail: nicholas.ayache@inria.fr

Sébastien Ourselin
Anthony Maeder
CSIRO ICT Centre, e-Health Research Centre
20/300 Adelaide St., Brisbane, Queensland 4000, Australia
E-mail: {sebastien.ourselin, anthony.maeder}@csiro.au

Library of Congress Control Number: 2007937392

CR Subject Classification (1998): I.5, I.4, I.3.5-8, I.2.9-10, J.3, J.6

LNCS Sublibrary: SL 6 – Image Processing, Computer Vision, Pattern Recognition, and Graphics

ISSN   0302-9743
ISBN-10 3-540-75756-2 Springer Berlin Heidelberg New York
ISBN-13 978-3-540-75756-6 Springer Berlin Heidelberg New York

This work is subject to copyright. All rights are reserved, whether the whole or part of the material is
concerned, specifically the rights of translation, reprinting, re-use of illustrations, recitation, broadcasting,
reproduction on microfilms or in any other way, and storage in data banks. Duplication of this publication
or parts thereof is permitted only under the provisions of the German Copyright Law of September 9, 1965,
in its current version, and permission for use must always be obtained from Springer. Violations are liable
to prosecution under the German Copyright Law.

Springer is a part of Springer Science+Business Media

springer.com

© Springer-Verlag Berlin Heidelberg 2007
Printed in Germany

Typesetting: Camera-ready by author, data conversion by Scientific Publishing Services, Chennai, India
Printed on acid-free paper   SPIN: 12175383   06/3180   5 4 3 2 1 0

Preface

The 10th International Conference on Medical Imaging and Computer Assisted Intervention, MICCAI 2007, was held at the Brisbane Convention and Exhibition Centre, South Bank, Brisbane, Australia from 29th October to 2nd November 2007.

MICCAI has become a premier international conference in this domain, with in-depth papers on the multidisciplinary fields of biomedical image computing, computer assisted intervention and medical robotics. The conference brings together biological scientists, clinicians, computer scientists, engineers, mathematicians, physicists and other interested researchers and offers them a forum to exchange ideas in these exciting and rapidly growing fields.

The conference is both very selective and very attractive: this year we received a record number of 637 submissions from 35 countries and 6 continents, from which 237 papers were selected for publication. Some interesting facts about the distribution of submitted and accepted papers are shown graphically at the end of this preface.

A number of modifications were introduced into the selection process this year.

1. An enlarged Program Committee of 71 members was recruited by the Program Chair and Co-chair, to get a larger body of expertise and geographical coverage.
2. New key words regrouped within 7 new categories were introduced to describe the content of the submissions and the expertise of the reviewers.
3. Each submitted paper was assigned to 3 Program Committee members whose responsibility it was to assign each paper to 3 external experts (outside of the Program Committee membership) who provided scores and detailed reports in a double blind procedure.
4. Program Committee members provided a set of normalized scores for the whole set of papers for which they were responsible (typically 27 papers). They did this using the external reviews and their own reading of the papers and had to complete missing reviews themselves. Program Committee members eventually had to provide a recommendation for acceptance of the top 35% of their assigned papers.
5. During a 2 day meeting of about 20 members of the Program Committee in Sophia-Antipolis, France, borderline papers were examined carefully and the final set of papers was accepted to appear in the LNCS proceedings. A top list of about 100 papers was scrutinized to provide the Program Chair and Co-chair with a list of 54 potential podium presentations.
6. From this list, the Program Chair and Co-chair selected 38 podium presentations to create a program with a reasonable number of oral sessions and spread of content.

7. Because 199 excellent contributions would be presented as posters, it was decided in consultation with the MICCAI Society Board to augment the time allocated to the poster sessions, and replace the oral poster teasers by continuous video teasers run on large screens during the conference.

The selection procedure was very selective, and many good papers remained among the 400 rejected. We received 9 factual complaints from the authors of rejected papers. A subcommittee of the Program Committee treated all of them equally, checking carefully that no mistake had been made during the selection procedure. In a few cases, an additional review was requested from an independent Program Committee member. In the end, all the original decisions were maintained, but some additional information was provided to the authors to better explain the final decision.

Seven MICCAI Young Scientist Awards were presented by the MICCAI Society on the last day of the conference. The selection was made before the conference by nominating automatically the 21 eligible papers with the highest normalized scores (provided by the Program Committee during the reviewing procedure), and regrouping them into the 7 main categories of the conference. A subgroup of the Program Committee had to vote to elect one paper out of 3 in each category.

The 2007 MedIA-MICCAI Prize was offered by Elsevier to the first author of an outstanding article in the special issue of the Medical Image Analysis Journal dedicated to the previous conference MICCAI 2006. The selection was organized by the guest-editors of this special issue.

We want to thank wholeheartedly all Program Committee members for their exceptional work, as well as the numerous external expert reviewers (who are listed on the next pages). We should also acknowledge the substantial contribution made towards the successful execution of MICCAI 2007 by the BioMedical Image Analysis Laboratory team at the CSIRO ICT Centre / e-Health Research Centre.

It was our pleasure to welcome MICCAI 2007 attendees in Brisbane. This was the first time the conference had been held in Australia, indeed only the second time outside of Europe/North America, the other being MICCAI 2002 in Japan. This trend will continue with MICCAI 2010, which is planned for Beijing. The vibrant sub-tropical river city of Brisbane with its modern style and world-class conference venue was a popular choice and a convenient point of departure for delegates who took the opportunity while there to see more of the Australian outback.

We thank our two invited keynote speakers, Prof. Peter Hunter from the Bioengineering Institute at the University of Auckland, New Zealand, and Prof. Stuart Crozier from Biomedical Engineering at the University of Queensland, Brisbane, whose excellent presentations were a highlight of the conference. We also acknowledge with much gratitude the contributions of Terry Peters, MICCAI 2007 General Co-Chair, whose strong connection with the MICCAI Society and past MICCAI conferences proved invaluable to us. We also note our thanks to our sponsors, without whose financial assistance the event would have been a far lesser one.

We look forward to welcoming you to MICCAI 2008, to be held 4-8 September in New York City, USA, and MICCAI 2009, scheduled to be held in London, UK.

October 2007

Nicholas Ayache
Sébastien Ourselin
Anthony Maeder

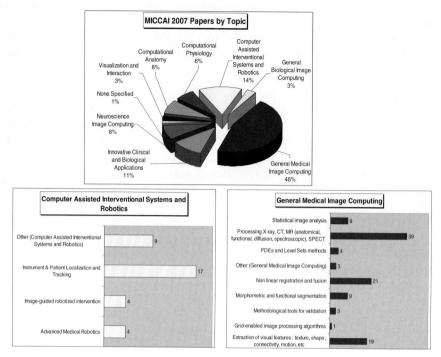

Fig. 1. View at a glance of MICCAI 2007 accepted submissions based on the declared primary keyword. A total of 237 full papers were presented.

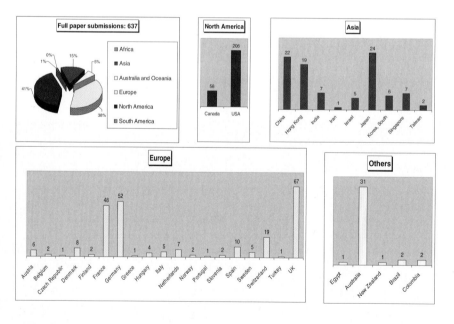

Fig. 2. Distribution of MICCAI 2007 submissions (637 in total) by continent

MICCAI Young Scientist Awards

The MICCAI Young Scientist Award is a prize of US$500 awarded to the first author (in person) for the best paper in a particular topic area, as judged by reviewing and presentation (oral or poster). At MICCAI 2007, up to 7 prizes were available, in the topic areas publicised in the conference CFP:

1. General Medical Image Computing
2. Computer Assisted Intervention Systems and Robotics
3. Visualization and Interaction
4. General Biological and Neuroscience Image Computing
5. Computational Anatomy
6. Computational Physiology
7. Innovative Clinical and Biological Applications

All current first author students and early career scientists attending MICCAI 2007 were eligible. The awards were announced and presented at the closing session of the conference on Thursday, 1st November 2007.

MICCAI 2005 Student Awards

Image Segmentation and Analysis: Pingkun Yan, "MRA Image Segmentation with Capillary Active Contour"

Image Registration: Ashraf Mohamed, "Deformable Registration of Brain Tumor Images via a Statistical Model of Tumor Induced Deformation"

Computer-Assisted Interventions and Robotics: Henry C. Lin, "Automatic Detection and Segmentation of Robot Assisted Surgical Motions"

Simulation and Visualization: Peter Savadjiev, "3D Curve Inference for Diffusion MRI Regularization"

Clinical Application: Srinivasan Rajagopalan, "Schwarz Meets Schwann: Design and Fabrication of Biomorphic Tissue Engineering Scaffolds"

MICCAI 2006 Student Awards

Image Segmentation and Registration: Delphine Nain, "Shape-Driven 3D Segmentation Using Spherical Wavelets"

Image Analysis: Karl Sjöstrand, "The Entire Regularization Path for the Support Vector Domain Description"

Simulation and Visualization: Andrew W. Dowsey, "Motion-Compensated MR Valve Imaging with COMB Tag Tracking and Super-Resolution Enhancement"

Computer-Assisted Interventions and Robotics: Paul M. Novotny, "GPU Based Real-Time Instrument Tracking with Three Dimensional Ultrasound"

Clincial Applications: Jian Zhang, "A Pilot Study of Robot-Assisted Cochlear Implant Surgery Using Steerable Electrode Arrays"

The 2007 MedIA-MICCAI Prize

This prize is awarded each year by Elsevier to the first author of an outstanding article of the previous MICCAI conference, which is published in the MICCAI special issue of the Medical Image Analysis Journal.

In 2006, the prize was awarded to T. Vercauteren, first author of the article:

Vercauteren, T., Perchant, A., Pennec, X., Malandain, G., Ayache, N.: Robust mosaicing with correction of motion distortions and tissue deformations for in vivo fibered microscopy. Med. Image Anal. 10(5), 673–692 (2006)

In 2005, the prize was awarded to D. Burschka and M. Jackowski who are the first authors of the articles:

Burschka, D., Li, M., Ishii, M., Taylor, R.H., Hager, G.D.: Scale invariant registration of monucular endoscopic images to CT-Scans for sinus surgery. Med. Image Anal. 9(5), 413–426 (2005)

Jackowski, M., Kao, C.Y., Qiu, M., Constable, R.T., Staib, L.H.: White matter tractography by anisotropic wave front evolution and diffusion tensor imaging. Med. Image Anal. 9(5), 427–440 (2005)

Organization

Executive Committee

General Chair   Anthony Maeder (CSIRO, Australia)
General Co-chair   Terry Peters (Robarts Research Institute,
                            Canada)
Program Chair   Nicholas Ayache (INRIA, France)
Program Co-chair   Sébastien Ourselin (CSIRO, Australia)

Program Committee

Elsa Angelini (ENST, Paris, France)
Simon R. Arridge (University College London, UK)
Leon Axel (University Medical Centre, USA)
Christian Barillot (IRISA, Rennes, France)
Margrit Betke (Boston University, USA)
Elizabeth Bullitt (University of North Carolina, Chapel Hill , USA)
Albert Chung (Hong Kong University of Science and Technology, China)
Ela Claridge (The University of Birmingham, UK)
Stuart Crozier (University of Queensland, Australia)
Christos Davatzikos (University of Pennsylvania, USA)
Marleen de Bruijne (University of Copenhagen, Denmark)
Rachid Deriche (INRIA, Sophia Antipolis, France)
Etienne Dombre (CNRS, Montpellier, France)
James S. Duncan (Yale University, USA)
Gary Egan (Howard Florey Institute, Australia)
Randy Ellis (Queens University, Canada)
Gabor Fichtinger (Johns Hopkins University, USA)
Alejandro Frangi (Pompeu Fabra University, Barcelona, Spain)
Guido Gerig (University of North Carolina, Chapel Hill, USA)
Polina Golland (Massachusetts Institute of Technology, USA)
Miguel Angel Gonzalez Ballester (University of Bern, Switzerland)
Richard Hartley (Australian National University, Australia)
David Hawkes (University College London, UK)
Pheng Ann Heng (The Chinese University of Hong Kong, China)
Robert Howe (Harvard University, USA)
Peter Hunter (The University of Auckland, New Zealand)
Tianzi Jiang (The Chinese Academy of Sciences, China)
Sarang Joshi (University of Utah, USA)

Leo Joskowicz (The Hebrew University of Jerusalem, Israel)
Hans Knustsson (Linkoping University, Sweden)
Rasmus Larsen (Technical University of Denmark, Denmark)
Boudewijn Lelieveldt (Leiden University Medical Centre, Netherlands)
Cristian Lorenz (Philips, Hamburg, Germany)
Frederik Maes (Katholieke Universiteit Leuven, Belgium)
Gregoire Malandain (INRIA, Sophia Antipolis, France)
Jean-Francois Mangin (CEA, SHFJ, Orsay, France)
Dimitris Metaxas (Rutgers University, New Jersey, USA)
Kensaku Mori (Mori Nagoya University, Japan)
Nassir Navab (TUM, Munich, Germany)
Poul Nielsen (The University of Auckland, New Zealand)
Wiro Niessen (Erasmus Medical School, Rotterdam, Netherlands)
Alison Noble (Oxford University, UK)
Jean-Christophe Olivo-Marin (Institut Pasteur, Paris, France)
Nikos Paragios (Ecole Centrale de Paris, France)
Xavier Pennec (INRIA, Sophia Antipolis, France)
Franjo Pernus (University of Ljubljana, Slovenia)
Josien Pluim (University Medical Center, Utrecht, Netherlands)
Jean-Baptiste Poline (CEA, SHFJ, Orsay, France)
Jerry L. Prince (Johns Hopkins University, USA)
Richard A. Robb (Mayo Clinic, College of Medicine, Rochester, Minnesota, USA)
Daniel Rueckert (Imperial College, London, UK)
Tim Salcudean (The University of British Columbia, Canada)
Yoshinobu Sato (Osaka University, Japan)
Achim Schweikard (Institute for Robotics and Cognitive Systems, Germany)
Pengcheng Shi (Hong Kong University of Science and Technology, China)
Stephen Smith (Oxford University, UK)
Lawrence Staib (Yale University, USA)
Colin Studholme (University of California, San Francisco, USA)
Gabor Székely (ETH, Zurich, Switzerland)
Russell Taylor (Johns Hopkins University, USA)
Jean-Philippe Thiran (EPFL, Lausanne, Switzerland)
Jocelyne Troccaz (CNRS, Grenoble, France)
Bram van Ginneken (University Medical Center, Utrecht, Netherlands)
Koen Van Leemput (HUS, Helsinki, Finland)
Baba Vemuri (University of Florida, USA)
Simon Warfield (Harvard University, USA)
Sandy Wells (Massachusetts Institute of Technology, USA)
Carl-Fredrik Westin (Westin Harvard University, USA)
Ross Whitaker (University of Utah, USA)
Chenyang Xu (Siemens Corporate Research, USA)
Guang Zhong Yang (Imperial College, London, UK)

MICCAI Board

Nicholas Ayache, INRIA, Sophia Antipolis, France
Alan Colchester, University of Kent, Canterbury, UK
James Duncan, Yale University, New Haven, Connecticut, USA
Gabor Fichtinger, Johns Hopkins University, Baltimore, Maryland, USA
Guido Gerig, University of North Carolina, Chapel Hill, North Carolina, USA
Anthony Maeder, University of Queensland, Brisbane, Australia
Dimitris Metaxas, Rutgers University, Piscataway Campus, New Jersey, USA
Nassir Navab, Technische Universität, Munich, Germany
Mads Nielsen, IT University of Copenhagen, Copenhagen, Denmark
Alison Noble, University of Oxford, Oxford, UK
Terry Peters, Robarts Research Institute, London, Ontario, Canada
Richard Robb, Mayo Clinic College of Medicine, Rochester, Minnesota, USA

MICCAI Society

Society Officers

President and Board Chair   Alan Colchester
Executive Director   Richard Robb
Executive Secretary   Nicholas Ayache
Treasurer   Terry Peters
Elections Officer   Karl Heinz Hoehne

Society Staff

Membership Coordinator   Gabor Székely, ETH, Zurich, Switzerland
Publication Coordinator   Nobuhiko Hata, Brigham and Women's
                               Hospital, Boston, USA
Communications Coordinator   Kirby Vosburgh, CIMIT, Boston, USA
Industry Relations Coordinator Tina Kapur, Brigham and Women's Hospital,
                               Boston, USA

Local Planning Committee

Sponsors and Exhibitors   Oscar Acosta-Tamayo
Registration and VIP Liaison   Tony Adriaansen
Tutorials and Workshops   Pierrick Bourgeat
Posters   Hans Frimmel, Olivier Salvado
Social Events   Justin Boyle
Technical Proceedings Support Jason Dowling
Professional Society Liaison   Brian Lovell
Webmaster   Jason Pickersgill & Josh Passenger
Student & Travel Awards   Olivier Salvado

Sponsors

CSIRO ICT Centre
e-Health Research Centre
Northern Digital, Inc.
Medtronic, Inc.
The Australian Pattern Recognition Society
CSIRO Preventative Health Flagship
Siemens Corporate Research
GE Global Research

Reviewers

Abend, Alan
Abolmaesumi, Purang
Acar, Burak
Acosta Tamayo, Oscar
Acton, Scott T.
Adali, Tulay
Aja-Fernández, Santiago
Alexander, Daniel
Allen, Peter
Alterovitz, Ron
Amini, Amir
An, Jungha
Andersson, Mats
Antiga, Luca
Ardekani, Babak
Ashburner, John
Atkins, Stella
Atkinson, David
Avants, Brian
Awate, Suyash
Aylward, Stephen
Azar, Fred S.
Azzabou, Noura
Babalola, Kolawole
Bach Cuadra, Meritxell
Baillet, Sylvain
Bajcsy, Ruzena
Bansal, Ravi
Bardinet, Eric
Barmpoutis, Angelos
Barratt, Dean
Bartoli, Adrien

Bartz, Dirk
Basser, Peter
Batchelor, Philip
Baumann, Michael
Bazin, Pierre-Louis
Beckmann, Christian
Beichel, Reinhard
Bello, Fernando
Benali, Habib
Berger, Marie-Odile
Bhalerao, Abhir
Bharkhada, Deepak
Bhatia, Kanwal
Bilston, Lynne
Birkfellner, Wolfgang
Bischof, Horst
Blanquer, Ignacio
Blezek, Daniel
Bloch, Isabelle
Bockenbach, Olivier
Boctor, Emad
Bodensteiner, Christoph
Bogunovic, Hrvoje
Bosch, Johan
Botha, Charl
Bouix, Sylvain
Boukerroui, Djamal
Bourgeat, Pierrick
Bresson, Xavier
Brummer, Marijn
Bucki, Marek
Buehler, Katja

Buelow, Thomas
Bueno Garcia, Gloria
Buie, Damien
Buzug, Thorsten
Caan, Matthan
Cai, Wenli
Calhoun, Vince
Camara, Oscar
Cameron, Bruce
Cammoun, Leila
Camp, Jon
Cardenas, Valerie
Carneiro, Gustavo
Carson, Paul
Cates, Joshua
Cathier, Pascal
Cattin, Philippe
Cavusoglu, Cenk
Celler, Anna
Chakravarty, Mallar
Chaney, Edward
Chang, Sukmoon
Chappelow, Jonathan
Chefd'hotel, Christophe
Chen, Jian
Chen, Ting
Chi, Ying
Chinzei, Kiyoyuki
Chiu, Bernard
Christensen, Gary
Chua, Joselito
Chui, Chee Kong
Chui, Yim Pan
Chung, Adrian
Chung, Moo
Chung, Pau-Choo
Cinquin, Philippe
Ciuciu, Philippe
Clarysse, Patrick
Clatz, Olivier
Cleary, Kevin
Cois, Constantine
Collins, Louis
Collins, David
Colliot, Olivier

Commowick, Olivier
Cootes, Tim
Corso, Jason
Cotin, Stephane
Coulon, Olivier
Coupe, Pierrick
Crouch, Jessica
Crum, William
D'Agostino, Emiliano
Dam, Erik
Dan, Ippeita
Darkner, Sune
Dauguet, Julien
Davis, Brad
Dawant, Benoit
De Craene, Mathieu
Deguchi, Daisuke
Dehghan, Ehsan
Delingette, Hervé
DeLorenzo, Christine
Deng, Xiang
Desai, Jaydev
Descoteaux, Maxime
Dey, Joyoni
Diamond, Solomon Gilbert
Dieterich, Sonja
Dijkstra, Jouke
Dillenseger, Jean-Louis
DiMaio, Simon
Dirk, Loeckx
Dodel, Silke
Dornheim, Jana
Dorval, Thierry
Douiri, Abdel
Duan, Qi
Duay, Valérie
Dubois, Marie-Dominique
Duchesne, Simon
Dupont, Pierre
Durrleman, Stanley
Ecabert, Olivier
Edwards, Philip
Eggers, Holger
Ehrhardt, Jan
El-Baz, Ayman

Ellingsen, Lotta
Elson, Daniel
Ersbøll, Bjarne
Fahmi, Rachid
Fan, Yong
Farag, Aly
Farman, Allan
Fenster, Aaron
Fetita, Catalin
Feuerstein, Marco
Fieten, Lorenz
Fillard, Pierre
Fiorini, Paolo
Fischer, Bernd
Fischer, Gregory
Fitzpatrick, J. Michael
Fleig, Oliver
Fletcher, P. Thomas
Florack, Luc
Florin, Charles
Forsyth, David
Fouard, Celine
Freiman, Moti
Freysinger, Wolfgang
Fripp, Jurgen
Frouin, Frédérique
Funka-Lea, Gareth
Gangloff, Jacques
Garnero, Line
Gaser, Christian
Gassert, Roger
Gavrilescu, Maria
Gee, James
Gee, Andrew
Genovesio, Auguste
Gerard, Olivier
Ghebreab, Sennay
Gibaud, Bernard
Giger, Maryellen
Gilhuijs, Kenneth
Gilmore, John
Glory, Estelle
Gobbi, David
Goh, Alvina
Goksel, Orcun

Gong, Qiyong
Goodlett, Casey
Goris, Michael
Grady, Leo
Grau, Vicente
Greenspan, Hayit
Gregoire, Marie
Grimson, Eric
Groher, Martin
Grunert, Ronny
Gu, Lixu
Guerrero, Julian
Guimond, Alexandre
Hager, Gregory D
Hahn, Horst
Hall, Matt
Hamarneh, Ghassan
Han, Xiao
Hansen, Klaus
Hanson, Dennis
Harders, Matthias
Hata, Nobuhiko
He, Huiguang
He, Yong
Heckemann, Rolf
Heintzmann, Rainer
Hellier, Pierre
Ho, HonPong
Hodgson, Antony
Hoffmann, Kenneth
Holden, Mark
Holdsworth, David
Holmes, David
Hornegger, Joachim
Horton, Ashley
Hu, Mingxing
Hu, Qingmao
Hua, Jing
Huang, Junzhou
Huang, Xiaolei
Huang, Heng
Hutton, Brian
Iglesias, Juan Eugenio
Jäger, Florian
Jain, Ameet

James, Adam
Janke, Andrew
Jannin, Pierre
Jaramaz, Branislav
Jenkinson, Mark
Jin, Ge
John, Nigel
Johnston, Leigh
Jolly, Marie-Pierre
Jomier, Julien
Jordan, Petr
Ju, Tao
Kabus, Sven
Kakadiaris, Ioannis
Karjalainen, Pasi
Karssemeijer, Nico
Karwoski, Ron
Kazanzides, Peter
Keil, Andreas
Kerdok, Amy
Keriven, Renaud
Kettenbach, Joachim
Khamene, Ali
Kier, Christian
Kikinis, Ron
Kindlmann, Gordon
Kiraly, Atilla
Kiss, Gabriel
Kitasaka, Takayuki
Knoerlein, Benjamin
Kodipaka, Santhosh
Konietschke, Rainer
Konukoglu, Ender
Korb, Werner
Koseki, Yoshihiko
Kozerke, Sebastian
Kozic, Nina
Krieger, Axel
Kriegeskorte, Nikolaus
Krissian, Karl
Krol, Andrzej
Kronreif, Gernot
Krupa, Alexandre
Krupinski, Elizabeth
Krut, Sébastien

Kukuk, Markus
Kuroda, Kagayaki
Kurtcuoglu, Vartan
Kwon, Dong-Soo
Kybic, Jan
Lai, Shang-Hong
Lambrou, Tryphon
Lamperth, Michael
Lasser, Tobias
Law, W.K.
Lazar, Mariana
Lee, Su-Lin
Lee, Bryan
Leemans, Alexander
Lekadir, Karim
Lenglet, Christophe
Lepore, Natasha
Leung, K. Y. Esther
Levman, Jacob
Li, Kang
Li, Shuo
Li, Ming
Liao, Shu
Liao, Rui
Lieby, Paulette
Likar, Bostjan
Lin, Fuchun
Linguraru, Marius George
Linte, Cristian
Liu, Yanxi
Liu, Huafeng
Liu, Jimin
Lohmann, Gabriele
Loog, Marco
Lorenzen, Peter
Lueders, Eileen
Lum, Mitchell
Ma, Burton
Macq, Benoit
Madabhushi, Anant
Manduca, Armando
Manniesing, Rashindra
Marchal, Maud
Marchesini, Renato
Marsland, Stephen

Martel, Sylvain
Martens, Volker
Martí, Robert
Martin-Fernandez, Marcos
Masood, Khalid
Masutani, Yoshitaka
McGraw, Tim
Meas-Yedid, Vannary
Meier, Dominik
Meikle, Steve
Melonakos, John
Mendoza, Cesar
Merlet, Jean-Pierre
Merloz, Philippe
Mewes, Andrea
Meyer, Chuck
Miller, James
Milles, Julien
Modersitzki, Jan
Mohamed, Ashraf
Monahan, Emily
Montagnat, Johan
Montillo, Albert
Morandi, Xavier
Moratal, David
Morel, Guillaume
Mueller, Klaus
Mulkern, Robert
Murgasova, Maria
Murphy, Philip
Nakamoto, Masahiko
Nash, Martyn
Navas, K.A.
Nelson, Bradley
Nichols, Thomas
Nicolau, Stephane
Niemeijer, Meindert
Nikou, Christophoros
Nimsky, Christopher
Novotny, Paul
Nowinski, Wieslaw
Nuyts, Johan
O'Donnell, Lauren
Ogier, Arnaud
Okamura, Allison

O'Keefe, Graeme
Olabarriaga, Silvia
Ólafsdóttir, Hildur
Oliver, Arnau
Olsen, Ole Fogh
Oost, Elco
Otake, Yoshito
Ozarslan, Evren
Padfield, Dirk
Padoy, Nicolas
Palaniappan, Kannappan
Pang, Wai-Man
Papademetris, Xenios
Papadopoulo, Théo
Patriciu, Alexandru
Patronik, Nicholas
Pavlidis, Ioannis
Pechaud, Mickael
Peine, William
Peitgen, Heinz-Otto
Pekar, Vladimir
Penney, Graeme
Perperidis, Dimitrios
Peters, Terry
Petit, Yvan
Pham, Dzung
Phillips, Roger
Pichon, Eric
Pitiot, Alain
Pizer, Stephen
Plaskos, Christopher
Pock, Thomas
Pohl, Kilian Maria
Poignet, Philippe
Poupon, Cyril
Prager, Richard
Prastawa, Marcel
Prause, Guido
Preim, Bernhard
Prima, Sylvain
Qian, Zhen
Qian, Xiaoning
Raaymakers, Bas
Radaelli, Alessandro
Rajagopal, Vijayaraghavan

Rajagopalan, Srinivasan
Rasche, Volker
Ratnanather, Tilak
Raucent, Benoit
Reinhardt, Joseph
Renaud, Pierre
Restif, Christophe
Rettmann, Maryam
Rexilius, Jan
Reyes, Mauricio
Rhode, Kawal
Rittscher, Jens
Robles-Kelly, Antonio
Rodriguez y Baena, Ferdinando
Rohlfing, Torsten
Rohling, Robert
Rohr, Karl
Rose, Chris
Rosen, Jacob
Rousseau, François
Rousson, Mikael
Ruiz-Alzola, Juan
Russakoff, Daniel
Rydell, Joakim
Sabuncu, Mert Rory
Sabuncu, Mert
Sadowsky, Ofri
Salvado, Olivier
San Jose Estepar, Raul
Sanchez Castro, Francisco Javier
Santamaria-Pang, Alberto
Schaap, Michiel
Schilham, Arnold
Schlaefer, Alexander
Schmid, Volker
Schnabel, Julia
Schwarz, Tobias
Seemann, Gunnar
Segonne, Florent
Sermesant, Maxime
Shah, Shishir
Sharma, Aayush
Sharp, Peter
Sharp, Greg
Shekhar, Raj

Shen, Hong
Shen, Dinggang
Shimizu, Akinobu
Siddiqi, Kaleem
Sielhorst, Tobias
Sijbers, Jan
Sinha, Shantanu
Sjöstrand, Karl
Sled, John
Smith, Keith
Soler, Luc
Sonka, Milan
Stewart, Charles
Stewart, James
Stindel, Eric
Stoel, Berend
Stoianovici, Dan
Stoll, Jeff
Stoyanov, Danail
Styner, Martin
Suetens, Paul
Sugita, Naohiko
Suinesiaputra, Avan
Sun, Yiyong
Sundar, Hari
Szczerba, Dominik
Szilagyi, Laszlo
Tagare, Hemant
Talbot, Hugues
Talib, Haydar
Talos, Ion-Florin
Tanner, Christine
Tao, Xiaodong
Tarte, Segolene
Tasdizen, Tolga
Taylor, Zeike
Taylor, Jonathan
Tek, Huseyin
Tendick, Frank
Terzopoulos, Demetri
Thévenaz, Philippe
Thirion, Bertrand
Tieu, Kinh
Todd-Pokropek, Andrew
Todman, Alison

Toews, Matthew
Tohka, Jussi
Tomazevic, Dejan
Tonet, Oliver
Tong, Shan
Tosun, Duygu
Traub, Joerg
Trejos, Ana Luisa
Tsao, Jeffrey
Tschumperlé, David
Tsechpenakis, Gavriil
Tsekos, Nikolaos
Twining, Carole
Urschler, Martin
van Assen, Hans
van de Ville, Dimitri
van der Bom, Martijn
van der Geest, Rob
van Rikxoort, Eva
van Walsum, Theo
Vandermeulen, Dirk
Ventikos, Yiannis
Vercauteren, Tom
Verma, Ragini
Vermandel, Maximilien
Vidal, Rene
Vidholm, Erik
Vilanova, Anna
Villa, Mari Cruz
Villain, Nicolas
Villard, Caroline
von Berg, Jens
von Lavante, Etienne
von Siebenthal, Martin
Vosburgh, Kirby
Vossepoel, Albert
Vrooman, Henri
Vrtovec, Tomaz
Wang, Defeng
Wang, Fei
Wang, Guodong
Wang, Yongmei Michelle
Wang, Yongtian
Wang, Zhizhou
Wassermann, Demian

Weese, Jürgen
Wegner, Ingmar
Wein, Wolfgang
Weisenfeld, Neil
Wengert, Christian
West, Jay
Westenberg, Michel
Westermann, Ruediger
Whitcher, Brandon
Wiemker, Rafael
Wiest-Daessle, Nicolas
Wigstrom, Lars
Wiles, Andrew
Wink, Onno
Wong, Ken
Wong, Kenneth
Wong, Stephen
Wong, Tien-Tsin
Wong, Wilbur
Wood, Bradford
Wood, Fiona
Worsley, Keith
Wörz, Stefan
Wšrn, Heinz
Wu, Jue
Xia, Yan
Xie, Jun
Xu, Sheng
Xu, Ye
Xue, Hui
Xue, Zhong
Yan, Pingkun
Yang, King
Yang, Lin
Yang, Yihong
Yaniv, Ziv
Yeo, Boon Thye
Yeung, Sai-Kit
Yogesan, Kanagasingam
Yoshida, Hiro
Young, Alistair
Young, Stewart
Yu, Yang
Yue, Ning
Yuen, Shelten

Yushkevich, Paul
Zacharaki, Evangelia
Zemiti, Nabil
Zerubia, Josiane
Zhan, Wang
Zhang, Fan
Zhang, Heye
Zhang, Hui
Zhang, Xiangwei

Zhang, Yong
Zheng, Guoyan
Zheng, Yefeng
Zhou, Jinghao
Zhou, Kevin
Zhou, Xiang
Ziyan, Ulas
Zollei, Lilla
Zwiggelaar, Reyer

Table of Contents – Part I

Image Segmentation and Classification

Image Guided Intervention and Robotics

General Medical Image Computing - I

Computer Assisted Intervention and Robotics - I

Computational Anatomy - I

Computational Physiology - I

Innovative Clinical and Biological Applications - I

Physiology and Physics-based Image Computing

Brain Atlas Computing

Simulation of Therapy

General Medical Image Computing - II

Computer Assisted Intervention and Robotics - II

Table of Contents – Part II

Computer Assisted Intervention and Robotics - II

Visualization and Interaction

Neuroscience Image Computing - I

Computational Anatomy - II

Innovative Clinical and Biological Applications - II

Spectroscopic and Cellular Imaging

Spatio-Temporal Registration

General Medical Image Computing - III

Computer Assisted Intervention and Robotics - III

General Biological Imaging Computing

Neuroscience Image Computing - II

Computational Anatomy - III

Computational Physiology - II

Innovative Clinical and Biological Applications - III

Geodesic-Loxodromes for Diffusion Tensor Interpolation and Difference Measurement*

Gordon Kindlmann[1], Raúl San José Estépar[1], Marc Niethammer[2], Steven Haker[1], and Carl-Fredrik Westin[1]

[1] Department of Radiology
[2] Department of Psychiatry, Brigham and Women's Hospital,
Harvard Medical School, USA
gk@bwh.harvard.edu

Abstract. In algorithms for processing diffusion tensor images, two common ingredients are interpolating tensors, and measuring the distance between them. We propose a new class of interpolation paths for tensors, termed *geodesic-loxodromes*, which explicitly preserve clinically important tensor attributes, such as mean diffusivity or fractional anisotropy, while using basic differential geometry to interpolate tensor orientation. This contrasts with previous Riemannian and Log-Euclidean methods that preserve the determinant. Path integrals of tangents of geodesic-loxodromes generate novel measures of over-all difference between two tensors, and of difference in shape and in orientation.

1 Introduction

Diffusion tensor imaging (DTI) can uniquely discern the directional microstructure of living tissue [1]. Certain mathematical attributes of diffusion tensors have established clinical value. The tensor trace is three times the bulk mean diffusivity (often referred to as apparent diffusion coefficient or ADC), and is used for rapid detection of ischemic stroke [2], and for detecting edema around brain lesions [3]. Fractional anisotropy (FA) indicates the directional dependence of diffusion, and is currently the mainstay of DTI applications, because FA changes are associated with many neurological or psychiatric conditions [4,5,6].

Recent work has created a sophisticated mathematical context for diffusion tensors, considered as elements of a Riemannian manifold with a particular affine-invariant metric, derived from statistical or information-theoretic considerations [7,8,9,10]. The Log-Euclidean approach is a computationally efficient close approximation [11]. These methods are rigorous in that they explicitly respect the positive-definiteness of diffusivity. A consequence is that the determinant $\det(\mathbf{D})$ is given especial importance, since its level-set $\det(\mathbf{D}) = 0$ delimits the region of positive-definite tensors. Riemannian and Log-Euclidean tensor interpolation guarantee monotonic interpolation of the determinant.

---

* This work supported by NIH grants U41-RR019703, P41-RR13218, R01-MH050740, and R01-MH074794. DTI data courtesy of Dr. Susumu Mori, Johns Hopkins University, supported by NIH R01-AG20012-01 and P41-RR15241-01A1.

N. Ayache, S. Ourselin, A. Maeder (Eds.): MICCAI 2007, Part I, LNCS 4791, pp. 1–9, 2007.
© Springer-Verlag Berlin Heidelberg 2007

We present a novel tensor interpolant, the *geodesic-loxodrome*, designed around clinically significant tensor properties. In navigation, loxodromes are paths of constant bearing. We generalize this to monotonically interpolate three tensor shape parameters, including tensor size and anisotropy. Geodesic-loxodromes are by definition the shortest path with the loxodrome properties, so they form geodesics on the manifold of tensors with fixed shape. In essence, geodesic-loxodromes are minimal-length paths between tensors that monotonically interpolate tensor shape. By computing tangents to geodesic-loxodromes and projecting out different components of the tangent, we create novel shape-specific and orientation-specific measures of the large-scale difference between tensors.

For these tasks, we have found it advantageous to treat diffusion tensors as elements of a vector space. Linear transforms on $\mathbb{R}^n$ constitute a vector space isomorphic to $\mathbb{R}^{n \times n}$ [12]. Though often viewed as a covariance matrix, a diffusion tensor $\mathbf{D}$ is also a linear transform on $\mathbb{R}^3$ with the essential physical property of mapping (by Fick's first law) concentration gradient vector ∇c to diffusive flux vector $\mathbf{j} = -\mathbf{D}\nabla c$ [1]. The set of *positive-definite* tensors is not a vector space (it is not closed under subtraction), but if one seeks merely to describe properties of given tensors, or to interpolate tensors in a convex manner, then the methods need not be explicitly designed around the positive-definiteness constraint.

2   Theoretical Background

Loxodromes are paths of constant bearing, or paths maintaining a fixed angle with north [13]. Stated another way, let $\mathbf{p}(\theta, \phi) = (r \cos(\theta) \sin(\phi),$ $r \sin(\theta) \sin(\phi), r \cos(\phi))$ be a parameterization of a radius-r globe in $\mathbb{R}^3$ with $\mathbf{p}(0,0)$ at the north pole. Then $\mathbf{n}(\mathbf{x}) = -\partial\mathbf{p}/\partial\phi|_{\mathbf{p}^{-1}(\mathbf{x})}$ is a tangent to the sphere, pointing north. Let $\widehat{\mathbf{n}}(\mathbf{x}) = \mathbf{n}(\mathbf{x})/|\mathbf{n}(\mathbf{x})|$. Then, a loxodrome with unit speed and bearing $\cos^{-1}(\alpha)$ is traced by a path $\gamma(t)$ on the globe for which:

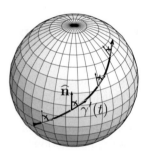

$$|\gamma'(t)| = 1 \ \text{ and } \ \gamma'(t) \cdot \widehat{\mathbf{n}}(\gamma(t)) = \alpha \ \text{ for all } t. \tag{1}$$

The path tangent $\gamma'(t)$ is also tangent to the sphere, and its constant inner product with $\widehat{\mathbf{n}}$ implies that $\gamma(t)$ moves northward (or southward) at a constant rate. Our geodesic-loxodromes similarly move along certain tensor shape parameters at a constant rate, thereby monotonically interpolating tensor shape. We now review the mathematics needed to define geodesic-loxodromes, including the theoretical distinction between tensor *shape* and *orientation*.

Notation.   The six-dimensional vector space of second-order symmetric tensors is notated Sym_3. Tensor contraction $\mathbf{A}:\mathbf{B} = \mathrm{tr}(\mathbf{A}\mathbf{B}^{\mathsf{T}})$ is an inner product on Sym_3, and the norm is $|\mathbf{D}| = \sqrt{\mathbf{D}:\mathbf{D}}$. The tensor $\mathbf{A}$ can be decomposed into isotropic and deviatoric parts, defined by $\overline{\mathbf{A}} = \mathrm{tr}(\mathbf{A})\mathbf{I}/3$ and $\widetilde{\mathbf{A}} = \mathbf{A} - \overline{\mathbf{A}}$, respectively. $\mathbf{I}$ is the identity tensor. SO_3 is the group of rotations on $\mathbb{R}^3$. The *group action* $\psi : \mathrm{SO}_3 \times \mathrm{Sym}_3 \mapsto \mathrm{Sym}_3, \psi(\mathbf{R}, \mathbf{D}) = \mathbf{R}\mathbf{D}\mathbf{R}^{\mathsf{T}}$ defines a mapping on

Sym_3 for each rotation $\mathbf{R}$ in SO_3. The *orbit* of $\mathbf{D}$ is $\text{SO}_3(\mathbf{D}) = \{\mathbf{R}\mathbf{D}\mathbf{R}^\mathsf{T} | \mathbf{R} \in \text{SO}_3\}$; informally it is all possible rotations of $\mathbf{D}$. The orbits of ψ partition Sym_3 into equivalence classes because SO_3 is a group. We can then say that tensors $\mathbf{A}$ and $\mathbf{B}$ have the same *shape* if they are on the same orbit $\text{SO}_3(\mathbf{A}) = \text{SO}_3(\mathbf{B})$, which is equivalent to saying they have the same three eigenvalues. A *tensor invariant* $J : \text{Sym}_3 \mapsto \mathbb{R}$ can be defined as a scalar-valued function of tensors that is constant on orbits: $\text{SO}_3(\mathbf{D}_0) = \text{SO}_3(\mathbf{D}_1) \Rightarrow J(\mathbf{D}_0) = J(\mathbf{D}_1)$. Trace $\text{tr}()$ and determinant $\det()$ are invariants, as are the tensor eigenvalues.

Just as scalar-valued functions over the vector space $\mathbb{R}^3$ have gradients with values in $\mathbb{R}^3$, tensor invariants have gradients with values in Sym_3[1]. Adapting the ∇ notation from vector calculus, we use $\nabla J(\mathbf{D})$ to represent the tensor-valued gradient of invariant J, evaluated at tensor $\mathbf{D}$. ∇J "points" in the direction along which J increases fastest. Deriving expressions for gradients of standard invariants is in continuum mechanics texts [14], for example $\nabla\text{tr}(\mathbf{D}) = \mathbf{I}$ and $\nabla\det(\mathbf{D}) = \det(\mathbf{D})\mathbf{D}^{-1}$. Any invariant J is constant on orbits of ψ, thus $\nabla J(\mathbf{D})$ is orthogonal at $\mathbf{D}$ to the orbit $\text{SO}_3(\mathbf{D})$. We can then say that near $\mathbf{D}$, $\nabla J(\mathbf{D})$ spans one degree of freedom in tensor shape. For tensors in Sym_3, shape has three degrees of freedom (because the three eigenvalues are independent), and we intend to define at each tensor $\mathbf{D}$ an orthonormal basis for shape variation.

Orthogonal Invariants. We build upon work by Ennis and Kindlmann that advocates sets of orthogonal invariants for DTI analysis [15]. Invariants J_1 and J_2 are said to be orthogonal if $\nabla J_1(\mathbf{D}) : \nabla J_2(\mathbf{D}) = 0$ for all $\mathbf{D}$. We adopt the same two sets of orthogonal invariants $\{K_i\}$ and $\{R_i\}$ as in [15], because they contain trace and FA, which we intend to preserve in our method:

$$
\begin{array}{ll}
K_1(\mathbf{D}) = \text{tr}(\mathbf{D}) & R_1(\mathbf{D}) = |\mathbf{D}| \\
K_2(\mathbf{D}) = |\widetilde{\mathbf{D}}| & R_2(\mathbf{D}) = \text{FA}(\mathbf{D}) = \sqrt{\dfrac{3\widetilde{\mathbf{D}}:\widetilde{\mathbf{D}}}{2\mathbf{D}:\mathbf{D}}} \\
K_3(\mathbf{D}) = \text{mode}(\mathbf{D}) & R_3(\mathbf{D}) = K_3(\mathbf{D}) = \text{mode}(\mathbf{D})
\end{array}
\tag{2}
$$

where $\text{mode}(\mathbf{D}) = 3\sqrt{6}\det(\widetilde{\mathbf{D}}/|\widetilde{\mathbf{D}}|)$. Both sets include measures of *size* (either trace K_1 or norm R_1) and of *anisotropy* (either eigenvalue standard deviation K_2 or fractional anisotropy R_2), and both use mode ($K_3 = R_3$) to distinguish linear (mode $= +1$) from planar (mode $= -1$) anisotropy. Trace (K_1) and FA (R_2) are not orthogonal, and so are in different invariant sets [15]. The determinant is another measure of size, but we are unaware of two complementary invariants that, with determinant, constitute an orthogonal invariant set. We restate from [15] the formulae for the tensor-valued gradients of K_i and R_i:

$$
\begin{array}{ll}
\nabla K_1(\mathbf{D}) = \mathbf{I} & \nabla R_1(\mathbf{D}) = \mathbf{D}/|\mathbf{D}| \\
\nabla K_2(\mathbf{D}) = \mathbf{\Theta}(\mathbf{D}) = \widetilde{\mathbf{D}}/|\widetilde{\mathbf{D}}| & \nabla R_2(\mathbf{D}) = \sqrt{\dfrac{3}{2}}\left(\dfrac{\mathbf{\Theta}(\mathbf{D})}{|\mathbf{D}|} - \dfrac{\widetilde{\mathbf{D}}|\mathbf{D}}{|\mathbf{D}|^3}\right) \\
\nabla K_3(\mathbf{D}) = \dfrac{3\sqrt{6}\mathbf{\Theta}(\mathbf{D})^2 - 3K_3(\mathbf{D})\mathbf{\Theta}(\mathbf{D}) - \sqrt{6}\mathbf{I}}{K_2(\mathbf{D})} & \nabla R_3(\mathbf{D}) = \nabla K_3(\mathbf{D}) .
\end{array}
\tag{3}
$$

---

[1] We omit the distinction between covariant and contravariant vectors as we use only orthonormal bases, whose orthonormality is preserved by our group action ψ [14].

We notate the normalized gradient of invariant J as $\widehat{\boldsymbol{\nabla}} J(\mathbf{D}) = \boldsymbol{\nabla} J(\mathbf{D})/|\boldsymbol{\nabla} J(\mathbf{D})|$. Thus, at each tensor $\mathbf{D}$, $\{\widehat{\boldsymbol{\nabla}} K_i(\mathbf{D})\}$ and $\{\widehat{\boldsymbol{\nabla}} R_i(\mathbf{D})\}$ form orthonormal bases for local shape variation: nearby tensors along those directions differ only in shape, not orientation, from $\mathbf{D}$. Note that tensor diagonalization is not required to compute either the invariants or their gradients.

3   Methods

Interpolation.   We define the *geodesic-loxodrome* $\boldsymbol{\gamma}(t)$ between $\mathbf{A}$ and $\mathbf{B}$ in Sym_3 as the *shortest* path satisfying (compare to Equation 1):

$$\boldsymbol{\gamma}(0) = \mathbf{A}, \quad \boldsymbol{\gamma}(l) = \mathbf{B}, \quad |\boldsymbol{\gamma}'(t)| = 1, \quad \text{and}$$
$$\boldsymbol{\gamma}'(t) : \widehat{\boldsymbol{\nabla}} J_i(\boldsymbol{\gamma}(t)) = \alpha_i \quad \text{for all } t \in [0, l], i \in \{1, 2, 3\} \tag{4}$$

where l and α_i are constants that characterize the path, and either $J_i = K_i$ or $J_i = R_i$. By using normalized invariant gradients ($\widehat{\boldsymbol{\nabla}} J_i$ instead of $\boldsymbol{\nabla} J_i$), $\boldsymbol{\gamma}(t)$ depends on the tensor shape degree of freedom parameterized by J_i, but not on the parameterization rate $|\boldsymbol{\nabla} J_i|$, which in general is not constant. $\boldsymbol{\gamma}(t)$ *linearly* interpolates invariants with constant-magnitude gradients (trace K_1, K_2, and norm R_1); other invariants are merely *monotonically* interpolated:

$$\frac{d}{dt} J_i(\boldsymbol{\gamma}(t)) = \boldsymbol{\gamma}'(t) : \boldsymbol{\nabla} J_i(\boldsymbol{\gamma}(t)) = \boldsymbol{\gamma}'(t) : \widehat{\boldsymbol{\nabla}} J_i(\boldsymbol{\gamma}(t)) |\boldsymbol{\nabla} J_i(\boldsymbol{\gamma}(t))| = \alpha_i |\boldsymbol{\nabla} J_i(\boldsymbol{\gamma}(t))|.$$

α_i is constant and $|\boldsymbol{\nabla} J_i(\boldsymbol{\gamma}(t))| \geq 0$, thus $\frac{d}{dt} J_i(\boldsymbol{\gamma}(t))$ has fixed sign, and $J_i(\boldsymbol{\gamma}(t))$ is monotonic. In particular, if $J_i(\mathbf{A}) = J_i(\mathbf{B})$ for some i, $J_i(\boldsymbol{\gamma}(t))$ is constant, and $\boldsymbol{\gamma}(t)$ lies in a level-set $\mathcal{L}_i$ of J_i. If $J_i(\mathbf{A}) = J_i(\mathbf{B})$ for all $i = 1, 2, 3$, then $\boldsymbol{\gamma}(t)$ lies within the intersection $\cap_i \mathcal{L}_i$. However, $\cap_i \mathcal{L}_i$ is exactly the orbit $\mathcal{O} = \mathrm{SO}_3(\mathbf{A}) = \mathrm{SO}_3(\mathbf{B})$ of ψ, because the three J_i determine the λ_i, and tensors with equal eigenvalues are on the same orbit. As $\boldsymbol{\gamma}(t)$ is by definition the shortest such path in $\mathcal{O}$, by the Hopf-Rinow-de Rham theorem it is a geodesic on $\mathcal{O}$ [16]. Space does not permit a proof, but conditions for the theorem are met because $\mathcal{O}$ is a closed subset of a complete metric space. We also note without proof that geodesics on $\mathcal{O}$ are not simply images under ψ of geodesics on SO_3, because the extrinsic curvatures of orbits are non-uniformly scaled by eigenvalue differences.

Distance Measurement.   A distance $d(\mathbf{A}, \mathbf{B})$ between $\mathbf{A}$ and $\mathbf{B}$ can be defined in terms of the geodesic-loxodrome $\boldsymbol{\gamma}(t)$ connecting them: $d(\mathbf{A}, \mathbf{B}) = \int_0^l |\boldsymbol{\gamma}'(t)| dt = l$. However, the normalized invariant gradients $\widehat{\boldsymbol{\nabla}} J_i$ can also decompose the path tangent $\boldsymbol{\gamma}'(t)$ into mutually orthogonal shape $\boldsymbol{\sigma}(t)$ and orientation $\boldsymbol{\omega}(t)$ tangents. From these we define shape d_{sh} and orientation d_{or} distances, which measure large-scale differences specifically in shape and orientation:

$$\boldsymbol{\sigma}(t) = \sum_i \boldsymbol{\gamma}'(t) : \widehat{\boldsymbol{\nabla}} J_i(\boldsymbol{\gamma}(t)) \widehat{\boldsymbol{\nabla}} J_i(\boldsymbol{\gamma}(t)) \rightarrow d_{sh}(\mathbf{A}, \mathbf{B}) = \int_0^l |\boldsymbol{\sigma}(t)| dt$$
$$\boldsymbol{\omega}(t) = \boldsymbol{\gamma}'(t) - \boldsymbol{\sigma}(t) \rightarrow d_{or}(\mathbf{A}, \mathbf{B}) = \int_0^l |\boldsymbol{\omega}(t)| dt \tag{5}$$

Implementation.   Our initial investigation of geodesic-loxodromes has focused on their theoretical definition and properties, rather than on a fast numerical solution. We describe here a brute-force gradient-descent scheme for updating vertices of a discretized polyline through Sym_3 (initialized with linear interpolation) so that it converges to the geodesic-loxodrome. For any vertex $\mathbf{D}_n$, let $\mathbf{D}^- = (\mathbf{D}_n + \mathbf{D}_{n-1})/2$ and $\mathbf{D}^+ = (\mathbf{D}_{n+1} + \mathbf{D}_n)/2$ be the (linearly) interpolated tensor values at the edge midpoints around $\mathbf{D}_n$, and let $\mathbf{T}^- = \mathbf{D}_n - \mathbf{D}_{n-1}$ and $\mathbf{T}^+ = \mathbf{D}_{n+1} - \mathbf{D}_n$ be the (non-normalized) tangents into, and away from, $\mathbf{D}_n$.

Then, $r_i(\mathbf{D}_n) = \mathbf{T}^+ : \widehat{\boldsymbol{\nabla}} J_i(\mathbf{D}^+) - \mathbf{T}^- : \widehat{\boldsymbol{\nabla}} J_i(\mathbf{D}^-)$ is the change in the projection of the path tangent onto $\widehat{\boldsymbol{\nabla}} J_i$, which is zero on a loxodrome, and $\kappa(\mathbf{D}_n) = |\mathbf{T}^+ - \mathbf{T}^-|$ is approximately proportional to the curvature at $\mathbf{D}_n$, which is minimized on a minimal-length path. Gradient descent on r_i^2 and κ^2 leads to the update rule $\mathbf{D}_n \leftarrow \mathbf{D}_n + \delta(\sum_i r_i(\mathbf{D}_n)\widehat{\boldsymbol{\nabla}} J_i(\mathbf{D}_n) + \mathbf{U} - \sum_i(\mathbf{U} : \widehat{\boldsymbol{\nabla}} J_i(\mathbf{D}_n))\widehat{\boldsymbol{\nabla}} J_i(\mathbf{D}_n))$, where $\mathbf{U} = \mathbf{D}_{n-1} - 2\mathbf{D}_n + \mathbf{D}_{n+1}$, and δ is the time increment. Note that the curve-shortening curvature flow along $\mathbf{U}$ is only allowed to act along the subspace (of orientation change) orthogonal to the $\widehat{\boldsymbol{\nabla}} J_i(\mathbf{D}_n)$. After all vertices have been so updated, vertices are moved along the polyline to enforce equi-distant spacing (constant-rate parameterization). Results here use a 100-point polyline with $\delta = 0.1$, converging sufficiently in about one second on a modern PC. Distances (Eq. 5) are computed by summing (over the polyline) the lengths of the segments (for $d(\mathbf{A}, \mathbf{B})$), or their projections onto the span of the local $\widehat{\boldsymbol{\nabla}} J_i$ (for $d_{sh}(\mathbf{A}, \mathbf{B})$), or the complements of these projections (for $d_{or}(\mathbf{A}, \mathbf{B})$).

4   Results

We demonstrate geodesic-loxodromes with glyphs and with plots of invariants along interpolation paths. Tensors are shown as superquadric glyphs [17]. For qualitative comparisons, the invariant plots (on the right side of the figures) are individually scaled (mode K_3 is also shifted). Figure 1 interpolates two linearly anisotropic tensors of different size and orientation. By their definitions, the first three methods monotonically interpolate *one* invariant: the tensor trace (K_1) with linear interpolation (Fig. 1(a)), and the tensor determinant with Riemannian [7,8,9,10] (Fig. 1(b)) and Log-Euclidean [11] (Fig. 1(c)) interpolation. By monotonically interpolating *three* orthogonal invariants, however, geodesic-loxodromes fully control tensor shape. In particular, the cylindrical shape is maintained in Fig. 1(d) by fixing the anisotropy type (tensor mode K_3).

Figure 2 interpolates two tensors with equal size (as measured by norm $R_1 = |\mathbf{D}|$), but unequal FA (R_2), mode (R_3), and orientation. As in Fig. 1, Riemannian results were very similar to Log-Euclidean, and so are not shown. Log-Euclidean interpolation (Fig. 2(a)) does not monotonically interpolate norm (R_1) or FA (R_2), and the wide range of mode (R_3) leads to planar anisotropy dissimilar to the endpoints. The geodesic-loxodrome (Fig. 2(b)), on the other hand, maintains the norm, and monotonically interpolates the other invariants. Though not part of the geodesic-loxodrome formulation, in this case the tensor determinant is also monotonically interpolated; the apparent lengthening is due to rotation.

Figure 3 demonstrates distance measures on a single slice of a DTI scan (pixel size 1.5^3mm). The cerebral spinal fluid (CSF) is bright in the tensor trace

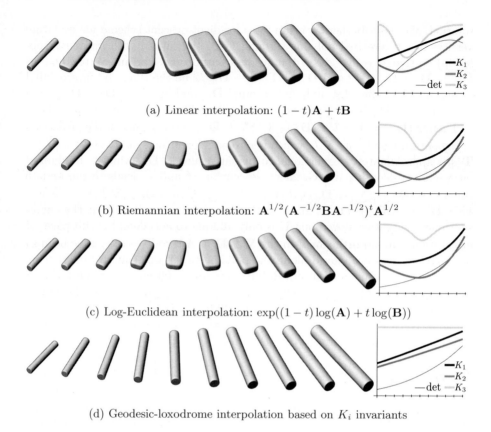

(a) Linear interpolation: $(1-t)\mathbf{A} + t\mathbf{B}$

(b) Riemannian interpolation: $\mathbf{A}^{1/2}(\mathbf{A}^{-1/2}\mathbf{B}\mathbf{A}^{-1/2})^t\mathbf{A}^{1/2}$

(c) Log-Euclidean interpolation: $\exp((1-t)\log(\mathbf{A}) + t\log(\mathbf{B}))$

(d) Geodesic-loxodrome interpolation based on K_i invariants

Fig. 1. Interpolations between two cylindrical tensors. Trace (K_1) is linearly interpolated in (a), and determinant is monotonically interpolated in (b) and (c). Geodesic-loxodromes (d) monotonically interpolate all K_i as well as (in this case) the determinant. Constancy of mode (K_3) wholly avoids planar anisotropy at intermediate values.

image (Fig. 3(a)), and the white matter is bright in the FA image (Fig. 3(b)), both of which show a square centered on a reference pixel in the corpus callosum splenium (left-right oriented linear anisotropy). Subsequent subfigures show measured distances between the tensors at each pixel and at the reference pixel. The linear (Fig. 3(c)), Log-Euclidean (Fig. 3(d)), and geodesic-loxodrome d distances (Fig. 3(e)) differ in brightness and contrast but are otherwise qualitatively similar. However, the geodesic-loxodrome shape distance d_{sh} (Fig. 3(f)) and orientation distance d_{or} (Fig. 3(g)) highlight different structures. The shape distance d_{sh} is consistently low throughout the white matter, since these voxels all have similar shape. The orientation distance d_{or}, on the other hand, is low in the gray matter, since there is little orientation change between isotropic and anisotropic tensors of comparable size. Within the white matter (where FA is highest), d_{or} successfully distinguishes between left-right and other orientations (where d_{or} is low and high, respectively). These results suggest that the novel shape and

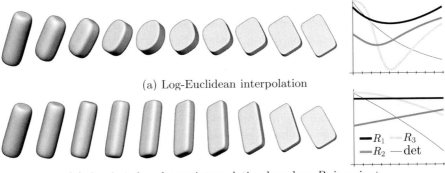

(a) Log-Euclidean interpolation

(b) Geodesic-loxodrome interpolation based on R_i invariants

Fig. 2. Log-Euclidean and geodesic-loxodrome interpolation between two tensors with equal R_1 (tensor norm). By monotonically interpolating FA (R_2) and anisotropy type (mode R_3), geodesic-loxodromes better maintain tensor shape during rotation.

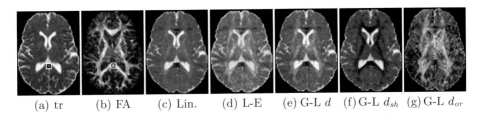

(a) tr   (b) FA   (c) Lin.   (d) L-E   (e) G-L d (f) G-L d_{sh} (g) G-L d_{or}

Fig. 3. DTI slice with distance measures. The tensor trace (a) and FA (b) images indicate (small square) the reference white-matter voxel to which distances are measured. Note that the geodesic-loxodrome shape distance d_{sh} (f) is low inside white matter.

orientation distance measures (d_{sh} and d_{or}) based on geodesic-loxodromes can better differentiate neuroanatomic structures than previous distance measures, highlighting their possible utility for segmentation.

5 Discussion and Future Work

This work was inspired by how the Riemannian and Log-Euclidean methods guarantee monotonic interpolation of a particular invariant, the determinant. Geodesic-loxodromes monotonically interpolate not one but three tensor invariants, which by their orthogonality completely determine tensor shape, and which by design include at least one clinically significant invariant, either trace (K_1) or FA (R_2). Choosing between $J_i = K_i$ or $J_i = R_i$ depends on desired path properties: the K_i are better if mean diffusivity ($K_1/3$) is an essential tissue parameter for the particular application, while R_i may be better if FA (R_2) values are fundamental, although the actual differences between using K_i and R_i are small. Our results highlight the importance of controlling anisotropy type (tensor mode) during interpolation, which is unaddressed by previous methods. Geodesic-loxodromes demonstrate the mapping of an intuitive distinction between shape and orientation into a mathematical formulation of interpolation and distance measurement. In this light, the most closely related previous work is by Chefd'hotel *et al.*, in which images of diffusion tensors are regularized by an "isospectral" flow that smoothes orientations but maintains shape [18].

We are uncertain whether geodesic-loxodromes are geodesics on some six-dimensional Riemannian manifold embedded in Sym_3. However, we believe it should be possible to generalize to geodesic-loxodromes the notion of a weighted *intrinsic mean* of multiple tensors on a Riemannian manifold [8,9,10], which would lead to a novel method of interpolating three-dimensional images of tensor samples. This requires fast numerical methods for computing geodesic-loxodromes and their exponential map counterparts (finding the geodesic-loxodrome given its starting point and initial tangent), which is our current focus. We are also studying how to apply our distance measures to segmentation, including optimizing a weighted combination of d_{sh} and d_{or} into a single distance measure.

References

1. Basser, P.J., Mattiello, J., Bihan, D.L.: Estimation of the effective self-diffusion tensor from the NMR spin-echo. J. Mag. Res. B B103(3), 247–254 (1994)
2. Sotak, C.H.: The role of diffusion tensor imaging in the evaluation of ischemic brain injury - A review. NMR in Biomedicine 15, 561–569 (2002)
3. Lu, S., Ahn, D., Johnson, G., Law, M., Zagzag, D., Grossman, R.I.: Diffusion-tensor MR imaging of intracranial neoplasia and associated peritumoral edema: Introduction of the tumor infiltration index. Neurorad. 232(1), 221–228 (2004)
4. Thomalla, G., Glauche, V., Koch, M A, Beaulieu, C., Weiller, C., Röther, J.: Diffusion tensor imaging detects early Wallerian degeneration of the pyramidal tract after ischemic stroke. NeuroImage 22(4), 1767–1774 (2004)
5. Salat, D.H., Tuch, D.S., Hevelone, N.D., Fischl, B., Corkin, S., Rosas, H.D., Dale, A.M.: Age-related changes in prefrontal white matter measured by diffusion tensor imaging. Annals of the New York Academy of Sciences 1064, 37–49 (2005)
6. Tuch, D.S., Salat, D.H., Wisco, J.J., Zaleta, A.K., Hevelone, N.D., Rosas, H.D.: Choice reaction time performance correlates with diffusion anisotropy in white matter pathways supporting visuospatial attention. Proc. Nat. Acad. Sci. 102(34), 12212–12217 (2005)
7. Batchelor, P.G., Moakher, M., Atkinson, D., Calamante, F., Connelly, A.: A rigorous framework for diffusion tensor calculus. Mag. Res. Med. 53(1), 221–225 (2005)
8. Fletcher, P.T., Joshi, S.: Riemannian geometry for the statistical analysis of diffusion tensor data. Signal Processing 87(2), 250–262 (2007)
9. Lenglet, C., Rousson, M., Deriche, R., Faugeras, O.: Statistics on the manifold of multivariate normal distributions: Theory and application to diffusion tensor MRI processing. J. Math. Imaging Vis. 25(3), 423–444 (2006)
10. Pennec, X., Fillard, P., Ayache, N.: A Riemannian framework for tensor computing. Int. J. Comp. Vis. 66(1), 41–66 (2006)
11. Arsigny, V., Fillard, P., Pennec, X., Ayache, N.: Log-Euclidean metrics for fast and simple calculus on diffusion tensors. Mag. Res. Med. 56(2), 411–421 (2006)

12. Hoffman, K., Kunze, R.: Linear Algebra, ch. 3,8. Prentice-Hall, Inc. Englewood Cliffs, NJ (1971)
13. Pearson, F.: Map Projection: Theory and Applications, ch. 8. CRC Press, Boca Raton, FL (1990)
14. Holzapfel, G.A.: Nonlinear Solid Mechanics. John Wiley and Sons, Ltd. England (2000)
15. Ennis, D.B., Kindlmann, G.: Orthogonal tensor invariants and the analysis of diffusion tensor magnetic resonance images. Mag. Res. Med. 55(1), 136–146 (2006)
16. Petersen, P.: Riemannian Geometry. Springer, Heidelberg (1997)
17. Ennis, D.B., Kindlman, G., Rodriguez, I., Helm, P.A., McVeigh, E.R.: Visualization of tensor fields using superquadric glyphs. Mag. Res. Med. 53, 169–176 (2005)
18. Chefd'hotel, C., Tschumperlé, D., Deriche, R., Faugeras, O.: Regularizing flows for constrained matrix-valued images. J. Math. Imaging Vis. 20(1–2), 147–162 (2004)

Quantification of Measurement Error in DTI: Theoretical Predictions and Validation*

Casey Goodlett[1], P. Thomas Fletcher[2], Weili Lin[3], and Guido Gerig[1,4]

[1] Department of Computer Science, University of North Carolina
[2] School of Computing, University of Utah
[3] Department of Radiology, University of North Carolina
[4] Department of Psychiatry, University of North Carolina

Abstract. The presence of Rician noise in magnetic resonance imaging (MRI) introduces systematic errors in diffusion tensor imaging (DTI) measurements. This paper evaluates gradient direction schemes and tensor estimation routines to determine how to achieve the maximum accuracy and precision of tensor derived measures for a fixed amount of scan time. We present Monte Carlo simulations that quantify the effect of noise on diffusion measurements and validate these simulation results against appropriate in-vivo images. The predicted values of the systematic and random error caused by imaging noise are essential both for interpreting the results of statistical analysis and for selecting optimal imaging protocols given scan time limitations.

1   Introduction

Diffusion tensor MRI (DT-MRI) has become a critical technology for studying white matter in-vivo. In clinical studies, derived tensor measures such as anisotropy measures or mean diffusivity are commonly used for voxel-wise and region-based statistical analysis [1]. In order to understand the significance of statistical analysis, the precision and accuracy of the measurements must be well understood. DT-MRI is particularly sensitive to error introduced by imaging noise for two reasons. First, since multiple diffusion-weighted images are needed, each individual image must be acquired relatively quickly, reducing the signal-to-noise ratio (SNR) for each image. Secondly, unlike structural MRI where intensities are primarily used to establish contrast between tissue types, DT-MRI measures quantitative physical properties requiring a more careful evaluation of noise. This paper both simulates the influence of Rician noise on tensor derived measures and evaluates the simulation against in-vivo experiments.

Several studies have investigated the effects of noise on tensor measurements through theory and Monte Carlo simulation [2,3,4]. Jones and Basser showed how

---

* This work is part of the National Alliance for Medical Image Computing (NA-MIC), funded by the National Institutes of Health through Grant U54 EB005149. The authors acknowledge support from the NIMH Silvio Conte Center for Neuroscience of Mental Disorders MH064065 as well as the National Alliance for Autism Research (NAAR) and the Blowitz-Ridgeway Foundation.

N. Ayache, S. Ourselin, A. Maeder (Eds.): MICCAI 2007, Part I, LNCS 4791, pp. 10–17, 2007.
© Springer-Verlag Berlin Heidelberg 2007

Rician noise tends to underestimate high values of the apparent diffusion coefficient (ADC) along gradient directions [5]. Basu, Fletcher, and Whitaker used the Rician noise model to demonstrate statistical bias and develop a regularization filter for diffusion-weighted images [6]. Fillard et al. combined a maximum likelihood (ML) tensor estimator with a regularization function to jointly smooth and estimate a tensor field [7]. This paper builds on previous work by combining a comparison of gradient direction schemes with tensor estimation methods to study the error in diffusion tensors given noisy image acquisition in a clinical framework. In this paper we work within the assumption of a single diffusion tensor model per voxel and do not consider high angular resolution diffusion imaging (HARDI). Our simulations show that increasing the number of gradient directions reduces the bias introduced by the orientation of the tensor. Furthermore, we demonstrate the increased variability caused by linear least squares estimation on sequences with many gradient directions. We also present a novel validation of the simulation with experiments using in-vivo data.

2   Methods

The estimated diffusion tensor can be understood as a function of observed diffusion-weighted MR intensities via the Stejskal-Tanner equation

$$S_i = S_0 \exp\left(-b\mathbf{g}_i \mathbf{D} \mathbf{g}_i^T\right). \tag{1}$$

Diffusion weighted images are acquired by computing the magnitude of the Fourier transform of a measured k-space signal. Pure Johnson noise in both the real and and imaginary components of k-space is well-approximated by a Gaussian distribution, and noise in the magnitude signal S_i is well characterized by a Rician distribution. A noisy measurement R of an underlying signal A in the diffusion-weighted image is a random variable given by

$$R = \sqrt{(A+X)^2 + Y^2}, \quad X, Y \sim N(0, \sigma^2), \tag{2}$$

where X and Y are Gaussian random variables. The probability density function for a Rician random variable R with true intensity A and noise variance σ^2 is

$$f(x|A, \sigma) = \frac{x}{\sigma^2} \exp\left(-\frac{x^2 + A^2}{2\sigma^2}\right) I_0\left(\frac{xA}{\sigma^2}\right), \tag{3}$$

where I_0 is the zero-order modified Bessel function of the first kind. The Rician distribution is equivalent to the Rayleigh distribution when $A = 0$, and converges to a Gaussian distribution as $\sigma/A \to 0$. For low signals the expected value of the measurement is greater than the true signal, $\mathrm{E}[R] > A$.

The apparent diffusion coefficient (ADC) in a direction $\mathbf{g}_i$ is measured in a voxel by the ratio of a baseline signal S_0 and an attenuated diffusion-weighted signal S_i. Because Rician random variables with low A have a positive bias, we are likely to observe a higher signal than the true intensity. Overestimation of an intensity S_i causes an underestimation of diffusion in the direction g_i because of

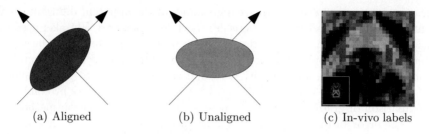

(a) Aligned   (b) Unaligned   (c) In-vivo labels

Fig. 1. Example of tensors with principal eigenvector aligned or unaligned with a gradient direction. Figure 1(c) shows the computed classes in in-vivo experiments.

the exponential decay in the Stejskal-Tanner equation (1). Measurements of low diffusion have lower attenuation and correspondingly less bias. The tendency to underestimate high ADC values causes two major challenges for reliable measurements in DTI. First, mean diffusivity is likely to be underestimated for regions with high diffusion. This is a particular problem in the cerebrospinal fluid (CSF), where the ADC is high in all directions. Secondly, anisotropy can be underestimated depending on the alignment of the principal diffusion direction of a highly anisotropic tensor with the gradient directions. As shown in Figure 1, the maximum measured ADC of a highly anisotropic tensor depends on the gradient direction sampling, and the bias in the measured FA value depends on the orientation of the tensor.

A minimum of six gradient images plus a baseline image are required to estimate the parameters of the diffusion tensor. Since diffusion-weighted images typically have low SNR, acquiring more images than the minimum seven is desirable to improve SNR and obtain more robust measures of diffusivity and anisotropy. To improve SNR, repetitions of gradient directions can be acquired and are typically processed by averaging of repetitions on-scanner or offline where corresponding images are registered and averaged. Alternatively, additional diffusion-weighted images can be acquired using more gradient directions, and the additional observations are combined in the tensor estimation. In images with multiple repetitions of the same gradient direction, the signals are typically averaged. However, the mean of the signals is a poor estimator of the true signal A, because of the bias in the Rician distribution. Averaging of the intensities across repetitions consequently tends to overestimate the signal and underestimate the ADC in voxels with low SNR.

For gradient schemes with more than the minimal number of gradient directions, several methods exist in the literature for estimating diffusion tensors from the diffusion-weighted images. The most common approach has been a linear least squares (LLS) estimator for the tensor parameters $\boldsymbol{\beta}$ from the log of the observed signal intensities $\mathbf{S}$ with baseline signal S_0. The matrix $\mathbf{X}$, which is Nx6, encapsulates the b-value and gradient directions.

$$\hat{\boldsymbol{\beta}}_{\text{lls}} = (\mathbf{X}^T\mathbf{X})^{-1}\mathbf{X}^T(\ln\mathbf{S} - \ln S_0). \tag{4}$$

To avoid the re-weighting penalties associated with the log, non-linear least squares (NLS) estimation optimizes the objective function

$$f_{\text{nls}}(\boldsymbol{\beta}) = ||\mathbf{S} - S_0 \exp(\mathbf{X}\boldsymbol{\beta})||^2 \tag{5}$$

on the diffusion-weighted signal. Our implementation uses Levenberg-Marquadt optimization. Salvador et al. proposed a weighted least squares (WLS) estimator

$$\hat{\boldsymbol{\beta}}_{\text{wls}} = (\mathbf{X}^T\mathbf{W}^2\mathbf{X})^{-1}(\mathbf{X}^T\mathbf{W}^2(\ln \mathbf{S} - \ln S_0)) \tag{6}$$

$$\mathbf{W} = \text{Diag}(\mathbf{X}\hat{\boldsymbol{\beta}}_{\text{lls}}) \tag{7}$$

based on the log Rician probability distribution [8]. Our implementation of this method uses iterative weight refinement until the tensor values converge.

An ML estimate of the diffusion tensor using the log-likelihood function of the Rician distribution was proposed by Fillard et al. [7]. We use a similar method that does not use a spatial regularization term or the log of the tensor matrix. The ML method explicitly accounts for the noise model and uses an estimate of the noise level computed from the background of the image. The ML estimation of tensor parameters is obtained by numerical optimization of the log-likelihood function

$$\log L(\boldsymbol{\beta}) = \sum_i \log\left(\frac{S_i}{\sigma^2}\right) - \frac{S_i^2 + S_0^2 e^{2X_i\boldsymbol{\beta}}}{2\sigma^2} + \log\left(I_0\left(\frac{S_i S_0^2 e^{2X_i\boldsymbol{\beta}}}{\sigma^2}\right)\right), \tag{8}$$

where X_i is a row of the matrix $\mathbf{X}$ and N is the number of gradient directions. Our implementation uses a gradient descent optimizer to maximize the objective function. We evaluate the different tensor estimation methods across several different gradient sampling schemes using a Monte Carlo framework for simulating the effect of imaging noise on derived properties.

3   Simulation

Our Monte Carlo simulations compute the distribution of estimated tensors from the predicted signal of a given true tensor with added Rician noise. The true tensor has a fixed trace of $2.1x10^{-3}mm^2/s$, which is a typical value for white matter. Several levels of anisotropy and orientation are simulated. The simulations use a b-value of $1000\ s/mm^2$, a noise level of $\sigma = 27$ estimated from the background of the image, and a baseline signal of 250.

The simulations show that positive bias of Rician noise at low signal level can lead to underestimation of FA and trace. Furthermore, the orientation of the tensor within the gradient fields correlates with the bias, and statistical comparison of structures with different fiber orientations is potentially biased. Many common clinical gradient schemes use the minimal six gradient directions and with these schemes the expected bias depends on the orientation of the fiber structure within the magnetic field. Figure 2 shows the bias and variability of the FA and trace of a fixed diffusion tensor as the tensor rotates in space relative

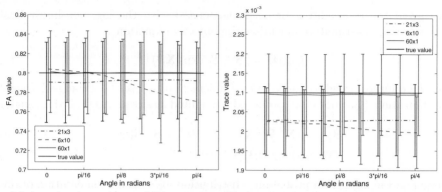

(a) Angular dependence of FA estimate   (b) Angular dependence of trace estimate

Fig. 2. The orientation dependence of estimated FA and trace under different sampling schemes. The horizontal axis ranges from the principal diffusion direction unaligned with any gradient direction for $x = 0$ to being perfectly aligned with one of the gradient directions for a rotation of $x = \pi/4$. The noise level is $\sigma = 27$ as determined from our collected data. Notice in the 6 direction scan the difference in mean estimated FA of .04 (5%) between the same tensor orientated at 0 and $\pi/4$ radians. Weighted least squares estimation was used for this simulation.

to a gradient direction. The simulations show that FA is substantially correlated with orientation. The trace estimate has less bias due to orientation, but the trace is underestimated in gradient schemes with repeated directions. Figure 3 shows the simulated distribution of FA, trace, and the Frobenius norm of the difference between the estimated and true tensor using a 60 direction protocol. Weighted least squares and maximum likelihood perform similarly, while linear least squares has more variability, non-linear least squares tends to have a lower estimate of trace.

The simulations demonstrate the bias due to orientation of tensor derived measures when using protocols with a minimal number of gradient directions. Furthermore, when protocols with many gradient directions are used linear least squares estimation can increase variability, and non-linear least squares estimation can underestimate trace. The simulations predict that the minimum error is introduced by using as many isotropic non-repeated gradient directions as possible with weighted or ML estimation methods.

4   Experiments and Validation

We acquired test sets of data under different imaging protocols to compare with the Monte Carlo simulations. Three sets of images of a single healthy adult volunteer were acquired on a Siemens Allegra 3T head-only scanner. The scanning time for each sequence was approximately 12 minutes. Diffusion weighted images were acquired with an isotropic resolution of $2x2x2mm$ resolution and image size 128x128x39. Three different sequences were used: 6 directions with 10

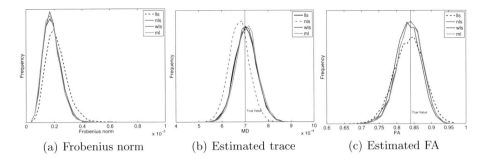

(a) Frobenius norm   (b) Estimated trace   (c) Estimated FA

Fig. 3. Distribution of estimated values in Monte Carlo simulations of a tensor with FA=0.8 using 10,000 repetitions and a 60 direction protocol: (a) the Frobenius norm of the difference between the estimated and true tensor, (b) the estimated trace, and (c) the estimated FA. The weighted, non-linear, and ML estimation techniques reduce the variance of estimated FA and decrease the Frobenius norm of the error in the estimated tensor. Non-linear least squares tends to underestimate the trace.

repetitions, 21 directions with 3 repetitions, and 60 directions with 1 repetition. All scans were of approximately equal time to demonstrate the trade-off between image repetition and acquiring more gradient directions. To eliminate bias from differences in the baseline images, the 14 acquired baseline images were registered to a T2 atlas using a rigid transformation and normalized mutual information. The baseline images were averaged to produce a common baseline image. The transformation from each baseline image to the atlas was also applied to the diffusion-weighted images in the corresponding set, and the gradient directions were corrected by the rotation component of the transformation. For sequences with repeated directions, the corresponding gradient directions were averaged. The noise level σ was estimated from the background of the images.

A white matter segmentation was created by co-registration of a T1 structural image to the averaged baseline image and applying a tissue segmentation tool. A label image was created from the six direction image by identifying voxels within the white matter segmentation which are highly aligned or highly unaligned with the closest gradient direction. The angle for each voxel is given by $\theta = \arccos(\min_i(\hat{e}_1 \cdot g_i))$, where $\hat{e}_1$ is the estimated principal eigenvector. In the six direction scan nearby gradients are separated by $pi/2$, and as a result the maximum angle between the principal eigenvector and the nearest gradient direction is $\pi/4$ so $\theta \in [0, \pi/4]$. The threshold for aligned tensors was $\theta < \pi/16$ and for unaligned tensors $\theta > 3\pi/16$. Figure 1(c) shows the labels overlaid on the FA image.

The difference between the histograms of FA for aligned and unaligned tensors decreases with an increase in the number of gradient directions as shown in Figure 4. Table 1 lists the mean difference between aligned and unaligned voxels using different gradient schemes and tensor estimation methods. The experimental results confirm the simulation prediction of underestimated anisotropy in tensors aligned in the six direction scan, because the difference decreases as

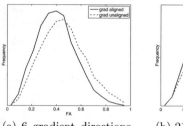

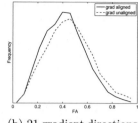

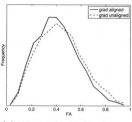

(a) 6 gradient directions with 10 repetitions   (b) 21 gradient directions with 3 repetitions   (c) 60 gradient directions with 1 repetition

Fig. 4. The histograms of estimated FA using weighted least squares estimation for aligned and unaligned tensors with (a) 6 gradient directions with 10 repetitions (b) 21 gradient directions with 3 repetitions and (c) 60 gradient directions with 1 repetition. Notice the significant reduction in difference between the two histograms as the number of gradient directions increases, because of a decrease in noise bias. Quantitative results are given in Table 1.

Table 1. Mean difference of FA values between aligned and unaligned voxels. The difference between the mean FA decreases with an increase in the number of gradient directions, confirming the simulation prediction that some of the difference is due to the choice of gradient sampling. All least squares methods are equivalent in the six direction scan because an exact solution exists.

	6 directions (10 reps)	21 directions (3 reps)	60 directions (1 reps)
LLS:	0.053	0.030	0.019
NLS:	0.053	0.032	0.020
WLS:	0.053	0.032	0.021
ML:	0.045	0.033	0.021

Table 2. Mean and variance of trace values in white matter across gradient sampling schemes and estimation methods. The six direction scan has the highest estimated trace. In the 21 and 60 direction scans the non-linear least squares method has a lower estimate of the trace than the other methods. The maximum-likelihood has the highest estimate of trace of all the methods.

	6 directions (10 reps)	21 directions (3 reps)	60 directions (1 reps)
LLS:	2.373e-03 (7.2071e-08)	2.304e-03 (7.7886e-08)	2.307e-03 (2.2293e-07)
NLS:	2.373e-03 (7.2071e-08)	2.289e-03 (7.7122e-08)	2.235e-03 (2.0839e-07)
WLS:	2.373e-03 (7.2071e-08)	2.307e-03 (7.8263e-08)	2.311e-03 (2.2847e-07)
ML:	2.472e-03 (8.5249e-08)	2.383e-03 (1.0698e-07)	2.326e-03 (2.4044e-07)

the number of gradient direction increases. The experimental estimate of tensor trace is higher for low directions images, which is different than the simulation prediction. The difference could be due to the assumption of a single tensor model in the simulation. We conclude that studies comparing different regions could be substantially biased by the orientation of the tissue within the magnetic field. Therefore studies relying on statistical analysis of anisotropy measures should use as many gradient directions as possible instead of repeating a minimum number of gradient directions. The results from the analysis of the in-vivo scans confirms the results of the simulation experiments.

5   Conclusions

In this paper we have evaluated the magnitude of error in DTI measurements caused by imaging noise through Monte Carlo simulations and in-vivo experiments. We have shown that low direction schemes introduce a statistical bias with a clinically relevant magnitude. Furthermore, we have shown that standard linear least squares tensor estimation introduces additional variability in tensor estimation. Understanding the magnitude of these two effects is critical for interpreting the results of statistical analysis. For new imaging studies these results indicate that scans with non-repeated isotropic gradient sampling should be preferred over protocols with a small number of repeated gradient directions, and that weighted least squares or ML tensor estimation should be preferred. Future work will extend the analysis to errors which are introduced by EPI distortion, subject motion, and inter-subject registration.

References

1. Kubicki, M., Park, H., Westin, C., Nestor, P., Mulkern, R., Maier, S., Niznikiewicz, M., Connor, E., Levitt, J., Frumin, M., Kikinis, R., Jolesz, F., McCarley, R., Shenton, M.: DTI and MTR abnormalities in schizophrenia: Analysis of white matter integrity. NeuroImage 26(3), 1109–1118 (2005)
2. Bastin, M.E., Armitage, P.A., Marshall, I.: A theoretical study of the effect of experimental noise on the measurement of anisotropy in diffusion imaging. Magn Reson Imaging 16(7), 773–785 (1998)
3. Jones, D.K.: The Effect of Gradient Sampling Schemes on Measures Derived From Diffusion Tensor MRI: A Monte Carlo Study. Magnetic Resonance in Medicine 51(4), 807–815 (2004)
4. Basser, P.J., Pajevic, S.: Statistical artifacts in diffusion tensor MRI (DT-MRI) caused by background noise. Magnetic Resonance in Medicine 44(1), 41–50 (2000)
5. Jones, D.K., Basser, P.J.: Squashing peanuts and smashing pumpkins: How noise distorts diffusion-weighted MR data. Magnetic Resonance in Medicine 52(5), 979–993 (2004)
6. Basu, S., Fletcher, P.T., Whitaker, R.: Rician Noise Removal in Diffusion Tensor MRI. In: Larsen, R., Nielsen, M., Sporring, J. (eds.) MICCAI 2006. LNCS, vol. 4190, pp. 117–125. Springer, Heidelberg (2006)
7. Fillard, P., Arsigny, V., Pennec, X., Ayache, N.: Clinical DT-MRI estimation, smoothing and fiber tracking with log-Euclidean metrics. In: ISBI 2006, Crystal Gateway Marriott, Arlington, Virginia, USA. LNCS, pp. 786–789 (2006)
8. Salvador, R., Peña, A., Menon, D.K., Carpenter, T.A., Pickard, J.D., Bullmore, E.T.: Formal characterization and extension of the linearized diffusion tensor model. Human Brain Mapping 24(2), 144–155 (2005)

In-utero Three Dimension High Resolution Fetal Brain Diffusion Tensor Imaging

Shuzhou Jiang[1], Hui Xue[1,2], Serena Counsell[1], Mustafa Anjari[1], Joanna Allsop[1], Mary Rutherford[1], Daniel Rueckert[2], and Joseph V. Hajnal[1]

[1] Imaging Sciences Department, MRC Clinical Sciences Centre, Hammersmith Hospital, Imperial College London, London, United Kingdom
[2] Department of Computing, Imperial College London, London, United Kingdom

Abstract. We present a methodology to achieve 3D high resolution *in-utero* fetal brain DTI that shows excellent ADC as well as promising FA maps. After continuous DTI scanning to acquire a repeated series of parallel slices with 15 diffusion directions, image registration is used to realign the images to correct for fetal motion. Once aligned, the diffusion images are treated as irregularly sampled data where each voxel is associated with an appropriately rotated diffusion direction, and used to estimate the diffusion tensor on a regular grid. The method has been tested successful on eight fetuses and has been validated on adults imaged at 1.5T.

1 Introduction

Fetal brain imaging by MRI is attracting increasing interest because it offers excellent contrast and anatomical detail. However, unpredictable fetal motion has led to the widespread use of single shot techniques that can freeze fetal motion for individual slices. An even greater challenge is *in-utero* Diffusion Weighted Imaging (DWI). Preliminary trials [1;2] have been performed in which for a few relatively thick slices, a b_0 image and diffusion weighted images with 3 directions of sensitization were acquired within a maternal breath hold time. These early experiments relied on the chance event of the fetus remaining still for all 4 sets of images so that apparent diffusion coefficients (ADC) could be calculated. Diffusion tensor imaging (DTI) offers the potential for more information than DWI particularly for tractography studies. However, DTI is even more challenging than DWI for fetal imaging [3], because it requires a b_0 image and at least 6 diffusion images that are sensitized in non-collinear directions for each slice studied. These extra images increase the minimum acquisition time so that the requirements for the maternal breath-hold become more onerous. Without a maternal breath-hold fetal motion combines with the mother's respiration to disrupt the spatial correspondence between component images required to calculate tensor properties.

Snapshot imaging with Volume Reconstruction (SVR) is a method developed to perform 3D high resolution and high SNR in-utero anatomical imaging of the fetal brain using dynamic scanning and image registration[4-6]. In this study we extended the SVR technique to DTI of the in-utero fetal brain and validated it using adult data.

N. Ayache, S. Ourselin, A. Maeder (Eds.): MICCAI 2007, Part I, LNCS 4791, pp. 18–26, 2007.
© Springer-Verlag Berlin Heidelberg 2007

2 Method and Implementation

We will restrict the discussion to structures that can be treated as rigid bodies undergoing an unknown motion and shall take the fetal brain as an exemplar of such structures. The scenario of interest involves motion that is fast enough to preclude self consistent whole brain imaging even with echo planar imaging (EPI) (typical time > 3 seconds), but slow enough to produce individual high quality 2D images (typical time < 100msec). The acquired slices consist of voxels which have a measured intensity $I(x,y,z)$ at prescribed positions in the scanner frame of reference, $\Omega_0(x,y,z)$. We now adopt a 3D Cartesian coordinate system $\Omega(x,y,z)$ fixed relative to the anatomy of interest. This coordinate frame moves relative to the scanner coordinate frame as the subject moves. The acquired voxel data are legitimate samples in Ω, but at unknown locations (x,y,z). Because of the motion, the samples $I(x,y,z)$ are irregularly spaced in Ω. Provided their locations can be determined and the samples are sufficiently dense throughout the region of interest in Ω, data interpolation can be used to generate a full representation on a regular Cartesian lattice in Ω. In the case of DTI data, the individual diffusion weighted slices have different contrast both relative to the b_0 images and to each other because of the effects of varying the direction of sensitization on anisotropic tissues such as white matter tracts. In addition the correct sensitization direction for each acquired slice must be maintained once it is correctly placed in the anatomical space. Successful reconstruction of a 3D representation of diffusion tensor matrix that can then be reformatted into any desired plane thus has 3 requirements:

1) Sufficient samples in Ω with at least 6 independent diffusion directions as well as a non-diffusion weighted (b=0) image to allow full representation of the anatomical structure.

2) Determination of the mapping from Ω_0 to Ω for each sample

3) Reconstruction of the diffusion tensor matrix D on a regular sampled 3D space given the scattered, irregularly spaced samples $I(x,y,z)$ that are each associated with an appropriately oriented diffusion gradient direction.

2.1 Achieving the Required Sample Density

In the proposed application the fetal brain to be imaged may move between acquisition of individual slice acquisitions. This causes uneven slice samples when viewed in the anatomical reference frame (Ω) and is likely to result in violation of the Nyquist sampling criterion at some locations. To avoid this problem the target volume in Ω_0 is repeatedly imaged by simply looping through all slice positions so that in the absence of motion each location is sampled with at least 6 different diffusion gradients multiple times. We refer to each complete set of slices spanning Ω_0 for the entire set of diffusion weighted images for different diffusion gradient directions plus one non diffusion weighted image as a loop. The number of loops required depends on the motion. In these experiments we used 3-4 loops each with 15 non-linear diffusion directions subject to the total scan duration being acceptable to the pregnant subjects.

2.2 Motion Compensation Through Slice to Volume Registration

A self consistent 3D b_0 image V0 is first reconstructed using the method described in [5;6]. Then each diffusion weighted slice is registered to the b_0 volume V0 using normalized mutual information (NMI)[7] as the cost function. Registration proceeds in a temporally hierarchical manner as follows: The data is first divided into temporally contiguous blocks each containing multiple slices that together provide full coverage of the volume of Ω_0 of interest (i.e. each loop is divided into 15 stacks of diffusion weighted images). Initially subject motion between slices in a stack is ignored, these stacks of slices are treated as 3D volumes and registered to the 3D b_0 volume V0 using rigid body transformations.

   Once the data is aligned, the size of temporally contiguous blocks is reduced so the data is divided into sub-packages that are temporally contiguous although the slices in each sub-package may not be spatially contiguous. These sub-packages are each registered to V0. The registration process involves moving the sub-package with V0 held fixed in space, but always interpolating the V0 intensity values to provide comparison intensity values. When the transformations ($T(\Omega_0 \rightarrow \Omega)$) of all sub-packages have been determined, the time scale is reduced again and the process repeated until each slice is treated in isolation.

   Followed the method in[5;6;8], a slice/stack-to-volume registration method based on a multi-start, multi-resolution approach using the Powell method to optimize each transformation parameter in turn was developed.

2.3 Reconstruction of the Diffusion Tensor Matrix

Using an anatomic coordinate system fixed relative to the reconstructed b_0 image volume V0, and given acquired diffusion sensitization direction g, rotation matrix R with respect to V0, and the corresponding intensity I_0 in V0 determined via cubic B-spline interpolation [9], the diffusion intensity I can be determined by:

$$I = I_0 * \exp(-bg'D_{Lab}g) = I_0 * \exp(-bg'(R'D_{Ana}R)g) \qquad (1)$$

D_{Lab} and D_{Ana} are the diffusion tensor matrix in laboratory and anatomic coordinate respectively, g is a unit vector in the direction of sensitization and b is the diffusion sanitization parameter in s/mm^2. We can further obtain a normalized logarithm value s using eq.(2) to prepare for later linear tensor fitting.

$$s = -\log(I/I_0)/b = g'(R'D_{Ana}R)g \qquad (2)$$

   Once aligned, we treat the data s as irregularly sampled with each voxel associated with an appropriately rotated diffusion direction, and use all the data to estimate the diffusion tensor D on a regular grid. For each scattered point $s_{scatter}$, we can use (3) to define its value, where the β_i are spatial coefficients associated with regularly sampled diffusion tensor matrix $D_{Ana;regular,i}$.

$$s_{scatter} = g'(R'D_{Ana;scatter}R)g = \sum_{i=1}^{N}\beta_i g'(R'D_{Ana;regular,i}R)g \qquad (3)$$

   We can then reconstruct the scattered diffusion tensor to a regular grid by solving a huge matrix equation, (4),

$$\overline{S}_{scatter} = M_R M_G * diag(M_S,M_S,M_S,M_S,M_S,M_S)*[D_{xx};D_{yy};D_{zz};D_{xy};D_{xz};D_{yz}] \qquad (4)$$

where $\bar{S}_{scatter}$ is a vector containing all the scattered points, M_R is a matrix specifying rotations R, M_G contains the diffusion gradient directions and M_S is a spatial interpolation matrix. They are all sparse. D_{xx} - D_{yz} are 6 independent parameters of the diffusion tensor. We use the Sparse Equations and Least SQuares Regression (LSQR)[10] method to solve for sparse matrix D_{xx} - D_{yz} , and then calculate its eigenvalues at each grid point to determine corresponding ADC and FA values. Nearest neighbor interpolation is used here to estimate the spatial coefficient β_i given dense sampling.

The 3×3 symmetric diffusion tensor matrix D should be positive definite. A further refinement using constraint minimization is performed to guarantee the positive definition of the diffusion matrix.

2.4 Fetal Scanning Protocol

Fetal brain images were acquired on a 1.5 T Philips Achieva scanner (Best, The Netherlands) using a 5 channel torso array with a spin echo EPI diffusion tensor sequence. Image matrix of 150×150, field of view of 300 mm and slice thickness 3 to 4 mm with slices centered every half slice thickness, i.e., 1.5 to 2mm were used depending on the maturity of the fetus. 60 slices covered the entire region of fetal brain. Slices were acquired in 2 packages and within each packages starting at one extreme end in an interleaved order to avoid slice cross-talk. We set the repeat time TR to be 12s to avoid spin history effects while TE is chosen to be the shortest possible (54ms) for the chosen b-value of 500 s/mm^2. Typical scanning time was 7 minutes for each loop of 15 diffusion directions with the SAR lower than 0.5W/kg. These studies were approved by Hammersmith Hospital Ethics Committee.

3 Verification Using Adult Data

Images of adult brains acquired with spin echo EPI were used to test the accuracy of slice-to-volume registration for diffusion data and the subsequent reconstruction. Two datasets were acquired using the same diffusion tensor imaging protocol at 1.5 T but with a SENSE head coil. Slice-to-volume registration accuracy is validated using similar experiment described in [4;5]. 819 single slices from both diffusion and non-diffusion weighted scans of the same subject were selected, and each was registered to the b_0 volume and compared with the gold standard volume-to-volume registration. The slice-to-volume registration was found to be accurate within ¼ voxel size.

In a second set of experiments an adult volunteer deliberately moved about once per second, including making head rotations around all three axis up to 30 degree. 4 loops of 15 direction DTI data were acquired with in-plane resolution 3mm×3mm, slice thickness 3.6 mm and -1.8mm slice gap. TR was 8 seconds while TE was 55ms which was the minimum for a b value 500 s/mm^2. For comparison, images were also acquired with the same protocol while the subject was still. All the slices that were not corrupted by in-plane motion were registered and reconstructed. Motion effects in the diffusion tensor data were easily identified because these generally caused

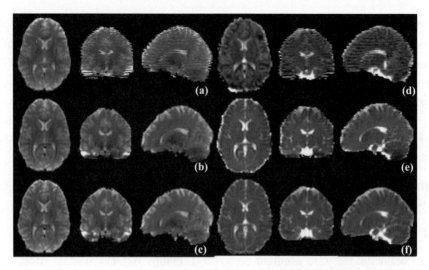

Fig. 1. Results for adult volunteer that deliberately moved during scanning: (a) is one loop of acquired transverse b=0 slices viewed in 3D, (d) is the reconstructed ADC map before motion correction. (b) and (e) are reconstructed b=0 volume and ADC map. (c) and (f) are corresponding volume from stationary gold standard.

catastrophic reconstruction failures with gross signal loss in part of the individual EPI slices. The results were then compared to the gold standard (stationary volunteer) data to evaluate the method.

For the moving subject DTI data, reconstruction fidelity was assessed visually using difference images and by calculating the mean absolute difference and its standard deviation (STD) between the gold standard and the reconstruction for b_0 volume, ADC and FA values. Region of Interest (ROI) measurements of both ADC and FA values are also performed.

A self-consistent 3D b_0 image volume was first reconstructed using the SVR method [5]. As displayed in Fig 1, the reconstructed B0 data is almost identical to the gold standard b_0 data that was acquired when the subject stayed still. The standard error, i.e., the square root of the residual mean square, between the reconstructed volume and the gold standard is 3.6%.

After motion correction and fitting of the diffusion tensor to the resulting scattered data, the reconstructed 3D ADC map (Fig. 1 (e)) shows clear consistency of ADC values. This contrasts with the corrupted ADC evaluation obtained without motion correction (Fig 1. (d)). When compared to the gold standard ADC values of the same subject, the result had a standard error of 5.6%. The 3D FA map as displayed in Fig. 2 (b) is quite close to the gold standard displayed in Fig. 2 (c) as well, and was found to achieve a standard error of 6.7%.

Furthermore, 8 Regions of Interest (ROI) measurement including Genu of Corpus Callosum (GCC), Splenium of Corpus Callosum (SCC), Posterior Limb of Internal Capsule (PLIC), Forceps major (FC), Anterior Limb of Internal Capsule (ALIC), Posterior region of Corona Radiate (PCR), Superior Longitudinal Fasciculus (SLF) and Superior region of Corona Radiate (SCR) on both ADC and FA values as displayed in Fig. 2(c) were performed for detailed validation. The reconstructed ADC and FA values were in excellent agreement with the gold standard (still subject) data in all 8 ROIs as listed in Table 1 and 2.

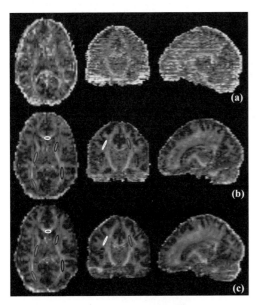

Table 1. ROI Measurement on ADC

	Rec ADC	GS ADC
SCC	0.75 ±0.05	0.78 ±0.11
PLIC	0.88 ±0.09	0.91 ±0.06
FC	0.88 ±0.09	0.88 ±0.09
GCC	0.89± 0.09	0.91 ±0.10
ALIC	0.80± 0.07	0.80 ±0.08
PCR	0.86± 0.04	0.84 ±0.04
SLF	0.81± 0.06	0.83 ±0.05
SCR	0.84 ±0.05	0.86 ±0.04

Table 2. ROI Measurement on FA ($\mu m^2 / ms$)

	Rec FA	GS FA
SCC	0.74 ± 0.11	0.75 ± 0.11
PLIC	0.64 ± 0.04	0.63 ± 0.04
FC	0.56 ± 0.09	0.57 ± 0.11
GCC	0.65 ± 0.09	0.63 ± 0.07
ALIC	0.56 ± 0.07	0.56 ± 0.09
PCR	0.56 ± 0.09	0.58 ± 0.11
SLF	0.52 ±0.10	0.53 ± 0.10
SCR	0.42 ±0.07	0.42 ± 0.04

Fig. 2. Results for adult volunteer that deliberately moved during scanning: FA maps. (a) is the FA map reconstructed directly before motion correction. (b) are the corresponding views of the FA maps reconstructed to a 3mm×3mm×1.8mm resolution image after registration and scattered diffusion tensor fitting. (c) are the corresponding views of the FA maps from the gold standard data from the stationary volunteer. 8 Regions of Interest (ROI) measurements on the ADC and FA maps from both the reconstructed data and the gold standard stationary subject data were performed. The ROI include samples in the GCC(while), SCC(orange), PLIC(red), FC(purple), ALIC(green) and PCR(blue) on the transverse view and SLF(white) and SCR(red) on the coronal orientation.

4 Results

Eight fetuses with gestational age between 24 and 34 weeks as listed in Table 3 and 4 were examined. Data from all the examinations have been successfully reconstructed.

4.1 Fetal Examples

Fig.3 shows data from a fetus of gestational age 26 weeks 5 days that had enlarged ventricles and agenesis of the corpus callosum. It was scanned with 15 diffusion gradient directions, and 4 loops of transverse images were acquired with 2mm in-plane resolution and 4mm (2mm slice separation) slice thickness. Approximately 25% of slices were corrupted because of extreme sensitivity to motion, and so had to be excluded. The acquired slice data is not consistent in space Fig. 3 (a). Final reconstruction achieved 2mm isotropic resolution in all three dimensions for b=0 images, as well as ADC and FA maps. Successful reconstruction of the 3D b=0 image volume shown in Fig. 3 (b) provides an accurate target for registering the diffusion weighted slices. After motion correction, the reconstructed 3D ADC map Fig. 3 (c) shows clearly consistent appearances of ADC values. Different tissue types can clearly be differentiated, i.e. WM, CSF and cortex on the FA map Fig. 3 (d). The FA calculation is less robust than ADC and the results show greater fluctuations. A high resolution anatomical volume acquired with T2-W single short Turbo Spin Echo (ssTSE) dynamic sequence was also reconstructed for comparison in Fig. 3 (e) with 1.25mm cubic resolution.

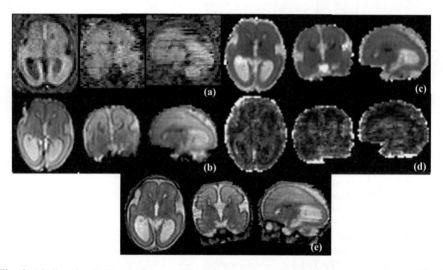

Fig. 3. 15-direction DTI of a fetus of 26 weeks plus 5 days. (a) is one loop of acquired fetal Diffusion transverse data viewed in Transverse, Coronal and Sagittal planes with 2 mm×2 mm in plane resolution, 4mm slice thickness and -2mm gap. (b)-(d) are corresponding reconstructed b0 image, ADC map and FA map respectively with 2mm cubic resolution. (e) is reconstructed anatomical data.

4.2 ROI Analysis for ADC and FA Values

Region of Interest (ROI) analysis was performed on all fetal subjects for 9 regions as shown in Table 3 and 4. ADC measurements could be made for all 8 subjects. 5 of them had FA maps of sufficient quality for measurement; while the rest 3 have much

Table 3. Region of Interest (ROI) Measurement of 8 Fetal Subject on ADC values ($\mu m^2 / ms$)

Diag.	GA	LtCSO	RtCSO	LtFrontalWM	RtFrontalWM	LfThalamus	RtThalamus	LtPLIC	RtPLIC	Genu
Normal	24.4	1.63±0.07	1.56±0.04	1.46±0.09	1.51±0.03	1.42±0.17	1.43±0.12	1.31±0.14	1.32±0.11	1.28±0.05
Mild VD	25.4	1.79±0.04	1.78±0.02	1.63±0.09	1.70±0.02	1.31±0.04	1.26±0.02	1.34±0.03	1.34±0.05	1.42±0.09
Agen CC	26.7	1.90±0.04	1.80±0.03	1.78±0.03	1.77±0.05	1.45±0.08	1.42±0.05	1.41±0.06	1.43±0.04	N/A
Mild UVD	27	1.82±0.06	1.61±0.03	1.63±0.13	1.73±0.10	1.33±0.14	1.41±0.08	1.17±0.16	1.29±0.12	1.43±0.12
Mild VD	30	1.91±0.09	1.89±0.08	1.90±0.11	1.93±0.03	1.36±0.06	1.18±0.08	1.42±0.11	1.25±0.04	1.33±0.16
Normal	31.3	1.52±0.08	1.73±0.14	1.89±0.09	1.86±0.05	1.24±0.05	1.35±0.05	1.21±0.06	1.22±0.09	1.45±0.17
Destructive	34	1.09±0.06	1.21±0.08	1.23±0.05	1.30±0.05	0.74±0.02	0.85±0.08	0.86±0.02	0.96±0.09	1.36±0.16
Agen CC	34.3	1.50±0.09	1.61±0.12	0.74±0.19	1.87±0.07	1.38±0.12	1.40±0.09	1.06±0.06	1.15±0.17	N/A

VD: ventricular dilation; Agen CC: Agenesis of the corpus callosum; UVD: unilateral ventricular dilation. Destructive: severe cerebellar hypoplasia.
Lt/Rt CSO: Left/Right Centrum Semiovale(Central); Lt/Rt FrontalWM: Left/Right Frontal White Matter; Lt/Rt Thalamus: Left/Right Thalamus; Lt/Rt PLIC: Left/Right Posterior Limb of Internal Capsule; Genu: Genu of Corpus Callosum.

Table 4. Region of Interest (ROI) Measurement of 5 Fetal Subject on FA values

Diag.	GA	LtCSO	RtCSO	LtFrontalWM	RtFrontalWM	LfThalamus	RtThalamus	LtPLIC	RtPLIC	Genu
Normal	24.4	0.16±0.02	0.14±0.02	0.18±0.03	0.25±0.03	0.17±0.04	0.15±0.03	0.27±0.01	0.23±0.04	0.43±0.04
Mild VD	25.4	0.12±0.01	0.11±0.02	0.18±0.03	0.20±0.04	0.22±0.05	0.13±0.04	0.25±0.04	0.29±0.05	0.40±0.11
Agen CC	26.7	0.10±0.03	0.11±0.04	0.16±0.03	0.16±0.04	0.14±0.03	0.19±0.06	0.27±0.08	0.37±0.06	N/A
Mild VD	30	0.16±0.06	0.15±0.07	0.15±0.05	0.12±0.04	0.25±0.06	0.20±0.09	0.35±0.04	0.28±0.06	0.51±0.09
Destructive	34	0.28±0.05	0.23±0.08	0.30±0.08	0.16±0.04	0.21±0.08	0.24±0.05	0.35±0.08	0.44±0.10	0.49±0.04

less good quality diffusion weighted raw images caused by severe motion to support robust FA calculation. Both ADC and FA have been shown to be age dependent in premature infants and to be changed by pathology [11]. Our fetal data, especially the normal subjects, are consistent with these *ex-utero* results.

5 Conclusion

We have described a methodology for diffusion tensor imaging of moving subjects by combining registered single shot 2D slices from sequential diffusion weighted scans. The method has been performed successfully on adults and especially on fetuses, for which no effective conventional diffusion tensor imaging method is currently available. The results allow fine structure of both ADC and FA maps to be clearly revealed potentially providing a means of monitoring microstructural development of the in-utero fetal brain for the first time. A future development that we would like to pursue is tractography of the fetal brain.

References

[1] Righini, A., et al.: Apparent diffusion coefficient determination in normal fetal brain: a prenatal MR imaging study. AJNR 24, 799–804 (2003)

[2] Prayer, D., et al.: MRI of normal fetal brain development. Eur.J.Radiol. 57(2), 199–216 (2006)

[3] Bui, T., et al.: Microstructural development of human brain assessed in utero by diffusion tensor imaging. Pediatr Radio 36, 1133–1140 (2006)

[4] Rousseau, F., et al.: A novel approach to high resolution fetal brain MR imaging. In: Duncan, J.S., Gerig, G. (eds.) MICCAI 2005. LNCS, vol. 3749, pp. 548–555. Springer, Heidelberg (2005)

[5] Jiang, S., et al.: A novel approach to accurate 3D high resolution and high SNR fetal brain imaging. In: ISBI 2006, pp. 662–665 (2006)

[6] Jiang, S., et al.: MRI of moving subjects using multi-slice Snapshot images with Volume Reconstruction (SVR): application to fetal, neonatal and adult brain studies. IEEE Tran. Medical Imaging 26(7), 967–980 (2007)

[7] Studholme, C., et al.: An overlap invariant entropy measure of 3D medical image alignment. Pattern Recognition 32(1), 71–86 (1999)

[8] Jenkinson, M., et al.: Improved optimization for the robust and accurate linear registration and motion correction of brain images. NeuroImage 17, 825–841 (2002)

[9] Lee, S., et al.: Scattered data interpolation with multilevel B-splines. IEEE Trans. Visualization Comput. Graph. 3, 228–244 (1997)

[10] Paige, C.C., et al.: LSQR: An Algorithm for Sparse Linear Equations and Sparse Least Squares. ACM Transactions on Mathematical Software (TOMS) 8(1), 43–71 (1982)

[11] Partridge, S.C., et al.: Diffusion tensor imaging: serial quantitation of white matter tract maturity in premature newborns. NeuroImage 22, 1302–1314 (2004)

Real-Time MR Diffusion Tensor and Q-Ball Imaging Using Kalman Filtering

C. Poupon[1,2], F. Poupon[1,2], A. Roche[1,2], Y. Cointepas[1,2],
J. Dubois[3], and J.-F. Mangin[1,2]

[1] CEA Neurospin - Bât. 145, 91191 Gif-sur-Yvette, France
cyril.poupon@cea.fr
[2] IFR49, 91191 Gif-sur-Yvette, France
[3] Faculté de médecine, Université de Genève, Switzerland

Abstract. Magnetic resonance diffusion imaging (dMRI) has become an established research tool for the investigation of tissue structure and orientation. In this paper, we present a method for real time processing of diffusion tensor and Q-ball imaging. The basic idea is to use Kalman filtering framework to fit either the linear tensor or Q-ball model. Because the Kalman filter is designed to be an incremental algorithm, it naturally enables updating the model estimate after the acquisition of any new diffusion-weighted volume. Processing diffusion models and maps during ongoing scans provides a new useful tool for clinicians, especially when it is not possible to predict how long a subject may remain still in the magnet.

1 Introduction

Magnetic resonance (MR) diffusion imaging has become an established technique for inferring structural anisotropy of tissues and mapping the white matter connectivity of the human brain [1]. The term diffusion refers to the Brownian motion of water molecules inside tissues that results from the thermal energy carried by these molecules. MR images can be sensitized to that physiological phenomenon from the application of a specific pair of well-known diffusion gradients together with a spin echo pulse sequence.

Technically, diffusion imaging requires the acquisition of a set of diffusion sensitized images from which molecules displacement probability is inferred. Several mathematical models have been designed, becoming more and more complex over the last decade while attempting to make less and less assumptions. In this paper, we focus on both the diffusion tensor (DTI) model (historically the first) introduced by Basser [2] and the Q-ball model (QBI) introduced by Tuch [3]. Despite the huge amount of assumptions (unrestricted environment, structural homogeneity within voxels), the DTI model is still widely used because it can be used in a clinically acceptable time (a few minutes for an entire brain coverage) and provides useful information to the clinicians about the average translational motion (apparent diffusion coefficient, ADC), the anisotropy of white matter structure (fractional anisotropy index, FA), and the RGB orientation map (RGB)). Today, clinical studies of brain pathologies (either neurodegenerative or psychiatric) involve statistical analysis of ADC and FA maps. Q-ball

N. Ayache, S. Ourselin, A. Maeder (Eds.): MICCAI 2007, Part I, LNCS 4791, pp. 27–35, 2007.
© Springer-Verlag Berlin Heidelberg 2007

belongs to the class of high angular resolution diffusion imaging (HARDI) models that aim at solving the partial voluming problem due to the existence of several putative populations of fibres within a voxel. Such models have been developed to address the inference of white matter connectivity mapping from the knowledge of local microstructural orientations of tissue.

Compared to DTI, QBI requires from five to ten times more diffusion gradient orientations with a higher b-value and therefore cannot be considered as reliable for clinical use for many reasons. First, clinical protocols generally involve different MR acquisitions (T1, T2, BOLD) limiting the time alloted to diffusion imaging. Second, the patient may move severely during the acquisition (a frequent situation for patients impaired with Huntington disease, Parkinson disease, schizophrenia), hence increasing the risk of aborting the scanning. The same problem arises for studies involving newborns who cannot be sedated: generally, less than 75% of the subjects can be exploited because they often wake up inside the magnet, due to the level of noise. The opposite situation is also true: the patient can be more cooperative than hypothesized first and it's worth starting with a high b-value DTI scan and continuing with a QBI scan if the patient is still.

This paper addresses the feasibility of real time DTI and QBI processing for displaying reconstructed associated maps during an ongoing scan. This will make it possible to start the scan estimating both models, to cancel the acquisition at any time, or to sustain the scanning when the subject is still in the magnet. If the scanning is stopped after too few diffusion gradient orientations, none of the model is exploitable. Then, according to the acquired number of orientations, either DTI model, QBI model or both can be obtained. To our knowledge, real time processing was previously addressed for BOLD functional imaging [4], but has never been proposed for diffusion imaging.

DTI and QBI models can be expressed in the light of the general linear model framework (GLM) assuming a white noise model. Among available techniques for solving least-squares linear regression models, the Kalman filter provides an appropriate answer to the real time requirement, as it is an incremental solver. After the acquisition of the entire volume for each diffusion gradient orientation, this filter can update DTI and QBI maps, provide variance of the estimate and can deliver an immediate feedback to the clinician or to the expert in cognitive neurosciences.

After introducing the linear models for DTI and QBI in section 2.1, we describe the Kalman filter-based algorithm implemented in section 2.2. Then we focus on the optimization of the diffusion gradient orientation set in section 2.3. In section 3, we give a setup of the realtime protocol used and we illustrate the technique using DTI and QBI MR data, before concluding.

2   Methods

2.1   Model Fitting Formulation

Let us consider the vector $\boldsymbol{m} = [m_1, ..., m_N]$, acquired during the acquisition corresponding to the diffusion-sensitized signal measured with the different diffusion gradient orientations at a given voxel in the scanned volume. The gradient orientations $\boldsymbol{o}_i$ are indexed by i corresponding to the time rank during the acquisition and are numbered from 1 to N. The choice of the orientation set will be discussed later in section 2.3. The magnitude of the sensitization is given by the b-value in s/mm^2. We also define m_0 corresponding to the unweighted signal measured with diffusion gradients off.

Tensor general linear model
The DT model states that the diffusion of water molecules can be considered as free, yielding a Gaussian probability density function characterized by a second order tensor $\boldsymbol{D}$. The signal attenuation observed when applying a diffusion gradient along the normalized direction $\boldsymbol{o} = [o_x, o_y, o_z]^T$ of the space and with sensitization b is exponential:

$$m = m_0 e^{-b\boldsymbol{o}^T \boldsymbol{D}\boldsymbol{o}} + \mu \tag{1}$$

where μ represent the acquisition noise that usually follows a Rician distribution. Taking the natural logarithm of this attenuation, we easily obtain the general linear model:

$$\boldsymbol{y} = \boldsymbol{B}\boldsymbol{d} + \boldsymbol{\epsilon} \tag{2}$$

where we define the measured vector of attenuations $\boldsymbol{y} = [y_1, ..., y_N]^T$, with $y_i = log(m_0/m_i)$ and $\boldsymbol{d} = [D_{xx}, D_{xy}, D_{xz}, D_{yy}, D_{yz}, D_{zz}]^T$ being the vector of the six unknown coefficients of the diffusion tensor. $\boldsymbol{B}$ is a $N \times 6$ matrix called the diffusion sensitization matrix, built from N rows $\boldsymbol{b}_1, ..., \boldsymbol{b}_N$ depending only on the diffusion gradient settings $\boldsymbol{b_i} = b_i[o_{x,i}{}^2, 2o_{x,i}o_{y,i}, 2o_{x,i}o_{z,i}, o_{y,i}{}^2, 2o_{y,i}o_{z,i}, o_{z,i}{}^2]$.

ϵ is the $N \times 1$ vector of errors $\epsilon_i = -ln(1+\mu e^{b_i \boldsymbol{o}_i{}^T \boldsymbol{D}\boldsymbol{o}_i}/m_0) \approx -\mu e^{b_i \boldsymbol{o}_i{}^T \boldsymbol{D}\boldsymbol{o}_i}/m_0$. Theoretically, the noise model depends on the unknowns as well as on the Rician noise μ, but we assume it is not far from a Gaussian distribution. Studying the true distribution of the noise must be done, but it is not the purpose of this paper that deals with the real-time aspect of the algorithm, even if the estimate is not statistically optimum.

Q-ball general linear model
The Q-ball model states that the orientation distribution function (ODF) $\psi(\boldsymbol{o}) = \int_0^\infty p(r\boldsymbol{o})dr$ that gives the likelihood of any orientation $\boldsymbol{o}$ can be obtained by sampling a sphere in the Q-space [3] which radius is set up by a high b-value (typically greater than $3000s/mm^2$) with a huge number of gradient orientations (from 160 to 500 according to the litterature). A good approximation of the ODF was proposed by Tuch using the Funk-Radon transform (FRT). In order to obtain $\psi(\boldsymbol{o}_i)$, the FRT integrates the MR signal along the equator of the given orientation $\boldsymbol{o}_i$.

A first linear model of the FRT has been published in [5] corresponding to the raw algorithm. More recently, Descoteaux et al [6] proposed an elegant reformulation of the FRT using the Funk-Hecke theorem for decomposing the ODF onto a symmetric, orthonormal and real spherical harmonics.

Let $\boldsymbol{c} = [c_1, ..., c_K]^T$ be the $K \times 1$ vector of coefficients c_j of the spherical harmonics decomposition of the ODF and is calculated from the reconstruction equation:

$$\boldsymbol{c} = \boldsymbol{P}\left(\boldsymbol{B}^T\boldsymbol{B} + \lambda\boldsymbol{L}\right)^{-1}\boldsymbol{B}^T\boldsymbol{m} \tag{3}$$

where $\boldsymbol{B}$ is a $N \times K$ matrix built from the modified spherical harmonics basis $B_{ij} = Y_j\left(\theta(\boldsymbol{o_i}), \phi(\boldsymbol{o_i})\right)$ (θ is the colatitude and ϕ is the azimuth of the diffusion gradient orientation $\boldsymbol{o_i}$), $\boldsymbol{L}$ is the $K \times K$ matrix of Laplace-Beltrami regularization operator, λ is the regularization factor, $\boldsymbol{P}$ is the $K \times K$ Funk-Hecke diagonal matrix with elements $P_{ii} = 2\pi P_{l(j)}(0)/P_{l(j)}(1)$ ($P_{l(j)}(x)$ is the Legendre polynomial of degree $l(j)$, see also [6] for the definition of $l(j)$)).

From the knowledge of the decomposition $\boldsymbol{c}$, we can obtain the ODF value for the orientation $\boldsymbol{o}$ calculating the composition (4):

$$\psi(\boldsymbol{o}) = \sum_{j=1}^{N} c_j Y_j\left(\theta(\boldsymbol{o}), \phi(\boldsymbol{o})\right) \tag{4}$$

The equation (3) can easily be reversed to get the general linear model:

$$\boldsymbol{m} = \boldsymbol{B}^+\boldsymbol{c} + \boldsymbol{\epsilon} \quad \text{with} \quad \boldsymbol{B}^+ = \left(\boldsymbol{P}\left(\boldsymbol{B}^T\boldsymbol{B} + \lambda\boldsymbol{L}\right)^{-1}\boldsymbol{B}^T\right)^{\dagger} \tag{5}$$

where $\boldsymbol{\epsilon}$ is the vector of Rician acquisition noise that we assume to be Gaussian in order to stay in the ordinary linear least square framework. The $()^{\dagger}$ stands for the Moore-Penrose pseudo-inverse operator. Further investigation must be done concerning this operator in order to prevent the apparition of negative items in the vector c when the spherical harmonics order is increased.

2.2 Kalman Filtering

The Kalman filter is a recursive solver that optimally minimize the mean square error of the estimation [7][8]. Because of its recursive nature, it is a suitable method for updating the DTI or QBI model parameters after the acquisition of each new diffusion-sensitized volume. Moreover, the Kalman filter provides, at each time frame, an estimated covariance of the parameter estimate that can be used to automatically stop the ongoing scan when the maximum variance falls below a minimum threshold.

In section 2.1, we obtained two general linear models for DTI and QBI of the form $\boldsymbol{y} = \boldsymbol{Ax} + \boldsymbol{\epsilon}$. The Kalman filter exploits any new measure y for updating the unknown parameters $\boldsymbol{x}$, usually called the state vector.

Assume that after the acquisition of rank i, a current estimate $\hat{\boldsymbol{x}}(i-1)$ is available. Given the new MR measurement $y(i)$ and the vector $\boldsymbol{a}(i) = [A_{i1}, ..., A_{iP}]^T$ corresponding to the ith row of the matrix $\boldsymbol{A}$, the innovation $\nu(i) = y(i) - \boldsymbol{a}(i)^T\hat{\boldsymbol{x}}(i-1)$ is calculated. The Kalman filter then updates the parameters using the recursion:

$$\begin{cases} \boldsymbol{k}(i) = \left(1 + \boldsymbol{a}(i)^T\boldsymbol{P}(i-1)\boldsymbol{a}(i)\right)^{-1}\boldsymbol{P}(i-1)\boldsymbol{a}(i) \\ \hat{\boldsymbol{x}}(i) = \hat{\boldsymbol{x}}(i-1) + \nu(i)\boldsymbol{k}(i) \\ \boldsymbol{P}(i) = \boldsymbol{P}(i-1) - \boldsymbol{k}(i)\boldsymbol{a}(i)^T\boldsymbol{P}(i-1) \end{cases} \tag{6}$$

where the vector $k(i)$ is usually called the Kalman gain. $P(i)$ represents an estimate of the normalized covariance matrix of x given the information at time i. The unnormalized covariance of $\hat{x}(i)$ is equal to $\hat{\sigma}(i)^2 P(i)$ using the recursion:

$$\hat{\sigma}(i) = \frac{i-1}{i}\left[\hat{\sigma}(i-1) + \nu(i)^2 \left(1 + a(i)^T P(i-1)a(i)\right)^{-1}\right] \tag{7}$$

The initial guesses $\hat{x}(0)$, $P(0)$ and $\hat{\sigma}(0)$ can be respectively set to the null vector, the identity matrix and zero.

2.3 Optimum Diffusion Gradient Orientation Set

Contrary to functional scans where the time order of the stimuli cannot be modified, diffusion scans can play the diffusion gradient orientation set in random order, provided it is a uniform distribution of the orientations in the tridimensional space, for obtaining an accurate tensor or Q-ball estimation.

The optimum orientation count is still debated in the litterature [9]. Increasing this number directly improves the SNR of the ADC, FA and ODF maps, at the price of a longer scan time and knowing that it is not always possible to predict how long a subject will remain still in the magnet. In order to reduce the risk of failure, we implemented the sequence of orientations proposed in [10], which yields the "best" spatial distribution of the orientations, should the acquisition be terminated before completion. This sequence consists in a series of small meaningful subsets of 14 uniform orientations, while all clusters complement each other with additional orientations. Figure 1 gives an example of 42 orientations divided into 3 subsets of 14 orientations. The distribution obtained from the 14 or 28 orientation subsets are more uniform with the optimum distribution than with the conventional distribution. This strategy has been applied only for DTI scanning, but can be also used for QBI scanning.

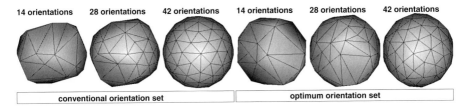

Fig. 1. Comparison of conventional and optimum sets of 42 orientations; meshes of the full distributions are represented as well as meshes corresponding to subsets restrained to the 14 or 28 first orientations; conventional set is more uniform than the optimum set when the full set is acquired, but less uniform when it is not complete; optimum set is to be prefered for real time scan that can be interrupted at any time

2.4 DTI and QBI Acquisition Settings

The real time diffusion Kalman filter was evaluated on an adult, under a protocol approved by the Institutional Ethical Committee. Two different acquisitions were performed using a DW Dual Spin Echo EPI technique on a 1.5T MRI system (ExciteII, GE Healthcare, USA) for validating both DTI and QBI solvers. Pulse sequence settings were $b = 700s/mm2$, 42 optimum gradient orientation set, matrix 128×128, 60 slices, $FOV = 24cm$, slice thickness $TH = 2mm$, $TE/TR = 66.2ms/12.5s$ for a DTI scan time of $9min48s$, and $b = 3000s/mm^2$, 200 conventional gradient orientation set, matrix 128×128, 60 slices, $FOV = 24cm$, slice thickness $TH = 2mm$, $TE/TR = 93.2ms/19s$ for a QBI scan time of $72min50s$.

3   Results

3.1   Real Time Standard Diffusion Maps

At each iteration of the DTI scan, an approximation of the diffusion tensor is available for each voxel of the brain. Therefore it is possible to process its eigensystem online and then to estimate the ADC / FA / RGB maps. Columns 1-3 of figure 2 depict the evolution of these maps during the ongoing scan. For comparison, the 4th column shows the result of a standard offline SVD analysis. There is no qualitative difference with the 3rd column processed using the Kalman filter.

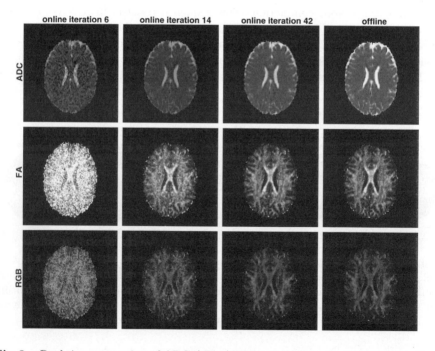

Fig. 2. Real time processing of ADC / FA / RGB maps using the DTI Kalman filter during an ongoing DTI scan at $b = 700s/mm^2$ with 42 diffusion gradient orientations; the columns 1/2/3 correspond to iteration 6, 14 and 42; the last column shows the result of the standard offline processing

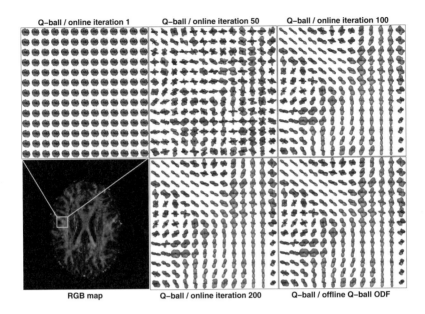

Fig. 3. Real time processing of a Q-ball ODF map using the QBI Kalman filter during an ongoing QBI scan at $b = 3000s/mm^2$ with 200 diffusion gradient orientations; the bottom row displays a RGB orientation map (left) on which is drawn a region of interest inside the white matter, containing fibre crossings and homogeneous voxels, and the corresponding map of Q-ball ODFs (right) processed with the offline routine; the top row shows iterations 1, 50 and 200 of the same ODF map calculated with the online Kalman filter

The use of an optimum orientation set speeds up the convergence of the estimation that can be considered exploitable by clinicians from the 14th iteration. The time required to perform one iteration of the DTI Kalman filter over the full brain is less than 8 seconds on a 3.2GHz linux station, which is lower than the repetition time $TR = 12.5s$ of the scan. Consequently, there is no addtional delay between two consecutive acquisitions, making this protocol truly real time.

3.2   Real Time Orientation Distribution Function Maps

The Q-ball online Kalman filter was used for processing ODFs during the ongoing QBI scan. A symmetrical spherical harmonics basis of order 8 was chosen and the Laplace-Beltrami regularization factor was set to 0.006 as proposed in [6]. The ODFs are reconstructed on 400 normalized uniform orientations. The QBI dedicated Kalman filter (5) provides, at each step and for each voxel of the brain, an estimate of the decomposition of the ODF on to a symmetric spherical harmonics basis from which it is easy to obtain the values for any orientation o of the space (equation (4)).

The top row on figure 3 shows the evolution of the ODF map during the Kalman recursion on a region of interest contained in the subcortical white matter, and exhibiting some fibre crossings as well as voxels with homogeneous fibre populations. As for DTI, there is no qualitive difference between the ODF maps obtained from the online Kalman filter or from the offline Q-ball algorithm given by equation (3). The choice for that order can be discussed, because there are 45 spherical harmonic coefficients to estimate, which represents a lot of unknown, and consequently requires a lot of iterations before to converge. A lower order would give nice results after less iterations.

The time required for performing one iteration of the QBI Kalman filter on a slice is almost 5 seconds, which is lower than the repetition time $TR = 19s$ of the scan. Obviously, it is more time consuming than DTI processing where the entire brain can be processed within 8 seconds. In the case of QBI, only 4 slice locations can be performed in real time. However, the C++ code can still be optimized and parallelized on a grid of processors, if the whole brain is to be processed in real time.

4   Conclusion

We have developed an incremental Kalman-filter based framework dedicated to real-time diffusion MR imaging. This framework address both diffusion tensor and Qball models, and enables processing the standard DTI / QBI maps, in real time during an ongoing scan. The methodology developed in this paper is very suitable for clinical use when a quick feedback is required during the acquisition or when the cooperation of the subject is not certain. More quantitative evaluations of the difference between online and offline reconstructions must be performed for validating this approach, as well as studying more deeply the underlying model of noise present in DTI and QBI data, which was not the main purpose of this paper. There is also a clear need to study the best trade-off between the iteration number, the wavevector number [11] , the regularization factor, and estimation order. A future extension of this work entails online fibre tracking. To that end, we plan to modify the diffusion Kalman filter in order to process incremental connectivity maps during ongoing diffusion scans.

References

1. LeBihan, D., Breton, E., Lallemand, D.: MR imaging of intravoxel incoherent motions: application to diffusion and perfusion in neurologic disorders. Radiology 161, 401–407 (1986)
2. Basser, P.J., Mattiello, J., Le Bihan, D.: Estimation of the effective self-diffusion tensor from the NMR spin echo. Journal of Magnetic Resonance 103, 247–254 (1994)
3. Tuch, D.: Diffusion MRI of complex tissue structure. PhD thesis, Harvard-MIT (2002)
4. Roche, A., Pinel, P., Dehaene, S., Poline, J.-B.: Solving incrementally the fitting and detection problems in fMRI time series. In: Barillot, C., Haynor, D.R., Hellier, P. (eds.) MICCAI 2004. LNCS, vol. 3217, pp. 719–726. Springer, Heidelberg (2004)
5. Tuch, D.: Q-ball imaging. Magn. Reson. Med. 52, 1358–1372 (2004)

6. Descoteaux, M., Angelino, E., Fitzgibbons, S., Deriche, R.: A fast and robust ODF estimation algorithm in Q-ball imaging. In: Proc. ISBI 2006, Arlington, USA, pp. 81–84 (2006)
7. Ayache, N.: Artificial vision for mobile robots. The MIT Press, Cambridge, USA (1991)
8. Welch, G., Bishop, G.: An Introduction to the Kalman Filter. In: SIGGRAPH 2001 course 8, In Computer Graphics, Annual Conference on Computer Graphics & Interactive Techniques, Cambridge, USA (1991)
9. Jones, D.: The effect of gradient sampling schemes on measures derived from diffusion tensor MRI: a Monte Carlo study. Magn. Reson. Med. 51, 807–815 (2004)
10. Dubois, J., Poupon, C., Lethimonnier, F., Le Bihan, D.: Optimized diffusion gradient orientation schemes for corrupted clinical DTI data sets. MAGMA 19, 134–143 (2006)
11. Khachaturian, M.-H., Wisco, J.-J., Tuch, D.: Boosting the sampling efficiency of q-Ball imaging using multiple wavevector fusion. Magn. Reson. Med. 57, 289–296 (2007)

Finsler Tractography for White Matter Connectivity Analysis of the Cingulum Bundle*

John Melonakos[1], Vandana Mohan[1], Marc Niethammer[2], Kate Smith[2], Marek Kubicki[2], and Allen Tannenbaum[1]

[1] Department of Electrical and Computer Engineering, Georgia Institute of
Technology, USA
jmelonak@ece.gatech.edu
[2] Psychiatry Neuroimaging Laboratory, Harvard Medical School, USA

Abstract. In this paper, we present a novel approach for the segmentation of white matter tracts based on Finsler active contours. This technique provides an optimal measure of connectivity, explicitly segments the connecting fiber bundle, and is equipped with a metric which is able to utilize the directional information of high angular resolution data. We demonstrate the effectiveness of the algorithm for segmenting the cingulum bundle.

1 Introduction

Since the advent of diffusion weighted magnetic resonance imaging (DW-MRI), a great amount of research has been devoted to finding and characterizing neural connections between brain structures. In this paper, we present a novel approach for the segmentation of white matter tracts based on Finsler active contours [1]. Furthermore, we show results of the algorithm for segmenting the cingulum bundle (CB).

Recently, tractography advances have been made which provide full brain optimal connectivity maps from predefined seed regions. These approaches can be subdivided into stochastic and energy-minimization approaches.

Stochastic approaches produce probability maps of connectivity between a seed region and the rest of the brain. Parker *et al.* developed PICo, a probabilistic index for standard streamline techniques [2]. Perrin *et al.* presented probabilistic techniques for untangling fiber crossings using q-ball fields [3]. In other work, Friman *et al.* proposed a method for probabilistically growing fibers in a large number of random directions and inferring connectivity from the resulting percentages of connections between seed and target regions [4]. While providing

* This work was supported in part by grants from NSF, AFOSR, ARO, MURI, MRI-HEL as well as by a grant from NIH (NAC P41 RR-13218) through Brigham and Women's Hospital. This work is part of the National Alliance for Medical Image Computing (NAMIC), funded by the National Institutes of Health through the NIH Roadmap for Medical Research, Grant U54 EB005149. Information on the National Centers for Biomedical Computing can be obtained from http://nihroadmap.nih.gov/bioinformatics.

N. Ayache, S. Ourselin, A. Maeder (Eds.): MICCAI 2007, Part I, LNCS 4791, pp. 36–43, 2007.
© Springer-Verlag Berlin Heidelberg 2007

a measure of connectivity between brain regions, these stochastic approaches do not provide an explicit segmentation of the fiber bundle itself.

Energy-minimization techniques have also been developed. Parker *et al.* proposed fast marching tractography which minimizes an energy based on both the position and direction of the normal to a propagating front [5]. O'Donnell *et al.* cast the tractography problem in a geometric framework finding geodesics on a Riemannian manifold based on diffusion tensors [6]. Similarly, Prados *et al.* and Lenglet *et al.* demonstrated a Riemannian based technique, GCM (Geodesic Connectivity Mapping), for computing geodesics using a variant of fast marching methods adapted for directional flows [7,8]. Jackowski *et al.* also find Riemannian geodesics using Fast Sweeping methods as given by Kao *et al.* [9,10,11]. In cases of high angular diffusion data, these Riemannian based approaches do not take advantage of the full directional resolution due to the loss of information incurred by the construction of diffusion tensors.

In this paper, we present a technique which provides an optimal measure of connectivity, explicitly segments the connecting fiber bundle, and is based on the richer Finsler metric. Rather than following the traditional approach of finding a large number of fibers (which individually have questionable meaning), clustering them, and then performing statistical analyses on the clusters, we present an alternative approach. We first find the optimal connection, which we term the *anchor tract*, on the Finsler manifold between the seed and target regions. Then, we initialize an expanding surface level set evolution on the anchor tract which grows until it stops at a local minima on the edge of the fiber bundle. Finally, since the fiber bundle extraction does not rely upon standard statistical measures, such as fractional anisotropy (FA), for the segmentation, we are free to use these measures to statistically compare fiber bundles in clinical studies.

In Section 2, we motivate our interest in segmenting the cingulum bundle. In Section 3, we describe the algorithm for extracting the anchor tracts. Then, in Section 4, we present our surface evolution algorithm for extracting the full cingulum bundle. Finally, in Section 5, we show results for extracting the anchor tracts and the corresponding cingulum bundle.

2   The Cingulum Bundle

The cingulum bundle is a 5-7 mm in diameter fiber bundle that interconnects all parts of the limbic system. It originates within the white matter of the temporal pole, and runs posterior and superior into the parietal lobe, then turns, forming a "ring-like belt" around the corpus callosum, into the frontal lobe, terminating anterior and inferior to the genu of the corpus callosum in the orbital-frontal cortex [12]. Because of its involvement in executive control and emotional processing, the cingulum bundle has been investigated in several clinical populations, including depression and schizophrenia. Previous studies, using DW-MRI, in schizophrenia, demonstrated decrease of FA in anterior part of the cingulum bundle [13,14], at the same time pointing to the technical limitations restricting these investigations from following the entire fiber tract.

3   Anchor Tracts on a Finsler Manifold

In this section, we present our algorithm for extracting the optimal path, or *anchor tract*, between two regions in the brain. In this formulation, the optimal path is defined with respect to a Finsler metric. In the case of data acquired with only 6 gradient directions, this reduces to a Riemannian metric because there are 6 independent elements of the diffusion tensor. However, in the case of high angular data, the Finsler metric is more flexible than the Riemannian metric as it is not restricted to an ellipsoidal diffusion profile which results from the Gaussian diffusion assumption.

In order to find the anchor tract, we construct a dynamic programming based approach which uses a Fast Sweeping method, see [15,10,11] for algorithmic details. Also, see the work by Jackowski *et al.* for a formulation of this algorithm based on the Riemannian metric [9]. For the sake of completeness, we include a brief overview of the algorithm.

For any given starting point $\boldsymbol{p}_0$, define the value function as the minimum cost for reaching a seed region $S \subset \mathbb{R}^n$ from $\boldsymbol{p}_0$. The resulting Hamilton-Jacobi-Bellman equation is

$$\begin{cases} 0 = \inf_{\hat{\boldsymbol{d}} \in S^{n-1}} \{ \ \psi(\boldsymbol{p}, \hat{\boldsymbol{d}}) + \nabla \mathcal{L}^*(\boldsymbol{p}) \cdot \hat{\boldsymbol{d}} \ \}, \\ \mathcal{L}^*(\boldsymbol{s}) = 0 \text{ for } \boldsymbol{s} \in S, \end{cases} \tag{1}$$

where ψ is the local cost at each point, $\boldsymbol{p}$, and for each direction, $\hat{\boldsymbol{d}}$, and $\mathcal{L}^*$ is the optimal Finsler length. Numerically, this equation may be solved via Fast Sweeping as shown in Algorithm 1.

Algorithm 1. Sweeping algorithm for the HJB equation (1)

Require: seed region S, direction-dependent local cost ψ
1: Initialize $\mathcal{L}^*(\cdot) \leftarrow +\infty$, except at starting points $s \in S$ where $\mathcal{L}^*(s) \leftarrow 0$
2: **repeat**
3:     **sweep** through all voxels $\boldsymbol{p}$, in all possible grid directions
4:         $\hat{\boldsymbol{d}}' \leftarrow \arg\min_{d \in S^{n-1}} f_{\mathcal{L}^*, \psi}(\boldsymbol{p}, \hat{\boldsymbol{d}})$
5:         **if** $f_{\mathcal{L}^*, \psi}(\boldsymbol{p}, \hat{\boldsymbol{d}}') < \mathcal{L}^*(\boldsymbol{p})$ **then** $\mathcal{L}^*(\boldsymbol{p}) \leftarrow f_{\mathcal{L}^*, \psi}(\boldsymbol{p}, \hat{\boldsymbol{d}}')$ and $\hat{\boldsymbol{d}}^*(\boldsymbol{p}) \leftarrow \hat{\boldsymbol{d}}'$ **end if**
6:     **end sweep**
7: **until** convergence of $\mathcal{L}^*$

The Fast Sweeping algorithm results in optimal connectivity maps and characteristic vectors at every point in the domain. The anchor tract is then determined by following the characteristic vectors from the target region back to the seed region, not by gradient descent as is standard in direction-independent schemes [16].

There are many numerical schemes which may be used to solve the Hamilton-Jacobi-Bellman equation given above. The number of sweeping iterations required by the Fast Sweeping algorithm depends upon the number of turns in the optimal path. Since neural tracts tend to have few total turns, the Fast Sweeping algorithm is efficient for extracting tracts. We also note that the connections of graph cuts and such directional metrics have been described in [17,18,19]. Of particular note, in [18] the explicit connection between Finsler distances and the flux methods of [20] is considered in some detail.

4   Level Set Fiber Bundle Segmentation

In this section, we discuss the level set surface evolution which we have used to extract the volumetric cingulum bundle. This level set surface is initialized on the anchor tract described in Section 3. By using the calculus of variations, the minimizing flow for a directional cost $\psi(\boldsymbol{p}, \hat{\boldsymbol{d}})$ is obtained as,

$$\Sigma_t = -\{\nabla_{\boldsymbol{p}}\psi \cdot N + Tr(\nabla_{\hat{\boldsymbol{d}}\hat{\boldsymbol{d}}}\psi) + (n-1)\psi H\}N, \tag{2}$$

where Σ is the evolving hypersurface, N is the outward unit normal to the hypersurface, and H denotes the mean curvature. A derivation of this flow can be found in [21]. The expression for the evolution of the level set function 'u' is obtained as,

$$u_t = \{\nabla_{\boldsymbol{p}}\psi \cdot \nabla u\} + \{Tr(\nabla_{\hat{\boldsymbol{d}}\hat{\boldsymbol{d}}}\psi) + (n-1)\psi H\} \parallel \nabla u \parallel. \tag{3}$$

We use the sparse field method of Whitaker *et al.* to efficiently implement this level set surface evolution [22]. We also use the angular interpolation algorithm presented by Tao *et al.* [23].

In order to find the edge of the cingulum bundle, we construct a cost, ψ, which aligns the tangent plane of the hypersurface with edges in the directions of diffusion of the image volume. To produce a measure of these diffusion edges, we compute the positional gradient of each diffusion direction. We then construct ψ as a function of these positional gradients.

Mathematically the form of the cost function that we desire to extremize can be written as follows.

$$\psi(\boldsymbol{p}, \hat{\boldsymbol{d}}) = \psi(\boldsymbol{p}, N(\boldsymbol{p})) = f(\nabla_{\boldsymbol{p}}\phi(\boldsymbol{p}, d_1)\cdot N, \nabla_{\boldsymbol{p}}\phi(\boldsymbol{p}, d_2)\cdot N \cdots \nabla_{\boldsymbol{p}}\phi(\boldsymbol{p}, \hat{\boldsymbol{d}}_{n_s})\cdot N) \tag{4}$$

where d_1 through d_{n_s} denote the n_s diffusion directions, ϕ denotes the DWI data, $N(\boldsymbol{p})$ denotes the normal to the hypersurface at position $\boldsymbol{p}$, and f is a linear function of the arguments.

There are many possible choices for the function ψ. In this paper, we choose ψ to be the following:

$$\psi = \{\frac{1}{n_s} \cdot \sum_{i=0}^{n_s} \frac{\nabla_{\boldsymbol{p}}\phi(\boldsymbol{p}, d_i) \cdot N(\boldsymbol{p})}{\parallel \nabla_{\boldsymbol{p}}\phi(\boldsymbol{p}, d_i) \parallel}\} - 1. \tag{5}$$

This cost ranges from [-1,0] and is maximized (at 0) when the normal to the hypersphere is aligned with the mean gradient direction.

5   Experiments and Results

In this section, we present segmentation results for anchor tracts of the right and left cingulum bundles of 12 schizophrenic and 12 normal patients. Further, we present a first implementation of the level set surface flow introduced in Section 4. Scans were acquired on a 3 Tesla GE system (General Electric Medical Systems, Milwaukee, WI). We acquired 51 directions with $b = 700\frac{s}{mm^2}$, 8 baseline scans with $b = 0\frac{s}{mm^2}$. The following scan parameters were used: TR 17000 ms, TE 78

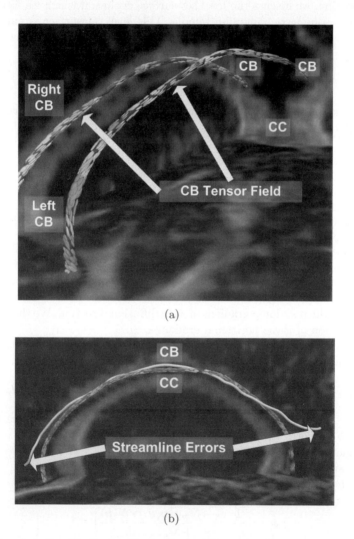

(a)

(b)

Fig. 1. Cingulum Bundle Anchor Tracts from: (a) detailed view of a normal control case, (b) streamline example on a schizophrenic case

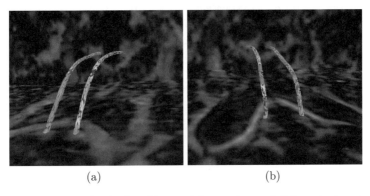

(a)   (b)

Fig. 2. Cingulum Bundle Anchor Tracts: (a) anterior and (b) posterior views of a normal control case

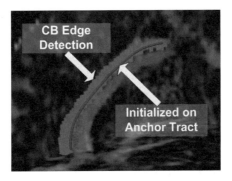

Fig. 3. Cingulum bundle level set segmentation result on a schizophrenic case

ms, FOV 24 cm, 144 x 144 encoding steps, 1.7 mm slice thickness. We acquired 81 axial-oblique slices parallel to the AC-PC line covering the whole brain.

Manually selected endpoints were provided by experts for each case. Masking is necessary to ensure that the tract does not take shortcuts through cerebral spinal fluid (CSF). We used a simple thresholding on the trace of the tensors to mask out CSF regions. Furthermore, we applied a threshold on strong left-right diffusion to mask out the corpus callosum which runs inferior to the cingulum bundle.

First, we show results of extracting the cingulum bundle anchor tract. In each figure, the tracts are superimposed upon the diffusion data which has been colored by direction (e.g. green signifies high anterior-posterior diffusion). The tensors, shown for convenience, are colored by FA. In Fig. 1, we depict the advantage of this algorithm in segmenting the cingulum bundle. The cingulum bundle curves around the ventricles on both the anterior and posterior ends. In Fig. 1(a), we show how the anchor tracts follow the smoothly varying tensor field around the bend of the ventricles. In Fig. 1(b), we share an example of a streamline based approach (freely available in the 3D Slicer tool) which fails in the same bend around the ventricles. This is the area where large tracts are joining the main bundle from both medial and lateral parts of the parietal lobes. Using the full directional data, our method is able to resolve the cingulum bundle in the presence of the merging fibers. In Fig. 2, we show anterior and posterior zoomed-out views of the anchor tracts.

Next, we show the result of an edge-based surface level set evolution on a portion of the cingulum bundle. We present here a proof of concept implementation of the theory from Section 4. In our experiment, the level set flow converged to the edge of the bundle as depicted in the image.

6   Conclusions and Future Work

In this work, we have introduced a novel approach for the segmentation of white matter tracts. We have shown an application of the method for the segmentation of the cingulum bundle. Given manually selected endpoints, the algorithm automatically extracts the cingulum bundle.

We have shown how the method was able to find centerlines, or *anchor tracts* of the cingulum bundle on 24 cases. We have also shown a first implementation of the edge-based level set surface extraction. In the future, we will run the edge-based level set segmentation on all 24 cases. We will also explore the use of other cost functions, especially region-based costs, for the level set segmentation. Finally, we will be able to compute statistics across the resulting segmented cingulum bundles for the population of schizophrenics and normal controls.

References

1. Melonakos, J., Pichon, E., Angenent, S., Tannenbaum, A.: Finsler active contours. IEEE Transactions on Pattern Analysis and Machine Intelligence, Preprint available online (2007)
2. Parker, G., Haroon, H., Wheeler-Kingshott, C.: A framework for a streamline-based probabilistic index of connectivity(PICo) using a structural interpretation of MRI diffusion measurements. Journal of Magnetic Resonance Imaging 18(2), 242–254 (2003)
3. Perrin, M., Poupon, C., Cointepas, Y., Rieul, B., Golestani, N., Pallier, C., Riviere, D., Constantinesco, A., Le Bihan, D.: Fiber tracking in Q-ball fields using regularized particle trajectories. Proc. of IPMI 2(3) (2005)
4. Friman, O., Farnebäck, G., Westin, C.: A Bayesian approach for stochastic white matter tractography. IEEE Transactions on Medical Imaging 25(8), 965 (2006)
5. Parker, G., Wheeler-Kingshott, C., Barker, G.: Estimating distributed anatomical connectivity using fast marchingmethods and diffusion tensor imaging. Medical Imaging, IEEE Transactions 21(5), 505–512 (2002)
6. O'Donnell, L., Haker, S., Westin, C.: New Approaches to Estimation of White Matter Connectivity in Diffusion Tensor MRI: Elliptic PDEs and Geodesics in a Tensor-Warped Space. In: Dohi, T., Kikinis, R. (eds.) MICCAI 2002. LNCS, vol. 2488, pp. 459–466. Springer, Heidelberg (2002)

7. Prados, E., Lenglet, C., Pons, J., Wotawa, N., Deriche, R., Faugeras, O., Soatto, S.: Control Theory and Fast Marching Techniques for Brain Connectivity Mapping. In: Proceedings of the 2006 IEEE Computer Society Conference on Computer Vision and Pattern Recognition, vol. 1, pp. 1076–1083 (2006)
8. Lenglet, C., Rousson, M., Deriche, R., Faugeras, O., Lehericy, S., Ugurbil, K.: A Riemannian Approach to Diffusion Tensor Images Segmentation. In: Christensen, G.E., Sonka, M. (eds.) IPMI 2005. LNCS, vol. 3565, pp. 591–602. Springer, Heidelberg (2005)
9. Jackowski, M., Kao, C., Qiu, M., Constable, R., Staib, L.: White matter tractography by anisotropic wavefront evolution and diffusion tensors imaging. Medical Image Analysis 9, 427–440 (2005)
10. Kao, C., Osher, S., Qian, J.: Lax–Friedrichs sweeping scheme for static Hamilton–Jacobi equations. Journal of Computational Physics 196(1), 367–391 (2004)
11. Kao, C., Osher, S., Tsai, Y.: Fast sweeping methods for static Hamilton-Jacobi equations. SIAM journal on numerical analysis 42(6), 2612–2632 (2005)
12. Schmahmann, J., Pandya, D.: Fiber Pathways of the Brain. Oxford University Press, Oxford (2006)
13. Kubicki, M., Westin, C., Nestor, P., Wible, C., Frumin, M., Maier, S., Kikinis, R., Jolesz, F., McCarley, R., Shenton, M.: Cingulate fasciculus integrity disruption in schizophrenia: a magnetic resonance diffusion tensor imaging study. Biological Psychiatry 54(11), 1171–1180 (2003)
14. Wang, F., Sun, Z., Cui, L.: Du, X., Wang, X., Zhang, H., Cong, Z., Hong, N., Zhang, D.: Anterior Cingulum Abnormalities in Male Patients With Schizophrenia Determined Through Diffusion Tensor Imaging (2004)
15. Pichon, E., Westin, C., Tannenbaum, A.: A Hamilton-Jacobi-Bellman approach to high angular resolution diffusion tractography. In: Duncan, J.S., Gerig, G. (eds.) MICCAI 2005. LNCS, vol. 3749, pp. 180–187. Springer, Heidelberg (2005)
16. Lin, Q.: Enhancement, extraction, and visualization of 3D volume data. Department of Electrical Engineering, Linköping University (2003)
17. Boykov, Y., Kolmorgorov, V., Cremers, D., Delong, A.: An integral solution to surface evolution PDEs via geo-cuts. In: Proceedings IEEE European Conference Computer Vision, pp. 409–422. IEEE Computer Society Press, Los Alamitos (2006)
18. Kolmorgorov, V., Boykov, Y.: What metrics can be approximated by geo-cuts or global optimization of length/area and flux. In: Proceedings IEEE International Conference Computer Vision, IEEE Computer Society Press, Los Alamitos (2003)
19. Boykov, Y., Kolmorgorov, V.: Computing geodesics and minimal surfaces via graph cuts. In: Proceedings IEEE International Conference Computer Vision, pp. 26–33. IEEE Computer Society Press, Los Alamitos (2003)
20. Vasilevsky, A., Siddiqi, K.: Flux maximizing geometric flows. IEEE PAMI 24, 1565–1579 (2002)
21. Pichon, E.: Novel methods for multidimensional image segmentation. PhD thesis, Georgia Institute of Technology (2005)
22. Whitaker, R.: A Level-Set Approach to 3D Reconstruction from Range Data. International Journal of Computer Vision 29(3), 203–231 (1998)
23. Tao, X., Miller, J.V.: A method for registering diffusion weighted magnetic resonance images. In: Larsen, R., Nielsen, M., Sporring, J. (eds.) MICCAI 2006. LNCS, vol. 4191, pp. 594–602. Springer, Heidelberg (2006)

Segmentation of Myocardial Volumes from Real-Time 3D Echocardiography Using an Incompressibility Constraint*

Yun Zhu[1], Xenophon Papademetris[2], Albert Sinusas[2],
and James S. Duncan[1,2]

[1] Department of Biomedical Engineering, Yale University
yun.zhu@yale.edu
[2] Department of Diagnostic Radiology, Yale University, USA

Abstract. Real-time three-dimensional (RT3D) echocardiography is a new imaging modality that presents the unique opportunity to visualize the complex three-dimensional (3-D) shape and the motion of left ventricle (LV) *in vivo*. To take advantage of this opportunity, automatic segmentation of LV myocardium is essential. While there are a variety of efforts on the segmentation of LV endocardial (ENDO) boundaries, the segmentation of epicardial (EPI) boundaries is still problematic. In this paper, we present a new approach of coupled-surfaces propagation to address this problem. Our method is motivated by the idea that the volume of the myocardium is close to being constant during a cardiac cycle and takes this tight coupling as an important constraint. We employ two surfaces, each driven by the image-derived information that takes into account the ultrasound physics by modeling speckle using shifted Rayleigh distribution while maintaining the coupling. By evolving two surfaces simultaneously, the final representation of myocardium is thus achieved. Results from 328 sets of RT3D echocardiographic data are evaluated against the outlines of three observers. We show that the results from automatic segmentation are comparable to those from manual segmentation.

1 Introduction

RT3D echocardiography, an emerging trend in ultrasound imaging, provides truly volumetric images to allow the assessment of cardiac anatomy and function. For quantitative analysis of these volumetric data, it is desirable to automatically outline the shape of LV throughout a cardiac cycle. While there have been a number of publications describing ultrasound image segmentation techniques (see [1] for an overview), most of the attention has been given to ENDO boundary segmentation. Limited work has been done to detect EPI contours that are equally important in the quantitative assessment of myocardial deformation, especially when a biomechanical model is applied.

---

* This work is supported by the grant 5R01HL082640-02.

N. Ayache, S. Ourselin, A. Maeder (Eds.): MICCAI 2007, Part I, LNCS 4791, pp. 44–51, 2007.
© Springer-Verlag Berlin Heidelberg 2007

The detection of EPI contours is more challenging than the detection of ENDO contours because the tissue/background contrast is lower than the blood pool/tissue contrast, resulting in the more ambiguous EPI boundaries, as shown in Figure 1. In addition, the speckle caused by the interference of energy from randomly distributed small scatters partially masks EPI boundaries. Furthermore, the EPI boundary is often occluded by other structures in the body such as the liver and the chest wall, that can have similar intensity to the myocardium. All these factors, when combined together, make EPI border detection an open problem.

There were some limited attempts to segment EPI boundaries [2][3][4]. These efforts, however, do not explicitly use the constraints due to myocardial structure. Our group previously developed a region-based approach to segment ENDO contours from rotational 3-D echocardiography [5]. In [6], we used coupled level sets to segment brain images. In this work, we extend our previous work to find EPI boundaries in RT3D echocardiography. Our method described in this paper is motivated by the nearly constant volume of the myocardium during the entire cardiac cycle and takes this property as an important constraint. By evolving ENDO- and EPI surfaces simultaneously, each driven by its own image derived region force while maintaining the coupling, a final representation of the ENDO- and EPI surface is thus achieved.

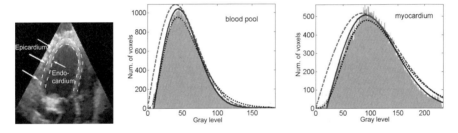

Fig. 1. The EPI contour is ambiguous while ENDO contour is clear

Fig. 2. Maximal likelihood fits of three models to RT3D echocardiographic data. Red: Rayleigh, Blue: Shifted Rayleigh, Black: Gamma.

2 Method

2.1 Statistical Modeling of Ultrasound Speckle

A number of statistical models, either theoretical or empirical, have been proposed. The Rayleigh distribution is the most popular model for fully developed speckle. Rician distribution, K-distribution, generalized K-distribution, homodyned K-distribution, and Rician Inverse of Gaussian distribution have also been considered. However, the analytical complexity of these complicated models is significant, particularly, when parameter estimation is required. Meanwhile,

Tao [7] proposed to use empirical models (Gamma, Weibull, Normal, and Log-Normal) to describe the distribution of gray levels in speckle.

In clinical echocardiography, a solid-state gel is sometimes placed in front of the transducer to fit the entire heart into the limited field of view, thus producing strong reverberation from the wall of the gel. In addition, ultrasound images can be very noisy, which makes the intensity distribution deviate from a pure Rayleigh distribution. To account for the speckle noise phenomena in the reverberation areas, we use a shifted Rayleigh distribution [8], a generalization of the Rayleigh distribution, to model the statistics of speckle. Using a shifted Rayleigh distribution, the probability of a voxel having intensity I is given as

$$\mathcal{P}\left(I;min,\alpha\right) = \frac{(I-min)\exp\left\{-\frac{(I-min)^2}{2\alpha^2}\right\}}{\alpha^2}, \text{ where } min \text{ and } \alpha \text{ are the parameters of}$$

the probability distribution function.

To justify the choice of this model, we compared it with the Rayleigh distribution and one empirical model, the Gamma distribution, by fitting the histograms of blood pool and myocardium of 111 sets of volumetric data using Maximum Likelihood Estimation (MLE), as shown in Figure 2. To quantify the comparison results, we used a goodness-of-fit technique and chose the Pearson chi-squared test to determine how well the images fit different distribution families. Suppose that we have n independent observations $x_1, x_2, ..., x_n$ to form a histogram of M bins. Let m_i be the number of observed points falling into bin i and $p_i = \int_{\text{bin}} p\left(x|\theta\right) dx$ be the probability of x falling into bin i, where θ is the vector of distribution's parameters. The statistics $\chi_s^2 = \sum_{i=1}^{M} \frac{(m_i - np_i)^2}{np_i}$ is therefore a measure of the deviation of samples from expectation. Pearson proved that the limiting distribution of χ_s^2 is a chi-squared distribution with degree of freedom of $M - L - 1$, where L is the number of the parameters estimated. Hence, the corresponding significance values of each fitting can be identified by finding the tail value of $\chi^2\left(M - L - 1\right)$, i.e. $p = \int_{\chi_s^2}^{+\infty} \chi^2\left(M - L - 1\right) dx$.

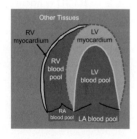

Fig. 3. The background (outside the dashed red line) is inhomogeneous

Table 1. The significance values of Model Fits for Blood Pool and Myocardium

	Rayleigh	shifted Rayleigh	Gamma
Blood pool	0.13	0.45	0.31
Myocardium	0.16	0.44	0.32

Table 1 shows the average significance values of fits in blood pool and myocardium. Our experiments show that shifted Rayleigh distribution has the largest significant value, and is thus chosen to model the speckle in RT3D echocardiographic images in our work.

2.2   Data Adherence Derivation

The strength of the signal due to the myocardial boundaries depends on the relative orientation of the border to transducer direction, and attenuation. Thus conventional intensity gradient-based methods have limited success in echocardiographic segmentation. A region-based deformable models, however, has shown promising performance in segmentation images with weak edges [9]. Let Ω be a bounded open subset of $\mathbb{R}^3$, and be partitioned by ENDO surface C^+ and EPI surface C^- into three regions - LV blood pool, LV myocardium, and background, which are denoted as Ω_1, Ω_2, and Ω_3 respectively. A region-based deformable model which maximizes the intensity homogeneity within each region can be defined as

$$L\left(C^+, C^-\right) = \log \mathcal{P}\left(I | C^+, C^-\right) = \sum_{l=1}^{3} \int_{\Omega_l} \log \mathcal{P}\left(I; min_l, \alpha_l\right) d\mathbf{x} \qquad (1)$$

where $\mathcal{P}\left(I; min_l, \alpha_l\right)$ is the shifted Rayleigh distribution. For $l = 1$, it models the distribution of speckle in LV blood pool. For $l = 2$, it models the distribution of speckle in LV myocardium.

While the histograms of speckle in blood pool and myocardium are unimodal, the background has a bimodal histogram, as shown in Figure 4. It is so because the background includes more than one tissue type (e.g. RV blood pool, RV myocardium, and other tissues)(as shown in Figure 3), and therefore modeling it with a single distribution would be insufficient. To tackle this problem, we use a mixture model and invoke EM algorithm to fit the background histogram. In Figure 4, we show the histogram of each region with the fitted shifted Rayleigh distribution function.

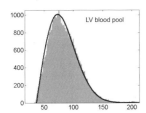 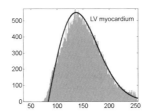 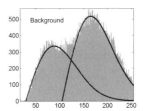

Fig. 4. The histograms of LV blood pool, LV myocardium, and background from RT3D echocardiographic data with estimated shifted Rayleigh distribution superimposed on them

2.3   Incompressibility Constraint

The myocardium is composed of cardiac muscle with specialized muscle fibers that act as a syncytium which contracts and relaxes spontaneously. Studies have shown that the volume of myocardium varies less than 5% during a cardiac cycle [10][11]. Papademetris has previously applied a biomechanical model with a Poisson ratio close to 0.5 to recover the motion of myocardium during a cardiac cycle [12]. In this work, we use this incompressibility constraint as an important constraint to help detect the EPI border. Since myocardium is only nearly incompressible, it is more reasonable to formulate this constraint in a probabilistic framework, rather than impose a deterministic constraint.

We assume that the volume of myocardium from a cardiac sequence has a Gaussian distribution $\mathcal{N}\left(V_0, \sigma_0^2\right)$

$$P\left(C^+, C^-\right) = \frac{1}{\sqrt{2\pi}\sigma_0} \exp\left\{-\frac{(V-V_0)^2}{2\sigma_0^2}\right\} \qquad (2)$$

where $V = \int_{\Omega_2} d\mathbf{x}$ is the volume of myocardium. Assuming that $0.025V_0$ is the maximum deviation extent (use $3\sigma_0$), we have the following relationship

$$3\sigma_0 = 0.025V_0 \qquad (3)$$

$$\sigma_0 = \frac{1}{120}V_0 \qquad (4)$$

2.4   Maximum a Posteriori Framework

To incorporate the data-derived information (section 2.2) and the incompressibility constraint (section 2.3) into a uniform framework, we formulate our problem in a Maximum A Posteriori (MAP) framework, which maximizes the posterior probability with the prior information of evolving surfaces.

$$\left(\hat{C}^+, \hat{C}^-\right) = \arg\max_{C^+, C^-} P\left(C^+, C^- | I\right) = \arg\max_{C^+, C^-} \underbrace{P\left(I | C^+, C^-\right)}_{\text{adherence to data}} \underbrace{P\left(C^+, C^-\right)}_{\substack{\text{incompressibility} \\ \text{constraint}}}$$

$$= \arg\max_{C^+, C^-} \left\{\sum_{l=1}^{3} \int_{\Omega_l} \log P\left(I; min_l, \alpha_l\right) d\mathbf{x} - \frac{(V-V_0)^2}{2\sigma_0^2}\right\} \qquad (5)$$

The maximization of equation 5 can then be identified by the coupled Euler-Lagrange equations

$$\frac{\partial C^+}{\partial t} = \left\{\log\frac{P\left(I; min_1, \alpha_1\right)}{P\left(I; min_2, \alpha_2\right)} - \frac{V-V_0}{\sigma_0^2}\right\}\mathbf{n}^+ \qquad (6)$$

$$\frac{\partial C^-}{\partial t} = \left\{\log\frac{P\left(I; min_2, \alpha_2\right)}{P\left(I; min_3, \alpha_3\right)} + \frac{V-V_0}{\sigma_0^2}\right\}\mathbf{n}^- \qquad (7)$$

where $\mathbf{n}^+$ and $\mathbf{n}^-$ are the normals of C^+ and C^- respectively.

3   Results

The RT3D echocardiographic data were acquired using a Philips SONOS 7500 machine. This system uses a 4-MHz matrix-array transducer which consists of

3000 miniaturized piezoelectric elements and offers steering in both azimuth and elevation of the beam, permitting real-time 3-D volumetric image acquisition and rendering.

We performed experiments on 22 sequences of RT3D echocardiographic data, and each sequence has 13-17 frames depending on the heart rate. Hence, we ran our algorithm with a total of 328 sets of volumetric data. Considering the intra- and inter- observer variability, we asked three experts, blind to each other, to independently outline the ENDO- and EPI contours of all the frames of image sequences. The average volume of myocardium in the first frame was taken to be the mean volume of myocardium in that sequence. Considering the temporal continuity of a cardiac sequence, our algorithm used the segmented contour of the current frame as an initial contour for the subsequent frame. It normally took 5-8 minutes to segment one frame with the size of $164 \times 164 \times 208$.

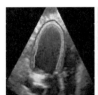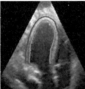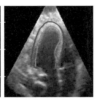   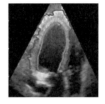

Fig. 5. Example of segmented ENDO and EPI contours from frames 2, 4, and 6 during cardiac systole   **Fig. 6.** Result without the incompressibility constraint

In Figure 5, we show the long axis view of segmented ENDO- and EPI contours at frames 2, 4, and 6 during cardiac systole. In Figure 6, we compare the results with and without the incompressibility constraint. It shows that, without incompressibility constraint, the EPI boundary leaked while the ENDO boundary was still located. Figure 7 shows an example of volumetric RT3D echocardiographic data with ENDO and EPI surfaces superimposed on it. Figure 8 shows a good correlation between the manually identified and automatic algorithm determined volume of myocardium when the incompressibility constraint was applied.

In addition, we computed two distance error metrics and two area error metrics, namely, mean absolute distance (MAD), Hausdorff distance (HD), the percentage of correctly segmented voxels(PTP), and the percentage of false positives(PFP). Let $A = \{\mathbf{a}_1, \mathbf{a}_2, ..., \mathbf{a}_n\}$, $B = \{\mathbf{b}_1, \mathbf{b}_2, ..., \mathbf{b}_m\}$, Ω_a be the region enclosed by C_a, and Ω_m be the region enclosed by C_m. We define MAD $= \frac{1}{2} \left\{ \frac{1}{n} \sum_{i=1}^{n} d(\mathbf{a}_i, B) + \frac{1}{m} \sum_{i=1}^{m} d(\mathbf{b}_i, A) \right\}$, HD $= \max \left(\max_i \{d(\mathbf{a}_i, B)\} + \max_j \{d(\mathbf{b}_j, A)\} \right)$, where $d(\mathbf{a}_i, B) = \min_j \|b_j - a_i\|$. We also define PTP $= \frac{\text{Volume}(\Omega_a \cap \Omega_m)}{\text{Volume}(\Omega_m)}$ and PFP $= \frac{\text{Volume}(\Omega_m) - \text{Volume}(\Omega_a \cap \Omega_m)}{\text{Volume}(\Omega_a)}$. While MAD represents the global disagreement between two contours, HD compares two contours locally.

Tables 2 and 3 compare the results from automatic segmentation to those from manual segmentation. Table 2 shows that ENDO boundaries were detected with

50   Y. Zhu et al.

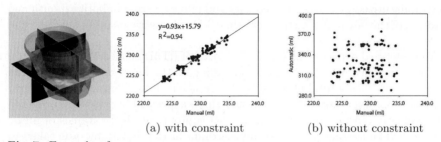

(a) with constraint   (b) without constraint

Fig. 7. Example of
segmented   ENDO **Fig. 8.** Linear regression analysis of myocardial volume with and
and EPI surfaces   without the incompressibility constraint

Table 2. Comparison automatic outline to three observers' outline of ENDO boundaries

	MAD(mm)	HD(mm)	PTP(%)	PFP(%)
Automatic-manual (with constraint)	1.45 ± 0.30	2.41 ± 0.47	96.21 ± 1.97	4.04 ± 1.90
Automatic-manual (without constraint)	1.50 ± 0.28	2.43 ± 0.59	95.71 ± 1.85	4.17 ± 1.80
Manual-Manual	1.30 ± 0.27	2.14 ± 0.52	96.34 ± 1.93	4.00 ± 1.84

Table 3. Comparison of automatic outline to three observers' outline of EPI boundaries

	MAD(mm)	HD(mm)	PTP(%)	PFP(%)
Automatic-manual (with contraint)	1.75 ± 0.50	2.90 ± 0.80	94.35 ± 1.02	5.46 ± 0.76
Automatic-manual (without constraint)	4.86 ± 1.86	6.87 ± 2.34	77.92 ± 6.97	21.14 ± 7.87
Manual-manual	2.56 ± 0.78	3.21 ± 0.96	94.89 ± 2.34	5.23 ± 0.80

sufficient accuracy even if the incompressibility constraint was not applied. This
is because the ENDO boundaries are relatively clear compared to the EPI boundaries. However, Table 3 shows that for EPI boundaries, when the incompressibility constraint was not applied, computer-manual MAD was 3.1mm larger than
manual-manual MAD and computer-manual PTP&PFP were $13\% - 17\%$ worse
than manual-manual PTP&PFP. This is because the EPI boundaries leaked
out without the constraint. When the incompressibility constraint was applied,
however, the automatic algorithm produced results with comparable accuracy
to a manual segmentation. Furthermore, we observed from Tables 2 and 3 that
the variability of manual-manual segmentation was smaller for ENDO than for
EPI. This is probably because EPI boundaries are more ambiguous for observers
to detect, which was also the reason we have multiple observers instead of a
single one.

4   Conclusion

In this paper, we presented a novel approach to segmenting the full myocardial volume from RT3D echocardiographic images using the incompressibility property that the volume of myocardium varies less than 5% during a cardiac cycle. Our experiments showed that computer-generated contours agreed with the observers' hand-outlined contours as much as the different observers agreed with each other. Future work includes the joint segmentation and motion analysis of echocardiographic sequences.

References

1. Noble, J.A., Boukerroui, D.: Ultrasound image segmentation: A survey. IEEE Trans. Med. Imag. 25(8), 987–1010 (2006)
2. Malassiotis, S., Strintzis, M.G.: Tracking the left ventricle in echocardiographic images by learning heart dynamics. IEEE Trans. Med. Imag. 8(3), 282–290 (1999)
3. Dias, J.M.B., Leitao, J.M.N.: Wall position and thickness estimation from sequences of echocardiographic images. IEEE Trans. Med. Imag. 15(1), 25–38 (1996)
4. Feng, J., Lin, W.C., Chen, C.T.: Epicardial boundary detection using fuzzy reasoning. IEEE Trans. Med. Imag. 10(2), 187–199 (1991)
5. Lin, N., Yu, W., Duncan, J.S.: Combinative multi-scale level set framework for echocardiographic image segmentation. Med. Imag. Analysis 9(4), 529–537 (2003)
6. Zeng, X., Staib, L.H., Schultz, R.T., Duncan, J.S.: Segmentation and measurement of cortex from 3d mr images using coupled surfaces propagation. IEEE Trans. Med. Imag. 18(10), 927–937 (1999)
7. Tao, Z., Tagare, H.D., Beaty, J.D.: Evaluation of four probability distribution models for speckle in clinical cardiac ultrasound images. IEEE Trans. Med. Imag. (11), 1483–1491 (2006)
8. Goodman, J.W.: Some fundamental properties of speckle. J. Opt. Soc. Amer. 66(11), 1145–1150 (1976)
9. Chan, T., Vese, L.: Active contours without edges. IEEE Trans. Imag. Proc. 10(2), 266–277 (2001)
10. Yin, F.C.P., Chan, C.C.H., Juddy, R.M.: Compressibility of perfused passive myocardium. Amer. J. Physiol. - Heart Circ. Physiol. 271(5), 1864–1870 (1996)
11. Liu, Y.H., Bahn, R.C., Ritman, E.L.: Dynamic intramyocardial blood volume: Evaluation with a radiological opaque marker method. Amer. J. Physiol. - Heart Circ. Physiol. 263(3), 963–967 (1992)
12. Papademetris, X., Sinusas, A., Dione, D.P., Constable, R.T., Duncan, J.S.: Estimation of 3d left ventricular deformation from 3d medical image sequences using biomechanical models. IEEE Trans. Med. Imag. 21(7), 786–800 (2002)

Localized Shape Variations for Classifying Wall Motion in Echocardiograms

K.Y. Esther Leung and Johan G. Bosch

Biomedical Engineering, Thoraxcenter, Erasmus MC, Rotterdam, The Netherlands
k.leung@erasmusmc.nl
http://www.erasmusmc.nl/ThoraxcenterBME

Abstract. To quantitatively predict coronary artery diseases, automated analysis may be preferred to current visual assessment of left ventricular (LV) wall motion. In this paper, a novel automated classification method is presented which uses shape models with localized variations. These sparse shape models were built from four-chamber and two-chamber echocardiographic sequences using principal component analysis and orthomax rotations. The resulting shape parameters were then used to classify local wall-motion abnormalities of LV segments. Various orthomax criteria were investigated. In all cases, higher classification correctness was achieved using significantly less shape parameters than before rotation. Since pathologies are typically spatially localized, many medical applications involving local classification should benefit from orthomax parameterizations.

1 Introduction

Coronary artery diseases are a major cause of death in the western world. Detection of wall-motion abnormalities of the left ventricle (LV), widely accepted as predictors for these diseases, is therefore of great clinical importance. To obtain quantitative measures of LV wall motion, automated analysis of LV wall motion may be preferred to currently visual, therefore qualitative, assessments. The goal of this study is to evaluate a new automated classification approach for detecting local wall-motion abnormalities. The method uses point-distribution models with localized variations obtained with orthomax rotations.

Point-distribution models, or shape models, are parametric representations of a set of shapes. These models have been used extensively in various medical image processing contexts, especially segmentation [1],[2]. Shape models are often built using Principal Component Analysis (PCA), which maximizes the variance of the input data. This results in models with global variations. Previously, PCA shape models of LV endocardial borders were used to classify global clinical parameters (e.g. LV volume) as well as local parameters (e.g. wall motion of LV segments) [3]. However, relatively many shape modes were needed to classify the *local* wall motion, because *global* shape parameters were used. We therefore hypothesize that models with local variations should be able to represent local wall motion using less shape modes.

Several methods for building more localized shape models have been proposed, including independent component analysis [4] and various sparse PCA methods

N. Ayache, S. Ourselin, A. Maeder (Eds.): MICCAI 2007, Part I, LNCS 4791, pp. 52–59, 2007.
© Springer-Verlag Berlin Heidelberg 2007

[5],[6]. Recently, Stegmann et al. [7] suggested a method using orthomax rotations, which seems particularly attractive due to its computational feasibility in high-dimensional spaces. The applicability for localized classification was mentioned in that paper, but has not yet been investigated.

To determine whether localized shape models can improve classification of local wall-motion abnormalities of the left ventricle, shape models were constructed using PCA and rotated according to the orthomax criterion. The varimax, quartimax, and factor-parsimony criteria were investigated. Classification correctness, the number of shape modes needed, and cluster representation were studied in the original and rotated shape space, for different proportions of retained variance.

2 Methods

2.1 Shape Modeling

Shape models of the LV endocardial contours were constructed using full-cycle 2D+time (2D+T) echocardiograms. By modeling the complete cardiac cycle, typical motion patterns associated with certain pathologies were included. More details of the model can be found in our previous work [8].

Each 2D+T shape was represented as a vector $\mathbf{x}$, consisting of 37 equally distributed landmark coordinates per phase. Sixteen cardiac phases were used for each shape. Shape models describing the main variations in a patient population were built using PCA: $\mathbf{x} = \bar{\mathbf{x}} + \mathbf{\Phi}\mathbf{b}$, where $\bar{\mathbf{x}}$ denotes the average shape, $\mathbf{\Phi} = (\phi_1|\dots|\phi_p)$ the $n \times p$ matrix of orthogonal shape eigenvectors or modes, and $\mathbf{b}$ a vector of shape coefficients. Any new shape can be approximated in the PCA space, spanned by the p orthogonal eigenvectors, using the pseudoinverse ($\mathbf{\Phi}^{-1}$) of the eigenvector matrix ($\mathbf{b} \approx \mathbf{\Phi}^{-1}(\mathbf{x} - \bar{\mathbf{x}})$).

To obtain a more compact model, only a proportion f of the total variance $V = \sum_{i=1}^{p} \lambda_i$ was retained: $\sum_{i=1}^{k} \lambda_i \geq fV$, where k denoted the number of eigenvectors with the largest eigenvalues λ_i.

2.2 Orthomax Rotations

Orthomax rotations were applied to the PCA shape models to produce models with localized spatial variations [7],[9]. Orthomax rotations are reparameterizations of the PCA space producing a simple basis. The orthogonal orthomax rotation matrix $\mathbf{R}$ is calculated by maximizing the criterion ξ:

$$\xi = \{\sum_{j=1}^{k}\sum_{i=1}^{n} G_{ij}^4 - \frac{\gamma}{n}\sum_{j=1}^{k}[\sum_{i=1}^{n} G_{ij}^2]^2\}/n \ , \tag{1}$$

where G_{ij} denotes the scalar element in the ith row and j^{th} column in the rotated eigenvector matrix $\mathbf{G} = \mathbf{\Phi}\mathbf{R}$, and γ is determined by the orthomax type. The shape coefficients after rotation $\mathbf{b}_R$ can be found with $\mathbf{b}_R = \mathbf{R}^{-1}\mathbf{b}$.

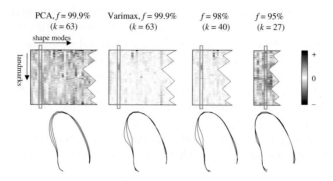

Fig. 1. Top row: eigenvector matrices of PCA and varimax-rotated shape model of the four-chamber. Bottom row: end-diastolic shape variations of the fifth mode, showing more localization for shape models with higher proportions of retained variance f.

Interestingly, the orthogonal orthomax criterion is equivalent to the Crawford-Ferguson criterion, which is a weighted sum of row and column complexity of the eigenvector matrix [10]. Therefore, orthomax rotations can be interpreted as a redistribution of the factor loadings of the eigenvector matrix so that each row or column has a minimal number of nonzero elements, i.e. columns or rows are as sparse as possible. The two extremes are quartimax ($\gamma = 0$) and factor parsimony ($\gamma = n$), favoring row sparsity and column sparsity respectively [9]. Varimax ($\gamma = 1$), a commonly-used type, resides somewhere in between [11]. When applied to a *shape* eigenvector matrix, the variation is emphasized in certain modes and spatial regions, whereas the variation is suppressed in other regions (see Fig. 1). In practice, complete row or column sparsity cannot be achieved because the shape model is restricted to the observed, physically allowed variations in the training shapes.

An important property to consider is the number of shape modes k. PCA modes with high eigenvalues describe global variation, whereas modes with low eigenvalues generally contain noise. Eliminating these noise modes before the orthomax rotation may lead to more representative local variations. However, if too many modes are removed, important information needed for classification may be lost. Also, a lower k generally results in less localized shape variations, because each mode must capture more variations (see Fig. 1). Therefore, different proportions of retained variance f were investigated : $f = 95\%$, 98%, 99% and 99.9% corresponding to $k = 27, 40, 48$, and 63 modes in the four-chamber (4C) model, and to $k = 25, 38, 46$, and 62 modes in the two-chamber (2C) model.

2.3   Wall-Motion Classification

Classification of wall-motion abnormalities was demonstrated on dobutamine stress echocardiography data from 129 unselected infarct patients [12]. The total data set was split randomly into a training set (TRN) of 65 patients and a testing set (TST) of 64 patients. Endocardial contours were drawn in the apical 4C and

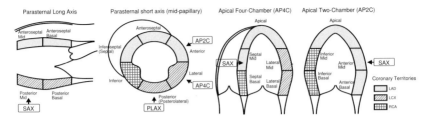

Fig. 2. 13-segment model of the left ventricle (LAD = left anterior descending artery, LCX = left circumflex artery, RCA = right coronary artery)

2C sequences using a semi-automated technique based on pattern matching, dynamic programming, and spatiotemporal geometric models [8]. 4C and 2C shape models were built with the image sequences in the TRN set [3]. Shape coefficients $\mathbf{b}$ and $\mathbf{b}_R$ were calculated for all data sets and used as predictor (or independent) variables in the classification.

Myocardial wall motion in these images was evaluated visually by consensus of two expert readers, independently of the shape models. Motion scores were assigned to each of the 13 LV segments (0 = normokinesia, 1 = hypokinesia, 2 = akinesia, 3 = dyskinesia; see Fig. 2). Wall-motion scores of each of the nine segments in the 4C and 2C views were grouped into a normal class (score = 0) and an abnormal (score > 0) class and used as the response (dependent) variables in the classification.

Two classification experiments were performed, representing an 'ideal' and a 'worst-case' situation. In both cases, the shape model was built on the TRN set. In the 'ideal' case, a leave-one-out approach was used where the classifier was trained on the TRN set but one sample and tested with that sample. This process was then repeated for all TRN samples. In the 'worst-case' situation, the classifier was trained on the whole TRN set and then tested on all TST cases. This resembled classification in the real-world: both shape model and classifier were trained from a limited training set and tested on completely 'new' shapes.

To assess the classification in the PCA and orthomax rotated space, cluster measurements were computed. Common measures of cluster compactness and cluster separation are the within-class scatter matrix $\mathbf{S}_W$ and the between-class scatter matrix $\mathbf{S}_B$ [13]. Since $\mathbf{S}_W$ and $\mathbf{S}_B$ are related to the variance of the point-cluster in each direction, a better measure of cluster quality is the ratio J of the trace of the two scatter matrices ([14], p. 311): $J = \frac{\text{tr}(\mathbf{S}_B)}{\text{tr}(\mathbf{S}_W)}$.

3   Results

Orthomax rotations were applied to 4C and 2C shape models, using an iterative method based on singular value decomposition [7], as implemented in Matlab (v. 7.0.4 (R14), 2005). Whereas PCA shape modes are ordered according to variance, thus exhibiting global variations in the first modes, orthomax modes show local variations in most modes (see Fig. 3).

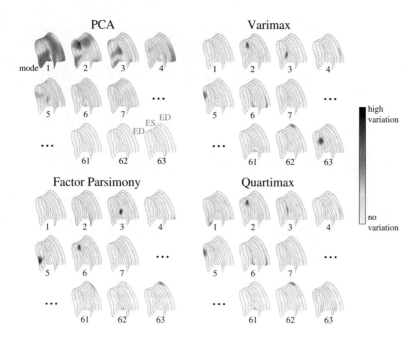

Fig. 3. Global PCA and localized orthomax-rotated modes of the 4C shape model, $f = 99.9\%$. Absolute displacements of the landmarks due to ± 3 SD model-variation are shown on the average 2D+T shape.

Shape parameters were used to predict the presence of wall motion abnormalities per LV segment. Classification was performed using the Linear Discriminant Analysis option in the statistical package SPSS (v. 11.0.1, 2001). Shape parameters were added using the 'stepwise' option, using the 'unexplained variance' criterion. Significantly less orthomax modes were needed than PCA modes, without compromising classification correctness (i.e. the proportion of segments correctly classified as normal or abnormal), regardless of the criterion used (Table 1). Also, models with higher f needed less shape modes during classification. The results per segment are given in Table 2 for the varimax criterion.

Fig. 4 shows cluster quality J (section 2.3) in PCA and varimax space. Clearly, classification in the varimax space gives larger J, i.e. better cluster separation, than in the PCA space in most cases.

4   Discussion and Conclusions

In this study, localized shape models of the left ventricle were generated using orthomax rotations. Using these localized shape models, significantly fewer parameters were needed for classifying segmental wall motion in 2D echocardiographic sequences, while preserving classification correctness. Best results were obtained using all PCA modes before rotations, probably as a result of a sparser rotated basis; apparently, the classification was not hampered by possible noise

Table 1. Classification correctness versus the number of shape modes used (mean±SD), for different proportions of retained variance f in the shape models, and different orthomax criteria. * denotes significantly ($p < 0.05$, paired t-test) less shape parameters than PCA.

	f	Classification correctness TRN L-1-O	TST	#parameters
PCA	99.9%	88.9 ± 5.9%	74.0±9.4%	8.0 ± 3.0
quartimax	99.9%	90.1 ± 5.2%	75.4±9.8%	5.6 ± 3.9*
factor parsimony	99.9%	89.4 ± 5.7%	76.3±10.3%	5.4 ± 3.2*
varimax	99.9%	91.1 ± 4.5%	76.5±10.5%	5.1 ± 3.2*
	99%	88.9 ± 5.9%	76.0±8.7%	5.7 ± 3.3*
	98%	87.7 ± 7.0%	75.8±9.5%	6.4 ± 3.5
	95%	86.3 ± 6.1%	76.3±9.0%	6.6 ± 3.7

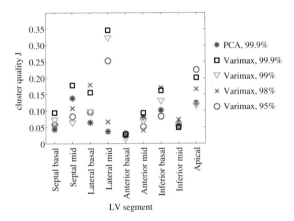

Fig. 4. Cluster quality J (see section 2.3) shows better cluster separation in varimax than PCA classification space, for different proportions of retained variance

in the higher PCA modes. Similar results were obtained for the quartimax, varimax, and factor parsimony criteria, probably because the reparameterizations are restricted by the allowable variations in the training set. The relatively large improvement in the lateral region may be due to the combination of the orthomax rotation and the variations in the TRN set, which by chance produced a sparser parameter representation for those segments.

Furthermore, the normal and abnormal wall motion classes were better separated in the orthomax parameter space than in the original PCA space. A clear relationship between the improvement in classification correctness, the number of shape modes used, and cluster quality could not be determined because of the small number of data sets in this study, but generally speaking, better classification can be expected in a better-defined parameter space. The cluster measurements revealed that there was still a reasonable amount of overlap of the classes. This may be partly due to the high variability of visual wall motion

Table 2. Classification correctness versus the number of PCA and varimax shape parameters used, for nine segments

		PCA $f = 99.9\%$				Varimax $f = 99.9\%$			
		Classification correctness			# para-meters	Classification correctness			# para-meters
View	Segment	TRN	L-1-O	TST		TRN	L-1-O	TST	
4C+2C	Apical	93.8%	81.3%		7	95.4%	85.9%		6
4C	Septal Basal	86.6%	70.3%		10	90.8%	64.1%		5
4C	Septal Mid	92.3%	73.4%		12	92.3%	73.4%		11
4C	Lateral Basal	86.2%	64.1%		8	90.8%	82.8%		2
4C	Lateral Mid	76.9%	69.8%		6	81.5%	71.4%		2
2C	Anterior Basal	95.4%	95.3%		3	96.9%	96.9%		2
2C	Anterior Mid	93.8%	74.6%		11	93.8%	76.2%		9
2C	Inferior Basal	84.6%	71.9%		5	90.8%	71.9%		5
2C	Inferior Mid	90.8%	65.6%		10	87.7%	65.6%		4
	mean	88.9%	74.0%		8.0	91.1%	76.5%		5.1
	SD	5.9%	9.4%		3.0	4.5%	10.5%		3.2

scoring. Regrettably, this variability could not be determined for this data set because the scoring was performed by consensus. In the future, we would like to use a more objective measure such as quantitative deformation parameters as the gold standard, rather than visual wall motion scores. The class overlap also suggests that better classification might be achieved with a nonlinear discriminant function, such as support vector machines.

While PCA modes are ordered according to variance, orthomax modes are naturally unordered. In future work, we would like to investigate categorization of modes more thoroughly, e.g. according to the locality of the shape variations [13]. This might allow us to preselect the shape modes for classification, instead of having the classifier do the selection.

Moreover, it would be interesting to compare the proposed orthomax method with other localization methods, such as independent component analysis [4] and sparse PCA methods [5],[6]. Recently, Frouin et al. [15] proposed an intensity-based method for detecting wall-motion abnormalities using factor analysis, which might also be used for rotating *shape* models to a predefined motion pattern. This is a subject of further investigation.

Finally, since pathologies are typically spatially localized, we anticipate many medical applications where sparse representations are preferred to the conventional PCA approach. The orthomax criterion is shown to be suitable for building these sparse representations with relative ease. Although not explored in this study, sparse texture models can be constructed in a very similar manner [7]. The direct cardiac application would be to examine myocardial thickening, which might also be a predictor of coronary disease. In the future, we would like to extend the method to coupled shape models of rest and stress stage cardiac contours, to investigate local differences in wall-motion.

Acknowledgments

Financial support from the Dutch Technology Foundation STW is gratefully acknowledged. We thank O. Kamp and F. Nijland for providing the patient data, G. van Burken for the data analysis support, and M. van Stralen, M. M. Voormolen, M. Sonka, and M. B. Stegmann for the useful discussions.

References

1. Cootes, T.F., Edwards, G.J., Taylor, C.J.: Active appearance models. IEEE Trans. Pattern Anal. Machine Intell. 23(6), 681–685 (2001)
2. Stegmann, M.B.: Generative interpretation of medical images. PhD thesis, Technical University of Denmark (2004)
3. Bosch, J.G., Nijland, F., Mitchell, S.C., Lelieveldt, B.P.F., Kamp, O., Reiber, J.H.C., Sonka, M.: Computer-aided diagnosis via model-based shape analysis: Automated classification of wall motion abnormalities in echocardiograms. Acad. Radiol. 12(3), 358–367 (2005)
4. Üzümcü, M., Frangi, A.F., Reiber, J.H.C., Lelieveldt, B.P.F.: Independent component analysis in statistical shape models. Proc. SPIE Med. Imag.: Image Processing 5032, 375–383 (2003)
5. Zou, H., Hastie, T., Tibshirani, R.: Sparse principal component analysis. tech. rep. Standford University (2004)
6. Sjöstrand, K., Stegmann, M.B., Larsen, R.: Sparse principal component analysis in medical shape modeling. SPIE Med. Imag.: Image Processing 6144, 61444X (2006)
7. Stegmann, M.B., Sjöstrand, K., Larsen, R.: Sparse modeling of landmark and texture variability using the orthomax criterion. SPIE Med. Imag.: Image Processing 6144, 61441G (2006)
8. Bosch, J.G., Mitchell, S.C., Lelieveldt, B.P.F., Nijland, F., Kamp, O., Sonka, M., Reiber, J.H.C.: Automatic segmentation of echocardiographic sequences by active appearance motion models. IEEE Trans. Med. Imag. 21(11), 1374–1383 (2002)
9. Browne, M.W.: An overview of analytic rotation in exploratory factor analysis. Multivar. Behav. Res. 36(1), 111–150 (2001)
10. Crawford, C.B., Ferguson, G.A.: A general rotation criterion and its use in orthogonal rotation. Psychometrika 35(3), 321–332 (1970)
11. Kaiser, H.F.: The varimax criterion for analytic rotation in factor analysis. Psychometrika 23(3), 187–200 (1958)
12. Nijland, F., Kamp, O., Verhorst, P.M.J., de Voogt, W.G., Bosch, H.G., Visser, C.A.: Myocardial viability: impact on left ventricular dilatation after acute myocardial infarction. Heart 87, 17–22 (2002)
13. Suinesiaputra, A., Frangi, A.F., Üzümcü, M., Reiber, J.H.C., Lelieveldt, B.P.F.: Extraction of myocardial contractility patterns from short-axis MR images using independent component analysis. In: Sonka, M., Kakadiaris, I.A., Kybic, J. (eds.) CVAMIA 2004. LNCS, vol. 3117, pp. 75–86. Springer, Heidelberg (2004)
14. Webb, A.R.: Statistical Pattern Recognition, 2nd edn. John Wiley & Sons, Ltd. Chichester (2002)
15. Frouin, F., Delouche, A., Raffoul, H., Diebold, H., Abergel, E., Diebold, B.: Factor analysis of the left ventricle by echocardiography (falve): a new tool for detecting regional wall motion abnormalities. Eur. J. Echocardiogr. 5(5), 335–346 (2004)

Image Guidance of Intracardiac Ultrasound with Fusion of Pre-operative Images*

Yiyong Sun[1], Samuel Kadoury[1], Yong Li[1], Matthias John[2], Jeff Resnick[3],
Gerry Plambeck[3], Rui Liao[1], Frank Sauer[1], and Chenyang Xu[1]

[1] Siemens Corporate Research, Princeton, NJ, USA
yiyong.sun@siemens.com
[2] Siemens Medical Solutions, Erlangen, Germany
[3] Siemens Medical Solutions, Mountain View, CA, USA

Abstract. This paper presents a method for registering 3D intracardiac echo (ICE) to pre-operative images. A magnetic tracking sensor is integrated on the ICE catheter tip to provide the 3D location and orientation. The user guides the catheter into the patient heart to acquire a series of ultrasound images covering the anatomy of the heart chambers. An automatic intensity-based registration algorithm is applied to align these ultrasound images with pre-operative images. One of the important applications is to help electrophysiology doctors to treat complicated atrial fibrillation cases. After registration, the doctor can see the position and orientation of the ICE catheter and other tracked catheters inside the heart anatomy in real time. The image guidance provided by this technique may increase the ablation accuracy and reduce the amount of time for the electrophysiology procedures. We show successful image registration results from animal experiments.

1 Introduction

Atrial fibrillation (AFib) is a leading cause of stroke. About 2.2 million people in US have AFib. There are 200,000 new cases in 2006. Current pulmonary vein ablation techniques are achieving success rates of 85% in curing paroxysmal AFib with low risk [1]. During pulmonary vein ablation, a soft thin flexible tube with an electrode at the tip is inserted through a large vein or artery in the groin and moved into the heart. This catheter is directed to the locations in the heart that produce AFib to burn them off. Currently many heart centers have the cathlabs performing pulmonary vein ablation of AFib on a regular basis.

Intracardiac echo (ICE) catheters are routinely used in many cathlabs for transseptal catheterization and left atrial procedures. It offers the unique advantage to visualize anatomy and hemodynamics while also providing the interventional cardiac electrophysiologist real time feedback on other catheters deployed in the heart [2]. However, the ultrasound image generated from the ICE catheter

---

* We would like to thank Wolfgang Wein, Norbert Strobel, and Ann Dempsey at Siemens, Dr. Rebecca Fahrig and Dr. Amin Al-Ahmad at Stanford University Medical Center for their support on this work.

N. Ayache, S. Ourselin, A. Maeder (Eds.): MICCAI 2007, Part I, LNCS 4791, pp. 60–67, 2007.
© Springer-Verlag Berlin Heidelberg 2007

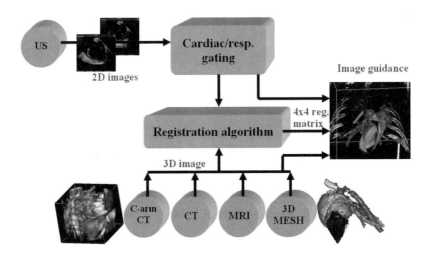

Fig. 1. System overview

has a limit field of view compared to other modalities such as fluoroscopy. Due to its flexibility, the image plane can drastically change. It requires a lot of experience and agility of the doctor to get familiar of operating the ICE catheter.

By fusing the 3D tracked ICE images with the pre-operative images such as CT, C-arm CT[1], or MR, doctor can see the position and orientation of the ICE catheter inside the heart in real time. Since multiple sensors can be tracked simultaneously, a tracked ablation catheter is automatically registered to the pre-operative image after completing the registration of the tracked ICE catheter. The image guidance provided by this technique can increase the ablation accuracy and reduce the amount of time for the electrophysiology (EP) procedures.

Figure 1 shows the framework of registering tracked ultrasound sequence to 3D images. In this paper particularly, we register it to C-arm CT data. The advantage of using C-arm CT data is the high resolution 3D image can be obtained inside the EP lab immediately before or during the intervention. Our method also applies to the conventional CT and MR pre-operative data. The background is presented in Section 2. Section 3 describes the method. Experimental results are showed in Section 4, followed by discussion in Section 5.

2   Background

The registration of intra-operative ultrasound images (US) and pre-operative CT/MR images has been proposed to aid the interventional and surgical procedures. Roche et al. [4] rigidly register 3D ultrasound with MR images using bivariate correlation ratio as similarity measure. Penney et al. [5] propose to register a set of ultrasound slices and a MR volume of a liver by converting

---

[1] CT-like images generated by C-arm system in the operating room [3].

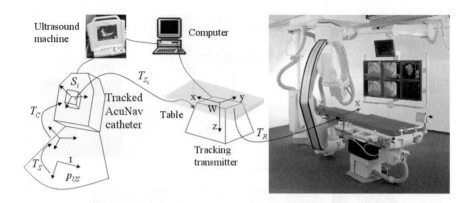

Fig. 2. System setup and transformations

them to vessel probability images. In [6], US and CT kidney images are rigidly registered. Wein et al. [7] register the ultrasound images to a CT scan on neck data of patients.

For EP applications, image integration using CartoMerge (Biosense Webster, Inc.) has been widely used, which is able to register a cloud of mapping points to the segmented surface of the pre-operative image [8,9]. In [10], a registration between cardiac CT data and ICE is described. A point-to-surface registration, by first extracting surface point sets of the left atrium from the ICE images, is used. However, these approaches all require the segmentation of either 3D data or the ultrasound image, which itself is a challenging problem and has a direct impact on the final registration accuracy.

There are several advantages of our system compared to the existing image integration solutions to EP applications. Our image-based registration method does not require segmenting ultrasound image or CT image, so it needs little user interaction. The registration does not need the mapping of heart chambers. Mapping usually takes time and may introduce error due to respiratory motion and chamber wall deformation from the pushing of the catheter. Besides cardiac gating, we also perform respiratory gating using a position sensor, which has been ignored in previous approaches. And with C-arm CT, the doctor can access all the necessary image modalities in the operating room.

3   Method

3.1   System Setup

Figure 2 shows the set up of the system. 3D images are acquired on an Angiographic C-arm system (AXIOM Artis, Siemens Medical Solutions). To image the left atrium of a patient we acquire images during 4 consecutive rotational 190° C-arm runs to get enough images to reconstruct a 3D image of one cardiac phase. Each run has 247 frames at a speed of 60 frames per second. The radiation dose is 1.2 μGy per frame. The images are reconstructed and processed on a PC workstation. For visualization purpose, the left atrium and other heart structures are segmented using dedicated software.

The images acquired by the ICE catheter (AcuNav, Siemens Medical Solutions) are transferred via a frame grabber card into the PC at 30 frames per second. To track the position of the ICE catheter tip we used a magnetic tracking system (Microbird, Ascension). Its position sensor has been integrated in the same tubing with the ultrasound transducer. The transmitter is installed under the table of the C-arm system, such that an ICE catheter above the table is within the operating range and can be tracked during an intervention. During ICE imaging we record the ECG signal of the patient, and track the position sensor at the ICE catheter tip and the other position sensor at the patient's chest (for respiratory motion correction) simultaneously.

Let us denote the coordinate system of the tracking device as W, and the coordinate system of the sensor when acquiring the ith ICE frame as S_i. The tracking device provides transformation matrix T_{S_i} of S_i relative to W. The position of an ICE image pixel in S_i is determined by a scaling matrix T_S and a transformation T_C provided by an offline calibration using the method described in [11]. An ICE image pixel $\boldsymbol{p}_{\mathrm{US}}$ is mapped to a point in CT coordinate system by $\boldsymbol{p}_{\mathrm{CT}} = T_R \cdot T_{S_i} \cdot T_C \cdot T_S \cdot \boldsymbol{p}_{\mathrm{US}}$, where T_R is the registration matrix to be estimated, as showed in Figure 2.

3.2   Cardiac and Respiration Motion Gating

Heart motion as well as respiratory motion are factors that influence the accuracy of registration. To eliminate the respiratory motion from the frames to be registered, the displacement in the Z axis of the second sensor placed on the patient's chest was analyzed. We pick the frames acquired without significant chest movement. To detect the respiratory rest phases, the position variance of the sensor in the Z axis during the previous 50 acquired frames is computed. If the variance is below a given threshold, the frames would be considered. The threshold can be adjusted during the ICE image acquisition. We further select the frames with a fixed time interval from the previous R-wave in the ECG signal for cardiac gating. Typically we get about 3 cardiac gated frames for each respiration. The doctor puts the ICE catheter in the right atrium and sweeps the ICE across the heart chambers. When a qualified frame is selected, the system notifies the doctor to proceed to another orientation or position.

3.3   Image Registration

The registration process computes a rigid transformation from the coordinate system of the tracking device to the C-arm CT space. Because the ultrasound only images the heart and the CT image contains the whole thorax of the subject, an initial alignment between them is needed before applying the automatic search for the six registration parameters. Since the tracking device is fixed under the table, an initial rotation can be estimated from the axes of the tracking

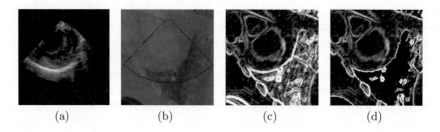

(a)   (b)   (c)   (d)

Fig. 3. Preprocessing of C-arm CT data to match ICE image. (a) 2D ICE image, (b) C-arm CT MPR image, (c) gradient image of (b), (d) after applying a mask on (c) for pixels whose intensity in (b) is higher than a threshold.

transmitter and the patient orientation of the C-arm CT data. An initial translation can be estimated by asking the user to either select a point in the 3D data corresponding to the tip location, or manually match the ICE frame and Multiplanar Reconstruction (MPR) of the 3D data. This estimation does not need to be very accurate. For example, if the segmentation of the C-arm CT data is available, the centroid of the right atrium segmentation can be used to initialize the registration.

The initial registration is followed by an automatic registration step. The registration parameters are optimized according to the similarity between the gated ICE images and its corresponding CT slices. Because ICE has high intensity at the chamber boundary and low intensity values inside the chamber, we use the gradient magnitude of the CT data in similarity computation. The gradient at each voxel of the CT volume is computed using 3D Sobel filter before applying the registration. Figure 3(a) to 3(c) show an ICE image, the corresponding CT slice, and the gradient magnitude on the CT slice. The high gradient magnitude outside the heart chamber can affect the accuracy of registration results because it does not appear in the ICE image. Therefore, a thresholding step is performed on the CT intensity image and the obtained mask is then applied to the gradient magnitude image, as showed in Figure 3(d). This threshold value can be adjusted interactively from the user interface.

We compute the Normalized Cross-Correlation (NCC) for each pair of the ICE image and the CT gradient magnitude slice. The sum of all NCC values is taken as the similarity measure, Similarity$(T_R) = \sum_{i=1}^{N} \text{NCC}(\text{US}_i, \text{CT}_i(T_R))$, where US$_i$ is the ith ICE image from the gated sequence of N images, CT$_i(T_R)$, is the resliced plane from the cardiac C-arm CT gradient magnitude data corresponding to US$_i$ and a given transformation T_R. We take the measure only for those pixels located inside the pre-defined fan shape of the ultrasound image.

We use the best neighbor method in the optimization. An initial step size is first chosen. In each iteration, all of the parameters are changed in turn with the step size and the value of similarity measure is computed. The change that causes the greatest improvement in the similarity measure is kept. This iteration continues until no change can give a better similarity measure. Then, the step size is reduced and above process is repeated again. We choose an initial step size 5.5 mm or 5.5 degree. They are then reduced by a factor of 2 when needed. The minimum step size for stop criterion is 0.1 mm or 0.1 degree. We also tested other optimization strategies such as Powell method and gradient decent method. However, we get the best result using the best neighbor method. This may be due to the existence of many local optima which makes the one dimensional search and gradient estimation, used in Powell and gradient decent methods, respectively, behave poorly.

4   Experimental Results

During the experiment on an anesthetized pig, 54 ICE sequences were saved while the physician was imaging the pig's heart chambers. The registration was performed offline. The size of C-arm CT volume is $512 \times 512 \times 444$. The data is downsampled by a factor of 2 on each dimension to speed up the registration process. From one of the image sequences, 18 frames were selected after cardiac and respiratory gating. The ICE images were captured in a resolution of 640×480. They are clipped and resized to 128×128 for the registration. Figure 4 shows the registration results in a side by side comparison with the corresponding C-arm CT MPR images. The registration procedure implemented in C++ took less than a minute on a system with an 2.8 GHz Intel P4 processor and 2 GB DDR memory.

The registration results were validated quantitatively by comparing chamber wall distance between 2D ICE image and 3D C-arm CT images. 29 ICE images covering the LA and LV were manually selected and segmented by an ultrasound image specialist using dedicated software. Figure 5(a) shows the LA segmentation on one ICE image. Four heart chambers in 3D C-arm CT image were segmented using a tool developed for cardiac CT data. The mask boundary of the 3D segmentations cut by the ICE image plane is displayed on the ICE image, as showed in Figure 5(b). We computed the shortest distance from each pixel on the 2D segmentation boundary to the 3D segmentation boundary for all 29 ICE images. The average distance is 3.14 ± 3.13 mm.

As another qualitative evaluation, we constructed a 3D ultrasound volume from a dense ICE sweeping and compared it with the registered 3D C-arm CT volume. Figure 5(c) and 5(d) show a side by side comparison of two volumes cut by the same clip plane, where the LA and LV matches well in two volumes.

Figure 6(a) shows a 2D ICE image of LA and the corresponding MPR slice of the C-arm CT image. In Figure 6(b), the ICE catheter is displayed in 3D showing the position and orientation of the ultrasound fan relatively to the segmented heart chambers. The ultrasound fan clipped the LA and the pulmonary veins can be clearly observed. Other tracked sensors can be displayed in the same coordinate system after the registration. For example, the red ball represents the location of the sensor on the chest. We also provide an endoscopic visualization of pre-operative data by setting up a perspective camera on the catheter tip, as showed in Figure 6(b). A clip plane is enabled to make the user directly see the region of interest.

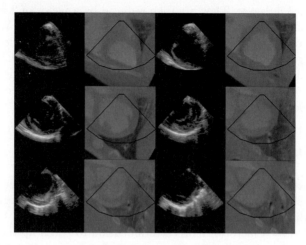

Fig. 4. A side by side comparison of the registered ICE images with C-arm CT MPR images

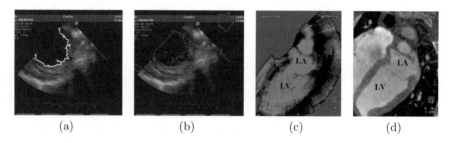

| (a) | (b) | (c) | (d) |

Fig. 5. Visual inspection of registration results. (a) 2D ICE image LA segmentation (yellow contour), (b) C-arm CT LA segmentation cut by the ICE image (red contour), (c) a cross-sectional image of the dense ICE acquisitions, (d) corresponding MPR of C-arm CT image after registration.

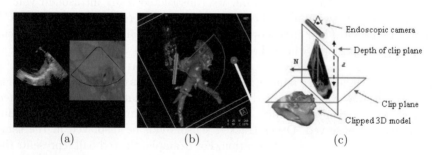

| (a) | (b) | (c) |

Fig. 6. (a) CT slice provides a bigger field of view on the anatomy, (b) ICE catheter and other tracked sensor (red ball) are displayed with 3D segmented heart chambers, (c) endoscopic view set up

5   Discussion and Future Work

We presented a method of registering ICE images and 3D C-arm CT data for EP applications. This framework also works with other pre-operative data such as CT and MR. Compared to previous works, our method performs both cardiac and respiratory gatings. And it does not require segmenting 3D data or ICE images. We showed good registration result on data acquired in animal experiments. Currently, the method still needs user interactions to choose proper threshold and provide initial alignment before applying the registration. Our next step is to make the registration process simpler and faster and validated by physicians in online case studies. It is also possible to estimate the respiratory motion from the position sensor on the ICE catheter instead of using an extra sensor on the patient chest. We believe the proposed method can help the physicians to learn and perform complex EP ablation procedures, improve the ablation accuracy, and reduce the EP procedure time.

References

1. Pappone, C., et al.: Atrial electroanatomic remodeling after circumferential radiofrequency pulmonary vein ablation: Efficacy of an anatomic approach in a large cohort of patients with atrial fibrillation. Circulation 104, 2539–2544 (2001)
2. Maloney, J., Burnett, J., Dala-Krishna, P., Glueck, R.: New directions in intracardiac echocardiography. Journal of Interventional Cardiac Electrophysiology 13, 23–29 (2005)
3. Lauritsch, G., Boese, J., Wigstrom, L., Kemeth, H., Fahrig, R.: Towards cardiac C-arm computed tomography. IEEE Trans. Med. Imaging 25(7), 922–934 (2006)
4. Roche, A., Pennec, X., Malandain, G., Ayache, N.: Rigid registration of 3D ultrasound with MR images: a new approach combining intensity and gradient information. IEEE Trans. Med. Imaging 20(10), 1038–1049 (2001)
5. Penney, G., Blackall, J., Hamady, M., Sabharwal, T., Adam, A., Hawkes, D.: Registration of freehand 3D ultrasound and magnetic resonance liver images. Med. Image. Anal. 8(1), 81–91 (2004)
6. Leroy, A.: Rigid registration of freehand 3D ultrasound and CT-scan kidney images. In: Proc. Medical Image Computing and Computer-Assisted Intervention, pp. 837–844 (2004)
7. Wein, W., Roper, B., Navab, N.: Automatic registration and fusion of ultrasound with CT for radiotherapy. In: Proc. Medical Image Computing and Computer-Assisted Intervention, pp. 303–311 (2005)
8. Sun, Y., et al.: Registration of high-resolution 3D atrial images with electroanatomical cardiac mapping: Evaluation of registration method. Proc. SPIE Medical Imaging 5744, 299–307 (2005)
9. Fahmy, T., et al.: Intracardiac echo-guided image integration. Journal of Cardiovascular Electrophysiology 18(3), 276–282 (2007)
10. Zhong, H., Kanade, T., Schwartzman, D.: Virtual Touch.: An efficient registration method for catheter navigation in left atrium. In: Proc. Medical Image Computing and Computer-Assisted Intervention, pp. 437–444 (2006)
11. Khamene, A., Sauer, F.: A novel phantom-less spatial and temporal ultrasound calibration method. In: Proc. Medical Image Computing and Computer-Assisted Intervention, pp. 65–72 (2005)

3D Reconstruction of Internal Organ Surfaces for Minimal Invasive Surgery

Mingxing Hu[1], Graeme Penney[1], Philip Edwards[2], Michael Figl[2], and David Hawkes[1]

[1] Centre for Medical Image Computing, University College London
[2] Department of Surgical Oncology and Technology, Imperial College London,
London, United Kingdom
{mingxing.hu,g.penney,d.hawkes}@ucl.ac.uk, {eddie.edwards,
m.figl}@imperial.ac.uk

Abstract. While Minimally Invasive Surgery (MIS) offers great benefits to patients compared with open surgery surgeons suffer from a restricted field-of-view and obstruction from instruments. We present a novel method for 3D reconstruction of soft tissue, which can provide a wider field-of-view with 3D information for surgeons, including restoration of missing data. The paper focuses on the use of Structure from Motion (SFM) techniques to solve the missing data problem and application of competitive evolutionary agents to improve the robustness to missing data and outliers. The method has been evaluated with synthetic data, images from a phantom heart model, and *in vivo* MIS image sequences using the da Vinci telerobotic surgical system.

1 Introduction

The past decade has witnessed significant advances on robotic assisted Minimally Invasive Surgery (MIS) evolving from early laboratory experiments to an indispensable tool for many surgeries. MIS offers great benefits to patients: the incisions and trauma are reduced and hospitalisation time is shorter. Robotic assisted techniques further enhance the manual dexterity of the surgeon and enable him to concentrate on the surgical procedure. Despite of all these advantages, MIS using an endoscope still suffers from a fundamental problem: the narrow field-of-view. As a result, the restricted vision impedes the surgeon's ability to collect visual information (locating landmarks, etc.) from the scenes and his/her awareness of peripheral sites.

A large amount of research work has been carried out which attempts to provide more 2D or 3D preoperative or intraoperative information to the surgeon. For example, Seshamani et al. presented an endoscopic mosaicing technique to display a broader field-of-view of the scene by stitching together images in a video sequence [1]. Unfortunately, the mosaicing results are only 2D images with larger scene areas, which lack any 3D information. In order to recover the 3D depth of a scene, Devernay proposed a five-step strategy to achieve 3D reconstruction of the operating field based on vision techniques [2]. More recently stereo-based techniques were proposed to reconstruct soft tissue structure in MIS, which can also track the temporal motion of the deformable surface [3, 4]. However, a drawback of these methods is that the images captured for 3D reconstruction are mainly from a fixed field-of-view, so they

N. Ayache, S. Ourselin, A. Maeder (Eds.): MICCAI 2007, Part I, LNCS 4791, pp. 68–77, 2007.
© Springer-Verlag Berlin Heidelberg 2007

cannot offer 3D information of peripheral scenes around the operating field. Exceptions to this are [5, 6], where a 3D map of the scene is built and camera movement is recovered based on the Simultaneous Localization and Mapping technique. However, they require long term repeatable landmarks to estimate the camera parameters, which are hard to obtain in dynamic scenes with soft tissue.

This paper tries to solve the 3D reconstruction problem of internal organ surface for MIS and makes the following contributions: (i) 3D structure is recovered from a moving vision system using Structure from Motion (SFM) techniques [7]. Feature points are detected and tracked when the camera system moves around the operating area. The 3D positions of these features are reconstructed to provide a broader field-of-view. Therefore, we can offer a wider operating scene with 3D information to the surgeon, which can be used for 3D-3D registration of the anatomy to the pre-operative data. We also want to emphasize that the proposed method is able to reconstruct 3D organ surface without any laser scanner or fiducial markers but only with endoscopic cameras. (ii) A Competitive Evolutionary Agent-based (CEA) algorithm is proposed to solve the missing data problem and improve robustness to outliers [8]. Features may move out of the field-of-view during the feature tracking so the missing data needs to be filled before estimating the 3D structure. Outliers obtained from bad location and false tracking, on the other hand, can distort the estimation to such a degree that the fitted parameters become arbitrary. The CEA algorithm is applied to remove outliers from the feature dataset, so as to minimize their effect on the whole estimation. The proposed technique is validated using a heart phantom with known 3D geometry and using *in vivo* data from totally endoscopic coronary artery bypass (TECAB) surgery with the da Vinci^{TM} system.

2 Material and Methods

2.1 Stereo Feature Tracking

The first step to reconstruct 3D structures during a MIS endoscopic procedure is to track image features as the cameras move. One of the well-known tracking methods is the Lucas-Kanade (LK) tracker [9], which we extended to a stereo framework. The LK tracker minimizes the sum of squared errors between two images I_k and I_{k+1} by altering the warping parameters $\mathbf{p}$ which are used to warp I_{k+1} to the coordinate frame of I_k. For a general motion model with transformation function $W(\mathbf{x}, \mathbf{p})$, the objective function is

$$\min \sum_{\mathbf{x}} [I_{k+1}(W(\mathbf{x};\mathbf{p}+\Delta\mathbf{p}))- I_k(\mathbf{x})]^2 \qquad (1)$$

This expression is linearized by a first order Taylor expansion on $I_{k+1}(W(\mathbf{x};\mathbf{p}+\Delta\mathbf{p}))$

$$\min \sum_{\mathbf{x}} \left[I_{k+1}(W(\mathbf{x};\mathbf{p}))+\nabla I_{k+1}\frac{\partial W}{\partial \mathbf{p}} - I_k(\mathbf{x}) \right]^2$$

Where ∇I_{k+1} is the image gradient vector and $\partial W/\partial \mathbf{p}$ is the Jacobian of the transformation function. In our stereo framework, the tracking process is extended to four directions, namely, two temporally consecutive directions, $Tr(I_k, I_{k+1})$ (where

$Tr(I_k, I_{k+1})$ denotes tracking from I_k to I_{k+1}) and $Tr(J_k, J_{k+1})$, and two corresponding (stereo) directions, $Tr(I_k, J_k)$ and $Tr(J_k, I_k)$, as shown in Fig. 1. Since the relative position of the stereoscopic cameras is fixed and remains unchanged during MIS surgery, we can use this to adapt the window size and initial position for feature tracking in the corresponding directions. Then features $\mathbf{x}_{I(k)}$ and $\mathbf{x}_{J(k)}$ are considered to be a stereo pair (two projections of a 3D point $\mathbf{X}$ from two viewpoints), if they satisfy

$$\varepsilon = \left\| \mathbf{x}_{I(k)} - \mathbf{x}'_{J(k)} \right\|_F + \left\| \mathbf{x}_{J(k)} - \mathbf{x}'_{I(k)} \right\|_F \leq \delta \tag{2}$$

where $\mathbf{x}'_I$ (or $\mathbf{x}'_J$) is the corresponding point of $\mathbf{x}_I$ (or $\mathbf{x}_J$) in image J (or I) and they are added to the feature dataset if the error ε is less than the threshold δ.

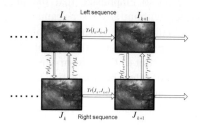

Fig. 1. Framework of stereo tracking

2.2 Structure from Motion with Missing Data

In the feature tracking process, it is possible that some features are only detected and tracked for few frames. These features cannot be used for reconstruction using conventional vision techniques [7, 11]. The missing data needs to be recovered before 3D reconstruction can be carried out.

Given a set of tracked feature points, their 2D and 3D locations can be related using the following matrix:

$$\underbrace{\begin{bmatrix} \lambda_1^1 \mathbf{x}_1^1 & \cdots & \lambda_n^1 \mathbf{x}_n^1 \\ \vdots & \ddots & \vdots \\ \lambda_1^m \mathbf{x}_1^m & \cdots & \lambda_n^m \mathbf{x}_n^m \end{bmatrix}}_{\mathbf{M}} = \underbrace{\begin{bmatrix} \mathbf{P}^1 \\ \vdots \\ \mathbf{P}^m \end{bmatrix}}_{\mathbf{P}} \underbrace{\begin{bmatrix} \mathbf{X}_1 & \cdots & \mathbf{X}_n \end{bmatrix}}_{\mathbf{X}} \tag{3}$$

where $\mathbf{x}_i^j = (x_i^j, y_i^j, 1)^T$ is the projection of 3D point $\overline{\mathbf{X}}_i = (X_i, Y_i, Z_i, 1)^T$ ($i = 1, \cdots, n$) onto the j-th ($j = 1, \cdots, m$) image plane. $\mathbf{P}^j$ is a 3×4 projective matrix of frame j, and λ_j^i is the projective depth, which can be computed using epipolar geometry [11]. The measurement matrix can be further factorized into shape and motion components, $\mathbf{P}$ and $\mathbf{X}$, by enforcing the rank four constraint. In the absence of missing data, the solution to this linearized problem is found as the $\mathbf{P}$ and $\mathbf{X}$ ($rank(\mathbf{P}) = rank(\mathbf{X}) = 4$) that minimize:

$$\min \mathbf{R}_e = \min_{\mathbf{P}, \mathbf{X}} \left\| \mathbf{M} - \mathbf{PX} \right\|_F^2 \tag{4}$$

where $\mathbf{R}_e$ is the residual between the model $\mathbf{PX}$ and the data $\mathbf{M}$.

However, in the presence of missing data, this is not the case. Recently Martinec and Pajdla proposed a structure recovery method [10], which modified the projective reconstruction in [11] with the Jacobs' linear fitting method [12]. The central idea is to apply a linear algebra operation to fit an unknown matrix $\mathbf{M}_r$ of a certain rank $r = 4$ to the incomplete noisy measurement matrix $\mathbf{M}$ by using a number of incomplete submatrices $\mathbf{S}$ (quadruplet of linear independent columns of $\mathbf{M}$). Since each submatrix $\mathbf{S}$ can provide some constraints, putting all the constraints together will generate much stronger constraints to the whole fitting problem. Readers are referred to [12] for further information about data filling techniques.

Ideally, each submatrix (quadruplet of the columns) should be considered, but the vast number of candidates makes the computation almost infeasible. In [10] a random selection of submatrices is used instead. This is a major drawback as it does not maximize the contributions of the submatrix samples to the whole problem. A system which allows more information to be obtained from each submatrix would be able to solve more difficult fitting problems given the limited amount of information. Moreover, if some outliers are included in $\mathbf{S}$, it may not contribute any useful information to the estimation, or even divert the whole estimation to some incorrect result.

2.3   Competitive Evolutionary Agents for 3D Reconstruction

In order to more effectively choose a selection of submatrices we employ a new approach based on competitive evolutionary agents to solve the 3D reconstruction problem with missing data and outliers. The agents represent a subset of the columns used to construct the submatrices. They carry out evolutionary behavior, such as reproduction and diffusion, to search for good samples from a large number of candidates. The quality of the submatrix is also supervised using a fitness function, which measures the amount of missing data and perturbation levels of noise and outliers.

Agent definition
Suppose that Ψ is the dataset representing all the columns of $\mathbf{M}$. Ψ may be viewed as a one-dimensional index to measurements of the feature points, and also as an environment in which the agents inhabit and evolve. Then the evolutionary agent can be defined as

$$Agent = \langle \mathbf{V}, \ a, \ F_{fitness}, \ fml, \ Rep, \ Diff, \ Die \rangle$$

where $\mathbf{V}$ is an r-dimensional position vector which denotes positions in Ψ and the value of its component V_k, $k = 1, \cdots, r$, is an index number within Ψ. a, $F_{fitness}$ and fml represents its internal behavior, i.e., agent age, fitness and family index respectively. Rep, $Diff$ and Die describe its external behavior, i.e., reproduction, diffusion and vanishing, respectively.

Fitness function
The value of the fitness function is mainly determined by the number and position of missing data and unknown depths. For example, for each agent we can construct a

submatrix $\mathbf{S}_t = \begin{bmatrix} \mathbf{s}_t^1 & \mathbf{s}_t^2 & \mathbf{s}_t^3 & \mathbf{s}_t^4 \end{bmatrix}$ using the selected quadruplet from $\mathbf{M}$, and $t \in T$ (T is a random set of indices). Then we calculate the number of rows without missing data n_{fill}^4, and the number of rows with one missing entry n_{fill}^3. Rows with more than one missing element are seldom considered, because they cannot provide good constraints for the relevant viewpoints. In this way a concise matrix $\hat{\mathbf{S}}_k$ is constructed with the rows of $\mathbf{S}_k$ containing either zero or only one missing element. Then the number of unknown depths in $\hat{\mathbf{S}}_k$, n_{depth}, is calculated. Matrix $\hat{\mathbf{S}}_k$ can be used for decomposition to provide constraints for matrix factorization. Therefore, the fitness function can be written as

$$F_{fitness} = n_{fill}^4 + \alpha_1 n_{fill}^3 - \alpha_2 n_{depth} \tag{5}$$

where $0 < \alpha_1, \alpha_2 \leq 1$ are the constants used to weight the data-missing level and depth-unknown level terms. Generally, the larger the fitness value, the fewer missing entries and unknown depths in the selected submatrix.

Evolutionary behavior

Evolutionary agents adapt to their environment by way of behavioral responses, namely, reproduction and diffusion. Letting $\Phi^{(g)}$ denote the set of active agents in generation g.

(1) Reproduction: Each active agent $\alpha^{(g)}$ will breed a finite number m_{br} of offspring agents $\alpha^{(g+1)}$. The differences between $\alpha^{(g)}$ and $\alpha^{(g+1)}$ primarily lie in the position vectors $\mathbf{V}^{(g)}$ and $\mathbf{V}^{(g+1)}$. Some elements of $\mathbf{V}^{(g)}$ are chosen and changed to a new index number selected randomly from Ψ by a random number generator. Then the fitness of the new generated agent is computed using equation (5), and compared with that of the siblings of the same family, $\alpha_{(l)}^{(g+1)}$ (where l denotes the family number). Only the agent with largest fitness value will survive and move on to the diffusion process.

(2) Diffusion: After the reproduction process, the successful agent $\alpha^{(g+1)}$ will compare its fitness with that of its parent $\alpha^{(g)}$. If the offspring has a fitness advantage, it will be appended to the agent set $A^{(g+1)}$, and its parent will become inactive and be removed from the evolutionary environment. If not, the offspring will be deleted and the age of its parent will be increased by one. In addition, if the age of an agent exceeds its life span, it will be removed from the environment.

2.4 Experimental Design

In order to assess and quantify the performance of the proposed method, a heart phantom made of silicone rubber (The Chamberlain Group, Great Barrington, MA, USA) was used, dimensions 6" (atria / apex) × 4" wide × 3.5" (anterior / posterior). Then the 3D surface of the phantom was reconstructed using the AlignRT (VisionRT, London, UK) system to provide the ground truth surface data. This enabled us to choose points from surface as ground truth data to evaluate the accuracy of the proposed method, or to register the reconstructed point cloud directly to the surface. In addition a CT scan of the heart phantom was also used (Philips MX8000 IDT 16 slice CT scanner: voxel size 1×1×2mm with 768×768×145 voxels). Fig. 2 shows the heart phantom, the 3D surface obtained from the AlignRT system and the 3D surface reconstructed from CT scan using the marching cubes algorithm implemented in VTK.

We have carried out experiments on three sets of data: synthetic test data, heart phantom data and *in vivo* data from endoscopic surgery. These sets of data and a description of the experiments are described in the following paragraphs.

The synthetic data was produced using 3D points $\underline{X}$ randomly selected from the 3D surface captured using the AlignRT system. These points were projected to twenty image planes with different rotation and translation parameters to generate sets of 2D image points. Two sets of experiments were then carried out:

(G1): Ten different ranges of Gaussian noise are added to the image measurements, with a zero mean and standard deviation varying from 0.5 to 5.0. The percentage of missing data was fixed at 20%.
(G2): The standard deviation of Gaussian noise was fixed at 2.0, and the percentage of missing data was varied from 10% to 60%.

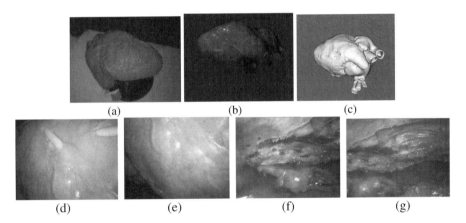

(a)   (b)   (c)

(d)   (e)   (f)   (g)

Fig. 2. Examples of experimental data: (a) Image of the heart model; (b) 3D surface reconstructed from AlignRT scanning; (c) 3D model reconstructed from CT scanning; (d) and (e) show the first and last frames of the image sequence of phantom heart; (f) and (g) show the first and last frames of the image sequence from TECAB surgery;

The da Vinci^{TM} robotic surgical system (Intuitive Surgical, Inc., Sunnyvale, CA, USA) was used to obtain images of the heart phantom. The heart phantom was placed on a bed and the endoscopic cameras were positioned approximately 40mm from the heart surface. Twenty images were selected from this set of data (every fifth frame) and the first and last frames captured from left camera are shown in Fig. 2 (d) and (e), respectively. Using these data our algorithm detected and tracked feature points over the image sequence. In total 401 features were detected and on average 48.8% of the data within the matrix $\mathbf{M}$ was missing.

Our *in vivo* data set consisted of endoscopic images from a TECAB surgical procedure using the da Vinci system. Fig. 2 (f) and (g) shows the first and last frames from the left sequence respectively. A surface was reconstructed from this data set. In total 397 features were detected and tracked and on average 45.8% of data within the matrix **M** was missing. In order to further improve the accuracy of the proposed method, a bundle adjustment technique [13] was also applied after data filling. This technique minimizes the RMS error, which is the mean squared distance between the observed image points and the reprojected image points $\hat{\mathbf{x}} = \mathbf{PX}$.

3 Experimental Results

3.1 Synthetic Data

In the noise testing experiment (G1), we ran 100 trials for each noise level. A graph of the result is shown in Fig. 3 (a). It can be seen that the CEA-based method performs better than the *M&P* method [10] over all the experiments. In particular, as the noise level increases ($\sigma = 4, 5$), the performance of our approach is affected less than the *M&P* method. Fig. 3 (b) displays the results of the missing-data testing (G2). We can see that the average error of CEA increases when the amount of missing data increases, but not as significant as that of the *M&P* method. This suggests that evolutionary agents can effectively select good samples from a vast pool of candidates, even when a large percentage of the elements are missing.

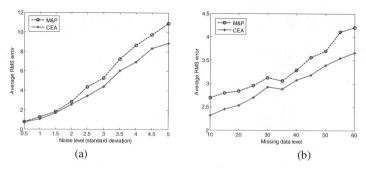

(a)   (b)

Fig. 3. Experimental results of synthetic data testing. (a) Average RMS error under different noise levels; (b) Average RMS error under different missing-data levels.

3.2 Phantom Model

Fig. 4 (a) and (b) illustrate the results of our data filling method. The measured features are marked with blue "o" and the reprojected points to those image planes are marked with red "x". In Fig. 4 (a), it can be seen that LK tracker lost the feature since the 7th frame, but using the proposed data filling method we can still "track" the feature in frames 8 and 9 and the recovered positions appear visually reasonable. Fig. 4 (c) displays the reconstructed 3D point cloud using the proposed technique. Since we did not have a gold standard transformation between the 3D points and our CT image, we used the Iterative Closet Point (ICP) [14] algorithm to register the 3D points to the surface derived from CT to obtain a measure of 3D reconstruction accuracy. Fig. 4 (d) shows the final position after ICP registration. Most of the points lie on or are close to the surface and the mean residual is around 1.87 mm. Moreover, using visual inspection we can see that the positions of 3D points are overlaid on the CT surface after ICP registration in roughly the correct position.

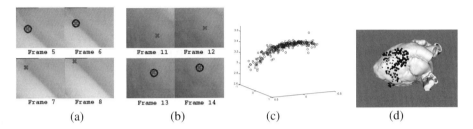

Fig. 4. Results using the heart phantom. (a) and (b) show the data filling results of two features; (c) and (d) display the reconstructed point cloud and its registration result to CT scan model.

3.3 *In vivo* Data

Fig. 5(a) shows the results of our missing data filling algorithm on the *in vivo* data, the feature point shown was not detected or tracked until the 9th frame, however our data filling method was able to accurately recover its position in frames 7 and 8.

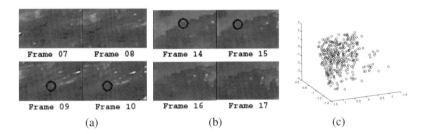

Fig. 5. Experimental results of *in vivo* data testing. (a) and (b) illustrate the data filling results of two features, respectively; (c) displays the reconstructed point cloud using the proposed method.

Unfortunately no ground truth 3D data was available for this patient. Instead we report the RMS surface reconstruction error. Before removing the outliers, the average RMS error for all the visible features was 3.977. This reduced to 1.535 after 65 outliers were detected and removed from the feature dataset. Finally the bundle adjustment technique was applied, after initialization using the output from the CEA method, and the error was further reduced to 1.040. Fig. 5 (c) shows the point cloud reconstructed from the endoscopic image sequence.

4 Discussion and Conclusions

In this paper we have introduced a new method to reconstruct a 3D surface of soft tissue structure with missing data for robotic assisted MIS surgery, which can provide a wider field-of-view of the operating area with 3D information. 3D structure of operating scenes is recovered from a moving stereoscopic vision system and a competitive evolutionary agent optimisation strategy is used to improve the robustness of the proposed technique to missing data and outliers. Our approach has been evaluated with both a heart phantom of known geometric structure and *in vivo* data from TECAB surgery. The results indicate the proposed method can handle both missing data and outliers, even when a large amount of missing data is involved in the estimation.

Efforts in the near future will focus on assessing reconstructed surface accuracy of the phantom heart with known gold standard position (for example, using some manually selected 3D points or attached fiducial markers). Our long term goal is to register the 3D information from optical images with the pre-operative data (CT or MRI) which will also be used as a ground truth for further *in vivo* testing of our method.

Acknowledgments. The authors would like to thank Dr. Fernando Bello for his help in obtaining the VisonRT data of the heart phantom. Special thanks also go to Tim Carter for data display and Dr. Gang Gao for ICP registration.

References

1. Seshamani, S., Lau, W., Hager, G.: Real-Time Endoscopic Mosaicking. In: Larsen, R., Nielsen, M., Sporring, J. (eds.) MICCAI 2006. LNCS, vol. 4190, pp. 355–363. Springer, Heidelberg (2006)
2. Devernay, F., Mourgues, F., Coste-Maniere, E.: Towards Endoscopic Augmented Reality for Robotically Assisted Minimally Invasive Cardiac Surgery. In: Proc. International Workshop on Medical Imaging and Augmented Reality, pp. 16–20 (2001)
3. Stoyanov, D., Darzi, F., Yang, A., Dense, G.-Z.: 3D Depth Recovery for Soft Tissue Deformation During Robotically Assisted Laparoscopic Surgery. In: Barillot, C., Haynor, D.R., Hellier, P. (eds.) MICCAI 2004. LNCS, vol. 3217, pp. 41–48. Springer, Heidelberg (2004)
4. Lau, W., Ramey, N., Corso, J., Thakor, N., Hager, G.: Stereo-Based Endoscopic Tracking of Cardiac Surface Deformation. In: Barillot, C., Haynor, D.R., Hellier, P. (eds.) MICCAI 2004. LNCS, vol. 3217, pp. 494–501. Springer, Heidelberg (2004)
5. Burschka, D., Li, M., Taylor, R., Hager, G.: Scale-Invariant Registration of Monocular Endoscopic Images to CT-Scans for Sinus Surgery, In: Proc. MICCAI. In: Barillot, C., Haynor, D.R., Hellier, P. (eds.) MICCAI 2004. LNCS, vol. 3217, pp. 413–421. Springer, Heidelberg (2004)
6. Mountney, P., Stoyanov, D., Davison, A., Yang, G.-Z.: Simultaneous Stereoscope Location and Soft-Tissue Mapping for Minimal Invasive Surgery. In: Larsen, R., Nielsen, M., Sporring, J. (eds.) MICCAI 2006. LNCS, vol. 4190, pp. 347–354. Springer, Heidelberg (2006)

7. Tomasi, C., Kanade, T.: Shape and Motion from Image Streams under Orthography: a Factorization Method. Int. J. Computer Vision 9(2), 137–154 (1992)
8. Hu, M.X., McMenemy, K., Ferguson, S., Dodds, G., Yuan, B.Z.: Epipolar geometry estimation based on evolutionary agents, Pattern Recognition (to be published)
9. Lucas, B., Kanade, T.: An Iterative Image Registration Technique with an Application to Stereo Vision. In: Proc. IJCAI, pp. 674–679 (1981)
10. Martinec, D., Pajdla, T.: Structure from Many Perspective Images with Occlusions. In: Heyden, A., Sparr, G., Nielsen, M., Johansen, P. (eds.) ECCV 2002. LNCS, vol. 2351, pp. 355–369. Springer, Heidelberg (2002)
11. Sturm, P., Triggs, B.: A Factorization based Algorithm for Multi-Image Projective Structure and Motion. In: Buxton, B.F., Cipolla, R. (eds.) ECCV 1996. LNCS, vol. 1065, pp. 709–720. Springer, Heidelberg (1996)
12. Jacobs, W.: Linear Fitting with Missing Data for Structure-from-Motion. Computer Vision and Image Understanding 82(1), 57–81 (2001)
13. Triggs, B., McLauchlan, P., Hartley, R., Fitzgibbon, A.: Bundle Adjustment: A Modern Synthesis. Vision Algorithm: Theory and Practice, 298–375 (2000)
14. Besl, P., McKay, N.: A Method for Registration of 3-D Shapes. IEEE Trans. on PAMI 14(2), 239–256 (1992)

Cardiolock: An Active Cardiac Stabilizer
First in Vivo Experiments Using a New Robotized Device

Wael Bachta[1], Pierre Renaud[2], Edouard Laroche[1], Jacques Gangloff[1],
and Antonello Forgione[3]

[1] LSIIT (UMR CNRS-ULP 7005), Strasbourg I University, France
{wael,laroche,jacques}@eavr.u-strasbg.fr
[2] LGeCo, INSA-Strasbourg, France
pierre.renaud@insa-strasbourg.fr
[3] IRCAD / EITS, University Hospital of Strasbourg, France
antonello.forgione@ircad.u-strasbg.fr

Abstract. Off-pump Coronary Artery Bypass Grafting (CABG) is still
today a technically difficult procedure. In fact, the mechanical stabilizers
used to locally suppress the heart excursion have been demonstrated to
exhibit significant residual motion. We therefore propose a novel active
stabilizer which is able to compensate for this residual motion. The interaction between the heart and a mechanical stabilizer is first assessed
in vivo on an animal model. Then, the principle of active stabilization,
based on the high speed vision-based control of a compliant mechanism,
is presented. In vivo experimental results are given using a prototype
which structure is compatible with a minimally invasive approach.

1 Introduction

The complex motion of the heart makes an off-pump CABG technically challenging. For example, the left anterior descending coronary artery may exhibit
an excursion of 12.5 mm whereas its diameter is in the order of 1 mm [1] and
the accuracy needed for suturing is in the range of 0.1 mm. Several passive mechanical stabilizers have been proposed to overcome this difficulty by reducing
the anastomosis site excursion. They have been evaluated through different experiments. In [2], the residual motion of the coronary artery stabilized with a
passive Medtronic Octopus device is assessed on 3 pigs using a camera coupled
with a laser sensor. The residual excursion in the direction perpendicular to the
cardiac tissue ranged between 0.5 mm and 2.6 mm. In [1], a 3D heart wall motion
analysis during stabilization has been carried out through experiments on ten
pigs. The reported systolic to diastolic heart motion is larger than 1.5 mm using
three different commercial passive devices. To our knowledge, only a very few
articles deal with the use of a mechanical stabilizer compatible with the even
more challenging minimally invasive off-pump CABG. In [3], the authors com-
municate the results of robot-assisted totally endoscopic CABG experiments on
human beings. One of the reported difficulties encountered by the surgeons is
the significant residual motion of the passive Medtronic EndoOctopus stabilizer
used during the tests.

N. Ayache, S. Ourselin, A. Maeder (Eds.): MICCAI 2007, Part I, LNCS 4791, pp. 78–85, 2007.
© Springer-Verlag Berlin Heidelberg 2007

All these authors point out the insufficient performances of commercially available stabilizers. Experimental results are then expressed in terms of residual motion, which is the end user point of view. Nevertheless, very few information is available about the forces encountered by the stabilizer due to the heart. In [4], in vivo assessment of the cardiac forces has been carried out to design a mechanical stabilizer. However, the relationship between the forces and the physiological motions, i.e. respiratory and cardiac motions, as well as the dynamics of the interaction between the stabilizer and the heart surface, are not studied in details.

In [5,6,7,8] robotic systems are considered to compensate for the heart motion during off-pump CABG. The principle is to synchronize a robotized tool holder with the anastomosis site movement. From a safety point of view, using one robot to simultaneously perform the surgeon gesture and the stabilization task may not be satisfying. The robot has to undergo high accelerations to track the heart motion. The kinetic energy of the robot is a danger for the patient, especially when the tool is in contact with the heart surface. Moreover, the extension of this approach to minimally invasive surgery (MIS) is not obvious. One solution consists in shrinking the size of the parts moving at high speed, e.g by using a miniature robot with endocavity mobilities. This is still a technical challenge.

In this paper a novel approach is proposed, which allows the separation of the stabilization and the surgical tasks. We introduce the principle of an active cardiac stabilizer that allows to actively suppress the residual motion. The fundamental principle of our approach is similar to some extent to vibration cancellation techniques. The architecture of this new active stabilizer, called Cardiolock, is furthermore compatible with MIS.

In section 2 an experimental analysis of the interaction between the cardiac muscle and a rigid non-actuated stabilizer is presented. High-speed vision, force measurements and biological signals have been synchronously recorded during in vivo experiments on a pig. These data are of great interest for understanding the stabilizer behavior and to improve the design of the active device. In section 3, the design and principle of the active stabilizer are presented. In vivo experiments with the developed prototype are then presented, showing its efficiency, before concluding on further developments of the stabilizer.

2   Experimental Evaluation of the Heart Contact Forces

In order to complete several publications focused on the heart motion analysis [9,10], we present here an experimental evaluation of the forces applied by a passively stabilized heart. This allows a better understanding of the interaction between the cardiac muscle and a mechanical stabilizer, and provides useful information for the design of a stabilizer.

2.1   The Experimental Setup

The experiment has been carried out on a 40 kg pig which underwent full sternotomy after receiving a general anesthesia. The ventilation tidal volume was

set to 600 ml with a frequency of 16 breaths/min. The recorded fundamental
heart frequency was 1.81 beats/sec. A custom rigid stabilizer held by a medical
robot was positioned on the myocardium (Fig.1). This stabilizer is composed of
a 10 mm diameter stainless steel beam and a distal device to access the thoracic
cavity. This distal device hosts a 6 degrees-of-freedom (DOF) ATI Nano-17 force
sensor, that has a resolution of 0.0125 N for the force and 0.0625 Nmm for the
torque. The stabilizer tip has been designed with a suction capability, and its
residual displacement is measured using the position of a visual marker in the
image of a 333 Hz high speed camera (DALSA CAD6) with a 256 × 256 CCD
grayscale sensor. A Navitar Precise Eye Zoom lens was used to get a resolution
of 128 pixels per mm in the experimental configuration. The ventilation was acquired through two unidirectional Honeywell Awm700 airflow sensors. The ECG
signal was acquired using a 3 leads ECG cable and an electrocardiograph Schiller
Cardiovit AT-6 (Fig.1). All the data acquisitions are synchronized on the camera
frame rate with a sofware running under Xenomai real time operating system.

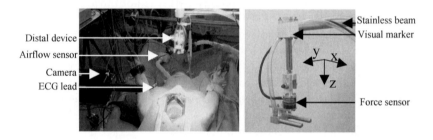

Fig. 1. The experimental setup and a close-up on the distal device

2.2   The Experimental Results

The figure 2 shows the obtained force and torque measured during one respiratory cycle for the biological parameters given above. The corresponding peak
to peak values are reported in Table 1. The most significant force component
is along the z axis, namely the anterior-posterior direction. The other force
components are however not negligible with a ratio around 3 between the force
components along x and z . Torque is of small amplitude, in the range of 15 Nmm.
    It is interesting to note (Fig.3) that the peaks of the 3 force components
do not occur simultaneously. Furthermore, even if the amplitude of the force
components in the x and y directions is lower than in the z direction, their

Table 1. The peak to peak force and torque values

	F_x (N)	F_y (N)	F_z (N)	T_x (Nmm)	T_y (Nmm)	T_z (Nmm)
with ventilation	1.2	1	3.8	13	20	13
without ventilation	0.8	1	2	12	12	10

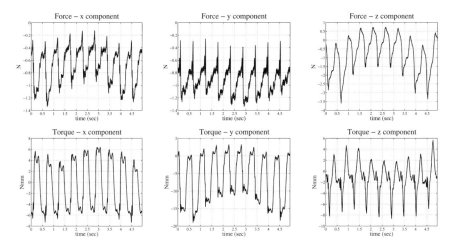

Fig. 2. Measurement of the force and torque components during one respiratory cycle

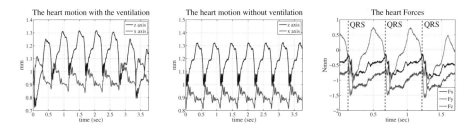

Fig. 3. From left to right: the heart motion with and without ventilation, and the heart contact force during 3 cardiac phases

transients are sharper. Figure 3 shows also that the force peaks are correlated with the physiological signals. Indeed, the peaks occur a short time (about 10 ms) after the QRS complex detection, i.e. during the systolic phase.

An acquisition without ventilation shows (Table 1) that the cardiac movement is responsible for half of the total force along the z axis, for the whole force along y and for almost the whole x component. While the remaining excursion of the stabilizer tip (Fig.3) in presence of ventilation is about 0.61 mm along the z axis and 0.3 mm along the x axis, it is reduced respectively to 0.3 mm and 0.19 mm when setting the ventilation off. The y direction corresponds to the beam axis and the displacement due to traction is therefore negligible.

One may notice that the force along z contains small positive values, indicating that the heart tries to pull the stabilizer. This is due to the stabilizer initial positioning. This positioning is therefore important since high positive force values could yield injuries to the the the myocardium.

3   The Active Heart Stabilizer

3.1   The Active Compensation Principle

The necessary stabilization accuracy can be estimated to 0.1 mm with respect to the $1 - 2$ mm diameter of the coronary arteries and the 0.1 mm diameter of the stitching thread. In a MIS context, the shape of a stabilizer should be a cylinder, of maximum external diameter between 10 and 12 mm, with a length approximately equal to 300 mm, so that any heart surface can be reached by insertion through a trocar. According to the elasticity theory, the distal stabilizer deflection due to the measured cardiac force exceeds the required precision. The experiments carried out in Section 2 with a passive stabilizer confirm this analysis, showing clearly the limits of passive stabilization. In fact the displacement could then reach 0.6 mm which is far beyond the necessary accuracy.

Therefore, we introduce the principle of an active stabilization. Indeed we propose an active system composed of an actuated cardiac stabilizer and an exteroceptive measurement. Using this feedback, the actuated stabilizer can be controlled in order to cancel the residual cardiac motion. Herein we use high speed visual feedback but any kind of exteroceptive measurement could be used.

3.2   The Current Design

At the current stage of development, the aim of the proposed prototype (Fig.4) is to compensate for the anastomosis site displacement in the anterior-posterior direction, since the maximum force and residual motion are encountered in that direction. The proposed device globally consists in two parts. A first active part is composed of a one DOF closed-loop mechanism remaining outside the patient body in a MIS context. The other part is a beam of 10 mm diameter and 300 mm length. This part, which dimensions are compatible with MIS, can be simply locked on the first part. Figure 4 shows that the closed-loop mechanism is composed of a piezo actuator (Cedrat Technologies) and three revolute compliant joints. Piezo actuation is adopted to obtain high dynamics and compliant joints are used to avoid backlash. The closed-loop mechanism is designed to transform the piezo actuator translation into a rotation of the beam, as described in Figure 5. For description purpose only, the compensation is then decomposed in two sequential steps: on the left side, one can see a magnified deflection due to an external load, and on the right side the cancellation of the tip displacement by modifying the geometry of the closed-loop mechanism. Further details on the methodology to select the mechanism architecture and dimensions are given in [11].

In a MIS context, asepsy can be obtained in two steps: the first external subsystem can be wrapped in a sterile bag and the other part can be sterilized using an autoclave. To be fully compatible with MIS, a distal end will need to be designed to provide more degrees of freedom for the the placement on the myocardium. Finally, the Cardiolock will probably be held by a surgical robot to handle the trocar constraint (e.g via a Remote Center of Motion mechanism).

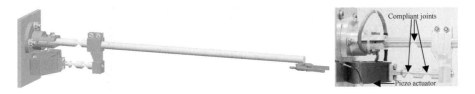

Fig. 4. The current prototype of the active stabilizer. On the left, a CAD global view and on the right the detail of the closed-loop mechanism on the current prototype.

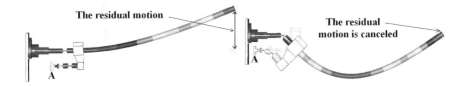

Fig. 5. A finite element analysis of the compensation. The actuator controls the horizontal position of the point A. Displacements are magnified for the sake of clarity.

3.3   High Speed Visual Servoing

The displacement of the stabilizer tip is caused by the piezo actuator action and by the external cardiac force. The measurement of this displacement is provided at 333 Hz by the high speed camera. Assuming small displacements, a linear model can be derived: $Y(z) = \mathbf{G}(z)U(z) - \mathbf{F}(z)D(z)$ where Y, U, D represent the z-transform of respectively the measured visual information, the actuator displacement, the cardiac force and $\mathbf{G}(z)$, $\mathbf{F}(z)$ are two transfer functions. The stabilization task consists in designing an appropriate feedback control law to cancel the displacement caused by the cardiac force, i.e reject the effects of $D(z)$ by controling $U(z)$. To do so, $\mathbf{G}$ has been first identified and $\mathbf{F}$ is constructed by approximation from the poles of $\mathbf{G}$ and an experimentally estimated static gain [11]. Since the previous model does not take into account the cardiac tissue mechanical properties, the control law must be robust with respect to modeling uncertainties. A H_∞ methodology is hence used to design the feedback controller, tuned to reject with high performances the cardiac force perturbation.

3.4   First in Vivo Results

The previous experimental setup was used to carry out some in vivo active stabilization experiments (Fig.6). The beam of the passive stabilizer was simply replaced by the novel actuated mechanism. The same distal device is used to provide an easy access to the thoracic cavity. Figure 7 reports the result of two stabilization tests. In both cases, the controller was switched on 6 seconds after the beginning of the experiment. The peak to peak heart excursion was then divided by 4. The RMS of the residual motion is 0.37 mm before activation of the active stabilization, which corresponds to the deflection measured in section 2,

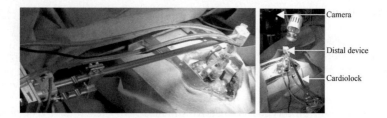

Fig. 6. The Cardiolock device during an experimental validation

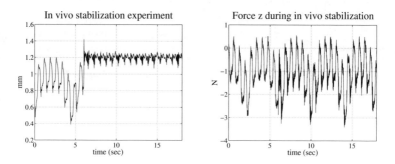

Fig. 7. In vivo stabilization results. On the left the measured motion, on the right the recorded contact force. The active stabilization starts after 6 seconds.

and 0.03 mm after activation. Since the frequency of the respiratory motion is low, it is completely suppressed, whereas the cardiac component is partially filtered. In the second experiment, the force along z was recorded (Fig.7). Only a slight variation of the force is observed. This may be explained by the little displacement, about 0.3 mm, imposed to the local area of interest in order to achieve the stabilization.

4   Conclusion

In this paper, a new robotized stabilizer, the Cardiolock device, has been proposed. After a detailed experimental assessment of the heart contact forces, stabilization experiments have been carried out showing promising performances. Future work will include a comparison of the proposed stabilizer with a commercial endoscopic stabilizer. A development of a multi DOF mechanism with the appropriate vision measurement will also be investigated in order to compensate for all possible residual motions.

References

1. Lemma, M., Mangini, A., Redaelli, A., Acocella, F.: Do cardiac stabilizers really stabilize? experimental quantitative analysis of mechanical stabilization. Interactive Cardiovascular and Thoracic Surgery (2005)

2. Cattin, P., Dave, H., Grunenfelder, J., Szekely, G., Turina, M., Zund, G.: Trajectory of coronary motion and its significance in robotic motion cancellation. European Journal of Cardio-thoracic Surgery 25 (2004)
3. Loisance, D., Nakashima, K., Kirsch, M.: Computer-assisted coronary surgery: lessons from an initial experience. Interactive Cardiovascular and Thoracic Surgery (2005)
4. Gilhuly, T., Salcudean, S., Ashe, K., Lichtenstein, S., Lawrence, P.: Stabilizer and surgical arm design for cardiac surgery. In: IEEE Int. Conf. on Robotics and Automation - ICRA (1998)
5. Thakral, A., Wallace, J., Tolmin, D., Seth, N., Thakor, N.: Surgical motion adaptive robotic technology (s.m.a.r.t): Taking the motion out of physiological motion. In: Niessen, W.J., Viergever, M.A. (eds.) MICCAI 2001. LNCS, vol. 2208, Springer, Heidelberg (2001)
6. Nakamura, Y., Kishi, K., Kawakami, H.: Heartbeat synchronization for robotic cardiac surgery. In: IEEE Int. Conf. on Robotics and Automation - ICRA 2 (2001)
7. Ginhoux, R., Gangloff, J., de Mathelin, M., Soler, L., Sanchez, M., Marescaux, J.: Beating heart tracking in robotic surgery using 500 hz visual servoing, model predictive control and an adaptive observer. In: IEEE Int. Conf. on Robotics and Automation - ICRA (2004)
8. Bebek, O., Cavusoglo, M.: Predictive control algorithms using biological signals for active relative motion canceling in robotic assisted heart surgery. In: IEEE Int. Conf. on Robotics and Automation - ICRA (2006)
9. Shechter, G., Resar, J., McVeigh, E.: Displacement and velocity of the coronary arteries: cardiac and respiratory motion. IEEE trans. on medical imaging (2006)
10. Cuvillon, L., Gangloff, J., de Mathelin, M., Forgione, A.: Toward robotized beating heart tecabg: assessment of the heart dynamics using high-speed vision. In: Int. Conf. on Medical Image Computing and Computer-Assisted Intervention (2005)
11. Bachta, W., Renaud, P., Laroche, E., Forgione, A., Gangloff, J.: Design and control of a new active cardiac stabilizer. In: IEEE/RSJ Int. Conf. on Intelligent Robots and Systems - IROS (2007)

Automated Segmentation of the Liver from 3D CT Images Using Probabilistic Atlas and Multi-level Statistical Shape Model

Toshiyuki Okada[1], Ryuji Shimada[1], Yoshinobu Sato[1], Masatoshi Hori[2], Keita Yokota[1], Masahiko Nakamoto[1], Yen-Wei Chen[3], Hironobu Nakamura[2], and Shinichi Tamura[1]

[1] Division of Image Analysis
[2] Department of Radiology,
Osaka University Graduate School of Medicine, Suita, Osaka, 565-0871, Japan
{toshi,yoshi}@image.med.osaka-u.ac.jp
[3] College of Information Science and Engineering, Ritsumeikan University, Japan

Abstract. An atlas-based automated liver segmentation method from 3D CT images is described. The method utilizes two types of atlases, that is, the probabilistic atlas (PA) and statistical shape model (SSM). Voxel-based segmentation with PA is firstly performed to obtain a liver region, and then the obtained region is used as the initial region for subsequent SSM fitting to 3D CT images. To improve reconstruction accuracy especially for largely deformed livers, we utilize a multi-level SSM (ML-SSM). In ML-SSM, the whole shape is divided into patches, and principal component analysis is applied to each patches. To avoid the inconsistency among patches, we introduce a new constraint called the adhesiveness constraint for overlap regions among patches. In experiments, we demonstrate that segmentation accuracy improved by using the initial region obtained with PA and the introduced constraint for ML-SSM.

1 Introduction

Segmentation of the liver from 3D data is a prerequisite for computer-assisted diagnosis and preoperative planning. Prior information of the liver, typically represented as statistical atlases, is useful for robust segmentation. Two types of statistical atlases, a statistical shape model (SSM) [1] and a probabilistic atlas (PA) [2], have been utilized to increase robustness of the segmentation.

A SSM is widely used for organ segmentation and its potential performance for liver segmentation has been shown [3][4]. However, previous methods using SSM [3][4] had the following problems: (1)There is essential limitation on reconstruction accuracy especially for diseased livers involving large deformations and lesions. (2) Good initialization is required to obtain proper convergence. One approach to overcome the first problem is to use multi-level SSM (ML-SSM) [5], in which the whole organ shape is divided into multiple patches, which are further subdivided at finer representation levels. One problem of ML-SSM is, however,

N. Ayache, S. Ourselin, A. Maeder (Eds.): MICCAI 2007, Part I, LNCS 4791, pp. 86–93, 2007.
© Springer-Verlag Berlin Heidelberg 2007

inconsistency among patches at finer levels. While previous work tried to solve the inconsistency problem [6], they did not apply the method to the liver, which has highly complex shape and large inter-patient variation. Another approach to address the first problem is to perform SSM fitting followed by shape constrained deformable model fitting [4]. However, shape constraints inherent in the liver are not embedded in the deformable model, and robustness against large deformation and lesions has not been verified. Further, the second problem has not been addressed in the previous studies. Heimann et al. reported that not a few cases failed to converge due to the initialization problem [4].

An alternative approach to represent prior information is probabilistic atlas (PA) [2], where the existence probability of the liver is assigned to each voxel position. Recently, prediction accuracy of PA was shown to improve using spatial standardization based on surrounding structures [7][8]. Zhou et al. showed that highly accurate segmentation was possible from non-contrasted CT images by using an automated method based on PA [8]. However, the datasets they used consisted of normal and a fraction of mildly diseased livers and did not verify the performance for severely diseased livers.

In this paper, we formulate an automated method for liver segmentation using both PA and ML-SSM. The features of our method are as follows: (1) Initialization for SSM fitting is automated using automated segmentation based on PA. (2) ML-SSM is used to improve reconstruction accuracy especially for largely deformed livers. (3) A new constraint is introduced to avoid inconsistency among patches at finer levels of ML-SSM. We experimentally evaluate the improvements of the performance by introducing the above features.

2   Methods

2.1   Spatial Standardization Using the Abdominal Cavity

Given training datasets, PA and ML-SSM are constructed. Before the construction, spatial standardization of the datasets is necessary. To do so, one CT dataset which was judged to have an average liver shape by a radiology specialist was selected as a standard patient, and its abdominal cavity is regarded as the standardized space to represent the standardized liver position and shape [7].

An individual patient dataset is mapped into the standardized patient space through nonrigid registration. We assume that the regions of the abdominal cavity and liver have already been manually segmented from 3D data. Let A_i and L_i denote the shapes of the i-th patient's abdominal cavity and liver, respectively, where $i = 0, 1, 2, ..., n - 1$. These shapes are represented by a 3D point dataset, which is the vertices of the decimated surface model generated from the manually segmented region of 3D data. Let A_0 be the abdominal cavity of the selected standard patient data. Let $T(\mathbf{x}; A_i)$ be the dense 3D deformation vector field generated by nonrigid registration between i-th patient and the standard patient so that the abdominal cavity A_i and A_0 are registered, where $\mathbf{x}$ is 3D position of the data. To generate the dense 3D deformation vector field, we use the point-based

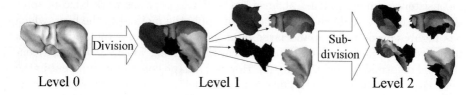

Fig. 1. Hierarchical division of the liver shape for multi-level statistical shape model

nonrigid registration method developed by Chui et al. [9]. The standardized liver shape L_i' of original shape L_i is given by $L_i' = \{\mathbf{x} + T(\mathbf{x}; A_i) | \mathbf{x} \in L_i\}$.

2.2   Constructing Statistical Atlases

Constructing probabilistic atlas. Let $B_i(\mathbf{x})$ be a binary image where value 1 is assigned to inside of standardized liver L_i' and value 0 to other regions. The probabilistic atlas, $P(\mathbf{x})$, standardized using the abdominal cavity shape is defined as the average of $B_i(\mathbf{x})$ over n patient datasets by $P(\mathbf{x}) = (1/n) \sum_{i=0}^{n-1} B_i(\mathbf{x})$.

Constructing multi-level statistical shape model. Let $L_0 \ (= L_0')$ be the liver shape of the standard patient. Let $\mathbf{v}_{0k} = (v_{0kx}, v_{0ky}, v_{0kz}) \ (k = 1, \cdots, m)$ denote the vertices of L_0, where m is the number of the vertices. Let $\mathbf{q}_0$ denote the concatenation of $\mathbf{v}_{0k}$, where $\mathbf{q}_0$ is a $3m$-dimensional vector. Point-based nonrigid registration [9] between the standard liver L_0 and individual liver L_i' is performed to determine the correspondences of the vertices between the individual and standard livers.

To construct a multi-level surface model, L_i is divided into N_1 sub-shapes (we call them "patches") [6]. These patches are recursively divided and multi-level surface model $L_{i\ell j}(j = 1, \cdots, N_\ell)$ is constructed (Fig. 1), where $L_{i\ell j}$ denotes j-th patch at level ℓ of i-th patient, and N_ℓ denotes the number of patches at level ℓ ($N_0 = 1$). Each $L_{i\ell j}(i = 0, \cdots, n-1)$ is normalized by its center of gravity. Let $\mathbf{q}_{i\ell j}$ denote concatenation of vertices of $L_{i\ell j}$. We assume that the adjacent patches at the same level overlap each other along their boundaries. These overlap regions are used to impose a constraint for eliminating inconsistency among patches, which will be described in the next subsection. From n datasets of each patch, $\mathbf{q}_{i\ell j}(i = 0, \cdots, n-1)$, the mean vector $\bar{\mathbf{q}}_{\ell j}$ is computed, and then principal component analysis (PCA) is applied for each patch independently to obtain eigenvectors $\Phi_{\ell j}$ corresponding to principal components. ML-SSM at level ℓ is defined as

$$\mathbf{q}_{\ell j}(\mathbf{b}_{\ell j}) = \bar{\mathbf{q}}_{\ell j} + \Phi_{\ell j}\mathbf{b}_{\ell j} \quad (j = 1, \cdots, N_\ell) \tag{1}$$

where $\mathbf{b}_{\ell j}$ is the shape parameter vector at level ℓ of j-th patch.

2.3   Segmentation of the Liver Using Statistical Atlases

The proposed segmentation method using PA and ML-SSM consists of the following steps:

1. Initial region extraction using voxel-based segmentation with PA [8].
2. Estimation of initial shape parameters by fitting SSM to the initial region.
3. Repeat the following multi-level segmentation processes until the finest level.
   (a) Repeat the following segmentation processes for a fixed number of times.
       i. Detection of edge points of the liver boundaries from CT data by searching along surface normals of current ML-SSM surface.
       ii. Estimation of shape parameters by fitting ML-SSM to the edge points.
   (b) Divide the current patches of ML-SSM into those at the next finer level.

In the following, details of step 1, step 2, and segmentation processes at step 3(a) are described.

Initial region extraction using voxel-based segmentation with PA. Abdominal CT data is spatially standardized by the method described in section 2.1 (Fig. 2(a)), and smoothed with an anisotropic diffusion filter [3]. For the standardization, the abdominal cavity region is extracted automatically unlike the training phase (The extraction method is briefly described in 3.1). The volume of interest (VOI) is defined as the region where probabilistic atlas $P(\mathbf{x})$ (Fig. 2(b)) is larger than threshold value T_{map}. Let $I(\mathbf{x})$ be the standardized and smoothed image. Likelihood image $Q(\mathbf{x})$ is given by $Q(\mathbf{x}) = \exp\left(-(I(\mathbf{x}) - \bar{I})^2/(2\sigma^2)\right)$, where $\bar{I}$ and σ are average intensity and standard deviation, respectively, which are estimated based on histogram analysis inside the VOI [8]. $Q(\mathbf{x})$ is defined as the Gaussian of $I(\mathbf{x})$ and it is the largest when $I(\mathbf{x})$ is the same as the average intensity $\bar{I}$. Given $Q(\mathbf{x})$ and $P(\mathbf{x})$, combined likelihood image $Q'(\mathbf{x})$ (Fig. 2(c)) is defined as $Q'(\mathbf{x}) = Q(\mathbf{x})P(\mathbf{x})$. Note that the voxel value of $Q'(\mathbf{x})$ is normalized between 0 and 1. The initial region is extracted by thresholding of $Q'(\mathbf{x})$ using a fixed threshold value followed by opening and closing (Fig. 2(d)).

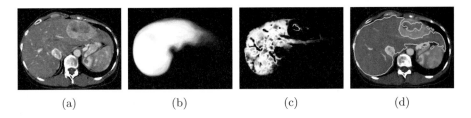

(a)   (b)   (c)   (d)

Fig. 2. Initial region segmentation processes using probabilistic atlas. (a) Standardized image. (b) Probabilistic atlas. (c) Combined likelihood image. (d) Extracted initial region (green contours).

Estimation of initial shape parameters. Let R be the surface model generated from initial region. Given R, we obtain the initial shape parameter $\mathbf{b}_0$ by iteratively minimizing

$$C_D(\mathbf{q}_0(\mathbf{b}_0); R) = \frac{1}{|\mathbf{q}_0(\mathbf{b}_0)|} \sum_{\mathbf{x} \in \mathbf{q}_0(\mathbf{b}_0)} w\left(d(\mathbf{x}, R)\right) d(\mathbf{x}, R)$$

$$+\frac{1}{|R|}\sum_{\mathbf{x}\in R} w\left(d\left(\mathbf{x}, \mathbf{q}_0(\mathbf{b}_0)\right)\right) d\left(\mathbf{x}, \mathbf{q}_0(\mathbf{b}_0)\right) \qquad (2)$$

where $d(\mathbf{x}, S)$ is the Euclidean distance between point $\mathbf{x}$ and surface S, and $|\cdot|$ denotes the number of vertices of surface model. Robust weight function $w(x)$ is used to deal with outliers due to large lesions [10]. $w(x)$ is defined as $w(x) = \begin{cases} 1 & \text{if } |x| \leq s \\ s/|x| & \text{if } |x| > s \end{cases}$ in which s is the robust standard deviation given by $s = \max\left(1.4826 \times \text{median}\{|d_k - \text{median}(d_k)|\}, 5.0 \text{ mm}\right)$, and d_k is residual in millimeters at each vertex.

Segmentation processes using ML-SSM. The edge points of the liver boundaries in CT images are detected from analysis of the CT value profile along the surface normal of the ML-SSM [3]. In this study, the parameters needed for profile analysis are automatically determined using the result of histogram analysis obtained in the initial region extraction processes.

Detected edge points are fitted to ML-SSM. Let P be the set of detected edge points from CT data. Let $\mathbf{q}_\ell$ and $\mathbf{b}_\ell$ denote concatenations of $\mathbf{q}_{\ell j}(\mathbf{b}_{\ell j})$ and $\mathbf{b}_{\ell j}$ $(j = 1, \cdots, N_\ell)$, respectively. Given P and level ℓ, we estimate the shape parameters $\mathbf{b}_\ell$ by minimizing

$$C(\mathbf{q}_\ell(\mathbf{b}_\ell); P) = C_D(\mathbf{q}_\ell(\mathbf{b}_\ell); P) + \lambda C_A(\mathbf{q}_\ell), \qquad (3)$$

where $C_D(\mathbf{q}_\ell(\mathbf{b}_\ell); P)$ is the sum of distances between model surface $\mathbf{q}_\ell$ and edge points P, and $C_A(\mathbf{q}_\ell)$ is the adhesiveness constraint for the overlap regions to eliminate the inconsistency among adjacent patches. Further, λ is a weight parameter balancing the two constraints. λ was determined experimentally. Letting $O_{\ell i}$ be the overlap regions, the cost functions of the adhesiveness constraint, $C_A(\mathbf{q}_\ell)$, is defined as

$$C_A(\mathbf{q}_\ell) = \frac{1}{m_\ell}\sum_{i=1}^{N_\ell}\sum_{\mathbf{x}\in O_{\ell i}} (\mathbf{x} - \mathbf{x}')^2, \qquad (4)$$

where $\mathbf{x}'$ is the point that corresponds to $\mathbf{x}$ in the overlap region of the adjacent patch.

3 Experimental Results

3.1 Experimental Conditions

28 abdominal CT datasets (slice thickness 2.5 mm, pitch 1.25 mm, FOV 350×350 mm^2, 512 × 512 matrix, 159 slices) were used. We randomly selected 8 datasets for evaluation, and others for training. The probabilistic atlas and ML-SSM were constructed from the 20 training datasets. A radiology specialist judged the livers were largely deformed due to disease in 9 datasets among the 20 training datasets. Also, the livers were largely deformed in 5 datasets among the 8 evaluation datasets.

Table 1. Evaluation results of segmentation accuracy. Averages of 8 datasets of Jaccard similarity measure and average distance [mm] (divided by slash) are shown in each experimental condition. The results of the proposed method are enhanced.

Initialization	Using segmentation with PA		Using average shape	
Adhesiveness constraint	$\lambda = 0$	$\lambda = 0.2$	$\lambda = 0$	$\lambda = 0.2$
Initial region	0.80 / 3.15		– / –	
Level 0	0.80 / 3.20		0.79 / 3.61	
Level 1	0.84 / 2.36	0.83 / 2.58	0.84 / 2.60	0.83 / 2.94
Level 2	0.79 / 2.48	**0.86 / 2.15**	0.79 / 2.73	0.85 / 2.54

(Jaccard similarity measure / Average distance [mm]).

While the abdominal cavity of the training data was manually segmented, that of the evaluation data was automatically extracted by combining the inner surface of the thoracic cage and the diaphragm surface approximated by a thin-plate spline surface fitted to the lung bottom [8].

The number of SSM vertices at level 0 was 2500. The finest level of ML-SSM was 2, that is, $\ell = 0, 1, 2$. The numbers of patches were 4 at level 1 and 16 at level 2. The threshold value T_{map} of probabilistic atlas $P(\mathbf{x})$ was set to 0.9. The weight parameter λ for the adhesiveness constraint was set to $\lambda = 0.2$. The iteration count of segmentation processes at each level was 10 times.

For comparison purpose, the experiments were also performed under the following conditions. (1) The adhesiveness constraint was not used, that is, $\lambda = 0$. (2) Instead of using the initial region obtained by voxel-based segmentation with PA, the average shape of the liver was used as the initial parameter of ML-SSM, that is, $\mathbf{b}_0 = \mathbf{0}$.

To evaluate segmentation accuracy, we used two types of measures, Jaccard similarity measure[11] and average distance. The former is defined as $|A \cap B|/|A \cup B|$, where A and B are the estimated region using ML-SSM and the corresponding manually segmented true region, respectively. The latter is the average of symmetric distances between the estimated and true surfaces [3].

3.2   Results

Table 1 summarizes the results of segmentation accuracy. When the weight parameter of the adhesiveness constraint was set to $\lambda = 0.2$, segmentation accuracy was improved as hierarchy level of ML-SSM increased. When $\lambda = 0.0$, however, segmentation accuracy was decreased at level 2. The average distance of the proposed method using segmentation with PA as the initial region was smaller than using the average shape although there was not significant difference in Jaccard similarity measure. These results show the usefulness of using the adhesiveness constraint and segmentation with PA as the initial region, both of which have been introduced in this paper.

Figure 3 shows the result of the proposed method for each dataset ($\lambda = 0.2$, using initial segmentation with PA). In all evaluation datasets, ML-SSM at

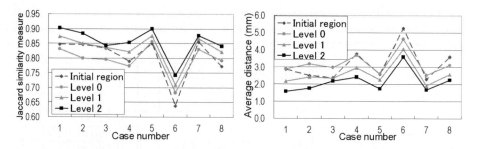

Fig. 3. Evaluation results of segmentation accuracy for each data by proposed method ($\lambda = 0.2$). Left: Jaccard similarity measure. Right: Average distance.

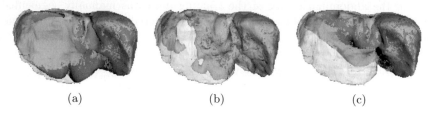

(a)   (b)   (c)

Fig. 4. Results of case 6. 3D surface models of the estimated shape (blue model) and the true shape (semitransparent white model) are superimposed so that their difference is easily understandable. (a) Region obtained by ML-SSM at level 2 using the proposed method. (b) Initial region obtained by voxel-based segmentation with PA. (c) Region obtained by ML-SSM at level 2 using average shape as initial region.

level 2 achieved the best results, and its Jaccard similarity measure and average distance were 0.86 ($\pm$ 0.05) and 2.15 ($\pm$ 0.62) mm on average, respectively.

Figure 4 shows the results of case 6, which had a large tumor (whose volume was more than 20 % of the whole liver) and large deformation. The estimated liver shape by ML-SSM at level 2 using the proposed method (Fig. 4(a)) was closer to the true shape than the initial region obtained by voxel-based segmentation with PA [8] (Fig. 4(b)) and the result by ML-SSM at level 2 when the average shape was used as an initial region (Fig. 4(c)).

4 Discussion and Conclusions

We have developed an automated segmentation method of the liver using statistical atlases. The proposed method was shown to improve segmentation accuracy for datasets including largely deformed livers by combining initial segmentation based on PA and subsequent ML-SSM fitting. We consider that the initial segmentation could capture boundary information even in deformed livers although not a few outlier boundaries were included. Subsequent ML-SSM fitting could deal with outlier boundaries to some extent, and further the edge detection accuracy was improved by hierarchization. Thus, the segmentation accuracy improved. We also demonstrate that the adhesiveness constraint was effective to deal with inconsistency at finer levels of ML-SSM. The accuracy was significantly degraded at the fine level (level 2) without the constraint.

In the current version of our method, automated extraction of the abdominal cavity is necessary for standardization of datasets to construct statistical atlases. Its extraction accuracy sometimes is insufficient. However, a circumscribed trapezoid of the thoracic cage, which is extracted in a highly stable manner [8], can be used for standardization instead of the abdominal cavity at the expense of slight degradation of the prediction accuracy of the constructed PA. As future work, we will evaluate the proposed segmentation approaches using different standardization methods including the above method. Further, we will evaluate the proposed approach by leave-one-out cross validation using large CT datasets.

References

1. Cootes, T.F., et al.: Active shape models - their training and application. Computer Vision and Image Understanding 61(1), 38–59 (1995)
2. Park, H., et al.: Construction of an abdominal probabilistic atlas and its application in segmentation. IEEE Trans. Med. Imaging 22(4), 483–492 (2003)
3. Lamecker, H., et al.: Segmentation of the liver using a 3D statistical shape model. Technical report, Zuse Institue, Berlin (2004)
4. Heimann, T., et al.: Active shape models for a fully automated 3D segmentation of the liver – an evaluation on clinical data. In: Larsen, R., Nielsen, M., Sporring, J. (eds.) MICCAI 2006. LNCS, vol. 4191, pp. 41–48. Springer, Heidelberg (2006)
5. Davatzikos, C., et al.: Hierarchical active shape models, using the wavelet transform. IEEE Trans. Med. Imaging 22(3), 414–423 (2003)
6. Zhao, Z., et al.: A novel 3D partitioned active shape model for segmentation of brain MR images. In: Duncan, J.S., Gerig, G. (eds.) MICCAI 2005. LNCS, vol. 3749, pp. 221–228. Springer, Heidelberg (2005)
7. Yokota, K., et al.: Construction of conditional statistical atlases of the liver based on spatial normalization using surrounding structures. In: Proceedings of Computer Assisted Radiology and Surgery (CARS), Osaka, Japan, pp. 39–40 (July 2006)
8. Zhou, X., et al.: Constructing a probabilistic model for automated liver region segmentation using non-contrast x-ray torso CT images. In: Larsen, R., Nielsen, M., Sporring, J. (eds.) MICCAI 2006. LNCS, vol. 4191, pp. 856–863. Springer, Heidelberg (2006)
9. Chui, H., et al.: A new point matching algorithm for non-rigid registration. Computer Vision and Image Understanding 89, 114–141 (2003)
10. Besl, P.J., et al.: Robust window operators. Machine Vision and Applications 2(4), 179–191 (1989)
11. Jaccard, P.: The distribution of the flora in the alpine zone. New Phytologist 11(2), 37–50 (1912)

Statistical and Topological Atlas Based Brain Image Segmentation

Pierre-Louis Bazin and Dzung L. Pham

Johns Hopkins University, Baltimore, USA

Abstract. This paper presents a new atlas-based segmentation framework for the delineation of major regions in magnetic resonance brain images employing an atlas of the global topological structure as well as a statistical atlas of the regions of interest. A segmentation technique using fast marching methods and tissue classification is proposed that guarantees strict topological equivalence between the segmented image and the atlas. Experimental validation on simulated and real brain images shows that the method is accurate and robust.

1 Introduction

The segmentation of medical images into separate structures and organs often requires the incorporation of a priori information. The use of statistical atlases is one approach for encoding spatial and intensity information for each structure, and may include relational information as well [1,2]. In a typical scenario, the atlas is transformed to match the image of interest, and a statistical classification method combines the atlas and image information to segment the structures. An alternative is to perform a non-rigid registration of a single atlas to the image with the appropriate structures segmented by mapping the segmentation labels [3,4,5]. Hybrid methods incorporating statistical atlas and non-rigid registration have also been proposed [6,7].

In all cases, the atlas introduces a bias toward images most similar to the atlas images. In addition, many of the global and regional topological properties of the structures are ignored in these representations. For example, segmented structures may become disjointed or connect freely with neighboring structures, irrespective of the underlying anatomy. Several methods have been proposed to preserve topology in the case of a single object [14,15] or multiple, separate objects [16,8]. However, none of these methods is able to preserve the topology of groups of objects. Even if the topology of two objects is invariant, the topology of the union of these objects is not constrained and can be arbitrary (see Fig. 1). This is an important issue when segmenting multiple structures, since the true anatomy typically follows strict topological relationships.

In this paper, we show that topological constraints on both the structures and their groups can be used to encode continuity and relationships without biasing shape. We present a strictly homeomorphic atlas-based segmentation algorithm and apply it to the segmentation of the major structures of the brain in magnetic resonance (MR) images. Our method employs only a coarse statistical atlas of the shape, deriving the segmentation predominantly from the image and topological constraints. In the case of homogeneous structures, intensity prior distributions can be ignored, making the framework largely independent of the imaging modality.

N. Ayache, S. Ourselin, A. Maeder (Eds.): MICCAI 2007, Part I, LNCS 4791, pp. 94–101, 2007.
© Springer-Verlag Berlin Heidelberg 2007

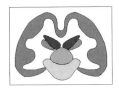 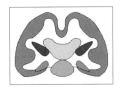

Fig. 1. Importance of the topology of groups: the individual structures in above images have the same topology, but the relationships between them are different, which corresponds to changes in the topology of groups (unions) of structures

The proposed algorithm significantly extends a topology-preserving tissue segmentation technique from our earlier work [8] by introducing several improvements. First, a statistical atlas and intensity relations are used to model objects with similar intensities. Second, a new topology preservation criterion is employed that maintains not only the topology of individual objects but also the topology of all groups of objects. With these improvements, the new approach is capable of segmenting more detailed structures, such as subcortical regions. Experiments on simulated and real images demonstrate the accuracy and robustness of the algorithm.

2   Methods

We seek to recover a set of K anatomical structures from a MR image. Given a priori information about the structures shape and topology, we build an atlas to guide the segmentation. The atlas is first aligned with the image to segment, then a segmentation technique based on tissue classification and topology-preserving front propagation adapts the segmentation from the atlas to fit the image data.

2.1   Statistical Atlas

The first component of our algorithm is a statistical atlas, which will help distinguish structures with similar intensities. The atlas is built from a set of N manual delineations of the structures of interest. For each image in the atlas, the delineation is rigidly aligned with the current atlas image, and a smooth approximation of the probabilities is accumulated. The smoothing replaces the step edge at the boundary of each structure in their binary delineation by a linear ramp over a band of size ε. The accumulated prior p_{jk} represents the probability of being inside each structure as a function of the distance to its boundary and its variability over the atlas images, similarly to sigmoid-based representations [9,10]. By taking all these factors into account, we expect to reduce the bias toward the mean shape of the atlas and allow the statistical atlas to only influence areas most likely to be inside each structure. Fig. 2 shows the statistical priors computed from 18 subjects. Later in Section 3, it will be seen that the results of our method do not greatly depend on the size of N.

During the segmentation, the statistical atlas must be registered to the image. We use a joint segmentation and registration technique [11] that alternates between estimating the segmentation given the current atlas position, and then maximizes the following correlation energy with respect to T given the current segmentation:

$$E_R(T) = \sum_{jk} p_{T(j)k}^q u_{jk}^q. \tag{1}$$

where T is a rigid or affine transformation, u_{jk} the membership function for structure k at point j defined in Section 2.3 and q a fuzziness factor used in the underlying fuzzy segmentation method (see Sec. 2.3). We use $q = 2$ in this work. The transformation is computed using a gradient ascent technique. The initial alignment is computed using a Gaussian pyramid, while a single scale is sufficient to refine the alignment during the segmentation.

2.2   Topological Atlas

The second component of our algorithm is an atlas of the structures' topology, encoded in a parcellation of the brain. Anatomical structures can have a very complex geometry, yet they all tend to have a very simple topology, such as that of a sphere or torus. Groups of tissues and organs in contact provide additional topological properties. For instance, it is often assumed that the cerebral cortex has a spherical topology, but this requires to group together cerebral gray and white matter, sub-cortical structures and ventricles.

Creation of an appropriate topology atlas is non-trivial: manual segmentations have arbitrary topology, and inferring topological properties from anatomical atlases is not straightforward. As we are interested in the major structures of the brain, we created an atlas for the following structures, based on statistical atlases and anatomy textbooks: cerebral gray matter (CRG), cerebral white matter (CRW), cerebellar gray matter (CBG), cerebellar white matter (CBW), brainstem (BS), ventricles (VEN), caudate (CAU), putamen (PUT), thalamus (THA) and sulcal cerebro-spinal fluid (CSF). Both the statistical and topology atlases are in the same coordinate space and are based on manual segmentations from the IBSR V2.0 dataset [12] with additional editing [8], as shown in Fig. 2.

2.3   Tissue Segmentation

To perform the segmentation, we extend the FANTASM (Fuzzy And Noise Tolerant Adaptive Segmentation Method) [13] approach. Given the original image I, FANTASM minimizes an energy function with respect to the membership functions u_{jk}, the gain field g_j, and the class centroids c_k. The gain field is a smoothly varying function that we model as a low degree polynomial (see [11]).

As with any tissue classification technique, difficulties arise if adjacent structures have the same or very close centroid values; the boundary between them becomes more sensitive to noise, and the boundaries with other structures may be shifted away because of their lower membership values. The additional information provided by a statistical atlas will help remedy this issue but will also lower the influence of the signal intensity and blur the segmentation in areas of large variability between individuals. Because we model the topology of the structures to segment, we can also make use of the relationship between them to lower the influence of competing intensity clusters in regions that

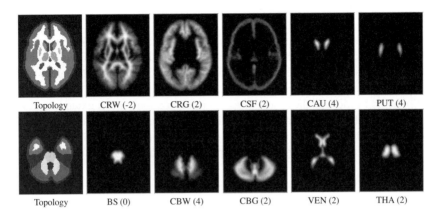

Fig. 2. The statistical and topological atlas: two slices from the topology atlas (left) and one from each structure prior (right). The Euler characteristic for each structure is given in parenthesis.

are spatially disconnected. We define global relationship sets $R_G(k)$ to be the structures in contact with k according to the topology atlas, and local relationship sets $R_L(j)$ to be structures in contact at the boundary closest to the point j in the current segmentation. The map $R_L(j)$ is obtained by searching for the structures in contact at all boundary points, and then propagating this information inside the volume (see example in Fig. 3, where each gray level represents a unique R_L).

We incorporate the atlas and relationship information into FANTASM, resulting in the following energy function:

$$E_S = \sum_{jk} \frac{u_{jk}^q}{r_{jk}} \|g_j I_j - c_k\|^2 + \frac{\beta}{2} \sum_{l \in N_j, m \neq k} \frac{u_{jk}^q}{r_{jk}} u_{lm}^q, + \frac{\gamma}{2} \sum_{m \neq k} \frac{w_{km}}{r_{jk}} u_{jk}^q p_{jm}^q \qquad (2)$$

The first term in (2) is the data driven term, the second term enforces smoothness on the memberships, and the third term controls the influence of the statistical atlas. The relationship function r_{jk} is defined to be

$$r_{jk} = \begin{cases} 1 & k \in R_L(j), \\ \frac{1}{2} & k \in R_G(l), l \in R_L(j) \\ 0 & \text{otherwise.} \end{cases} \qquad (3)$$

The atlas weights w_{km} is defined as

$$w_{km} = \frac{s_w \max_{ln} |c_l - c_n|^2}{s_w \max_{ln} |c_l - c_n|^2 + |c_k - c_m|^2} \qquad (4)$$

and is close to one when $c_k \simeq c_m$ but goes to zero when $c_k \neq c_m$. The relationship function penalizes against class configurations that are inconsistent with the topology atlas. For pixel classes that do not touch any classes near pixel j, r_{jk} is set to zero, and the configuration possesses infinite energy. The atlas weights allow the priors to influence the segmentation only where the intensity contrast between structures is low.

2.4   Topology-Preserving Fast Marching Segmentation

The energy function of (2) is used to compute membership functions for each structure in a fashion similar to FANTASM [13]. In addition, we compute a "hard" segmentation that is derived from the memberships but is constrained to be homeomorphic to the topology template.

We recently introduced the *digital homeomorphism criterion* that extends the binary case to multiple objects and guarantees that the atlas and segmented image are related by a homeomorphism in both the continuous and digital domain [17]. This improvement is essential as it allows a more truthful representation of the anatomy than previous methods.

The segmentation itself is performed using two successive iterations of a fast marching front propagation technique, first thinning the structures into a skeleton-like object and then growing the structures back to find the optimal boundary, using a minimal path strategy [18,8]. The speed function of the fast marching is a function of the memberships:

$$f^- = (1 - \alpha)u_{jk} + \alpha\kappa_{jk}$$
$$f^+ = (1 - \alpha)(1 - u_{jk}) + \alpha(1 - \kappa_{jk}) \tag{5}$$

where κ_{jk} is a measure of the curvature of the boundary for structure k at j normalized in $[0, 1]$ and α a weighting parameter. f^- is used in the thinning algorithm, f^+ in the growing algorithm. The thinning is stopped when the volume remaining inside each structure is below a given fraction of the original volume (in this work, 1/3 of the volume). The digital homeomorphism criterion is checked at all steps, ensuring that the topology of all structures and groups are preserved at all times.

The complete algorithm is as follows:

1. *Align atlases to image and set initial segmentation to the topological atlas.*
2. *Build the local relationship map R_L from the current segmentation.*
3. *Compute the memberships u_{jk}, centroids c_k and the inhomogeneity field g_j.*
4. *Thin structures using the fast marching algorithm with f^-.*
5. *Grow back the structures using f^+ and update the segmentation.*
6. *Refine the alignment of the atlases.*
7. *Loop to step 2 until convergence.*

The convergence criterion is the relative amount of change in the energy E per iteration, which typically becomes lower than 10^{-3} in 10 to 20 iterations in the following experiments (approximatively 45 to 60 minutes). The overall complexity of the algorithm is $O(N \log N) + O(KN)$, with N the size of the image and K the number of structures. Parameters were determined empirically and fixed for all experiments.

3   Experiments and Validation

3.1   Simulated Images

A first set of experiments was conducted with the Brainweb phantom [19]: several levels of noise and field inhomogeneity were simulated for T1 and T2-weighted modalities and the corresponding images segmented. Because the original Brainweb ground truth is only concerned with the three major tissue classes (gray matter, white matter, cerebro-spinal fluid), we performed a manual segmentation to separate cerebellum/brainstem, cerebrum, and grouped sub-cortical structures. The results from the segmentation were grouped accordingly (CAU, PUT and THA as sub-cortical structures SUB, BS and CBW as CBS), and the difference measured with the Dice overlap measure ($D(A,B) = \frac{2A \cap B}{A+B}$), see Table 1. Euler characteristic were found identical for all segmentations, as expected.

Table 1. Dice coefficients for the Brainweb dataset, for varying noise (N) and inhomogeneity (I)

Modality	N / I	Tissues			Structures					
		WM	GM	CSF	CRW	CRG	CBS	CBG	SUB	VEN
T1	N 0%, I 0%	0.953	0.935	0.884	0.963	0.941	0.767	0.895	0.850	0.897
	N 1%, I 0%	0.951	0.934	0.884	0.961	0.940	0.766	0.896	0.849	0.897
	N 3%, I 0%	0.947	0.928	0.882	0.957	0.934	0.762	0.892	0.845	0.896
	N 3%, I 20%	0.947	0.927	0.880	0.957	0.933	0.761	0.896	0.846	0.896
	N 3%, I 40%	0.947	0.918	0.880	0.956	0.931	0.765	0.898	0.842	0.898
	N 5%, I 0%	0.938	0.919	0.876	0.948	0.923	0.755	0.888	0.836	0.896
	N 5%, I 20%	0.938	0.919	0.877	0.948	0.923	0.754	0.891	0.839	0.896
	N 5%, I 40%	0.939	0.919	0.876	0.949	0.922	0.754	0.893	0.838	0.896
	N 7%, I 0%	0.927	0.906	0.869	0.937	0.909	0.745	0.884	0.828	0.894
	N 9%, I 0%	0.916	0.895	0.862	0.926	0.897	0.737	0.877	0.820	0.893
T1	Mean	0.940	0.921	0.877	0.950	0.925	0.756	0.891	0.839	0.896
	St.Dev.	0.007	0.013	0.012	0.011	0.014	0.010	0.006	0.010	0.001
T2	Mean	0.902	0.887	0.879	0.912	0.891	0.724	0.871	0.797	0.856
	St.Dev.	0.019	0.020	0.007	0.020	0.023	0.013	0.009	0.020	0.014
Euler characteristic		-2	6	2	-2	2	0	2	6	2

The Brainweb 'ground truth' has arbitrary topology and our segmentation will always deviate from it because of the topological constraints it follows (the Euler characteristics for the Brainweb WM,GM and CSF tissue classes are 6, -1750 and -174 respectively). Despite this, the segmentation is very close to the Brainweb ground truth almost everywhere. The larger difference in CBS is due to the mean intensity of the brainstem, which is between the WM and GM intensities considered in Brainweb, and thus is not segmented as a homogeneous region in the ground truth. The topology enforces continuity for each structure, resulting in a segmentation very robust to high noise levels. The segmentation results for T1 and T2 images are similar, despite the signal differences between the modalities.

3.2   Real Images

We tested the algorithm on the IBSR dataset, where we could compare each label individually (see Fig. 3). Because we used the same dataset to create the atlas, we performed four different evaluations. In the first, all 18 images from the dataset were used to create the atlas, whereas the second, third and fourth atlases respectively used the first 8, 3 and 1 images of the dataset. We also compared the results with the segmentation obtained by performing a non-rigid registration with HAMMER [4] and transferring the object labels. The overlap with the original segmentation is computed as before (see Table 2).

The sulcal CSF is grouped with CRG and CBG in the IBSR segmentation, thus the overlap with the original ground truth are lowered for CRG and CBG and irrelevant for CSF. The algorithm recovers all structures with an accuracy significantly higher than

Table 2. Dice coefficients for the IBSR dataset

						Structures				
		CRW	CRG	BS	CBW	CBG	CAU	PUT	THA	VEN
Atlas 01-18	Mean	0.887	0.816	0.847	0.846	0.840	0.797	0.761	0.775	0.832
	St.Dev.	0.012	0.049	0.016	0.026	0.030	0.037	0.030	0.054	0.048
Atlas 01-08	Mean	0.886	0.816	0.848	0.843	0.845	0.798	0.755	0.765	0.832
	St.Dev.	0.012	0.048	0.019	0.027	0.028	0.039	0.034	0.056	0.049
Atlas 01-03	Mean	0.883	0.826	0.843	0.846	0.848	0.799	0.743	0.763	0.831
	St.Dev.	0.015	0.041	0.022	0.026	0.028	0.040	0.043	0.052	0.051
Atlas 01	Mean	0.879	0.832	0.853	0.839	0.859	0.794	0.744	0.760	0.833
	St.Dev.	0.018	0.038	0.016	0.038	0.024	0.043	0.044	0.051	0.051
HAMMER	Mean	0.788	0.782	0.744	0.763	0.848	0.740	0.599	0.773	0.662
	St.Dev.	0.032	0.038	0.059	0.042	0.032	0.039	0.071	0.046	0.078

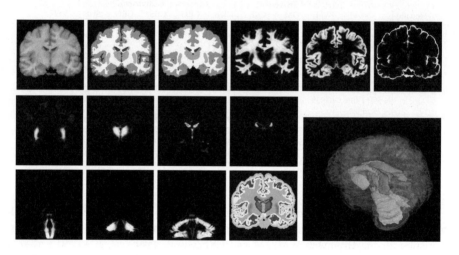

Fig. 3. Example of segmentation from the IBSR dataset. From left to right, top to bottom: original image, computed segmentation, manual segmentation, membership functions for CRW, CRG, CSF, PUT, THA, VEN, CAU, BS, CBW, CBG, relation map R_L, 3D rendering.

the non-rigid registration approach and similar to the reported inter-rater scores of [2]. The overlap is somewhat lower for the sub-cortical structures, due to their smaller size, non-constant intensities, and inaccurate boundaries. The results are mostly independent of the number of images used to generate the atlas, indicating that precise prior information about shape and location is not required by the algorithm.

4   Conclusion

In this paper, we presented a new framework for the segmentation of multiple structures in MR images. By combining topology constraints with smooth atlas priors, we are able to recover the main structures of the brain, both cortical and sub-cortical. The proposed algorithm is modality-independent, robust to high levels of noise and inhomogeneity, and the influence of spatial priors is limited, reducing the bias inherent to atlas-based methods. More importantly, the framework guarantees a strict homeomorphism between all groups of structures in the atlas and the segmented images, allowing an accurate representation of the anatomy that may be readily used for cortical unfolding and diffeomorphic shape analysis applications.

References

1. Leemput, K.V., Maes, F., Vandermeulen, D., Suetens, P.: Automated model-based tissue classification of MR images of the brain. IEEE Trans. Medical Imaging 18(10), 897–908 (1999)
2. Fischl, B., Salat, D.H., Busa, E., Albert, M., Dieterich, M., Haselgrove, C., van der Kouwe, A., Killiany, R., Kennedy, D., Klaveness, S., Montillo, A., Makris, N., Rosen, B., Dale, A.M.: Whole brain segmentation: Automated labeling of neuroanatomical structures in the human brain. Neuron 33, 341–355 (2002)
3. Christensen, G.E., Joshi, S.C., Miller, M.I.: Volumetric transformation of brain anatomy. IEEE Trans. Medical Imaging 16(6), 864–877 (1997)
4. Shen, D., Davatzikos, C.: Hammer: Hierarchical attribute matching mechanism for elastic registration. IEEE Trans. Medical Imaging 21(11) (2002)
5. Rohde, G.K., Aldroubi, A., Dawant, B.M.: The adaptive bases algorithm for intensity-based nonrigid image registration. IEEE Trans. Medical Imaging 22(11), 1470–1479 (2003)
6. Ciofolo, C., Barillot, C.: Brain segmentation with competitive level sets and fuzzy control. In: Proc. Int. Conf. Information Processing in Medical Imaging, Glenwood Springs (2005)
7. Pohl, K.M., Fisher, J., Levitt, J.J., Shenton, M.E., Kikins, R., Grimson, W.E.L., Wells, W.M.: A unifying approach to registration, segmentation and intensity correction. In: Proc. Int. Conf. Medical Image Computing and Computer-Assisted Intervention, Palm Springs (2005)
8. Bazin, P.L., Pham, D.: Topology-preserving tissue classification of magnetic resonance brain images. IEEE Trans. Medical Imaging 26(4), Special Issue on Computational Neuroanatomy (2007)
9. Rousson, M., Xu, C.: A general framework for image segmentation using ordered spatial dependency. In: Proc. Int. Conf. Medical Image Computing and Computer-Assisted Intervention, Copenhagen (2006)
10. Pohl, K.M., Fisher, J., Shenton, M.E., McCarley, R.W., Grimson, W.E.L., Kikins, R., Wells, W.M.: Logarithm odds maps for shape representation. In: Proc. Int. Conf. Medical Image Computing and Computer-Assisted Intervention, Copenhagen (2006)
11. Pham, D., Bazin, P.L.: Simultaneous registration and tissue classification using clustering algorithms. In: Proc. Int. Symposium on Biomedical Imaging, Arlington (2006)
12. Worth, A.: Internet brain segmentation repository (1996), http://www.cma.mgh.harvard.edu/ibsr/
13. Pham, D.L.: Spatial models for fuzzy clustering. Computer Vision and Image Understanding 84, 285–297 (2001)
14. Malandain, G., Bertrand, G., Ayache, N.: Topological segmentation of discrete surfaces. Int. J. Computer Vision 10(2), 183–197 (1993)
15. Han, X., Xu, C., Prince, J.L.: A topology preserving level set method for geometric deformable models. IEEE Trans. Pattern Analysis and Machine Intelligence 25(6), 755–768 (2003)
16. Mangin, J.F., Frouin, V., Bloch, I., Regis, J., Lopez-Krahe, J.: From 3d magnetic resonance images to structural representations of the cortex topography using topology preserving deformations. J. Mathematical Imaging and Vision 5, 297–318 (1995)
17. Bazin, P.L., Ellingsen, L., Pham, D.: Digital homeomorphisms in deformable registration. In: Proc. Int. Conf. Information Processing in Medical Imaging, Kerkrade (2007)
18. Li, H., Yezzi, A., Cohen, L.: 3d brain segmentation using dual-front active contours with optional user interaction. Int. J. Biomedical Imaging, 1–17 (2006)
19. Collins, D.L., Zijdenbos, A.P., Kollokian, V., Sled, J.G., Kabani, N., Holmes, C., Evans, A.: Design and construction of a realistic digital brain phantom. IEEE Trans. Medical Imaging 17(3) (1998)

A Boosted Segmentation Method for Surgical Workflow Analysis

N. Padoy[1,2], T. Blum[1], I. Essa[3], H. Feussner[4], M-O. Berger[2], and N. Navab[1]

[1] Chair for Computer Aided Medical Procedures (CAMP), TU Munich, Germany
[2] LORIA-INRIA Lorraine, Nancy, France
[3] College of Computing, Georgia Institute of Technology, Atlanta, USA
[4] Chirurgische Klinik und Poliklinik, Klinikum Rechts der Isar, TU Munich, Germany
Nicolas.Padoy@cs.tum.edu

Abstract. As demands on hospital efficiency increase, there is a stronger need for automatic analysis, recovery, and modification of surgical workflows. Even though most of the previous work has dealt with higher level and hospital-wide workflow including issues like document management, workflow is also an important issue within the surgery room. Its study has a high potential, e.g., for building context-sensitive operating rooms, evaluating and training surgical staff, optimizing surgeries and generating automatic reports.

In this paper we propose an approach to segment the surgical workflow into phases based on temporal synchronization of multidimensional state vectors. Our method is evaluated on the example of laparoscopic cholecystectomy with state vectors representing tool usage during the surgeries. The discriminative power of each instrument in regard to each phase is estimated using AdaBoost. A boosted version of the Dynamic Time Warping (DTW) algorithm is used to create a surgical reference model and to segment a newly observed surgery. Full cross-validation on ten surgeries is performed and the method is compared to standard DTW and to Hidden Markov Models.

1 Introduction and Related Work

Workflow analysis related to business processes like document and record management, patient throughput and scheduling within hospitals, has been a well-established topic over the last decade[1].In recent years, workflow monitoring inside the Operating Room (OR) has gained more attention[2,3]. Automatic recovery and analysis of a surgical workflow will help designing future ORs, specialized for certain surgeries and capable of providing context-sensitive user interfaces as well as automatic report generation and monitoring. Furthermore, systems dedicated to the training and the evaluation of the surgical staff may also benefit from automatic workflow analysis.

High-level approaches deal with abstract representation of surgeries. Jannin et al. present in [4] a Unified Modeling Language (UML) diagram for multimodal neurosurgical procedures. They use it to improve multimodal information management as well as surgical planning. This model was further used in Raimbault

N. Ayache, S. Ourselin, A. Maeder (Eds.): MICCAI 2007, Part I, LNCS 4791, pp. 102–109, 2007.
© Springer-Verlag Berlin Heidelberg 2007

et al.[5] to build a database of surgical cases, which can be queried to take benefit from past surgical experience. In [6], Neumuth et al. propose a system using business processes modeling to formalize and facilitate the abstract recording of a huge amount of surgeries by an operator in the surgical room. While such works pave the way for the statistical analysis of surgical workflow, they do not provide a direct representation in terms of surgical signals, as would be required for monitoring.

Other approaches focus on the analysis of dedicated surgical gestures. In [7], based on the torque/force signals provided by the Da Vinci robot, Lin et al. propose a method to recognize the elementary movements of a suturing task. Linear discriminants analysis is used in combination with a Bayes classifier to segment the motion. In Rosen et al.[8] the statistics of a surgical movement are analyzed for surgeon evaluation. The torque/force signals of the laparoscopic instruments recorded during a suturing task are learned with Hidden Markov Models (HMMs) in order to classify the skill level of the performing surgeon. To assess the quality of a surgical movement, Leong et al.[9] use the 3D trajectory of tracked laparoscopic instruments. The view invariant representations of the trajectories are evaluated with HMMs.

We present a complementary approach with an objective of automatically segmenting a *complete* surgery into phases using *live* signals from the OR. Our method is based on the temporal synchronization of multidimensional feature vectors to an average reference surgery. The algorithm is evaluated on the example of laparoscopic cholecystectomy, whose goal is to remove the gallbladder. This is a rather common but also complex surgery comprising many surgical phases. Even though the surgery depends in the details on the patient's anatomy, the surgeon follows a protocol consisting of 14 phases starting with the insertion of the trocars up till the suturing phase. These phases are illustrated in table 1.

While our algorithm is not limited to the use of a certain kind of features, we use binary vectors indicating instrument presence during the surgery. Many other signals would be available from the OR. However, we focus in this work on the usage of the surgical tools since it describes well the underlying workflow of a laparoscopic operation. The method is based on a modification of the Dynamic Time Warping (DTW) algorithm, which is applied with an adaptive distance measure. The measure is defined from the discriminative power of each instrument with respect to the current surgical phase, estimated by AdaBoost[10]. Widely used for feature selection[11], AdaBoost provides a natural way for feature weighting. This information is combined with temporal synchronizations to create an average model out of labeled training surgeries. Finally, the adaptive version of DTW is used to synchronize an unsegmented surgery to the model. Using this synchronization, labels from the average model can be carried over to an unsegmented surgery.

In an early work[12], DTW was used to synchronize several surgeries together in order to create an average model without any a-priori knowledge. The focus was set on surgical synchronization and results were evaluated in terms of simultaneous video visualization. For segmentation, we present in this work a

Table 1. The fourteen phases labeling each surgery

1	CO2 inflation	8	Liver Bed Coagulation 1
2	Trocar Insertion	9	Packaging of Gallbladder
3	Dissection Phase 1	10	External Gallbladder Retraction
4	Clipping Cutting 1	11	External Cleaning
5	Dissection Phase 2	12	Liver Bed Coagulation 2
6	Clipping Cutting 2	13	Trocar Retraction
7	Gallbladder Detaching	14	Abdominal Suturing

learning-based method. This new approach shows significant improvements and is evaluated with a complete cross-validation on a set of 10 surgeries. It is also compared to standard DTW without weights and to HMMs.

2   Methods

2.1   Overview

We first introduce the representation of the acquired signals in section 2.2. It is followed by the derivation of the weights per instrument and phase in section 2.3. The Adaptive Dynamic Time Warping (ADTW) algorithm is introduced in section 2.4. In the same section we describe its use for the segmentation of a new surgery. Finally, the computation of the average surgical model is presented in section 2.5.

2.2   Instrument Signals

In minimally-invasive surgeries the instruments strongly correlate with the underlying surgical workflow. To record the surgical actions during the procedure, instrument presence is acquired for $K = 17$ laparoscopic instruments and represented as a multivariate time series $\mathbb{I}$ where $\mathbb{I}_t \in \{0,1\}^K$:

$$\mathbb{I}_{t,k} = 1 \quad \textbf{iff} \quad \text{instrument } k \text{ is used at time } t$$

The instrument signals for an exemplary operation are displayed in fig. 1(a). The vertical lines display the segmentation in phases. While several phases can be simply characterized by a few instruments, in the others the relation phase/instruments is more complicated (for instance for phases 3 to 7). This is well illustrated by fig. 1(b) where the self-similarity matrix of the temporal vector sequence is displayed. The similarity matrix M is here defined by $m_{t_1,t_2} = exp^{-d(\mathbb{I}_{t_1}, \mathbb{I}_{t_2})}$. The phases are marked by vertical and horizontal lines on the matrix. For phases involving very specific instruments, a distinctive block appears on the diagonal, while for phases involving the same instruments blocks are harder to identify. Note the distinctive blocks bottom-right off the diagonal for the liver bed coagulation phases, indicating their strong correlation as they use almost the same instruments (phases 8 and 12).

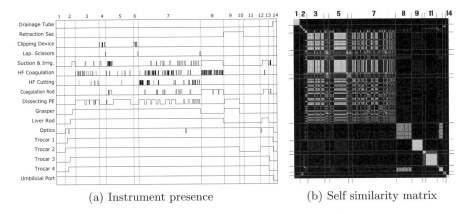

(a) Instrument presence

(b) Self similarity matrix

Fig. 1. Temporal sequence of instrument vectors for one surgery, and its self similarity matrix, showing the amount of instrument usage similarity between all phases

2.3 Weighting Method

The instruments occurring within a phase vary and are generally not sufficient to characterize the phase, as the temporal sequence of actions often plays a decisive role. But the instruments can be weighted to reflect their ability to discriminate between neighboring phases. When synchronizing a surgery to the average reference model, using those weights, the ADTW algorithm will put a higher priority on the most significant instruments for each phase.

AdaBoost[10] builds a strong classifier out of a sum of weak classifiers. They are iteratively chosen to optimally classify weighted training data and are themselves weighted accordingly. For each phase p, a strong classifier trying to classify all the instrument vectors of the phase with respect to all the vectors of the neighboring phases is built. By choosing the pool of weak classifiers to be simply related to the instruments, weights for the instruments can be naturally derived from the strong classifier.

The weak classifiers are chosen to perform the classification based on the presence/absence of a single instrument: a simple weak learner $C_{n,x}$ classifies an instrument vector according to whether the state of the instrument n within the vector is equal to x. AdaBoost selects at each step i a classifier C_{n_i,x_i} and a weight α_i to construct the strong classifier:

$$SC = \sum_i \alpha_i C_{n_i,x_i}$$

The variable n_i and x_i indicate the instrument and its state that were selected at step i. As the algorithm reweights the data that was hard to classify, the selected weak classifiers are the most important for the classification. The weights are obtained by looking at the influence of each instrument k within the strong classifier:

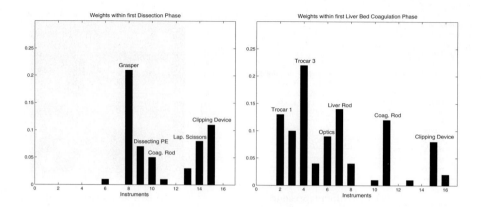

Fig. 2. Instrument weights computed for the first dissection phase (phase 3) and the first liver bed coagulation phase (phase 12)

$$ w_k = \left| \sum_{n_i=k, x_i=1} \alpha_i - \sum_{n_i=k, x_i=0} \alpha_i \right| $$

They are then normalized to one. As they are computed for each phase, this leads to weights $w_k^{(p)}$, for all phase p and instrument k. Depending on the phase, the convergence of AdaBoost requires a few to several dozens of steps. As some phases are very short, better results are obtained by classifying the phases with respect to the two previous and the two next phases. Fig. 2 displays the computed weights for two phases. In the first dissection phase, the three most significant instruments are found to be the grasper, which has to be present, and the clipping device and laparoscopic scissors, which have to be absent. In the first liver bed coagulation phase, they are the trocar 1 and 3 as well as the liver rod, which all have to be present.

2.4   Adaptive DTW

The Dynamic Time Warping algorithm[13] is both a time-invariant similarity measure and a method to synchronize two time series by finding a non-linear warping path. It has to warp each point in one time series onto at least one point in the other time series while respecting the temporal order. This is done in a way to minimize the sum of the distances between all points that are warped onto each other. It has been applied in various domains to synchronize series of application-dependent feature vectors[14,15]. As the length of a phase varies highly between different OPs, depending on the patient anatomy and the surgeon ability, the synchronization of a surgery to the model is also highly non-linear.

Traditional DTW computes the distance between the two series with a fixed distance function. As our reference time series is segmented in phases, we propose to use a distance function which is phase-dependent, so as to involve mainly instruments which are discriminative for a phase.

We define for each phase p the weighted distance d_p between instrument vectors v_1 and v_2:

$$d_p(v_1, v_2) = \sqrt{\sum_{k=1}^{k=K} w_k^{(p)} (v_{1,k} - v_{2,k})^2}$$

To compute the ADTW, within the dynamic time warping algorithm the distance function corresponding to the known phase of the reference series is used.

By warping an unsegmented surgery onto a segmented reference surgery, we can carry over the segmentation. As reference we use a model of an average surgery whose creation is described below.

2.5 Average Model Computation

Out of all training surgeries $\mathbb{O}_1 \ldots \mathbb{O}_n$ an average surgery is computed. Let $\mathbb{P}_{ij}$ be the ith phase from surgery $\mathbb{O}_j$. The average phase $\overline{\mathbb{P}_i}$ is constructed as follows. Out of $\mathbb{P}_{i1} \ldots \mathbb{P}_{in}$ the phase with length closest to the average length of this phase is chosen as initial average $\overline{\mathbb{P}_i}$. Next $\mathbb{P}_{i1} \ldots \mathbb{P}_{in}$ are warped onto $\overline{\mathbb{P}_i}$ using DTW with the weighted distance d_i of the current phase. Next, $\overline{\mathbb{P}_i}$ is updated by taking the average of the warped versions of $\mathbb{P}_{i1} \ldots \mathbb{P}_{in}$.

These two steps are repeated iteratively until convergence of $\overline{\mathbb{P}_i}$. In the final step, the average surgery is built by simply concatenating all average phases $\overline{\mathbb{P}_1} \ldots \overline{\mathbb{P}_{14}}$. While the training surgeries only consist of boolean values, stating whether an instrument is in use, the average can also contain non-boolean values. These can be interpreted as the probability of an instrument to be used at this moment.

3   Experiments and Results

For the experiments we use 10 surgeries of a cholecystectomy, labeled with 14 phases as described in the previous sections. One surgeon did 9 of the surgeries, where some parts have been performed by assistants. The 10th surgery has been done completely by another surgeon from the same school. A complete cross-validation has been performed, each time using 9 surgeries to compute weights with AdaBoost and construct the average surgery. The remaining surgery is then segmented using the three following algorithms for comparison: ADTW, standard DTW and HMMs. The standard DTW method is similar to ADTW, but all weights are set to be constant and equal. The labeled training information is thus only used in the creation of the reference model. For HMMs, the same amount of a-priori information is provided: left-right HMMs with fourteen states are used and trained on the labeled surgeries. The transition model is computed so that the expected state duration matches the average phase duration of the 9 surgeries in the training set. The observation model is computed from the usage frequency of each instrument within each phase, assuming instrument independence as this yields the best results. To evaluate the quality of the segmentation, we compute the following errors:

Table 2. Mean of the computed errors on all cross-validation tests

	overall error	mean error per phase	max error per phase	skipped phases
HMM	8.9%	10.1%	60.9%	0.5
standard DTW	0.8%	0.9%	10.9%	0
ADTW	0.3%	0.3%	4.5%	0

- **overall error**: percentage of wrong segmentation labels in the complete surgery
- **mean error per phase**: percentage of wrong segmentation labels within a phase, mean on the 14 phases
- **max error per phase**: percentage of wrong segmentation labels within a phase, maximum on the 14 phases
- **skipped phases**: number of phases that have no overlap with their ground-truth.

The mean results on all cross-validation tests are displayed in table 2. The segmentation with HMMs provided the worst results. As a few phases are skipped in several surgeries, leading to a *max error per phase* of 100%, the resulting *max error per phase* in the table is very high. However, they still recognise 91.1% of the labels, with a time resolution of a second. None of standard DTW and ADTW provided skipped phases, but ADTW outperforms in mean DTW without adaptive weights by a factor greater than 2. It yields a very accurate segmentation for *all* phases, as the mean *max error per phase* is below 5%. The max *max error per phase* is 13.6% for ADTW, while it is 40.2% for standard DTW. Moreover, experiments with the 10 surgeries show the errors to decrease faster with ADTW than with standard DTW when the size of the training set grows. Finally, the surgery carried out by the second surgeon obtained also very good segmentation results.

4   Discussion and Conclusion

In this paper we presented a reliable way to automatically recognize the workflow of a laparoscopic operation using only little training data. We have shown that the laparoscopic instruments provide enough information to automatically segment fourteen procedural phases of laparoscopic cholecystectomies with a high success rate. To this end the laparoscopic instruments used in each phase are analyzed with AdaBoost and weighted according to their discriminative power. An adaptive dynamic time warping algorithm using those weights synchronizes the workflow to a reference model, yielding the segmentation.

While the segmentation is automatic after acquisition of the input information, up-to-now not all input signals are obtained automatically for practical reasons. Automatic signal acquisition is for example currently possible for instruments like the coagulation/cutting device or the optics. With the use of sensors, it would also be possible to get it for the others.

Experiments were carried out on 10 cholecystectomies and cross-validation proved the algorithm to outperform both standard DTW and HMMs. These results are very promising and we believe they can apply to other kinds of laparoscopic surgeries. Examples of valuable by-products of this research are the automatic reporting of a surgical operation and/or the evaluation and comparison of trainees. Future work will focus on selecting appropriate input information that can be obtained automatically, so as to provide a fully automatic system and pave the way for surgical monitoring.

Acknowledgments. This research is partially funded by Siemens Medical Solutions.

References

1. Dazzi, L., Fassino, C., Saracco, R., Quaglini, S., Stefanelli, M.: A patient workflow management system built on guidelines. In: AMIA 1997, pp. 146–150 (1997)
2. Herfarth, C.: 'lean' surgery through changes in surgical workflow. British Journal of Surgery 90(5), 513–514 (2003)
3. Cleary, K., Chung, H.Y., Mun, S.K.: Or 2020: The operating room of the future. Laparoendoscopic and Advanced Surgical Techniques 15(5), 495–500 (2005)
4. Jannin, P., Raimbault, M., Morandi, X., Gibaud, B.: Modeling surgical procedures for multimodal image-guided neurosurgery. In: Niessen, W.J., Viergever, M.A. (eds.) MICCAI 2001. LNCS, vol. 2208, pp. 565–572. Springer, Heidelberg (2001)
5. Raimbault, M., Morandi, X., Jannin, P.: Towards models of surgical procedures: analyzing a database of neurosurgical cases. In: Med. Imaging, SPIE, pp. 97–104 (2005)
6. Neumuth, T., Strauß, G., Meixensberger, J., Lemke, H.U., Burgert, O.: Acquisition of process descriptions from surgical interventions. In: Bressan, S., Küng, J., Wagner, R. (eds.) DEXA 2006. LNCS, vol. 4080, pp. 602–611. Springer, Heidelberg (2006)
7. Lin, H.C., Shafran, I., Murphy, T.E., Okamura, A.M., Gregory, D., Hager, D.D.Y.: Automatic detection and segmentation of robot-assisted surgical motions. In: Duncan, J.S., Gerig, G. (eds.) MICCAI 2005. LNCS, vol. 3749, pp. 802–810. Springer, Heidelberg (2005)
8. Rosen, J., Solazzo, M., Hannaford, B., Sinanan, M.: Task decomposition of laparoscopic surgery for objective evaluation of surgical residents' learning curve using hidden markov model. Comput Aided Surg. 7(1), 49–61 (2002)
9. Leong, J., Nicolaou, M., Atallah, L., Mylonas, G., Darzi, A., Yang, G.Z.: HMM Assessment of Quality of Movement Trajectory in Laparoscopic Surgery. In: Larsen, R., Nielsen, M., Sporring, J. (eds.) MICCAI 2006. LNCS, vol. 4190, pp. 752–759. Springer, Heidelberg (2006)
10. Freund, Y., Schapire, R.E.: A decision-theoretic generalization of on-line learning and an application to boosting. In: Vitányi, P.M.B. (ed.) EuroCOLT 1995. LNCS, vol. 904, pp. 23–37. Springer, Heidelberg (1995)
11. Viola, P., Jones, M.J.: Robust real-time face detection. IJCV 57(2), 137–154 (2004)
12. Ahmadi, S.A., Sielhorst, T., Stauder, R., Horn, M., Feussner, H., Navab, N.: Recovery of surgical workflow without explicit models. In: Larsen, R., Nielsen, M., Sporring, J. (eds.) MICCAI 2006. LNCS, vol. 4190, pp. 420–428. Springer, Heidelberg (2006)
13. Sakoe, H., Chiba, S.: Dynamic programming algorithm optimization for spoken word recognition. IEEE Trans. Acoust. Speech Signal Process. 26(1), 43–49 (1978)
14. Darrell, T., Essa, I.A., Pentland, A.: Task-specific gesture analysis in real-time using interpolated views. IEEE Trans. PAMI 18(12), 1236–1242 (1996)
15. Kassidas, A., MacGregor, J.F., Taylor, P.A.: Synchronization of batch trajectories using dynamic time warping. AIChE Journal 44(4), 864–875 (1998)

Detection of Spatial Activation Patterns as Unsupervised Segmentation of fMRI Data

Polina Golland[1], Yulia Golland[2], and Rafael Malach[3]

[1] Computer Science and Artificial Intelligence Laboratory, MIT, USA
[2] Department of Psychology, Hebrew University of Jerusalem, Israel
[3] Department of Neurobiology, Weizmann Institute of Science, Israel

Abstract. In functional connectivity analysis, networks of interest are defined based on correlation with the mean time course of a user-selected 'seed' region. In this work we propose to simultaneously estimate the optimal representative time courses that summarize the fMRI data well and the partition of the volume into a set of disjoint regions that are best explained by these representative time courses. Our approach offers two advantages. First, is removes the sensitivity of the analysis to the details of the seed selection. Second, it substantially simplifies group analysis by eliminating the need for a subject-specific threshold at which correlation values are deemed significant. This unsupervised technique generalizes connectivity analysis to situations where candidate seeds are difficult to identify reliably or are unknown. Our experimental results indicate that the functional segmentation provides a robust, anatomically meaningful and consistent model for functional connectivity in fMRI.

1 Introduction and Motivation

In this paper we propose and demonstrate a new approach to detection and analysis of spatial patterns of activation from fMRI data. Functional connectivity analysis [4] is widely used in fMRI studies for detection and analysis of large networks that co-activate with a user-selected 'seed' region of interest. Time course correlation typically serves as a measure of similarity with the mean time course of the selected seed region. Since no alternative hypothesis for correlation values is formulated, the user must select a threshold, or significance level, used in rejecting the null hypothesis that assumes zero correlation. This approach is highly useful for analyzing experiment-specific fMRI data, but integration across different runs or across subjects is challenging due to high variability of inter-voxel correlation values across scans. Furthermore, in some studies it is unclear how to select the seed region, and we would instead prefer to discover the interesting 'seeds' and the associated networks in an unsupervised way. To eliminate the sensitivity of the analysis to the seed and threshold selection and to generalize the method to situations when candidate seeds are not immediately obvious, we propose to simultaneously estimate an optimal partition of the volume into a set of disjoint networks and the representative time courses associated with these networks. This formulation gives rise to an unsupervised segmentation algorithm

N. Ayache, S. Ourselin, A. Maeder (Eds.): MICCAI 2007, Part I, LNCS 4791, pp. 110–118, 2007.
© Springer-Verlag Berlin Heidelberg 2007

that, very much like EM-segmentation of anatomical scans[19], estimates segmentation labels by fitting a mixture density to the image data. The algorithm adaptively determines the threshold for assigning a voxel to a network based on the similarity of that voxel to the representative time courses, eliminating the need for subject-specific threshold selection.

Our approach is based on a model that parcelates the brain into disjoint subregions. Principal Component Analysis (PCA) and Independent Component Analysis (ICA) [3] provide an alternative model of functional connectivity that treats the data as a linear combination of components, i.e., spatial maps with associated time courses. The physiological evidence for either model is yet to be established, but we find the parcellation model more appealing in explaining functional organization, in particular when we extend the model to multiple scales.

ICA, PCA and clustering have been extensively explored in the contexts of regression-based detection [1, 2, 7, 8, 9, 13, 14, 16, 17]. Application of clustering in fMRI analysis has traditionally focused on grouping voxels into small, functionally homogeneous regions in paradigm-based studies [8, 13, 17]. In contrast, we aim to construct a top-down representation of global patterns of activation spanning the entire brain. Recently, clustering was also demonstrated in application to full-brain scans in rest state [5, 18], revealing anatomically meaningful regions of high functional coherency. Unlike prior work in clustering of fMRI data [8, 13, 17, 18], we do not aim to determine the optimal number of systems in the decomposition. Instead, our experience shows that active browsing of the segmentation results across several levels of resolution (system size) in the anatomical region of interest is substantially more instructive than considering flat parcellations generated for a fixed, large number of clusters. In addition, we perform clustering on the original time courses, replacing the dimensionality reduction step used in [18] by the constrained signal model that effectively fold the dimensionality reduction into the estimation process. The resulting algorithm is simple to implement and analyze, yet it produces highly stable results across runs and subjects.

ICA offers an unsupervised component-based decomposition of the spatiotemporal fMRI data, but the interpretation of the resulting component maps remains challenging. In particular, the method produces a flat decomposition into a large number of spatially sparse, typically non-overlapping, components which are often treated as a segmentation of the volume. We find it natural to explicitly formulate the problem of characterizing the spatial patterns of coactivation as segmentation of the fMRI volume. This model is well matched to the questions of interest in exploratory analysis of fMRI data, in addition to producing anatomically meaningful results that are easy to interpret as partitions of the cortex into systems.

2   Unsupervised Segmentation of fMRI Data

Classical correlation-based connectivity analysis assumes a user-specified hypothesis, for example through a selection of a seed region. In contrast, we formulate the problem of characterizing connectivity as a partition of voxels into subsets that are well characterized by N_s representative hypotheses, or time courses, $\mathbf{m}_1, \ldots \mathbf{m}_{N_s}$ based on the similarity of their time courses to each hypothesis. We model the fMRI signal $\mathbf{Y}$ at each voxel as generated by the mixture $p_{\mathbf{Y}}(\mathbf{y}) = \sum_{s=1}^{N_s} \lambda_s p_{\mathbf{Y}|S}(\mathbf{y}|s)$ over N_s conditional likelihoods $p_{\mathbf{Y}|S}(\mathbf{y}|s)$ [15]. λ_s is the prior probability that a voxel belongs to system $s \in \{1, \ldots, N_s\}$. Following a commonly used approach in fMRI analysis, we model the class-conditional densities as normal distributions centered around the system mean time course, i.e., $p_{\mathbf{Y}|S}(\mathbf{y}|s) = \mathcal{N}(\mathbf{y}; \mathbf{m}_s, \Sigma_s)$. The high dimensionality of the fMRI data makes modeling a full covariance matrix impractical. Instead, most methods either limit the modeling to estimating variance elements, or model the time course dynamics as an auto-regressive (AR) process. At this stage, we take the simpler approach of modeling variance and note that the mixture model estimation can be straightforwardly extended to include an AR model. Unlike separate dimensionality reduction procedures, this approach follows closely the notions of functional similarity used by the detection methods in fMRI. In other words, we keep the notion of co-activation consistent with the standard analysis and instead redefine how the co-activation patterns are represented and extracted from images.

We employ the EM algorithm [6] to fit the mixture model to the fMRI signals from a set of voxels, leading to a familiar set of update rules:

$$\tilde{p}^n(s|\mathbf{y}_v) = \frac{\lambda_s^n \mathcal{N}(\mathbf{y}_v; \mathbf{m}_s^n, \Sigma_s^n)}{\sum_{s'} \lambda_{s'}^n \mathcal{N}(\mathbf{y}_v; \mathbf{m}_{s'}^n, \Sigma_{s'}^n)}, \qquad \lambda_s^{n+1} = \frac{\sum_v \tilde{p}^n(s|\mathbf{y}_v)}{V}$$

$$\mathbf{m}_s^{n+1} = \frac{\sum_v \tilde{p}^n(s|\mathbf{y}_v)\mathbf{y}_v}{\sum_v \tilde{p}^n(s|\mathbf{y}_v)}, \qquad \Sigma_s^{n+1}(t,t) = \frac{\sum_v \tilde{p}^n(s|\mathbf{y}_v)(\mathbf{y}_v(t) - \mathbf{m}_s^{n+1}(t))^2}{\sum_v \tilde{p}^n(s|\mathbf{y}_v)}$$

where $\tilde{p}^n(s|\mathbf{y}_v)$ is the estimate of the posterior probability that voxel v belongs to system s, and $\{\lambda_s^n, \mathbf{m}_s^n, \Sigma_s^n\}_{s=1}^{N_s}$ are the model parameter estimates at step n of the algorithm. As mentioned above, we model the covariance matrix as a diagonal matrix. To ensure that we properly explore the non-convex space of the solutions, we perform multiple runs (10 in our experiments) of the algorithm using different random initializations and select the solution that corresponds to the maximum likelihood of the data. We initialize each run by randomly selecting N_s voxels and using their time courses as an initial guess for the cluster means.

When the algorithm converges, $\tilde{p}(\cdot|\mathbf{y}_v)$ represents probabilistic segmentation. The exponential form of class-conditional densities, combined with high dimensionality of the input space, leads to essentially binary posterior probabilities (in our experience, fewer than 1% of voxels is assigned a posterior probability that is more than 10^{-3} away from 0 or 1). Unlike anatomical segmentation, atlas-based approaches are not applicable to this problem, since the instantaneous properties of fMRI signals vary substantially across runs, and little is known about spatial organization of the functional activity we should expect to see as a result of segmentation. Consequently, we perform the segmentation in a fully unsupervised fashion.

To summarize the results of the segmentation across subjects, we must make sure that the labels assigned to the same anatomical system agree across subjects. We employ an approximate algorithm that matches the label assignments in pairs of subjects with the goal of maximizing the number of voxels with the same label in both subjects until convergence. In practice, this algorithm quickly (1-2 passes over all subjects) finds the correct label permutation in each subject.

3   Experimental Results

We demonstrate our approach on a study of functional connectivity that included 7 subjects. We used previously collected fMRI scans in a large set of visual experiments, from simple localizer tasks to viewing continuous stimuli (movies), as well as a rest scan. The total amount of fMRI data per subject was close to one hour. In the movie viewing experiments, the functional connectivity analysis revealed two systems: the stimulus-dependent system that contained sensory-motor cortexes and was strongly correlated with the seed region in the visual cortex and the 'intrinsic' system that showed little correlation with the visual seed, but exhibited high intra-system correlation [11].

The functional scans were pre-processed for motion artifacts, manually aligned into the Talairach coordinate system, detrended (removing linear trends in the baseline activation) and smoothed (8mm kernel). We experimented with different amount of smoothing and observed that is had very little effect on the resulting decompositions. We restricted the analysis to the voxels in the cortical segmentation mask in the corresponding anatomical scans and chose to visualize the resulting decompositions on the inflated surface of the cortex, as well as using a flattened representation of both hemispheres. Functional segmentations extracted for the same subject in different visual experiments varied little in the anatomical boundaries of the detected systems even though the details of the systems' time course dynamics changed substantially across experiments. This is in line with the current theories of the functional organization of the brain that postulate anatomically stationary regions whose changing activation dynamics drives the cognitive processes. Using all the data in a single segmentation resulted in a more repeatable segmentation when compared across subjects, suggesting that increasing the amount of fMRI data stabilizes the estimation process. The experimental results reported in the remainder of this section are based on all available data for each subject.

Fig. 1a shows the 2-system partition extracted in each subject independently of all others. It also displays the boundaries of the intrinsic system determined through the traditional seed selection, showing good agreement between the two partitions. In contrast to the difficulties associated with the subject-specific threshold selection in group analysis within the standard functional connectivity framework, the clustering-based decomposition produces highly repeatable maps that do not involve subject-specific adjustments. Fig. 1c shows a group-level label map that summarizes the maps from Fig. 1a, further illustrating the stability of the decomposition. We emphasize that no sophisticated group-wise

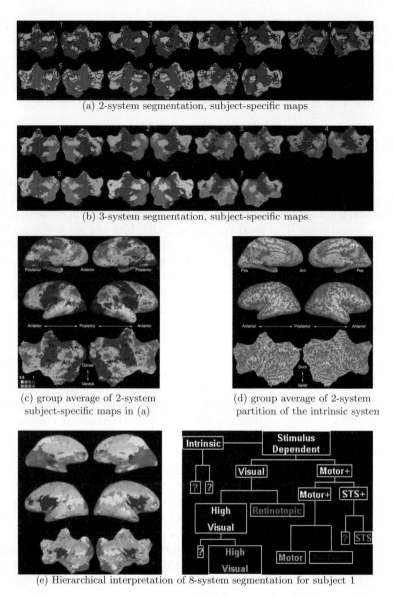

(a) 2-system segmentation, subject-specific maps

(b) 3-system segmentation, subject-specific maps

(c) group average of 2-system
subject-specific maps in (a)

(d) group average of 2-system
partition of the intrinsic system

(e) Hierarchical interpretation of 8-system segmentation for subject 1

Fig. 1. Functional segmentation examples. (a,b) Subject-specific segmentation results for two and three systems respectively (flattened view). Green: intrinsic system, blue: stimulus-driven cortex, red: visual cortex. Solid lines show the boundaries of the intrinsic system determined through seed selection. (c) Group average of the subject-specific 2-system maps. Color shading shows the proportion of subjects whose clustering agreed with the majority label. (d) Group average of the subject-specific segmentation of the intrinsic system into two sub-systems. Only voxels consistently labeled across subjects are shown. (e) Subject-specific segmentation into a large number of systems. Browsing of all preceding levels (not shown here) revealed the hierarchy displayed on the right. Colors show matching systems in the image (left) and labels in the hierarchy (right).

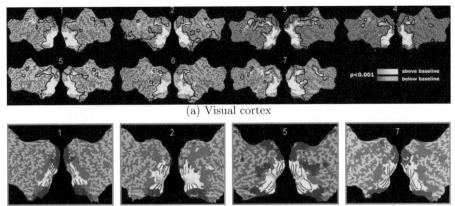

(a) Visual cortex

(b) Segmentation of the visual cortex: retinotopical cortex (yellow),
peripheral visual areas (blue) and high visual areas (red).

Fig. 2. Comparison with the regression-based detection. (a) Color shows the statistical parametric map; solid lines indicate the boundaries of the visual system obtained through clustering. (b) 3-system segmentation of the visual cortex for subjects 1,2,5,7. Only the posterior half of the flattened view is shown for each subject. The black lines indicate the boundaries of V1-V4 regions.

registration was performed; no information was shared across subjects during segmentation. Subsequent subdivision of the cortical gray matter into three systems produced the results in Fig. 1b. With the exception of one subject, the 3-system segmentation reveals visual cortex. In subject 7, the visual cortex separated in segmentation into 4 systems (shown in the figure). Fig. 1e shows an example of subject-specific segmentation into 8 systems and its hierarchical interpretation that was constructed by a neuroscientist through interactive browsing of the increasingly detailed segmentations (not shown here). While the final segmentation map in Fig. 1e would be difficult to interpret if it were considered as a stand-alone flat parcellation, a collection of segmentations into an increasingly large number number of systems makes interpretation exceedingly easy. The nested nature of the segmentation results suggests future work in hierarchical representations that capture and exploit this property to improve detection and interpretation.

Since the original study aimed to characterize the intrinsic system, we also performed a subdivision of just that system in each subject. Interestingly, this subdivision produced a stable partition across subjects; the corresponding group-level map is shown in Fig. 1d. The overlap of the smaller sub-systems is weaker than that of the intrinsic system, but it clearly represents a coherent division of the intrinsic system. We are currently investigating neuroanatomical and functional characteristics of the two new sub-areas.

We also provide preliminary validation of the method by comparing the resulting parcellations with well known partitions in the visual cortex. Fig. 2a compares the boundaries of the visual system identified through clustering (red

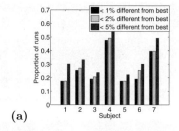 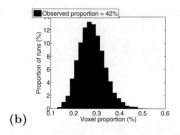

(a)   (b)

Fig. 3. Performance statistics. (a) Proportion of runs that resulted in the segmentation that was close to the best (max likelihood) segmentation. (b) Null hypothesis distribution for the number of voxels that showed perfect agreement across all subjects.

cluster in Fig. 1b) with the statistical parametric map (SPM) from a block-design visual localizer experiment. The regions of reduced activation in the SPM correspond to the well known suppression of activation in the intrinsic system (anterior of the visual cortex; outside the visual system) and the reduction in the signal often observed in the peripheral visual areas (posterior cortex; included in the visual system). We can see that the two methods agree on the location of the boundary between the visual cortex and the adjacent areas. We emphasize that the segmentation method had no access to the protocol regressor from the visual experiments. Further subdivision of the visual system revealed the central-peripheral partition that separates retinotopic areas (V1 through V4) from the peripheral visual areas and the retinotopic-high partition that separates the retinotopic cortex from the high visual areas. These two fundamental organizational principles have been extensively studied using a set of techniques, including fMRI [12]. Fig. 2b compares the results of segmentation with the retinotopical mapping available for four subjects in our study. The solid lines indicate the extent and the boundaries of the retinotopic areas obtained in a separate fMRI experiment [12]. We can see that the segmentation accurately estimated the boundaries between the retinotopic areas (yellow), the high visual areas (red) and the peripheral areas (blue) using fMRI data from a diverse set of experiments which were not specifically tailored for retinotopic mapping.

To test the robustness of the EM algorithm in this application, we ran the segmentation for 100 different random iterations and examined the resulting maps. We sorted the resulting segmentations by the value of the corresponding data likelihood. Using the best result as a reference, Fig. 3a shows the number of resulting segmentations that varied from the best segmentation by less than 1%, 2% and 5% respectively. We observe that a reasonable proportion of the runs (from 15% to 50%) produced segmentations that are very close to the best one. Similar to other hill-climbing optimization problems, our goal is not to ensure that all runs result in a good solution, but rather than sufficiently high proportion of random initializations leads to a good solution. To quantify the significance of the agreement across subjects, we ran permutation tests. In each iteration of the test, the voxel locations were permuted, the best relabeling across subjects was estimated and the proportion of voxels that achieved perfect agreement across subjects was recorded. When comparing the observed proportion in the real data with the histograms created in the permutation test for 10^5 iterations (Fig. 3b), we note that the result is dramatically significant under this null hypothesis. Our future work includes developing more realistic null hypotheses that maintain spatial statistics of labels observed in the estimated segmentations.

4   Conclusions

We proposed and demonstrated a novel approach to characterizing global spatial patterns of co-activation in fMRI. The analysis produces hierarchical decompositions of the gray matter into a set of regions with increasingly consistent functional activity. By explicitly decoupling inter-subject variability in the spatial pattern of activation from the time course variability, our approach overcomes the need for subject-specific threshold selection often necessary in the standard methods for group analysis of fMRI data. In contrast to component-based analysis, the proposed method provides an intuitive model of cortical parcellation into systems and leads naturally to a hierarchical formulation that we plan to explore in the future. We provide initial validation of the method by comparing the detected systems with the previously known divisions of cortical areas. We also demonstrate an application of the method to detect novel functional partitions.

Acknowledgements. This research was supported in part by the NIH NIBIB NAMIC U54-EB005149, NCRR NAC P41-RR13218 and NCRR mBIRN U24-RR021382 grants, by the NSF CAREER grant 0642971 to P. Golland and by Morris and Barbara Levinson Professorial Chair and ISF Center of Excellence the Dominique Center, the Benozyio Center for Neuro-Degeneration to R. Malach.

References

[1] Baumgartner, R., et al.: Fuzzy clustering of gradient-echo functional MRI in the human visual cortex. J. Magnetic Resonance Imaging 7(6), 1094–1101 (1997)

[2] Beckmann, C.F., Smith, S.M.: Tensorial Extensions of Independent Component Analysis for Group FMRI Data Analysis. NeuroImage 25(1), 294–311 (2005)

[3] Bell, A.J., Sejnowski, T.J.: An information-maximization approach to blind separation and blind deconvolution. Neural Computation 7, 1129–1159 (1995)

[4] Biswal, B., et al.: Functional connectivity in the motor cortex of resting human brain using echo-planar MRI. Magnetic Resonance in Medicine 34, 537–541 (1995)

[5] Cordes, D., et al.: Hierarchical clustering to measure connectivity in fMRI resting-state data. Magnetic Resonance Imaging 20(4), 305–317 (2002)

[6] Dempster, A., Laird, N., Rubin, D.: Maximum likelihood from incomplete data via the EM algorithm. Series B 39(1), 1–38 (1977)

[7] Fadili, M.J., et al.: A multistep Unsupervised Fuzzy Clustering Analysis of fMRI time series. Human Brain Mapping 10(4), 160–178 (2000)

[8] Filzmoser, P., Baumgartner, R., Moser, E.: A hierarchical clustering method for analyzing functional MR images. Magnetic Resonance Imaging 10, 817–826 (1999)

[9] Friston, K.J., et al.: Functional connectivity: the principle component analysis of large (PET) data sets. J. Cereb. Blood Flow Metab. 13, 5–14 (1993)

[10] Friston, K.J.: Functional and effective connectivity: a synthesis. Human Brain Mapping 2, 56–78 (1994)

[11] Golland, Y., et al.: Extrinsic and intrinsic systems in the posterior cortex of the human brain revealed during natural sensory stimulation. Cereb. Cortex 17, 766–777 (2007)

[12] Grill-Spector, K., et al.: A sequence of early object processing stages revealed by fMRI in human occipital lobe. Human Brain Mapping 6(4), 316–328 (1998)

[13] Goutte, C., et al.: On clustering fMRI time series. Neuroimage 9(3), 298–310 (1999)

[14] McKeown, M.J., et al.: Analysis of fMRI data by blind separation into spatial independent components. Human Brain Mapping 6, 160–188 (1998)

[15] McLachlan, G.J., Basford, K.E.: Mixture models. Inference and applications to clustering. Dekker (1988)

[16] Moser, E., Diemling, M., Baumgartner, R.: Fuzzy clustering of gradient-echo functional MRI in the human visual cortex. J. Magnetic Resonance Imaging 7(6), 1102–1108 (1997)

[17] Thirion, B., Faugeras, O.: Feature Detection in fMRI Data: The Information Bottleneck Approach. Medical Image Analysis 8, 403–419 (2004)

[18] Thirion, B., Dodel, S., Poline, J.B.: Detection of signal synchronizations in resting-state fMRI datasets. NeuroImage 29, 321–327 (2006)

[19] Van Leemput, K., et al.: Automated model-based tissue classification of MR images of the brain. IEEE TMI 18(10), 897–908 (1999)

Robotic Assistance for Ultrasound Guided Prostate Brachytherapy

Gabor Fichtinger[1], Jonathan Fiene[1], Christopher W. Kennedy[1], Gernot Kronreif[2], Iulian Iordachita[1], Danny Y. Song[1], E. Clif Burdette[3], and Peter Kazanzides[1]

[1] The Johns Hopkins University, Baltimore, Maryland, USA
[2] PROFACTOR Research and Solutions GmbH, Seibersdorf, Austria
[3] Acoustic Medsystems, Inc., Urbana-Champaign, IL, USA
gabor@cs.jhu.edu

Abstract. We present a robotically assisted prostate brachytherapy system and test results in training phantoms. The system consists of a transrectal ultrasound (TRUS) and a spatially co-registered robot integrated with an FDA-approved commercial treatment planning system. The salient feature of the system is a small parallel robot affixed to the mounting posts of the template. The robot replaces the template interchangeably and uses the same coordinate system. Established clinical hardware, workflow and calibration are left intact. In these experiments, we recorded the first insertion attempt without adjustment. All clinically relevant locations were reached. Non-parallel needle trajectories were achieved. The pre-insertion transverse and rotational errors (measured with Polaris optical tracker relative to the template's coordinate frame) were 0.25mm (STD=0.17mm) and 0.75^{o} (STD=0.37^{o}). The needle tip placement errors measured in TRUS were 1.04mm (STD=0.50mm). The system is in Phase-I clinical feasibility and safety trials, under Institutional Review Board approval.

1 Introduction

Transrectal ultrasound (TRUS) guided brachytherapy is an effective treatment for low-risk prostate cancer [1], but many implants continue to fail or cause adverse side effects. The procedure entails permanently implanting radioactive seeds into the prostate. It is commonly believed that pinpoint accuracy in executing a pre-operative implant plan should lead to good dosimetry. However, as two decades of practice have demonstrated, this is not achieved by all clinicians. Instead of enforcing a pre-operative plan, intra-operative dosimetry and in-situ optimization have been receiving increasing attention [2]. This approach, however, demands precise localization of the implanted needles and seeds [3], which assumes exquisite spatial and temporal synchronization of the needle insertion and imaging tasks. The needles and seeds can be localized in TRUS, the dose field analyzed, and finally the remainder of the implant can be optimized. Needle positions are often rearranged to avoid overdosing and/or seeds added to fill cold spots. This, however, is a repetitive manual process that is prone to human operator errors and consumes valuable time in the operating room. Time delays may allow for increased edema that may change the anatomy and

N. Ayache, S. Ourselin, A. Maeder (Eds.): MICCAI 2007, Part I, LNCS 4791, pp. 119–127, 2007.
© Springer-Verlag Berlin Heidelberg 2007

thereby negatively impact outcome. It is expected that intra-operative dosimetry can resolve these problems. This function, however, requires spatial and temporal synchronization of the actions of imaging, needle insertion, and needle/seed tracking. In current systems that attempt on-line dosimetry, these steps are performed sequentially by the physician who handles TRUS and needles together with the medical physicist who operates the treatment planning system (TPS). Motorizing the TRUS [4] and adapting the ultrasound phase/focus [5] have been shown to possess excellent potential in volume imaging and needle tracking. Hence the outstanding issue appears to be synchronizing needle action with ultrasound imaging. We first considered optical or electromagnetic (EM) tracking, but they turned out to be clinically impractical for a plethora of well known problems, such as lack of sight for optical trackers and field distortions for EM trackers; leaving us with some form of robotic assistance. Several medical robots have been proposed previously for prostate brachytherapy [6,7,8,9,10] which strive to increase the accuracy of needle placement by transforming the workflow into a process we call "surgical CAD/CAM" [10]. Unfortunately, they add a great deal of complexity to the procedure and alter current hardware, calibration, and workflow standards. Our approach is different in that it adheres to the established standards of care, while also providing all practical benefits of robotic assistance. The novelty of our work lays in the adaptation and integration of existing robotic hardware in a simple and inherently safe manner.

2 System Design

The system consists of a central computer running the FDA-approved Interplant® TPS (CMS Inc., St. Louis, MO); a TRUS imager (B&K Medical, 6.5MHz); an AccuSeed implant stand with digital probe positioner (also by CMS); and a small parallel needle guidance robot, as shown in Figure 1(left). We adapted a light weight parallel robot that rests on the mounting posts of the conventional template, as seen in Figure 1(right). The robot and the template are interchangeable during the procedure, as they are mounted in the same location and are calibrated to operate in the same coordinate frame. Thus, the unique feature of our system is retaining the existing clinical setup, hardware and workflow. In the case of a malfunction or even a slight suspicion of it, the physician can revert to the conventional template-based manual procedure without interruption. The robot is controlled by a standalone computer, thereby preserving the integrity of the FDA-approved Interplant system originally developed by Burdette Medical. The TRUS unit and the encoded stepper produce temporally and spatially tagged image streams for the TPS. In the experiments reported in this paper, an anthropomorphic mannequin was positioned supine, with a standard brachytherapy implant training phantom (CIRS Inc, Norfolk, VA) built into its perineum, as shown in the pictures of Figure 4.

The robot was originally developed for image-guided needle biopsy [11] and was customized by the manufacturer (PROFACTOR GmbH, Seibersdorf, Austria) to our specifications. The robot consists of two 2D Cartesian motion stages arranged in a parallel configuration (Figure 2). The xy stage provides planar motion relative to the mounting posts, in the plane that corresponds to the face of the template. The workspace of ±4cm in each direction is sufficient to cover the prostate with a generous margin. The $\alpha\beta$ stage rides on the xy stage, with a workspace of ±2cm. The xy and $\alpha\beta$ stages hold a pair of carbon fiber fingers that are manually locked into place during setup. A passive needle guide sleeve is attached between the fingers using free-moving ball joints. We decided against active needle driving. Instead, the robot functions as a fully encoded stable needle guide, through which the physician manually inserts the needle into the patient. The physician thus retains full control and natural haptic sensing, while

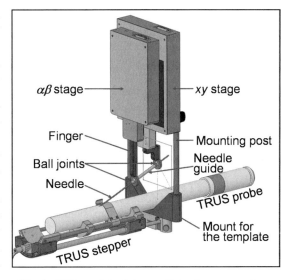

Fig. 1. CAD model of the parallel robot mounted over the TRUS probe on the mounting posts of the template

the needle is being observed in live transverse and sagittal TRUS, ensuring exquisite control of the insertion depth relative to the target anatomy. If necessary, the insertion depth can also be encoded as in Seidl *et al.* [12], thus fully eliminating any practical need for active needle driving.

When the $\alpha\beta$ stage is in motion, the guide sleeve performs 2D rotation about the ball joint on the finger attached to the xy stage. Needle angulation offers manifold advantages over the conventional template guidance where all needles were forced to

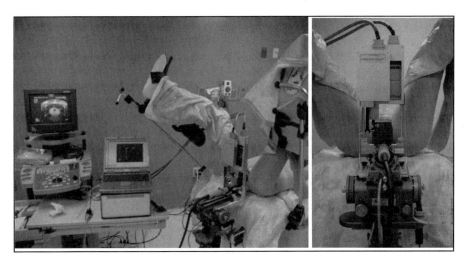

Fig. 2. System setup in the OR (left) and a closer view of the robot from the physician's perspective (right). Observe how the standard clinical hardware and setup are fully preserved.

be parallel. Vertical angulation allows for avoidance of pubic arch interference, as seen in Figure 4(left). This happens when part of the prostate is hidden behind the pubic bone, which in contemporary practice can make patients with large prostates (>55cc) ineligible for brachytherapy. Additionally, biaxial angulation can account for anatomical asymmetries better than parallel needles, thereby yielding more conformal dose. The rotational workspace is a ±20° cone, sufficient to provide the required features. The length of the current needle guide sleeve is 70mm, providing steady support for the needle against buckling and slipping on the skin. While the guide sleeve takes up a longer length of the needle than the original template, it allows for shorter carbon fiber fingers that are stiffer and thus more accurate. If the needle guide length proves to be a clinical problem, we will redesign the fingers to reduce the length of the sleeve. The guide's diameter is slightly above 18G, to accommodate standard brachytherapy needles without friction and play. (Note that the sleeve can be made to fit a needle of arbitrary size, such as a biopsy gun.) The disposable sleeve can be snapped in and out of the ball joints by hand. The robot is covered with a sterile plastic drape during the procedure; only the fingers and the guide sleeve are sterilized.

The robot weighs 1,300g. Its dimensions in home position are 140 x 180 x 65 mm. Although it exerts some torque on the template posts, the load is bilaterally distributed over the stepper base with a supporting bracket, a precaution that prevents the robot from bending over the TRUS probe. The bracket can be seen Figure 4.

The robot control: The robot control architecture is shown in Figure 3. Low-level robot control is performed on a DMC-2143 controller board and AMP-20341 linear power amplifier (Galil Motion Control, Rocklin, CA, USA), which are connected via Ethernet to the laptop PC that runs the Robot GUI (Graphical User Interface) and the Interplant application software processes. Communication between these two processes is provided by a socket (UDP) connection. This required a minor modification to the Interplant software to add a "robot control" menu that invokes a small set of methods, defined in a dynamically loaded library (DLL), to initialize the robot, query its position, and move it to a new position. The DLL transmits these requests, via the socket connection, to the Robot GUI, which then invokes the appropriate methods in the Robot Class.

Since the Robot GUI is in a separate process, it can also interact with the user directly; in particular, it updates the robot position/status display and accepts motion commands from the user.

In the current system, this is used to set the needle orientation because these two degrees of freedom are not controlled by the Interplant software. As noted in Figure 3, most of the custom software created for this project is written in C++ or Python. There is also a small safety loop that compares the primary position sensors (incremental encoders) to the secondary position sensors (incremental encoders).

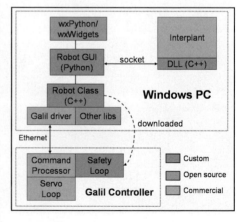

Fig. 3. The robot control architecture

This is written in a Galil-specific interpreted language and is downloaded to the controller during initialization.

The calibration of the robot is identical to that of the conventional manual system and uses the same software kit and water tank. In essence, we move the needle tip inside the tank in a known trajectory by precise motion of the robot (serving as ground truth) and we also mark the needle positions in sagittal and transverse TRUS. Then by maximizing the similarity between the observations and ground truth, we obtain a transformation matrix between the TRUS and robot coordinate frames. Unlike any previous brachytherapy robot, ours does not require calibration before each procedure because the robot remains calibrated as long as its mounting remains calibrated to the TRUS.

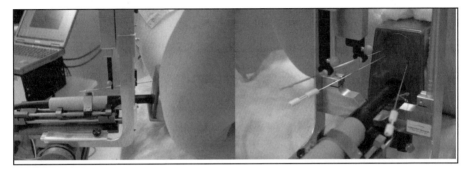

Fig. 4. Insertion of angulated needles. The needle is slanted upward to reach behind the pubic arch (left). Laterally slanted therapy needle in the presence of stabilizer needles (right).

The clinical workflow begins with segmenting the anatomy in TRUS and creating an implant plan. Bilateral stabilization needles may also be inserted. For each implant needle, the coordinates of the desired needle location are sent to the robot. The robot moves the needle guide onto the entry point over the perineum and orients it to the desired angle. The current Interplant dosimetry package does not support slanted needles, but the robot has this functionality. The physician inserts the preloaded needle or seed gun (such as Mick applicator) into the guide sleeve, and enters the needle into the desired depth while observing its progress in the live TRUS. The TPS has a near perfect estimate of the expected location of the needle in TRUS and a visual outline of the planned needle position is superimposed onto the spatially registered TRUS. The TPS processes the image to locate the needle and the operator may apply manual correction. The TPS then updates the dosimetry based upon the inserted needle position. The physician can make manual correction to the needle before approving the position and releasing the payload, or the physician may opt to pull out the needle without releasing the seeds. Only after correct needle position is confirmed, the physician will retract the needle and release the seeds. During the retraction of the needle, live TRUS images are acquired, wherein shadows of the seeds appear as they are released from the needle. The TPS processes the image to locate the seeds being dropped and the operator may also apply manual correction. Once the seeds are located, the computer promptly calculates a full dosimetry, using the seeds already implanted in their actual delivered locations, combined with the contribution of the remaining planned seeds. At this time, the physician can modify the remainder of the implant plan to compensate for cumulative deviations from the original plan. The cycle of execution is repeated with the next needle until satisfactory dosimetric coverage is achieved, which is the overall objective of the procedure.

3 Experiments and Results

We evaluated the prototype system in phantom trials. The robot fits in the neutral space over the perineum (Figure 1), without obstructing the swing space for a C-arm if one is present. The robot executed the designed ranges of motions. The Cartesian stage safely covered the axial dimensions of the prostate with generous margin. The function of needle angulation was also tested. Figure 4(left) depicts sufficient vertical angulation to point the needle behind the pubic arch while Figure 4(right) demonstrates vertical and lateral angulation. Note that unlike in any previous brachytherapy robot system, the implant needles can be inserted in the presence of bilateral stabilizer needles commonly used for reducing prostate motion during needle

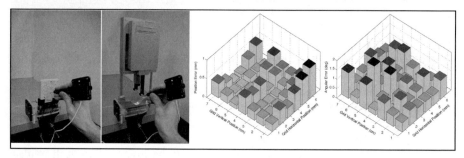

Fig. 5. Comparison of needle guidance between template and robot with Polaris tracker (left). Error bars for the translation (middle) and rotation (right) differences.

insertion [13]. In the case of collision, the distal finger gently deflects the stabilizer away, without causing tissue injury, while the physician is standing by to prevent the stabilization needle from being accidentally caught in the robot finger. (This issue will be studied further in a forthcoming Phase-I safety trial.)

We measured the accuracy of robotic needle positioning relative to the template. The robot, as mentioned earlier, is registered to the TRUS and the TPS commands address the robot in template coordinates. We performed 42 parallel positioning movements (7 rows of 6 columns, spaced 1 cm apart) in the z-axis with the robotic system and then manually with the template. We measured the positions of the corresponding template hole and the robotic needle guide before

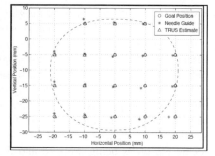

Fig. 6. Accuracy of robotically guided needle insertion relative to TRUS

insertion with a calibrated ballpoint pointer (Traxtal Inc, Toronto, ON) tracked by a Polaris tracker (Northern Digital, Waterloo, ON), as seen in Figure 5(left). The error bars in Figure 5(middle) show a mean location error of 0.25mm (STD=0.17mm) which is less than the stated accuracy of the tracker. We also measured the accuracy of needle angulation relative to the z-axis. We performed 42 robotic positioning movements (7 rows of 6 columns, spaced 1 cm apart, in random angles between the extremes). We measured the angle of the guide sleeve by pivoting on both ends with the calibrated tracker pointer. The error bars shown in Figure 5(right) display a mean rotation error of $0.75°$ (STD=$0.37°$), comparable with the accuracy of tracking.

We also measured the accuracy of robotic needle positioning followed by needle insertion into the phantom, relative to TRUS. We inserted 18 parallel needles along the z axis, marked their locations in TRUS and measured the location of the guide sleeve with the Polaris. As shown in Figure 6, all needles landed close to their goal, with a mean error of 1.04mm (STD=0.50mm). Locations near the prostate edge show somewhat larger errors attributed to slight needle deflection, which is still generously sufficient for brachytherapy. Placement accuracy of slanted needles suggested similar results, but we note that while slanted needles are currently not used in the dose planner, they are useful for adding individual seeds to patch up cold spots.

The apparatus allows for natural haptic feedback, but similarly to current template based practice, this feeling may be somewhat compromised by friction forces caused by needle bending and sliding forces. Lateral stabilization needles [13] provide some relief, as Podder *et al.* demonstrated in recent *in-vivo* needle force measurements [14].

In testing dynamic dosimetry, standard needles were inserted into a phantom. The moving needle was captured in live TRUS. A typical screen shot is shown in Figure 7, where the needle appears in the sagittal image as a white line. The expected seed positions relative to the needle tip are marked with squares. These squares were then used as initial search regions for localizing the seeds upon releasing them into the prostate. The resulting dose display was instantly updated so the clinician could follow the buildup of therapy dose, relative to the anatomy. Color-coded isodose lines seen around the needle are updated as the seeds are captured.

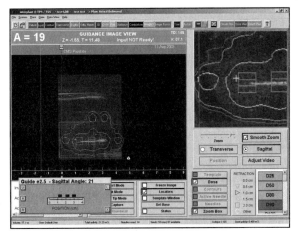

Fig. 7. Dynamic dosimetry screen from Interplant. The needle and seeds are captured in TRUS images as they are being inserted, while the resulting dose display is updated.

4   Conclusion

The robotic assistant provides needle placement accuracy equivalent to that of conventional templates while offering much greater flexibility, owing to its biaxial needle angulation and continuum Cartesian needle spacing. It is a digitally encoded system that allows for synchronized imaging and image-based needle/seed tracking, thereby opening the way for online dosimetry and implant optimization. These features were achieved without causing interference with established clinical hardware, workflow, or calibration standards. This is especially important as commercial potential and clinical viability in contemporary medicine are inseparable issues. Engineering development will continue with motorizing the TRUS base which already performs optical encoding of the stepper, making such a process relatively straightforward. Note that the system is functional without such motorization of the TRUS probe, though it requires some degree of manual adjustment during needle insertion and seed release, which from the dosimetric point of view is only an issue of convenience.

This work has been supported by DoD PC-050042, DoD PC050170, NIH 2R44 CA099374-02, and the NSF Engineering Research Center for Computer Integrated Surgical Systems and Technology under NSF EEC-9731748.

References

1. Zelefsky, M.J., Hollister, T., Raben, A., et al.: Five-year biochemical outcome and toxicity with transperineal CT-planned permanent I-125 prostate implantation for patients with localized prostate cancer. Int. J. Radiat. Oncol. Biol. Phys. 47, 1261–1266 (2000)
2. Zelefsky, M.J., Yamada, Y., Marion, C., et al.: Improved conformality and decreased toxicity with intraoperative computer-optimized transperineal ultrasound-guided prostate brachytherapy. Int. J. Radiat. Oncol. Biol. Phys. 55, 956–963 (2003)
3. Nag, S., Ciezki, J.P., Cormack, R., et al.: Intraoperative planning and evaluation of permanent prostate brachytherapy: Report of the American brachytherapy society. Int. J. Radiat. Oncol. Biol. Phys. 51, 1420–1430 (2001)
4. Wan, G., Wei, Z., Gardi, L., et al.: Brachytherapy needle deflection evaluation and correction. Med. Phys. 32, 902–909 (2005)
5. Okazawa, S., Ebrahimi, R., Chuang, J., et al.: Methods for segmenting curved needles and the needle tip in real-time ultrasound imaging. Medical Image Analysis, vol. 10(3), pp. 330–342. Elsevier Science Inc. New York (2006)
6. Fichtinger, G., Burdette, E.C., Tanacs, A., et al.: Robotically assisted prostate brachytherapy with transrectal ultrasound guidance-Phantom experiments. Brachytherapy 5(1), 14–26 (2006)
7. Wei, Z., Wan, G., Gardi, L., et al.: Robot-assisted 3D-TRUS guided prostate brachytherapy: System integration and validation. Med. Phys. 31, 539–548 (2004)
8. Yu, Y., Podder, T., Zhang, Y., et al.: Robot-Assisted Prostate Brachytherapy. In: Larsen, R., Nielsen, M., Sporring, J. (eds.) MICCAI 2006. LNCS, vol. 4190, pp. 41–49. Springer, Heidelberg (2006)
9. Phee, L., Yuen, J., Xiao, D., et al.: Ultrasound Guided Robotic Biopsy of the Prostate. International Journal on Humanoid Robotics 3(4), 463–483 (2006)
10. Fichtinger, G., DeWeese, T.L., Patriciu, A., et al.: Robotically Assisted Prostate Biopsy And Therapy With Intra-Operative CT Guidance. Journal of Academic Radiology 9(1), 60–74 (2002)
11. Kettenbach, J., Kronreif, G., Figl, M., et al.: Robot-assisted biopsy using ultrasound guidance: initial results from in vitro tests. Eur. Radiol. 15, 765–771 (2005)

12. Seidl, K., Fichtinger, G., Kazanzides, P.: Optical Measurement of Needle Insertion Depth. In: IEEE International Conference on Biomedical Robotics, Pisa, Italy (February 15-19, 2006)
13. Taschereau, R., Pouliot, J., Roy, J., et al.: Seed misplacement and stabilizing needles in transperineal permanent prostate implants. Radiother Oncol. 55, 59–63 (2000)
14. Podder, T., Clark, D., Sherman, J., Fuller, D., Messing, E., Rubens, D., Strang, J., Brasacchio, R., Liao, L., Ng, W.S., Yu, Y.: Vivo motion and force measurement of surgical needle intervention during prostate brachytherapy. Med. Phys. 33(8), 2915–2922 (2006)

Closed-Loop Control in Fused MR-TRUS Image-Guided Prostate Biopsy

Sheng Xu[1], Jochen Kruecker[1], Peter Guion[2], Neil Glossop[3], Ziv Neeman[2], Peter Choyke[2], Anurag K. Singh[2], and Bradford J. Wood[2]

[1] Philips Research North America, Briarcliff, NY 10510, USA
{sheng.xu,jochen.kruecker}@philips.com
[2] National Institutes of Health, Bethesda, MD 20892, USA
[3] Traxtal Inc, Toronto, ON M5V 2J1, Canada

Abstract. Multi-modality fusion imaging for targeted prostate biopsy is difficult because of prostate motion during the biopsy procedure. A closed-loop control mechanism is proposed to improve the efficacy and safety of the biopsy procedure, which uses real-time ultrasound and spatial tracking as feedback to adjust the registration between a preoperative 3D image (e.g. MRI) and real-time ultrasound images. The spatial tracking data is used to initialize the image-based registration between intraoperative ultrasound images and a preoperative ultrasound volume. The preoperative ultrasound volume is obtained using a 2D sweep and manually registered to the MRI dataset before the biopsy procedure. The accuracy of the system is 2.3±0.9 mm in phantom studies. The results of twelve patient studies show that prostate motion can be effectively compensated using closed-loop control.

Keywords: motion compensation, prostate biopsy, image registration.

1 Introduction

Prostate cancer is the most common non-skin cancer and the second leading cause of cancer death among American men [1]. Transrectal ultrasound (TRUS) guided needle biopsy is the most frequently used method for diagnosing prostate cancer due to its real-time nature, low cost, and simplicity [2]. However, the use of ultrasound (US) to detect prostate cancer is limited by its relatively poor image quality and low sensitivity and specificity for prostate cancers. It is difficult to use US for targeted biopsy guidance because most cancers are not visible sonographically. Magnetic resonance imaging (MRI) is superior for visualizing the prostate anatomy and focal lesions suspicious for prostate cancer. However, MRI imaging is costly and the magnetic environment makes interventional procedures more complex thus making MRI imaging unsuitable as an intra-procedural modality for routine biopsy guidance.

Since preoperative MRI and real-time US complement each other, it is desirable to fuse them and take advantage of the superior visualization of MRI images in TRUS guided biopsy [3]. Several systems have been presented in literature for image fusion

N. Ayache, S. Ourselin, A. Maeder (Eds.): MICCAI 2007, Part I, LNCS 4791, pp. 128–135, 2007.
© Springer-Verlag Berlin Heidelberg 2007

of preoperative MRI (or CT) images and real-time US images [4][5]. In these systems, the ultrasound probe is tracked by a localizer that assigns a global coordinate system to the US images. The registration between the MRI image and the localizer is obtained using fiducial markers before the surgical intervention. After both MRI and US are registered to the localizer, multi-planar reconstruction of the MRI image can be computed and overlaid on the 2D US image in real-time.

It should be noted that these systems only work well if the target is static relative to the fiducial markers. Unfortunately, the prostate moves considerably in the pelvic cavity for several reasons: First, the patient often moves involuntarily due to pain or pressure related to the needle insertion; Second, the transrectal ultrasound probe itself can move and distort the prostate. Finally, respiratory motion of the patient may shift the prostate [6]. It is apparent that skin fiducials are not very useful for the motion correction. In our earlier work [7], gold seeds were implanted into the prostate. This approach was abandoned because very few seeds could be identified in both MRI and US. Without intraoperative feedback to account for prostate motion, the system features an open-loop control mechanism. Since the prostate is a very small organ, the motion can easily result in loss of accuracy in the MRI/US fusion display, leading to inaccurate needle insertions when using the fused display for targeted biopsies. Sometimes, MRI and US images can be completely disconnected from each other, making the MRI image useless for surgical navigation.

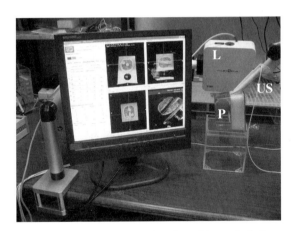

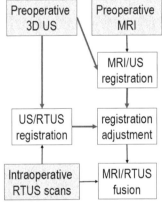

Fig. 1. System components: localizer (L), tracked ultrasound probe (US) and prostate phantom (P)

Fig. 2. Closed-loop control using feedback from real-time ultrasound (RTUS)

2 Methods

A closed-loop control system is proposed to account for prostate motion. The system uses intraoperative feedback to adjust the initial static registration between the MR and US images. The primary components of the system are shown in Figure 1.

2.1 Clinical Workflow

The prostate MRI image is acquired first and transferred to a workstation. An endorectal coil is used to improve the MRI image quality and simulate the force of the ultrasound probe through the rectal wall although the degree of deformation is not exact. The MRI image can be obtained at any time before the biopsy. The patient is then positioned on an examination table and the 2D TRUS probe with tracking sensors is placed in the rectum. At the beginning of the TRUS procedure, the operator performs a 2D axial sweep (prostate base to apex) such that the series of 2D ultrasound images covers the entire volume of the prostate. The images and corresponding tracking data from the tracking sensors are transferred to the workstation in real-time. Based on these images and tracking data, a preoperative ultrasound volume is immediately reconstructed on the workstation [8]. Since all the 2D ultrasound images are tracked, the position and orientation of the reconstructed ultrasound volume can be determined in the tracking space. The MR image and ultrasound volume are then spatially aligned by manually adjusting a rigid-body transformation [7]. During the needle insertion and specimen acquisition, the operator manually holds the 2D probe to scan the prostate. Spatial tracking of the ultrasound probe, together with registering MRI image with the tracking coordinate system, enables real-time fusion of the live ultrasound image with the spatially corresponding multi-planar reconstruction (MPR) from the MRI scan. When prostate motion results in misalignment between the US and MR images, image-based registration between the real-time 2D ultrasound images and the preoperative ultrasound volume is carried out. The registration result is used to recover the correct MRI/US fusion image in the presence of prostate motion.

2.2 Closed-Loop Control

The closed-loop control is achieved by registering the real-time ultrasound images (RTUS) to the preoperative ultrasound volume as shown in Figure 2. The red arrows represent the closed loop. After the preoperative ultrasound volume is reconstructed, its position is fixed relative to the localizer, and can be used as a reference for motion compensation. As described in equation 1, the system uses feedback from the real-time scans to adjust the initial registration between the MRI image and the preoperative ultrasound volume, allowing for motion compensation of the prostate.

$$T_{MRI \rightarrow RTUS} = T_{\text{Pr}op\ US \rightarrow RTUS} \bullet T_{MRI \rightarrow \text{Pr}op\ US} \tag{1}$$

where $T_{MRI \rightarrow \text{Pr}op\ US}$ is the initial manual registration between the preoperative US and MRI images carried out before the biopsy procedure; and $T_{\text{Pr}op\ US \rightarrow RTUS}$ is a transformation determined by the online image registration between the real-time ultrasound images and the preoperative ultrasound volume.

It seems that the localizer plays no role in equation 1, meaning that in theory the closed-loop control can be achieved without the tracking system. However, the ultrasound transducer is held manually in any arbitrary position and orientation. The online image registration between the preoperative ultrasound volume and the real-time images can be extremely difficult if the spatial relationship between them is completely unknown. In addition, equation 2 requires the image-based registration to be conducted in real-time, which is very computationally expensive for current computers. The advantage of using the tracking system is that the registration only needs to be carried out when significant prostate motion occurs. In addition, the tracking system allows the transformation between the preoperative ultrasound volume and the RTUS imaging plane to be computed, thus providing a good starting point ($\hat{T}_{\mathrm{Pr}\,op\,US \rightarrow RTUS}$ in equation 2) to initialize the image registration.

$$\hat{T}_{\mathrm{Pr}\,op\,US \rightarrow RTUS} = T_{Localizer \rightarrow RTUS\ plane} \bullet T_{\mathrm{Pr}\,op\,US \rightarrow Localizer} \qquad (2)$$

2.3 RTUS/US Registration

It is initially assumed that the prostate is in the same location as it was during the 2D sweep, therefore the transformation between the current ultrasound image and the preoperative ultrasound volume can be estimated in equation 2. The image-based registration takes the estimate as a starting point and performs numerical optimization. Since the starting point is determined by the tracking system and independent from the registration results of any other frames in history, it is always valid whether the processing of earlier frames succeeded or not. Given that the image registration may fail due to a lack of texture information, having an independent and robust starting point for each frame is critical.

The image registration algorithm is based on minimizing the sum-of-squared differences (SSD) between the current ultrasound image and the preoperative ultrasound volume. SSD is an attractive similarity measure for online registration because the mathematical formulation of SSD allows the objective function to be efficiently optimized using standard optimization algorithms such as the Gauss-Newton or the Levenberg-Marquardt algorithm.

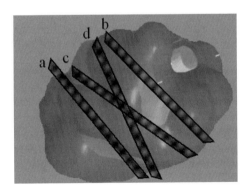

Since the spatial tracking of the ultrasound probe assigns a physical location in space to each image pixel, the 2D image is actually a single slice 3D image, allowing volume-to-volume registration to be conducted. However, the registration of the single slice volume is very sensitive to noise because there are many local minima along the off-plane direction, decreasing the algorithm's efficacy. It is therefore desirable to use more image frames for the registration. As an example illustrated in Figure 3, four ultrasound image frames are registered to the preoperative volume

Fig. 3. Selected image frames for 2.5D to 3D registration

together. These four frames are selec-ted from a series of image frames in a short time period (e.g. 3 seconds). Since the probe is held manually, it is unlikely that the probe will be absolutely static. The motion of the operator can help to cover more prostate tissue in the off-plane direction. Using spatial tracking of the probe, two frames with the furthest translational distance are selected from the image series (Figure 3, a and b). The other two frames (Figure3, c and d) are selected due to their most different orientations. The registration between these frames and the ultrasound volume can be categorized as 2.5D to 3D registration. The objective function of the registration is

$$O(\mu) = \sum_{k=1}^{N} \sum_{(x,y)} \left[I_k(x, y) - V(T_{k,\mu}(x, y, 0)) \right]^2 \qquad (3)$$

where N is the number of frame used in the registration, I_k is the kth 2D frame, V is the preoperative ultrasound volume, T is a transformation model between I_k and V, and μ is a parameter vector. In our current implementation, a rigid-body transformation with six degrees of freedom (DOFs) is used to model prostate motion in the objective function. Other transformation models with higher DOFs (e.g. affine, quadratic etc...) may be able to account for some prostate deformation. However, the registration's robustness may be sacrificed. One interesting feature of our system is that the tracking error of the localizer (e.g. metal distortion) and the calibration error of the probe can be automatically corrected because of the direct image registration,

3   Experiments and Results

Both phantom and patient studies were carried out to evaluate the system. A 2D endo-cavity probe (C9-5, Philips Medical Systems, Andover, MA) was used to acquire 2D US images. The probe was tracked by attaching a disposable CIVCO (Kalona, IA) biopsy guide equipped with custom tracking sensors (Traxtal Inc., Toronto, Canada). The US images were captured using a frame-grabber card (Winnov, Sanata Clara, CA) and processed using custom software on a workstation with two 3.7 GHz Dual Core Intel® Xeon® CPUs. The 2D sweep took 10 to 24 seconds. The reconstruction of the preoperative ultrasound volume took approximately 15 seconds using a speed enhanced algorithm and parallel computing [9]. The manual registrations between the MRI and ultrasound volumes were obtained in two to four minutes based on pre-segmented MRI images and some presets of prostate orientations [7]. The 2.5D/3D registration algorithm took about 15 seconds to compensate for prostate motion. The entire ultrasound procedure took approximately 15 minutes in patient studies.

3.1 Phantom Study

The system's accuracy was validated in a phantom study. A 6-DOF reference tracker was attached to a prostate biopsy phantom (CIRS, Norfolk, VA, USA). The global coordinate system was fixed on the phantom tracker and dynamic reference tracking [10] was used. Therefore, the prostate was static relative to the reference tracker. After the US volume was reconstructed, the 2.5D/3D registrations were carried out to measure the prostate's position. An artificial error of 5 to 15 mm was introduced to the starting point of the registration. The error was uniformly distributed in 3D space. As an example shown in Figure 4, the registration starting point (Figure 4.c) was significantly different from the intraoperative image (Figure 4.a). Since the prostate was static in the reference coordinate system, a correct registration should recover the initial position. Figure 4.b shows the corresponding image of Figure 4.a in the US volume after the registration. The registration error of each voxel was defined as the distance from the recovered position to its original position. A total of twenty measurements were taken in the experiment, resulting in an error of 2.3±0.9 mm.

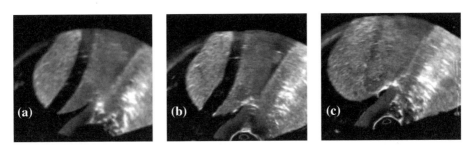

Fig. 4. Example of 2.5D/3D registration. (a) real-time ultrasound; (b) registration result of (a) in the reconstructed preoperative ultrasound volume; (c) initial starting point of the registration.

3.2 Patient Studies

The system was evaluated in patient studies from three perspectives. The capture range of the 2.5D/3D registration was first tested. Figure 5 shows the objective function near the global minimum with respect to two translation parameters, giving an indication of the smoothness of the objective function and the likely capture range.

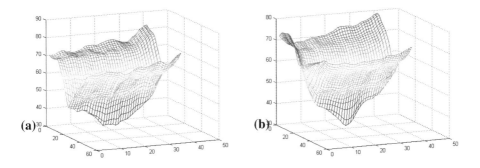

Fig. 5. Two-dimensional plots of the objective function near the global minimum with respect to two translation parameters. (a) is the result of registering one image frame. (b) is the result of registering four image frames. The grid unit is 1 mm.

Figure 5 (a and b) are the results of registering one frame and four frames respectively. It can be observed that using more image frames results in a smoother objective function. The numerical optimization is therefore less likely to be trapped by local minima, making the registration more robust.

With the 2.5D/3D registration, the closed-loop control system was able to prospectively compensate for prostate motion in patient studies. As an example shown in

Figure 6, the MRI volume is transformed to the 2D US image space. The red contours are the intersections of the prostate surface with the real-time US image. The segmentation was based on the MRI image and obtained before the biopsy procedure. After significant prostate motion was observed (Figure 6.b) in the image fusion, the image-based motion compensation was executed. As shown in Figure 6.c, the motion between the US and MRI images was well compensated.

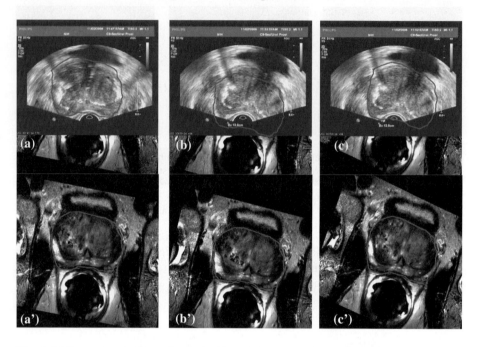

Fig. 6. Motion compensation using 2.5D/3D registration. The red contours show the prostate segmentation in MRI image. The 3D MRI volume is pre-registered to a 3D ultrasound volume that is not shown. Top row: RTUS overlaid on MRI. Bottom row: MRI images. (a) and (a') are the initial registration without patient motion; (b) and (b') are the deteriorated registration after patient motion; and (c) and (c') are the registration after motion compensation.

The ultrasound image series and probe motion in patient studies were also recorded for retrospective analysis. A total of twelve patient studies were analyzed. At the time point of the motion compensation, one ultrasound image and two MR images (one each before and after the motion compensation) were saved for each patient. The prostate was then segmented from these 2D images by a radiologist and a radiation oncologist. The prostate segmentations of the MR images before and after the motion compensation were compared to the corresponding ultrasound segmentation respectively. The overlapping area of the MR and ultrasound segmentations was calculated. The results were normalized with the prostate's area of the ultrasound image. The analysis shows that the overlapping of the prostate between the MR and ultrasound images was 75% ± 19% before the motion compensation and 94% ± 5% after the motion compensation. The difference is statistically significant based on the students-t test (p<0.01).

4 Discussion and Conclusions

This paper has presented a motion compensation system for prostate biopsy procedures using closed-loop control. The system takes advantages of both ultrasound and MRI imaging. Real-time fusion of MRI and ultrasound images can be obtained in presence of prostate motion. The tracking error of the localizer can be automatically accounted for using the image-based registration. Since only preoperative MRI images and 2D ultrasound scans are used, the system does not tie up MRI machine time for interventional procedures, providing a lower cost solution for MR guided prostate biopsy procedures. Patient studies show that the system is promising for clinical use.

The registration between the preoperative MRI and US images is currently done manually because it is the most reliable approach and the registration time seems to be clinically acceptable. It has been noticed that the physician can use the time needed for registration to examine the patient. However, robust and automatic MRI/US registration should be explored, since it is almost impossible to account for prostate deformation manually. The limitation of the current system is that the 2.5D/3D registration time is not negligible. Therefore, the system is more effective for correcting large bulk motion than continuous motion.

References

1. American Cancer Society: Prostate Cancer, Statistics for 2007 (2007)
2. Fichtinger, G., Krieger, A., Susil, R.C., Tanacs, A., Whitcomb, L.L., Atalar, E.: Transrectal prostate biopsy inside closed MRI scanner with remote actuation, under real-time image guidance. In: Dohi, T., Kikinis, R. (eds.) MICCAI 2002. LNCS, vol. 2489, pp. 91–98. Springer, Heidelberg (2002)
3. Kaplan, I., Oldenburg, N.E., Meskell, P., Blake, M., Church, P., Holupka, E.J.: Real time MRI-ultrasound image guided stereotactic prostate biopsy. Magn. Reson Imaging 20(3), 295–299 (2002)
4. Schlaier, J.R., Warnat, J., Dorenbeck, U., Proescholdt, M., Schebesch, K.M., Brawanski, A.: Image fusion of MR images and real-time ultrasonography: evaluation of fusion accuracy combining two commercial instruments, a neuronavigation system and a ultrasound system. Acta Neurochir (Wien) 146(3), 276–277 (2004)
5. Krücker, J., Xu, S., Viswanathan, A., Shen, E., Glossop, N., Wood, B.J.: Clinical evaluation of electromagnetic tracking for biopsy and radiofrequency ablation guidance. Int. J. CARS 1, 169–171 (2006)
6. Malone, S., Crook, J.M., Kendal, W.S., et al.: Respiratory-induced prostate motion: Quantification and characterization. Int. J. Radiat. Oncol. Biol. Phys 48, 105–109 (2000)
7. Kruecker, J., Xu, S., Glossop, N., Guion, P., Choyke, P., Singh, A., Wood, J.B.: Fusion of real-time trans-rectal ultrasound with pre-acquired MRI for multi-modality prostate imaging. SPIE Medical Imaging 2007 (2007)
8. Trobaugh, J.W., Trobaugh, D., Richard, W.D.: Three dimensional imaging with stereotactic ultrasonography. Comput. Med. Imaging. Graph 18(5), 315–323 (1994)
9. Xu, S., Kruecker, J., Glossop, N., Wood, B.J.: Speed Enhanced Construction of 3D Free-Hand Ultrasound. Computer Assisted Radiology and Surgery. Berlin, Germany (2007)
10. Glossop, N., Hu, R., Dix, G., Behairy, Y.: Registration methods for percutaneous image guided spine surgery. Computer Assisted Radiology and Surgery (1999)

Simulation and Fully Automatic Multimodal Registration of Medical Ultrasound

Wolfgang Wein[1,2], Ali Khamene[1], Dirk-André Clevert[3], Oliver Kutter[2], and Nassir Navab[2]

[1] Imaging & Visualization Department
Siemens Corporate Research, Princeton, NJ, USA
{wolfgang.wein,ali.khamene}@siemens.com
[2] Chair for Computer Aided Medical Procedures (CAMP)
Technische Universität München, Germany
{wein,kutter,navab}@cs.tum.edu
[3] Department of Clinical Radiology,
University Hospitals Munich-Grosshadern, Germany
dirk.clevert@med.uni-muenchen.de

Abstract. The fusion of 3D freehand ultrasound with CT and CTA has benefits for a variety of clinical applications, however a lot of manual work is usually required for correct registration. We developed new methods that allow one to simulate medical ultrasound from CT in real-time, reproducing the majority of ultrasonic imaging effects. The second novelty is a robust similarity measure that assesses the correlation of a combination of multiple signals extracted from CT with ultrasound, without knowing the influence of each signal. This serves as the foundation of a fully automatic registration, which aligns a freehand ultrasound sweep with the corresponding 3D modality using a rigid or an affine transformation model, without any manual interaction. We also present the used initialization, global and local parameter optimization schemes, and validation on abdominal CTA and ultrasound imaging of 10 patients.

1 Introduction

Conventional 2D ultrasound systems can be equipped with position sensing to perform 3D acquisitions of arbitrary size, and to obtain spatial information during the exam. The fusion of such 3D freehand ultrasound imaging with tomographic modalities can, among many other applications, improve the diagnostic value (e.g. for assessment of indeterminate lesions, therefore the term *Diagnostic Fusion*), and integrate anatomic and planning information for interventional navigation of needle procedures. This requires that the target anatomy is precisely registered in ultrasound and the pre-operative modality. Doing so in an automated manner is very challenging, and an active area of research. in [1], image-based registration of MRI to 3DUS is achieved by using both MRI intensity and gradient information in a similarity criterion based on Correlation Ratio. Automatic registration on a single kidney CT/US data using Correlation Ratio

N. Ayache, S. Ourselin, A. Maeder (Eds.): MICCAI 2007, Part I, LNCS 4791, pp. 136–143, 2007.
© Springer-Verlag Berlin Heidelberg 2007

as well, here by enhancing the CT intensities with major boundaries, is done in [2]. In [3], both MRI and US are remapped to an intermediate vessel probability representation using training data sets, then cross-correlation is used as similarity measure. In [4], a multi-component similarity measure involving weighted Mutual information is used on CT intensities and edge maps for rigid alignment with freehand ultrasound of the head and neck.

The mentioned methods all require manual initialization of the registration transformation, some need manual frame selection as well. In our work, we present a simulation of ultrasound from CT, which is realistic enough to allow a stable registration, yet is computationally efficient at the same time. This has the side effect that the simulation can be used by physicians or sonographers in training to get a feeling for the accessibility and optimal orientations even before the ultrasound exam, or the ultrasound-guided intervention. Besides, a novel similarity measure is developed, which is invariant to missing simulation details, hence having smooth properties and a global maximum at the correct alignment.

2   Simulation of Ultrasound from CT

An ultrasound wave is partly reflected whenever a change in acoustic impedance is encountered in the imaged tissue. The acoustic impedance $Z = \rho c$ depends on the tissue density ρ and the speed of sound c. Ultrasound machines assume a constant $c = 1540 m/s$ in human soft tissue, while a significantly different speed of sound occurs e.g. in air and bone. The ratio of an ultrasound wave intensity reflected at a tissue interface with different acoustic impedances Z_1 and Z_2 is $(Z_2 - Z_1)^2/(Z_2 + Z_1)^2$, given a specular interface with angle of incidence equal to the angle of reflection. The diffuse reflection, reflected straight back to the ultrasound transducer depends on the angle:

$$\Delta r(Z_1, Z_2, \theta) = (\cos \theta)^n \left(\frac{Z_2 - Z_1}{Z_2 + Z_1} \right)^2 \tag{1}$$

$$t(Z_1, Z_2) = 1 - \left(\frac{Z_2 - Z_1}{Z_2 + Z_1} \right)^2 = \frac{4 Z_2 Z_1}{(Z_2 + Z_1)^2} \tag{2}$$

The exponent n describes the heterogenity on the interface, causing the amount of reflection to be more or less narrow around the perpendicular of the tissue interface. We lack detailed physical knowledge from CT, hence we use $n = 1$, as it produces good results and simplifies the equations. The transmitted intensity $t(Z_1, Z_2)$ does not depend on the angle of incidence,if refraction is neglected.

The X-Ray attenuation μ measured by a CT scanner is approximately proportional to the tissue density, see e.g. [5] for a reference table. As tissue density is in turn proportional to acoustic impedance, we can directly derive the an incremental acoustic intensity reflection from it:

$$\Delta r(\boldsymbol{x}, \boldsymbol{d}) = \left(\boldsymbol{d}^T \frac{\nabla \mu(\boldsymbol{x})}{|\nabla \mu(\boldsymbol{x})|} \right)^n \left(\frac{|\nabla \mu(\boldsymbol{x})|}{2\mu(\boldsymbol{x})} \right)^2 \tag{3}$$

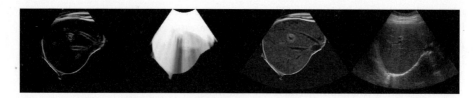

Fig. 1. Simulation of ultrasonic effects from CT, from left to right: Reflection r, transmission t, simulation $r + p$, original ultrasound. 3-dimensional Perlin noise has been added to the occluded part of the simulation.

$$\text{for } n = 1: \quad \Delta r(\boldsymbol{x}, \boldsymbol{d}) = \left(\boldsymbol{d}^T \nabla\mu(\boldsymbol{x})\right) \frac{|\nabla\mu(\boldsymbol{x})|}{(2\mu(\boldsymbol{x}))^2} \tag{4}$$

$$t(\boldsymbol{x}) = 1 - \left(\frac{|\nabla\mu(\boldsymbol{x})|}{2\mu(\boldsymbol{x})}\right)^2 \tag{5}$$

$\mu(\boldsymbol{x})$ is the CT attenuation value at position $\boldsymbol{x}$, $\nabla\mu(\boldsymbol{x})$ its spatial derivative. $\boldsymbol{d}$ is a unit vector denoting the direction of the ultrasound wave propagation, the scalar multiplication with the normed CT gradient vector yields the angular dependency equivalent to $cos(\theta)$. The ultrasound wave intensity is reduced according to $t(\boldsymbol{x})$ at each tissue interface, while $\Delta r(\boldsymbol{x}, \boldsymbol{d})$ contributes to the wave intensity detected by the probe. Integrating over this reflection and transmission behavior yields for any depth along a scanline:

$$I(\boldsymbol{x}) = I_0 \exp\left(-\int_0^{\lambda_x} \left(\frac{|\nabla\mu(\boldsymbol{x_0} + \lambda\boldsymbol{d})|}{2\mu(\boldsymbol{x_0} + \lambda\boldsymbol{d})}\right)^2 d\lambda\right) \left(\boldsymbol{d}^T \nabla\mu(\boldsymbol{x})\right) \frac{|\nabla\mu(\boldsymbol{x})|}{(2\mu(\boldsymbol{x}))^2} \tag{6}$$

where I_0 is the original intensity of the ultrasound pulse, we define it as $I_0 = 1$. In addition, we apply a log-compression with one parameter a, which amplifies smaller reflections (resembling the Dynamic Range knob on the ultrasound machine), yielding the resulting value of the simulation:

$$r(\boldsymbol{x}) = (log(1 + aI(\boldsymbol{x})))(log(1 + a)) \tag{7}$$

For a linear array probe, the integral in equation 6 can be computed efficiently by traversing the columns in the simulated ultrasound image from top to bottom while updating the transmitted intensity based on the interpolated CT intensity and gradient values. For curvilinear arrays, we compute the image row-wise from top to bottom, while using an auxiliary channel storing the remaining transmitted ultrasound wave intensity (starting with 1 in the first row). For every pixel, this transmission value is retrieved by linear interpolation from two pixels in the above row, according to the ultrasound ray angle derived from the curvilinear geometry.

This provides a means to simulate large-scale ultrasonic reflection at tissue boundaries, and the related shadowing effects at strong interfaces like bone. However, individual tissue types have specific echogeneity and speckle patterns

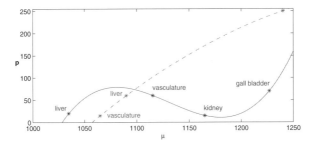

Fig. 2. Intensity mapping p for CT (red, dashed) and portal-venous CTA (blue) soft tissue. Note that the liver-vasculature relation is inverted in the two modalities.

by themselves, based on the microscopic tissue inhomogenities. There is no simple relationship between tissue echogeneity and CT hounsfield units, therefore we add an intensity mapping $p(\boldsymbol{x})$ (further described in section 3.2) on a narrow soft-tissue range to the simulated large-scale reflection $r(\boldsymbol{x})$. Figure 1 depicts the simulation result for a transversal liver image.

3 CT-Ultrasound Registration

3.1 Automatic Frame Selection

Since we simulate ultrasound imaging effects with respect to the probe geometry, the original B-mode scan planes of the sweep have to be used rather than a 3D reconstruction. Neighboring frames of the freehand sweep contain similar information, hence we use always the one out of n frames that has the highest image entropy. This assures that frames which contain unique fine vascularity, that can be located in CT as well, are picked for registration. If two neighboring frames have the highest entropy out of their group of n, only one of them (again with the highest entropy) is used. Furthermore, a threshold is used to discard frames at the beginning and end of the sweep with little structures. In our experiments, n=3 was used, resulting in 15-22 frames per sweep for registration.

3.2 Idealized Intensity Prior

It seems appropriate to use statistical similarity metrics like Mutual Information (MI) and Correlation Ratio (CR) for assessing the correspondence of original CT and ultrasound intensities. In their general formulation, however, they do not work well for our registration problem, since there are too many possible configurations where the Joint Entropy is minimal (for MI), or the intensities from one image can be predicted well from the other one (for CR). At correct alignment of CT and US, they typically produced only a small local optimum. Known approaches for restricting the possible intensity distributions are distance metrics to Joint Histograms learnt from correct registrations (e.g. Kullback-Leibler-Distance), as well as bootstrapping parameters for a polynomial intensity mapping in the actual registration process itself [1]. In both cases, very important information is disregarded, as e.g. small vascularity is essential for a correct registration within the liver, but due its appearance on a relatively small fraction of the image content, it would neither affect a Joint Histogram or a least-squares estimate of a polynomial intensity mapping. Since CT attenuation measurements are mostly reproducible, we define a mapping function $p(\mu)$ based on a number of correspondences (liver tissue, liver vasculature, kidney, gall bladder) between CT/CTA intensities and tissue echogeneity in ultrasound, see figure 2.

3.3   Similarity Measure

In a Correlation Ratio framework, the registration transformation parameters are modified in order to maximize

$$CR = 1 - \frac{\sum_{x \in \Omega}(U(x) - f(\mu(T(x))))^2}{|\Omega|\mathrm{Var}(I)} \tag{8}$$

with f denoting the mapping function which estimates the intensities of the image U from the transformed image μ. If a linear mapping $f(\mu) = \alpha\mu + \beta$ is assumed, equation 8 can be directly related to the common Normalized Cross-Correlation (NCC) similarity metric.

For a pixel intensity in the ultrasound image, it is unknown how much the contribution of large-scale reflections and general tissue echogeneity is. Hence both the mapped CT intensity $p(\mu)$ and the simulated reflection r have to be integrated in a correlation framework with the ultrasound intensity. Using the notation $p_i = p(\mu(T(\boldsymbol{x_i}))), r_i = r(T(\boldsymbol{x_i})), u_i = U(\boldsymbol{x_i})$ for the intensity triple at a certain voxel, we define the intensity function as

$$f(\boldsymbol{x_i}) = \alpha p_i + \beta r_i + \gamma \tag{9}$$

The unknown parameters α, β and γ then have to minimize

$$\left\| M \begin{pmatrix} \alpha \\ \beta \\ \gamma \end{pmatrix} - \begin{pmatrix} u_1 \\ \vdots \\ u_n \end{pmatrix} \right\|^2 \quad \text{with } M = \begin{pmatrix} p_1 & r_1 & 1 \\ \vdots & \vdots & \vdots \\ p_n & r_n & 1 \end{pmatrix} \tag{10}$$

Therefore the solution is

$$\begin{pmatrix} \alpha \\ \beta \\ \gamma \end{pmatrix} = (M^T M)^{-1} M \begin{pmatrix} u_1 \\ \vdots \\ u_n \end{pmatrix} = \begin{pmatrix} \sum p_i^2 & \sum p_i r_i & \sum p_i \\ \sum p_i r_i & \sum r_i^2 & \sum r_i \\ \sum p_i & \sum r_i & n \end{pmatrix}^{-1} \begin{pmatrix} \sum p_i u_i \\ \sum r_i u_i \\ \sum u_i \end{pmatrix} \tag{11}$$

Direct inversion of the symetric matrix $M^T M$ results in a closed-form solution for the parameters. They are then inserted in equation 8 to yield a novel registration similarity metric, which we denote *Linear Correlation of Linear Combination (LC^2)*. It assesses the correlation of ultrasound intensities u_i and a

Table 1. Registration results on 10 patient data sets in terms of the Fiducial Registration Error (FRE) as root mean square (RMS) values in mm

Patient	no. points	manual	pt-based	rigid	affine	remarks
1	8	13.8	9.0	17.0	11.4	strong compresson at top
2	7	16.8	10.0	14.4	8.5	
3	11	10.6	8.9	12.0	11.2	10cm renal tumor
5	5	10.0	8.4	15.5	8.7	kidney
6	7	8.0	6.2	10.7	9.9	
7	11	9.1	6.5	10.8	9.3	pt-based reg. visually bad
9	15	4.2	3.5	7.6	6.8	rigid and affine reg. excellent
11	8	11.1	5.6	8.2	8.2	
13	5	11.6	10.7	13.4	12.3	
14	13	6.6	5.4	7.8	8.0	

linear combination with unknown weights of signals p_i, r_i extracted from CT. The value of LC^2 is constant with respect to brightness and contrast changes of the ultrasound image (as NCC), but also independent to how much of the two described physical effects contributes to the image intensities. The latter is important, since e.g. hepatic vasculature or the gall bladder is represented mostly by p (different intensities due to echogeneity in ultrasound, no borders), while large-scale tissue interfaces correspond to r (strong edge in ultrasound, comparable intensities on both sides).

We compute equations 11 and 8 for every ultrasound frame in the set, and use the mean of the results as cost function.

3.4   Optimization Strategy

A rough initial estimate of the orientation is obtained from the tracking setup. The large-scale translation is determined by performing a brute-force scan of the translation space. On the configuration which yields the highest similarity measure value (for a number of similar high results, the one closest to a reasonable preset translation is used), a local optimization of the translation is executed using a Simplex-based non-linear optimizer [6]. Successively, all six parameters of the rigid transformation are refined. As an optional last step, an optimization is executed on all rigid and three selected affine transformation parameters. These are the two scaling parameters and the one shearing of the sagittal plane, since respiratory motion mainly causes deformation in that plane [7].

4   Results

An abdominal diagnostic fusion study was performed on 10 patients with various pathology. Our freehand ultrasound system uses an Ascension MicroBird magnetic tracking system with a Siemens Sequoia ultrasound machine and progressive RGBS video fed into a PC with frame grabber. The position sensor was

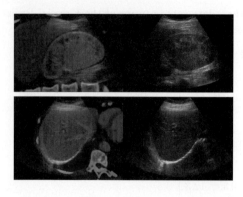 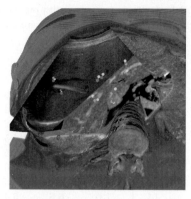

Fig. 3. Left: kidney of patient 5, rigid reg. and liver of patient 6, affine reg. Right: Registered liver of patient 9 with fiducial points (yellow=CT, green=initial US, red=registered US), an oblique CT plane and contextual cutaway volume rendering [9] of CT.

affixed to the transducer using hot-melt adhesive, a method based on [8] was used to determine the calibration. We used the portal-venous phase CTA scans on a dual-source Siemens Somatom Definition scanner, and transversal liver ultrasound sweeps (except for one patient, where a kidney sweep was chosen) for evaluation of the algorithm.

After manually aligning each of the data sets, a physician selected 5-15 point correspondences on anatomical landmarks, including portal & hepativ vein, biliary duct, aorta vena cava and heart atrium. Table 1 lists the RMS distances after manual alignment, point-based rigid registration according to [10], and rigid & semi-affine registration using our methods. The automatic registration converges correctly for all patients with an execution time of $\sim$ 20 seconds. At the initial estimate (before the translation search), the FRE was between $11 - 62mm$. The errors after automatic alignment are in the same range of the manual ones, but larger than the residual errors after point-based registration. Since all of the registrations seem visually correct (some results are depicted in figure 3), we assume to have a fairly large uncertainty in the definition of point correspondences, especially in cranio-caudal direction. This confirms that manual CT-ultrasound registration is error-prone, as it usually reduces the problem to definition of points on 2D-planes, or manually aligning a single 2D plane (as in use in existing products for interventional CT-US navigation) - not guaranteeing a correct matching in 3D. If affine registration is used, displacements mostly on the top of the images are further reduced (often a large shift of the gall bladder was decreased), accounting for the majority of errors caused by probe pressure, breathing and different patient setup. We expect that the FRE values (all $< 2cm$) represent an upper bound for a target registration error (TRE) on liver lesions (which we did not define in the scope of this study due to difficult locatability of relevant clinical targets in most of the data).

Regarding the diagnostic value of the study, reading of the registered CT/US data could exclude a number of suspicions on a total of five patients, including partial portal vein thrombosis, acute inflammation of the gall bladder and infiltration of renal cancer into liver tissue.

5 Discussion and Conclusion

We have presented a system for fully automatic alignment of a single freehand ultrasound sweep with CT and CTA data. We expect this to greatly increase the acceptance of multimodal fusion for a number of clinical applications, since it provides a simple workflow and enables more precise registration. Further clinical studies on diagnostic and interventional fusion using the described method are underway. A local variant of the developed LC^2 measure is possible by averaging over smaller overlapping patches, which can further increase the robustness with respect to ultrasound imaging artifacts not covered by the simulation, as well as user adjustments on the ultrasound machine. Besides, LC^2 can easily be extended to handle a larger number of signals from both modalities. Real-time compensation of respiratory motion and deformable mapping techniques will be investigated as well, based on the proposed methods.

References

1. Roche, A., Pennec, X., Malandain, G., Ayache, N.: Rigid registration of 3D ultra-sound with MR images: a new approach combining intensity and gradient information. IEEE Trans. Med. Imag. 20, 1038–1049 (2001)
2. Leroy, A., Mozer, P., Payan, Y., Troccaz, J.: Rigid registration of freehand 3D ultrasound and CT-Scan kidney images. In: Barillot, C., Haynor, D.R., Hellier, P. (eds.) MICCAI 2004. LNCS, vol. 3216, p. 837. Springer, Heidelberg (2004)
3. Penney, G., Blackall, J., Hamady, M., Sabharwal, T., Adam, A., Hawkes, D.: Registration of freehand 3D ultrasound and magnetic resonance liver images. Medical Image Analysis 8, 81–91 (2004)
4. Wein, W., Röper, B., Navab, N.: Automatic registration and fusion of ultrasound with CT for radiotherapy. In: Duncan, J.S., Gerig, G. (eds.) MICCAI 2005. LNCS, vol. 3750, pp. 303–311. Springer, Heidelberg (2005)
5. Schneider, U., Pedroni, E., Lomax, A.: The calibration of CT hounsfield units for radiotherapy treatment planning. Phys. Med. Biol. 41, 111–124 (1996)
6. Press, W.H., Teukolsky, S.A., Vetterling, W.T., Flannery, B.P.: Numerical Recipes in C, 2nd edn. CRC Press, Inc. (1992)
7. Rohlfing, J.T., Maurer, C.R.: Modeling liver motion and deformation during the respiratory cycle using intensity-based nonrigid registration of gated MR images. Medical Physics 31, 427–432 (2004)
8. Rousseau, F., Hellier, P., Barillot, C.: Confhusius: A robust and fully automatic calibration method for 3D freehand ultrasound. Medical Image Analysis 9 (2005)
9. Burns, M., Haidacher, M., Wein, W., Viola, I., Groeller, E.: Feature emphasis and contextual cutaways for multimodal medical visualization. In: EuroVis 2007 Proceedings (2007)
10. Walker, M., Shao, L., Volz, R.: Estimating 3-D location parameters using dual number quaternions. CVGIP: Image Understanding, 358–367 (1991)

Medical and Technical Protocol for Automatic Navigation of a Wireless Device in the Carotid Artery of a Living Swine Using a Standard Clinical MRI System

Sylvain Martel[1], Jean-Baptiste Mathieu[1], Ouajdi Felfoul[1], Arnaud Chanu[1],
Eric Aboussouan[1], Samer Tamaz[1], Pierre Pouponneau[1], L'Hocine Yahia[2],
Gilles Beaudoin[3], Gilles Soulez[3], and Martin Mankiewicz[1]

[1] NanoRobotics Laboratory, Department of Computer Engineering and Institute of
Biomedical Engineering, École Polytechnique de Montréal (EPM), Campus de l'université de
Montréal, P.O. Box 6079, Station Centre-ville, Montréal (Québec), Canada H3C 3A7
[2] Laboratoire d'Innovation et d'Analyse de la Bioperformance (LIAB), École Polytechnique
de Montréal, Montréal, (Québec), Canada
[3] CHUM-Hôpital Notre-Dame Département de radiologie, Pavillon Lachapelle (CHUM)
Bureau C-1077 1560 Sherbrooke est Montréal (Québec) Canada H2L 4M1
{Sylvain.Martel,Jean-Baptiste.Mathieu,Ouajdi.Felfoul,
Arnaud.Chanu,Eric.Aboussouan,Samer.Tamaz,Pierre.Pouponneau,
L'Hocine Yahia,Martin.Mankiewicz}@polymtl.ca,
{Gilles.Beaudoin,Gilles.Soulez}@umontreal.ca

Astract. A 1.5 mm magnetic sphere was navigated automatically inside the carotid artery of a living swine. The propulsion force, tracking and real-time capabilities of a Magnetic Resonance Imaging (MRI) system were integrated into a closed loop control platform. The sphere was released using an endovascular catheter approach. Specially developed software is responsible for the tracking, propulsion, event timing and closed loop position control in order to follow a 10 roundtrips preplanned trajectory on a distance of 5 cm inside the right carotid artery of the animal. Experimental protocol linking the technical aspects of this *in vivo* assay is presented. In the context of this demonstration, many challenges which provide insights about concrete issues of future nanomedical interventions and interventional platforms have been identified and addressed.

Keywords: Magnetic resonance imaging, wireless, tracking, control, *in vivo* assay.

1 Introduction

The possibility of controlling magnetic particles using external magnetic fields opens the way for many medical applications. This potential has been acknowledged for many years now as, back in 1965, aneurism embolization studies were based on micron sized iron powders spatially confined with magnetic tipped catheters [1]. Ever since, magnetic drug delivery carriers have evolved and are now composed of state of the art nanoparticles such as stealth magnetoliposomes or smart polymer based

N. Ayache, S. Ourselin, A. Maeder (Eds.): MICCAI 2007, Part I, LNCS 4791, pp. 144–152, 2007.
© Springer-Verlag Berlin Heidelberg 2007

magnetic particles [2-5]. Targeting of these particles is still performed using external magnets or magnetized needles or catheters. Magnetic targeting would greatly benefit from an increase of the role of computerized platforms to achieve automated control over the spatial distribution of the particles.

Stereotaxis for example proposes a computerized steering platform for catheters. Their magnetic tipped catheters can be steered using actuated external magnets [6]. Orientation of the catheters is controlled by computerized platform acting on the tilt angle of the external magnets. Proper corrective action is computed based on tracking information from X-ray projection images.

Computer controlled magnetic guidance platforms able to navigate magnetic particles to target the deepest recesses of the human body are currently under development.

In [7,8], magnetic microdevices are navigated *in vitro* using a custom built coil apparatus relying on Helmholtz and Maxwell pairs. Optical tracking methods provide simple and effective solutions for the needs of theses applications. As a matter of fact, these microdevices are developed for future surgical procedures in transparent media such as the vitreous humor.

Optical tracking methods cannot be used for endovascular applications. In this environment, using medical imaging scanners to obtain tracking feedback data is mandatory. In addition to being widespread in hospitals, MRI scanners provide a magnetic actuation method without depth limitation [9,10], real-time interventional software architecture [12], X-Ray free unparalleled soft tissue contrast and high precision and high sensitivity tracking [11]. These positive features make the use of MRI systems as a core element for novel interventional platforms a very promising approach.

In vivo computerized navigation of a 1.5 mm sphere in the carotid artery of a living swine was achieved through proper integration of the different components of a clinical MRI system [13].

This paper presents the integration issues and the medical and technical protocol involved in achieving this proof of concept. It begins with a description of the system architecture followed by the experimental protocol (animal preparation, tracking, trajectory planning). Real-time *in vivo* navigation is then described followed by sphere release and retrieval techniques.

2   System Overview

The interventional procedure is executed using a standard clinical MRI system (Siemens Magnetom Avanto 1.5T, Erlangen, Germany) with real-time feedback capabilities. A ferromagnetic sphere is propelled in the vascular network of a living swine through the application of magnetic gradient pulses using standard imaging magnetic gradient coils already present on all MRI systems [9, 13]. A comprehensive custom software environment for the control, propulsion and tracking is responsible for the device navigation in the swine [11] with a feedback control frequency of 24 Hz. An overview of the real-time pulse sequence used for the device navigation is illustrated on Fig.1.

For the device to be continuously navigated across a given path, a feedback loop must be present in order to provide a control loop between the decision element, in our case the reconstruction computer, and the execution element, the MRI scanner itself. The real-time feedback capabilities allow the modification of pulse sequence events such as RadioFrequency (RF) pulses, magnetic gradient or ADC on the fly. The developed dedicated software architecture depicted in Fig.1 consists of a path planning module, a tracking module, propulsion and controller module, and a central agent.

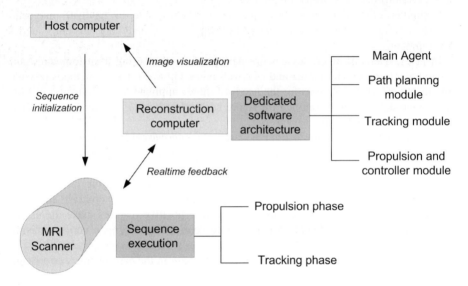

Fig. 1. Overview of the computer architecture incorporated in the standard Siemens environment. The host computer is responsible for the real-time sequence compilation and initialization before being sent for execution on the scanner. This computer also serves as the visualization computer after the image reconstruction step is over. The MRI scanner is the actual hardware that runs the pulse sequence for data acquisition. Finally, the reconstruction computer is responsible for the image generation after the data acquisition step on the scanner is done. In the presented dedicated software environment, a feedback loop exists between the reconstruction computer and the MRI scanner which allows the pulse sequence to be modified on the fly.

All these modules are located in a reconstruction routine in the reconstruction computer. A sequence environment is responsible for the application of the tracking sequence and the propulsion sequence which is executed by the scanner. The reconstruction routine is mainly responsible for the command generation in order to propel the device in a given direction based on the actual position and pre-computed trajectory. Since the device is moved using the magnetic gradient coils already present on the MRI system, the computed command calculated inside the propulsion and controller module is a magnetic gradient amplitude and direction to be applied in the next pulse sequence propulsion phase. The real-time MRI pulse sequence developed is a successive repetition of a propulsion phase which consists of the application of a magnetic gradient oriented in space with a given amplitude and an off-resonance tracking phase based on [12]. An overview of the pulse sequence is illustrated in Fig.2.

The image calculation environment consists of two simultaneous running processes. The first process contains the control module which computes the required command to be applied in the next propulsion phase of the real-time sequence. This process is called up through the real-time feedback loop trigger located in the sequence described above. The second process is the tracking module and is called up from the tracking phase of the sequence. It is responsible for the device position computation based on the acquired data of the sequence tracking sequence.

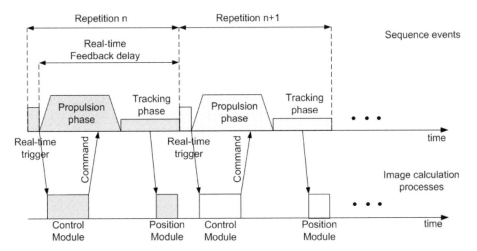

Fig. 2. Overview of the real-time sequence and the image calculation processes for the navigation of the magnetic sphere. A sequence kernel composed of a real-time trigger event, a propulsion phase event and a tracking event is repeated over time. The real-time trigger event starts the control module process for the command generation and the tracking phase calls up the position module process for the device position calculation.

Projections taking advantage of the magnetic field being induced by the sphere are used for tracking [11]. Following the application of a non-selective off-resonance RF pulse, only the spins surrounding the device are excited. Readout gradient are then used to acquire three orthogonal projections that are processed by the tracking module. Once computed, the position is stored for the next command computation in the control module. A central agent is responsible for the overall modules interactions and for the command sending to the running pulse sequence.

The real-time feedback delay depicted in Fig.2 is the minimum time allowed for the command computation and transmission. It is set by the user prior to the intervention. Below this delay, the command computation cannot be completed and the sequence is aborted. Since the sequence tracking phase duration is fixed and lasts 22 ms for a 3D positioning scheme, the propulsion phase delay is thus only dependent on the real-time feedback delay and is equal to the real-time feedback delay minus the tracking delay. A longer propulsion phase translates into a longer force application time on the device but also in a shorter operating control frequency. Moreover, a longer propulsion phase means a longer contribution time of the magnetic gradient coils which could lead to a heating threshold overshoot, preventing the sequence execution.

3 Interventional Protocol

3.1 Animal Preparation

In vivo experiments are performed on a 25 kg domestic swine under general anaesthesia (Pentobarbital). This assay study is pre-approved by the animal care and use committee. One 6-F, 80 cm long introducer catheter (Cook, Bloomington, Indiana) is inserted through a right femoral approach into the proximal portion of the right carotid artery under fluoroscopic guidance (HICOR/ACOM-TOP, Siemens, Erlangen, Germany). A short 5-F introducer is also positioned in the left femoral artery and a 5 mm × 18 mm angioplasty balloon (AV100, Medtronic, Santa Rosa, CA) is advanced under fluoroscopic guidance in the distal portion of the right common carotid artery (10 cm downstream to the tip of the long introducer) over a 0.018" guide wire. The long introducer is used as the release route for the magnetic sphere to be controlled whereas the balloon catheter is used to control the flow and eventually block the sphere in order to facilitate its retrieval upon completion of the control experiments.

The swine is placed in the MRI scanner. A spine with a body array coils are used to collect the MRI signal. The animal is inserted feet first supine and centered inside the MRI bore with respect to its carotid artery. The 6-F inner dilator catheter of the long introducer catheter is used to push a chrome steel sphere inside the long introducer. The sphere is brought in pre-release position 15 mm before the distal tip of the long introducer using a color marking on the inner dilator as a visual landmark. The balloon catheter is inflated to prevent the sphere from being carried away in case of unplanned problems. The real time MRI sequence is then started and the sphere can be released by pushing the dilator all the way through the long introducer. Once the sphere is released, its movement is dealt with by the control sequence which objective is to navigate it by following the waypoints. After travelling through all of the waypoints, the control sequence is turned off and the tracking data history is saved.

3.2 Tracking

Since tracking of the ferromagnetic sphere relies on its magnetic signature, it is critical not to have any other magnetic source present in the imaging volume. An off-resonance imaging sequence is used to verify that the volume of interest is free from magnetic perturbation that can interfere with the tracking phase.

The volume is screened to ensure that there is no magnetic perturbation. The device is introduced inside the arteries attached to a catheter and brought as close as possible to the operating region. The tracking sequence is then executed in order to fine tune its parameters like the offset RF frequency, the flip angle and bandwidth per pixel. These parameters depend in fact on the magnetic characteristic and size of the device being used as well as the background tissues where the acquisition is done.

3.3 Angiography, Path Planning and Registration

Once the animal has been tested for magnetic perturbations, a roadmap of the environment and the trajectory for the sphere are determined. First step of the process implies imaging the Region Of Interest (ROI) using a standard MRI angiographic sequence with gadoteridol (ProHance, Bracco Diagnostics, Mississauga, Canada). Threshold filtering is applied on the 3D scan to allow better visualization of the target region before the path-planning step.

In order to determine the path the device will follow, waypoints are placed in the acquired volume (Fig. 3). Eleven waypoints consisting of three coordinates with a back and forth trajectory between the last two coordinates, are set. The next procedure implies transforming these points in the global MRI coordinates axis of reference. The registration software developed as a combination of an MRI sequence and a Matlab script is used to analyze the device position, transform the waypoints coordinates to the MRI frame of reference and display the result over the image acquired earlier. Synchronisation of the waypoint trajectory file with the real actual position of the sphere in reference to the isocenter of the MRI is then performed [14].

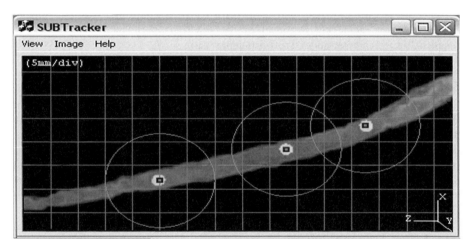

Fig. 3. 3D volume of the carotid artery of the swine filtered at 50% of the image scalar intensity range. Dots show the waypoints the sphere followed, circles show the precision regions of radius φ .

4 Endovascular Navigation

4.1 Real-Time Navigation

Once the waypoints are in the correct axis coordinate system, they are saved in a path file containing all the 3D positions to be reached during the intervention. Before the sequence is started, the waypoints list is loaded into memory in the control module for fast access during the operation. During the execution, the device's position coordinates computed through the tracking module process are compared with the next waypoint to be reached. If the error distance between the bead and the waypoint is comprised in a circle of radius φ centered on the waypoint's position (Fig.3.), the waypoint is considered to be reached and the next waypoint is loaded for the destination. The circle radius was set to $\varphi = 10$ mm prior to the intervention.

Real-time navigation of the ferromagnetic sphere in the carotid artery of the swine requires a proper real-time feedback delay to be chosen in order to allow both a sufficient propulsion power and a sufficient operating frequency to ensure stability and efficiency for the control loop. Prior to the *in vivo* intervention, many navigation experiments in MRI phantoms have been realized in order to empirically obtain the optimal real-time feedback delay. A feedback delay of 41 ms was chosen for the *in vivo* intervention, leading to a propulsion phase delay of 19 ms considering a fixed tracking time of 22 ms. The total sequence repetition time is thus 30.6 ms leading to an achievable operation frequency of 24 Hz for autonomous navigation. This operation frequency is adequate for device navigation through the selected trajectory described in 3.3. A real-time imaging sequence provided by Siemens (Trufi-irttt) is used to monitor the introduction of the sphere through the long introducer. The real-time control program is then started, deals with the position of the sphere through the 11 waypoints of the trajectory and stabilizes it on the last one. A maximum velocity of 13 cm/s was achieved. Retrieval of the sphere is performed using a custom magnetic tipped catheter under Trufi-irttt supervision.

5   Conclusion

It was demonstrated that MRI systems provide all the components for implementing a medical device navigation platform (actuation method, imaging of biological tissues, device tracking and computer feedback). The methodology described in the previous sections identifies the main aspects and constraints related with future nanomedical interventional protocols. It addresses the aspects of system architecture design, fast and precise tracking technique, path planning, coordinate system registration as well as device release and recovery.

The long term objective of the project is the spatial control of an agglomeration of magnetic micro/nano devices for targeted delivery of drugs and biosensors. Such agglomeration will be injected as a bolus of a magnetic colloidal suspension that will be carried by the blood flow and guided using external magnetic gradients.

Both the methodology and navigation platform will have to be adapted for that purpose. Due to the scaling laws of magnetic propulsion, special hardware components will have to be developed to generate sufficient magnetophoretic velocity for the micro/nano particles [10]. The tracking scheme will likely change from an Off resonance excitation based technique to a more sensitive T2* contrast method while the injected bolus will get dilute when spreading in the vascular bed. A learning control algorithm will have to be implemented in order to determine an optimal steering gradient combination for targeting. Other improvements will arise from the refinement of the protocol and methods with time and usage. As a matter of fact, in its current state, the protocol that was described in this paper can take several hours to be executed. Many steps during the procedure will have to be made automatic before it can gain acceptance from the physicians. Short terms applications of this navigation platform can also be envisioned since small modifications of clinical MRI systems would allow them to navigate readily available medical instruments such as catheters with minimum investment from hospitals.

References

1. Alksne, J.F., Fingerhunt, A.G.: Magnetically controlled metallic thrombosis of intracranial aneurysms. Bull. Los Angeles Neurol. Soc. 30, 153–155 (1965)
2. Alexiou, C., Arnold, W., Hulin, P., Klein, R.J., Renz, H., Parak, F.G., Bergemann, C., Lubbe, A.S.: Magnetic mitoxantrone nanoparticle detection by histology, X-ray and MRI after magnetic tumor targeting. Journal of Magnetism and Magnetic Materials 225(1-2), 187–193 (2001)
3. Babincova, M., Cicmanec, P., Altanerova, V., Altaner, C., Babinec, O.: AC-magnetic field controlled drug release from magnetoliposomes: Design of a method for site-specific chemotherapy. Bioelectrochemistry 55(1-2), 17–19 (2002)
4. Morales, M.A., Jain, T.K., Labhasetwar, V., Leslie-Pelecky, D.L.: Magnetic studies of iron oxide nanoparticles coated with oleic acid and Pluronic block copolymer. Journal of Applied Physics 97(10) (2005)
5. Viroonchatapan, E., Ueno, M., Sato, H., Adachi, I., Nagae, H., Tazawa, K., Horikoshi, I.: Preparation and characterization of dextran magnetite-incorporated thermosensitive liposomes: an on-line flow system for quantifying magnetic responsiveness. Pharm Res. 12, 1176–1183 (1995)
6. Stereotaxis. Stereotaxis Home. Page last accessed: 20/03/2007, http://www.stereotaxis.com/
7. Yesin, K.B., Exner, P., Vollmers, K., Nelson, B.J.: Design and control of in-vivo magnetic microrobots. In: Duncan, J.S., Gerig, G. (eds.) MICCAI 2005. LNCS, vol. 3749, pp. 819–826. Springer, Heidelberg (2005)
8. Yesin, K.B., Vollmers, K., Nelson, B.J.: Modeling and control of untethered biomicrorobots in a fluidic environment using electromagnetic fields. International Journal of Robotics Research 25(5-6), 527–536 (2006)
9. Mathieu, J.-B., Beaudoin, G., Martel, S.: Method of propulsion of a ferromagnetic core in the cardiovascular system through magnetic gradients generated by an MRI system. IEEE Transactions on Biomedical Engineering 53(2), 292–299 (2006)
10. Mathieu, J.-B., Martel, S.: Magnetic Steering of Iron Oxide Microparticles Using Propulsion Gradient Coils in MRI. In: Proceedings of 28th Annual International Conference of the IEEE in Engineering in Medicine and Biology Society EMBS; New York City, USA (2006)
11. Felfoul, O., Mathieu, J.-B., Beaudoin, G., Martel, S.: MR-tracking Based on Magnetic Signature Selective Excitation. IEEE Transactions On Medical Imaging. (Accepted, to be published ref# TMI-2006-0769) (2007)
12. Chanu, A., Aboussouan, E., Tamaz, S., Martel, S.: Sequence Design and Software Environment for Real-time Navigation of a Wireless Ferromagnetic Device using MRI System and Single Echo 3D Tracking. In: Proceedings of 28th Annual International Conference of the IEEE in Engineering in Medicine and Biology Society EMBS; New York City, USA pp. 1746–1749 (2006)

13. Martel, S., Mathieu, J.-B., Felfoul, O., Chanu, A., Aboussouan, E., Tamaz, S., Pouponneau, P., Beaudoin, G., Soulez, G., Yahia, L.H., Mankiewicz, M.: Automatic navigation of an untethered device in the artery of a living animal using a conventional clinical magnetic resonance imaging system. Applied Physics Letters 90, 114105 (2007)
14. Aboussouan, E., Martel, S.: High precision absolute positioning of medical instruments in MRI systems. In: Proceedings of 28th Annual International Conference of the IEEE in Engineering in Medicine and Biology Society EMBS, August. 30 - September 3, New York City, USA, pp. 743–746 (2006)

Improving the Contrast of Breast Cancer Masses in Ultrasound Using an Autoregressive Model Based Filter*

Etienne von Lavante and J. Alison Noble

Department of Engineering Science, University of Oxford, UK

Abstract. The assessment and diagnosis of breast cancer with ultrasound is a challenging problem due to the low contrast between cancer masses and benign tissue. Due to this low contrast it has proven to be difficult to achieve reliable segmentation results on breast cancer masses. An autoregressive model has been employed to filter out of the backscattered RF-signal from a tissue harmonic image which is not degraded by harmonic leakage. Measurements on the filtered image have shown a significant (up to 45 %) increase in contrast between cancer masses and benign tissue.

1 Introduction

Ultrasonic imaging has become an indispensable tool used in diagnosis of cancer masses during breast cancer diagnosis. However, despite its central role in breast cancer diagnosis, even for skilled radiologists it is still a challenging problem to correctly diagnose and measure cancer masses. This challenge is reflected in the high number of false positive cancer diagnoses made, leading to roughly half of all biopsies made being unnecessary. The main cause of the high uncertainty in ultrasonic cancer diagnosis is strong image artifacts characteristic to ultrasound imagery, such as attenuation, speckle, shadowing and general low contrast.

It is hoped to decrease the uncertainty of the cancer diagnosis with the help of automated medical image segmentation. However, due to the highly variable nature of cancer masses in both shape and image texture, segmentation methods based on statistical priors such as [1,2] have not shown as much promise as in other areas of medical image analysis. Other recent methods, such as those based on a Bayesian frameworks [3,4] or local image statistics [5], fail to segment cancer masses reliably. The problem these methods face is that, unlike with cysts, the contrast between cancer masses and surrounding tissue is very low and speckle is the predominant image feature. Therefore one question is whether it is possible to develop an enhancement method specifically aimed at enhancing cancer masses.

Recent advances in signal processing have reduced the effect of speckle on the overall image appearance with the introduction of new techniques such as dynamic beam focussing and tissue harmonic imaging. However, speckle still

---

* Research supported by UK EPSRC Grant GR-S94575 01.

N. Ayache, S. Ourselin, A. Maeder (Eds.): MICCAI 2007, Part I, LNCS 4791, pp. 153–160, 2007.
© Springer-Verlag Berlin Heidelberg 2007

remains the predominant texture feature in any ultrasound B-mode image. A lot of research has gone into speckle reducing filters, with one of the most recent ones being the Speckle Reducing Anisotropic Filter [6] derived from the Frost and Lee filters [7,8]. Despite their general effectiveness in reducing speckle, they tend to oversmooth the image, and are consequently rarely used for diagnostic breast ultrasound.

For breast cancer diagnosis the only clinically used method which appears to considerably increase the contrast between cancer masses and surrounding tissue is tissue harmonic imaging [9]. This method can be regarded as one of the current state of the art filtering techniques, which is usually implemented by using finite impulse filters (FIR). This therefore suggests that one should take advantage of the principles of tissue harmonic imaging and filtering in the frequency domain to develop a novel filter which will increase the general contrast of breast cancers.

1.1   Tissue Harmonic Imaging

Due to the nonlinear nature of tissue, the back scattered signal from an ultrasound pulse interacting with its target will contain, besides the fundamental frequency band of the emitted pulse, also higher harmonics of this band. These higher harmonics are mostly generated due to the peaks of transmitted pulse traveling faster than the troughs due to tissue having different velocities for sound wave propagation in compressed tissue as opposed to relaxed tissue. This effect causes very weak harmonics which are accumulated as the emitted ultrasound pulse propagates through tissue [10]. Hence, the signal received at the ultrasound transducer is made up of the fundamental frequency generated by direct reflections of the ultrasound pulse at tissue interfaces and inhomogeneities, and the higher harmonics generated by the tissue itself, called here the tissue harmonic signal.

There are two principal methods for harmonic imaging, the first one is based on using the pulse inversion technique [11], and the other one is by the application of FIR filters to retrieve the fundamental harmonic and second harmonic from the received signal. While the pulse inversion technique is effective in reducing the effects of harmonic leakage from the fundamental harmonic, it has the major disadvantage of halving the effective frame rate and being more susceptible to motion artifacts. Hence, for tissue harmonic imaging the FIR method is preferred despite its problem of harmonic leakage to the fundamental harmonic affecting the higher harmonics [12], which adds additional noise to these harmonics.

2   Method

One way to overcome the effects of harmonic leakage is to develop a linear predictive model of the emitted pulse and then, using parametric spectral estimation, to both estimate the spectral content of the emitted pulse and the remaining tissue harmonic signal. If one has found a good parametric model, the advantages of using such a model compared to Fourier Transform based methods is its ability to detect peaks at superresolution, greater resistance to spectral ringing and reduced computational complexity. In several articles [13,14] an autoregressive (AR) model of the received RF-signal has been used to estimate various tissue parameters from ultrasound data. The output $y(n)$ of such an AR-model of order M is defined as the output of the following linear filter driven by white Gaussian noise $\eta(n)$:

$$y(n) = \eta(n) - \sum_{k=1}^{M} a(k)y(n-k) \tag{1}$$

where $a(k)$ are the AR coefficients of an order M AR-model. Intuitively, most users of ultrasound devices regard the B-mode image as a two dimensional representation of the power of the reflected signal of an insonified target. With this observation and using the model in (1) one can directly compute the power spectral density (PSD) $P_{yy}(f)$, and consequently the power of the signal, as:

$$P_{yy}(f) = \frac{r_p}{\|1 + \sum_{k=1}^{M} a(k)e^{-2j\pi fk}\|^2} \tag{2}$$

In linear predictive modeling this model will correspond to an all-poles model, whose power spectrum will be a series of peaks, corresponding to the AR coefficients $a(k)$, among a general flat noise level, whose power is defined by the residual r_p. The received signal of the emitted pulse can be modelled very closely by an all-poles model, as its power spectrum is, by design, a Gaussian bell-curve. Any noise in the received RF-signal will be due to non-linear interaction of this pulse with tissue, hence corresponding to the signal of the tissue harmonics, as described in the previous section. Using this model, the power of the received tissue harmonic signal is defined by the residue r_p, which can be directly displayed to yield an estimation of the tissue harmonic signal without the noise introduced by harmonic leakage.

In its current implementation $a(k)$ and r_p are estimated from RF-data using Burg's iterative algorithm [15], using an AR-model order of seven, following the recommendation from [13]. Experiments have shown that the results are very robust to the chosen AR-model order. As the resulting residue signal has still a very high dynamic range, the dynamic range has been compressed by applying the Gamma-Brightness correction function, as it is used in analogue screens, to the data before displaying it:

$$P_{yy\text{new}} = P_{yy} \exp(1/\gamma) \qquad \text{with } \gamma = 4.5 \tag{3}$$

The value for the parameter $\gamma = 4.5$ was experimentally chosen to give, in the experiment, a sufficient contrast to detect subtle image details in the filtered image. The value for this variable is image dependent and will vary between 3.5 and 5.0 depending on the desired contrast and viewing preferences of the user.

3   Methods for Evaluation

Unfortunately, due to the cross-patient variability of ultrasound data one cannot compare directly the image statistics of ultrasound data across individual image sets. However, despite these variations, the relative difference of statistics measured between cancer regions and "normal" tissue regions remain remarkably similar across multiple data sets. Hence, in order to evaluate any improvements the filtering technique has on the ability to distinguish cancer masses from healthy tissue, the following procedure was used: various image classifiers computed from a region within the cancer mass and a region of healthy tissue with fully developed speckle were compared in each image. For each image, the contrast to noise ratio (CNR) of each classifier was computed as:

$$CNR = \frac{\|\mu_c - \mu_h\|}{\sqrt{\sigma_c^2 + \sigma_h^2}} \qquad (4)$$

where μ_c and μ_h are the mean of the classifier in the cancer and healthy tissue regions, and σ_c and σ_h are the standard deviation of the classifier in the cancer and healthy tissue regions, respectively. Having calculated both the CNR of the filtered image CNR_f and the original B-mode data CNR_b, one can calculate the percentage fractional improvement of the classifier $frac_{imp}$ as:

$$frac_{\text{imp}} = (CNR_f / CNR_b) * 100 \qquad (5)$$

3.1   Intensity Based Statistics

Using the above method, one can directly compute and compare the general grayscale contrast between cancer masses and healthy tissues. Furthermore, one can also compute the SNR of both the cancer region SNR_c and healthy region SNR_h by [16]:

$$SNR = \bar{I}/\sigma_I \qquad (6)$$

with $\bar{I}$ being the mean intensity and σ_I being the standard deviation of the intensity of the region of interest. However, as the physical principles causing speckle cannot be removed, one should not expect any significant improvement of the SNR by filtering the image, and it will remain by definition close to unity. The main purpose of the SNR is to judge the degree to which speckle is fully developed in the region of interest.

3.2   Texture Measures

Due to the texture created by speckle, any trained clinician will not evaluate a region of interest solely on its image intensity, but rather on the general appearance of image texture. Hence, the 1st order statistics give an incomplete picture of the quality of the filtered image. One of the texture based metrics chosen for the validation of this method is the Neighbourhood Gray-Level Difference

Matrix (NGTDM) [17] and the metrics derived from this statistic. The details on how to populate the NGTDM matrix $s(i)$ can be read in [17]. Using this matrix one can calculate the contrast f_{cont}, busyness f_{busy}, complexity f_{comp} and coarseness f_{coar} of a texture.

3.3 Frequency Domain Analysis

As with all applications of linear predictive modeling, a very important question is the applicability of the employed AR-model to the data. Here the power spectral density (PSD) from a 256 pixel window of a patch with fully developed speckle and of a cancer mass is estimated using a Periodogram. This PSD is then compared to the PSD obtained by estimating (2) over the same data windows.

4   Results and Discussion

4.1   Experimental Set-Up

Since tissue phantoms cannot reproduce the subtleties of real diagnostic ultrasound data, and the main advantage of harmonic imaging is the ability to identify more subtle features, it was chosen to base all experiments solely on already recorded patient data. All data was recorded during a breast cancer study, on an Analogic AN-2300 with a BK-Medical 8805 probe using a centre frequency of 4.0 MHz, and recording the RF-data at a sampling frequency of 40 MHz. From the datasets recorded during this study 25 cancer cases were arbitrarily chosen and analysed using the methods described in Section 3.

4.2   Power Spectrum Analysis

Regarding Fig. 1 proves that the current AR-model indeed estimates with high precision the main harmonics of the backscattered RF-signal. The AR-model also closely follows the frequency shift of the backscattered signal, which is very significant with approximately 2MHz at the cancer patch, and 1MHz at the other one. In terms of power, the difference between the AR-model and the Periodogram is larger in the speckle patch than in the cancer mass patch. Hence, using the model from Section 2 one would expect a stronger r_p signal from the speckle patch. As this is indeed the case in Fig. 4.3, one can conclude that the model developed here has its validity on real life data, despite the AR-model also following the second harmonic and a non-harmonic peak in the speckle signal.

4.3   Discussion of Experimental Data

As can be seen in Fig. 2, when comparing the filtered image to classical B-mode, the quality of the image has been significantly improved. In the filtered image Fig. 4.3 spiculations from the cancer mass are much more pronounced,

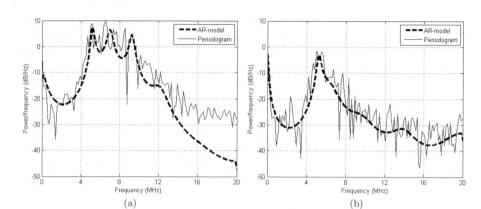

Fig. 1. comparison of the power spectral density estimated by the employed AR-model and using an Periodogram. Both PSD where computed over 256 data point Hamming window. a) Was computed over a patch with fully developed speckle, b) over a cancer mass.

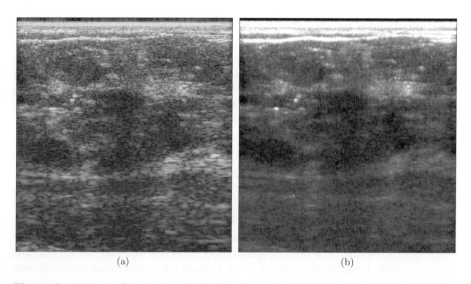

Fig. 2. the image quality improvement is easily noticable between the classical B-Mode image a) and the filtered image b)

and the overall size of the mass appears a bit larger. As cancer masses tend to appear in ultrasound B-Mode images smaller than their true mass, this difference could be of clinical significance. The visual impression is also strongly supported by the image intensity based statistics, with the fractional improvement of the CNR being on average 145%. This large improvement in the CNR was found for almost all images. However there were still some images, such as the first set displayed in 2, where there was no improvement. Surprisingly, the SNR improved noticeably with an average fractional improvement of the SNR_c being 105% and the SNR_h being 118%. As it can be seen in Table 1 the results of the texture measures are more ambiguous. Here, only the contrast f_{cont} and coarseness f_{coar} classifiers have shown consistent results, as the individual values for the busyness f_{busy} and complexity f_{comp} measures have shown a too large variance across the set of images to make any conclusions possible. It appears that these two measures do not well describe the image textures found in ultrasound data. The improvement of the contrast measure of the NGTDM in the filtered was caused by the reduction of speckle inside most cancer regions, producing a very low contrast texture compared to surrounding tissue. The reduction of speckle inside most cancer regions is also responsible for the improvement of coarseness CNR, as the coarseness of the cancer texture in the filtered image has been reduced by a factor of 10, while the coarseness of the surrounding tissue still remains similar to the values for the B-mode data.

Table 1. Experimental Results

	$mean_{bm}$	$mean_{filt}$	σ_{bm}	σ_{filt}	$frac_{imp}$
CNR	0.817	1.187	0.052	0.129	145%
SNR_c	0.94	0.99	0.017	0.014	105%
SNR_h	0.98	1.16	0.008	0.025	118%

	CNR_{bm}	CNR_{filt}	$frac_{imp}$
f_{busy}	0.226	0.49	216%
f_{cont}	2.65	7.89	297%
f_{coar}	0.094	2.387	2539%
f_{comp}	1.33	1.27	95%

5   Conclusion

Both visual inspection and quantitative analysis have shown that the filtered image has in the majority of the datasets a much higher contrast between the cancer masses and its surrounding tissue. This contrast has shown by visual inspection on many cancer masses an improved ability to discern its shape and size. Regarding the quantitative analysis, the improvement of the image intensity CNR is a notable result. This encourages the possibility of developing a more robust breast cancer segmentation algorithm, which is currently work in progress. The algorithm is not computationally demanding, and could be readily implemented in real time on current hardware. Hence, the next step of our research is to implement this filter on to an ultrasound machine, to assess the degree to which the measured increase in contrast and the subjective image improvement effect the diagnosis of breast cancer in clinical practice.

References

1. Xie, J., et al.: Segmentation of kidney from ultrasound images based on texture and shape priors. IEEE Trans. Med. Imag. (1), 45–57 (2005)
2. Zhan, Y., et al.: Deformable segmentation of 3-d ultrasound prostate images using statistical texture matching method. IEEE Trans. Med. Imag. (3), 256–272 (2006)
3. Boukerroui, D., et al.: Segmentation of ultrasound images - multiresoloution 2d and 3d algorithm. . . . Pattern Recognition Letters (4), 779–790 (2003)
4. Xiao, G.: 3-D Free-hand Ultrasound Imaging and Image Analysis of the Breast. PhD thesis, University of Oxford (2001)
5. Madabhushi, A., et al.: Combining low-, high-level and empirical domain knowledge for automated segmentation. . . . IEEE Trans. Med. Imag. (2), 632–645 (2003)
6. Yu, Y., Acton, S.: Speckle reducing anisotropic diffusion. IEEE Trans. Image Proc. (11), 1260–1270 (2002)
7. Frost, V.S., et al.: A model for radar images and its application for adaptive digital filtering. . . . IEEE Trans. Pat. Analy. Mach. Intel. 4(2), 157–165 (1982)
8. Lee, J.S.: Digtial image enhancement and noise filtering by using local statistics. IEEE Trans. Pat. Analy. Mach. Intel. 2(2), 165–168 (1980)
9. Tranquart, F., et al.: Clinical use of ultrasound tissue harmonic imaging. Ultrasound Med. Bio. 25(6), 889–894 (1999)
10. Starritt, H.C., et al.: The development of harmonic distortion in pulsed finite-amplitude ultrasound passing through liver. Physics Med. Bio. 31, 1401–1409 (1986)
11. Simpson, D.H., et al.: Pulse inversion doppler: A new method for detecting non-linear echoes from mircobubble. . . . In: Proc IEEE Ultras Symp, pp. 1597–1600. IEEE Computer Society Press, Los Alamitos (1997)
12. Shen, C., Li, P.: Harmonic leakage and image quality degradation in tissue harmonic imaging. IEEE Trans. Ultras. Fer. Freq. Cont. 48(3), 728–736 (2001)
13. Gorce, J., et al.: Processing radio frequency ultrasound images: A robust method for local spectral features estimation. . . . IEEE Trans. Ultra. Fer. Freq. Cont. (12), 1704–1719 (2002)
14. Wear, K.A., et al.: Application of autoregressive spectral analysis to cepstral estimation. . . . IEEE Trans. Ultra. Fer. Freq. Cont. (1), 50–58 (1993)
15. Press, W., Teukolsky, S., Vetterling, W., Flannery, B.: Numerical Recipes in C++. Cambridge University Press, Cambridge (2002)
16. Burckhardt, C.B.: Speckle in ultrasound b-mode scans. IEEE Trans Sonics Ultras 25(1) (1978)
17. Amadasun, M., King, R.: Textural features corresponding to textural properties. IEEE Trans Systems Man and Cybern 19(5), 1264–1274 (1989)

Outlier Rejection for Diffusion Weighted Imaging

Marc Niethammer[1,2,3], Sylvain Bouix[1,2,3], Santiago Aja-Fernández[2],
Carl-Fredrik Westin[2], and Martha E. Shenton[1,3]

[1] Psychiatry Neuroimaging Laboratory
[2] Laboratory of Mathematics in Imaging,
Brigham and Women's Hospital, Harvard Medical School, Boston MA, USA
[3] Laboratory of Neuroscience, VA Boston Healthcare System, Brockton MA, USA
{marc,sylvain,santi,westin,shenton}@bwh.harvard.edu

Abstract. This paper introduces an outlier rejection and signal reconstruction method for high angular resolution diffusion weighted imaging. The approach is based on the thresholding of Laplacian measurements over the sphere of the apparent diffusion coefficient profiles defined for a given set of gradient directions. Exemplary results are presented.

1 Motivation and Background

Diffusion weighted imaging (DWI) has become an increasingly popular imaging technique in neuroscience as it provides insight into the architecture of brain white matter. The imaging technology is ever improving and high angular and spatial resolutions are now possible. However, acquiring many gradient directions and small voxel sizes requires fast imaging techniques such as Echo Planar Imaging (EPI), and these are usually prone to various artifacts and often have low signal to noise ratios. The most common artifacts associated with diffusion EPI are susceptibility artifacts and geometric distortions due to gradient induced eddy currents. Less common, but critical to DWI are strong signal drops introduced by patient motion or scanner table vibrations [1].

Preprocessing of DWI data is thus beneficial when dealing with such data. Typically, diffusion data acquired through EPI receives the following processing steps [2]. First, geometric distortions induced by eddy currents are corrected using affine coregistration to the baseline image. Second, the image may be filtered for noise. Finally, diffusion tensors are estimated at each image location. Image intensity artifacts, like strong signal drops, are sometimes taken into account by a robust tensor estimator based on an outlier rejection mechanism [3,2]. While these methods are powerful, they assume Gaussian diffusion profiles, thus removing some of the benefits of high angular resolution DWI. Various methods exist for noise removal and direct estimation of diffusion profiles for high angular resolution DWI acquisitions (e.g. [4]), however these methods do not explicitly address the rejection of outliers. A robust estimation method in analogy to the work in [3] could be constructed for a richer class of diffusion profiles. We instead present an outlier rejection algorithm that is not tied to any diffusion model,

N. Ayache, S. Ourselin, A. Maeder (Eds.): MICCAI 2007, Part I, LNCS 4791, pp. 161–168, 2007.
© Springer-Verlag Berlin Heidelberg 2007

makes minimal assumptions about the process of magnetic resonance (MR) diffusion, and allows for the use of subsequent processing methods without the need for explicit outlier handling.

2   Outlier Rejection Approach

Fig. 1 shows an extreme outlier example, where whole slices for gradient directions exhibit signal intensities that are too low. Since dark values indicate large diffusion, linear least squares tensor estimation may result in incorrect directional information due to dropped slices. Our hypothesis is that at a voxel location, the signal associated with neighboring gradient directions should be relatively smooth on the sphere and that outlier signals exhibit sudden changes which can be detected (Fig. 1(a) and (b)). We quantify this measure of smoothness by the Laplacian, on the sphere, of the apparent diffusion coefficients (ADC). We seek to find voxels exhibiting a large Laplacian (Fig. 1(b)) and replace them by interpolating the values of their neighbors on the sphere. Our processing pipeline decomposes into the following steps: (i) affine registration of the DWI volumes to the baseline volume to account for patient movement and eddy currents. This is done using the FSL package[1]; (ii) noise filtering of the aligned volumes (Sec. 2.1); (iii) Laplacian computation of the ADC profile on the sphere for every voxel location (Sec. 2.2); (iv) thresholding of the Laplacian profile to declare outliers

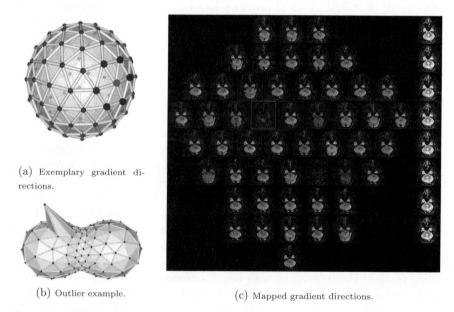

(a) Exemplary gradient directions.

(b) Outlier example.

(c) Mapped gradient directions.

Fig. 1. Exemplary outliers, relation to the gradient directions, and an example diffusion profile with an outlier

[1] http://www.fmrib.ox.ac.uk/fsl/

(Sec. 2.3); and (v) replacement of image information of potential outliers by sphere-neighborhood-interpolated values (Sec. 2.4).

2.1 Noise Filtering

Since the proposed outlier rejection methodology is based on the computation of the Laplacian (a second derivative) noise filtering is an essential pre-processing step to ensure that noise effects will not dominate the Laplacian results as derivative operators amplify noise. Unlike direct filtering of a diffusion profile (e.g. [4]), our noise filtering is not based on a diffusion model, but performed separately on each individual baseline and gradient volumes. A Linear Minimum Mean Square Error Estimator respecting the Rician noise model is used for the filtering [5]. The filtering is performed slice by slice. The estimator is

$$\widehat{A_{ij}^2} = \langle M_{ij}^2 \rangle - 2\sigma_n^2 + K_{ij}(M_{ij}^2 - \langle M_{ij} \rangle^2),$$

with $K_{ij} = 1 - \frac{4\sigma_n^2 \left(\langle M_{ij}^2 \rangle - \sigma_n^2 \right)}{\langle M_{ij}^4 \rangle - \langle M_{ij}^2 \rangle^2}$, where $(\cdot)_{ij}$ denotes position (i,j), M_{ij} is the image

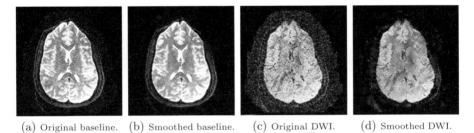

(a) Original baseline.   (b) Smoothed baseline.   (c) Original DWI.   (d) Smoothed DWI.

Fig. 2. Smoothing before Laplacian calculations helps removing the noise without greatly affecting the ability to detect outliers. In accordance with the Rician noise model dark areas are smoothed more than bright areas.

intensity magnitude, A_{ij} the noise-free image intensity magnitude, $\widehat{(\cdot)}$ denotes estimated quantities, $< \cdot >$ is the sample estimated value operator, and σ_n is the noise standard deviation of the Rician noise model[2]

$$p(M|A, \sigma_n) = \frac{M}{\sigma_n^2} e^{-\frac{M^2 + A^2}{2\sigma_n^2}} I_0 \left(\frac{AM}{\sigma_n^2} \right) h(M),$$

where $I_0(\cdot)$ is the 0th order modified Bessel function and $h(\cdot)$ is the Heaviside step function. The estimated noise-free image intensity magnitude is given by $\sqrt{\widehat{A_{ij}^2}}$. While not strictly fulfilling the noise-model after one filtering step, the filtering methodology may be run recursively [5] (for a number of iteration steps) by

---

[2] We refer the reader to [5] for a detailed description of how σ_n is automatically estimated, and how the noise is filtered.

replacing image magnitudes by their estimated noise-free magnitudes and then applying the filter to these results.

Fig. 2 shows an exemplary smoothing result for an axial baseline slice and an axial slice of a DWI volume. As expected from the Rician noise model assumption, dark areas are smoothed to a greater extent. Noise filtering was done with an estimation and filtering neighborhood of 7 by 7. Fifteen iterations were executed, running the algorithm to steady state. To demonstrate that filtering in the volume domain suggests beneficial effects on Laplacian computations (see Sec. 2.2 on how to compute the Laplacian) Fig. 3 shows a two-dimensional log-histogram, displaying the log-frequency of Laplacian-ADC pairs. Clearly, noise filtering tightens the distribution and results in less pronounced Laplacian-tails of the distribution.

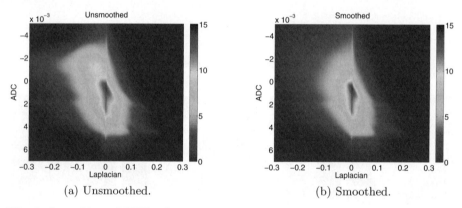

(a) Unsmoothed.   (b) Smoothed.

Fig. 3. Smoothing of DWI volumes reduces the likelihood of obtaining large Laplacian values, suggesting beneficial noise removal properties for the computation of local diffusion profiles

2.2   Laplace-Beltrami Computations

Given a set of unit norm gradient direction $\{g_i\}$, we compute the convex hull, M, of the set of points given by the gradient directions and its antipodal pairs $\mathcal{P} = \{g_i, -g_i\}$ to establish neighborhood relations between the gradient directions and to induce a spherical surface triangulation based on the specified gradient directions. To find severe outliers we compute the Laplacian of the ADCs over the sphere. This can be accomplished by means of the *Laplace-Beltrami* operator Δ_{lb}.

At a given point $p_i \in \mathcal{P}$ one can define a discretized version of Δ_{lb} of the form

$$\Delta_{lb} p_i = \sum_{j \in \mathcal{N}(i)} w_{ij} \left(p_j - p_i \right),$$

where $\mathcal{N}(i)$ denotes the one-ring neighborhood set of vertex $\boldsymbol{p}_i$, i.e., all vertices that are directly connected to $\boldsymbol{p}_i$, and w_{ij} are positive weighting constants given by the discretization scheme, [6]. We use the weighting scheme proposed by Meyer et al. [7]

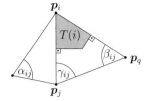

$$w_{ij} = \frac{1}{A_M(\boldsymbol{p}_i)} \frac{\cot\alpha_{ij} + \cot\beta_{ij}}{2}, \qquad (1)$$

Fig. 4. Illustration of the weight computation for the discretization of the Laplace-Beltrami operator on a triangulated mesh

where $A_M(\boldsymbol{p}_i)$ denotes the local surface patch of $\boldsymbol{p}_i$ and α_{ij} and β_{ij} are the angles of the triangles opposite the edge (i,j), see Fig. 4 for an illustration. $A_M(\boldsymbol{p}_i)$ is computed as $A_M(\boldsymbol{p}_i) = \sum_{T(i)} \overline{A}(T(i))$, where $T(i)$ denotes the triangles containing vertex i and

$$\overline{A}(T(i)) = \begin{cases} \frac{1}{8}\left(\|\boldsymbol{p}_i - \boldsymbol{p}_q\|^2 \cot\gamma_{ij} + \|\boldsymbol{p}_i - \boldsymbol{p}_j\|^2 \cot\beta_{ij}\right) & \text{if } T(i) \text{ is non-obtuse,} \\ \text{area}(T(i))/2 & \text{if } T(i) \text{ is obtuse at } i, \\ \text{area}(T(i))/4 & \text{otherwise.} \end{cases}$$

Using the same discretization weights, we compute the Laplacian of the ADCs on the sphere by applying the discretized Δ_{lb} to the ADCs associated to the individual gradient directions and their antipodal pairs $\Delta_{lb} a(\boldsymbol{p}_i) = \sum_{j \in \mathcal{N}(i)} w_{ij} \left(a(\boldsymbol{p}_j) - a(\boldsymbol{p}_i)\right)$, where the ADC is given as $a(\boldsymbol{p}_i) = -\frac{1}{b}\log\frac{S(\boldsymbol{p}_i)}{S_0}$, with S_0 the non-diffusion-weighted baseline image intensity, b the b-value and $S(\boldsymbol{p}_i)$ the DWI intensity of the gradient direction associated with the vertex $\boldsymbol{p}_i$.

2.3 Thresholding to Define Outliers

Once the Laplacian of the ADCs over the sphere has been computed for the whole image volume based on the noise-filtered DWIs, thresholds to declare a measurement as an outlier need to be established. Only large deviations from the norm (decreases as well as increases) should be picked up by the methodology. To define this thresholding region, we create two-dimensional histograms for a number of DWI reference volumes. The histograms measure the frequency of (ADC, Laplacian of ADC) pairs. The histograms for the reference DWI acquisitions are summed up and subsequently smoothed with a Gaussian filter to account for sparse histogram sampling.

Data resulting in negative ADC values are always flagged as outliers and only voxels inside the brain are considered[3]. For all other data, Laplacian thresholds are established for every ADC value. These fixed thresholds are then being applied to newly acquired data. A simple outlier rejection method [8] based on the interquartile range is used; more sophisticated methodologies are conceivable. Specifically, given the observed Laplacian values ($l(ADC)$) for an ADC value,

---

[3] A coarse brain mask was created by simple intensity thresholding.

the Laplacian outlier thresholds are defined as

$$l_{min}(ADC) = Q_l - \frac{3}{2}\text{IQR}, \quad l_{max}(ADC) = Q_u + \frac{3}{2}\text{IQR}, \quad \text{IQR}(ADC) = Q_u - Q_l,$$

where Q_l and Q_u denote the lower and the upper quartiles of $l(ADC)$ and IQR is the interquartile range; see Fig. 5 for an example. All values that are either smaller than l_{min} or larger than l_{max} for their Laplacian values are classified as outliers. In this way only extreme values will be considered as outliers.

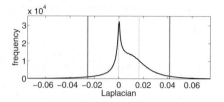

Fig. 5. Example Laplacian histogram for a fixed ADC range. Dotted lines indicate the lower and upper quartiles, solid (red) lines indicate the thresholds l_{min} and l_{max} respectively.

2.4   Interpolation

Measurements declared as outliers are replaced by smoothly interpolated values based on neighborhood information. Specifically, $(a(\boldsymbol{p}_i))_t = \Delta_{lb}a(\boldsymbol{p}_i)$, is run to steady state, while keeping all values that are not declared as outliers at their original value throughout the evolution. The ADCs are then mapped back to image intensities.

3   Results

We present two experiments, both of which work with data acquired on a GE 3T scanner, using an EPI sequence with 51 gradient sensitized directions, 8 baselines and a b value of 700 $\frac{s}{mm^2}$. The voxel size is 1.7mm^3. Fig. 1 shows an extreme outlier example, where whole slices for gradient directions exhibit signal intensities that are too low. Fig. 6 shows the result of such dropped slices on tensor estimation. Since dark values indicate large diffusion, linear least squares tensor estimation may result in incorrect directional information due to dropped slices. The outlier rejection scheme markedly improves this estimation. Fig. 7 shows results for a less severe, more localized artifact. The resulting reconstruction of the image intensity values is more consistent with its neighborhood and visually sensible.

4   Conclusion

We presented a framework for outlier rejection in high angular DWI that does not depend on a specific diffusion model. The method only relies on the weak assumption that measurements in neighboring directions should be similar. We measure this similarity by computing the Laplacian of the ADC on the sphere and find appropriate thresholds to detect and replace outliers. Currently only a simple outlier detection method is used. Future work will look into alternative

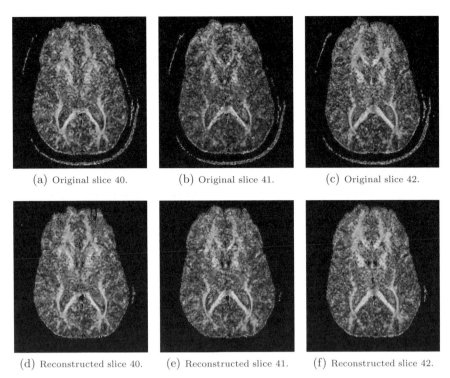

(a) Original slice 40.   (b) Original slice 41.   (c) Original slice 42.

(d) Reconstructed slice 40.   (e) Reconstructed slice 41.   (f) Reconstructed slice 42.

Fig. 6. Color by orientation from linear least squares tensor estimation with and without outlier rejection. A signal intensity drop can cause major misestimations of diffusion direction (b). After reconstruction, the artifactual blue coloring due to outliers in (b) is replaced by sensible values in (e) through interpolation of ADC on the sphere.

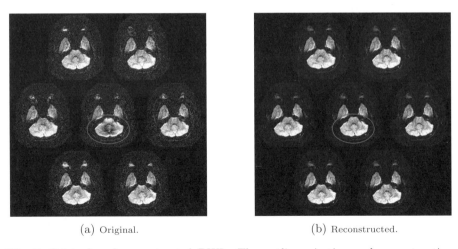

(a) Original.   (b) Reconstructed.

Fig. 7. Original and reconstructed DWIs. The outlier rejection and reconstruction methodology succeeds in reconstructing corrupted image information (inside red ellipse) based on the neighboring direction information (the images surrounding the center image).

outlier detection methodologies. We will also be introducing spatial neighbor-hood information for the outlier rejection, do an extensive validation of the methodology and will in particular focus on the reconstruction aspect of diffusion profiles that do not follow the tensor model.

Acknowledgements

This work was supported in part by a Department of Veteran Affairs Merit Award (SB,MS,CFW), a Research Enhancement Award Program (MS), and National Institute of Health grants R01 MH50747 (SB,MS), K05 MH070047 (MS), U54 EB005149 (MN,SB,MS), R01 MH074794 (CFW), and P41 RR13218 (CFW). We thank the anonymous reviewers for their suggestions.

References

1. Bernstein, M.A., King, K.F., Zhou, X.J.: Handbook of MRI pulse sequences. Elsevier, Amsterdam (2004)
2. Mangin, J.-F., Poupon, C., Clark, C.A., Bihan, D.L., Bloch, I.: Distortion correction and robust tensor estimation for MR diffusion imaging. Medical Image Analysis 6, 191–198 (2002)
3. Chang, L.-C., Jones, D.K., Pierpaoli, C.: RESTORE: Robust estimation of tensors by outlier rejection. Magnetic Resonance in Medicine 53, 1088–1095 (2005)
4. Descoteaux, M., Angelino, E., Fitzgibbons, S., Deriche, R.: Apparent diffusion coefficients from high angular resolution diffusion imaging: Estimation and applications. Magnetic Resonance in Medicine 56, 395–410 (2006)
5. Aja-Fernandez, S., Lopez, C.A., Westin, C.F.: Filtering and noise estimation in magnitude MRI and Rician distributed images. IEEE Transactions on Image Processing (submitted 2007)
6. Xu, G.: Convergent discrete Laplace-Beltrami operators over triangular surfaces. In: Proceedings of the Geometric Modeling and Processing Conference, pp. 195–204 (2004)
7. Meyer, M., Desbrun, M., Schröder, P., Barr, A.H.: Discrete differential-geometry operators for triangulated 2-manifolds. In: Proceedings of VisMath 2002 (2002)
8. Hoaglin, D.C., Iglewicz, B., Tukey, J.W.: Performance of some resistant rules for outlier labeling. Journal of the American Statistical Association 81, 991–999 (1986)

Generating Fiber Crossing Phantoms Out of Experimental DWIs

Matthan Caan[1,2], Anne Willem de Vries[2], Ganesh Khedoe[2], Erik Akkerman[1], Lucas van Vliet[2], Kees Grimbergen[1], and Frans Vos[1,2]

[1] Department of Radiology, Academic Medical Center, University of Amsterdam, NL
[2] Quantitative Imaging Group, Delft University of Technology, NL
m.w.a.caan@tudelft.nl

Abstract. In Diffusion Tensor Imaging (DTI), differently oriented fiber bundles inside one voxel are incorrectly modeled by a single tensor. High Angular Resolution Diffusion Imaging (HARDI) aims at using more complex models, such as a two-tensor model, for estimating two fiber bundles.

We propose a new method for creating experimental phantom data of fiber crossings, by mixing the DWI-signals from high FA-regions with different orientation. The properties of these experimental phantoms approach the conditions of real data. These phantoms can thus serve as a 'ground truth' in validating crossing reconstruction algorithms. The angular resolution of a dual tensor model is determined using series of crossings, generated under different angles. An angular resolution of 0.6π was found in data scanned with a diffusion weighting parameter b=1000 s/mm^2. This resolution did not change significantly in experiments with b=3000 and 5000 s/mm^2, keeping the scanning time constant.

1 Introduction

In the last decade, specifications of MR-scanners have increasingly improved. Consequently, Diffusion Weighted Images (DWIs) can be acquired at higher resolution and with better image quality. A more precise analysis of the diffusion profile of water in the human brain has thus become possible. This diffusion process is modeled by a rank-two symmetric positive-definite tensor [1], describing both the average distance and the orientation of the displacement. Anisotropic diffusion is associated with white matter structures, whereas isotropic diffusion is generally related to grey matter and cerebral spinal fluid. The Fractional Anisotropy (FA) has been introduced as a distance measure to an isotropic tensor [2], which is of use in analyzing changes in white matter integrity. The first eigenvector of the diffusion tensor represents the orientation of fibrous white matter structures, which can be tracked throughout the image volume [3]. Such tractography is of practical interest for pre-operative planning. Additionally, studies to brain diseases are increasingly using fiber tracts as features in analysis [4].

Still, the minimal size of a voxel in a DWI is orders of magnitude higher than the diameter of the individual axons. Only macroscopic brain properties

N. Ayache, S. Ourselin, A. Maeder (Eds.): MICCAI 2007, Part I, LNCS 4791, pp. 169–176, 2007.
© Springer-Verlag Berlin Heidelberg 2007

can therefore be described. What is more, it is likely that multiple fiber bundles are crossing inside a single voxel, due to the partial volume effect. Multiple anisotropic diffusion processes in different directions are then modeled as a single process, introducing a severe bias in the tensor estimation. Consequently, regions of crossing fibers have to be excluded from comparative studies to brain diseases using tensor properties. Additionally, the measured principal diffusion direction is ill-defined and not related to the underlying anatomical structure. Fiber tracking based on a single tensor fit will erroneously connect distinct tracts or be terminated in a crossing. A dual tensor fit in regions of crossing fibers is thus indispensable for correctly tracking fibers through the brain.

Several solutions were proposed for overcoming the crossing-fiber problem. Non-parametric methods aim to find the probability density function of the spin diffusion displacement. For instance, q-ball imaging was proposed [5] for calculating diffusion orientations from High Angular Resolution Diffusion Images (HARDI). Parametric methods include a two-tensor model for analyzing the diffusion signal [5,6,7]. This work was continued by using spherical harmonics to characterize anisotropy [8], which was elsewhere shown to be related to the coefficients of higher order tensors [9]. Recently, high angle fiber crossings were reconstructed in clinical data with a diffusion weighting parameter $b = 1000s/mm^2$ [10].

In order to validate the reconstruction of crossings, various experiments with simulated data have been performed. For instance, data with additive uncorrelated Gaussian noise was simulated [11]. Scanning artifacts and patient movement are thereby ignored. Additionally, using a spinal chord, an experimental crossing phantom was created [12]. Still, a ground truth is missing for properly facilitating a validation of crossings found in the human brain.

We propose a new method for generating fiber crossing phantoms out of experimental data, containing realistic imaging artifacts. These phantoms can serve as a 'ground truth' in validating algorithms aiming to resolve crossing fibers. Series of crossings, generated under different angles, give insight into the precision that can be achieved in estimating the fiber bundle orientations. Therefore, a restricted two-tensor model is fitted on the projected data onto the plane of the crossing. Included in our analysis is the influence of the diffusion weighting parameter b on the angular resolution.

Finally, the relevance of a proper modeling of crossing fiber regions is demonstrated. Streamlines generated through a crossing are shown to erroneously depict the fiber paths. Using a dual tensor model, it is shown that the FA of two crossing fibers bundles can be distinctively estimated.

2   Method

2.1   Experimental Phantom Data

Signal. The MR-signal measured in a certain voxel contains the contributions of the individual underlying volume fractions of different tissue. Dependent on the heterogeneity of the local tissue, more or less distinct fractions are present within a voxel. A summation of the fractions is assumed to correctly model the acquired MR-signal. This assumption is justified by the fact that there is no reason to expect inherent phase signal differences within a voxel. Previously, this summability was for instance silently used in [13], where an MR-signal is Monte Carlo simulated by aggregating a number of spins per voxel. And as an illustration, the figures 1b and 2b can be compared, showing that adjacent perpendicular fiber bundles contribute equally to the signal of the intermediate voxel, inducing partial voluming.

We now propose to mix voxels out of experimental Diffusion Weighted Images (DWIs) whose FA is high enough to assume a single fiber bundle inside. Thus we are able to generate fiber crossings with different known properties, derived from single tensor fits of the individual parts. Here, only two voxels are mixed; dependent on the application even a higher number of orientations could be combined.

By using this approach, most known and unknown imaging artifacts that are present in real data are included in the phantoms. A realistic validation of a crossing reconstruction algorithm of interest has thus become possible.

Noise. Diffusion is measured as an attenuated signal, such that noise is expected to significantly affect the acquired images. This noise follows a Gaussian distribution, added independently to both the real and imaginary part of the signal. DWIs, being magnitude images with relatively low SNR, are thereby containing Rician noise [14]. The noise in the generated phantom data now yields the sum of two Rician noise processes. Following the central limit theorem, this noise distribution can be expected to slightly tend back towards Gaussian. For simplicity, a Gaussian noise model is now used in reconstructing the generated crossing fibers.

2.2   Two-Tensor Model

In the case of two fiber orientations in a single voxel, distinction between these orientations is needed. We model the diffusion process of two fibers as the sum of two Gaussian distributions with different diffusion tensors, $\mathbf{D}^1$ and $\mathbf{D}^2$, closely following [15]. Note that this model intuitively closely relates to the way the experimental phantoms are generated. Without loss of generality, the two fibers are assumed to reside in the (x, y)-plane. The equation that models the MR-signal then becomes:

$$S(\tilde{\mathbf{g}}) = S_0 \left(f \exp(-b\tilde{\mathbf{g}}^T \mathbf{D}^1 \tilde{\mathbf{g}}) + (1 - f) \exp(-b\tilde{\mathbf{g}}^T \mathbf{D}^2 \tilde{\mathbf{g}}) \right), \tag{1}$$

with

$$\mathbf{D}^{1,2} = \begin{pmatrix} D_{xx}^{1,2} & D_{xy}^{1,2} & 0 \\ D_{xy}^{1,2} & D_{yy}^{1,2} & 0 \\ 0 & 0 & D_z \end{pmatrix}, \tag{2}$$

where f is the volume fraction of the first tensor D_z is the same for both tensors. The gradient directions $\mathbf{g}$ are rotated to $\tilde{\mathbf{g}}$, such that the fiber bundles are

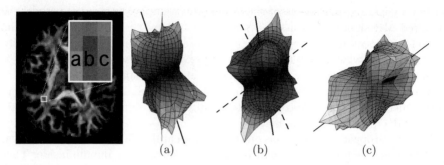

Fig. 1. Axial slice of the FA with logarithmic signal profiles of three adjacent voxels (a-c), measured at b=3000 mm/s^2. Solid lines represent single tensor fits, dashed lines dual tensor fits to the data. Note the correspondence between the dashed lines in (b) and the solid lines in (a) and (c).

situated in the (x, y)-plane. The tensor components $D_{xz}^{1,2}$ and $D_{yz}^{1,2}$ are assumed to be negligible and are thus set to zero. Moreover, the diffusion in the direction perpendicular to the plane of interest is assumed to be equal for both fibers, i.e. the smallest eigenvalues of both tensors are equal. The data is therefore projected onto this direction. As a reference, the normal to the plane spanned by the principal diffusion directions in the voxels, used to generate the crossing, is used.

In measuring the diffusion profile of a crossing fiber, proper contrast is needed between the signal contributions of both fibers. Theoretically, altering the diffusion weighting parameter b highly influences this contrast. In figure 2a, a logarithmic signal profile ($\ln S_0 - \ln S(\mathbf{g})$) of a crossing fiber is computed for different b-values. The iso-lines further away from the origin (corresponding to high b) reveal more information about the crossing than the iso-lines near the origin. However, in measured data noise increasingly distorts measurements at higher b-values.

The angular resolution for different b-values will be determined in generated experimental phantoms, using the dual tensor method. The minimal angle between fiber bundles that can be estimated is defined at the point where both the bias and variance clearly start increasing.

3   Results

DTI-data of four healthy volunteers, between 20 and 30 years of age, were acquired on a Philips Intera 3.0 Tesla MRI scanner (Philips Intera, Philips Medical Systems, Best, The Netherlands) by means of a spin-echo EPI sequence. The diffusion weighting was along 92 three-fold tessellated icosahedric gradient directions. Other parameters were: TE 84 msec, TR 7912 msec, b=1000, 3000 and 5000 s/mm^2 , FOV 220 mm, scan matrix 112 x 110, image matrix 128 x 128, slice thickness 3mm. Eddy current induced distortion was visually inspected to be negligible.

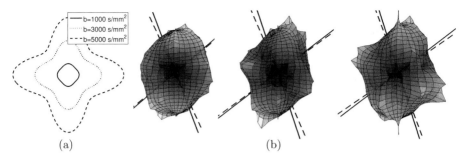

(a)   (b)

Fig. 2. (a) Computed logarithmic signal profiles for two perpendicular tensors with typical white matter properties [16] and (b) measured profiles after mixing voxels a and c in figure 1, for b=1000, 3000 and 5000 s/mm^2 respectively. Solid lines represent single tensor fits before mixing, dashed lines dual tensor fits to the data after mixing. The profiles are scaled for proper visualization.

Only voxels for which FA > 0.6 were included. 1000 pairs of voxels were chosen to generate a uniform distribution of angles between the bundles in these voxels in the range $[0, \pi/2]$. Next, the measured signals S of these pairs were mixed, forming the crossing fiber phantoms.

For illustration purposes, logarithmic signal profiles of three adjacent voxels measured at b=3000 s/mm^2 are displayed in figure 1. Here, the superior longitudinal fasciculus (a) and posterior corona radiata (c) are crossing (b). Logarithmic signal profiles after mixing DWIs of voxels a and c in figure 1 for b=1000, 3000 and 5000 s/mm^2 are given in figure 2b.

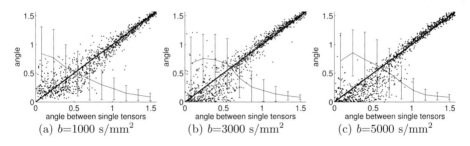

(a) b=1000 s/mm^2 (b) b=3000 s/mm^2 (c) b=5000 s/mm^2

Fig. 3. Scatter plot of the estimated angle between the principal directions in the generated crossing fiber, as function of the angle between the single tensors. The diagonal solid bold line refers to ground truth. The solid line with errorbars denotes the error and standard deviation in the projection direction. Crossings were generated by mixing DWIs of two voxels with FA$>$0.6, for b=1000, 3000 and 5000 s/mm^2 (a,b,c).

Optimization was performed based on the interior-reflective Newton method (Matlab, Mathworks) [17]. A quadratic regularization term for the volume fraction f was added to the cost function, with a scaling factor of 0.2 around the mean value 0.5. The results of fitting the generated crossing fibers for b=1000,

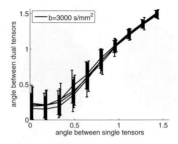

Fig. 4. Estimated mean angle with errorbars denoting the standard deviation, as function of the input angle for $b=3000$ s/mm^2 for four datasets of healthy individuals.

3000 and 5000 s/mm^2 are displayed in figure 3. The reproducibility of the method was analyzed by computing the angular deviation with respect to the input angle for data with $b=3000$ s/mm^2 of four healthy individuals, depicted in figure 4.

An angular resolution of 0.6π was found, for both $b=1000$, 3000 and 5000 s/mm^2. Reproducible results in four subjects were achieved.

Finally, a single streamline was generated in the body of the corpus callosum, passing through the crossing with the corticospinal tract [3]. This streamline incorrectly follows the indermediate orientation of the two fiber bundles. A dual tensor fit was performed along this tract, and estimated fiber bundle orientations were plotted. The decreased FA and increased planar tensor component c_p of the single tensor indicate the presence of a crossing. This is confirmed by the higher FAs of the dual tensors along the tract. The results of this experiment are given in figure 5.

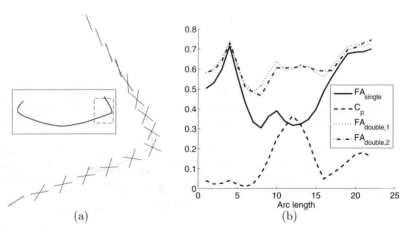

Fig. 5. (a) Selected part of a single streamline in the body of the corpus callosum (inset), with solid lines representing the principal directions after a dual tensor fit, and (b) anisotropy measures based on single (FA$_{single}$, c_p) and dual tensor fit (FA$_{dual,1}$, FA$_{dual,2}$) along this tract

4 Discussion

We propose a new method for creating experimental phantom data of fiber crossings, by mixing the DWI-signals from high FA-regions with different orientation. The properties of these experimental phantoms approach the conditions of real data. These phantoms can thus serve as a 'ground truth' in validating crossing reconstruction algorithms. In this paper, the angular resolution of a dual tensor model is determined. Series of crossings, generated under different angles, give insight into the precision that can be achieved in estimating the fiber bundle orientations. Not only are the results based on realistic imaging artifacts, but also can the reconstructed fiber orientations be compared to a ground truth, being the single tensor fits on the individual voxels.

An equal angular resolution of 0.6π was found, for both $b=1000$, 3000 and 5000 s/mm^2. A higher resolution for higher b-values was to be expected, due to more non-linear behaviour of the diffusion profile. Apparently, the decreased SNR in high b-value data (with constant scanning time), due to a stronger signal attenuation, strongly affected the algorithm's performance. Using a Rician noise model in a Maximum Likelihood estimator might reduce the bias in the reconstructed angle. The error in the estimated projection direction clearly increases for lower input angles, resulting in an ill-defined crossing fiber plane. Nevertheless, the deviation in estimated output angles did not decrease significantly when the correct projection direction was used instead.

Future work consists of acquiring DTI-data at b-values around 1000 s/mm^2, to determine the optimal b-value in maximizing the angular resolution in the reconstruction of crossing fibers. Building a theoretical model will aid in choosing proper values for b and other imaging parameters, the number of repetitive measurements and gradient directions. Eventually, tractography with increased precision and an unbiased anisotropy estimation will lead to an improved analysis of both healthy and pathological brain data.

Instead of generating phantoms out of magnitude data, the real and imaginary part of the DWIs could be individually mixed. A Gaussian noise model could then be obtained in both parts, making even more realistic experimental phantoms. However, phase distortions, between and within acquisitions, hamper usage of the complex data. Until now, no correction method for these distortions is available.

The proposed validation method is expected to be useful in various crossing reconstruction algorithms. As a result, crossing fiber regions can be reliably included in clinical studies to brain diseases.

Acknowledgments

The involvement of M.W.A. Caan took place in the context of the Virtual Laboratory for e-Science project (http://www.vl-e.nl/), is supported by a BSIK grant from the Dutch Ministry of Education, Culture and Science (OC&W) and is part of the ICT innovation program of the Ministry of Economic Affairs (EZ).

References

1. Basser, P., Mattiello, J., Bihan, D.L.: Estimation of the effective self-diffusion tensor from the NMR spin echo. J. Magn. Reson. B(103), 247–254 (1994)
2. Basser, P.: Inferring microstructural features and the physiological state of tissues from diffusion-weighted images. NMR Biomed. 8, 333–334 (1995)
3. Blaas, J., Botha, C., Peters, B., Vos, F., Post, F.: Fast and reproducible fiber bundle selection in dti visualization. In: Proc. IEEE Visualization, pp. 59–64 (2005)
4. Corouge, I., Fletcher, P.T., et al.: Fiber tract-oriented statistics for quantitative diffusion tensor MRI analysis. Med. Im. Anal. 10, 786–798 (2006)
5. Tuch, D.: Diffusion MRI of complex tissue structure. PhD thesis (2002)
6. Frank, L.: Anisotropy in high angular resolution diffusion-weighted MRI. Magn. Reson. Med. 45, 935–939 (2001)
7. Kreher, B., Schneider, J., et al.: Multitensor approach for analysis and tracking of complex fiber configurations. Magn. Res. Med. 54, 1216–1225 (2005)
8. Frank, L.R.: Characterization of anisotropy in high angular resolution diffusion-weighted MRI. Magn. Reson. Med. 47, 1083–1099 (2002)
9. Özarslan, E., Mareci, T.H.: Generalized diffusion tensor imaging and analytical relationships between diffusion tensor imaging and high angular resolution diffusion imaging. Magn. Reson. Med. 50, 955–965 (2003)
10. Peled, S., Friman, O., et al.: Geometrically constrained two-tensor model for crossing tracts in DWI. Magn. Reson. Med. 24, 1263–1270 (2006)
11. Alexander, D., Barker, G., et al.: Optimal image parameters for fiber-orientation estimation in diffusion MRI. NeuroImage 27, 357–367 (2005)
12. Assaf, Y., Freidlin, R., et al.: New modeling and experimental framework to characterize hindered and restricted water diffusion in brain white matter. Magn. Reson. Med. 52, 965–978 (2004)
13. Anderson, A.W.: Theoretical analysis of the effects of noise on diffusion tensor imaging. Magn. Reson. Med. 46, 1174–1188 (2001)
14. Gudbjartsson, H., Patz, S.: The Rician distribution of noise MRI data. Magn. Res. Red. 910–914 (1995)
15. Peled, S., Westin, C.F.: Geometric extraction of two crossing tracts in DWI. Proc. Intl. Soc. Mag. Reson. Med. 13, 1 (2005)
16. Pierpaoli, C., Jezzard, P., et al.: Diffusion tensor MR imaging of the human brain. Radiology 201, 637–648 (1996)
17. Coleman, T.F., Li, Y.: An interior trust region approach for nonlinear minimization subject to bounds. SIAM J. Optim. 6, 418–445 (1996)

Motion and Positional Error Correction for Cone Beam 3D-Reconstruction with Mobile C-Arms

C. Bodensteiner[1], C. Darolti[2], H. Schumacher[3], L. Matthäus[1],
and A. Schweikard[1]

[1] Institute of Robotics and Cognitive Systems, University of Lübeck, Ger
[2] Institute for Signal Processing, University of Lübeck, Ger
[3] Institute of Mathematics, University of Lübeck, Ger
bodensteiner@rob.uni-luebeck.de

Abstract. CT-images acquired by mobile C-arm devices can contain artefacts caused by positioning errors. We propose a data driven method based on iterative 3D-reconstruction and 2D/3D-registration to correct projection data inconsistencies. With a 2D/3D-registration algorithm, transformations are computed to align the acquired projection images to a previously reconstructed volume. In an iterative procedure, the reconstruction algorithm uses the results of the registration step. This algorithm also reduces small motion artefacts within 3D-reconstructions. Experiments with simulated projections from real patient data show the feasibility of the proposed method. In addition, experiments with real projection data acquired with an experimental robotised C-arm device have been performed with promising results.

1   Introduction

Modern mobile C-arm devices allow for intraoperative 3D-reconstruction. Unfortunately, compared to conventional (fixed) CT-scanners, 3D-reconstructions from these devices show greater artefacts due to hardware tradeoffs required for mobile usage. Inconsistencies caused by noise, mechanical flex, geometric distortions, patient motion and errors in positioning the C-arm affect the 3D-reconstruction results. In this paper we present a method to compensate for positioning error inconsistencies in projection data. This approach is also capable of eliminating small motion artefacts within 3D-reconstructions by modelling them as a virtual x-ray camera repositioning.

Forward projection registration algorithms have been successfully used to compensate for motion in SPECT imaging [1]. Inspired by this work, we now combine a conventional rigid 2D/3D-registration algorithm with an iterative reconstruction algorithm. To our best knowledge, this approach has not been used for cone beam 3D-reconstruction before.

We use the averaging nature of algebraic 3D-reconstruction techniques to correct the position and orientation of the acquired projections by means of registration. In the 2D/3D-registration step, 3D-transformations of the positions of the x-ray cameras are calculated to minimize a distance measure between the

N. Ayache, S. Ourselin, A. Maeder (Eds.): MICCAI 2007, Part I, LNCS 4791, pp. 177–185, 2007.
© Springer-Verlag Berlin Heidelberg 2007

acquired projections and a set of forward projections. The forward projections are digital reconstructed radiographs (DRR) generated from the previously re-constructed volume through virtual x-ray cameras at new positions. As a result, an iterative reconstruction scheme arises which is robust with respect to small positional error and rigid motion artefacts.

2   Method

Cone beam 3D-reconstruction with algebraic methods can be formulated as the following linear least-squares problem: find $f \in \mathbf{R}_+^n$ such that

$$R\left(f\right) = \|Af - b\| = min! \qquad (1)$$

where A denotes a projection-operator (also called system matrix) simulating the cone beam projections, f the reconstruction volume, n the image size, and b the measured projections. In a first step only positional errors of the C-arm device are considered. Assuming that x-ray camera transformations can be modeled as 3D rigid object motion transformations, this leads to the following minimization problem:

$$J\left(\begin{array}{c} f \\ \varPhi \end{array}\right) = \sum_{i=1}^{M} \|A_i f(\varPhi_i) - b_i\| = min! \qquad (2)$$

Here A_i denotes the i-th part of the projection operator simulating one cone beam projection image b_i, M the number of acquired projection images and $\varPhi_i$ the 3D rigid motion transformation of the reconstructed object with six degrees of freedom. An equation similiar to Eqn.(2) is minimized in an iterative procedure to compensate for motion in SPECT imaging [2]. Our approach is to first solve Eqn.(1) with a reconstruction algorithm. In a second step the motion parameters of Eqn.(2) are estimated with a rigid 2D/3D-registration algorithm by employing an appropriate distance measure [3]. The motion parameters are then used to correct the x-ray camera positions. In the next iteration, the reconstruction algorithm uses the information from the corrected projections to compute a new least-squares solution with respect to all projection equations given in Eqn.(1). This procedure is then iteratively repeated until some convergence criteria are fulfilled. The corrected projection positions obtained with this method represent an equal or better projection geometry with respect to the used distance measure, since we initialize the registration algorithm with the projection positions given by the C-arm device. For reasons of clarity and completeness a short description of the employed reconstruction algorithm and details of the 2D/3D-registration algorithm are given.

2.1   3D-Reconstruction Algorithm

The algebraic reconstruction technique (ART) was used for 3D-reconstruction. Let $g_i(\lambda; b; \cdot), G(\lambda; b; \cdot) : \mathbf{R}^n \to \mathbf{R}^n$ be the applications of:

$$g_i(\lambda; b; f) = f - \lambda \frac{\langle f, a_i \rangle - b_i}{\|a_i\|^2} a_i, i = 1, \cdots, m, \qquad (3)$$

$$G(\lambda; b; f) = (g_1 \circ \cdots \circ g_m)(\lambda; b; x), \tag{4}$$

where a_i denotes the i-th row of the system matrix A and b_i the i-th element of the measured projection image. Letting λ denote a relaxation parameter, the algorithm of Kaczmarz calculates a limit point for the following iteration equation:

$$f^0 \in \mathbf{R}^n; \quad k = 0, 1, 2, ...; \quad f^{k+1} = G(\lambda; b; f^k). \tag{5}$$

Censor et. al [4] proved that for sufficiently small values of λ the algorithm converges to a least squares solution of a weighted version of Eqn.(1). This technique has the advantage that it is able to employ a former reconstruction result in order to compute a new least squares solution. For further details and enhancements regarding the reconstruction of inconsistent projection data we refer to [5].

2.2   2D/3D-Registration

2D/3D-registration algorithms are conventionally used to find the transformation between intraoperative 2D radiographs and a preoperative CT-volume. In our application we have two significant advantages over conventional 2D/3D-registration scenarios, since the imaged object does not change and we have a good initialization of the position in case of positional error correction. The main building blocks of these algorithms are the distance measure and the optimization scheme [3]. We only consider intensity based distance measures which do not require prior segmentation. We tested the sum of squared distances (SSD) for minimizing the positional inconsistencies. We also tested a gradient-based correlation distance measure [3]. In this case, the cost function to be optimized $C = \frac{1}{2}(C_x + C_y)$ is calculated as the average of the normalized cross correlations of the partial derivatives of the projection and DRR image intensities. $Pr_x(x, y) = \frac{\partial Pr(x,y)}{\partial x}$ and $Pr_y(x, y) = \frac{\partial Pr(x,y)}{\partial y}$ denote the partial derivatives of image intensities, and $\overline{Pr_x}$ and $\overline{Pr_y}$ denote their mean values.

$$C_x = \frac{\sum_{x,y}(Pr_x(x, y) - \overline{Pr_x})(Drr_x(x, y) - \overline{Drr_x})}{\sqrt{\sum_{x,y}(Pr_x(x, y) - \overline{Pr_x})^2}\sqrt{\sum_{x,y}(Drr_x(x, y) - \overline{Drr_x})^2}} \tag{6}$$

The gradient cost function seems to be more robust with respect to positional inconsistencies in the data. In addition, problems caused by different image generation processes of DRRs and real projections are resolved as well.

The optimization was carried out in a hierarchical multi-level approach: a pyramid of images is constructed by down-sampling and filtering the image at multiples of 2 and the optimization is run for each level of the pyramid. This allows for a robust and fast optimization, since evaluating the cost function at lower levels is computationally very cheap.

The values of the cost functions for transformation parameters varying around the optimum found by the 2D/3D-registration algorithm have been plotted in Fig. 1. They all show a relatively smooth, monotonically increasing function with a unique maximum and an appropriate convergence range in the vicinity of the found value. Also, one can see that out-of-plane parameters (here the x-deviation) usually cannot be determined as accurately as other parameters due to the projection geometry [6]. A variant of the Hooke-Jeeves pattern-search [7] was used as an optimization-scheme. To avoid double function evaluations the function values were cached in a hash table as described in [8].

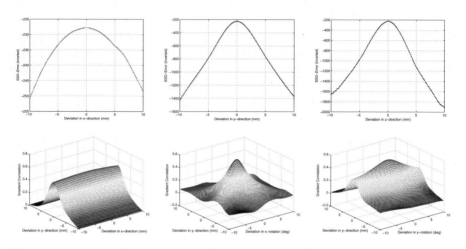

Fig. 1. Cost function values for the proximal femur experiment as a function of deviation from the optimal value found by the 2D/3D-registration algorithm. The upper row shows the values of SSD distance measure for deviations of the translational parameters (x, y, z). The lower row shows the values of gradient cost function for deviations of two transformation parameters: $(x, y), (y, \theta_x), (y, \theta_y)$.

2.3   Implementation Details and Computation Time

All algorithms were implemented in C++ and parallelized with OpenMP [9]. When using several processor cores, a almost linear speedup has been observed since all employed algorithms are inherently parallel. The registration of one projection image (Fig. 3, 568^2 pixel) took around 30s-40s for a 256^3 volume and 3 image pyramid levels. For fast DRR generation a shear warp factorization algorithm [6] was used. A typical complete registration iteration on our test system (Dual Xeon 5160, 16 GB Ram) took around 780s for a 256^3 dataset and 100 projections (568^2). One iteration of our software based reconstruction algorithm (double precision) took around 180s. To allow for intraoperative usage, a clear reduction of computation time must be obtained. Since DRR generation is the most time consuming part of the registration algorithm, our future implementation will make use of GPU based algorithms (e.g. 3D texture based DRR generation, GPU based reconstruction algorithms).

The entries of the system matrix A were determined by discretizing the ray beam with a trilinear interpolation coefficient approach [10]. The reconstruction volume was also optimized by a block structure such as to speed up memory access in order to enable a fast set up of the system matrix equations [10].

2.4   Clinical- and C-Arm Projection Data Experiments

We generated DRR's (100 projections, 568x568, 180 degree angle range) from a clinical dataset (512x512x200) of a distal femur bone. After resampling the dataset to an isotrope 256^3-grid, we perturbed all camera positions T_{World}^{Cam} to $T_{World}^{pertCam}$ (max $\pm$10mm, max $\pm$1deg). The perturbed projections were generated from a different DRR generator as the one employed in the registration process in order to simulate the different image generation process. In a first experiment we measured the registration accuracy by registering 400 perturbed DRRs to the original volume. The euler angle representation of the deviation matrix Tm was used for evaluation.

$$Tm_{regCam}^{Cam} = T_{regCam}^{World} T_{World}^{Cam} \tag{7}$$

We applied the iterative correction process to the perturbed data and in each step, we ran 5 ART-iterations to reconstruct the object. The projections where then iteratively registered to the previous reconstruction result.

The real projection data was acquired with a robotized experimental C-arm [11] from Ziehm-Imaging (Fig. 2). The position of the C-arm is known from the direct kinematics. In addition this C-arm can be arbitrarily positioned to a point in its working space by computing the inverse kinematics solution described in [12].

In the first experiment a sawbone model of the proximal femur was imaged in a planar angular orbit (50 projections, 568x568, 180 degree angle range). A sequential ART algorithm with a small relaxation parameter ($\lambda = 0.25$) was used for reconstruction. After 6 ART-iterations per step, the original projection images were registered to the reconstruction result, and subsequently a new reconstruction was started.

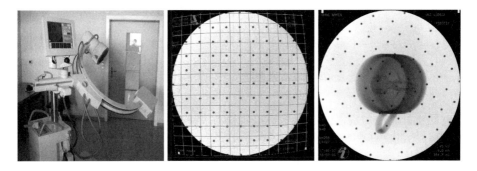

Fig. 2. Left: the robotized C-arm prototype. Middle: determination of the geometrical distortions using bi-variate polynomials. Right: projection image of the rat skull lying in a cup with calibration grid.

In a second experiment we imaged a rat skull (60 projections, 568x568, 135 degree angle range). In this experiment, the geometric distortion was corrected using bi-variate polynomials of degree five [8]. The coefficients were determined using a calibration object placed on the image intensifier (Fig. 2). This step becomes obsolete for the next version of the robotized C-arm device which will be equipped with digital flat panel detector technology, where no geometrical distortions occur.

3   Results

The registration accuracy of the clinical data experiment showed medium rotational deviations of 0.137 (x), 0.0134 (y) and 0.07 (z) degree and medium translational deviations of 0.05 (x), 0.70 (y), 0.35 (z) mm. In addition the visualization of the 2D/3D-registration results showed a clear positional error reduction (Fig. 3). In order to evaluate the correction algorithm results, we used the reconstruction residual (1), which is a direct measure for inconsistencies in the projection data. For the clinical dataset (Fig. 6) the residual dropped from initially 17019 to 7421 after 10 complete iterations (original data 2375).

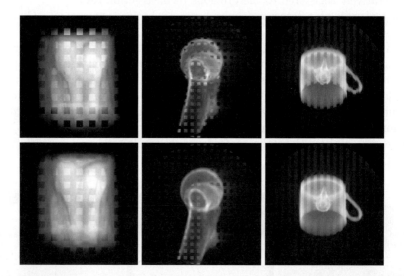

Fig. 3. Registration of one projection image with its DRR (top row unregistered) of the clinical distal femur bone (left), the sawbone proximal femur bone (middle) and the rat skull lying in a small cup (right)

Fig. 5 shows the reconstruction residual of the proximal femur experiment. The residual declines after each reconstruction-registration step. This gives evidence that the calculated positions lead to a more consistent reconstruction and in succession to a more accurate registration. In the rat skull experiment, a fast decline of the residiual could be observed, due to the prior removal of geometric distortions. Also a siginficant improvement in reconstruction quality could be observed after one iteration (Fig. 4) of the proposed correction scheme.

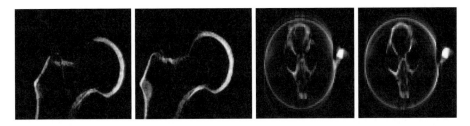

Fig. 4. Reconstructed slices from a proximal femur sawbone model and a rat skull. The respective left slice shows the uncorrected reconstruction result. Artefacts appearing as doubled, blurred edges and holes are significantly reduced by the iterative correction process (sawbone 7 iterations, rat skull 1 iteration).

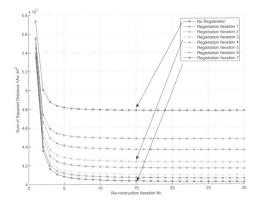

Fig. 5. Plot of the reconstruction residual (proximal femur experiment) in dependency of the reconstruction and registration iterations

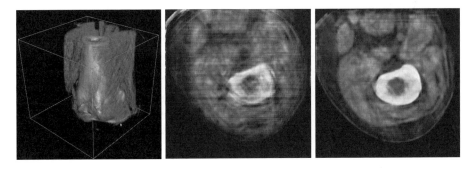

Fig. 6. Results from the clinical dataset of the distal femur. Reconstruction from original data, the volume rendering is clipped and visualized with a modified opacity function (left). Axial slice from the initial reconstruction from perturbed data (middle). Same slice after 10 iterations of the proposed algorithm (right).

4   Discussion

In this paper we have implemented a new method for positional error and motion compensation by integrating a 2D/3D-registration algorithm into a cone beam 3D-reconstruction framework. In all experiments, the inconsistencies were clearly reduced resulting in significantly improved reconstructions. In the case of simulated projections, perturbing the projection data has the effect that the position and orientation of the original object is also slightly modified. This disturbes a simple comparison. We plan to perform a rigid registration of the two volumes to allow for a direct comparison of the reconstruction results. The effect of slight positional changes of the reconstructed object due to the correction process can be also an issue for intraoperative navigation applications, since the reconstruction result is sometimes directly used for registration free navigation. To allow an intraoperative usage, the registration and reconstruction time must be in the range of two minutes. This is achievable by using GPU based algorithms and modern parallel hardware. Another important issue is registration accuracy. When performing position correction the use of subsequent projection image subsets should improve registration accuracy and robustness. Also slight changes of intrinsic x-ray camera parameters should be taken into account to model the twisting and bending of the C-arm.

References

1. Lee, K.J., et al.: Use of forward projection to correct patient motion during SPECT imaging. Physics in Medicine and Biology 43, 171–187 (1998)
2. Schumacher, H., Fischer, B.: A new approach for motion correction in SPECT imaging. In: Bildverarbeitung fuer die Medizin (2007)
3. Penney, G., Weese, J., Little, J.A., et al.: A comparison of similarity measures for use in 2d-3d medical image registration. In: Medical Image Computing and Computer-Assisted Intervention p. 1153 (1998)
4. Censor, Y., Gordon, D., Gordon, R.: Strong underrelaxation in kaczmarz's method for inconsistent systems. Numer. Math. 41, 83–92 (1983)
5. Popa, C., Zdunek, R.: Kaczmarz extended algorithm for tomographic image reconstruction from limited-data. Mathematics and Computers in Simulation 65, 579–598 (2004)
6. Weese, J., Goecke, R., Penney, G., Desmedt, P., Buzug, T., Schumann, H.: Fast voxel-based 2d/3d registration algorithm using a rendering method based on the shear-warp factorization. In: Proceedings of SPIE, pp. 802–810 (1999)
7. Parker, D.: An empirical investigation of the global behavior of several pattern search algorithms. In: Technical Report, Department of Computer Science - University of North Carolina (1999)
8. Dotter, M.: Flouroskopiebasierte Navigation zur intraoperativen Unterstuetzung orthopaedischer Eingriffe. PhD thesis, Technische Universitaet Muenchen (2006)
9. Chandra, R., Menon, R., Daqum, L., et al.: Parallel Programming in OpenMP. Morgan Kaufmann, San Francisco (2001)

10. Mueller, K.: Fast and accurate three-dimensional reconstruction from cone-beam projection data using algebraic methods. PhD thesis, Ohio State University (1998)
11. Binder, N., Bodensteiner, C., Matthaeus, L., et al.: Image guided positioning for an interactive c-arm fluoroscope. In: Computer Assisted Radiology and Surgery (CARS) (2006)
12. Matthaeus, L., Binder, N., Bodensteiner, C., et al.: Closed form inverse kinematic solution for fluoroscopic c-arms. Advanced Robotics 21 (2007)

Cortical Hemisphere Registration Via Large Deformation Diffeomorphic Metric Curve Mapping

Anqi Qiu[1] and Michael I. Miller[2]

[1] Division of Bioengineering, National University of Singapore
[2] Center for Imaging Science, Johns Hopkins University

Abstract. We present large deformation diffeomorphic metric curve mapping (LDDMM-Curve) for registering cortical hemispheres. We showed global cortical hemisphere matching and evaluated the mapping accuracy in five subregions of the cortex in fourteen MRI scans.

1 Introduction

Computational algorithms have been developed to compare anatomical shape and functions of the brain in subjects with and without neuropsychiatric disease using high-resolution magnetic resonance (MR) imaging datasets. The most popular approach for making such comparisons is to first spatially normalize brain structures and carry functions (e.g. cortical thickness, functional response) using atlas coordinates, and then to perform hypothesis testing in the atlas. We call this approach an extrinsic analysis since it depends on the relation between individual brains and the atlas. This is a powerful approach allowing us to study a large number of populations. Due to high variability of the brain anatomy across subjects, the spatial normalization becomes a crucial step because its accuracy directly influences statistical testing being inferred. Therefore, there has been great emphasis by groups on the study of the brain coordinates via vector mapping.

Cortical hemisphere registration driven by sulcal and gyral curves has been paid a great attention since sulci and gyri preserve the sulco-gyral pattern of the cortex. Specially, the brain is functionally partitioned by the sulci whose variability has been shown relative to clinical stages (e.g [1]). Compared to landmark points, the sulcal and gyral curves are one-dimensional higher manifolds and partially incorporate the geometry of the cortex. As comparing with image mapping based on intensity, the sulcal and gyral curves indirectly incorporate the intensity information since they lie at the boundary of the gray and white matters or gray matter and cerebrospinal fluid (CSF). And these curves also incorporate anatomical labeling information that is missing in the intensity-based image matching methods. As comparing with mappings of images and cortical surfaces, the vector mapping of the curves has less computation as well as itself has its own valuable clinical applications. However, due to high variability of brain structures across subjects, a desirable curve matching algorithm for brain

N. Ayache, S. Ourselin, A. Maeder (Eds.): MICCAI 2007, Part I, LNCS 4791, pp. 186–193, 2007.
© Springer-Verlag Berlin Heidelberg 2007

registration has to be able to handle cases, for instance, the initial and ending points of two curves do not necessarily correspond to the same structures and one curve can be a part of the other.

Our group has focused on a diffeomorphic metric mapping of anatomical coordinates in the setting of Large Deformation Diffeomorphic Metric Mapping (LD-DMM). The basic diffeomorphic metric mapping approach provides one-to-one, smooth with smooth inverse transformations acting on the ambient space. Thus, connected sets remain connected, disjoint sets remain disjoint, and the smoothness of features such as curves and surfaces is preserved. Specially, it places the set of anatomical shapes into a metric space for understanding anatomical structures across subjects. The LDDMM approach has been adapted to landmarks, images, and tensors [2,3,4].

We present the LDDMM-Curve mapping algorithm for registering cortical hemisphere. We show that such a mapping approach does not require exact correspondence information in the sense that paired curves on two anatomies can be represented by unequal number of points and one can be partial of the other or partially overlap with the other. We applied this approach to fourteen MRI datasets and evaluated them in five subregions of the cortex.

2   Large Deformation Diffeomorphic Metric Curve Mapping (LDDMM-Curve)

2.1   Vector-Valued Measure and Its Norm

Since a curve is a geometric object, it cannot be uniquely reconstructed based on the locations of a set of points. We consider that our curve embedded in $\mathbb{R}^3$ is a one-dimensional manifold in the sense that the local region of every point on the curve is equivalent to a line which can be uniquely defined by this point and the tangent vector at this location. In our curve mapping setting, we incorporate both the location information of points and their tangent vectors.

Assume curve C is discretized into a sequence of points $\mathbf{x} = (x_i)_{i=1}^n$. If $x_n = x_1$, then curve C is closed. We thus approximate curve C by a sequence of points and tangent vectors, $C = (c_{\mathbf{x},i}, \tau_{\mathbf{x},i})_{i=1}^n$, where $c_{\mathbf{x},i} = \frac{x_{i+1}+x_i}{2}$ is the center of two sequent points and $\tau_{\mathbf{x},i} = x_{i+1} - x_i$ is the tangent vector at $c_{\mathbf{x},i}$. One can associate curve C with a specific measure μ_C given by sum of vector-valued Diracs, $\mu_C = \sum_{i=1}^{n-1} \tau_{\mathbf{x},i} \delta_{c_{\mathbf{x},i}}$ such that μ_C acts on the smooth vector w in the form of $(\mu_C|w) = \sum_{i=1}^{n-1} \tau_{\mathbf{x},i} \cdot w$. Its norm is defined as

$$\|\mu_C\|_{W^*}^2 = \|\sum_{i=1}^{n-1} \tau_{\mathbf{x},i} \delta_{c_{\mathbf{x},i}}\|_{W^*}^2 = \sum_{i=1}^{n-1} \sum_{j=1}^{n-1} k_W(c_{\mathbf{x},i}, c_{\mathbf{x},j}) \, \tau_{\mathbf{x},i} \cdot \tau_{\mathbf{x},j}, \quad (1)$$

where k_W is the kernel in a reproducing kernel Hilbert space W of smooth vectors and W^* is the dual of W. The theoretical derivation of this norm can be found elsewhere [5]. Roughly, the more rounded the curve is, the higher energy it possesses, since flat shaped parts of the curve tend to vanish.

We assume that curves C and S are discretized by point sequences $\mathbf{x} = (x_i)_{i=1}^{n}$ and $\mathbf{y} = (y_j)_{j=1}^{m}$, the sequence of transformed points $\mathbf{z} = (\phi(x_i))_{i=1}^{n}$ gives a discretization of the deformed curve $\phi \cdot C$. The closeness of $\phi \cdot C$ and S can be quantified via the norm of the difference between their measures in Hilbert space W^*, a matching functional $D(\phi \cdot C, S)$, given by

$$D(\phi \cdot C, S) = \| \sum_{i=1}^{n-1} \tau_{\mathbf{z},i} \delta_{c_{\mathbf{z},i}} - \sum_{j=1}^{m-1} \tau_{\mathbf{y},j} \delta_{c_{\mathbf{y},j}} \|_{W^*}^2 , \qquad (2)$$

which is explicitly

$$D(\phi \cdot C, S) = \sum_{i=1}^{n-1}\sum_{j=1}^{n-1} k_W(c_{\mathbf{z},i}, c_{\mathbf{z},j}) \tau_{\mathbf{z},i} \cdot \tau_{\mathbf{z},j} - 2 \sum_{i=1}^{n-1}\sum_{j=1}^{m-1} k_W(c_{\mathbf{z},i}, c_{\mathbf{y},j}) \tau_{\mathbf{z},i} \cdot \tau_{\mathbf{y},j}$$

$$+ \sum_{i=1}^{m-1}\sum_{j=1}^{m-1} k_W(c_{\mathbf{y},i}, c_{\mathbf{y},j}) \tau_{\mathbf{y},i} \cdot \tau_{\mathbf{y},j} . \qquad (3)$$

The first and last terms are intrinsic energies of the two curves. The middle term gives penalty to mismatching between tangent vectors of S and those of $\phi(C)$. The explicit form of $D(\phi \cdot C, S)$ suggests that it does not require equal number of points on the two curves. One can be a part of the other or partially overlapped with the other. Optimal matching between curves will be defined via minimization of a functional composed of the matching term D and optionally a regularization term to guarantee smoothness of the transformations. Next we need to propose a model for deformation maps ϕ.

2.2   Variational Formulation of the LDDMM-Curve Mapping

We assume that shapes can be generated one from the other via a flow of diffeomorphisms, solutions of ordinary differential equations $\dot{\phi}_t = v_t(\phi_t), t \in [0,1]$ with $\phi_0 = $ id the identity map, and associated vector fields $v_t, t \in [0,1]$. We compute pairs C, S, such that there exists a diffeomorphism ϕ transforming one to the other $\phi_1 \cdot C = S$ at time $t = 1$. The metric distance between shapes is the length of the geodesic curves $\phi_t \cdot C, t \in [0,1]$ through the shape space generated from C connecting to S. The metric between two shape C, S takes the form

$$\rho(C,S)^2 = \inf_{v_t: \dot{\phi}_t = v_t(\phi_t), \phi_0 = \text{id}} \int_0^1 \|v_t\|_V^2 dt \quad \text{such that } \phi_1 \cdot C = S . \qquad (4)$$

where $v_t \in V$, a Hilbert space of smooth vector fields with norm $\| \cdot \|_V$. In practice, the metric ρ and the diffeomorphic correspondence $\phi = \phi_1$ between the pair of curves (C, S) is calculated via a variational formulation of the "inexact matching problem". We associate for each pair of curves (C, S), a norm-squared cost $D(\phi_1 \cdot C, S)$; then the variational problem requires minimization of the functional

$$J(v_t) = \inf_{v_t: \dot{\phi}_t = v_t(\phi_t), \phi_0 = \text{id}} \gamma \int_0^1 \|v_t\|_V^2 dt + \sum_{p=1}^{P} D(\phi_1 \cdot C^{(p)}, S^{(p)}) , \qquad (5)$$

where $D(\phi_1 \cdot C^{(p)}, S^{(p)})$ is given in (3) for the pth pair of curves $\{C^{(p)}, S^{(p)}\}$. P indicates the number of paired curves considered in the mapping. For the simplicity of notation.

To ensure that the resulting solutions to (5) are diffeomorphisms, v_t must belong to a space, V, of regular vector fields [6,7], for $t \in [0,1]$ with $\int_0^1 \|v_t\|_V dt < \infty$. We model V as Hilbert space with an associated kernel function k_V. Define the trajectories $x_i(t) := \phi_t(x_i)$ for $i = 1, \ldots, n$. Then the general solution to this variational problem can be written in the form of

$$v_t(x) = \sum_{i=1}^{n} k_V(x_i(t), x)\alpha_i(t) , \tag{6}$$

where $\alpha_i(t)$ are referred to as *momentum vectors*, which are analogous to the momentum in fluid mechanics. These momentum vectors can be computed from trajectories $x_i(t)$ by solving the system of linear equations

$$\frac{dx_i(t)}{dt} = \sum_{j=1}^{n} k_V(x_j(t), x_i(t))\alpha_j(t), \qquad i = 1, \ldots, n. \tag{7}$$

2.3 Spline Interpolation of Deformation

Assume x to be a point on a cortical surface. We would like to apply the deformation on x based on $\hat{v}_t$ found from the LDDMM-Curve mapping. Starting from any arbitrary state $\hat{v}_t$ of the time-dependant vector fields, let us find the optimal vector fields v_t that keep trajectories $x_i(t) = \phi_t(x_i)$, where x_i is a point on curve C in (5), unchanged. This is a classical interpolation problem in a Hilbert space setting, which finds vector fields that minimize the V-norm and satisfy for each time t and each $1 \leq i \leq n$ the constraint $v_t(x_i(t)) = \dot{x}_i(t)$ where $x_i(t)$ are the fixed trajectories. The solution to this interpolation is expressed as a linear combination of spline vector fields involving the kernel operator k_V as given in (6) and its associated trajectory can be computed by (7). The spline interpolation of deformation in space of V guarantee diffeomorphism.

3 Experiments

3.1 Subjects, MRI Acquisition, and Data Processing

Fourteen subjects were randomly selected from schizophrenia and bipolar disorder studies in the Division of Psychiatric Neuroimaging at Johns Hopkins University School of Medicine. MRI scans were acquired using 1.5 T scanner and MPRAGE sequence (repetition time = 13.40 ms, echo time = 4.6 ms, flip angle = $20°$, number of acquisition = 1, matrix 256×256) with 1 mm^3 isotropic resolution across the entire cranium.

The cortical surfaces at the boundary between the gray matter and white matter were generated by freesurfer [8]. Sulcal curves are well observed in the cortical surface. We delineated six sulcal curves and five brain outline curves on each cortical surface via a semi-automated method [9]. As shown in Figure 1, the six curves include three of them in the lateral view, the superior frontal sulcus, the central sulcus, the Sylvian fissure, and three in the medial view, the sulcus on the top of corpus callosum, the parieto-occipital fissure, and the calcarine sulcus. These six sulcal curves are selected because they are either the sulci segmenting the brain into functional distinct regions or major sulci in the brain lobe. The five brain outline curves are labeled from the inferior to the superior and from the posterior to the anterior as numbered in Figure 1(B). To define each curve, we manually selected a pair of starting and ending points and then the dynamic programming procedure automatically tracked the curve between the two points along the sulcus (for six sulcal curves) or the gyrus (for five brain outlines) [9]. During the LDDMM-Curve mapping, the eleven curves of one subject were chosen as template curves to map to target curves of other surfaces via the LDDMM-Curve algorithm. Finally, the optimal deformation was applied for transforming the cortical surfaces back to the template surface coordinates. In our experiments, kernels of $k_V(x, y)$ and $k_W(x, y)$ were radial with the form $e^{-\frac{|y-x|^2}{\sigma^2}} id$, where id is a 3×3 identity matrix. σ_V and σ_W represent the kernel sizes of k_V and k_W, respectively. They were experimentally adjusted as $\sigma_V = 100$ and $\sigma_W = 5$.

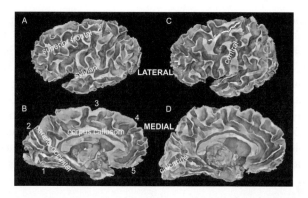

Fig. 1. Panels (A,B) respectively show a surface in the lateral and medial views. Panel (C,D) shows another example. Six sulci and five brain outlines are labeled on each surface.

3.2 Examples

Figure 2 illustrates two cortical surfaces deformed to the template surface coordinates via the LDDMM-Curve mapping algorithm. The template surface is in yellow and the two surfaces to be deformed are in green. The top rows of panels (A,B) indicate that the green surfaces are roughly in the same orientation as the yellow template surface before the mapping. However, the superior region and occipital lobe on the green surfaces are clearly not aligned with those on the template. Moreover, the sulco-gyral patterns are mismatched between the green and yellow template surfaces. We illustrate the mapped green surfaces superimposed with the template surface in the bottom rows of panels (A,B). Clearly, the overall structure of the green surfaces are well deformed to the shape of the template.

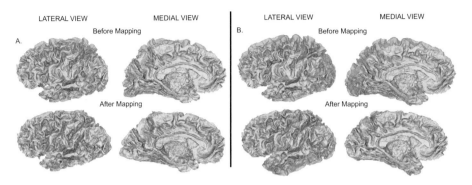

Fig. 2. Panels (A,B) respectively show one example of mapping surfaces using curves. The template surface is in yellow, while the other surfaces are in green. The top row of each panel illustrates the template superimposed with the target before the mapping; the bottom row shows after the mapping. The left and right columns are respectively show the lateral and medial views of the cortical surfaces.

3.3   Evaluation of the Mapping

There are two ways to evaluate the spatial normalization procedure, including measurements quantifying the mismatching of two objects as a direct evaluation method [10] as well as shape classification and group analysis of functional responses, e.g. [11] as an indirect evaluation method. We validate our mapping results via the direct evaluation method. We calculate the cumulative distribution of distances between the deformed targets and the template to quantify their closeness. We call this as *surface distance graph* from surface T to surface S, defined as the percentage of vertices on a template surface T having the distance to a surface S less than d mm. Let v_{s_i} and v_{t_i} respectively be vertices on surfaces S and T. The distance of v_{t_i} to S is defined by $d_{t_i} = \min_{v_{s_i} \in S} \|v_{s_i} - v_{t_i}\|$, where $\|\cdot\|$ is the Euclidean distance in R^3. The surface distance graph is the cumulative distribution of d_{t_i}. Since this measurement is sensitive to the folding structure, we chose five subregions of the cortex containing major sulci to be evaluated, as shown in Figure 3(A,B).

Panels (C-G) of Figure 3 shows the surface distance graphs for five subregions of the cortex that respectively contain the superior frontal sulcus, the central sulcus, the sylvian fissure, the calcarine sulcus, as well as the parieto-occipital fissure. The black curves are surface distance graphs corresponding to each individual original surface; the red curve is the average graph among them. Similarly, the gray curves are surface distance graphs corresponding to each individual deformed surface; the green curve is the average graph among them. These five panels show that the mean average surface distance graph after the

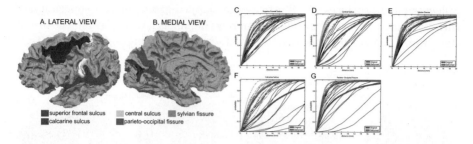

Fig. 3. Panels (A,B) respectively show the lateral and medial views of the template surface with colored subregions of the cortex. Panels (C-G) show surface distance graphs for each subregion of the cortex with gray lines corresponding to the deformed surfaces and black lines associated with the original surfaces. The red and green lines are the mean surface distance graphs before and after the mapping.

mapping is shifted to the top of one before the mapping, which indicates that these five structures were driven to the place close to their corresponding locations on the template. Compared to the spread of the surface distance graphs among the original surface, the graphs become much close to each other after the mapping, which suggests the removal of anatomical variation across subjects.

4   Conclusion

We present the LDDMM-Curve mapping algorithm in the discrete case to mapping multiple pairs of curves for cortical hemisphere registration. The relevant approach has been developed for dealing with geometric objects of surfaces in the LDDMM setting [12]. Both the LDDMM curve and surface mappings represent geometric curves or surfaces as vector-valued measure whose norm serves as a matching functional in the LDDMM variational formulation. Both of the approaches are powerful tools for brain registration. However, one deals with curve configuration and the other handles surface configuration. Compared to the surface mapping approach, the curve mapping has its own advantage of less computation. And also the selection of curves is often supervised and provides additional labeling information. The choice of the mapping algorithms depends on the interest of applications. For instance, to differentiate functional activations on the two banks of a sulcus, the LDDMM-Curve mapping would be a better choice since the LDDMM-Surface mapping does not incorporate anatomical label information.

Several curve mapping algorithms exist for the brain registration [13,1], which require the intermediate spherical step of deforming the cortex to a spherical representation. However, this intermediate step itself introduces a large distortion that does not consistently appear across subjects. Such mapping induced distortion can result in significant loss of power in extraction of structural information. In addition to that, the deformation may not be directly applied to the natural image space. However, our approach does not require an intermediate spherical representation of the brain and directly works on the natural coordinates of curves, which potentially provide better matching.

Acknowledgments

The work reported here was supported by grants: NIH R01 MH064838, NIH R01 EB00975, NIH P20 M071616, NIH P41 RR15241, and NSF DMS 0456253. The authors would like to thank Dr. J. Tilak Ratnanather and Dr. Barta for providing the data.

References

1. Thompson, P.M., Schwartz, C., Lin, R.T., Khan, A.A., Toga, A.W.: Three–dimensional statistical analysis of sulcal variability in the human brain. J. Neurosci. 16(13), 4261–4274 (1996)
2. Joshi, S., Miller, M.I.: Landmark matching via large deformation diffeomorphisms. IEEE Trans. Image Processing 9(8), 1357–1370 (2000)
3. Beg, M.F., Miller, M.I., Trouvé, A., Younes, L.: Computing large deformation metric mappings via geodesic flows of diffeomorphisms. International Journal of Computer Vision 61(2), 139–157 (2005)
4. Cao, Y., Miller, M., Winslow, R., Younes, L.: Large deformation diffeomorphic metric mapping of vector fields. IEEE Trans. Med. Imag. 24, 1216–1230 (2005)
5. Glaunès, J., Trouvé, A., Younes, L.: Modeling planar shape variation via hamiltonian flows of curves. In: Krim, H., Yezzi, A., (eds.) Statistics and Analysis of Shapes, Birkhauser (2006)
6. Trouvé, A.: An infinite dimensional group approach for physics based models (1995), Technical report electronically available at http://www.cis.jhu.edu
7. Dupuis, P., Grenander, U., Miller, M.I.: Variational problems on flows of diffeomorphisms for image matching. Quaterly of Applied Math. 56, 587–600 (1998)
8. Fischl, B., Sereno, M.I., Dale, A.M.: Cortical surface-based analysis II: inflation, flattening, and a surface-based coordinate system. NeuroImage 9, 195–207 (1999)
9. Ratnanather, J.T., Barta, P.E., Honeycutt, N.A., Lee, N., Morris, N.G., Dziorny, A.C., Hurdal, M.K., Pearlson, G.D., Miller, M.I.: Dynamic programming generation of boundaries of local coordinatized submanifolds in the neocortex: application to the planum temporale. NeuroImage 20(1), 359–377 (2003)
10. Vaillant, M., Qiu, A., Glaunès, J., Miller, M.I.: Diffeomorphic metric surface mapping in subregion of the superior temporal gyrus. accepted by NeuroImage (2007)
11. Miller, M.I., Beg, M.F., Ceritoglu, C., Stark, C.: Increasing the power of functional maps of the medial temporal lobe by using large deformation diffeomorphic metric mapping. Proc. Natl. Acad. Sci. 102, 9685–9690 (2005)
12. Vaillant, M., Glaunès, J.: Surface matching via currents. In: Christensen, G.E., Sonka, M. (eds.) IPMI 2005. LNCS, vol. 3565, pp. 381–392. Springer, Heidelberg (2005)
13. Vaillant, M., Davatzikos, C.: Hierarchical matching of cortical features for deformable brain image registration. In: Kuba, A., Sámal, M., Todd-Pokropek, A. (eds.) IPMI 1999. LNCS, vol. 1613, pp. 182–195. Springer, Heidelberg (1999)

Tagged Volume Rendering of the Heart

Daniel Mueller[1], Anthony Maeder[2], and Peter O'Shea[1]

[1] Queensland University of Technology, Brisbane, Australia
d.mueller@qut.edu.au
[2] e-Health Research Centre, CSIRO ICT Centre, Brisbane, Australia

Abstract. We present a novel system for 3-D visualisation of the heart
and coronary arteries. Binary tags (generated offline) are combined with
value-gradient transfer functions (specified online) allowing for interactive visualisation, while relaxing the offline segmentation criteria. The
arteries are roughly segmented using a Hessian-based line filter and the
pericardial cavity using a Fast Marching active contour. A comparison
of different contour initialisations reveals that simple geometric shapes
(such as spheres or extruded polygons) produce suitable results.

1 Introduction

It is often overlooked that segmentation is integral to volume visualisation [1].
In the case of indirect volume rendering ('surface rendering') the segmentation
takes the form of isosurface extraction using Marching Cubes [2] prior to the
actual rendering. In the case of direct volume rendering (DVR) the segmentation
is typically achieved during the rendering process ('online') via a lookup table
('transfer function'). Various online segmentation algorithms for DVR have been
discussed in the literature [3,4,5,6]. Kniss et al. [4] advocated the use of two-
dimensional transfer functions dependent on pixel value and gradient magnitude,
in which the user interactively specifies the function using a number of widgets.
Tzeng et al. [5] proposed an approach using a machine learning algorithm (such
as a support vector machine) applied to each pixel in the image.

However, such online methods suffer from a number of drawbacks. Firstly,
as discussed by Hadwiger et al. [7], 2-D transfer functions can not typically
distinguish between objects with similar characteristics. Secondly, online segmentation unnecessarily constrains the choice of algorithm. Take for example
3-D texture rendering: the segmentation method must be implemented on the
graphics hardware in real-time, currently precluding whole classes of algorithms
(including active contour methods). Tagged volume rendering addresses these
shortfalls using a number of *a priori* segmented binary masks ('tags') which are
assigned separate transfer functions [7,8,9].

To date much of the work regarding tagged volume rendering has fixated on
generic matters: there has been little focus on the applicability of the methods.
In contrast, this paper presents the material from an applications perspective
centred around the visualisation of the heart. For diagnostic and treatment planning purposes, radiologists and surgeons require means to visualise the coronary
arteries from multi-slice spiral computed tomography angiography (MS-CTA)

N. Ayache, S. Ourselin, A. Maeder (Eds.): MICCAI 2007, Part I, LNCS 4791, pp. 194–201, 2007.
© Springer-Verlag Berlin Heidelberg 2007

images. However, this task is non-trivial for various reasons: unwanted structures (such as the thoracic cage) clutter the regions of interest; and the contrast agent highlights the coronary arteries (as desired), but also portions of the ventricles, atria, aorta, and pulmonary arteries. As such, the traditional DVR approach using value-gradient transfer functions is insufficient for this application.

In this paper we apply tagged volume rendering to the problem. We utilise Hessian-based line filters for segmenting the coronary arteries [10] and propose the use of an active contour method [11] for segmenting the pericardial cavity. A suitable speed function is derived for controlling the expansion of the active contour. We experiment with various mechanisms for specifying the initial contour, and conclude that simple geometric shapes (such as spheres or extruded polygons) produce suitable results. Finally the three *a priori* segmented volumes (heart, arteries, and surrounds) are used as tags within a rendering scheme facilitating per-tag transfer functions. The proposed system is demonstrated using a number of clinically obtained *in vivo* datasets.

2   Method

The proposed system consists of two main steps: (1) the offline segmentation of binary tags, and (2) the online refinement of structures within these tags using traditional value-gradient transfer functions. This two-stage approach provides for online interactivity while promoting relaxed criteria for the offline segmentation. Furthermore, the offline segmentation can be performed on down-sampled volumes (which decreases the execution time) without affecting quality.

2.1   Tagged Volume Rendering

We implement generic direct volume rendering using 3-D texture mapping [4]. In this approach, 3-D textures are uploaded to the graphics processing unit (GPU). At the application level, the rendering system slices the uploaded 3-D textures using view-aligned polygons. This 'proxy-geometry' tri-linearly interpolates the textures at any given viewing angle. A small program ('shader') is applied to each potential pixel ('fragment'), acting as a post-interpolative transfer function.

For tagged volume rendering, a tag image is also uploaded to the GPU, the value of which switches on or off per-object transfer functions. In the original method [7], each tag represented an exact binary object to be classified (using a 1-D transfer function), resulting in the need to linearly filter tag boundaries to achieve appropriate resolution at the pixel level. Higuera et al. [8] extended this approach by adding a smoothing mechanism to create near-continuous tags.

We introduce an assumption (different from [7,8]) which simplifies the concept of a tag: we assume a tag is a mask guaranteeing to *include* structures of interest, but not *exactly* delineate them. Similar to Svakhine et al. [9, Sec. 3], we then apply value-gradient transfer functions to each object. As a result, the tag texture can be interpolated using a simple nearest-neighbour scheme and the complexity of pixel-resolution boundary filtering is avoided altogether.

2.2   Line Filtering for Vessel Segmentation

We use the line enhancement filter proposed by Sato et al. [10] to segment the coronary arteries. The response of a 1-D line filter is as follows:

$$R(\boldsymbol{x}, \sigma_f) = \left[-\frac{d^2}{dx^2} G(\boldsymbol{x}, \sigma_f) \right] * I(\boldsymbol{x}) \qquad (1)$$

where $*$ denotes convolution, $I(\boldsymbol{x})$ is the input image, and $G(\boldsymbol{x}, \sigma_f)$ is the Gaussian function. This filter can be extended to multiple dimensions using the Hessian matrix $\nabla^2 I(\boldsymbol{x})$. The eigenvalues $\lambda_1(\boldsymbol{x})$, $\lambda_2(\boldsymbol{x})$, $\lambda_3(\boldsymbol{x})$ (where $\lambda_1(\boldsymbol{x}) > \lambda_2(\boldsymbol{x}) > \lambda_3(\boldsymbol{x})$) of the Hessian can then be used to derive a line similarity measure (see [10, Sec. 2.1] for full details).

For our application we tune the filter to capture a single line width ($\sigma_f = 0.7$). After applying the filter, the final binary tag is extracted using region growing: for each dataset two seeds were placed in the left and right coronary arteries, and an intensity threshold specified to exclude non-vascular structures.

2.3   Fast Marching for Heart Segmentation

The Fast Marching method is a computationally efficient scheme for computing the propagation of an active contour [11]. In this scheme the front always expands outwards; that is, the speed function $F > 0$. The position of the front can be characterized by the arrival function $T(\boldsymbol{x})$ and reduces to the non-linear partial differential equation:

$$\|\nabla T\| F = 1 \qquad (2)$$

Fast Marching methods are advantageous because they implicitly handle topological changes and are computationally efficient (when implemented using heap sort algorithms). The method returns the arrival function $T(\boldsymbol{x})$, from which the contour at any desired arrival time can be obtained.

We propose the use of Fast Marching for segmenting the structures comprising the heart. The pericardial cavity — in which the heart resides — acts as a boundary restricting the propagation of the contour. In this sense the Fast Marching method can be seen as a form of boundary-regulated region growing.

Speed Function
As Sethian [11, pp. 4] states, the challenge is to specify a suitable speed function F. We propose an edge-based speed function:

$$F(I(\boldsymbol{x})) = \begin{cases} SIG(\ RGM(I(\boldsymbol{x}))\ ); & I(\boldsymbol{x}) > t_l \\ 0; & \text{otherwise} \end{cases} \qquad (3)$$

$$RGM(I(\boldsymbol{x})) = \left\| \nabla (\ G(\boldsymbol{x}, \sigma_g) * I(\boldsymbol{x})\ ) \right\| \qquad (4)$$

$$SIG(I(\boldsymbol{x})) = \left[1 + \exp\left(\frac{-I(\boldsymbol{x}) - \beta}{\alpha} \right) \right]^{-1} \qquad (5)$$

where RGM is the gradient magnitude computed using recursive filters which approximate convolution with the first derivative of a Gaussian, and SIG is the non-linear monotonic sigmoid mapping function. The proposed speed function F varies between $[0, 1]$ and depends on four parameters: σ_g, the aperture of the Gaussian convolution kernel; α, the width of the sigmoid function; β, the centre of the sigmoid function; and t_l, a global threshold which suppresses air in the lungs. It was empirically found these parameters could assume constant values across all the datasets: $\sigma_g = 0.5$, $\alpha = -10$, $\beta = 10$, and $t_l = -250$.

In most cases the proposed speed function is adequate, however the results can be improved by pre-processing the datasets. Firstly, we employed an edge-preserving denoising technique: the curvature flow method discussed in [11, Ch. 16] with time-step $t_{cf} = 0.1$ and iterations $n_{cf} = 10$ is adequate. Next, in order to suppress artificial boundaries caused by structures containing contrast agent, a global intensity threshold ($t_c \approx 125$) was applied. Finally, in cases with thin pericardium and pleura, the sternum must be reinserted to prevent contour leakage. This can be achieved using an intensity-based region growing operation seeded anywhere in the sternum. Fig. 1 depicts this pre-processing pipeline.

Initial Contour
The initial contour plays an important role in the final arrival function. For our application it is important to quickly and easily specify an initial contour likely to propagate evenly to the pericardium. We therefore devised a simple experiment comparing three initial contour specification methods:

Point Landmarks: The user places n_p points centrally and evenly within the pericardial cavity. This is the typical method for specifying the initial contour for Fast Marching methods [12]. It should be noted that it is difficult to ensure an even spread of these points.

Spherical Landmarks: The user places n_s spheres centrally within the pericardial cavity. Each sphere is positioned and sized such that its volume does not enter unwanted structures (except the lungs). See the first row in Fig. 2.

Extruded Polygon: The user positions n_g points ($n_g \geq 3$) describing a polygon on the sagittal plane. The polygon is extruded along the plane between $[z_{start}, z_{end}]$. As with the spheres, the specified volume is not allowed to enter unwanted structures (except the lungs). See the second row in Fig. 2.

To exclude portions of the initial contours in the lungs, the initial images were masked using the same threshold as the speed function (ie. $t_l = -250$). An ROC-like analysis comparing these methods is presented in the next section.

Obtaining the Final Contour
Because the tag will be refined using a gradient-based transfer function, it is important that material boundaries are included in the final contour. To achieve this we eroded the arrival function with a ball structuring element (radius $= 2$), denoted $T_e(\boldsymbol{x})$. The optimal arrival time (t_a) can be found using a number of mechanisms: (a) interactive thresholding of the arrival function, (b) the arrival time at a user specified point, or (c) the maximum or average arrival time of a group of points. Once the desired arrival time is determined, the final binary volume can be extracted by applying a binary threshold ($0 < T_e(\boldsymbol{x}) < t_a$).

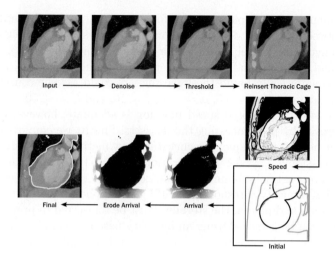

Fig. 1. This flow diagram depicts the data preparation and use of the Fast Marching method for segmenting structures within the pericardial cavity

3   Results

3.1   Data

For this study five datasets were chosen to represent anatomical variability. The first two datasets (A & B) exhibited severe calcific atherosclerosis and aortic calcification, typifying patients with advanced ischemic heart disease. The other datasets (C, D & E) displayed early indicators of heart disease: mild atherosclerosis in the coronary arteries. Dataset A is from an open-data initiative supported by the National Library of Medicine [13]. Datasets B-E were acquired in a hospital setting using contrast-enhanced, ECG-gated, 40-slice spiral computed tomography angiography (Brilliance 40, Philips Medical Systems, MA, USA)[1].

3.2   Initial Contour

An ROC-like analysis was performed to compare the three contour initialisation methods. As previously discussed, the binary tags have an inherent flexibility: they are not required to exactly delineate objects. To reflect this in our analysis — rather than comparing with manually segmented volumes — the results were compared with a number of point landmarks. For each dataset 100 points were placed in desired structures (eg. aorta, left and right coronary arteries, ventricles, and atria) and 100 points in undesired structures (eg. spine, sternum, ribs, diaphragm, and liver). A true positive occurred when a desired point fell inside the resultant segmentation; and similarly, a true negative occurred when an undesired point fell outside the resultant segmentation. This scheme allowed for

[1]   Thanks to Dr Richard Slaughter, The Prince Charles Hospital, Brisbane, Australia.

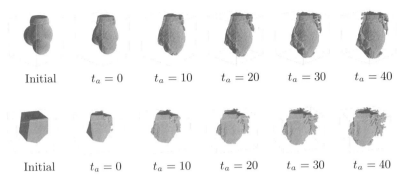

Fig. 2. Two of the contour initialisation methods at various arrival times (t_a). First row: Dataset C, four spherical landmarks. Second row: Dataset A, five-sided extruded polygon.

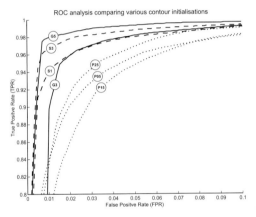

Fig. 3. ROC analysis comparing various contour initialisations. Spheres (S) and extruded polygons (G) performed slightly better than point landmarks (P).

'fuzzy' structures — such as the pericardium — which may either be included or excluded in the resultant segmentation without affecting the measure.

Different settings were used to generate a range of initial contours: for point landmarks $n_p = \{5, 10, 15, 20, 25\}$, for spherical landmarks $n_s = \{1, 2, 3, 4, 5\}$, and for extruded polygons $n_g = \{3, 4, 5, 6, 7\}$. The classifier discrimination threshold was the arrival threshold (t_a). The results from each dataset were linearly interpolated to create a common abscissa and then averaged.

The ROC curves depicted in Fig. 3 indicate that all of the contour initialisation methods produce good results (all curves tend towards the $[0, 1]$ point). The geometric shapes (spheres and extruded polygons) performed slightly better than point landmarks, most likely because they provided a better initial estimate of the desired contour. As such, the tags for the following renderings were generated using $n_g = 7$, with t_a computed using an interactive binary threshold.

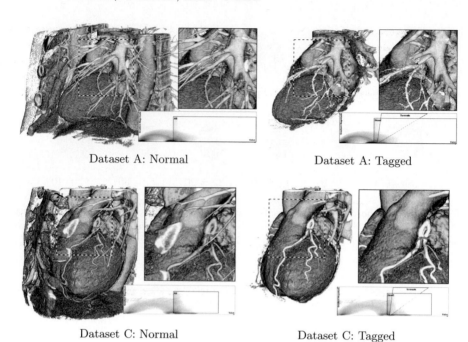

Dataset A: Normal   Dataset A: Tagged

Dataset C: Normal   Dataset C: Tagged

Fig. 4. Resultant images using the normal and tagged volume rendering approaches. In the tagged method the heart and coronary arteries are assigned different transfer functions (inset, lower right). For a colour version of this figure see: http://eprints.qut.edu.au/archive/00008156/

3.3   Final Renderings

The offline segmentation was implemented using the Insight Toolkit (ITK) [12] and the volume rendering using OpenGL and OpenGL Shading Language (GLSL) on a desktop computer (Intel Pentium D, 2×3.0 GHz processors, 2 GB RAM, NVIDIA GeForce 8800 GTX, 768 MB VRAM). The value image was represented using 16-bits, while the gradient magnitude and tag images were represented using 8-bits. The datasets were down-sampled (256^3) using linear interpolation for the tag segmentation and ROC analysis, and then the tag returned to full size ($\approx 512^3$) using nearest-neighbour interpolation for rendering.

Each tag image was processed in roughly 7 minutes: 3 min for vessel segmentation, 2 mins for pre-processing, 1 min for computing the speed function, and 1 min for Fast Marching. Each scene was rendered with a 512^2 viewport at interactive framerates: ≈ 15 fps with an interactive sampling rate ($r = 0.5$) and ≈ 5 fps with a high quality sampling rate ($r = 2.0$). Fig. 4 depicts normal and tagged results from two of the datasets (A & C). The advantage of tagged rendering over the normal approach is self evident: the coronary arteries are more easily distinguished on account of the removed clutter and improved contrast.

4   Conclusion

We presented a novel system for tagged volume rendering of the heart. The system is comprised of two stages: offline segmentation of the coronary arteries and pericardial cavity; followed by the online application of gradient-value transfer functions to refine the tags. This two-stage approach provides for interactivity while promoting relaxed segmentation criteria. An ROC-like analysis of the active contour method (used for segmenting the pericardial cavity) showed that simple geometric shapes (such as spheres or extruded polygons) offer good trade-offs between simplicity, sensitivity, and specificity. The proposed system is useful for diagnosis and treatment planning of ischemic heart disease.

References

1. Udupa, J.: Three-dimensional rendering in medicine: some common misconceptions. In: Medical Imaging: Visualization, Display, and Image-Guided Procedures, San Deigo, USA, SPIE, vol. 4319, pp. 660–670 (2001)
2. Lorensen, B., Cline, H.: Marching cubes: A high resolution 3D surface construction algorithm. In: Computer Graphics and Interactive Techniques, pp. 163–169. ACM Press, New York (1987)
3. Pfister, H., Lorensen, B., Bajaj, C., Kindlmann, G., Schroeder, W., Avila, L., Raghu, K., Machiraju, R., Lee, J.: The transfer function bake-off. IEEE Computer Graphics and Applications 21(3), 16–22 (2001)
4. Kniss, J., Kindlmann, G., Hansen, C.: Multidimensional transfer functions for interactive volume rendering. IEEE Transactions on Visualization and Computer Graphics 8(3), 270–285 (2002)
5. Tzeng, F., Lum, E., Ma, K.: An intelligent system approach to higher-dimensional classification of volume data. IEEE Transactions on Visualization and Computer Graphics 11(3), 273–284 (2005)
6. Weber, G., Dillard, S., Carr, H.: Topology-controlled volume rendering. IEEE Transactions on Visualization and Computer Graphics 13(2), 330–341 (2007)
7. Hadwiger, M., Berger, C., Hauser, H.: High-quality two-level volume rendering of segmented data sets on consumer graphics hardware. In: Visualization, pp. 301–308. IEEE Computer Society Press, Los Alamitos (2003)
8. Higuera, F.V., Hastreiter, P., Naraghi, R., Fahlbusch, R., Greiner, G.: Smooth volume rendering of labelled medical data on consumer graphics hardware. In: Medical Imaging: Visualization, Image-Guided Procedures, and Display. SPIE, vol. 5744, pp. 13–21 (2005)
9. Svakhine, N., Ebert, D.: Illustration motifs for effective medical volume illustration. IEEE Computer Graphics and Applications 25(3), 31–39 (2005)
10. Sato, Y., Nakajima, S., Shiraga, N., Atsumi, H., Yoshida, S., Koller, T., Gerig, G., Kikinis, R.: Three-dimensional multi-scale line filter for segmentation and visualization of curvilinear structures in medical images. Medical Image Analysis 2(2), 143–168 (1998)
11. Sethian, J.: Level Set and Fast Marching Methods. Cambridge Press, Cambridge (1999)
12. Ibanez, L., Schroeder, L., Ng, W., Cates, L.: J.: The ITK Software Guide: The Insight Segmentation and Registration Toolkit. Kitware, Inc. (2007)
13. Holmes, D., Workman, E., Robb, R.: The NLM-Mayo Image Collection. The Insight Journal, special issue: MICCAI Open Science Workshop pp. 1–8 (August 2005)

One-Class Acoustic Characterization Applied to Blood Detection in IVUS

Sean M. O'Malley[1], Morteza Naghavi[2], and Ioannis A. Kakadiaris[1]

[1] Computational Biomedicine Lab, University of Houston; Houston, TX
[2] Association for Eradication of Heart Attack; Houston, TX

Abstract. Intravascular ultrasound (IVUS) is an invasive imaging modality capable of providing cross-sectional images of the interior of a blood vessel in real time and at normal video framerates (10-30 frames/s). Low contrast between the features of interest in the IVUS imagery remains a confounding factor in IVUS analysis; it would be beneficial therefore to have a method capable of detecting certain physical features imaged under IVUS in an automated manner. We present such a method and apply it to the detection of blood. While blood detection algorithms are not new in this field, we deviate from traditional approaches to IVUS signal characterization in our use of 1-class learning. This eliminates certain problems surrounding the need to provide "foreground" and "background" (or, more generally, n-class) samples to a learner. Applied to the blood-detection problem on 40 MHz recordings made *in vivo* in swine, we are able to achieve ~95% sensitivity with ~90% specificity at a radial resolution of ~600 μm.

1 Introduction

Intravascular ultrasound (IVUS) is currently the gold-standard modality for intravascular imaging. However, the use of this imagery has been hampered by the fact that some tasks remain difficult as a result of the indistinguishability of certain features under IVUS. To help alleviate these problems, a number of computational methods have been proposed over the last decade which aim to detect or characterize one or more features in the IVUS image (e.g., plaque components [1], contrast agents [2], or blood [3]). Digitally enhancing the contrast between a feature and its background allows easier manual interpretation as well as improved computer-aided analysis. For instance, blood detection may serve as a pre-processing step for segmentation of the luminal border.

Our contribution in this paper is to investigate the feasibility of 1-class learning to the problem of distinguishing a single feature imaged under IVUS. In particular, we apply this to the problem of blood detection. The primary advantage to our approach is the fact that "background" samples need never be provided. In our case, as well as others in the field, the background can consist of a wide variety of other imaged tissues. As such, providing suitable background samples for training may be labor-intensive and subjective. With 1-class learning, we circumvent this problem by ignoring the background during training.

N. Ayache, S. Ourselin, A. Maeder (Eds.): MICCAI 2007, Part I, LNCS 4791, pp. 202–209, 2007.
© Springer-Verlag Berlin Heidelberg 2007

Instead, training only requires samples of the foreground class which, in general, can be obtained relatively easily from expert annotations. In practical terms, our method has an advantage over luminal-border segmentation methods in that it is not inherently tied to only detecting luminal blood. For example, we intend to apply this framework to detect extra-luminal blood as well, specifically in the microvascular network known to feed the coronary arteries and plaques [4].

An apparent disadvantage to our approach is that it need not necessarily work at all: as the learner is never exposed to negative examples, it could naively classify every sample as positive and give a 100% true-positive rate along with a 100% false-positive rate. Features which provide little distinguishing power between foreground and background will also result in a high false-positive rate. This being the case, our study has two goals: to describe how the recognizer framework may be applied to problems such as that of blood detection under ultrasound, and to examine specific features for accomplishing this. In Sec. 2 we provide background on the problems surrounding our task. In Sec. 3, we discuss our contribution. We conclude with results (Sec. 4) and a discussion (Sec. 5).

2   Background

Intravascular ultrasound: The IVUS catheter consists of either a solid-state or a mechanically-rotated transducer which transmits a pulse and receives an acoustic signal at a discrete set of angles over each radial scan. Commonly, 240 to 360 such one-dimensional signals are obtained per (digital or mechanical) rotation. The envelopes of these signals are computed, log-compressed, and then geometrically transformed to obtain the familiar disc-shaped IVUS image (Fig. 1). However, most of our discussion will revolve around the original polar representation of the data. That is, stacking the 1-D signals we obtain a 2-D frame in polar coordinates. Stacking these frames over time, we obtain a 3-D volume $I(r, \theta, t)$ where r indicates radial distance from the tranducer, θ the angle with respect to an arbitrary origin, and t the time since the start of recording (i.e., frame number). The envelope and log-compressed envelope signals we will represent by I_e and I_l respectively. Note that I contains real values while I_e and I_l are strictly non-negative. The I_l signal represents the traditional method of visualizing ultrasound data, in which log compression is used to reduce the dynamic range of the signal in order for it to be viewable on standard hardware. This signal is the basis for texture-based characterization of IVUS imagery. The signal I has a large dynamic range and retains far more information, including the frequency-domain information lost during envelope calculation. This "raw" signal is the basis for more recent radiofrequency-domain IVUS studies [1,5].

One-class learning: The backbone of our method is the 1-class support vector machine (SVM); a widely-studied 1-class learner or "recognizer." The problem of developing a recognizer for a certain class of objects can be stated as a problem

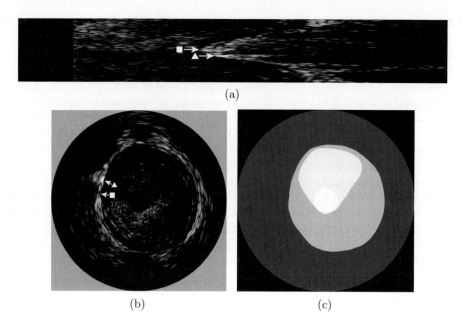

Fig. 1. (a) The log-compressed envelope of the IVUS signal in polar format. The r axis is horizontal (the origin being at the left, at the catheter) and the θ axis vertical (of arbitrary origin). (b) The same signal after Cartesian transformation. The arrows marked $\triangle$ and $\square$ (provided for orientation only) are positioned similarly in the polar and Cartesian spaces. (c) Diagram of the features of interest (from the center outward: the catheter, blood, plaque, and adventitia and surrounding tissues).

of estimating the (possibly high-dimensional) PDF of the features characterizing those objects, then setting a probability threshold which separates in-class objects from all other out-of-class objects. This threshold is necessary since, as learning does not make use of out-of-class examples, the in-class decision region could simply cover the entire feature space, resulting in 100% true- and false-positive rates. Following the approach of Schölkopf et al. [6], we denote this threshold as $\nu \in (0, 1)$. We note that as the learner is never penalized for false positives (due to its ignorance of the negative class), it is essential that the PDF's of the positive and negative classes be well-separated in the feature space.

The other parameter of interest is the width, γ, of the SVM radial basis function (i.e., $k(\mathbf{x}, \mathbf{x}') = \exp(-\gamma \|\mathbf{x} - \mathbf{x}'\|^2)$ for a pair of feature vectors $\mathbf{x}$ and $\mathbf{x}'$). Properties of a good SVM solution include an acceptable classification rate as well as a low number of resulting support vectors. A high number of support vectors relative to the number of training examples is not only indicative of overfitting, but is computationally expensive when it comes to later recognizing a sample of unknown class. A further discussion of the details of SVM operation is outside the scope of this paper; the unfamiliar reader is encouraged to consult the introduction by Hsu et al. [7].

3   Materials and Methods

3.1   Data Acquisition and Ground Truth

Ungated intravascular ultrasound sequences were recorded at 30 frames/s *in vivo* in the coronary arteries of five atherosclerotic swine. The IVUS catheter's center frequency was 40 MHz. Each raw digitized frame set $I(r, \theta, t)$ consists of 1794 samples along the r axis, 256 angles along the θ axis, and a variable number of frames along t (usually several thousand). The envelope I_e and log-envelope I_l signals were computed offline for each frame.

For training and testing purposes, a human expert manually delineates three boundaries in each image: one surrounding the IVUS catheter, one surrounding the lumen, and one surrounding the outer border of the plaque (as in Fig. 1(c)). The blood within the lumen is used as the positive class in training and testing. As our goal is to separate blood from all other physical features, we use the relatively blood-free tissue of the plaque as the negative class in testing. For most of these studies we have ignored the adventitia and surrounding tissues; in many cases this region contains blood-containing vessels and/or is difficult to reliably interpret.

3.2   Features

We investigate two classes of features: those intended to quantify speckle (i.e., signal randomness in space and time) and those based on frequency-domain spectral characterization. The former are traditionally used for blood detection and the latter for tissue characterization. These features[1] are defined for a 3-D signal window of dimensions $r_0 \times \theta_0 \times t_0$ as follows:

$$F_\alpha = \frac{1}{r_0 \theta_0} \sum_{i=1}^{r_0} \sum_{j=1}^{\theta_0} \text{stddev}[I(i, j, \cdot)] \tag{1}$$

$$F_\beta = \frac{1}{r_0 \theta_0 t_0} \sum_{i=1}^{r_0} \sum_{j=1}^{\theta_0} \sum_{k=1}^{t_0} |I(i, j, k)| \tag{2}$$

$$F_\delta = \frac{1}{r_0 \theta_0} \sum_{i=1}^{r_0} \sum_{j=1}^{\theta_0} \text{corr}[I(i, j, \cdot)] \tag{3}$$

$$F_\epsilon = \frac{1}{t_0} \sum_{k=1}^{t_0} \text{stddev}[I(\cdot, \cdot, k)] \tag{4}$$

$$F_\zeta = \sum_{i=1}^{\lceil r_0/2 \rceil} \sum_{j=1}^{\lceil \theta_0/2 \rceil} \sum_{k=1}^{\lceil t_0/2 \rceil} ijk\hat{I}(i, j, k) \tag{5}$$

$$F_\eta = \frac{F_\zeta}{\sum_{i=1}^{\lceil r_0/2 \rceil} \sum_{j=1}^{\lceil \theta_0/2 \rceil} \sum_{k=1}^{\lceil t_0/2 \rceil} \hat{I}(i,j,k)} \tag{6}$$

$$F_\iota = \text{FFT}\{\text{mean\_signal}[I]\}, \tag{7}$$

---

[1] These features were inspired by the principles behind temporal averaging in ultrasound (e.g., [8]) and tissue characterization (e.g., [1]).

where stddev($\cdot$) returns the sample standard deviation of the samples in its argument and corr($\cdot$) returns the correlation coefficient of its argument compared to a linear function (e.g., a constant signal), returning a value on $[-1, +1]$. The function $\hat{I}$ indicates the magnitude of the Fourier spectrum of I. Function FFT($\cdot$) computes the magnitude of the Fourier spectrum of its vector input (the vector result will be half the length of the input due to symmetry) and mean_signal($\cdot$) takes the mean of the θt IVUS signals in the window, producing one averaged 1-D signal.

The features represent measures of temporal (F_α and F_δ) and spatial (F_ϵ) speckle, a measure of signal strength (F_β), measures of high-frequency signal strength (F_ζ and, normalized by total signal strength, F_η), and a vector feature consisting of the raw backscatter spectrum (F_ι). In practice, this final feature is windowed to retain only those frequencies within the catheter bandwidth ($\sim$20-60 MHz in our case). Each feature, with the exceptions of (F_ζ, F_η, F_ι), are computed on I_e and I_l in addition to I. Hence, features (F_α, F_β, F_δ, F_ϵ) actually consist of vectors of three values. Feature (F_ι) consists of a vector that varies according to the sampling rate and bandwidth of the IVUS system.

Samples are extracted by setting a fixed window size (r_0, θ_0, t_0) and, from a set of consecutive IVUS frames (i.e., a volume) for which associated manually-created masks are available, placing the 3-D window around each sample in the volume. If this window does not overlap more than one class, the above features are computed for that window and associated with the class contained by it. To improve the scaling of the feature space, each feature of the samples used for training are normalized to zero mean and unit variance. The normalization values are retained for use in testing and deployment.

3.3   Training and Testing Scheme

In general, given a set of positive S_+ and negative S_- samples (from the lumen and plaque respectively), which typically represent some subset of our seven features, a grid search over γ and ν is performed to optimize a one-class SVM (Fig. 2). Optimization in this case aims to obtain an acceptable true positive rate on S_+, true negative rate on S_-, and low number of support vectors. In order to avoid bias, at every (γ, ν) point on the grid, 5-fold cross-validation is used. That is, the recognizer is trained on one-fifth of S_+ and tested on the remaining four-fifths of S_+ and all of S_- (the negative class is never used in training).

As feature selection is especially critical in a one-class training scenario, we will gauge the performance of each feature individually. More elaborate feature selection schemes (e.g., genetic algorithms) could be employed, but as one of our goals is to determine which features individually best characterize the blood, we will not investigate this issue here.

4   Results

In each case described here, thirty frames were manually segmented into "blood" and "non-blood" for training and testing purposes. (This number was deemed sufficient as the backscatter properties of the blood should not change significantly

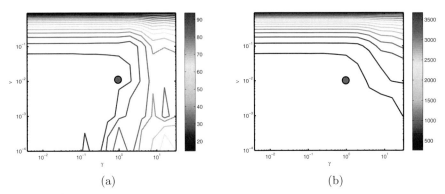

Fig. 2. SVM optimization over ν and γ. Contour maps represent (a) blood true-positive rate and (b) support vector count. The marker at $(\gamma = 1, \nu = 0.01)$ indicates a true-positive rate for blood of 97.1% and 101 support vectors. Similar plots (not shown) are made to show the false-positive rate in the plaque, in order to aid optimization.

over the course of recording.) For each of our seven features, we obtained the best possible results using the training method described previously. Specifically, we chose the parameters ν and γ such that there was a true-positive rate (sensitivity) of ~98%, where possible, and a minimal false-positive rate. (The 98% value was chosen arbitrarily to be a reasonable level.) The number of support vectors at this point is indicative of the generalization power of the feature; however, this information was not used for optimization purposes except as a sanity check, as a large number of support vectors is indicative of overfitting. A final parameter to be mentioned is the window size for feature extraction. In previous experiments we determined a reasonable tradeoff between window size and spatial accuracy to be $(r_0, \theta_0, t_0) = (255, 13, 13)$; this equates to a radial resolution of ~600 μm, angular resolution of ~18°, and temporal resolution of ~0.4 s. In all experiments presented here we use this window size.

We describe the results from one case in detail and two in summary. For Case 1, Table 1 summarizes the results for each feature for a typical sequence. To determine whether the performance of a particular feature was mainly due to that feature's application to a specific form of the data (i.e., either the raw signal, its envelope, or its log-compressed envelope), this table also lists the results of subdividing three of the highest-accuracy features into their components and performing experiments on these alone. Results from additional cases were similar as we employed the same hardware and the same type of subject (i.e., swine). In Case 2 as in Case 1, we classified blood against non-blood (i.e., plaque tissue) to obtain results of 97%/82.3%/2.8% (sensitivity, specificity, support vector fraction). In Case 3, we classified blood against manually-selected adventitial tissue to obtain results of 95.3%/100%/4%.

It should be noted that in all cases, the blood content of the extra-luminal tissue we compare against can affect specificity in an unknown manner. The high specificity of Case 3 is probably due to our choosing as our non-blood class

Table 1. Statistics relating the classification accuracy obtained by each feature with respect to true/false (T/F) positives/negatives (P/N). Positive/negative examples used: 8737/9039. Sensitivity is defined as TP/(TP + FN); specificity as TN/(TN + FP). Support vectors (SV) are listed as an absolute value and as a percentage of the number of (positive) examples used for training. Also shown are statistics relating the classification accuracy obtained by features F_α, F_ϵ, and F_ζ when they are applied to only one type of signal: the original*, envelope†, and log-envelope‡.

Feature	TP	FP	TN	FN	Sensitivity	Specificity	SV (%)
F_α	8644	705	8334	93	98.9	92.2	106 (1.2)
F_β	8727	3868	5171	10	99.9	57.2	17 (0.2)
F_δ	8649	8796	243	88	99.0	2.69	102 (1.2)
F_ϵ	8716	2	9037	21	99.8	100	33 (0.4)
F_ζ	8653	1264	7775	84	99.0	86.0	98 (1.1)
F_η	8600	2334	6705	137	98.4	74.2	246 (2.8)
F_ι	5010	27	9012	3727	57.3	99.7	8083 (92.5)
F_α^*	8404	3446	5593	333	96.2	61.9	271 (3.1)
$F_\alpha^\dagger$	8064	2811	6228	673	92.3	68.9	391 (4.5)
$F_\alpha^\ddagger$	8094	2552	6487	643	92.6	71.8	373 (4.3)
F_ϵ^*	7838	3488	5551	899	89.7	61.4	271 (3.1)
$F_\epsilon^\dagger$	7623	2962	6077	1114	87.2	67.2	187 (2.1)
$F_\epsilon^\ddagger$	7542	1860	7179	1195	86.3	79.4	191 (2.2)
F_ζ^*	8576	3241	5798	161	98.2	64.1	163 (1.9)
$F_\zeta^\dagger$	8591	3264	5775	146	98.3	63.9	160 (1.8)
$F_\zeta^\ddagger$	8417	3277	5762	320	96.3	63.7	147 (1.7)

extra-luminal tissues which were likely to be blood-free. In Cases 1 and 2 we used the entire plaque region as our negative class, in spite of the fact that this region may in reality contain detectable blood.

5   Discussion and Conclusion

Our highest performance was obtained using features which attempt to directly measure the amount of variability ("speckle") present in the signal, either temporally (F_α), spatially (F_ϵ), or in the frequency domain (F_ζ, F_η). Direct learning from the Fourier spectrum tended to perform poorly (F_ι). This is likely because one-class learning is ill-suited to determining the subtle differences in frequency spectra between the backscatter of various features imaged under ultrasound.

The performance of these features as applied to a single signal type (e.g., F_α^*) tended to be poorer than the results obtained otherwise (e.g., F_α). However, this trend does not extend to increased performance when a larger number of features are combined during training. For instance, we found that using all features except F_ζ together results in prohibitively poor specificity (<20%). This is an expected result for one-class SVMs, as their performance will degrade with the inclusion of features in whose spaces the objects of interest are poorly separated.

In the experiments described here, training and testing were performed on each sequence independently. A topic of future investigation is whether a recognizer trained on one sequence will have similar accuracy when applied to another (for instance, a sequence recorded in a different subject). We also plan to perform histological validation to determine the true accuracy of our approach when applied to the detection of extra-luminal blood. To achieve our ultimate goal of visualizing the microvasculature, we will also attempt to increase the resolution of our method to near the diameter of the vasa vasorum ($\sim$50-200 μm) [4].

Acknowledgements. We would like to thank S. Carlier (CRF; New York, NY) and E. Falk (Aarhus Univ. Hospital; Aarhus, Denmark) for their valuable assistance with data acquisition, and all the members of the Ultimate IVUS team for their input. This work was supported in part by NSF Grant IIS-0431144 (IAK) and a NSF Graduate Research Fellowship (SMO). Any opinions, findings, conclusions or recommendations expressed in this material are the authors' and may not reflect the views of the NSF.

References

1. Nair, A., Kuban, B.D., Tuzcu, E.M., Schoenhagen, P., Nissen, S.E., Vince, D.G.: Coronary plaque classification with intravascular ultrasound radiofrequency data analysis. Circulation 106, 2200–2206 (2002)
2. Goertz, D.E., Frijlink, M.E., Tempel, D., van Damme, L.C.A., Krams, R., Schaar, J.A., ten Cate, F.J., Serruys, P.W., de Jong, N., van der Steen, A.F.W.: Contrast harmonic intravascular ultrasound: A feasibility study for vasa vasorum imaging. Invest Radiol. 41, 631–638 (2006)
3. Hibi, K., Takagi, A., Zhang, X., Teo, T.J., Bonneau, H.N., Yock, P.G., Fitzgerald, P.J.: Feasibility of a novel blood noise reduction algorithm to enhance reproducibility of ultra-high-frequency intravascular ultrasound images. Circulation 102, 1657–1663 (2000)
4. Gössl, M., Malyar, N.M., Rosol, M., Beighley, P.E., Ritman, E.L.: Impact of coronary vasa vasorum functional structure on coronary vessel wall perfusion distribution. Am. J. Physiol. Heart. Circ. Physiol. 285, H2019–H2026 (2003)
5. Nair, A., Kuban, B.D., Obuchowski, N., Vince, D.G.: Assessing spectral algorithms to predict atherosclerotic plaque composition with normalized and raw intravascular ultrasound data. Ultrasound Med. Biol. 27, 1319–1331 (2001)
6. Schölkopf, B., Platt, J.C., Shawe-Taylor, J., Smola, A.J., Williamson, R.C.: Estimating the support of a high-dimensional distribution. Neural. Comput. 13, 1443–1471 (2001)
7. Hsu, C.W., Chang, C.C., Lin, C.J.: A practical guide to support vector classification. Technical report, Dept. of Computer Science and Information Engineering, National Taiwan University (2004)
8. Pasterkamp, G., van der Heiden, M.S., Post, M.J., ter Haar Romeny, B.M., Mali, W.P.T.M., Borst, C.: Discrimination of the intravascular lumen and dissections in a single 30-MHz US image: Use of "confounding" blood backscatter to advantage. Radiology 187, 871–872 (1993)

Phase Sensitive Reconstruction for Water/Fat Separation in MR Imaging Using Inverse Gradient

Joakim Rydell[1,2], Hans Knutsson[1,2], Johanna Pettersson[1,2],
Andreas Johansson[2], Gunnar Farnebäck[2], Olof Dahlqvist[1,3],
Peter Lundberg[1,3], Fredrik Nyström[4], and Magnus Borga[1,2]

[1] Center for Medical Image Science and Visualization (CMIV)
[2] Department of Biomedical Engineering, Linköping University, Sweden
[3] Department of Medicine and Care, Linköping University, Sweden
[4] Department of Endocrinology and Metabolism, Linköping University, Sweden

Abstract. This paper presents a novel method for phase unwrapping for phase sensitive reconstruction in MR imaging. The unwrapped phase is obtained by integrating the phase gradient by solving a Poisson equation. An efficient solver, which has been made publicly available, is used to solve the equation. The proposed method is demonstrated on a fat quantification MRI task that is a part of a prospective study of fat accumulation. The method is compared to a phase unwrapping method based on region growing. Results indicate that the proposed method provides more robust unwrapping. Unlike region growing methods, the proposed method is also straight-forward to implement in 3D.

1 Introduction

In MRI, reconstructed images are in general complex valued, but usually only the magnitude of the signal is saved and the resulting image is therefore real valued and positive. In many MRI applications, however, image analysis based on complex valued data dramatically improves the ability to acquire accurate estimates of physiological parameters. In some of these applications the analysis may be improved if an unwrapped phase field of the complex images is also accurately determined. The actual phase of the MRI signal may depend on hardware and experimental parameters such as the main B0 field homogeneity, echo time (TE), receiver and excitation coil sensitivity, but also on the choice of pulse sequence and tissue dependent factors.

One particular example were phase unwrapping can be very useful is in quantitative imaging of fat, something that is useful in obesity studies. In this paper, we present a novel phase unwrapping method and show how it can be used for quantitative fat imaging. The method is compared to an established method [1] on images obtained in a fat accumulation study.

There is a tremendous increase in the prevalence in obesity worldwide. It is well known that obesity, in particular the male abdominal fat accumulation

N. Ayache, S. Ourselin, A. Maeder (Eds.): MICCAI 2007, Part I, LNCS 4791, pp. 210–218, 2007.
© Springer-Verlag Berlin Heidelberg 2007

(apple shape) pattern is associated with high risk for development of type 2 diabetes, high blood pressure, and disturbed cholesterol levels. It is generally considered that the unfavorable prognosis in sedentary subjects with abdominal obesity is due to large amounts of intra abdominal fat [2]. However, this theory has not earlier been tested in prospective studies. The work presented here is a part of such an ongoing study of the impact on intra abdominal fat accumulation by fast food based weight gain combined with reduced physical activity.

2   Background

Differentiating tissues that mainly contain water from fat tissues in the abdomen is often performed using heavily T1 weighted images as these provide high contrast between fat tissues with short T1 and surrounding tissue [2,3]. Unfortunately this approach is very sensitive to partial volume effects as the tissue types are often not well separated. Donnelly et al evaluated segmentation of imaging data acquired using several different techniques. Results from a phantom modeling abdominal water and fat content showed that the fat volume fraction of the tissue is consequently underestimated using fat segmentation of T1 weighted images [4]. A better solution is to image the water and fat content both separately and together, by the application of constant level appearance (CLEAR) image reconstruction. This method removes the effect of inhomogeneous sensitivity profiles of the acquisition coils. Using this technique the estimated fat content is virtually independent on voxel size as well as partial volume effects as no classification of the voxels into water/fat is needed.

The two-point Dixon technique [5] enables the separation of water and fat signals in each individual voxel by signal acquisition using two different TEs in a gradient echo imaging sequence. At TE_1 the water and fat signal are measured $180°$ out of phase, and at TE_2 they are detected in phase. Without any other phase variations than those caused by the different resonance frequencies of water and fat, both the in phase and out of phase images would be real valued. In the image acquired at TE_2, where water and fat are in phase, both components would contribute to positive signal values, i.e. $I_2 = w + f$. In the out of phase image, I_1, water would contribute with positive values while fat contributes with negative values, i.e. $I_1 = w - f$. Then the water component could be obtained as $(I_1 + I_2)/2$ and the fat could be obtained as $(I_2 - I_1)/2$. However, due to experimental factors, the complex phase varies across the images. Because of the spatially varying phase offset, both images are complex:

$$I_1 = (w - f)e^{i\phi_1} \qquad (1)$$
$$I_2 = (w + f)e^{i\phi_2} \qquad (2)$$

where ϕ_1 and ϕ_2 are spatially varying phase fields. Hence the images need phase correction before the water and fat images can be calculated. In the in phase image, I_2, correcting the phase variations is easy. Since the water and fat components (w and f) are both positive, $w + f$ is also always positive and the corrected image $\tilde{I}_2$ is simply obtained as the magnitude of I_2; $\tilde{I}_2 = \|I_2\| = w + f$. However, since the sign of $w - f$ is unknown, the out of phase image I_1 can not be corrected in the same way. Instead an estimate of the phase field ϕ_1 is needed. When that field is known, a corrected image $\tilde{I}_1$ can be calculated as

$$\tilde{I}_1 = I_1 e^{-i\tilde{\phi}_1} \approx w - f \tag{3}$$

where $\tilde{\phi}_1$ is the estimate of the true phase field ϕ_1.

$\tilde{\phi}_1$ can be estimated in several different ways, a few of which are presented in [6,7,8]. In section 3.3 a method by Ma [1] is described along with the proposed method for calculating $\tilde{\phi}_1$.

3   Materials and Methods

3.1   Material

After ethical approval, we recruited 12 healthy lean males and 6 females as volunteers. The participants had to be willing to accept an increase in body weight of 5-15 % and to eat at least two fast food-based meals a day, preferably at well known fast food restaurants such as McDonald's and Burger King, for four weeks. All subjects continually had contact with dieticians during the study. The dietary advice was individually adjusted to result in an intake corresponding to doubling the caloric need. Physical activity was not to exceed 5000 steps per day. If a study subject reached a weight-gain of 15 % he or she terminated the study as soon as possible. The subjects were 26 ± 6.6 years old and the mean increase in body weight was 10 %. The corresponding change in body-mass index was from 21.9 ± 1.9 to $23.9 \pm 2.2 \text{kg/m}^2$. Five of the 18 subjects reached the maximal 15 % increase in body weight.

3.2   Data Acquisition

Images of the 18 subjects were acquired before and after the study, using a 1.5 Tesla Philips Achieva MR-scanner (R2). A four element sensitivity encoding (SENSE) body coil was positioned to provide as high signal to noise ratio (SNR) as possible from the level of the diaphragm to the bottom of the pelvis. No SENSE acceleration was used, i.e. the SENSE coil was only used to obtain a high SNR. Magnitude and phase images were acquired separately from two different stacks using a field of view (FOV) of 290×410 mm, 5 mm slice thickness, 40 slices and 1.6×1.6 mm in-plane resolution. The images were obtained at two different TEs using a multi-slice spoiled fast gradient echo pulse sequence. The first acquisition was obtained using $TE_1 = 2.3$ ms with the fat and water signals $180°$ out of phase, and the second using a $TE_2 = 4.6$ ms with the fat and water in phase. The repetition time (TR) was 286 ms. Data was collected using breath-hold technique. CLEAR reconstruction, which removes the effect of acquisition coil inhomogeneities, was used.

3.3   Data Processing

Two methods for phase unwrapping have been implemented: a method based on region growing by Ma [1] and the proposed method. The method by Ma has been implemented for comparison with the proposed technique and is presented in more detail in the following section. The section after that presents the proposed method. Each of these methods provides an estimate $\tilde{\phi}_1$ of the phase field, which is used to calculate a corrected out of phase image $\tilde{I}_1$ according to equation 3. It should be noted that neither of the methods is limited to water/fat separation. These methods solve the more general phase unwrapping problem, and are useful also for other applications where phase sensitive reconstruction is needed.

Region Growing Based Phase Unwrapping. A number of methods for phase correction of images acquired using a two-point or three-point Dixon technique are based on tracking the phase evolution with a region growing algorithm [6,7]. The method presented by Ma in [1] uses both phase and amplitude information to make the region growing process more robust. It performs phase correction by traversing the image pixel by pixel and for each pixel determines whether it mostly contains water or fat. Two phase-gradient maps, G_x and G_y, representing the phase difference in the x and y directions respectively, in combination with multiple pixel stacks, are used to determine the order in which the pixels are traversed. The idea is to choose the order according to the amount of phase variation in the image. Pixels with lower variation should be visited before pixels with higher variations to obtain a more robust processing.

To initiate the algorithm nine empty pixel stacks, one for each $10°$ interval from $0°$ to $90°$, are created. The phase-gradient maps are computed as the phase difference between two neighboring pixels along the x and y axes, respectively. An arbitrary pixel in the image is chosen as initial seed and put onto a pixel stack to start region growing. The following three steps are then repeated until all pixels have been checked:

1. Select the seed from the lowest non empty pixel stack.
2. Visit the four nearest neighbors, if not already visited, and place them onto the pixel stacks according to their G_x or G_y value, depending on from which direction the pixel is visited. If the value is in the $0°$-$10°$ interval the pixel is placed on the first pixel stack, if the value is in the $10°$-$20°$ interval it is placed on the second stack, etc.
3. Finally the phase value of the seed pixel is determined based on the neighboring pixels that have already been checked. If the phase difference between the seed pixel and a summation of already visited pixels within a defined boxcar region exceeds $90°$ the sign of the seed pixel is flipped.

When the current seed pixel has been checked a new one is chosen as described in step one. The result of the region growing process is a complex image without the phase discontinuities caused by the fat-water boundaries. Therefore the phase in each pixel of the resulting image describes the phase due to the local field inhomogeneity.

Inverse Gradient Method. We propose the following estimation procedure:

1. Calculate a synthetic in phase image I_1^* as

$$I_1^* = \|I_1\|e^{i\,2\arg(I_1)} \tag{4}$$

   In I_1^* the phase at each pixel will be twice the phase in I_1, which means that signals from water and fat will be in phase. The phase error due to magnetic field inhomogeneities will be twice as large as ϕ_1.
2. Find the gradient of the phase of I_1^*, i.e. a vector field describing how the phase of I_1^* changes with a small step in the x or y direction.
3. Divide the gradient field by 2. This is needed since the gradient is estimated from I_1^*, where the phase varies twice as fast as in I_1.
4. Use normalized convolution [9] to interpolate the gradient field in regions where the phase estimates can be expected to be very noisy.
5. Integrate the gradient field to obtain $\tilde{\phi}_1$, the estimate of the phase error ϕ_1. The integration procedure is described below. The integration problem is only solved in the image region corresponding to the body of the patient. Thus random phase variations outside the interesting region do not affect the resulting phase estimate.

At a first glance it may not be obvious that differentiating the phase and then integrating it again will have any effect on the final result. The rationale behind this operation is that while the phase itself contains discontinuities where it wraps from $-\pi$ to π, the gradient field is smooth. Integrating the gradient field yields an unwrapped phase which is not constrained to the interval $[-\pi, \pi]$. Hence the unwrapped phase can be divided by two without the ambiguities which arise when the number of multiples of 2π is unknown.

The reason for using the synthetic in phase image I_1^* with more rapid phase variation instead of the original out of phase image is that I_1 has phase discontinuities at the boundaries between water and fat. Such discontinuities adversely affect the estimate of the phase gradient. When the in phase image is used for estimating the phase, no discontinuities between different tissue types exist. It might be argued that the actual in phase image I_2 should be used instead of the synthetic image I_1^*. However, the phase variation in I_2 is not always exactly twice as fast as that in I_1 and thus the synthetic image I_1^* is needed for correcting I_1.

In regions where the signal intensity is very low, the phase of I_1^* is uncertain. Such regions include air filled cavities in the body and regions near boundaries between fat and water. In I_1 regions near such boundaries have low signal strength since the out of phase signals from water and fat cancel. Hence I_1^*, which is derived from I_1, also suffers from signal loss in those regions. Normalized convolution is used to interpolate the phase gradient in uncertain regions.

Integration of the phase gradient field $\mathbf{g}$ over a bounded and connected domain Ω is done by finding the scalar function ϕ whose gradients in a least squares sense are closest to $\mathbf{g}$ over Ω. It can be shown by calculus of variations [8,10] that ϕ satisfies a Poisson equation with inhomogeneous Neumann boundary conditions,

$$\begin{cases} \Delta \phi(\mathbf{x}) = \nabla \cdot \mathbf{g}(\mathbf{x}), & \text{all } \mathbf{x} \in \Omega, \\ \frac{\partial \phi}{\partial n}(\mathbf{x}) = \mathbf{n} \cdot \mathbf{g}(\mathbf{x}), & \text{all } \mathbf{x} \in \partial \Omega. \end{cases} \tag{5}$$

This partial differential equation needs to be solved numerically. There are off-the-shelf solvers available [11] but usually they are limited to rectangular domains Ω and sometimes also to simpler boundary conditions than the inhomogeneous Neumann. The limitation to rectangular domains can be worked around by solving the problem on a rectangular bounding box and iteratively updating the gradients outside Ω but this comes at a computational cost and can under some circumstances introduce systematic errors in the solution. Instead we have developed our own very efficient solver based on the full multi-grid method [12] which works directly on the specified domain. We have implemented the solver in 2D and 3D as a C code mex file for Matlab, and made it available for free download[1].

Because of the interpolation and the noisy phase estimates, the gradient field obtained after step 4 above is not guaranteed to be conservative. This means that the phase difference between two points in the image may be different depending on the choice of path between the points. Hence the integrated phase correction field is not perfect. To overcome this problem the algorithm is iterated approximately 10 times. Figures 1a and 2a show two examples of uncorrected images I_1. Corrected images $\tilde{I}_1$ are shown in figures 1f and 2f. In figures 1e and 2e intermediate results after one iteration are shown.

As can be seen in figures 1f and 2f, there is almost no phase variation within water or fat after the correction. However, the phase angles of water and fat are not necessarily $0°$ and $180°$, respectively, but instead any two complex angles $180°$ apart. Finding these angles and compensating for the constant phase offset is easy and yields a real valued image. One problem remains, though: there may still be a phase offset of $180°$, i.e. fat and water may be interchanged. However, it is known that the strongest signal originates from fat. Hence the sign of the corrected image is flipped if the signal with the largest magnitude is positive. After this final correction, we obtain $\tilde{I}_1 = w - f$ and the pure water and fat images can be calculated according to the equations in section 2.

The proposed method is related to the method presented by Song et al in [8], but that method is based on a three-point Dixon acquisition, i.e. it uses a third image, acquired at another echo time, to estimate the phase correction. In contrast, the proposed method estimates the phase correction using only the out of phase image I_1 and a synthetic in phase image derived from this image. This is necessary in order to be able to process these data sets since the phase error ϕ_1 can not be derived from the in phase image I_2 (see above). Another difference is that the method by Song solves the Poisson equation in a sequence of regions with consistent phase, while the proposed method solves the equation directly using a fast multi-grid solver.

---

[1] http://www.isy.liu.se/~gf/software/

4   Results

Figure 1 demonstrates the result for a slice from one data set. The uncorrected out of phase image is shown along with images corrected by phase estimates from the method based on region growing and from the proposed method. Fat and water images calculated according to the equations in section 2, using the corrected images $\tilde{I}_1$ and $\tilde{I}_2$, are also shown. The differences in the result for the two methods are minimal for this slice.

The slice in figure 2 is a more difficult case. The amount of phase wrap is much larger for this slice. The differences between the two methods are still not very large, but can be seen in some regions. A close-up of one of the regions in figure 2 where the differences are quite obvious is shown in figure 3. The first thing one notices is that the region belonging to the patient's arm has been classified differently by the two methods. This is, however, not relevant for measuring the abdominal fat. A more relevant difference is that a part of the subcutaneous fat, next to the arm, has obviously been misclassified by the

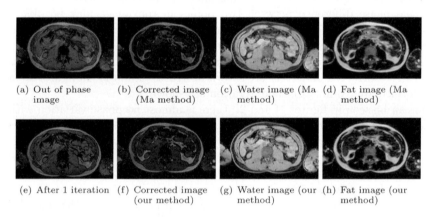

(a) Out of phase   (b) Corrected image   (c) Water image (Ma (d) Fat image (Ma
    image   (Ma method)   method)   method)

(e) After 1 iteration (f) Corrected image   (g) Water image (our (h) Fat image (our
                         (our method)   method)   method)

Fig. 1. Images from data set 1

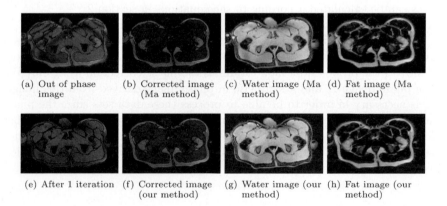

(a) Out of phase   (b) Corrected image   (c) Water image (Ma (d) Fat image (Ma
    image   (Ma method)   method)   method)

(e) After 1 iteration (f) Corrected image   (g) Water image (our (h) Fat image (our
                         (our method)   method)   method)

Fig. 2. Images from data set 2

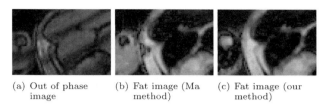

| (a) Out of phase | (b) Fat image (Ma | (c) Fat image (our |
| image | method) | method) |

Fig. 3. Close-up of a region in data set 2 to highlight the difference between the methods that occur in some regions

region growing method (visible as a darker area in this image) while our method has classified the region correctly. The resulting images have been qualitatively evaluated with good results. Extensive quantitative evaluation using phantoms will be performed in the near future.

5 Discussion

The experiments show that the two methods generate similar results, although there are regions in the data where differences occur. This is in some cases a result of parameter settings. The parameters for the region growing method were initially set equal to the ones used in [1]. These were found not to be optimal and were therefore changed to generate better results. Despite this, misclassifications such as that shown in the second example above occurs. It is possible to correct this by changing the parameters. This, however, results in errors in other slices and data sets. Since the proposed method estimates the phase iteratively, exact parameter selection is less crucial than for the region growing method. This makes the proposed method well suited for fully automatic processing of large data sets such as that acquired in the fat accumulation study.

In some slices, particularly in the presence of large air-filled cavities between anatomic structures, two-dimensional methods (both ours and the region growing method) may both fail, interchanging fat and water. An advantage of the presented method is that it is trivially extensible to three-dimensional correction, while this is rather difficult with region growing-based approaches. Preliminary results indicate that three-dimensional correction using the presented method alleviates the problems near air cavities.

The computational cost of the presented method is slightly higher than that of the region growing. Processing one two-dimensional image using our method takes approximately 5 seconds on a 2.4 GHz PC while our implementation of the region growing method takes approximately 3 seconds.

References

1. Ma, J.: Breath-hold water and fat imaging using a dual-echo two-point dixon technique with an efficient and robust phase-correction algorithm. Magnetic Resonance in Medicine 52(2), 415–419 (2004)

2. Fishbein, M., Mogren, C., Gleason, T., Stevens, W.: Relationship of hepatic steatosis to adipose tissue distribution in pediatric nonalcoholic fatty liver disease. J. Pediatr. Gastroenterol. Nutr. 42(1), 83–88 (2006)
3. Liou, T.H., Chan, W., Pan, L., Lin, P., Chou, P., Chen, C.: Fully automated large-scale assessment of visceral and subcutaneous abdominal adipose tissue by magnetic resonance imaging. International Journal of Obesity 30(5), 844–852 (2006)
4. Donnelly, L., O'Brien, K., Dardzinski, B.: Using a phantom to compare MR techniques for determining the ratio of intraabdominal to subcutaneous adipose tissue. American journal of roentgenology 180(4), 993–998 (2003)
5. Dixon, W.: Simple proton spectroscopic imaging. Radiology 153(1), 189–194 (1984)
6. Szumowski, J., Coshow, W., Li, F., Quinn, S.: Phase unwrapping in the three-point dixon method for fat suppression MR imaging. Radiology 192, 555–561 (1994)
7. Akkerman, E., Maas, M.: A region-growing algorithm to simultaneously remove dephasing influences and separate fat and water in two-point dixon imaging. In: Proceedings of the ISMRM Annual Meeting, Nice, France, ISMRM, p. 649 (1995)
8. Song, S.M.H., Napel, S., Pelc, N.J., Glover, G.H.: Phase unwrapping of MR phase images using Poisson equation. IEEE Transaction on Image Processing 4(5), 667–676 (1995)
9. Knutsson, H., Westin, C.F.: Normalized and differential convolution: Methods for interpolation and filtering of incomplete and uncertain data. In: Proceedings of IEEE Computer Society Conference on Computer Vision and Pattern Recognition, pp. 515–523 (1993)
10. Horn, B.K.P., Brooks, M.J.: The variational approach to shape from shading. Computer Vision, Graphics, and Image Processing 33, 174–208 (1986)
11. Press, W.H., Flannery, B.P., Teukolsky, S.A., Vetterling, W.T.: Numerical Recipes. Cambridge University Press, Cambridge (1986)
12. Wesseling, P.: An Introduction to Multigrid Methods. Wiley & Sons, New York (1992)

LOCUS: LOcal Cooperative Unified Segmentation of MRI Brain Scans

B. Scherrer[1,2], M. Dojat[1], F. Forbes[3], and C. Garbay[2]

[1] INSERM U836-UJF-CEA-CHU (Grenoble Institute of Neuroscience)
[2] LIG (Laboratoire d'Informatique de Grenoble), CNRS UMR 5217 (MAGMA)
[3] INRIA, Laboratoire Jean Kuntzmann, Universite de Grenoble (MISTIS)

Abstract. We propose to carry out cooperatively both tissue and structure segmentations by distributing a set of *local* and *cooperative* models in a unified MRF framework. Tissue segmentation is performed by partitionning the volume into subvolumes where local MRFs are estimated in cooperation with their neighbors to ensure consistency. Local estimation fits precisely to the local intensity distribution and thus handles nonuniformity of intensity without any bias field modelization. Structure segmentation is performed via local MRFs that integrate localization constraints provided by *a priori* general fuzzy description of brain anatomy. Structure segmentation is not reduced to a postprocessing step but cooperates with tissue segmentation to gradually and conjointly improve models accuracy. The evaluation was performed using phantoms and real 3T brain scans. It shows good results and in particular robustness to nonuniformity and noise with a low computational cost.

1 Introduction

MRI brain scan segmentation is a challenging task and has been widely addressed in the last 15 years. Difficulties in automatic segmentation arise from various sources including the size of the data, the low contrast between tissues, the limitations of available *a priori* knowledge, local perturbations such as noise or global perturbations such as intensity nonuniformity. Current approaches share three main characteristics: first, tissue and structure segmentations are considered as two separate tasks whereas they are clearly linked. Second, for a robust to noise segmentation, the Markov Random Field (MRF) probabilistic framework is classically used to introduce spatial dependencies between voxels [1,2]. Third, tissue models are generally estimated globally through the entire volume and do not reflect spatial intensity variations within each tissue, due mainly to biological tissue properties and to MRI hardware imperfections. Only the latter is generally addressed, modeled by the introduction of an explicit so called "bias field" model to estimate. Local segmentation is an attractive alternative. The principle is to compute models in various subvolumes to fit better to local image properties. However, the few local approaches proposed to date are clearly limited: they use local estimation as a preprocessing step only to estimate a bias field model [3], a training set for statistical local shape modelling [4], redondant information to

N. Ayache, S. Ourselin, A. Maeder (Eds.): MICCAI 2007, Part I, LNCS 4791, pp. 219–227, 2007.
© Springer-Verlag Berlin Heidelberg 2007

ensure consistency and smoothnesss between local estimated models [5,6], or an atlas providing a priori local spatial information [7] greedily increasing computational cost. We present in this paper an original LOcal Cooperative Unified Segmentation (LOCUS) approach which 1) performs tissue and structure segmentation by distributing a set of cooperating local MRF models through the volume, 2) segments structures by introducing prior localization constraints in a MRF framework and 3) ensures local models consistency and tractable computational time via specific cooperation and coordination mechanisms.

2   Method

2.1   MRF Segmentation

We consider a finite set of N voxels $V = \{1,...N\}$ on a regular 3-D grid. Our aim is to assign each voxel i to one of K classes considering the observed greylevel intensity y_i at voxel i. Both observed intensities and unknown classes are considered to be random fields denoted respectively by $\mathbf{Y} = \{Y_1,...,Y_N\}$ and $\mathbf{Z} = \{Z_1,...,Z_N\}$. Each random variable Z_i takes its value in $\{e_1,...,e_K\}$ where e_k is a K-dimensional binary vector corresponding to class k. Only the kth component of this vector is non zero and is set to 1. In a traditionnal Markov model based segmentation framework, it is assumed that the conditional field $\mathbf{Z}$ given $\mathbf{Y} = \mathbf{y}$ is a Markov random field, ie. $p(\mathbf{z}\,|\,\mathbf{Y} = \mathbf{y}, \boldsymbol{\Phi}) = W_{y,\Phi}^{-1} \exp(-H(\mathbf{z}\,|\,\mathbf{y}, \boldsymbol{\Phi}))$, where $H(\mathbf{z}\,|\,\mathbf{y}, \boldsymbol{\Phi})$ is an energy function depending on some parameters $\boldsymbol{\Phi} = (\Phi_y, \Phi_z)$ and given by:

$$H(\mathbf{z}\,|\,\mathbf{y}, \boldsymbol{\Phi}) = H(\mathbf{z}\,|\,\Phi_z) - \sum_{i \in V} \log p(y_i\,|\,z_i, \Phi_y). \tag{1}$$

This energy is a combination of two terms: the first term is a regularization term that accounts for spatial dependencies between voxels. Denoting by $\mathcal{N}(i)$ the neighbors of voxel i and by ${}^t z_i$ the transpose of vector z_i, we will consider a Potts model with external field:

$$H(\mathbf{z}\,|\,\Phi_z) = \sum_{i \in V} \left({}^t z_i v_i - \frac{\beta}{2} \sum_{j \in \mathcal{N}(i)} {}^t z_i z_j \right). \tag{2}$$

The second summation in (2) tends to favor neighbors that are in the same class when β is positive. This β parameter accounts for the strengh of spatial interaction. Other parameters are the v_i's that are K-dimensional vectors defining the so-called external field. In this case $\Phi_z = \{v_1,...,v_N, \beta\}$. The v_i's can be related to a priori weights accounting for the relative importance of the K classes at site i. The introduction of these extra parameters in the standard Potts model enables us to integrate a priori knowledge on classes. The second term in (1) is a data-driven term based on intensities. For MRI we generally consider Gaussian probability density functions for each k, $p(y_i\,|\,z_i = e_k, \Phi_y) = g_{\mu_k, \sigma_k}(y_i)$, with $\Phi_y = \{\mu_k, \sigma_k, k = 1...K\}$. Segmentation is then performed according to the

Maximum A Posteriori principle (MAP) by maximizing over $\mathbf{z}$ the probability $p\left(\mathbf{z}\,|\mathbf{y},\varPhi\right)$. This requires the evaluation of an intractable normalizing constant $W_{\mathbf{y},\varPhi}$ and the estimation of the unknown parameters $\varPhi$. A standard approach is to use EM-based algorithms to globally estimate the parameters through the entire volume. We propose in the next subsection a LOcal and Cooperative version of EM (LOC-EM) for local segmentation approaches.

2.2   Local Cooperative Tissue Segmentation (LOCUS-T)

We partition the volume into a set of C non-overlapping local subvolumes $V_c, c \in C$ and distribute one local MRF model M_c per subvolume. We consider $K = 3$ tissue classes: CSF (Cephalo-Spinal Fluid), GM (Grey Matter) and WM (White Matter). The hidden tissue classes t_i's take their values in $\{e_1, e_2, e_3\}$ respectively for classes $\{e_{CSF}, e_{GM}, e_{WM}\}$. Each local MRF model M_c is defined by the Gibbs distribution of energy (see Section 2.1):

$$H^c(\mathbf{t}\,|\mathbf{y},\varPhi^c) = \sum_{i \in V_c}\left[{}^t t_i \lambda_i^c - \frac{\beta^c}{2}\sum_{j \in \mathcal{N}(i)}{}^t t_i t_j - \log p\left(y_i\,\big|t_i,\varPhi_y^c\right)\right], \qquad (3)$$

where the parameters $\varPhi^c = \left\{\varPhi_t^c, \varPhi_y^c\right\}$ have to be estimated. However, the external field denoted by $\{\lambda_1^c, ...\lambda_N^c\}$ is not estimated but used to incorporate information coming from structure segmentation to perform cooperation. $\varPhi_t^c$ reduces then to $\{\beta^c\}$, while $\varPhi_y^c$ are the estimated parameters of the local Gaussian tissue intensity models. The MRF model M_c introduces spatial dependencies between voxels in its subvolume V_c, providing *consistent neighboring labels*. Because the estimation is local, some tissue classes are likely to be under-represented in some subvolumes, leading to poor model estimations with a classical EM scheme. We propose a LOcal and Cooperative version of EM (LOC-EM) for spatially organized subvolumes to ensure a *global consistency of local models*. We denote by $\mathcal{N}(M_c)$ the set of MRF models neighbouring M_c and introduce in EM a set of cooperation and coordination mechanisms as follows:

Cooperation between M_c and $\mathcal{N}(M_c)$
- *Model Checking:* we compute for each M_c a model $\widetilde{M_c}$ averaging the models of $\mathcal{N}(M_c)$. Then, for each class k, we compute the KullBack-Leibler distance $\mathcal{D}_k^c$ between intensity models of M_c and $\widetilde{M_c}$.
- *Model Correction:* if $\mathcal{D}_k^c$ is larger than a given threshold, we compute the corrected mean and variance of class k from a linear combination of intensity models in M_c and $\widetilde{M_c}$ using $\mathcal{D}_k^c$ to determine the linear coefficients.
- *Model Interpolation:* from local estimations in neighbouring subvolumes we get then one intensity model per voxel by using cubic splines interpolation between corrected models of M_c and of $\mathcal{N}(M_c)$. This results in a non-stationary field-like approach and has the advantage to ensure smooth model variation between neighboring subvolumes and to intrinsically handle nonuniformity of intensity inside each subvolume.

Coordination between MRF models

- *System starting:* each local EM enters in idle mode after its local initialization. A global intensity model is computed using the Fuzzy C-Mean algorithm and then only the MRF models closest to the global model are activated.
- *Knowledge spreading:* when the EM algorithm for M_c is stabilized, its neighbors are activated to perform estimation in turn. For already stabilized EM, model checking is performed. If it results in model correction and model interpolation, the corresponding EM are restarted to take into account the updated models modifications.

2.3 Cooperative Tissue and Structure Segmentation (LOCUS-TS)

We extend the approach above to segment both tissues and structures. We currently consider $L = 9$ subcortical structures: the ventricular system, the Frontal Horns, the Caudate Nuclei, the Thalamus, and the Putamens. For each target structure l we define a local Markov model M_l that labels voxels of its subvolume V_l in $K = 2$ classes referred to as *structure* and *background*. Denoting by $\mathbf{s} = \{s_i, i \in V_l\}$ the hidden classes, the energy function of M_l is given by:

$$H^l\left(\mathbf{s} \,|\mathbf{y}, \Psi^l\right) = \sum_{i \in V_l} \left[{}^t s_i \alpha_i^l - \frac{\beta^l}{2} \sum_{j \in \mathcal{N}(i)} {}^t s_i s_j - \log p\left(y_i \,|s_i, \Psi_{y,i}^l\right) \right], \qquad (4)$$

with $\Psi^l = \left\{\beta^l, \alpha_i^l, \Psi_{y,i}^l, i \in V_l\right\}$ and $s_i \in \{e_1, e_2\} = \{e_B, e_S\}$ for a voxel of the background or a voxel belonging to structure l.

Integration of prior localization constraints in the MRF

Automatic structure segmentation cannot rely only on radiometry information because intensity distributions of grey nuclei are largely overlapping. *A priori* knowledge should be introduced. A recent way to provide it is to describe brain anatomy with generic fuzzy spatial relations [8,9]. Three kind of relations are generally considered: distance, symmetry and orientation relations. They are expressed as 3D fuzzy maps to take into account the generic nature of the provided knowledge. Each subcortical structure is described by a set of such generic fuzzy spatial relations provided by a brain anatomist. Fusion operators between fuzzy sets are then used to combine the knowledge provided by each spatial relation and provide a generic Fuzzy Localization Map (FLM) of the structure in the volume. The FLM f^l of structure l is used in two ways: first it dynamically provides the structure subvolume V_l containing the structure l by a simple thresholding. Second, it can be integrated as an *a priori* anatomical knowledge in the MRF framework via the external field $\{\alpha_i, i \in V_l\}$. We denote by f_i^l the value of f^l at voxel i and propose to introduce the prior fuzzy knowledge of the FLM as relative prior weights for each voxel i, by setting $\alpha_i^l = {}^t[\alpha_i^l(e_B), \alpha_i^l(e_S)]$ to $\alpha_i^l = \gamma \,{}^t[-\log\left(1 - f_i^l\right), -\log f_i^l]$, where $\gamma > 0$ adjusts the influence of the external field. When $f_i^l \approx 0$, voxel i is unlikely to belong to the structure.

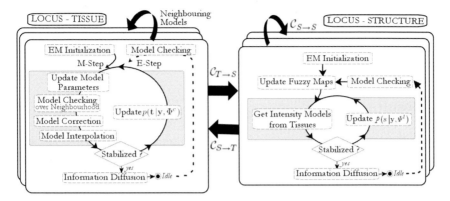

Fig. 1. Cooperative LOCUS-TS approach: for tissues (left), a LOC-EM cycle is distributed to each subvolume. For structures (right), each structure subvolume is associated to an EM cycle which cooperates with tissues.

It follows $\alpha_i^l(e_B) < \alpha_i^l(e_S)$ which favors in (4) the *background* class. When $f_i^l \approx 1$, voxel i is likely to belong to the structure. In that case $\alpha_i^l(e_B) > \alpha_i^l(e_S)$ and the class *structure* is favored.

Cooperation and coordination mechanisms between MRF models
Let $\mathcal{C}_{T \to S}(l)$ (resp. $\mathcal{C}_{S \to T}(c)$) denotes the tissue (resp. structure) subvolumes that overlap with the structure subvolume V_l (resp. tissue subvolume V_c). $\mathcal{C}_{S \to S}(l)$ denotes structures using l as a reference in a spatial relation. MRF models cooperate to make the segmentations gradually more accurate as described below.
- *Structure segmentation starting:* Structure models wait for their corresponding tissue models convergence to start their segmentation with sufficient reliable tissue knowledge.
- *Updating structure models via tissue models:* each structure l being composed of a single tissue $T^l \in \{e_{CSF}, e_{GM}, e_{WM}\}$, we do not estimate intensity models of class *structure* and class *background*. We rather compute them from tissue intensity models by setting for $i \in V_l$:

$$\begin{cases} p\left(y_i \,\middle|\, s_i = e_S, \Psi_{y,i}^l\right) = p\left(y_i \,\middle|\, t_i = T^l, \Psi_{y,i}\right) \\ p\left(y_i \,\middle|\, s_i = e_B, \Psi_{y,i}^l\right) = \max_{t \in \{e_{CSF}, e_{GM}, e_{WM}\}} p\left(y_i \,\middle|\, t_i = t, \Psi_{y,i}\right) \end{cases},$$

so that improvements in tissue intensity models estimation are dynamically taken into account by structure models.
- *Feedback of Structure Segmentation on Tissue Segmentation:* conversely, results from structure models are integrated in the tissue model via the external field λ^c (see Eq. 3). We express it as the disjunctive fusion over l of posteriori probabilities $p\left(\mathbf{s} \,\middle|\, \mathbf{y}, \Psi^l\right)$ coming from structures l of $\mathcal{C}_{S \to T}(c)$. It follows that structure segmentation is not reduced to a second step but is combined to tissue segmentation to improve their performances.

- *Updating Fuzzy Maps:* when the segmentation of structure l is updated the structure models of $\mathcal{C}_{S \to S}(l)$ take it into account by re-computing their spatial relations with respect to l, making the knowledge gradually more accurate.

A synthetic view of our approach is given in Fig 1.

3   Results

The evaluation was performed using both phantoms and real 3T brain scans. We choose not to estimate the β parameter but considered it as $\beta = 1/T$ with T a decreasing temperature. Experimentally $T : 10 \to 5$ provided good results. We first quantitatively compared LOCUS-T to two well known approaches, FAST [2] of FSL and SPM5 [10], with the Dice similarity metric on the BrainWeb phantoms with 40% of nonuniformity and different noise values (see Fig. 2). Fig. 3 shows a visual evaluation on a very high bias field real 3T brain scan[1]. Fig. 3 shows that SPM5 failed, probably due to the use of a priori information hard to match with a surface coil brain acquisition. Next, we evaluated the cooperative tissue and structure segmentations. Three experts have manually segmented on BrainWeb the left caudate nucleus, the left putamen and the left thalamus, from which we computed a ground truth segmentation using STAPLE [11].

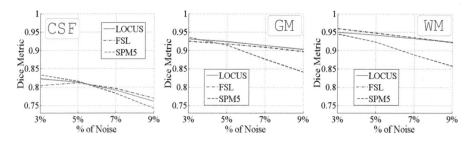

Fig. 2. Comparison of LOCUS-T, FSL and SPM5 on the BrainWeb phantoms

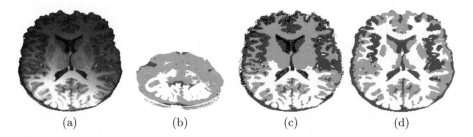

(a)   (b)   (c)   (d)

Fig. 3. Tissue segmentations provided by SPM5 (b), FSL (c) and LOCUS-T (d)

---

[1] This image was acquired with a surface coil which provides a high sensitivity in a small region (here the occipital lobe) for functional imaging applications.

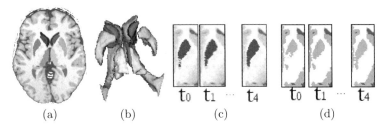

Fig. 4. Segmentation by LOCUS-TS on BrainWeb(a), 3D reconstruction(b), gradual improvement of putamen segmentation(c) and corresponding tissue segmentation(d)

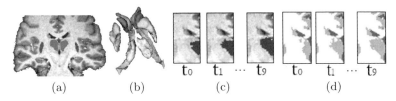

Fig. 5. Segmentation by LOCUS-TS on a real 3T image(a), 3D structure reconstruction(b), gradual improvement of thalamus segmentation(c) and tissue segmentation(d)

Fig. 4 illustrates the gradual improvements of tissue and structure segmentations provided by LOCUS-TS. At the first convergence (time t_0) of EM, the Dice index is respectively 0.76, 0.77 and 0.72 for the caudate nucleus, the putamen and the thalamus. At the end, it reaches 0.76, 0.79 and 0.80. Fig. 5 shows qualitative evaluation of LOCUS-TS on a real 3T brain scan.

4   Discussion

Classical global approaches require to estimate an explicit bias field model to take into account the tissue intensity inhomogeneities [10,12] due to MRI hardware imperfections. This model relies on the non realistic assumption of a single multiplicative bias field affecting all tissue classes equally. In contrast, the local estimation of MRF parameters in different subvolumes intrinsically handles the different sources of tissue intensity inhomogeneities. Our approach, with specific cooperation mechanisms between local models, appears to be an elegant and time efficient way to ensure global consistency of local models for tissue segmentation. It shows a significantly higher robustness to noise when compared to SPM5 (see Fig. 2), and more generally comparable results for a reduced computing time, namely, approximately 4min for LOCUS-T and respectively 8min and 14min for FSL and SPM5 on a 4Ghz Pentium, 1Go RAM. It illustrates that easy-to-segment subvolumes converge quickly, allowing the system to focus on other areas. LOCUS-T appears to be robust to very high intensity inhomogeneities as well (see Fig. 3), while SPM5, which uses an a priori atlas, fails in the segmentation and FSL does not estimate a correct bias field. In addition, instead of considering structure segmentation as a postprocessing, we propose to combine tissue and structure segmentations in a cooperative way: tissue and structure models are mutually updated, making both models gradually more accurate and providing optimal results (see Fig. 4 and 5). Improvements are particularly significant for structures such as thalamus or putamen for which contrast to noise ratio is low (see Dice index improvement in Section 3). As regards the additional use of a priori anatomical knowledge, standard structure segmentation approaches rely on a global atlas. Atlas warping methods are classicaly time consuming and more or less limited due to inter-subject variability. [7] introduced an atlas knowledge via the interaction energy term in a MRF. To be tractable, this solution considers that only the first order conditional dependence is important. This simplifying assumption, which reduces the Markov property, is not required with our approach. We consider instead an *a priori* description of brain anatomy based on fuzzy spatial relations. This was introduced in [8] with a region-based approach, while it is used in [9] in a deformable model framework. However, the image preprocessing steps required make this approach difficult to apply on high field images, with high intensity nonuniformity, or on non homogeneous structures such as putamen. Our solution consists in introducing fuzzy localization constraints as relative prior weights for each voxel in the MRF framework via an external field term. It does not suffer from such difficulties as can be illustrated on structures such as putamen, and is still time efficient (10 to 15min). Note that currently LOCUS segments only a subset of the 37 structures segmented by the method proposed in [7]. To conclude, the robustness and modularity of our LOCUS approach appear as interesting features when handling complex segmentation tasks. Efficiency is improved both in term of results quality and computing time.

References

1. Van Leemput, K., et al.: Automated model-based tissue classification of MR images of the brain. IEEE Trans. Med. Imag. 18(10), 897–908 (1999)
2. Zhang, Y., Brady, M., Smith, S.: Segmentation of brain MR images through a hidden Markov random field model and the expectation-maximisation algorithm. IEEE Trans. Med. Imag. 20(1), 45–47 (2001)
3. Shattuck, D.W., et al.: Magnetic resonance image tissue classification using a partial volume model. NeuroImage 13(5), 856–876 (2001)
4. Pohl, K.M., et al.: Logarithm odds maps for shape representation. In: Larsen, R., Nielsen, M., Sporring, J. (eds.) MICCAI 2006. LNCS, vol. 4191, pp. 955–963. Springer, Heidelberg (2006)
5. Rajapakse, J.C., Giedd, J.N., Rapoport, J.L.: Statistical approach to segmentation of single-channel cerebral MR images. IEEE TMI 16(2), 176–186 (1997)
6. Zhu, C., Jiang, T.: Multicontextual fuzzy clustering for separation of brain tissues in magnetic resonance images. NeuroImage 18(3), 685–696 (2003)
7. Fischl, B., et al.: Whole brain segmentation: automated labeling of neuroanatomical structures in the human brain. Neuron 33(3), 341–355 (2002)
8. Barra, V., Boire, J.Y.: Automatic segmentation of subcortical brain structures in MR images using information fusion. IEEE Trans. Med. Imag. 20(7), 549–558 (2001)

9. Colliot, O., et al.: Integration of fuzzy spatial relations in deformable models - Application to brain MRI segmentation. Pat. Rec. 39(8), 1401–1414 (2006)
10. Ashburner, J., Friston, K.: Unified segmentation. NeuroImage 26, 839–851 (2005)
11. Warfield, S.K., Zou, K.H., Wells, W.M.: Simultaneous truth and performance level estimation (STAPLE): An algorithm for the validation of image segmentation. IEEE Trans. Med. Imag. 23(7), 903–921 (2004)
12. Wells, W.M., Grimson, W.E.L., Kikinis, R., Jolesz, F A: Adaptative segmentation of MRI data. IEEE Trans. Med. Imag. 15(4), 429–442 (1996)

Spline Based Inhomogeneity Correction for ^{11}C-PIB PET Segmentation Using Expectation Maximization

Parnesh Raniga[1,3], Pierrick Bourgeat[1], Victor Villemagne[2], Graeme O'Keefe[2], Christopher Rowe[2], and Sébastien Ourselin[1]

[1] BioMedIA Lab, e-Health Research Centre, CSIRO ICT Centre,
Brisbane, Australia
[2] Department of Nuclear Medicine and Centre for PET, Austin Hospital,
Melbourne, Australia
[3] School of Electrical and Information Engineering, The University of Sydney,
Sydney, Australia

Abstract. With the advent of biomarkers such as ^{11}C-PIB and the increase in use of PET, automated methods are required for processing and analyzing datasets from research studies and in clinical settings. A common preprocessing step is the calculation of standardized uptake value ratio (SUVR) for inter-subject normalization. This requires segmented grey matter (GM) for VOI refinement. However ^{11}C-PIB uptake is proportional to amyloid build up leading to inhomogeneities in intensities, especially within GM. Inhomogeneities present a challenge for clustering and pattern classification based approaches to PET segmentation as proposed in current literature.

In this paper we modify a MR image segmentation technique based on expectation maximization for ^{11}C-PIB PET segmentation. A priori probability maps of the tissue types are used to initialize and enforce anatomical constraints. We developed a Bézier spline based inhomogeneity correction techniques that is embedded in the segmentation algorithm and minimizes inhomogeneity resulting in better segmentations of ^{11}C-PIB PET images. We compare our inhomogeneity with a global polynomial correction technique and validate our approach using co-registered MRI segmentations.

1 Introduction

With the recent development of Pittsburg Compound B (^{11}C-PIB) [1], a PET biomarker that binds to beta amyloid plaques ($A\beta$), it is now possible to observe *in-vivo* one of the major histopathological landmarks of Alzheimer's disease (AD). ^{11}C-PIB PET is now being tested worldwide in large studies aimed at tracking and better understanding the pathogenesis of AD with the hope that it could lead to early diagnosis. Processing and analyzing the large datasets generated by the studies is too resource intensive to perform manually and is inherently irreproducible prompting the need for automated techniques.

N. Ayache, S. Ourselin, A. Maeder (Eds.): MICCAI 2007, Part I, LNCS 4791, pp. 228–235, 2007.
© Springer-Verlag Berlin Heidelberg 2007

However, the acquisition and reconstruction of PET images place many constraints and pose many challenges. PET image resolution is comparatively lower than traditional imaging modalities such as Magnetic Resonance Imaging (MRI) and Computed Tomography. The resulting partial volume effects (PVE) cause blurring of anatomical regions, loss of detail and of strong edge information. Alongside these factors the distribution of $A\beta$ plaques varies considerably between individuals producing large inhomogeneities within the grey matter (GM) in ^{11}C-PIB PET images.

Because of the physiological and chemical differences between the different tissue types of the brain, quantitative analysis in neuroimaging relies on an accurate segmentation of brain tissues into its constituents, GM, white matter (WM) and cerebrospinal fluid (CSF). Notably for the analysis of ^{11}C-PIB PET images where AD pathologies and hence tracer uptake is confined to GM, an accurate segmentation is crucial for further analysis. Segmentation results are used to perform inter tissue comparison such as the ratio of uptake in GM to WM and for refinement of volume or regions of interest (VOI or ROI). We use the segmentations to refine cerebellar GM masks for standardized uptake value ratio (SUVR) calculations. Although MR image segmentation can be used instead, MR images are not always acquired as they represent a substantial cost burden [2].

There have been several approaches proposed in literature for segmentation of neuro-PET images. Pattern classification approaches such as those proposed in [3], [4] and [5] use tissue time activity curves (TTAC) derived from dynamic Flurodeoxyglucose (^{18}F-FDG) PET images. However, inhomogeneity in ^{11}C-PIB PET tracer uptake as compared to the relatively homogeneous ^{18}F-FDG uptake cause misclassifications and an inaccurate segmentation. Mykkänen et al. used simplex meshes and dual surface minimization (DSM) for the segmentation of ^{18}F-FDG and ^{11}C-Raclopride [6]. Tohka [7] conducted a study of DSM and other methods including generalized gradient vector field based active contours. A reliance on strong GM-WM boundaries which are not present in ^{11}C-PIB due to the inhomogeneities will result in inaccurate segmentation using these algorithms.

To compensate for the lack of detail and strong edge information, a priori data such as prior probability maps can be used similarly to the approach of Van Leemput et al., which has been validated on MR images [8]. We adopted and extended this approach by including an intensity inhomogeneity correction step that takes into account local changes within the GM. Anatomical priors are used as initialization and constraints in the algorithm improving robustness and accuracy and are advantageous over other initialization techniques such as thresholding and clustering for ^{11}C-PIB as they are data independent.

The inhomogeneity correction is performed using bi-cubic Bézier spline patches. Using spline patches allows for constraints such as smoothness and spatial consistency to be easily incorporated into the spline model. Splines provide a general framework within which tracer and physiology models can be embedded for greater accuracy and robustness. A similar approach, using thin plate splines,

was taken by [9] for inhomogeneity correction in MR images with the assumption
of low frequency global variations. Sample voxels, through which the spline was
fit were determined either by an observer or through a pre-classification step. As
discussed later in Section 2.2 these are not valid and are illustrated by our results
(see Section 4). Validation of our approach was performed using Dice similarity coefficient (DSC) [10] for the obtained PET segmentations as compared to
segmented co-registered MR images of the same patient.

2   Method

2.1   Data and Acquisition

For testing and validation of our algorithm we used a subset of scans from a study
the application of ^{11}C-PIB PET for early diagnosis. The subset consists of 35
patients of which 10 were clinically diagnosed with AD, 12 with Mild Cognitive
Impairment (MCI) and 13 were Normal Controls (NC). The AD group consisted
of 5 males and 5 females, mean age 74±9 yrs, the MCI group consisted of 6 males
and 6 females, mean age 72±10 yrs and the NC group consisted of 5 males and
8 females, mean age 72±6 yrs. Each patient underwent a 20 min PET scan, 40
minutes post injection and an SPGR T1-weighted MR scan. All PET scans were
128 by 128 voxels and 90 slices.

2.2   Tissue Classification

In van Leemput's tissue classification algorithm for MR images [8], voxel's intensities for the different tissue classes are modeled as Gaussian distributions in a
Gaussian finite mixture model. Parameters of the model are estimated from the
data and a priori probability maps in an iterative manner within a maximum
likelihood - expectation maximization (ML-EM) framework. A priori probability maps for GM, WM and CSF, which are registered to the image, are used
as initialization and as anatomical constraints. A Markov random field (MRF)
is included within the algorithm to ensure consistent results as voxels in the
neighborhood of a particular voxel contribute to its classification.

A bias field correction scheme is used in the algorithm to correct for the
intensity inhomogeneities that are present in MR images due to fluctuations
in magnetic fields of scanners. These inhomogeneities are modeled as smoothly
varying polynomials the coefficients of which are calculated by fitting intra-class
residuals using least squares. When fourth order polynomials are used, only
slow, global intensity changes can be modeled and corrected. The use of higher
order polynomials would result in extreme computation costs. Correction of local,
high intensity changes such as those found in GM of ^{11}C-PIB requires higher
degrees of freedom which are accommodated by piecewise spline functions. As
MR bias fields affect intensities in all the tissue types equally, coefficients for the
polynomials are calculated using information from all the tissue types, however
^{11}C-PIB inhomogeneities are confined only to GM, therefore at each iteration our
spline based approach only considers voxels with a high probability of being GM.

2.3   Inhomogeneity Correction

Considering both local and global changes, we modified van Leemput's algorithm by replacing the bias field correction step with an inhomogeneity correction step based on bi-cubic Bézier patches. A set of patches are tiled on each slice of the image and serve to subdivide the image and to interpolate correction coefficients, it should be noted that the patches may be set arbitrarily and this setting simplifies implementation. This allows us to approximate variability to a much higher degree than the polynomial based correction (PBC) used for MR image bias field correction.

A bi-cubic Bézier patch consists of 16 control points in three-dimensional space forming a surface that intersects each of the points. Intermediate points lying on the surface are calculated by interpolation. We use the patches to divide each slice of the image into regions and the third dimension of the control points is used to interpolate correction coefficients. It should be noted that although we use spline surfaces to decrease computation, this is still a fully three-dimensional approach as we use information from neighbors in three dimensions in calculating correction coefficients. Control points of each of the patches is uniformly spaced within the patch, with neighboring patches sharing control points along their common edges thus preserving continuity and smoothness.

After each slice has been subdivided into patches, the following steps are taken at each iteration :

- Mean intensity ($\mu P_{i,j,k}$) of voxels that have high probability of belonging to GM are calculated for each patch.
- The correction coefficient (CC) of each patch is set to the difference between the global GM mean (μG) and the GM mean of the patch($\mu P_{i,j,k}$) that is to (μG - $\mu P_{i,j,k}$).
- Intensity correction control points of each patch are set to weighted average of the CCs in 3×3×3 neighborhood, with patches geometrically closer having a linearly higher weighting.
- For each voxel that has high probability of belonging to GM, a voxel correction coefficient (VCC) is calculated by interpolating the control points of the corresponding patch and added to the voxels intensity.

These steps have the effect of normalizing means of local regions and since we restrict the correction to GM only, it normalizes GM means within local regions reducing the inhomogeneities present in ^{11}C-PIB images leading to better segmentations.

2.4   Experiments and Validation

Validation was performed using the DSC [10] between the PET Segmentation and the corresponding MR Segmentation as used in [11]. The PET segmentations considered were the spline based correction (SBC), the polynomial based correction (PBC) and the PBC constrained to only GM (PBC-GM). The effects of parameters such as the number of spline patches per slice were also tested with segmentations conducted using grids of 8×8, 16×16 and 32×32 patches per slice. For registration of the a priori probability maps, we used a robust, multi-modal block-matching algorithm [12].

3   Results

Results of the experiments and validation are presented below. Table 1 presents mean DSC for GM PET segmentations as compared to co-registered MR approaches using SBC with grids of 8 by 8, 16 by 16 and 32 by 32 patches per slice. Mean DSCs for the PBC and GM-PBC for GM segmentations are also presented. Table 2 presents the DSCs for WM segmentation. The results show that using grids with fewer patches results in lower mean GM DSCs and slightly higher mean WM DSCs. Compared to PBC and GM-PBC, mean GM DSCs for SBC were higher, significantly so for a grid of 32 by 32 patches per slice. WM mean DSC were comparable between the approaches but those using a 32 by 32 grid were lower. SBC segmentations are also more consistent with similar DSCs for AD, MCI and NC patient types.

Table 1. Mean DSC ± standard deviation of the ^{11}C-PIB PET GM segmentations with regards to the MR segmentation for SBC using 8×8, 16×16 and 32×32 grids and PBC and GM-PBC

Classification	SBC 8×8	SBC 16×16	SBC 32×32	PBC	GM-PBC
AD	0.55±0.05	0.58±0.05	0.6±0.05	0.53±0.05	0.52±0.04
MCI	0.57±0.05	0.60±0.05	0.62±0.05	0.56±0.05	0.56±0.05
NC	0.57±0.04	0.59±0.05	0.62±0.04	0.56±0.04	0.55±0.04

Table 2. Mean DSC ± standard deviation of the ^{11}C-PIB PET WM segmentations with regards to the MR segmentation for SBC using 8×8, 16×16 and 32×32 grids and PBC and GM-PBC

Classification	SBC 8×8	SBC 16×16	SBC 32×32	PBC	GM-PBC
AD	0.66±0.02	0.65±0.02	0.63±0.03	0.65±0.02	0.66±0.01
MCI	0.67±0.03	0.66±0.03	0.63±0.05	0.67±0.04	0.67±0.03
NC	0.66±0.03	0.65±0.03	0.63±0.03	0.66±0.03	0.67±0.01

Figures 1 and 2 presents axial slices from MR and ^{11}C-PIB PET scans along with segmented GM and WM masks of AD and NC patients using SBC with a 32 by 32 grid. Figure 3 presents MR and ^{11}C-PIB PET segmentations using SBC, PBC and GM-PBC. Notice the over segmentation of WM and under segmentation of GM using PBC and GM-PBC. Also, notice the similarity between PBC and GM-PBC. Segmentations were also performed without correction but as both the quantitative (DSC around 0.3 for GM and 0.5 for WM) and qualitative results significantly lower, they have been excluded for brevity.

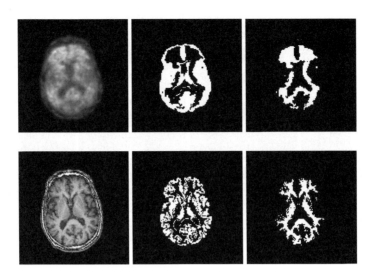

Fig. 1. Transaxial slices of ^{11}C-PIB PET (top row) and MR (bottom row) scans with original scan (column one) GM (column two) and WM (column three) segmentations of an AD patient

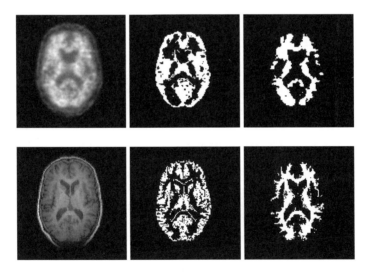

Fig. 2. Transaxial slices of ^{11}C-PIB PET (top row) and MR (bottom row) scans with original scan (column one), GM (column two) and WM (column three) segmentations of a NC patient

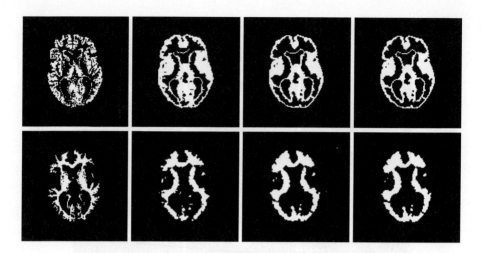

Fig. 3. Transaxial slices of ^{11}C-PIB PET and MR scans of an AD patient, with GM (top row) and WM (bottom row) segmentations. Column one are the MR segmentations, column two are PET segmentations using SBC and a 32 by 32 grid, column three are PET segmentations using PBC and the fourth column are PET segmentations using GM-PBC.

4   Discussion

GM segmentations produced by SBC had higher DSCs than those produced by PBC and GM-PBC. However, the DSCs for WM segmentations were lower. On inspection of the data, we noticed that the PBC and GM-PBC approaches tended to under segment GM and over segment WM as illustrated in Figure 3. This was especially true of AD patients with plaque build up in the frontal lobes where GM structures with medium-high uptake were segmented as WM. The PBC approaches also have a tendency to converge to the a priori probability maps, as there is too much variability for correct classification.

The need for a more local approach is illustrated by the results of SBC using grids of 8 by 8 and 16 by 16 patches per slice. DSCs for GM segmentations increased as the grid sizes were increased and those of WM segmentations decreased. Inspection of the segmentations revealed that using fewer patches per slice resulted in over segmentation of WM and under segmentation of GM as was with PBC and GM-PBC. Since grids with more patches have more degrees of freedom, they are able to better model the local changes.

To further improve the results of the segmentation, models of tracer uptake based on patient type and/or neuropsychological tests can be integrated into the inhomogeneity correction step. Better a priori data and template will not only improve registration of the PET images to the templates but also the segmentation itself. The technique presented could be applied to other tracers where there is inhomogeneity in uptake in either the GM or WM.

5   Conclusion

We have presented a novel approach to inhomogeneity correction and segmentation of ^{11}C-PIB images and validated it against co-registered, segmented MR images of the same patient and compared it against a global polynomial based correction approach. Our approach produced good GM segmentations with similar DSCs irrespective of patient classifications. The polynomial based approach tended to under segment the WM and over segmenting GM and were sensitive to patient types thus sensitive to inhomogeneity. Using different number of patches per slice, we have illustrated the need for techniques that correct on a local scale, which our approach does.

Since we are using an iterative EM approach and splines for inhomogeneity correction, we can embed models for different patients types and will be exploring this in the future. We are also investigating the use of a priori data and templates that are suited to the different patient types.

References

1. Klunk, W.E., Engler, H., et al.: Imaging brain amyloid in Alzheimer's disease with Pittsburgh compound-B. Ann. Neurol. 55(3), 306–319 (2004)
2. Raniga, P., Bourgeat, P., et al.: PIB-PET segmentation for automatic SUVR normalization without MR information. In: ISBI, pp. 348–351. IEEE, Washington DC (2007)
3. Wong, K.P., Feng, D., et al.: Segmentation of dynamic PET images using cluster analysis. IEEE Trans. Nucl. Sci. 49, 200–207 (2002)
4. Brankov, J.G., Galatsanos, N.P., et al.: Segmentation of dynamic PET or fMRI images based on a similarity metric. IEEE Trans. Nucl Sci. 50, 1410–1414 (2003)
5. Chen, J.L., Gunn, S.R. et al.: Markov random field models for segmentation of PET images. In: IPMI, Davis, CA, USA, June 18-22, 2001 pp. 468–474 (2001)
6. Mykkänen, J., Tohka, J., et al.: Automatic extraction of brain surface and midsagittal plane from PET images applying deformable models. Comput Methods Programs Biomed 79(1), 1–17 (2005)
7. Tohka, J.: Surface extraction from volumetric images using deformable meshes: A comparative study. In: ECCV, pp. 350–364 (2002)
8. Van Leemput, K., Maes, F., et al.: Automated model-based tissue classification of MR images of the brain. IEEE Trans. Med. Imaging. 18(10), 897–908 (1999)
9. Dawant, B.M., Zijdenbos, A.P., Margolin, R.A.: Correction of intensity variations in MR images for computer-aided tissue classification. IEEE Trans. Med. Imaging. 12, 770–781 (1993)
10. Dice, L.: Measures of the amount of ecologic association between species. Ecology 26, 297–302 (1945)
11. Kim, J., Cai, W., Feng, D., Eberl, S.: Segmentation of VOI from multidimensional dynamic PET images by integrating spatial and temporal features. IEEE Trans Inf. Technol. Biomed. 10, 637–646 (2006)
12. Ourselin, S., Roche, A., et al.: Reconstructing a 3D structure from serial histological sections. IVC 19, 25–31 (2001)

Hyperspherical von Mises-Fisher Mixture (HvMF) Modelling of High Angular Resolution Diffusion MRI*

Abhir Bhalerao[1] and Carl-Fredrik Westin[2]

[1] Department of Computer Science, University of Warwick, Coventry CV4 7AL
abhir.bhalerao@dcs.warwick.ac.uk
[2] Laboratory of Mathematics in Imaging, Harvard Medical School, Brigham and
Womens Hospital, Boston MA 02115
westin@bwh.harvard.edu

Abstract. A mapping of unit vectors onto a 5D hypersphere is used
to model and partition ODFs from HARDI data. This mapping has a
number of useful and interesting properties and we make a link to interpretation of the second order spherical harmonic decompositions of
HARDI data. The paper presents the working theory and experiments
of using a von Mises-Fisher mixture model for directional samples. The
MLE of the second moment of the HvMF pdf can also be related to fractional anisotropy. We perform error analysis of the estimation scheme in
single and multi-fibre regions and then show how a penalised-likelihood
model selection method can be employed to differentiate single and multiple fibre regions.

1 Introduction

The directional dependence of diffusion of water molecules in brain white matter
is the basis of DWI and a widely adopted non-invasive method for elucidating
white matter fibre directions and, through tractography, inferring connectivity
between brain regions [1]. DWI involves the acquisition of a set of images, in a
small number of directions, and reconstructing the Gaussian diffusion by estimating the diffusion tensor. For regions containing a bundle of fibres all oriented
in the same direction, the diffusion tensor model can characterise local *apparent*
diffusion with as few as 6 directions. In the regions where the fibres bifurcate,
cross or are adjacent to white-matter surfaces, the single tensor model is insufficient. High angular resolution diffusion imaging (HARDI) [2] can detect more
precisely the variation of diffusion along different directions. For a given (larger)
set of gradient directions, HARDI imaging can be analysed to produce samples
of a pdf of diffusion over the surface of a sphere – the radial marginal of the pdf
of the particle displacements. However, characterisation of the local geometry

---

* This work is partly funded by NIH Grants R01MH074794 and P41RR13218. We are
also grateful to Ulas Ziyan at CSAIL MIT, and Gordon Kindlmann (LMI) for their
help and insights into this work.

N. Ayache, S. Ourselin, A. Maeder (Eds.): MICCAI 2007, Part I, LNCS 4791, pp. 236–243, 2007.
© Springer-Verlag Berlin Heidelberg 2007

given such measurements, called the orientation distribution function or ODF, is much less clear than in diffusion tensor imaging.

Frank [3] proposed the use of spherical harmonics (SH) to characterize the local geometry of the diffusivity. A notable finding of his was that single fibre regions show up in the 2nd order harmonics set: Y_2^{-2}, Y_2^{-1}, Y_2^0, and Y_2^1, Y_2^2, whilst the order 4 functions can add further information about multiple fibre regions. He made proposals for the separation of these regions according to the prominence of a particular channel. In this work, we show the relationship between the projection of ODF samples on to the same basis set and that a particular linear combinations of the second order projections are just components of the rank tensor mapping. Thus a way to determine the principal diffusion direction (PDD) when using SHs to model and reconstruct the HARDI data is revealed.

Since the ODF is a distribution function, a natural way to model it is by pdfs. However, commonly used Gaussian models do not extend to the sphere in a straightforward way because of the problem of "wrapping" of 3D angles modulo π and 2π. McGraw [4] used the von Mises-Fisher (vMF) distribution to parameterise the ODF. To capture the structure of multiple fibre voxels, they fitted a mixture of vMF density functions with pairs of antipodal modes, with directions $\{\boldsymbol{\mu}_1, -\boldsymbol{\mu}_1, \boldsymbol{\mu}_2, -\boldsymbol{\mu}_2\}$, and went on to give expressions for scalar metrics of the parameterization (entropy), and distance metrics between pairs of mixtures using Riemannian Exp and Log maps for the purposes of interpolation. We build on this work by considering only unimodal and bimodal mixtures through a mapping of samples drawn from the ODF to a 5D representation which is free from the ambiguities associated with sign flips of vectors direction in 3D. This alleviates the need for introducing pseudo-modes into the fit. Such a representation of orientation was originally proposed by Knutsson [5] and has been used for filtering and optical flow analysis in vision. Recently Rieger and van Vliet [6] presented new insights into such orientation spaces and their properties. We show that these properties are important to measurements in diffusion imaging.

2   Theory

2.1   Hyperspherical von Mises-Fisher Distributions (HvMF)

The von Mises-Fisher (vMF) is the analog of the Gaussian distribution on a sphere and is parameterised by a principal direction (the mean direction $\boldsymbol{\mu}$) and a *concentration* parameter, κ. These distributions extends to arbitrary dimensions, p, though rarely are hyperspherical vMFs considered:

$$g_p(\boldsymbol{x}|\boldsymbol{\mu}, k) = c(\kappa)e^{\kappa \boldsymbol{\mu}^T \boldsymbol{x}}, \qquad c(\kappa) = \frac{\kappa^{p/2-1}}{((2\pi)^{p/2} I_{p/2-1}(\kappa))}, \qquad (1)$$

where the normalisation factor, $c(\kappa)$, contains a Bessel function of the first kind to a fractional order. g_p is bell-shaped with the general form $e^{b\cos(\psi)}$, where the exponent will have the range $[-b, b]$ and ψ is the angle difference between the *direction* of the sample $\boldsymbol{x}$ and the mean direction $\boldsymbol{\mu}$. A set of vectors which point more or less in the same direction would have a vMF pdf which is unimodal and symmetric around the mean direction. The relationship between the spread, b, and the variance or second-moment of the samples is less straightforward and non-linear. However, larger b values *concentrate* the probability mass around the mean direction.

2.2 A Double-Angle Representation for 3D Orientation

In directional statistics, antipodal vectors are regarded as the same. This ambiguity is elegantly removed in 2D by *angle doubling* or, in general, by taking outer products to form 2nd order tensors i.e. $x \to xx^T$ where $x = (x_1, x_2, x_3) \in \mathbb{R}^3$. The dimensionality of this space can be reduced by restricting the trace of this tensor to be 1 to produce the 5D mapping [5,6]. In spherical polar coordinates,

$$M_5(r, \theta, \phi) \to r(s, t, u, v, w), \tag{2}$$
$$s = \sin^2 \theta \cos 2\phi, \qquad t = \sin^2 \theta \sin 2\phi,$$
$$u = \sin 2\theta \cos \phi, \qquad v = \sin 2\theta \sin \phi, \qquad w = \sqrt{3}(\cos^2 \theta - \frac{1}{3}).$$

Although not explained in [6], we cannot robustly solve for (θ, ϕ) given any two coefficients in M_5. To accurately invert the mapping therefore, we have to reconstitute the implied tensor, xx^T, and calculate the direction of its principal eigen vector:

$$M_5^{-1} : r(s, t, u, v, w) \to r(\theta, \phi), \qquad xx^T = \begin{pmatrix} s + x_2^2 & \frac{t}{2} & \frac{u}{2} \\ \frac{t}{2} & x_3^2 - \frac{s + w\sqrt{3}}{2} & \frac{v}{2} \\ \frac{u}{2} & \frac{v}{2} & \frac{w\sqrt{3}+1}{3} \end{pmatrix}. \tag{3}$$

We note also that the above 5D mapping is equivalent to weighted amounts of selected 2nd order spherical harmonic basis functions:

$$(s, t, u, v, w) = (\frac{1}{3}Y_2^2, 8Y_2^{-2}, \frac{2}{3}Y_2^1, 4Y_2^{-1}, \frac{2}{\sqrt{3}}Y_2^0). \tag{4}$$

This is used below to estimate PDD directly from projections of HARDI samples.

2.3 Maximum Likelihood Estimates of HvMF Parameters

HvMF pdfs are parameterised by two parameters: the mean μ and the concentration parameter κ. These can be used to model the apparent diffusion of homogeneous fibre regions.

Given a set of independent sample vectors, $x_i, i = 1..n$, believed to be from $g_p(x|\mu, \kappa)$, the maximum likelihood estimate of the mean is obtained by the sum of the vectors divided by the length of the sum. It can be shown that the MLE of the concentration parameter, κ, is then obtained as follows:

$$r = \sum_i^n x_i, \qquad \hat{\mu} = \frac{r}{\| r \|}, \qquad \hat{\kappa} = A^{-1}(\bar{R}) \approx \frac{\bar{R}p - \bar{R}^3}{1 - \bar{R}^2}, \qquad \bar{R} = \frac{1}{n}\hat{\mu}^T r \tag{5}$$

where $A(\kappa) = I_{p/2}(\kappa)/I_{p/2-1}(\kappa)$, is the ratio of modified Bessel functions of the first kind to fractional orders (see Sra [7]).

2.4   Mixture Modelling: Fitting by EM and Model Selection

A HvMF mixture allows the modelling of more than one principal direction but an algorithm such as Expectation Maximization (EM) is needed to perform the parameter estimation. If we now assume that a set of samples, $\boldsymbol{x}_i, i = 1...n$, are now drawn from a m-mode mixture distribution,

$$G_p(\boldsymbol{x}|w, \Theta) = \sum_j^m w_j g_p(\boldsymbol{x}|\Theta_j) \tag{6}$$

with a convex set of weights, $\sum_j^m w_j = 1$ and each mode is parameterised by $\Theta_j = \{\boldsymbol{\mu}_j, \kappa_j\}$, then it can be shown that MLE for the mixture are given by the update equations (abbreviating notation for brevity):

$$\hat{\mu}_j^{t+1} = \frac{\sum_i^n P_{ij}^t \hat{\kappa}_{ij}^t \boldsymbol{x}_i}{\| \sum_i^n P_{ij}^t \hat{\kappa}_j^t \boldsymbol{x}_i \|} \qquad A(\hat{\kappa}_j^{t+1}) = \frac{\sum_i^n P_{ij}^t \boldsymbol{x}_i^T \boldsymbol{\mu}_j^t}{\sum_i^n P_{ij}^t} \qquad \hat{w}_j^{t+1} = \frac{1}{n} \sum_i^n P_{ij}^t \tag{7}$$

The posterior value at step t, P_{ij}^t, is calculated in the usual way for an EM algorithm from the expectation of the data, $\boldsymbol{x}_i$ given the current weights and parameter estimates, w_j, Θ^t.

Given a MLE fit to the samples, a parsimonious way to determine what number of modes m is best, is to use a model selection criterion such as the Akaike information criterion (AIC). The AIC is a number based on the log-likelihood of the data penalised by the number of parameters used to model the distribution. Thus, for the HvMF, for m modes, we have $m(p+2)$ parameters altogether (remembering the mean is p-dimensional). To select the model, we minimize for m

$$AIC(m) = -2 \sum_i^n \log G_p(x_i|\hat{w}, \hat{\Theta}) + 2m(p+2). \tag{8}$$

For our purposes, only $AIC(1)$ and $AIC(2)$ need be compared to select between single or multi-fibre regions.

2.5   Relationships Between Variance of ODF and a Measure of Anisotropy

The ML estimate of variance of the transformed set of samples, $\boldsymbol{X}_i \in \mathbb{S}^5$, can be used to characterise the anisotropy of the a Rank 1 tensor estimate. The ML estimate of variance in $\mathbb{S}^5$ is given by $1 - \bar{R}$ (from equation 5). $\bar{R}$ is the variation along the mean $\boldsymbol{\mu}$, while the spread is the perpendicular projection of the vector of length $n\bar{R}$ along $\hat{\boldsymbol{\mu}}$ (figure 1):

$$\boldsymbol{r} = n\bar{R}\boldsymbol{\mu}, \qquad var(\boldsymbol{X}) = \| \boldsymbol{I} - \boldsymbol{r}\boldsymbol{r}^T \|. \tag{9}$$

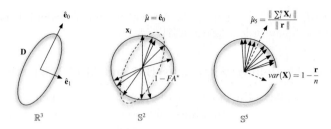

Fig. 1. This figure relates the common tensor diffusion model (left) with the mapping from the ODF (middle) and the 5D orientation mapping (right). Notice we have the ambiguity resulting from vectors in $\mathbb{R}^3$ being used to describe diffusion. The reason this is problematic is that diffusion requires a tensor quantity for its correct characterisation. The sign problem is resolved in the 5D space where all the vectors are concentrated around one direction.

We can define a modified fractional (FA) anisotropy related to standard FA:

$$FA = \sqrt{\frac{3}{2}}\frac{\| D - \frac{traceD}{3}I \|}{\| D \|}, \qquad FA^\star = \frac{\| \sum_i^n xx^T - \lambda_1 e_1 e_1^T \|}{\| \sum_i^n xx^T \|}. \qquad (10)$$

where $\| . \|$ is the tensor norm. The geometric interpretation of $FA^\star$ is that in FA the average diffusion in all directions is removed from the tensor to make it traceless, whereas only the diffusion in the principal direction, $\lambda_1 e_1 e_1^T$ is taken away in FA*. So, FA* will be larger than FA when $\lambda_1 \gg \lambda_2, \lambda_3$ but smaller when $\lambda_1 \approx \lambda_2, \lambda_3$[1].

3   Experiments and Discussion

We synthesized noisy ODFs from apparent diffusion of a tensor model with $S_0 = 1$ and $b = 700$ s/mm^2 with the approximate q-ball reconstruction technique outlined in [8]. These ODFs were then randomly sampled to give $x_i, i = 1..1024$. Then having used M_5, we performed 10 iterations of EM according to the ML update steps outlined above. In the illustrative results in figure 2 and the error analyses (figure 2), we used the same number of modes (m) as the number of synthesizing tensors used (ie. $m = 1$ or $m = 2$). For moderate SNR ratios, e.g. SNR = 64, the fitting is robust. Error analysis for $m = 1$ indicates that even in low SNRs the average estimation stays below 10°. For the two tensor case, we plotted the minimum angle error between either principal axis and either HvMF modal direction (4 possible correspondences are tried). The average of the minimum and maximum errors, which is an upper bound on this error, was then plotted.

We used HARDI data containing 120 gradient directions with $b = 700$s/mm^2 for further experiments. The ML estimates of the M_5 mean (of the HvMF eqn. 5) was used to create a PDD map (by decomposing the reconstituted tensor eqn. 3).

[1] $\star$ as it symbolises the spread of the vectors.

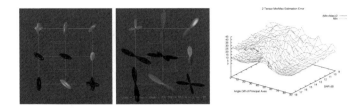

Fig. 2. HvMF fitting to samples drawn from noisy single and two tensor diffusion models (1024 samples used for EM estimation with SNR = 64dB). Tensor eccentricity is fixed at $(1, \frac{1}{3}, \frac{1}{3})$. Left figure depicts the single and muti-tensor voxels. Centre figure shows vHMF pdfs as isosurface: $xG(x|\Theta)$. Right figure, angle errors plot between two closest matching directions.

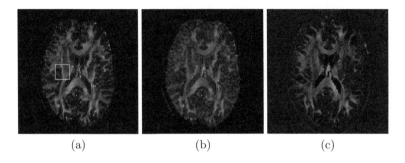

(a)   (b)   (c)

Fig. 3. Comparison of FA maps and PDDs obtained in different ways: (a) Standard FA with PDD shown in colours from a tensor fit to data (roi region used used below); (b) FA* produced using rank 1 spread measure (see equation 10); (c) FA from reconstituted tensor given 2nd order spherical harmonic basis expansion. Data contains 120 HARDI measurements (b is 700 s/mm^2). Note the similarities of all three maps which are obtained in different ways.

This map was weighted by the FA* and compared with coloured PDD and FA obtained by a standard least-squares tensor fitting (figures 3(a) and (b)). The resultant maps are indistinguishable other than, as expected, FA* being slightly greater in isotropic regions. Figure 3(c) shows estimates of PDD and FA obtained from HARDI data by the identity in equation 4. The HARDI measurements were interpolated using a cosine weighting kernel and then integrated with the 2nd order SH basis set, Y_2^m, by Monte Carlo integration. The coefficient images were then combined and a tensor reconstituted using the inverse M_5 mapping to yield the PDD and FA. The results are identical to FA of a standard tensor fit.

The images in figure 4 show 3D visualisations of a region from 1 slice of HARDI data showing the HvMF model selected fits to each voxel in comparison with single tensor fitting near the ventricle boundary. Qualitatively the results appear to be satisfactory but it is hard to judge whether the model selection is sensible. The HvMF is detecting planar and isotropic diffusion but by generally

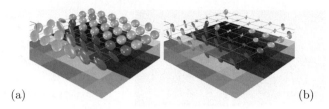

(a)   (b)

Fig. 4. Model selection by AIC on HvMF mixtures: (a) Single tensor estimates in small region on white-matter/CSF boundary; (b) HvMF estimates in same boundary region as in (a)

      (a)   (b)   (c)

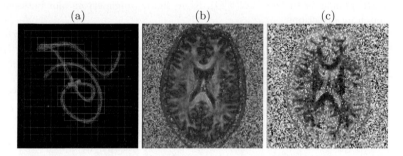

Fig. 5. (a) 2D synthetic example using vMF model selection (white=2) (yellow=1). (b) Log-likelihood of unimodal fit of H-vMF. (c) Log-likelihood of bimodal fit of H-vMF weighted by normalised squared difference in weights of two modal amplitudes (see text).

under fitting the data and preferring bimodal fits over a unimodal fit with small κ (note for $\kappa = 0$, the distribution is uniform). The AIC might be responsible as it less severe at penalising free parameters than say the Bayesian Information Criterion (BIC). It might be also that including a single parameter uniform component, $\frac{w_0}{4\pi}$, as part of the mixture to model will filter out the background low probabilities. 2D synthetic data was proceed in figure 5 where each region was labelled as either unimodal (yellow) or bimodal (white): all crossing regions are correctly labelled white. In figures 5(a) and (b) the voxel log-likelihoods after HvMF fitting are shown for the two cases. As expected, in (a), the fit is good in places where the fibre bundles generally lie and the map resembles a map of FA. In figure 5(b), we weighted the log-likelihood by the amplitudes of the normalised squared difference between the two principal modes: $(w_0 - w_1)^2/(w_0 + w_1)^2$ which will weight down those regions where their is a dominant mode. The results show that complementary regions to (a) are favoured by the bimodal fitting. Overall, the results indicate that some form of decision based selection may be necessary for better discrimination than achieved here, as reported recently by Peled et al. [9], if HvMF fitting was to be used in multi-tensor tractography. Such investigations are on-going.

4   Conclusions

We have described a probability model for high angular diffusion data. A 5D orientation mapping which resolves the inherent ambiguities in describing directional samples on a sphere is employed. This enables us to describe general ODFs in a natural and continuous way. In other words, we take advantage of the tensor mapping that respects that diffusion is bidirectional without having to resort to a Gaussian model. We also outlined the connection between spherical harmonic analysis of HARDI samples and our orientation space and how PDD calculations are equivalent. Our analyses indicate that this could be a fruitful approach for partitioning single and multi-fibre diffusion from HARDI data.

References

1. Weickert, J., Hagen, H.: Visualization and Processing of Tensor Fields. Springer, Heidelberg (2006)
2. Tuch, D.S., Reese, T.G., Wiegell, M.R., Makris, N., Belliveau, J.W., Weeden, V.J.: High angular resolution diffusion imaging reveals intravoxel white matter fiber heterogeneity. Magnetic Resonance in Medicine 48(4), 577–582 (2002)
3. Frank, L.R.: Characterization of Anisotropy in High Angular Resolution Diffusion-Weighted MRI. Magnetic Resonance in Medicine 47, 1083–1099 (2002)
4. McGraw, T., Vemuri, B., Yezierski, B., Mareci, T.: Segmentation of High Angular Resolution Diffusion MRI Modeled as a Field of von Mises-Fisher Mixtures. In: Leonardis, A., Bischof, H., Pinz, A. (eds.) ECCV 2006. LNCS, vol. 3953, pp. 461–475. Springer, Heidelberg (2006)
5. Knutsson, H.: Producing a continuous and distance preserving 5-d vector repesentation of 3-d orientation. In: Proceedings of IEEE Computer Society Workshop on Computer Architecture for Pattern Analysis and Image Database Management, pp. 18–20. IEEE Computer Society Press, Los Alamitos (1985)
6. Rieger, B., van Vliet, L.J.: Representing Orientation in n-Dimensional Spaces. In: Petkov, N., Westenberg, M.A. (eds.) CAIP 2003. LNCS, vol. 2756, pp. 17–24. Springer, Heidelberg (2003)
7. Sra, S., Dhillon, I.S.: Modeling Data using Directional Distributions. Technical report, Department of Computer Sciences, University of Texas (2002)
8. Bergman, O., Kindlmann, G., Lundervold, A., Westin, C.F.: Diffusion k-tensor Estimation from Q-ball Imaging Using Discretized Principal Axes. In: Larsen, R., Nielsen, M., Sporring, J. (eds.) MICCAI 2006. LNCS, vol. 4191, pp. 268–275. Springer, Heidelberg (2006)
9. Peled, S., Friman, O., Jolesz, F., Westin, C.-F.: Geometrically constrained two-tensor model for crossing tract in DWI. Magnetic Resonance Imaging 24, 1263–1270 (2006)

Use of Varying Constraints in Optimal 3-D Graph Search for Segmentation of Macular Optical Coherence Tomography Images

Mona Haeker[1,2], Michael D. Abràmoff[1,3], Xiaodong Wu[1],
Randy Kardon[3], and Milan Sonka[1,3]

Departments of [1]Electrical & Computer Engineering,
[2]Biomedical Engineering, and
[3]Ophthalmology & Visual Sciences, The University of Iowa,
Iowa City, IA 52242, USA
{mona-haeker, milan-sonka}@uiowa.edu

Abstract. An optimal 3-D graph search approach designed for simultaneous multiple surface detection is extended to allow for varying smoothness and surface interaction constraints instead of the traditionally used constant constraints. We apply the method to the intraretinal layer segmentation of 24 3-D optical coherence tomography (OCT) images, learning the constraints from examples in a leave-one-subject-out fashion. Introducing the varying constraints decreased the mean unsigned border positioning errors (mean error of 7.3 ± 3.7 μm using varying constraints compared to 8.3 ± 4.9 μm using constant constraints and 8.2 ± 3.5 μm for the inter-observer variability).

1 Introduction

Optical coherence tomography (OCT) is becoming an increasingly important modality for the noninvasive assessment of a variety of ocular diseases such as glaucoma, macular edema, and macular degeneration. For assessment of the macular region of the retina, one common scanning protocol involves the acquisition of six linear radial scans in a spoke pattern centered at the fovea (Fig. 1). Although the intraretinal layers are visible on such images, commercially-available quantitative assessment of such scans is currently limited to providing thickness measurements for one layer (e.g., the total retinal thickness on macular scans). Because the intraretinal layers may be affected differently by disease, an intraretinal segmentation approach is needed to enable quantification of individual layer properties, such as thickness or texture. While a few reported approaches for macular intraretinal segmentation exist in the literature (e.g., [1]), such approaches have been two-dimensional in nature.

To address this need, we have previously reported an optimal 3-D graph search approach for the intraretinal layer segmentation of macular scans [2, 3]. The approach is based on the optimal graph search method reported by Wu and Chen [4] and the extension to the multiple surface case by Li *et al.* [5]. In these approaches [4, 5], the surface segmentation problem is transformed into that of

N. Ayache, S. Ourselin, A. Maeder (Eds.): MICCAI 2007, Part I, LNCS 4791, pp. 244–251, 2007.
© Springer-Verlag Berlin Heidelberg 2007

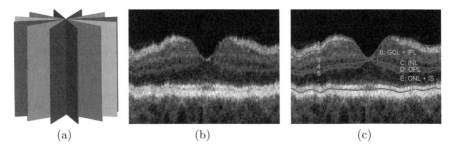

(a)   (b)   (c)

Fig. 1. Intraretinal layers on macular OCT images. (a) Schematic of six linear radial scans acquired during fast macular scanning protocol. Each color corresponds to one 2-D scan. (b) Example composite scan at one angular scan location. (c) Labeling of seven surfaces and corresponding six intraretinal layers on the 2-D composite scan.

finding a minimum-cost closed set in a constructed vertex-weighted geometric graph. Such a 3-D graph search method is well-suited for intraretinal layer segmentation for a variety of reasons. Perhaps the most important include 1) the ability to find an *optimal* set of surfaces with respect to a cost function in 3-D and 2) the ability to find multiple surfaces simultaneously. Note that even though the approach in [4,5] ultimately finds surfaces by finding a minimum-cost *s-t* cut in a constructed graph, it is fundamentally different than the "graph cut" methods of Boykov *et al.* (e.g., [6]).

However, in its original formulation, the 3-D optimal graph search method employs surface feasibility constraints that are constant in each direction. For example, the smoothness constraints for a particular surface $f(x, y)$ are represented by two parameters, Δ_x and Δ_y, reflecting the allowed change in surface height when moving from one neighboring surface point to the next in the x-direction and y-direction, respectively. Similarly, the surface interaction constraints (reflecting the allowed minimum and maximum distances between surface pairs) are constant. More flexibility in constraining surfaces to particular shapes would be obtained if varying constraints were allowed. Such a change would especially be important for surfaces in which the needed constraints are expected to change based on location (e.g., the foveal region in OCT images).

In this work, we show how the optimal 3-D graph search may be extended to handle *varying* surface smoothness and surface interaction constraints. We then show how to learn such constraints from a training set and apply the method to the intraretinal layer segmentation of macular OCT images.

2 Optimal 3-D Graph Search with Varying Constraints

The optimal 3-D graph search approach is designed to solve what we will call the "multiple surface segmentation problem." In very general terms, the multiple surface segmentation problem can be thought of as an optimization problem with the goal being to find the set of surfaces with the minimum cost such that the found surface set is feasible. Thus, there are two major components to the problem specification: 1) the specification of the constraints to require surface set feasibility and 2) the formalization of the cost of a set of surfaces. The first step in the graph search approach is to construct a graph such that the minimum-cost closed set of the graph corresponds to the set of surfaces with the minimum cost. (A closed set is a subset of the vertices of a graph such that no directed edges leave the set.) This is done by 1) ensuring that there is a one-to-one correspondence between each closed set in the constructed graph and each feasible surface set and 2) ensuring that the cost of each closed set in the graph corresponds (within a constant) to the cost of a set of (feasible) surfaces. Then the actual minimum-cost closed set is found by finding minimum-cost s-t cut in a closely related graph [4, 5]. In this section, we describe the surface set feasibility constraints and costs in more detail, also briefly showing how each component is represented in the constructed graph.

2.1   Surface Set Feasibility with Varying Constraints

Consider a volumetric image $I(x, y, z)$ of size $X \times Y \times Z$. We focus on the case in which each surface of interest can be defined with a function $f(x, y)$ mapping (x, y) pairs to z-values. Associated with each (x, y) pair is a column of voxels in which only one of the voxels — the voxel at $(x, y, f(x, y))$ — intersects the surface. Each column also has a set of neighbors. We use a "4-neighbor" relationship in which the set of neighbors for the column associated with (x, y) are the columns associated with $(x + 1, y)$, $(x - 1, y)$, $(x, y + 1)$, and $(x, y - 1)$.

In prior work, a single surface is considered feasible if the difference in z-values of neighboring surface points is less than or equal to a constant parameter (Δ_x in x-direction, Δ_y in y-direction). For example, for neighboring columns $\{(x, y), (x + 1, y)\}$ in the x-direction, this requires that

$$-\Delta_x \leq f(x, y) - f(x + 1, y) \leq \Delta_x. \tag{1}$$

A similar constraint exists for neighbors in the y-direction.

In this work, we allow the smoothness constraints to vary as a function of the column neighborhood pair. For a given neighborhood pair $\{(x_1, y_1), (x_2, y_2)\}$, the constraint becomes:

$$-\Delta^u_{\{(x_1, y_1),(x_2, y_2)\}} \leq f(x_1, y_1) - f(x_2, y_2) \leq \Delta^l_{\{(x_1, y_1),(x_2, y_2)\}}, \tag{2}$$

where $\Delta^u_{\{(x_1, y_1),(x_2, y_2)\}}$ reflects the maximum allowed increase in z-value when moving on a surface from column (x_1, y_1) to column (x_2, y_2) and $\Delta^l_{\{(x_1, y_1),(x_2, y_2)\}}$ reflects the maximum allowed decrease in z-value.

For a set of surfaces, additional constraints are added to model the desired relationships between the surfaces. For example, it may be known that one surface is always above another surface and that the distance between the surfaces is at least δ^l voxels, but no more than δ^u voxels (note the notational difference in δ used for surface interaction constraints and Δ used for smoothness constraints). Again, in prior work, these constraints were constant. In this work, we allow these constraints to be a function of (x, y) so that in principle, a different interaction constraint can be used for each column.

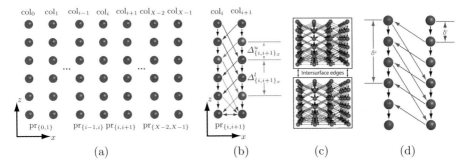

Fig. 2. Graph representation of feasibility constraints. (a–b) Surface smoothness constraints (shown only in x-direction using simplified notation). (c–d) Intersurface edges are added between the surface subgraphs to enforce the surface interaction constraints.

Graph representation. The structure of the constructed graph reflects the feasibility constraints. The graph is constructed in a similar manner as reported in [5] with the exception that the edges of the graph must take into account the varying constraints. First, one graph is created for each surface to be found. Then, intracolumn and intercolumn edges are added to enforce the surface smoothness constraints (Fig. 2(a-b)). Finally, the individual graphs are connected with intersurface edges to enforce the surface interaction constraints (Fig. 2(c-d)).

2.2   Cost of a Feasible Surface Set

We use the surface set cost formulation as presented in [3]. For completeness, we briefly review this formulation. Given a set of n non-intersecting surfaces $\{f_1(x,y),\ f_2(x,y),\ \ldots,\ f_n(x,y)\}$, the surfaces naturally divide the volume into $n+1$ regions (Fig. 3). Assuming the surfaces are labeled in "increasing" order, the regions can be labeled $R_0, \ldots, R_n$, where R_i reflects the region that lies between surface i and surface $i+1$ (with region boundary cases R_0 and R_n being defined as the region with lower z-values than surface 1 and the region with higher z-values than surface n, respectively). Each voxel can thus have $2n+1$ real-valued costs associated with it: n on-surface costs corresponding to the unlikeliness of belonging to each surface and $n+1$ in-region costs associated with the unlikeliness of belonging to each region. Let $c_{\mathrm{surf}_i}(x,y,z)$ represent the on-surface cost function associated with surface i and $c_{\mathrm{reg}_i}(x,y,z)$ represent the in-region cost function associated with region i. Then, the cost $C_{\{f_1(x,y),f_2(x,y),\ldots,f_n(x,y)\}}$ associated with the set of surfaces can be defined as

$$C_{\{f_1(x,y),f_2(x,y),\ldots,f_n(x,y)\}} = \sum_{i=1}^{n} C_{f_i(x,y)} + \sum_{i=0}^{n} C_{R_i}\,, \qquad (3)$$

where

$$C_{f_i(x,y)} = \sum_{\{(x,y,z)|z=f_i(x,y)\}} c_{\mathrm{surf}_i}(x,y,z) \quad \text{and} \quad C_{R_i} = \sum_{(x,y,z)\in R_i} c_{\mathrm{reg}_i}(x,y,z)\,.$$

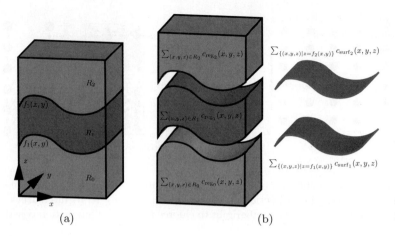

Fig. 3. Example schematic cost of two surfaces for the multiple surface segmentation problem. The two surfaces divide the volume into three regions.

Note that $C_{f_i(x,y)}$ reflects the cost associated with voxels on surface i and C_{R_i} reflects the cost associated with voxels belonging to region i.

Graph representation. The cost of each vertex in the graph is set such that the cost of each closed set corresponds to the cost (within a constant) of the set of surfaces. (The cost of a closed set is the summation of the costs of all the vertices.) The weight $w_i(x, y, z)$ of each vertex $(i = 1, 2, \ldots, n)$ can be defined as the summation of a term related to the on-surface costs $(w_{\mathrm{on-surf}_i}(x, y, z))$ and a term related to the in-region costs $(w_{\mathrm{in-reg}_i}(x, y, z))$:

$$w_i(x, y, z) = w_{\mathrm{on-surf}_i}(x, y, z) + w_{\mathrm{in-reg}_i}(x, y, z) . \tag{4}$$

For on-surface costs, the cost of each vertex is assigned the on-surface cost of the corresponding voxel minus the on-surface cost of the voxel below it [4,5]:

$$w_{\mathrm{on-surf}_i}(x, y, z) = \begin{cases} c_{\mathrm{surf}_i}(x, y, z) & \text{if } z = 0 \\ c_{\mathrm{surf}_i}(x, y, z) - c_{\mathrm{surf}_i}(x, y, z - 1) & \text{otherwise} \end{cases} . \tag{5}$$

For in-region costs, the cost of each vertex is assigned the in-region cost of the region below the surface associated with the vertex minus the in-region cost of the region above the surface associated with the vertex:

$$w_{\mathrm{in-reg}_i}(x, y, z) = c_{\mathrm{reg}_{i-1}}(x, y, z) - c_{\mathrm{reg}_i}(x, y, z) . \tag{6}$$

3   Application to Intraretinal Layer Segmentation

3.1   Segmentation Overview

To increase the signal to noise ratio on the macular OCT images, up to six raw macular series are first aligned and registered together using the methods described in [2]. This results in a composite 3-D scan for each eye. Then, for each composite 3-D OCT image, the seven surfaces are found in two groups using the optimal graph search approach: first, surfaces 1, 6, and 7 are found simultaneously. Then surfaces 2, 3, 4, and 5 are simultaneously determined. The cost functions are the same as we previously reported in [3]. Basically, the surfaces in the first group use on-surface costs based on image gradient and localized regional information, while the surfaces in the second group use in-region costs based on fuzzy membership values determined from image intensity.

3.2   Learning the Constraints

For each subject, the smoothness and surface interaction constraints are learned in a leave-one-subject-out fashion. For purposes of learning the varying smoothness constraints for each surface, it may be easiest to think of each pair of neighboring columns $\{(x_1, y_1), (x_2, y_2)\}$ as having its own constraint that needs to be learned separately. The basic idea is use manual tracings in the training set to determine the mean and standard deviation of how the z-value changes when moving from column (x_1, y_1) to column (x_2, y_2). Let $\overline{d}$ reflect the mean deviation (i.e., the mean of $f(x_1, y_1) - f(x_2, y_2)$ from the reference standard) and σ reflect the standard deviation. Then, to allow for 99% of the expected changes in z-value when moving from column (x_1, y_1) to column (x_2, y_2) (assuming a normal distribution), the two parameters of the smoothness constraint, $\Delta^l_{\{(x_1,y_1),(x_2,y_2)\}}$ and $\Delta^u_{\{(x_1,y_1),(x_2,y_2)\}}$ can be set as follows:

$$\Delta^l_{\{(x_1,y_1),(x_2,y_2)\}} = \overline{d} + 2.6 * \sigma \quad \text{and} \quad \Delta^u_{\{(x_1,y_1),(x_2,y_2)\}} = -(\overline{d} - 2.6 * \sigma) . \quad (7)$$

In this work, varying surface interaction constraints are used only in the simultaneous segmentation of the interior surfaces 2, 3, 4 and 5. The varying constraint is computed for the following surfaces pairings: 1-2, 2-3, 3-4, 4-5, and 5-6. For each surface pairing, the minimum distance between the surfaces at each column is set as the mean leave-one-out thickness minus 2.6 times the standard deviation (but truncated so as not to go below 0). Similarly, the maximum distance between the surfaces at each column is set as the mean leave-one-out thickness plus 2.6 times the standard deviation.

3.3   Experimental Methods

The intraretinal layer segmentation algorithm using varying constraints is applied to the composite 3-D images from fast macular scans from 12 subjects (24 eyes) with unilateral chronic anterior ischemic optic neuropathy. In addition, for comparison purposes, the algorithm is also applied to the same images using the constant smoothness and surface interaction constraints reported in [3]. Each composite 3-D image is comprised of six scans, each 128×1024 pixels. The physical width and height of the 2-D raw scans (and thus also the composite scans) is 6 mm $\times$ 2 mm, resulting in a pixel size of approximately 50 μm (laterally) $\times$ 2 μm (axially). One raw scan from each eye is independently traced by two human experts with the average of the two tracings being used as the reference standard. Borders that are not considered visible are not traced. The algorithmic result on the corresponding composite 2-D scan is converted into the coordinate system of the raw scan (inversely transforming the alignment/registration) and the mean unsigned border positioning errors for each border are computed. The unsigned border positioning errors are also computed using one observer as a reference standard for the other.

4   Results

The computed unsigned border positioning errors are summarized in Table 1. The smallest errors are consistently obtained for the variation of the algorithm using both varying smoothness and varying surface interaction constraints. For example, the overall (all surfaces combined) mean unsigned border positioning error is 7.3 ± 3.7 μm using both varying smoothness and varying interaction constraints and 8.3 ± 4.9 μm using constant constraints. These results compare favorably with the overall mean inter-observer variability of 8.2 ± 3.5 μm and the reported 9–10 μm axial resolution of the scanner system. The systematic improvement caused by introducing the varying constraints is at the 10% level overall. Even more noticeable differences occur in cases in which image information is locally ambiguous. Fig. 4 shows an example improvement.

Table 1. Summary of mean unsigned border positioning errors[†]

		Algorithm vs. Avg. Observer	
Border	Obs. 1 vs. Obs. 2	Varying S & I	Constant S & I
1	5.9 ± 1.2	4.6 ± 1.6	5.1 ± 2.3
2[‡]	6.3 ± 1.0	10.9 ± 4.3	11.2 ± 5.0
3[‡]	9.1 ± 3.7	8.9 ± 4.4	10.2 ± 4.9
4[‡]	7.6 ± 2.0	8.6 ± 1.9	12.0 ± 4.5
5	9.4 ± 3.9	8.3 ± 2.9	9.7 ± 5.4
6	7.6 ± 2.4	3.0 ± 1.0	3.6 ± 2.5
7	11.4 ± 4.7	7.6 ± 2.2	7.8 ± 2.2
Overall	8.2 ± 3.5	7.3 ± 3.7	8.3 ± 4.9

[†] Mean $\pm$ SD in μm for 24 scans.
[‡] Errors were not computed for those scans in which boundary was determined to not be visible by at least one observer.

5   Discussion and Conclusion

We have presented a method for the incorporation of varying constraints to the optimal 3-D graph search approach. In applying varying constraints to the intraretinal layer segmentation of optical coherence tomography images we

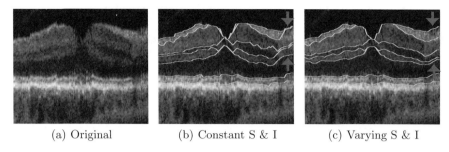

| (a) Original | (b) Constant S & I | (c) Varying S & I |

Fig. 4. Example improvement in segmentation result by using varying constraints

obtained a quantitative improvement in the results. Qualitatively, the varying constraints seemed to help the most in cases where the image information was less certain. In these cases, the constraints helped to ensure that a segmentation with a more feasible shape would be obtained. Thus, in addition to improving the cost function, incorporating varying constraints is another means of improving the segmentation for applications using the optimal 3-D graph search.

References

1. Cabrera Fernández, D., Salinas, H.M., Puliafito, C.A.: Automated detection of retinal layer structures on optical coherence tomography images. Opt. Express 13(25), 10200–10216 (2005)
2. Haeker, M., Sonka, M., Kardon, R., Shah, V.A., Wu, X., Abràmoff, M.D.: Automated segmentation of intraretinal layers from macular optical coherence tomography images (651214). In: Pluim, J.P.W., Reinhardt, J.M. (eds.) Proc. of SPIE Medical Imaging 2007: Image Processing. SPIE, vol. 6512, 651214 (2007)
3. Haeker, M., Wu, X., Abràmoff, M.D., Kardon, R., Sonka, M.: Incorporation of regional information in optimal 3-D graph search with application for intraretinal layer segmentation of optical coherence tomography images. In: Karssemeijer, N., Lelieveldt, B. (eds.) IPMI 2007. LNCS, vol. 4584, pp. 607–618. Springer, Heidelberg (2007)
4. Wu, X., Chen, D.Z.: Optimal net surface problems wih applications. In: Widmayer, P., Triguero, F., Morales, R., Hennessy, M., Eidenbenz, S., Conejo, R. (eds.) ICALP 2002. LNCS, vol. 2380, pp. 1029–1042. Springer, Heidelberg (2002)
5. Li, K., Wu, X., Chen, D.Z., Sonka, M.: Optimal surface segmentation in volumetric images – a graph-theoretic approach. IEEE Trans. Pattern Anal. Machine Intell. 28(1), 119–134 (2006)
6. Boykov, Y., Jolly, M.P.: Interactive organ segmentation using graph cuts. In: Delp, S.L., DiGoia, A.M., Jaramaz, B. (eds.) MICCAI 2000. LNCS, vol. 1935, pp. 276–286. Springer, Heidelberg (2000)

Automatic Segmentation of Bladder and Prostate Using Coupled 3D Deformable Models

María Jimena Costa*, Hervé Delingette, Sébastien Novellas,
and Nicholas Ayache

{Jimena.Costa,Herve.Delingette,Sebastien.Novellas,Nicholas.Ayache}
@sophia.inria.fr

Abstract. In this paper, we propose a fully automatic method for the coupled 3D localization and segmentation of lower abdomen structures. We apply it to the joint segmentation of the prostate and bladder in a database of CT scans of the lower abdomen of male patients. A flexible approach on the bladder allows the process to easily adapt to high shape variation and to intensity inhomogeneities that would be hard to characterize (due, for example, to the level of contrast agent that is present). On the other hand, a statistical shape prior is enforced on the prostate. We also propose an adaptive non–overlapping constraint that arbitrates the evolution of both structures based on the availability of strong image data at their common boundary. The method has been tested on a database of 16 volumetric images, and the validation process includes an assessment of inter–expert variability in prostate delineation, with promising results.

Keywords: prostate, bladder, 3D segmentation, coupled deformable models, CT.

1 Introduction

An essential part of a successful conformal radiotherapy treatment planning procedure is the accurate contouring of target volumes and organs at risk.

Because of the difficulty to accurately and reliably delineate structures in medical images, this task has traditionally been assigned to medical experts. However, manual editing is not only tedious but particularly prone to errors.

Semi–automatic or interactive approaches for segmentation allow the pratician to have better control over the segmentation process [1,2]. However, they remain time consuming and, especially for large databases, an automatic approach is desirable.

The segmentation of pelvic structures is a particularly difficult task since it involves soft tissues that present a very large variability in shape, size and intensity, the latter depending on the presence (partial or total) or absence of a contrast agent. The task is even more challenging in the case of prostate cancer, since, in this case, the characteristics of the organs at risk (bladder, rectum) are

---

* www-sop.inria.fr/asclepios/personnel/Jimena.Costa/

N. Ayache, S. Ourselin, A. Maeder (Eds.): MICCAI 2007, Part I, LNCS 4791, pp. 252–260, 2007.
© Springer-Verlag Berlin Heidelberg 2007

highly variable and have an important influence on the shape and location of the target organ itself (prostate).

After a short review of previous work, we present a novel framework for the localization and coupled segmentation of the prostate and bladder in CT images.

2   Previous Work

2.1   Un–coupled Bladder and Prostate Segmentation

Registration Approaches. These methods have been tested for CT bladder [3] and prostate [4] segmentation. Heavy variations in soft tissue (shape, size, intensity) are difficult to capture by these approaches, but they remain quite useful for initialization purposes.

Mathematical Morphology Approaches. Variations of these approaches have been tested in [5, 6]. They are easy to automate and can be quickly tuned and computed, but they are strongly dependent on the quality of the image.

Shape Deformation Approaches. Deformable models are quite flexible, since they can include shape priors [7, 1, 8], atlas initialization [9], fuzzy criteria [10] and multiple structure deformation [7]. *Explicit models* have been used for both prostate [11, 12] and bladder [10] segmentation. *Implicit models* have also been used to this end (see [8] for prostate and [13] for bladder segmentation).

Other Approaches. Other approaches include neural networks [2], radial searching [14], polar transform based methods [15] and genetic algorithms [16, 17], among others.

2.2   Multiple Structure Segmentation

Overlap penalization is proposed for both explicit [18] and implicit [7] models. In both cases, overlaps are punished in terms of energy minimization. The first approach couples multiple active contours in 2D video sequences through a unique energy function. The second presents a Bayesian inference framework where a shape prior can be applied on any of the structures. Neither approach is able to handle non–characterizable intensity inhomogeneities within structures.

Statistical shape and appearance model approaches are used in [11, 19, 20, 21, 22], among others. In [20], a segmentation method using both an intensity prior based on intensity profiles at each point and a geometric typicality (shape prior) is proposed. In [19, 21, 22], a perfect partition of the image into classes of similar intensities or textures is achieved. However, these techniques treat objects sharing similar image characteristics as a single item; thus, topological constraints between them cannot be enforced in the absence of a clear delimitation of the structures (for example, in a non–contrasted bladder and prostate case).

In fact, the approaches that we have found in the literature impose quite strong shape and/or appearance constraints on the structures involved.

The methods are therefore restricted to homogenous structures, or structures with characterizable inhomogeneities, which is not always the case in our database of images. We are thus motivated to propose a fully automatic framework for coupled bladder–prostate segmentation using explicit deformable models and a non–overlapping constraint. The method adjusts itself to different kinds of bladder (homogenous, different levels of inhomogeneities). The characteristics of the interface between both structures in the image are taken into account in this constraint. Since the prostate shows a much better statistical coherency in shape among patients than the bladder ([7]), a prostate shape prior is enforced.

3   Our Approach to Bladder Segmentation

In order to put the CT images in a common reference frame, locally affine registration [23] is performed on the pelvic bone structures (since they show lower variability than smooth tissues) and then interpolated to the soft tissues in the image. This allows us to perform the same cropping process on all the images, and to have a first localization of the target organs.

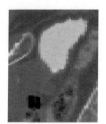 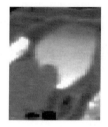 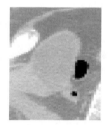 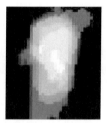

Fig. 1. Different types of bladders make the segmentation task challenging. From left to right, homogenous contrasted bladder, non–homogenous bladder and homogenous non–contrasted bladder (sagittal views). The rightmost image shows the variability in bladder shape and size, even in registered images (sagittal view).

The bladder is first located and classified as homogenous or non–homogenous, contrasted or non–contrasted (Figure 1) using a modified version of the region growing approach with highly contrasted voxels located within a zone of low intensity variability as seed points. Then, the segmentation begins by computing an approximation of the structure through mathematical morphology operations. A simplex mesh is deformed to fit this approximation. If the structure is not homogenous, the model is divided into zones that correspond to those found in the image data. The segmentation is later refined and smoothed using the bladder in the CT image itself. This process is illustrated in Figure 2. A more detailed explanation and validation of this method was presented in [24].

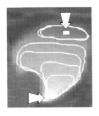 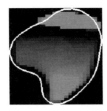 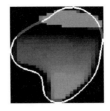 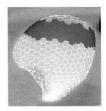

Fig. 2. Progression of modified region growing algorithms for a non–homogenous bladder, in order to generate a binary approximation of the structure. Seed points are indicated by arrows (left). An initial model is then deformed over the resulting approximation, and eventually divided into zones (if required by structure intensity inhomogeneities). The segmentation is then refined using the original, grey level image.

4 Our Approach to Prostate Segmentation

4.1 Prostate Localization

We use prior information on prostate localization, which has been computed based on the expert's segmentations of the structure in our database images. These images had previously been placed in a common frame of reference for bladder segmentation purposes using a non–rigid registration approach (see section 3).

4.2 Shape Statistics

The shape of the prostate across large patient population shows statistical coherency [7], but the image data is often not sufficient to establish the outline of this structure, it is helpful to incorporate shape prior knowledge. We built a shape model of the prostate from a database of training samples (CT images and their corresponding segmentations of the prostate performed by an expert). An initial deformable model was used to fit the manual segmentations of the prostates in the database, thus assuring a point correspondence between the models. A mean shape model and its principal deformation modes were computed using a Principal Component Analysis approach.

4.3 Intensity Information

We obtain initial information about the intensity of the prostate in each image from a small region inside the target structure. We define this region around a starting point located inside the mean shape model. We choose, among all the potential starting points, one located in a neighbourhood showing little intensity variance within a previously computed interval in Hounsfield units.

4.4 Initial Prostate Model Deformation

At each time step t, the position of vertex V_i in the prostate model is computed according to Equation 1.

$$V_i^{t+1} = V_i^t + \lambda(\alpha(f_i^{PCA}) + \beta(f_i^{ext}) + \delta(f_i^{int})) + (1 - \lambda)(f_i^{global}) \qquad (1)$$

where V_i^t and V_i^{t+1} are the positions of vertex i at time t and $t+1$, respectively. Parameter λ is a *locality* parameter: we start with $\lambda = 0$, a purely global (rigid + affine) deformation, and move progressively towards a more local deformation ($0 < \lambda < 1$). The influences of f^{PCA} (the PCA–based regularization force), f^{ext} (an image force that enforces intensity homogeneity within the structure) and f^{int} (internal regularization force) are weighted by parameters α, β and δ, respectively. Their values have been set to 0.4, 0.3 and 0.3.

The force f^{PCA} pulls the current model $\mathcal{S}$ towards $\mathcal{S}_S$, a "smooth" surface that belongs to the space spanned by the computed PCA modes of variation (for regularization purposes) and f^{ext} pulls it towards $\mathcal{S}_I$, an estimated target surface corresponding to the boundaries of the anatomical structure in the image. If we assume that the normal $\mathbf{n}(\mathbf{u})$ to the current surface $\mathcal{S}(\mathbf{u})$ is oriented outwards, the image guided term $\mathcal{S}_I(\mathbf{u})$ can be computed at each iteration as $\mathcal{S}(\mathbf{u}) + s_\star \, \mathbf{n}$ as

$$s_\star = \arg \min_{s \in [-L;L]} \sum_{v=-L}^{v=L} G_\sigma(|v - s|) * f(\mathcal{I}(\mathcal{S}(\mathbf{u}) + v \, \mathbf{n}), \mu, \sigma, sgn(v - s)) \qquad (2)$$

where s is the position of each vertex of the final mesh we want to evaluate, $-L$ and L are bounds on s, v is the position of the voxels along the normal of the mesh at vertex s, and $f(i, \mu, \sigma, sgn)$ is a confidence estimation. This confidence is a piecewise constant function that serves to increase or decrease the energy term, depending on the values of two expressions: $|\frac{\mathcal{I}(\mathcal{S}(\mathbf{u})) - \mu}{\sigma}| \leq 2$ and $sgn(v - s)$. For example, if the first term is false (i.e., the voxel's intensity is not compatible with the intensities found inside the structure) and the second term is true (i.e. the voxel is located inside the mesh), a positive penalization value is added to the energy term. Function G_σ defines a weight for the voxels that are taken into account at each iteration step; it may be a Gaussian p.d.f., a generalized rectangle function, or a combination of the two. The parameters are fully adjustable, to penalize more (or less) a non-homogeneity inside the structure or zone.

Once this strict deformation process stabilizes, we bring prostate–bladder model interaction into the game.

5   Context–Dependent Coupled Deformation

We present a coupled segmentation framework in which an asymmetric, non–overlapping constraint is enforced.

The non–overlapping of the structure models is achieved through the use of a specifically designed force to each mesh in the coupled deformation process (inspired by ([25])). At each deformation step, the areas enclosed by both the prostate and bladder models are checked for intersection. If such an intersection exists, a new elastic force, proportional to the distance maps to the meshes, is added to both models in order to drive them appart.

If the prostate–bladder interface is sufficiently "clear" (as in the case of contrasted bladders), we apply a symmetric non–overlapping force to both models.

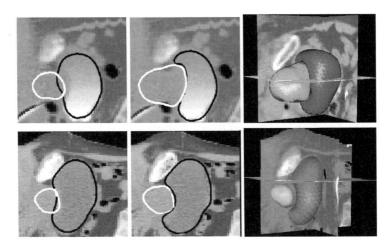

Fig. 3. Examples of the effect of the non–overlapping constraint in both partially clear (first row) and fuzzy (second row) prostate–bladder interfaces. From left to right, the independent evolution of prostate and bladder models, their coupled evolution with our non–overlapping constraint, and a 3D view of the result.

If, on the other hand, the interface is blurry, a higher priority is given to the model that contains the most information (like a shape prior), which is, in our case, the prostate mesh.

Our proposed asymmetric, context dependent non–overlapping constraint comprises interaction forces between the prostate and bladder meshes (F_{PoB} and F_{BoP}). To this end, the prostate shape model, the bladder model (F_{BoP}) and the strength of the border between the two in the image ($f(||\bigtriangledown I||)$) are taken into account, as shown by equations 3 and 4.

$$F_{BoP} = -\eta_P * ((\bigtriangledown Dmap_B)/||\bigtriangledown Dmap_B||) * (Dmap_B - \tau_B) * f(||\bigtriangledown I||) \quad (3)$$

$$F_{PoB} = -\eta_B * ((\bigtriangledown Dmap_P)/||\bigtriangledown Dmap_P||) * (Dmap_P - \tau_P) * (1 - f(||\bigtriangledown I||)) \quad (4)$$

where

$$f(||\bigtriangledown I||) = \begin{cases} \frac{||\bigtriangledown I||}{\vartheta}, & if||\bigtriangledown I|| \leq \vartheta \text{ (i.e., zone with low contrast)} \\ 1, & if||\bigtriangledown I|| > \vartheta \text{ (i.e., zone with high contrast)} \end{cases}$$

Parameters η_P and η_B weight the strength of the repulsion force, $Dmap_B$ and $Dmap_P$ are the distance maps to the bladder and prostate models, respectively, τ_B and τ_P are thresholds chosen on the distance maps (to establish a minimum distance between the models, if desired), $||\bigtriangledown I||$ is the norm of the image gradient, and ϑ is a threshold on the image gradient value to distinguish contrasted from non–contrasted prostate–bladder interfaces.

6   Results and Perspectives

The automatic segmentation algorithm was applied to a database of 16 CT images of the lower abdomen of male patients. The results were compared to experts' segmentations of bladder and prostate (the manual segmentation sets used for training and validation are disjoint). Figure 4 shows the obtained sensitivities and positive predictive values: the average sensitivity / positive predictive value is 0.81 / 0.85 for the bladder, and 0.75 / 0.80 for the prostate.

Image	Bladder Sensit.	PPV	Prostate Sensit.	PPV
1	0.82	0.94	0.73	0.99
2	0.87	0.95	0.86	0.92
3	0.88	0.94	0.75	0.91
4	0.86	0.89	0.95	0.72
5	0.89	0.97	0.72	0.81
6	0.86	0.86	0.79	0.81
7	0.91	0.96	0.86	0.87
8	0.87	0.85	0.82	0.94

Image	Bladder Sensit.	PPV	Prostate Sensit.	PPV
9	0.87	0.93	0.76	0.84
10	0.88	0.84	0.85	0.84
11	0.91	0.93	0.80	0.89
12	0.82	0.77	0.72	0.89
13	0.69	0.92	0.79	0.64
14	0.82	0.79	0.89	0.82
15	0.94	0.97	0.79	0.90
16	0.85	0.97	0.74	0.77

Fig. 4. Sensitivity and Positive Predictive Value results of the automatic segmentation of the bladder (left) and prostate (right) with respect to the one performed by an expert

For the validation of the prostate segmentations, we were able to assess the inter–expert variability thanks to a database of 5 CT images in which the prostates had been segmented by 3 different experts. We used the STAPLE [26] algorithm to compute a mean expert segmentation, and compared both the manual (expert) and automatic segmentations with respect to this mean. The results (Figure 5) show that the automatic segmentations are not far from the ones performed by the experts.

The results are promising, in spite of the low saliency (sometimes even indistinguishability) of the prostate in the images. The bladder–prostate interface

Image	Expert 1 Sensit.	PPV	Expert 2 Sensit.	PPV	Expert 3 Sensit.	PPV	Automatic Sensit.	PPV
1	0.82	0.87	0.98	0.80	0.94	0.91	0.71	0.98
5	0.80	0.99	0.99	0.64	0.90	0.96	0.72	0.85
6	0.82	0.89	0.96	0.75	0.99	0.97	0.81	0.81
9	0.92	0.95	0.98	0.69	0.77	0.98	0.66	0.92
10	0.91	0.91	0.96	0.96	0.97	0.84	0.89	0.79

Fig. 5. Sensitivity and Positive Predictive Value of both the expert and automatic segmentations of the prostate, with respect to the computed mean expert segmentation using the STAPLE [26] algorithm.

is correctly found. As the experts have confirmed, the prostate border that is not shared with the bladder is difficult to delineate, since there is little or no image information in this zone. This introduces some variability in the figures. We will continue to investigate this, and we would also like to incorporate multi-sequence analysis with MR and CT images, in order to have a better visibility of the prostate. Eventually, we will include the rectum in the joint segmentation process, since it is also an organ at risk during prostate cancer radiotherapy.

The work described in this article was performed in collaboration with Dosisoft, in the framework of the European Integrated Project MAESTRO, funded by the European Commission.

References

1. Freedman, D., Zhang, T.: Interactive graph cut based segmentation with shape priors. In: CVPR 2005, vol. 1, pp. 755–762. IEEE, Washington, DC, USA (2005)
2. Lee, C., Chung, P.: Identifying abdominal organs using robust fuzzy inference model. In: ICNSC 2004, vol. 2, pp. 1289–1294. IEEE, Washington, DC, USA (2004)
3. Unal, G., Slabaugh, G.: Coupled pdes for non-rigid registration and segmentation. In: CVPR 2005, vol. 1, pp. 168–175. IEEE, Washington, DC, USA (2005)
4. Malsch, U., Thieke, C., Bendl, R.: Fast elastic registration for adaptive radiotherapy. In: Larsen, R., Nielsen, M., Sporring, J. (eds.) MICCAI 2006. LNCS, vol. 4191, pp. 612–619. Springer, Heidelberg (2006)
5. Camapum, J., Silva, A., Freitas, A., et al.: Segmentation of clinical structures from images of the human pelvic area. In: SIBGRAPI 2004, pp. 10–16. IEEE Computer Society, Washington, DC, USA (2004)
6. Mazonakis, M., Damilakis, J., Varveris, H., et al.: Image segmentation in treatment planning for prostate cancer using the region growing technique. Br. J. Radiol. 74(879), 243–248 (2001)
7. Rousson, M., Khamene, A., Diallo, M., et al.: Constrained surface evolutions for prostate and bladder segmentation in ct images. In: Liu, Y., Jiang, T., Zhang, C. (eds.) CVBIA 2005. LNCS, vol. 3765, pp. 251–260. Springer, Heidelberg (2005)
8. Broadhurst, R., Stough, J., Pizer, S., et al.: Histogram statistics of local model-relative image regions. In: Olsen, O.F., Florack, L.M.J., Kuijper, A. (eds.) DSSCV 2005. LNCS, vol. 3753, pp. 72–83. Springer, Heidelberg (2005)
9. Ripoche, X., Atif, J., Osorio, A.: A 3d discrete deformable model guided by mutual information for medical image segmentation. In: Proceedings of the Medical Imaging Conference 2004, SPIE (2004)
10. Bueno, G., Martínez-Albalá, A., Adán, A.: Fuzzy-snake segmentation of anatomical structures applied to ct images. In: ICIAR (2), pp. 33–42 (2004)
11. Freedman, D., Radke, R., Zhang, T., et al.: Model-based multi-object segmentation via distribution matching. In: CVPRW 2004, vol. 1, p. 11. IEEE Computer Society, Washington, DC, USA (2004)
12. Dam, E., Fletcher, P.T., et al.: Prostate shape modeling based on principal geodesic analysis bootstrapping. In: Barillot, C., Haynor, D.R., Hellier, P. (eds.) MICCAI 2004. LNCS, vol. 3217, pp. 1008–1016. Springer, Heidelberg (2004)
13. Tsai, A., Yezzi, A.J., et al.: A shape-based approach to the segmentation of medical imagery using level sets. IEEE TMI 22(2), 137–154 (2003)

14. Xu, W., Amin, S., Haas, O., et al.: Contour detection by using radial searching for ct images. In: 4th EMBS Special Topic Conference, pp. 346–349. IEEE Computer Society, Washington, DC, USA (2003)
15. Zwiggelaar, R., Zhu, Y., et al.: Semi-automatic segmentation of the prostate. In: IbPRIA pp. 1108–1116 (2003)
16. Cosío, F.A.: Prostate segmentation using pixel classification and genetic algorithms. In: MICAI, pp. 910–917 (2005)
17. Ghosh, P., Mitchell, M.: Segmentation of medical images using a genetic algorithm. In: GECCO 2006, pp. 1171–1178. ACM Press, New York (2006)
18. Zimmer, C., Olivo-Marin, J.C.: Coupled parametric active contours. IEEE Trans. Pattern Anal. Mach. Intell. 27(11), 1838–1842 (2005)
19. Paragios, N., Deriche, R.: Geodesic active regions: a new paradigm to deal with frame partition problems in computer vision. JVCIR 13(1/2), 249–268 (2002)
20. Pizer, S.M., Fletcher, P.T., Joshi, S., Gash, A.G., Stough, J., Thall, A., Tracton, G., Chaney, E.L.: A method and software for segmentation of anatomic object ensembles by deformable m-reps. Med. Phys. 32(5), 1335–1345 (2005)
21. Vese, L.A., Chan, T.F.: A multiphase level set framework for image segmentation using the mumford and shah model. Int. J. Comput. Vision 50(3), 271–293 (2002)
22. Yezzi Jr, A., Tsai, A., Willsky, A.: A fully global approach to image segmentation via coupled curve evolution equations. JVCIR 13(1/2), 195–216 (2002)
23. Commowick, O., Arsigny, V., Costa, J., et al.: An efficient locally affine framework for the registration of anatomical structures. In: ISBI 2006, Arlington, Virginia, USA (2006)
24. Costa, M., Delingette, H., Ayache, N.: Automatic segmentation of the bladder using deformable models. In: ISBI 2007, Arlington, Virginia, USA (2007)
25. Pitiot, A., Delingette, H., Thompson, P.M., Ayache, N.: Expert knowledge guided segmentation system for brain MRI. NeuroImage 23(supplement 1), S85–S96 (2004) Special Issue: Mathematics in Brain Imaging
26. Warfield, S.K., Zou, K.H., Wells. III, W.M.: Simultaneous truth and performance level estimation (staple): an algorithm for the validation of image segmentation. IEEE TMI 23(7), 903–921 (2004)

Characterizing Spatio-temporal Patterns for Disease Discrimination in Cardiac Echo Videos

T. Syeda-Mahmood[1], F. Wang[1], D. Beymer[1], M. London[2], and R. Reddy[3]

[1] IBM Almaden Research Center, San Jose, CA, USA
[2] UCSF Veterans Hospital, San Francisco, CA, USA
[3] Mediciti Hospital, Hyderabad, India

Abstract. Disease-specific understanding of echocardiographic sequences requires accurate characterization of spatio-temporal motion patterns. In this paper we present a method of automatic extraction and matching of spatio-temporal patterns from cardiac echo videos. Specifically, we extract cardiac regions (chambers and walls) using a variation of multiscale normalized cuts that combines motion estimates from deformable models with image intensity. We then derive spatio-temporal trajectories of region measurements such as wall motion, volume and thickness. The region trajectories are then matched to infer the similarities in disease labels of patients. Validation results on patient data sets collected from many hospitals are presented.

1 Introduction

Analyzing the spatio-temporal regional motion patterns of the heart is important for cardiac disease discrimination. This problem is complicated by the heart's non-rigid motion, involving twists, rotations, and contractions. Furthermore, the poor imaging quality of 2D echo videos due to low contrast, speckle noise, and signal dropouts cause problems in interpretation. Thus, new methods for robust extraction of spatio-temporal regional motion patterns are needed.

In this paper we present a method of automatic extraction and matching of spatio-temporal patterns from cardiac echo videos. Specifically, we extract cardiac regions (chambers and walls) using a variation of multi-scale normalized cuts that combines motion estimates with image intensity. We then extract spatio-temporal trajectories of region measurements such as wall motion, volume, thickness, etc. In order to compare the regional measurements across diseases, the underlying regions must be brought into correspondence. For this, we use the framework of active shape models. The region trajectories are then compared to differentiate disease labels of videos. Validation results on patient data sets collected from many hospitals are presented.

While there is considerable work in cardiac echo region segmentation and tracking [1], not much work exists for automatic disease discrimination. An earlier work on diagnosis validation using video similarity [2] used features from the entire heart region, restricting its use in characterizing region-specific diseases.

The work reported here builds on the considerable literature for optical flow-based methods [3,4,5,6], spatial region segmentation methods [7] and deformable

N. Ayache, S. Ourselin, A. Maeder (Eds.): MICCAI 2007, Part I, LNCS 4791, pp. 261–269, 2007.
© Springer-Verlag Berlin Heidelberg 2007

shape models [8] (to perform a non-rigid alignment of shapes). Optical flow-based segmentation works poorly for cardiac regions due to the low quality of the echo videos and non-smooth heart motion. Spatial region segmentation [7], on the other hand, frequently results in under-segmentation due to the poor resolution in the echo video. While regional measurements are frequently used by physicians to diagnose diseases, many of these require human intervention for region annotation. In our approach, we attempt to automate the extraction of many of these regional measurements. Also, while many of the regional measurements are taken at snapshots in time (e.g. end of systole), our regional measurements capture variations within a heart cycle and can serve as a new diagnostic tool for physicians that is complementary to the existing measurements based on AHE guidelines.

2   Region Extraction

We extract cardiac regions using a variant of multi-scale normalized cuts. Specifically, let $G = (V, E, W)$ be a graph, with the pixels as graph nodes V, and edges in E connecting pairs of neighboring pixels. Let the weight W associated with each edge be based on the intensity and motion at each pixel. The normalized cut algorithm uses the normalized cut criterion [9] to partition the pixels into self-similar regions. Recently, Coor et al. [10] improved the efficiency of normalized cuts using a scale-space implementation. We adapt the multiscale normalized cuts to use a weighting function that combines image intensity with motion information so that nearby pixels with similar intensity values and motion are likely to belong to one object. The revised weighting function is given below:

$$W_I(i,j) = e^{-||X_i - X_j||/\delta_x - ||I_i - I_j||/\delta_I - ||V_i - V_j||/\delta_V} \tag{1}$$

where X_i denotes pixel location, I_i and V_i are image intensity and the motion at pixel location i.

We estimate motion by treating each successive pairs of intensity image frames as surfaces $(x, y, I(x, y))$ and finding a deformable surface model that warps one frame into the next as described in the Demons algorithm [11]. The resulting deformation field gives a consistent set of directional velocity vectors, sampling motion densely in both space and time.

Fig.1 illustrates cardiac region segmentation using the modified multilevel normalized cuts combining intensity and motion information. Fig.1a,b show adjacent frames of an echo video. Using Demons algorithm, a zoomed-in portion of the motion field is illustrated in Fig.1d. In the echo video, the inward and outward pull of the muscles in the different chambers and septal wall can be clearly captured in the resulting deformation field. By comparison, the optical flow field shows haphazard motion inconsistent with the actual observed motion in the echo videos (Fig.1e). Fig. 1c shows the results of using normalized cut-based segmentation based on intensity alone. Finally, Fig.1f shows the normalized cut result using both intensity and motion recovered from deformable registration. As can be seen, the combined use of intensity and motion information has resulted in improved delineation of chamber and septal wall boundaries.

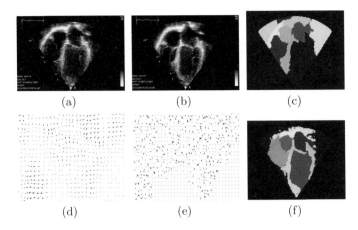

Fig. 1. Grouping results for echocardiogram frames using modified graph decomposition algorithm. (See text for details.)

3   Spatio-temporal Regional Measurements

We now discuss the extraction of spatio-temporal region trajectories. Using the deformable surfaces model of motion field, we can establish correspondence between pixels in adjacent fields as described in Section 2. Using this correspondence and the pixel label given by the segmentation step, we obtain the spatio-temporal trajectories of cardiac regions by tracking these regions across a heart beat cycle. To compare echo videos of similar patients, we extract meaningful measurements from the regions based on AHE guidelines. Specifically, we measure the following:

Volumetric trajectory $V(t)$: The atrial and ventricular volumes are one of the best diagnostic parameters to be measured for various cardiovascular diseases including myocardial infarction. For example, the change in ventricular volume through the heart beat cycle gives a good indication of the contractile performance, and any impairments can affect the temporal trajectory. We measure this simply as the area of the segmented regions obtained from Section 2 focusing on the cardiac chambers. The temporal trajectories allow the changing volume and hence the 2D + time aspects of the shape to be better modeled.

Translational Displacement $X(t)$: The extent of displacement is also a good indicator for many diseases such as hypertrophy, cardiomyopathy, etc. For example, hypokinesia patients often depict smaller septal wall motion. Thus the total extent of displacement as well as the instantaneous displacement of regions such as septal walls within a heart beat cycle can be a good indication of diseases.

Total Motion $M(t)$: The displacement feature measures the horizontal component of the full 3D motion of the heart regional volumes. To capture the overall motion of the heart region better, we use the average velocity curve described in [2]. The average velocity curve preserves a common sense of perceived motion per direction and is obtained by averaging the speed and direction of the velocity vectors at each pixel in the region within each frame.

By taking the projection of the average velocity curve along x, y, and t, we can obtain three additional region features. In particular, the projection onto x, y gives the total extent of planar motion of the region and is a good indication of the mechanical performance of the corresponding anatomical region.

4   Disease Discrimination from Regional Trajectories

We now turn to the problem of disease similarity inference by a match of the regional trajectories described above. Due to the variabilities introduced by anatomical differences, viewpoint variations, imaging quality, and segmentation errors, we expect the regional feature trajectories to show considerable variation even for patients within the same disease category. However, we expect to derive higher order statistics from the trajectories that make the comparison meaningful. Furthermore, the trajectories of corresponding regions (e.g. left ventricle to left ventricle) must be compared, so we chose to model the structure of the heart using an active shape model. Echo videos from patients with similar disease are then brought into alignment with the active shape model. The labels associated with the regions in the training stage are then used to infer the region correspondence.

4.1   Region Correspondence Using Active Shape Models

In active shape models [8], the shape of an object is represented by a set of feature points on the object, usually chosen to sample object contours at regular intervals. Given the locations of n feature points $f_1, f_2, \ldots, f_n$, the shape vector $\mathbf{s}$ concatenates the (x, y) coordinates of all feature points, $\mathbf{s} = [x_1, y_1, \ldots, x_n, y_n]^T$. For the heart, we have initially focussed on the apical four chamber view (Fig. 2). The feature points are centered around the mitral valve (point group mv), interventricular septum (ivs), interatrial septum (ias), and the lateral wall (lvl). We chose not to trace the entire boundary of the left ventricle because the apex is often not visible due to the ultrasound zoom and transducer location. Wall boundaries are annotated on both the inner and outer sections.

Image texture is represented by image patches centered around the feature locations. Given a shape with n features, the texture vector $\mathbf{t}$ concatenates the pixels from all the patches into one long vector.

We used a standard implementation of active shape models (ASMs) as described in [8] with a few enhancements. The training images for the active shape model were obtained from echo video sequences of patients with different diseases and different video frames within a heart beat cycle to capture the range of spatial and temporal variations of the heart structure. Cardiac cycle clips from apical four chamber (A4C) views were manually extracted from sample echo video. Each patient has at least two cycles extracted, with the first used for ASM training, and the remainder used for testing. The extracted cardiac cycles

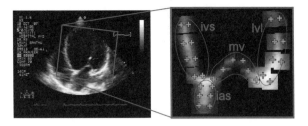

Fig. 2. Our active shape model contains 28 features in four groups centered about the mitral valve region. The right image shows the mean texture for the 28 feature patches.

are synchronized on frame 0 using the peak of the R wave as seen in the echo video's ECG lead.

Unlike most manual initializations for fitting active shape models to new images, we used an automatic initialization method where a distance-to-eigenspace method is first used to generate seed ASM initializations. The seed locations are then refined and evaluated using a coarse-to-fine pyramid approach.

Once we have fit the ASM model to a new image, corresponding regions are determined by simply associating the region label of the projected points of the active shape model with the underlying pixels.

4.2 Matching Regional Trajectories

Once the corresponding regions are identified, we normalize the trajectories to make them invariant to various artifacts of imaging. We normalize for heart rate differences by extracting a single heart cycle from the video starting from the peak of the R-wave as a common reference point (using the ECG signal embedded in the video). We also report all measurements in cm instead of image coordinates, which makes the trajectories invariant to effects of scale (zoom-in or out). This is done by using the 10 cm calibration markers on the left and right sides of the echo sector. Finally, we match trajectories of videos with the same viewpoint to make the comparison meaningful (e.g. 4AC to 4AC). Since the regional measurements used (area, extent of motion, etc.) are not affected by rotation, or translation, and since scale is accounted by keeping the centimeter unit, the trajectories are invariant to similarity transformations as well.

The regional measurements capture different aspects of cardiac regions. Hence, we measure their similarities differently as described below:

Volumetric trajectories: The distance between two volumetric trajectories $V_1(t)$ and $V_2(t)$ is given by

$$D(V_1, V_2) = \sum_i (V_{n1}(i) - V_{n2}(i))^2 \qquad (2)$$

where $V_{n1}(i) = \frac{V_1(i)}{Max(V_1)}$ and $V_{n2}(i) = \frac{V_2(i)}{Max(V_2)}$. By normalizing the regional volume, we factor out the effects of absolute volume and focus on trajectory shape. To use absolute volumes, further calibration will be needed.

Horizontal displacement: For the displacement trajectory $X(t)$, we measure the total motion of these curves by integrating the speed vector $|dX(t)/dt|$ over the cardiac cycle. Thus, given two displacement trajectories $X_1(t), X_2(t)$, the distance between them is given by

$$D(X_1, X_2) = | \int \left| \frac{dX_1(t)}{dt} \right| dt - \int \left| \frac{dX_2(t)}{dt} \right| dt | . \qquad (3)$$

Total motion: For the total motion trajectory, we measure the area under the curve. The difference between two projected motion trajectories $M_1(t), M_2(t)$ is

$$D(M_1(t), M_2(t)) = | \int \int M_1(x(t), y(t)) dx, dy - \int \int M_2(x(t), y(t)) dxdy | \qquad (4)$$

5   Results

To verify our conjecture that the trajectories of regional features are useful in inferring disease similarity, we experimented with a number of public cardiac echo data sets, namely, the GE Vivid online medical library, the Yale Medical School library, and data collected by cardiologists from various hospitals in India. The data sets depicted over 500 heart beat cycles chosen from over 50 patients with a number of cardiac diseases including cardiomyopathy, hypokinesia, mitral regurgitation, hypertrophy, etc. The echo videos from hospitals came with diagnoses as well as the common regional measurements such as wall thickness and ventricular volumes which were used as ground truth for testing our algorithms.

5.1   Disease Discrimination Using Regional Trajectories

We first illustrate the discrimination of diseases through regional trajectories. Fig. 3 shows the regional trajectories for patients with different disease labels. In the first row of Fig. 3, the two images on the left show videos of normal patients taken from the GE Vivid online library collection, while the third and fourth image show videos of patients diagnosed with asynchronous LV motion and left bundle-branch block respectively. The trajectories of the corresponding left ventricular volumes are shown in the second row of Fig. 3. The x-y projected motion trajectories of the intra-ventricular septum are shown in last row of Fig. 3. The volumetric trajectories show that the ventricular volume is minimum at roughly the midpoint of the cardiac cycle showing the symmetry of movement, while the diseases cases show asymmetry when the ventricular volume minimum is reached. In the projected motion trajectories, overall displacement of the IVS is much contained as seen by the small area spanned by the trajectories, whereas the diseased cases show a much larger area of total displacement.

The distance measures between each of the regional trajectories for the videos in Fig. 3 are shown below in Eqn. 5. Here the rows and columns correspond to the videos depicted in the first row of Fig. 3 respectively. As can be seen in each case, the normal videos are more similar in the distance metrics used than the abnormal cases.

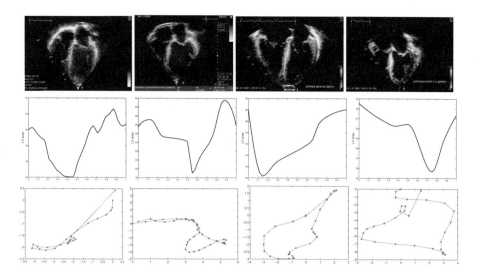

Fig. 3. Feature plots of four sample videos from GE Vivid online medical library. (see text for details).

$$\text{MSE Distance} = \begin{pmatrix} 0 & 1.9728 & 2.4524 & 3.4176 \\ 1.9728 & 0 & 3.3106 & 2.9627 \\ 2.4524 & 3.3106 & 0 & 3.3013 \\ 3.4176 & 2.9627 & 3.3013 & 0 \end{pmatrix} \qquad (5)$$

Using the total motion measurement, the total motion values for the 4 echo videos in square millimeter are $0.13, 0.55, 1.79, 1.16$ respectively. Thus even using this measure, the normal videos are deemed similar and are discriminable from the abnormal ones.

5.2 Disease Similarity Using Septal Motion

To further evaluate the validity of regional trajectories, we conducted a focused study on one of the regional measurements, namely, the displacement of the septal wall, as an indicator for disease. As the left ventricle (LV) expands and contracts, the septal wall shows a cyclic motion. In the case of motion abnormalities such as hypokinesia, the septal motion is considerably reduced.

To perform this study, we used a collection of echocardiogram videos from 20 cardiology patients from a hospital in India. The cardiologists capture the echo video in their normal clinical setting, and echo findings and disease diagnoses are included as text reports. Thus, we are able to divide the patients by any cardiac disease of interest – in this case, there were 14 patients diagnosed with hypokinesia in the septal wall, and 6 patients with normal motion of the septum.

Fig. 4, left, shows four example displacement curves $X(t)$, two for patients with a normal septum, and two for patients with a hypokinetic septum. The time axis in these plots have been normalized to one heart cycle. Qualitatively

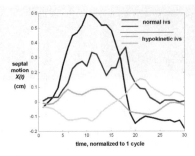 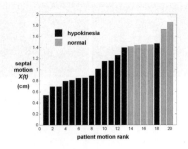

Fig. 4. Left: The motion displacement $X(t)$ for four patients, 2 normal ones and 2 with ivs hypokinesia; Right: the patients sorted by their septal motion

from the plots of $X(t)$, it is easy to see that the normal cases have much more motion displacement than the hypokinetic cases. Finally, we evaluated the effectiveness of the displacement measure for discriminating between patients with and without hypokinesia. Fig. 4, right, shows the result of ranking echo videos based on the displacement metric of Equation 3. As can be seen, the displacement trajectory can be used to discriminate the hypokinesia patients from the normal patients. The one outlier (patient 18) is due to a tracking error during trajectory formation when the lateral walls go out of view, biasing the septum tracking and increasing the septal motion estimate.

6   Conclusions

In this paper, we presented novel methods of automatic extraction and matching of spatio-temporal patterns from cardiac echo videos. The region trajectories are then matched to infer the similarities in disease labels of patients. Validation results on patient data sets collected from many hospitals were presented.

References

1. Dydenko, I., Jamal, F., Bernard, O., D'Hooge, J., Magnin, I.E., Friboulet, D.: A level set framework with a shape and motion prior for segmentation and region tracking in echocardiography. Medical Image Analysis 10(2), 162–177 (2006)
2. Syeda-Mahmood, T.F., Yang, J.: Characterizing normal and abnormal cardiac echo motion patterns. Computers in Cardiology 33, 725–728 (2006)
3. Gheissari, N., Bab-Hadiashar, A.: Motion analysis: Model selection and motion segmentation. In: ICIAP 2003, vol. 00, pp. 442–447 (2003)
4. Cremers, D., Soatto, S.: Motion competition: A variational framework for piecewise parametric motion segmentation. In: IJCV 2005, vol. 62(3), pp. 249–265 (2005)
5. Tagare, H.: Shape-based nonrigid correspondence with application to heart motion analysis. IEEE Trans. Med. Imaging 18(7), 570–579 (1999)
6. Papademetris, X., Sinusas, A.J., Dione, D.P., Duncan, J.S.: 3d cardiac deformation from ultrasound images. In: Taylor, C., Colchester, A. (eds.) MICCAI 1999. LNCS, vol. 1679, pp. 420–429. Springer, Heidelberg (1999)

7. Zerhouni, E., Parish, D., Rogers, W., Yang, A., Shapiro, E.: Human heart: Tagging with mr imaginga method for noninvasive assessment of myocardial motion. Radiology 169(1), 59–63 (1988)
8. Cootes, T.F., Taylor, C.J., Cooper, D.H., Graham, J.: Active shape models their training and application. Comput. Vis. Image Underst. 61(1), 38–59 (1995)
9. Shi, J., Malik, J.: Motion segmentation and tracking using normalized cuts. In: ICCV 1998, Washington, DC, USA, p. 1154 (1998)
10. Cour, T., Benezit, F., Shi, J.: Spectral segmentation with multiscale graph decomposition. In: CVPR 2005, Washington, DC, USA pp. 1124–1131 (2005)
11. Thirion, J.P.: Image matching as a diffusion process: an analogy with maxwell's demons. Medical Image Analysis 2(3), 243–260 (1998)

Integrating Functional and Structural Images for Simultaneous Cardiac Segmentation and Deformation Recovery⋆

Ken C.L. Wong[1], Linwei Wang[1], Heye Zhang[1], Huafeng Liu[2],
and Pengcheng Shi[3,1]

[1] Department of Electronic and Computer Engineering,
Hong Kong University of Science and Technology, Hong Kong
{eewclken,maomwlw,eezhy,eeship}@ust.hk
[2] State Key Laboratory of Modern Optical Instrumentation,
Zhejiang University, Hanzhou, China
liuhf@zju.edu.cn
[3] School of Biomedical Engineering, Southern Medical University, Guangzhou, China

Abstract. Because of their physiological meaningfulness, cardiac phys-iome models have been used as constraints to recover patient information from medical images. Although the results are promising, the parameters of the physiome models are not patient-specific, and thus affect the clinical relevance of the recovered information especially in pathological cases. In view of this problem, we incorporate patient information from body surface potential maps in the physiome model to provide a more patient-specific while physiological plausible guidance, which is further coupled with patient measurements derived from structural images to recover the cardiac geometry and deformation simultaneously. Experiments have been conducted on synthetic data to show the benefits of the framework, and on real human data to show its practical potential.

1 Introduction

In order to describe the physiology of the heart, cardiac physiome models have been developed from invasive or *in vitro* experiments of anatomy, biomechanics, and electrophysiology. These models typically comprise an electrical propagation model (E model), an electromechanical coupling model (EM model), and a biomechanical model (BM model), which are connected together through a cardiac system dynamics. Because of their physiological meaningfulness, phys-iome models have been posed as model constraints to recover patient cardiac information from medical images. In the recently proposed cardiac kinematics recovery framework [1], given the image-derived motion information at salient features such as heart boundaries, the cardiac kinematics of the patient is recovered through the guidance of the physiome model with improved physiological

⋆ This work is supported in part by the China National Basic Research Program (973-2003CB716100), and the Hong Kong Research Grants Council (CERG-HKUST6151/03E).

N. Ayache, S. Ourselin, A. Maeder (Eds.): MICCAI 2007, Part I, LNCS 4791, pp. 270–277, 2007.
© Springer-Verlag Berlin Heidelberg 2007

plausibility. The physiome model has also been used for recovering the local myocardial contractility from known displacement, with the aid of a relatively detailed anatomical heart model derived from patient's structural images [2]. Nevertheless, regardless of the promising potentials of the physiome models, most parameters used by these algorithms are not patient-specific, and thus the clinical relevance may be reduced especially under pathological conditions. Furthermore, following the spirit of [3], the segmentation and the deformation recovery tasks should be unified into a coherent process for more consistent and appropriate results.

In view of these problems, we propose a framework for simultaneous cardiac segmentation and deformation recovery, guided by a physiome model specified by information from body surface potential maps (BSPMs). Using the meshfree method [4], the heart is represented by a set of nodes bounded by surface elements, and simultaneous segmentation and deformation recovery is achieved by evolving the nodes through the physiome model and medical images. Adopting the recently proposed algorithm [5], the transmembrane potentials (TMPs) are recovered from BSPMs to give the patient-specific excitation sequence of the myocytes. This sequence is transformed into active contraction stresses through the EM model to provide the patient-specific physiological guidance for the recovery. On the other hand, a voxel matching algorithm based on comparing voxel similarities between two consecutive structural cardiac images is utilized to provide displacements of the boundary nodes as image-derived measurements. These BSPM-derived active stresses and image-derived measurements are coupled together through state-space equations composed of cardiac system dynamics, and filtering is applied to recover the cardiac geometry and deformation simultaneously in a statistically optimal sense. With this algorithm, functional images (BSPMs) are integrated with structural images through the physiome model to benefit both segmentation and deformation recovery. Experiments have been conducted on synthetic data to show the advantages of our framework, also on real human data to show its practical potentials.

2   Methodology

With the recent biological and technical breakthroughs, models describing cardiac physiology across different spatiotemporal scales are available, and appropriate models should be chosen depending on the specific purposes of the applications. As our proposed framework aims at recovering patient cardiac information from medical images, the cardiac physiome model being used should be able to capture the most significant cardiac physiological phenomena while ensure the computational feasibility of the complicated inverse problem. In consequence, we have chosen the FitzHugh-Nagumo model as the E model [5], a simple ordinary differential equation described in [2] as the EM model, and an anisotropic, elastic material model as the BM model [1]. These models are connected together through the total Lagrangian (TL) cardiac system dynamics to describe the relatively complete macroscopic physiology of the heart [1].

Using this physiome model as the central link, our proposed framework consists of three parts: integrating BSPMs with the physiome model to provide a relatively patient-specific physiological guidance, the voxel matching algorithm providing displacements of boundary nodes as image-derived measurements, and the state-space filtering framework coupling the measurements with the physiome model for simultaneous recovery of cardiac geometry and deformation.

2.1   Integrating BSPMs with Physiome Model

As described in the introduction, the physiome models used by the previous efforts are not patient-specific [1,2]. In order to partially address this problem, we utilize the algorithm proposed in [5] to recover TMPs from patient's BSPMs.

The algorithm consists of a spatiotemporal 3D TMP evolution model described via FitzHugh-Nagumo-like reaction-diffusion equations [1]:

$$\begin{cases} \frac{\partial \mathbf{U}_e}{\partial t} = -\mathbf{M}_e^{-1}\mathbf{K}_e\mathbf{U}_e + c_1\mathbf{U}_e(1 - \mathbf{U}_e)(\mathbf{U}_e - a) - c_2\mathbf{U}_e\mathbf{V}_e \\ \frac{\partial \mathbf{V}_e}{\partial t} = b(\mathbf{U}_e - d\mathbf{V}_e) \end{cases} \tag{1}$$

where $\mathbf{U}_e$ and $\mathbf{V}_e$ are vectors of TMPs and recovery variables. $\mathbf{M}_e$ and $\mathbf{K}_e$, constructed based on the meshfree method, account for the intercellular coupling of electrical propagation. a, b, $c1$, $c2$ and d are parameters defining the shapes of the action potentials.

To relate the observed BSPs with TMPs, the TMP-BSP projection model for the system-observation process follows the quasi-static electromagnetism:

$$\mathbf{\Phi} = \mathbf{H}_e\mathbf{U}_e \tag{2}$$

where $\mathbf{\Phi}$ represents BSPs and $\mathbf{H}_e$ is the transfer matrix obtained via a boundary element integral with embedded meshfree approximation.

Concerning about the *system uncertainties* of the TMP evolution model and *observation errors* of the measurements (BSPMs), (1) and (2) are written into state-space representations:

$$\mathbf{x}_e(t + \Delta t_e) = F_e(\mathbf{x}_e(t)) + \omega_e(t + \Delta t_e) \tag{3}$$

$$\mathbf{y}_e(t + \Delta t_e) = \tilde{\mathbf{H}}_e\mathbf{x}_e(t + \Delta t_e) + \nu_e(t + \Delta t_e) \tag{4}$$

where $\mathbf{x}_e(\cdot) = \begin{bmatrix} \mathbf{U}_e^T(\cdot) & \mathbf{V}_e^T(\cdot) \end{bmatrix}^T$ is the state vector and $\mathbf{y}_e(t + \Delta t_e) = \mathbf{\Phi}(t + \Delta t_e)$ is the observation vector. $F_e(\cdot)$ is the transition function in correspondence with the E model (1) and $\tilde{\mathbf{H}}_e = [\mathbf{H}_e \ \mathbf{0}]$. $\omega_e(t + \Delta t_e)$ and $\nu_e(t + \Delta t_e)$ are mutually independent vectors with zero-mean and known covariances, representing additive system uncertainties and observation errors.

With (3) and (4) available, unscented Kalman filtering described in [5] can be used to recover TMPs from patient BSPMs in a statistically optimal sense. Fig. 1 shows an example for the difference between TMPs obtained solely from the E model (Fig. 1(a)) and those recovered from BSPMs (Fig. 1(c)).

---

[1] In order to preserve the typical notations while avoiding confusion, some notations of the E model and the BM model are added with right subscripts e and m respectively.

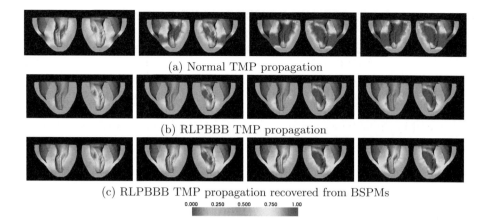

(a) Normal TMP propagation

(b) RLPBBB TMP propagation

(c) RLPBBB TMP propagation recovered from BSPMs

0.000   0.250   0.500   0.750   1.00

Fig. 1. Synthetic data. Volumetric TMP propagations at the beginning of ventricular excitations: depolarization at 1.5, 2.7, 5.4, 7ms (from left to right).

The recovered TMPs are then transformed into active contraction forces of the myocytes through the EM model [2], providing patient-specific physiological guidance to the recovery process through the cardiac system dynamics.

2.2 Extracting Motion Measurements from Structural Images

A voxel matching algorithm is used to provide displacements of the nodes representing the cardiac boundaries as the image-derived measurements.

Every boundary node is assumed to be lying on a voxel (source voxel) representing the heart boundary in the image at time t (source image), and searching for a corresponding voxel (target voxel) in the image at time $t + \Delta t$ (target image). Every source voxel is given a searching window, within which the target voxel is the one which has the minimum value of:

$$p = p_{edginess}[\alpha \ p_{appearance} + \beta \ p_{shape}] \tag{5}$$

where $p_{edginess}$ is related to segmentation, $p_{appearance}$ and p_{shape} are related to motion tracking. α and β are selected to reflect the varying data constraints at different parts of the heart at different time frames.

As the new positions of the boundary nodes in the target image need to be on the voxels representing the heart boundaries for segmentation purpose, $p_{edginess}$ has the form:

$$p_{edginess} = 1/(1 + \|\nabla I\|) \tag{6}$$

where $\|\nabla I\|$ is the magnitude of the image intensity gradient.

$p_{appearance}$ is the Gaussian weighted sum of the squared intensity difference between the voxel patches centered at the source voxel and the candidate target voxel respectively, thus it is related to the appearance similarity [6]. p_{shape} is

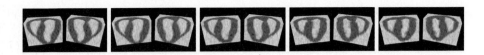

Fig. 2. Synthetic data. Structural images converted from synthetic heart deformations under RLPBBB condition (during systole, at 0, 60, 120, 180, and 240 ms).

calculated in the same way as $p_{appearance}$, with the squared intensity difference replaced by the bending energy [7]:

$$E_{bending} = 0.5 \left[\left(\kappa_{1,source} - \kappa_{1,target} \right)^2 + \left(\kappa_{2,source} - \kappa_{2,target} \right)^2 \right] \quad (7)$$

where $\kappa_{1,source}$, $\kappa_{1,target}$, $\kappa_{2,source}$, and $\kappa_{2,target}$ are the principal curvatures of the isointensity surfaces in the source and target images [8]. Thus, p_{shape} accounts for the shape coherence. As a result, the target voxel is lying on the heart boundary with similar appearance and/or shape to the source voxel.

The displacements of the boundary nodes become the image-derived measurements, providing patient's information for the recovery process.

2.3   Simultaneous Cardiac Segmentation and Deformation Recovery

In order to perform simultaneous cardiac segmentation and deformation recovery by evolving the node set representing the heart, state-space equations composed of the cardiac system dynamics is necessary to couple the BSPM-derived active stresses of section 2.1 with the image-derived measurements of section 2.2. The cardiac system dynamics represented by the TL formulation is in the form [1]:

$$\,_0^t\mathbf{M}_m \,^{t+\Delta t}\ddot{\mathbf{U}}_m + \,_0^t\mathbf{C}_m \,^{t+\Delta t}\dot{\mathbf{U}}_m + \,_0^t\tilde{\mathbf{K}}_m \Delta\mathbf{U}_m = \,^{t+\Delta t}\mathbf{R}_c + \,^{t+\Delta t}\mathbf{R}_b - \,_0^t\mathbf{R}_i \quad (8)$$

where $\,_0^t\mathbf{M}_m$ and $\,_0^t\mathbf{C}_m$ are the mass and damping matrices, and $\,_0^t\tilde{\mathbf{K}}_m$ is the strain incremental stiffness matrix which contains the internal stresses, the material and deformation properties of the BM model at time t. $\,^{t+\Delta t}\mathbf{R}_c$ is the force vector containing the BSPM-derived active stresses, $\,^{t+\Delta t}\mathbf{R}_b$ is the force vector for enforcing boundary conditions, and $\,_0^t\mathbf{R}_i$ is the force vector related to the internal stresses at time t. $\,^{t+\Delta t}\ddot{\mathbf{U}}_m$, $\,^{t+\Delta t}\dot{\mathbf{U}}_m$ and $\Delta\mathbf{U}_m$ are the respective nodal acceleration, velocity and incremental displacement vectors at time $t + \Delta t$. The BSPM-derived active stresses is now connected with the cardiac kinematics through this cardiac system dynamics.

While the BSPM-derived active stresses provide a relatively patient-specific physiological guidance to the recovery process, however, most parameters of the physiome model still not coincide with the physiological properties of the patient, and thus introduce the *system uncertainties*. On the other hand, the cardiac images cannot provide perfect measurements of the patient, and thus introduce the *observation errors*. In order to compromise the patient measurements and the physiome model with each other, a statistical filtering framework is required

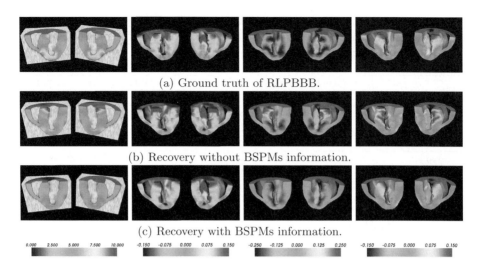

(a) Ground truth of RLPBBB.

(b) Recovery without BSPMs information.

(c) Recovery with BSPMs information.

Fig. 3. Synthetic data. Geometry and kinematics at 180ms, defined on a cylindrical coordinate system (r, θ, z), with the long axis of the left ventricle as the z-axis. Left to right: displacement magnitude map overlapped with image, radial strain map, circumferential strain map and radial-circumferential strain map.

to couple them together. As a result, (8) is rewritten as a TL-updated state-space equation which performs nonlinear state (displacements) prediction [1]:

$$\mathbf{x}_m(t + \Delta t_m) = \mathbf{F}_m(t)\mathbf{x}_m(t) + \mathbf{R}(t + \Delta t_m) + \omega_m(t + \Delta t_m) \qquad (9)$$

where $\mathbf{x}_m(t) = {}^t\mathbf{U}_m$ and $\mathbf{x}_m(t + \Delta t_m) = {}^{t+\Delta t_m}\mathbf{U}_m$ are the state vectors, containing the nodal displacements at time t and $t + \Delta t_m$, the kinematics we want to recover. $\mathbf{F}_m(t)$ is the transition matrix comprised by the ${}^t_0\mathbf{M}_m$, ${}^t_0\mathbf{C}_m$ and ${}^t_0\tilde{\mathbf{K}}_m$ matrices. $\mathbf{R}(t + \Delta t_m)$ is the input vector which contains the right hand side of (8). $\omega_m(t + \Delta t_m)$ is the zero-mean, additive, and white system uncertainties.

Furthermore, as described in section 2.2, the measurements are the image-derived, patient-specific displacements of the boundary nodes. In order to relate these measurements with the kinematics we want to recover, they are defined to be a subset of the state vector added by the zero-mean, additive, and white observation errors $\nu_m(t + \Delta t_m)$. Then the measurement vector $\mathbf{y}_m$ becomes:

$$\mathbf{y}_m(t + \Delta t_m) = \mathbf{H}_m\mathbf{x}_m(t + \Delta t_m) + \nu_m(t + \Delta t_m) \qquad (10)$$

where $\mathbf{H}_m$ is the measurement matrix containing only 0 and 1.

With the BSPM-derived active stresses ${}^{t+\Delta t}\mathbf{R}_c$ embedded in (9) and the image-derived measurement vector $\mathbf{y}_m$ in (10), Kalman filtering procedures can be performed to evolve the whole node set representing the heart in a statistically optimal sense [1]. In consequence, the patient cardiac geometry and deformation are recovered simultaneously.

Table 1. Synthetic data. Deviations of the recovered kinematics against the ground truth. Strains ($\epsilon_{\alpha\beta}$) are calculated under a cylindrical coordinate system (r, θ, z), with the long axis of the left ventricle as the z-axis.

	Without BSPMs information	With BSPMs information
$\mathbf{U}_m$ (in mm)	0.9907±1.0800	0.9760±1.0430
ϵ_{rr}	0.0341±0.0498	0.0296±0.0434
$\epsilon_{\theta\theta}$	0.0302±0.0501	0.0272±0.0388
ϵ_{zz}	0.0447±0.4329	0.0383±0.1741
$\epsilon_{r\theta}$	0.0236±0.0373	0.0221±0.0330
$\epsilon_{\theta z}$	0.0212±0.0574	0.0192±0.0282
ϵ_{zr}	0.0215±0.0550	0.0193±0.0334

3   Experiments

3.1   Synthetic Data

In order to show the benefits of our proposed framework, experiments have been conducted on synthetic data. Using the heart-torso model with geometry and cardiac fiber architecture adopted from [9] and [10], a specific pathological condition involving the right and left posterior fascicle branch bundle block (RLPBBB) has been studied. The major effect of the block is the disruption of the normal, coordinated and simultaneous distribution of the electrical signal to the two ventricles, which thus contract sequentially rather than simultaneously. The abnormal TMP propagation is shown against its normal counterpart in Fig. 1 (with 500ms in one cardiac cycle) . The simulated BSPMs are mapped from the TMPs with 10dB SNR white Gaussian noises added. The cardiac deformations are also converted into a gray scale structural image sequence of 50 frames with image size 75x75x16, added by 10dB SNR white Gaussian noises so that the information provided are sparse and noisy (Fig. 2). These synthetic data are used as inputs to our experiments.

Cardiac geometry and kinematics are recovered using the physiome model without BSPMs information and our proposed framework. Fig. 1(c) shows the TMP propagation recovered from BSPMs, which is similar to the RLPBBB case and substantially different from the normal case. From the color maps shown in Fig. 3, it can be seen that the geometry and kinematics recovered using our proposed algorithm are closer to the ground truth. This is because complementary information from both BSPMs and structural images are utilized. The same conclusion can be made through the numerical results shown in Table 1.

3.2   Human Data

Experiments on a normal human cardiac MR image sequence have been conducted to show that our proposed framework is applicable to real data with complicated structures. The image sequence contains 20 frames of a cardiac cycle. Each 3D image frame contains 8 image slices, with 10mm inter-slice spacing, in-plane resolution of 1.56mm/voxel, and temporal resolution of 43ms/frame

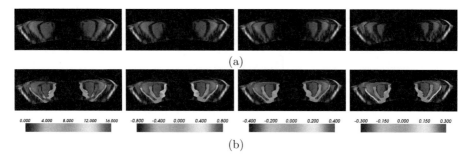

(a)

(b)

Fig. 4. (a). MR image sequence of a normal human heart during systole (frame #1, #3, #5, #7). (b). Recovered geometry and kinematics using the proposed algorithm (frame #5). Left to right: displacement magnitude map, radial strain map, circumferential strain map, and radial-circumferential strain map.

(Fig. 4(a)). The initial meshfree representation of the heart is obtained by segmentation of the first image frame (end of diastole), and fibers are mapped from the fiber architecture of the heart model from the University of Auckland [1,10]. Since the BSPMs of the patient are not available, synthetic BSPMs are currently used. Geometry and kinematics recovered using our proposed framework are shown in Fig. 4(b). Further experiments on diseased human and animal hearts are ongoing for further verifications.

References

1. Wong, K.C.L., Zhang, H., Liu, H., Shi, P.: Physiome model based state-space framework for cardiac kinematics recovery. In: Larsen, R., Nielsen, M., Sporring, J. (eds.) MICCAI 2006. LNCS, vol. 4190, pp. 720–727. Springer, Heidelberg (2006)
2. Sermesant, M., Moireau, P., Camara, O., Sainte-Marie, J., Andriantsimiavona, R., Cimrman, R., Hill, D.L.G., Chapelle, D., Razavi, R.: Cardiac function estimation from MRI using a heart model and data assimilation: Advances and difficulties. Medical Image Analysis 10(4), 642–656 (2006)
3. Paragios, N., Deriche, R.: Geodesic active contours and level sets for the detection and tracking of moving objects. IEEE TPAMI 22(3), 266–280 (2000)
4. Liu, G.: Meshfree Methods. CRC Press (2003)
5. Wang, L., Zhang, H., Shi, P., Liu, H.: Imaging of 3D cardiac electrical activity: a model-based recovery framework. In: Larsen, R., Nielsen, M., Sporring, J. (eds.) MICCAI 2006. LNCS, vol. 4190, pp. 792–799. Springer, Heidelberg (2006)
6. Anandan, P.: A computational framework and an algorithm for the measurement of visual motion. IJCV 2(3), 283–310 (1989)
7. Duncan, J., Lee, F., Smeulders, A., Zaret, B.: A bending energy model for measurement of cardiac shape deformity. IEEE TMI 10(3), 307–320 (1991)
8. Thirion, J., Gourdon, A.: Computing the differential characteristics of isointensity surface. Computer Vision and Image Understanding 61(2), 190–202 (1995)
9. MacLeod, R., Johnson, C., Ershler, P.: Construction of an inhomogeneous model of the human torso for use in computational electrocardiography. In: IEEE EMBS, pp. 688–689 (1991)
10. Nash, M.: Mechanics and material properties of the heart using an anatomically accurate mathematical model. PhD thesis, University of Auckland (1998)

Statistical Shape Modeling Using MDL Incorporating Shape, Appearance, and Expert Knowledge

Aaron D. Ward and Ghassan Hamarneh

Medical Image Analysis Lab,
School of Computing Science, Simon Fraser University, Canada
{award,hamarneh}@cs.sfu.ca
http://mial.cs.sfu.ca/

Abstract. We propose a highly automated approach to the point correspondence problem for anatomical shapes in medical images. Manual landmarking is performed on a *small subset* of the shapes in the study, and a machine learning approach is used to elucidate the characteristic *shape and appearance* features at each landmark. A classifier trained using these features defines a cost function that drives key landmarks to anatomically meaningful locations after MDL-based correspondence establishment. Results are shown for artificial examples as well as real data.

1 Introduction

In the study of the relationship between anatomical shapes and pathological conditions, it is useful to explore and quantify anatomical shape variability. To this end, the *point correspondence problem* must be solved: a mapping must be established between points that represents an anatomically meaningful correspondence, to ensure meaningful shape statistics. The Minimum Description Length (MDL) approach to this problem has received considerable attention in the research community [1]. Briefly, this approach is a means of evaluating a chosen point correspondence by measuring the information theoretic cost of transmitting the shape model resulting from the correspondence. A previous study revealed that the MDL approach exceeds other current approaches in its agreement with landmarks placed by a human expert [2]. However, for correspondences established between human brain ventricles, this study found that the mean disagreement between landmarks placed by MDL and expert landmarks was ≈ 4 mm; a significant error. Row 1 of figure 2 illustrates this problem; although the established correspondence appears good according to the coloured visualization, highlighting specific point correspondences reveals errors at the peak apexes, particularly at the small peak. Since this peak represents little information content, MDL's cost function tends to de-emphasize it.

The fundamental issue here is that *saliency is not necessarily encoded by an information theoretic compactness measure.* There exists research into integrating geometry into the MDL process [3,4]. The idea behind these approaches is to

N. Ayache, S. Ourselin, A. Maeder (Eds.): MICCAI 2007, Part I, LNCS 4791, pp. 278–285, 2007.
© Springer-Verlag Berlin Heidelberg 2007

represent the shapes in terms of some geometric measurement such as curvature, and run MDL on this representation. These approaches are steps in the right direction and speak to the need for the integration of geometric information with MDL. However, they suffer the shortcomings of the arbitrary choice of geometric features and their uniform use throughout the object surface, failing to consider that different surface points may be characterized by different features.

We propose the use of expert knowledge, in the form of a *small set* of land-marked training examples, to guide the selection of *shape and appearance* features. These features are used in guiding MDL-based point correspondence to solutions that correspond with human intuitions of point saliency. Since we expect that human anatomists establish meaningful point correspondence based both on local shape and appearance information (from the underlying medical images), we acquire *shape and appearance* information about the points chosen by the user during the training phase. We *automatically learn*, for each landmark, the specific shape and appearance features that best distinguish the landmark. We then use the learned features to guide the process of correspondence establishment toward a solution that agrees with human intuition. There exists an abundance of expert knowledge about anatomically meaningful landmarks, and our philosophy is that this information should not be ignored in a landmarking approach.

2 Methods

2.1 Method Overview

At a high level, the overall process used in this work consists of two steps, given by the boxes in figure 1: (1) acquiring knowledge about distinguishing shape and appearance features for each expert-chosen landmark ("Training"), and (2) applying that knowledge to drive the point correspondence process toward a better solution ("Correspondence via MDL + landmark features").

The goal of the *training step* is to find, for each landmark chosen by the user, a set of shape and appearance features that, when utilized in the point correspondence process, (1) drives landmarks toward anatomically meaningful targets as indicated by the user, and (2) reduces as much as possible the chances of a landmark being driven toward a wrong target having similar shape and appearance features to those indicated by the user. The high-level process used in training is to select a subset of shape and appearance features (in a subset, some features are used and some not) that best satisfies the above criteria. To this end, we have designed a cost function that evaluates each subset. The cost function is a combination of two types of errors: a *target error* ϵ_t and a *basin width error* ϵ_b. ϵ_t, for a given subset of features, is inversely related to the accuracy with which a classifier selects target contour points in the training set as belonging to the class of expert-labelled landmarks. Ideally, the classifier would select *only* the expert-selected points as targets, yielding $\epsilon_t = 0$. ϵ_b measures, for a given subset of features, the spacing between detected targets along the contour. Ideally, this spacing should be as large as possible in order to eliminate confusion between

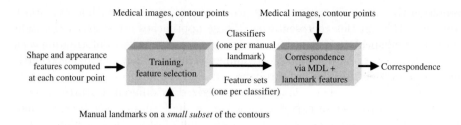

Fig. 1. The overall process followed in this work. See text for details.

targets during correspondence establishment, when landmarks are driven toward the nearest targets.

The goal of the *correspondence establishment step* is to find a point correspondence resulting in a shape model that is *as compact as possible while still anatomically meaningful*. To this end, we iteratively minimize the MDL cost function until convergence, which provides a good initialization for a subsequent minimization of a new cost function derived from the classifiers and feature subsets learned during training. This new cost function drives key landmarks to anatomically meaningful locations, according to information gained in training.

2.2   Training

Here, we explain the training step in more detail. Given a set of medical images and contour points lying on the boundaries of segmentations of an object of interest on each medical image, we manually collect n landmarks $l_{ij}, i \in \{1, \dots, n\}, j \in \{1, \dots, m\}$ on each of *a small number m* training examples. To this end, we present the user with not only the object contours, but also with the underlying medical images. The rationale for this is that the user may select points based on both shape and appearance features of the object.

Next, for each landmark, we train a classifier, *using the best possible subset of shape and appearance features* to distinguish the landmark as best as possible from all of the other points on the training objects' contours. The result is n different classifiers, one for each landmark. For the moment, we treat the feature selection problem [5] of choosing the best possible subset of features as a black box; we will return to it in section 2.4.

2.3   Correspondence Establishment

Given a set of classifiers (one per landmark) and feature subsets (one per classifier), each classifier assigns each contour point on *all* contours to one of two classes: points similar to the landmark chosen by the user (which we shall denote class U), and all of the other contour points (class $\tilde{U}$). For illustrative purposes here, we represent curve points parameterized from beginning to end as strings of digits. For example, curve 0000000000000000 has 16 points, each labelled with a zero. We denote points belonging to U with ones and points belonging to $\tilde{U}$ with zeros. Consider, for illustrative purposes, a case where a classifier, for one land-mark, given a curve and feature subset outputs 0000001110000000 (indicating that three points on the curve are similar to the user's chosen landmark). We need a function such that, given a position x on the curve, the cost function returns the distance to the point best matching the features of the user's chosen landmark. To do this, we first thin the cluster of ones, yielding 0000000100000000. We then take the distance transform of the result, yielding 7654321012345678. We denote the result of this distance transform, for landmark i on curve j as $c_{ij}(x)$. Thus $c_{ij}(x)$ is a function for landmark i on a shape j that drives landmarks to points similar to user landmarks. Consider a case where MDL deposits a landmark at a location x_0, 3 positions away from the correct target on the curve; $c_{ij}(x_0) = 3$. An energy minimization procedure using a cost function based on $c_{ij}(x)$ will thus drive points to the bottoms of the *basins* given by the cost functions $c_{ij}(x)$. More specifically, once MDL converges, we locate, on the first contour, the points m_{i1} corresponding to l_{i1}, $\forall i = 1 \ldots n$, as well as their corresponding points m_{ij} in all of the other contours. We then continue energy minimization using the following cost function based on $c_{ij}(x)$: $\epsilon_e = \sum_{i=1}^{n} \sum_{j=1}^{m} c_{ij}(m_{ij})$. Using the de-scription length as the cost function in an energy minimization scheme intended to establish point correspondence results in a remarkably good, but imperfect, point correspondence. This good point correspondence serves as an excellent initialization for a gradient descent optimization of ϵ_e.

2.4   Feature Selection

Here, we explain our approach to feature selection during the training step. We use a cost function to evaluate each subset, and choose the subset with the lowest cost. The cost function is a combination of a *target error* $\epsilon_t(p, i)$ and a *basin width error* $\epsilon_b(p, i)$, for a subset p and a given landmark i.

The classifier is trained using all of the user's selected points in class U, and all other points in class $\tilde{U}$. For example, consider 5 training shapes, each with 100 contour points. Consider a feature subset involving curvature and its first derivative. We thus have 500 points in 2D feature space, 5 of which (chosen by the user) are in U, the remainder in $\tilde{U}$. A classifier is trained on this data, attempting to find a decision boundary that best separates the two classes. All points are then reclassified into classes U and $\tilde{U}$ according to this classifier (in the ideal case, the point classifications do not change, but this is unlikely with real data).

The subset is then assessed according to the output of the classifier. The tar-get error is defined as $\epsilon_t(p, i) = \sum_{j=1}^{m} d(l_{ij}, \hat{u}_{ij})$, where $d(p, q)$ is the geodesic distance along the object contour between points p and q, and $\hat{u}_{ij}$ is the geodesi-cally nearest point in class U on the contour to l_{ij}. For example, if the user's selected landmark i (indicated with a 1) is 0000000100000000 and a classifier trained using subset p yields a classification of 0000000000100000 on shape j (the 1 is 3 positions away from the user's landmark), then $d(l_{ij}, \hat{u}_{ij}) = 3$. If the classification were identical to the user's selection, 0000000100000000, then $d(l_{ij}, \hat{u}_{ij}) = 0$. This measure indicates how far the classifier, given a shape subset, will move a landmark *off target*. The basin width error is defined as $\epsilon_b(p,i) = \sum_{j=1}^{m} \left(\frac{N_p}{2} - d(\hat{u}_{ij}, u_{ij}) \right)$, where N_p is the number of points on the longest contour in the training set (and thus the maximum basin width error is $\frac{N_p}{2}$) and u_{ij} is the geodesically nearest point in class U on the contour to $\hat{u}_{ij}$. For example, if the user's selected landmark i is 0000000100000000 and a classifier trained using subset p yields a classification of 010000010000100 on shape j, $d(\hat{u}_{ij}, u_{ij}) = 5$. A classification of 0001000101000000 yields $d(\hat{u}_{ij}, u_{ij}) = 2$. Clearly the former is to be preferred over the latter; the latter results in a possibly confusing minimum value of ϵ_e during correspondence establishment. For each subset p for a landmark i, we compute an overall error measure $\epsilon(p,i)$, which combines $\epsilon_b(p,i)$ and $\epsilon_t(p,i)$:

$$\operatorname*{argmin}_{p} \epsilon(p,i) = \begin{cases} \epsilon_t(p,i) + \frac{\epsilon_b(p,i)}{\frac{N_p}{2}+1} & \text{if } \exists \epsilon_t(p,i) < t \wedge \exists \epsilon_b(p,i) < \frac{N_p}{2} - t \\ \frac{\epsilon_t(p,i)}{\alpha(\epsilon_t(p,i)-t)+1} + \epsilon_b(p,i) & \text{otherwise} \end{cases}$$

(1)

In equation 1, t is a threshold specifying desired quantities for $\epsilon_t(p,i)$ and $\epsilon_b(p,i)$. The basic idea is that if $\epsilon_t(p,i)$ and $\epsilon_b(p,i)$ are sufficiently small, it is desirable for $\epsilon_t(p,i)$ to dominate the cost function; it is a hard constraint that we choose the subset with the smallest value of $\epsilon_t(p,i)$ in this case. If this condition is not met, then the cost function becomes a nonlinear combination of $\epsilon_t(p,i)$ and $\epsilon_b(p,i)$ such that the dominance of $\epsilon_t(p,i)$ diminishes as $\epsilon_t(p,i)$ grows. This avoids the choice of subsets with relatively large $\epsilon_t(p,i)$ and small $\epsilon_b(p,i)$ in cases where the smallest possible $\epsilon_t(p,i) \geq t$. The rate at which the dominance of $\epsilon_t(p,i)$ diminishes is directly proportional to α, which was set to 10^{-2} for all experiments in this paper. The threshold t can be set automatically by iterating MDL until convergence and then computing the maximum geodesic distance between any landmark and its correct position given by the training data.

Shape features used in our experiments include curvature, the absolute value of the first derivative of curvature, and the local area integral invariant [6]. Appearance features include the average image intensity in a circular region centered at each contour point, the average intensity along a segment extending normal to the contour *into* the object, and the average intensity along a segment extending normal to the contour *out of* the object. Each feature was computed at a variety of scales, and equation 1 was minimized by brute force. Note that our method does not dictate the specific choices of these features; the features used in this paper are chosen to exemplify the effectiveness of the method.

3   Results

Figure 2 qualitatively compares our method to the performance of standard MDL on rectangles (bottoms cut off for space considerations) with two protruding peaks, one small and one large. Row 1 of figure 2 shows MDL's performance, and row 2 shows the performance of our algorithm trained using a single example with two training points, indicated by the gray diamonds. For the small

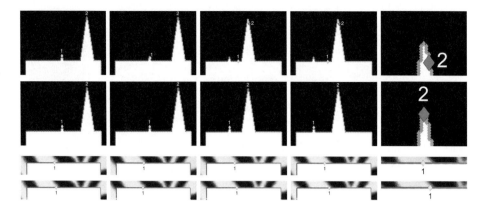

Fig. 2. Comparison of correspondences established by MDL (rows 1 and 3) with those established by our method (rows 2 and 4) on artificial examples. Corresponding points have the same colour (see electronic version). The points of interest are indicated by diamonds in different shades of gray, with numbers indicating correspondence.

peak, minimization of equation 1 resulted in the selection of curvature and the absolute value of its derivative as features, as expected. Interestingly, for the large peak, curvature features were not selected; the local area integral invariant was chosen instead, because this feature differentiates the large peak from the small peak, thus yielding a lower $\epsilon_b(p, i)$ error. Figure 2 also shows the performance of MDL versus our method for establishing correspondence on a rectangle (bottoms cut off for space considerations), with a point of interest defined by texture. Not surprisingly, standard MDL fails to do this (row 3) since it does not use appearance information (mean correspondence error 4). Our method (row 4) established perfect correspondence using the average local intensity value.

Figure 3 qualitatively compares standard MDL to our method on the corpus callosum (CC; a brain structure), as segmented from MR images. Row 1 shows the result from standard MDL, with diamonds indicating corresponding points of interest. These points should lie on the tip of the rostrum (the apex of the "hook" of the CC on the anterior side; see dark gray diamond in row 2, column 1), and at the interface between the CC and the fornix, which emanates below the CC in the middle of its body (see light gray diamond in row 2, column 1). In training, the system chose curvature and the absolute value of its derivative as features characterizing the rostrum, and the average intensities along segments normal to the contour emanating into and out of the object to characterize the fornix. Training was performed on 5 examples, with testing on 15 (4 examples shown due to space constraints). Figure 3 also compares standard MDL to our method for a point of interest on the right brain ventricle as segmented from MR images. The third row shows standard MDL, and the fourth row shows our method. Training was performed on 5 examples, with testing on 14 (4 examples shown). Features selected for this point were curvature and its derivative, and the local area integral invariant.

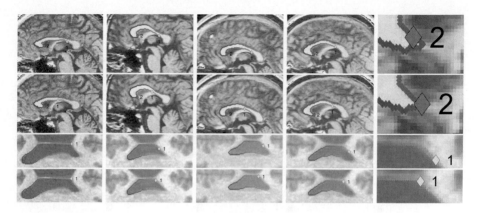

Fig. 3. Comparison of correspondences established by MDL (rows 1 and 3) with those established by our method (rows 2 and 4) on anatomically meaningful points on the corpus callosum and ventricles. Corresponding points have the same colour (see electronic version). The points of interest are indicated by diamonds in different shades of gray, with numbers indicating correspondence.

Table 1 shows training times, correspondence times, and mean geodesic landmark errors (defined as the mean of the geodesic distances between landmarks and their correct, manually-landmarked locations). Note that the correspondence times shown for our method include the time required to perform the MDL-based optimization. Our method shows a decrease in landmarking error, and training and correspondence execute reasonably quickly (on a 2.4Ghz AMD Opteron CPU). Note that for the ventricles, the mean error for our method is skewed by outliers; the median error for standard MDL is 6.0 pixels, compared to a median error of 1.5 pixels for our method.

Table 1. Training and correspondence times, and errors, shown as (standard MDL, our method). LP = large peak, SP = small peak, R = rostrum, F = fornix.

	Training (mm:ss)	Correspondence (mm:ss)	Error (pixels)
Two peaks	(NA, 01:12)	(00:27, 01:17)	(3.40, 0.00), LP
			(10.0, 0.00), SP
Texture	(NA, 00:48)	(00:27, 00:57)	(4.00, 0.00)
CC	(NA, 03:42)	(02:07, 11:30)	(1.20, 0.65), R
			(4.50, 1.90), F
Ventricle	(NA, 01:20)	(00:55, 02:10)	(5.30, 3.20)

4   Conclusions

We have demonstrated the efficacy of a hybrid system for point correspondence establishment, using cost functions measuring model compactness (MDL) and deviation from anatomically meaningful landmarks indicated by the user.

Although there exist previous approaches incorporating machine learning [7], to the best of our knowledge, ours is the first incorporation of machine learning to elicit local, characteristic features of anatomically meaningful points, and to make use of those features in a MDL-based approach to the correspondence problem. We demonstrate our approach on artificial and real data, showing that it runs reasonably quickly, and automatically reports the features that best characterize each chosen point. A general conclusion that can be drawn from this work is that description length alone is an insufficient criterion for establishing anatomically meaningful correspondences between shapes. It is evident from our results that a correspondence resulting from a shape model with larger than minimum description length yields a more meaningful correspondence. We hypothesize that the explanation for this observation is that the MDL criterion fails to capture all types of features which are *salient* to humans. Features which are insignificant in terms of their effect on the cost of transmitting the shape model are more likely to be ignored by a purely MDL-based shape correspondence method. Future work involves augmenting this system with more features, testing different types of classifiers, and using a more intelligent approach to minimize equation 1 to handle a larger number of features, including saliency features [8], for example. This approach also requires validation on large data sets with ground truth expert correspondences. We are also exploring the extension of this work to 3D, which involves 2D definitions of the geodesic distances used to compute ϵ_t and ϵ_b, and trivial 2D definitions of the thinning and distance transform operations (on surfaces) used to define ϵ_e. Also, the integration of the optimization of the MDL cost function and ϵ_e is being explored with the aim of producing a fully hybrid approach. It is also of interest to explore the utility of this approach in elucidating parts of the decision process used by experts to locate landmarks on medical images, by discerning characterizing shape and appearance features not obvious to the layperson or medical trainee.

References

1. Davies, R., et al.: A minimum description length approach to statistical shape modeling. IEEE TMI 21(5), 525–537 (2002)
2. Styner, M., et al.: Evaluation of 3D correspondence methods for model building. In: Taylor, C.J., Noble, J.A. (eds.) IPMI 2003. LNCS, vol. 2732, pp. 63–75. Springer, Heidelberg (2003)
3. Thodberg, H., et al.: Adding curvature to minimum description length shape models. BMVC 2, 251–260 (2003)
4. Heimann, T., et al.: Implementing the automatic generation of 3D statistical shape models with ITK. In: Open Science Workshop at MICCAI, Copenhagen (2006)
5. Guyon, et al.: An introduction to variable and feature selection. Journal of Machine Learning Research 3, 1157–1182 (2003)
6. Manay, S., et al.: Integral invariants for shape matching. IEEE PAMI 28(10), 1602–1618 (2006)
7. Pitiot, A., et al.: Learning shape correspondence for n-D curves. IJCV 71(1), 71–88 (2007)
8. Kadir, T., et al.: Scale, saliency and image description. IJCV 45(2), 83–105 (2001)

False Positive Reduction in Mammographic Mass Detection Using Local Binary Patterns

Arnau Oliver, Xavier Lladó, Jordi Freixenet, and Joan Martí

Institute of Informatics and Applications - University of Girona
Campus Montilivi, Ed. P-IV, 17071, Girona, Spain
{aoliver,llado,jordif,joanm}@eia.udg.es

Abstract. In this paper we propose a new approach for false positive reduction in the field of mammographic mass detection. The goal is to distinguish between the true recognized masses and the ones which actually are normal parenchyma. Our proposal is based on Local Binary Patterns (LBP) for representing salient micro-patterns and preserving at the same time the spatial structure of the masses. Once the descriptors are extracted, Support Vector Machines (SVM) are used for classifying the detected masses. We test our proposal using a set of 1792 suspicious regions of interest extracted from the DDSM database. Exhaustive experiments illustrate that LBP features are effective and efficient for false positive reduction even at different mass sizes, a critical aspect in mass detection systems. Moreover, we compare our proposal with current methods showing that LBP obtains better performance.

1   Introduction

Breast cancer is one of the most devastating and deadly diseases for women in their 40s. It is estimated that between one in eight and one in twelve women will develop breast cancer during their lifetime [1]. The most used method to detect breast cancer is mammography, because it allows the detection of the cancer at its early stages, a crucial issue for a high survival rate. The introduction of digital mammography gave the opportunity of increasing the number of commercial Computer-Aided Detection systems to help radiologists to interpret and diagnose mammograms. During the last decade several algorithms have been proposed for the automatic mass detection purpose [2]. However, the main drawback of these methods is the high number of obtained false positives [3]. A false positive is a region being normal tissue but interpreted by the automatic algorithm as a suspicious one. The so called false positive reduction algorithms try to solve this drawback, i.e. given a Region of Interest (RoI) – a sub-image containing the suspicious region – the aim is to validate whether it contains a real lesion or it is only a region depicting normal parenchyma.

Different algorithms have been proposed so far for such a task. For instance, the work of Sahiner et al. [4] consisted in extracting a huge set of features, selecting the most discriminative ones using genetic algorithms, and then classifying by using linear classifiers or neural networks. A similar strategy was used by Christoyianni et al. [5], who extracted gray-level, texture, and features related

N. Ayache, S. Ourselin, A. Maeder (Eds.): MICCAI 2007, Part I, LNCS 4791, pp. 286–293, 2007.
© Springer-Verlag Berlin Heidelberg 2007

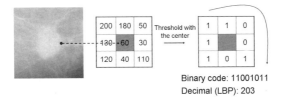

Fig. 1. Example of the basic LBP operator

to independent component analysis to train a neural network. Qian et al. [6] analyzed the implementation of an adaptive module to improve a Kalman-filter based neural net using features obtained from a wavelet decomposition. The works of Chang et al. [7] and Tourassi et al. [8] were based on directly comparing a new RoI image with all the RoI images in the database. In the first one, the gray level and the shape were used as a likelihood measure, while on the second one the similarity was based on mutual information. A different strategy was recently proposed by Oliver et al. [9,10], who adapted the eigenfaces approach to the mass detection problem.

In this paper we propose an alternative approach to perform mass false positive reduction by using the textural properties of the masses. The idea of our proposal is inspired by the recent work of Ahonen et al. [11] in which Local Binary Patterns (LBP) are successfully applied to the face recognition problem. In our work, we propose the use of LBP operators [12] to characterize micropatterns (i.e. edges, lines, spots, flat areas) and preserve at the same time the spatial structure of the mass. To our knowledge this is the first attempt to use LBP in the field of mammographic mass detection. Once the LBP characterization is done, we use Support Vector Machines to classify the RoIs between real masses and normal parenchyma. We perform experiments on a complete set of 1792 RoIs extracted from the DDSM database, evaluating the results when using different RoI image sizes, and when using different ratios of number of RoIs depicting masses and RoIs depicting normal tissue in the database. The obtained results and the comparison with previous works demonstrate the validity of our approach for reducing false positives.

The rest of the paper is organized as follows. Section 2 briefly presents the LBP as a texture descriptor. Section 3 describes our approach for mass false positive reduction. Experimental results are presented in Section 4. Finally, the paper ends with conclusions.

2   Local Binary Patterns (LBP)

The original LBP operator was introduced by Ojala et al. [13] with the idea to perform gray scale invariant two-dimensional texture analysis. The LPB operator labels the pixels of an image by thresholding the neighborhood (i.e. 3×3) of each pixel with the center value and considering the result of this thresholding as a binary number. Figure 1 shows an example of how to compute a LBP code. When all the pixels have been labeled with the corresponding LBP codes, the histogram of the labels is computed and used as a texture descriptor. Initially, the limitation of this basic LBP operator was its small 3×3 neighborhood since it can not deal with dominant features with large scale structures. Due to this fact, the operator was later extended to use neighborhoods of different sizes [12]. The idea of this operator is the detection of local binary patterns at circular neighborhoods of any quantization of the angular space and at any spatial resolution. Therefore, it is possible to derive the operator for a general case based on a circularly symmetric neighborhood of P members on a circle of radius R. In addition to evaluating the performance of individual operators of a particular configuration (P, R), one could analyze and combine responses of multiple operators realized with different parameters (P, R).

Another extension of LBP was the use of the so called uniform patterns [12]. A LBP is called uniform if it contains at most two bitwise transitions from 0 to 1 or vice versa when the binary string is considered circular. For example, 000011100 and 11100011 are uniform patterns. As stated by Ojala et al., the uniform patterns account for nearly 90% of all patterns in the $(8, 1)$ neighborhood and for about 70% in the $(16, 2)$ neighborhood in texture images. In this paper, we shall refer the uniform LBP operator as $LBP_{P,R}^{u2}$, where the subscript represents using the operator in a (P, R) neighborhood and the superscript $u2$ indicates using uniform patterns.

As in the original work of Ojala et al. the histogram of the labeled image $f_l(x, y)$ is used as a descriptor. We can define this histogram as

$$H_i = \sum_{x,y} I(f_l(x, y) = i), \qquad i = 0, \ldots, n - 1 \tag{1}$$

where n is the number of different labels produced by the LBP operator, and $I(A) = 1$ when A is true, while $I(A) = 0$ when A is false.

This discrete occurrence histogram of the uniform patterns computed over an image or an image region contains information about the distribution of the local micro-patterns such as edges, spots and flat areas, and has been demonstrated to be a very powerful texture descriptor.

3   Using LBP for Mammographic False Positive Reduction

In this work, we are dealing with mammographic images and in particular with the mass false positive reduction problem. Inherently to these images, texture and its spatial information play a key role in correctly detecting the masses. Due to this fact, we base our approach on the use of LBP for representing salient micro-patterns, and an adaptation of these descriptors for preserving also the spatial structure of the masses. The idea of our proposal has been inspired by the recent work of Ahonen et al. [11] in which LBP is used to perform face recognition. Our general procedure consists in using the LBP texture descriptor to build several local descriptions of the RoI and combining them into a global description. Afterwards, this global LBP descriptor is the one used to reduce the

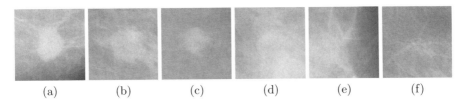

(a)   (b)   (c)   (d)   (e)   (f)

Fig. 2. Examples of RoIs: (a-c) RoIs with masses; (d-f) RoIs without masses

false positives, classifying the RoIs between true masses and normal tissue (see Figure 2 for examples of RoIs).

Initially, the RoI image – which contains the suspicious mass – is divided into several local regions. See Figure 3 for an example of a mass image divided into 5×5 rectangular regions. Notice that one could use different divisions of different size and shape. From these regions, texture descriptors are independently extracted using LBP and then concatenated to form a global description of the RoI based on the textural information of each region and its spatial distribution. Observe that we could also analyze and combine responses of multiple LBP operators realized with different parameters (P, R). For example, the computation of a set of different LBP operators for some specific regions with higher probability to contain mass information may improve the quality of the final RoI descriptor. This is illustrated in Figure 3 where the internal 3×3 regions (showed in a dark gray level) are used to compute different LBP operators. Note that a higher weight into the final descriptor is given for these regions. This point will be further discussed in the experimental section.

Following our methodology, the basic LBP histogram is extended into a spatially enhanced histogram which encodes both the local region appearance and the spatial relations (global geometry) of the mass. The RoI image is divided into m small regions $R_0, R_1, \ldots, R_m$ and the spatially enhanced histogram is defined as

$$H_{i,j} = \sum_{x,y} I(f_l(x,y) = i), \quad (x,y) \in R_j \qquad (2)$$

where $i = 0, \ldots, n - 1$, $j = 0, \ldots, m - 1$. In this histogram, the RoI is described on three different levels of locality: the labels for the histogram contain the pixel-level texture patterns, the labels are summed over a small region to produce information on a regional level and finally the regional histograms are concatenated to build a global description of the mass.

The final step of our proposal is the mass classification. For this purpose we use the well-known Support Vector Machines (SVM) technique [14] which performs an implicit mapping of data into a higher dimensional feature space, where linear algebra and geometry can be used to separate data. For our specific problem, SVM with a polynomial kernel is used to provide a membership between RoIs depicting a true mass and RoIs depicting normal parenchyma. In the experimental section we will compare the results obtained by using SVM with those obtained using a Nearest Neighbor (NN) classifier.

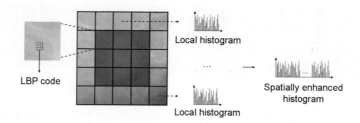

Fig. 3. Strategy for computing the LBP descriptor of an image

4   Experimental Results

Our approach has been evaluated using a database of 1792 RoIs extracted from
the DDSM mammographic database [15]. From this set, 256 depicted a true
mass, while the rest 1536 were normal, but suspicious tissue. According to the
size of the lesion, we use six different groups of RoI images, corresponding to the
following mass sizes intervals: $< 10 \ mm^2, (10 - 60) \ mm^2, (60 - 120) \ mm^2, (120 -
190) \ mm^2, (190 - 270) \ mm^2, > 270 \ mm^2$. The number of masses in each interval
were 28, 32, 37, 57, 69, and 33, respectively. Note we are dealing with different
lesion sizes, an important aspect for correctly classifying the masses.

The evaluation of our experiments is done by using a leave-one-out strategy
and Receiver Operating Characteristics (ROC) analysis. In the leave-one-out
methodology, a specific input RoI is selected and classified according to the
model obtained by training the system with the remaining RoIs in the database.
This procedure is repeated until all the RoIs have been used as an input image.
The SVM classifier provides a numerical value related to the membership of each
class. Thus, varying the threshold of this membership it is possible to generate a
ROC curve [16]. In such analysis, widely used in the medical field, the graphical
curve represents the true positive rate as a function of the false positives rate. The
percentage value under the curve (known as Az) is an indication for the overall
performance of the observer, and is typically used to analyze the performance
of the algorithms.

In order to perform a more global evaluation we compute the Az value for
different ratios of number of RoIs depicting masses and number of RoIs depicting
normal tissue (from ratio 1/1 to ratio 1/6). The idea of analyzing these different
ratios is twofold: firstly, to evaluate the performance of our method on different
levels of difficulty, and secondly, to compare our proposal with existing methods. Notice that previous works only provide results for specific ratios. Hence,
analyzing all these ratios will enable the comparison with them.

As explained in Section 3, some parameters may be optimized in order to
obtain the final LBP descriptor. For instance, the number of regions in which a
RoI image is divided or the parameters (P, R) used to obtain the LBP responses.
With the aim of choosing the number of divisions, we tested the performance of
LBP on three different configurations (3×3, 5×5 and 7×7 regions) for all the RoI
image sizes, all ratios, and using the basic $LBP_{8,1}^{u2}$ operator. The best result was

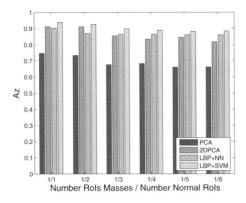

Fig. 4. Az values obtained with the methods PCA, 2DPCA, LBP+NN and LBP+SVM. Each Az value is the mean computed from the results of different RoI image sizes.

obtained when dividing each RoI image into 5×5 square regions and computing LBP operators for each one. Note that each region size depended on the original RoI image size. Using this configuration we obtained an overall mean Az value of 0.882 ± 0.051. With the aim of improving these results and obtaining a more accurate description of the central area, we added a new set of LBP operators for the 3×3 central regions. In particular, we computed two new LBP responses varying the radius R according to each RoI image size (i.e. $R = 1, 4$ and 6 was used for the first RoI image size). The global descriptor was then obtained concatenating the 43 histograms of all the regions and LBP operators. For this new configuration, an overall mean Az value of 0.906 ± 0.043 was obtained. Note that better results were obtained when including LBP operators with different radius R in the central regions. We then repeated the same experiment varying also the quantization of the angular space P in the basic LBP computation, using $LBP_{8,1}^{u2}$, $LBP_{8,2}^{u2}$, and $LBP_{16,2}^{u2}$. Similar results were obtained, although, $LBP_{8,1}^{u2}$ provided the best overall mean results for different RoI image sizes and ratios. This was the final descriptor we used for our experiments since it provided a good trade-off between performance and feature vector length.

Figure 4 shows the obtained mean Az values for each specific ratio when testing our proposal at different RoI image sizes. We include a quantitative comparison with the recent works of Oliver et al. [9,10], using our database of RoIs. While the first approach is based on using standard PCA, the second introduced a variation on their previous work by using the 2DPCA method [17] instead of the standard PCA technique (we shall refer to these methods as PCA and 2DPCA, respectively). Observe that the performance of our proposal was clearly better than the PCA method. The results were also better than the 2DPCA approach, specially for the cases in which we had smaller ratios 1/4, 1/5 and 1/6. Note also that the use of 2DPCA itself allowed to obtain better results than the original PCA approach. Using PCA we obtained an overall mean Az value of 0.686 ± 0.095 for different RoI image sizes and ratios, using 2DPCA

Table 1. Az comparison of different methods dealing with mass false positive reduction. We detail the number of RoIs and ratio used in the original works. We also include the results obtained with our LBP+SVM approach.

	Sahiner [4]	Qian [6]	Chang [7]	Tourassi [8]	Oliver [9]	LBP+SVM	
RoIs	672	800	600	1465	588	512	1024
Ratio	1/3	1/3	1/1	$\cong 1/1$	1/2	1/1	1/3
Az	0.90	0.86	0.83	0.87	0.83	0.94	0.90

the Az value was 0.868 ± 0.087, while using our LBP approach with SVM the Az value was 0.906 ± 0.043. Note that we also show the results of LBP when using a Nearest Neighbor (NN) classifier, obtaining an overall mean Az value of 0.871 ± 0.036. Observe that LBP with NN provided better performance than 2DPCA for smaller ratios, although the best results were provided by LBP with SVM. Regarding to the behavior when varying the RoI image sizes, we observed that LBP with SVM provided better and more constant results than PCA and 2DPCA methods (see the standard deviations).

We also include in Table 1 a qualitative comparison – in terms of Az value – with the rest of the approaches described in Section 1. Note that our efforts were concentrated on obtaining the same ratio of masses used in their experiments. However, we want to clarify that not all the methods used the same databases and therefore our aim is only to provide a general view of the performance of our LBP approach with respect to different strategies. For instance, the works of Chang et al. [7] and Tourassi et al. [8], which used a ratio 1/1, obtained Az values of 0.83 and 0.87 respectively. Note that for this ratio better performances were clearly obtained using our proposal. Similar behavior was observed for the works which used the ratios 1/2 and 1/3. Observe that the difference between the performance reported in the original PCA work of Oliver et al. (Az of 0.83) and the ones showed in our quantitative comparison (Az value of 0.69) is due to the use of different RoI image databases and their particular level of difficulty (the database used in [9] had less images and only 4 different RoI image sizes).

5   Conclusions

In this paper we have presented a novel method for mass false positive reduction based on textural features. First of all, a global descriptor for each RoI is obtained by analyzing its spatial textural information. Our approach divides a RoI image into small regions and computes local texture descriptions using local binary patterns. The combination of these local descriptors in a spatially enhanced histogram provides our final feature descriptor. Afterwards, these descriptors are used to classify the RoIs between true masses and normal parenchyma. Our experiments have shown firstly that LBP features are effective and efficient for false positive reduction at different RoI image sizes, and secondly than even when using different ratios of number of RoIs with masses and number of RoIs with normal tissue it is possible to obtain reliable results.

Acknowledgments

This work was partially supported by grants TIN2006-08035 and IdIBGi-UdG 91060080.

References

1. Bray, F., McCarron, P., Parkin, D.M.: The changing global patterns of female breast cancer incidence and mortality. Breast Cancer Research 6, 229–239 (2004)
2. Rangayyan, R.M., Ayres, F.J., Desautels, J.E.L.: A review of computer-aided diagnosis of breast cancer: Toward the detection of subtle signs. Journal of the Franklin Institute 344(3–4), 312–348 (2007)
3. Nishikawa, R.M., Kallergi, M.: Computer-aided detection, in its present form, is not an effective aid for screening mammography. Med. Phys 33, 811–814 (2006)
4. Sahiner, B., Chan, H.P., Wei, D., Petrick, N., Helvie, M.A., Adler, D.D., Goodsit, M.M.: Image feature selection by a genetic algorithm: Application to classification of mass and normal breast tissue. Med. Phys 23, 1671–1684 (1996)
5. Christoyianni, I., Koutras, A., Dermatas, E., Kokkinakis, G.: Computer aided of breast cancer in digitized mammograms. Comp. Med. Imag. and Graph. 26, 309–319 (2002)
6. Qian, W., Sun, X., Song, D., Clarke, R.A.: Digital mammography - wavelet transform and kalman-filtering neural network in mass segmentation and detection. Acad. Radiol. 8(11), 1074–1082 (2001)
7. Chang, Y.H., Hardesty, L.A., Hakim, C.M., Chang, T.S., Zheng, B., Good, W.F., Gur, D.: Knowledge-based computer-aided detection of masses on digitized mammograms: A preliminary assessment. Med. Phys 28(4), 455–461 (2001)
8. Tourassi, G.D., Vargas-Vorecek, R., Catarious, D.M., Floyd, C.E.: Computer-assisted detection of mammographic masses: A template matching scheme based on mutual information. Med. Phys 30(8), 2123–2130 (2003)
9. Oliver, A., Martí, J., Martí, R., Bosch, A., Freixenet, J.: A new approach to the classification of mammographic masses and normal breast tissue. IAPR Int. Conf. on Patt. Rec. 4, 707–710 (2006)
10. Oliver, A., Lladó, X., Martí, J., Martí, R., Freixenet, J.: False positive reduction in breast mass detection using two-dimensional PCA. In: Lect. Not. in Comp. Sc., vol. 4478, pp. 154–161 (2007)
11. Ahonen, T., Hadid, A., Pietikainen, M.: Face detection with local binary patterns: Application to face recognition. IEEE Trans. Pattern Anal. Machine Intell. 28(12), 2037–2041 (2006)
12. Ojala, T., Pietikainen, M., Maenpaa, T.: Multiresolution gray-scale and rotation invariant texture classification with local binary patterns. IEEE Trans. Pattern Anal. Machine Intell. 24(7), 971–987 (2002)
13. Ojala, T., Pietikainen, M., Harwood, D.: A comparative-study of texture measures with classification based on feature distributions. Patt. Rec. 29(1), 51–59 (1996)
14. Vapnik, V.: Statistical Learning Theory. John Wiley & Sons, New York (1998)
15. Heath, M., Bowyer, K., Kopans, D., Moore, R., Kegelmeyer, P.J.: The Digital Database for Screening Mammography. In: Int. Work. on Dig. Mammography, pp. 212–218 (2000)
16. Metz, C.E.: Evaluation of digital mammography by ROC analysis. In: Int. Work. on Dig. Mammography, pp. 61–68 (1996)
17. Yang, J., Zhang, D., Frangi, A.F., Yang, J.: Two-dimensional PCA: a new approach to appearance-based face representation and recognition. IEEE Trans. Pattern Anal. Machine Intell. 26(1), 131–137 (2004)

Fuzzy Nonparametric DTI Segmentation for Robust Cingulum-Tract Extraction

Suyash P. Awate, Hui Zhang, and James C. Gee

Department of Radiology, University of Pennsylvania, Philadelphia, PA 19104, USA
{awate,gee}@mail.med.upenn.edu,huiz@seas.upenn.edu

Abstract. This paper presents a novel segmentation-based approach for fiber-tract extraction in diffusion-tensor (DT) images. Typical tractography methods, incorporating thresholds on fractional anisotropy and fiber curvature to terminate tracking, can face serious problems arising from partial voluming and noise. For these reasons, tractography often fails to extract thin tracts with sharp changes in orientation, e.g. the *cingulum*. Unlike tractography—which disregards the information in the tensors that were previously tracked—the proposed method extracts the cingulum by exploiting the statistical coherence of tensors in the entire structure. Moreover, the proposed segmentation-based method allows *fuzzy* class memberships to optimally extract information within partial-volumed voxels. Unlike typical fuzzy-segmentation schemes employing Gaussian models that are biased towards ellipsoidal clusters, the proposed method *models the manifolds* underlying the classes by incorporating nonparametric data-driven statistical models. Furthermore, it exploits the nonparametric model to capture the *spatial continuity and structure* of the fiber bundle. The results on real DT images demonstrate that the proposed method extracts the cingulum bundle significantly more accurately as compared to tractography.

1 Introduction

Diffusion tensor (DT) magnetic resonance (MR) imaging allows us to differentiate the cerebral white/gray-matter structures such as the corpus callosum, thalamic nuclei, cingulum, etc. Extraction of these structures is of key interest in clinical studies concerning schizophrenia, Parkinson's disease, and Alzheimer's disease [1,2,3,4,5]. The driving clinical application for this paper is to investigate whether there are changes in the anterior cingulum in cocaine users that are associated with decreased gray-matter concentration in the same region [6].

The efficacy of tract-extraction methods on DT images can be severely limited by noise and partial-voluming artifacts. For instance, tractography methods often fails to extract the cingulum [3,4]—a thin tract that undergoes sharp changes in orientation and severe partial-volume contamination from the highly-anisotropic corpus callosum and the highly-isotropic ventricles lying adjacent to it (Figure 1). Tractography methods, which incorporate thresholds on the fractional anisotropy (FA) and fiber curvature to terminate tracking, can also consistently underestimate the size of fiber bundles [7].

N. Ayache, S. Ourselin, A. Maeder (Eds.): MICCAI 2007, Part I, LNCS 4791, pp. 294–301, 2007.
© Springer-Verlag Berlin Heidelberg 2007

Alternative approaches for extracting structures from DT images rely on segmentation approaches. Unlike tractography that disregards the information in the tensors that were previously tracked, segmentation approaches exploit the coherence of tensors in the entire structure of interest. Moreover, segmentation methods that allow fuzzy class memberships optimally extract information within partial-volumed voxels—crisp segmentations incorrectly account for this information towards the representation of a single class. In these ways, segmentation schemes can be more robust to DT-image artifacts.

Previous work in DTI segmentation employs Gaussian models that may not effectively model the tensor statistics because they are inherently biased towards ellipsoidal clusters. Fundamental anatomical characteristics of fiber bundles make fibers change their orientation *significantly*, e.g. cingulum (Figure 1), as they connect different structures. Thus, tensors in fiber bundles inherently lie on *manifolds* that do not conform to Gaussian models that are characterized by the mean. For instance, tensors in U-shaped/C-shaped bundles, that include tensors which start and end at similar orientations, must lie on a closed manifold.

This paper makes several contributions. It proposes a novel scheme based on fuzzy segmentation for extracting fiber bundles, e.g. cingulum, relying on a *nonparametric* statistical framework. The proposed method does not impose strong parametric tensor models, but adapts its models to arbitrary tensor probability density functions (PDFs), and the underlying manifolds, in data-driven ways. It extends the nonparametric model to capture the *spatial continuity and structure* of the fiber bundle. The *fuzzy* framework optimally extracts information from partial-volumed voxels. Results on real DT images show that the proposed method extracts the cingulum significantly more accurately than tractography.

2   Related Work

Typical methods for crisp and fuzzy segmentation [8,9,10] rely on representing each class by *only a single point* in the feature space (the class mean) and measure class membership based on the Euclidean/Mahalanobis distance to the class mean. Such approaches, however, (a) bias the segmentation towards ellipsoidal clusters in feature space and (b) do *not* yield themselves easily in capturing the spatial structure of the fiber bundle in the image. Nonparametric modeling approaches for crisp structural-MR segmentation [11,12] address the concern in (a), but not in (b). The proposed method: (i) generalizes class representation in fuzzy methods to the manifold underlying the class, (ii) extends a data-driven nonparametric scheme to adaptively infer the spatial structure of the fiber bundle in the image, and (iii) extracts information from partial-volumed tensors in a principled manner by incorporating fuzzy class memberships.

Segmentation methods entail quantifying distances between tensors that respect the group structure of the Riemannian DT space [13,14,1,15]. Lenglet *et al.* [1] use an affine-invariant Riemannian metric and model each class by a single Gaussian. Wang and Vemuri [2] use a piecewise-smooth Mumford-Shah framework to capture the spatial variations in tensors across a bundle. In contrast, the proposed method relies on nonparametric models and optimally extracts information from partial-volumed voxels using fuzzy class memberships.

The extraction of the cingulum tract, a key component of the limbic system that is relevant to memory and emotion, holds significance in many clinical studies relating to schizophrenia. Gong *et al.* [4] employ tractography to extract the cingulum bundle to study the left-right asymmetry in the structure. Their tractography results, however, clearly shows fibers "leaking" out of the cingulum. Concha *et al.* [3], acknowledging the impracticality of tractography for cingulum extraction, *divide* the cingulum into 3 parts (anterior, superior, descending) and perform tractography *independently* in each of these parts. In each part, they include tracts that pass through manually-selected regions-of-interest in the start, middle, and end of the part. The proposed method, on the other hand, extracts the cingulum in a simple, systematic, and optimal manner.

3   Nonparametric Statistical Diffusion-Tensor Modeling

This section describes the statistical formulation underlying the proposed nonparametric modeling technique. It starts by describing a generic kernel-based modeling scheme, that is independent of the particular metric associated with the Riemannian space. It then presents an appropriate tensor metric to considerably simplify the scheme, from a practical viewpoint, while maintaining the mathematical soundness of the framework.

We use kernel-based nonparametric PDF estimation based on a Parzen-window scheme in Riemannian space. For DT data, the kernel functions are smooth functions of the Riemannian geodesic distance on the tensor manifold. The mathematical expression for the Parzen-window tensor-PDF estimate is consistent with the expression of the usual (Euclidean) PDF estimate—it also relies on the intuitive notion of a kernel function having the largest value at the datum and monotonically-decreasing values with increasing distance from the datum. In the Riemannian case, each datum is the intrinsic mean of the associated kernel for sufficiently small bandwidths. We now describe this scheme.

Let $\mathcal{M}$ be a compact Riemannian manifold without boundary, of dimension D, with an associated metric-tensor g. The metric tensor induces an inner product on the manifold that generates the geodesic distance function $d_g(\cdot, \cdot)$ between two entities on $\mathcal{M}$. Let Z be a random variable on the probability space $(\Omega, \mathcal{A}, P)$ that takes values in $\mathcal{M}$. Let $\{z_1, z_2, \ldots, z_n\}$, where each $z_i \in \mathcal{M}$, be an independently-drawn and identically-distributed random sample derived from the PDF $P(Z)$. Let $K(Z)$ be a nonnegative and sufficiently-smooth kernel function. Then, the *consistent* nonparametric PDF estimate is [16]:

$$\hat{P}(z) = \frac{1}{N} \sum_{i=1}^{N} \frac{1}{\theta_{z_i}(z)} \frac{1}{\sigma^D} K\left(\frac{d_g(z, z_i)}{\sigma} \right),\tag{1}$$

where σ is the bandwidth associated with the kernel and $\theta_a(b)$ is the quotient of the canonical measure of the Riemannian metric $\exp_a^* g$ on $T_a(\mathcal{M})$ by the

Lebesgue measure of the Euclidean structure g_a on $T_a(\mathcal{M})$. We choose $K(\cdot)$ as the standard-Normal PDF: $K(\beta) = (1/(2\pi)^{D/2}) \exp(-\beta^2/2)$.

To evaluate the probability at any one point z we need to, in general, compute $\theta_{z_i}(z)$ separately for all the points z_i in the Parzen-window sample. This can become cumbersome, depending on the particular Riemannian tensor metric employed. The recently-proposed Log-Euclidean metric [14], in contrast to the affine-invariant Riemannian metric [13,1,15], induces a Riemannian space having zero curvature by mapping the DT space of 3×3 symmetric positive-definite matrices in an isomorphic, diffeomorphic, and *isometric* manner to the associated *Euclidean* vector space of 3×3 symmetric matrices. This mapping is precisely the matrix logarithm (denoted $\log_M$), i.e. $d_g(z, z_i) = \| \log_M(z) - \log_M(z_i) \|_{\text{Frobenius}}$ and $\theta_{z_i}(z) = 1$. The Parzen-window PDF estimate then simplifies to $\hat{P}(z) = (1/N) \sum_{i=1}^{N} G(z; z_i, \sigma)$, where $G(z; z_i, \sigma)$ is a multidimensional isotropic Gaussian (mean z_i and variance along each dimension σ^2) in the Riemannian space with $d_g(\cdot, \cdot)$ as the geodesic distance measure. Essentially, this scheme maps the diffusion tensors, using the matrix logarithm, to a Euclidean space and, in turn, computes probabilities using standard Parzen-window estimation in that space.

4   Fuzzy Segmentation with Manifold-Based Models

This section proposes a fuzzy-segmentation framework for fiber-tract extraction. It extracts tracts by iteratively optimizing an information-theoretic objective function and relying on nonparametric class models.

Our goal is to segment the image into $\mathcal{C}$ different classes ($c = 1, 2, \ldots, \mathcal{C}$). For extracting a single fiber bundle, $\mathcal{C} = 2$. These classes are distinguished by their respective PDFs $\{P_c(\cdot)\}_{c \in \mathcal{C}}$. The segmentation problem is, in a way, equivalent to that of deducing these PDFs.

Voxels in a fuzzy-segmentation framework can be *members* of more than one class—a standard notion in fuzzy set theory that does *not* constrain entities to belong to one set alone. We incorporate this notion using the fuzzy-membership functions that we define next. Consider $\mathcal{C}$ random variables $\{F_c : \mathcal{M} \to \Re\}_{c \in \mathcal{C}}$ that give a class-membership value for each element $\mathbf{z} \in \mathcal{M}$ belonging to class c. For all voxels t and all classes c, we want $0 \leq F_c(\mathbf{z}_t) \leq 1$ and $\sum_{c=1}^{\mathcal{C}} F_c(\mathbf{z}_t) = 1$. Under these constraints, we define the optimal fuzzy segmentation as:

$$\underset{\{F_c(\cdot)\}_{c=1}^{\mathcal{C}}}{\operatorname{argmax}} \sum_{c=1}^{\mathcal{C}} \left(\int_{\mathcal{M}} F_c(\mathbf{z}) P_c(\mathbf{z}) \log P_c(\mathbf{z}) d\mathbf{z} - \alpha \int_{\mathcal{M}} F_c(\mathbf{z}) \log F_c(\mathbf{z}) d\mathbf{z} \right). \quad (2)$$

The first term of the energy in (2) is a *modified* Shannon's entropy that allows each observation $\mathbf{z} \in \mathcal{M}$ to contribute some amount to the entropy of every class c that is proportional to its membership in class c—partial-volumed voxels would contribute to the descriptions of multiple classes. α is a user-controlled parameter that controls the degree of fuzziness/softness imposed on the segmentation.

The method of Lagrange multipliers—and the short-hand terms F_{ct} and P_{ct} for $F_c(\mathbf{z}_t)$ and $P_c(\mathbf{z}_t)$, respectively— gives the objective function as:

$$\mathcal{J} = \sum_{c=1}^{C} \sum_{t \in \mathcal{T}} \left[F_{ct} \log P_{ct} - \alpha F_{ct} \log F_{ct} \right] + \sum_{t \in \mathcal{T}} \lambda_t \left[\sum_{c=1}^{C} F_{ct} - 1 \right], \qquad (3)$$

where $\{\lambda_t\}_{t \in \mathcal{T}}$ is the set of Lagrange multipliers.

The proposed method modifies the nonparametric statistical model in [16] so as to exploit the prior information that the tract is a *spatially-continuous* entity in the image-coordinate space and, subsequently, to infer the *spatial structure* of the tract. We do this by augmenting the tensor-valued feature space by the 3D-coordinate space of the voxels. To include spatial information, we define the probabilities by P_{ct} as: $P_{ct} = (1/|\mathcal{S}_c|) \sum_{s \in \mathcal{S}_c} G(\mathbf{z}_t; \mu_{cs}, \sigma_c) G(t; \nu_{cs}, \rho_c)$, where the tensors $\{\mu_{cs}\}_{s \in \mathcal{S}_c}$, voxel locations $\{\nu_{cs}\}_{s \in \mathcal{S}_c}$, and bandwidths σ_c and ρ_c together model the PDF for class c in the *augmented feature space* $< \mathcal{M}, \mathcal{T} >$. This PDF captures: the manifold(s) underlying the tensor data in the tract, the variability of the tensors around the manifold(s), and the spatial continuity of the tract. For all classes, σ_c is a penalized maximum-likelihood estimate for the Parzen-window PDF of the entire image $\mathbf{z}_{t \in \mathcal{T}}$ [17]. We use $\rho_c = 1$.

We need to maximize $\mathcal{J}$ with respect to F_{ct}, μ_{cs}, ν_{cs}, and λ_t. Solving the Karush-Kuhn-Tucker (KKT) necessary conditions for optimality gives the update for the fuzzy memberships $F_{ct}(\forall s \in \mathcal{S}_c, \forall c = 1, 2, \ldots, C)$ as:

$$F_{ct} = \frac{(P_{ct})^{1/\alpha}}{\sum_{c=1}^{\mathcal{C}} (P_{ct})^{1/\alpha}}. \qquad (4)$$

Observe that, as expected, a large probability P_{ct} for voxel t to be in class c produces a correspondingly larger membership value F_{ct} of that voxel in class c. $\alpha \to \infty$ implies $F_{ct} \to 1/|\mathcal{C}|$; a completely fuzzy segmentation. For $\alpha \to 0$, $F_{ct} \to 1$ if class c with the largest P_{ct}; otherwise $F_{ct} \to 0$.

The updates for the class parameter $\mu_{cs}(\forall s \in \mathcal{S}_c, \forall c = 1, 2, \ldots, C)$ are:

$$\mu_{cs} = \frac{\sum_{t \in \mathcal{T}} F_{ct} \frac{G(\mathbf{z}_t; \mu_{cs}, \sigma_c) G(t; \nu_{cs}, \rho_c)}{P_{ct}} \mathbf{z}_t}{\sum_{t \in \mathcal{T}} F_{ct} \frac{G(\mathbf{z}_t; \mu_{cs}, \sigma_c) G(t; \nu_{cs}, \rho_c)}{P_{ct}}}; \nu_{cs} = \frac{\sum_{t \in \mathcal{T}} F_{ct} \frac{G(\mathbf{z}_t; \mu_{cs}, \sigma_c) G(t; \nu_{cs}, \rho_c)}{P_{ct}} t}{\sum_{t \in \mathcal{T}} F_{ct} \frac{G(\mathbf{z}_t; \mu_{cs}, \sigma_c) G(t; \nu_{cs}, \rho_c)}{P_{ct}}}$$

where the updated parameters μ_{cs} and ν_{cs} are weighted averages of the tensors $\mathbf{z}_t$ and voxel locations t, respectively. Observe that the weights take values between 0 and 1. The implementation is numerically stable because by construction, $0 \leq F_{ct} \leq 1$ and $0 \leq G(\mathbf{z}_t; \mu_{cs}, \sigma_c) G(t; \nu_{cs}, \rho_c)/P_{ct} \leq 1$. For the application in this paper, the iterative optimization method took about 4 iterations to converge; each iteration taking about 5 minutes using unoptimized Matlab code.

5   Results, Validation, and Discussion

We obtain real DT images: $128 \times 128 \times 40$ voxels; voxel size $1.7 \times 1.7 \times 3$ mm; single-shot spin-echo diffusion-weighted echo-planar imaging; 12 images per subject; 12 isotropically-distributed diffusion-encoding directions (b=1000 s/mm^2).

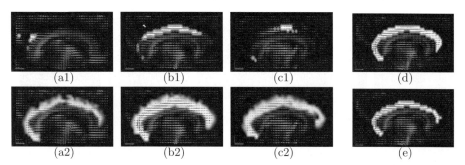

Fig. 1. The extracted cingulum, seen as the white background in the glyph-based color-coded DT visualization (sagittal slices), using: (a1)-(c1) tractography, and (a2)-(c2) proposed fuzzy-segmentation-based approach (white $\Rightarrow$ fuzzy membership value $F_{ct} = 1$, black $\Rightarrow F_{ct} = 0$, gray $\Rightarrow 0 < F_{ct} < 1$). (d) A manual segmentation (crisp) for the slice in (b1) or (b2) superimposed on the DT image. (e) An initialization (1 slice only; slice in (b1)or (b2)) for the segmentation superimposed on the DT image.

For extracting each cingulum in the brain, we obtained an initial (crisp) segmentation, on just a *single sagittal slice* of the cingulum, by thresholding tensors that: (i) have high FA (to separate white matter from the rest of the brain) and (ii) are orientated along anterior-posterior or inferior-superior directions. We manually remove voxels in the initialization (one slice) that clearly belonged to other far-off tracts, e.g. the fornix lying inferior to the corpus callosum [3].

Figure 1(a)–(c) shows the results of a standard tractography technique for the tract extraction using two regions-of-interest in the superior part of the cingulum. It is clear that tractography fails to extract the cingulum—a thin tract with sharp changes in orientation. On the other hand, Figure 1(d)–(f) shows that the proposed fuzzy segmentation approach—that exploits the statistical coherence of tensors in the entire structure—performs significantly better. Figure 2 shows the result, on another real DT image. For validation and quantitative comparison, we obtain two manual (crisp) segmentations by using interactive software to delineate color-coded scalar FA images—the color at each voxel is derived from the orientation of the tensor at that voxel. The Dice overlap metrics (averaged

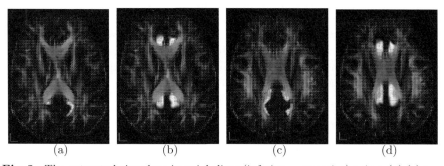

Fig. 2. The extracted cingulum in axial slices (inferior $\rightarrow$ superior) using: (a),(c) tractography, and (b),(d) proposed fuzzy-segmentation-based approach

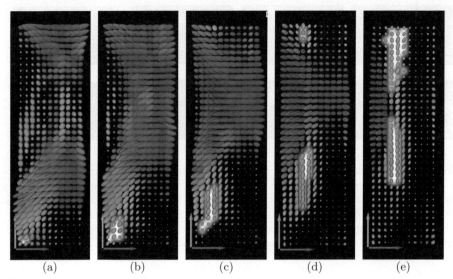

(a)   (b)   (c)   (d)   (e)

Fig. 3. Effect of partial voluming on tractography: (a)-(e) show regions near the cingulum/corpus-callosum interface in consecutive axial slices (inferior → superior)

over the two manual segmentations) for these two DT images were: (i) 0.63 and 0.60 for the proposed method (after thresholding the fuzzy membership values F_{ct} with a value of 0.5) and (ii) 0.32 and 0.33 for tractography.

Figure 3 shows enlarged axial views of the tractography result near the interface of the corpus callosum (red) and the cingulum (green). Significant partial voluming in this region, worsened by the low inter-axial-slice resolution, leads to a change in the orientation of the cingulum tensors. Thus, many cingulum tensors are no longer aligned with the direction of the cingulum tract, but rather have deviated orientations (brown) towards the orientation of the corpus callosum. Such phenomena cause fiber tracking, which uses thresholds on FA and curvature, to either: (i) wander far away from the desired cingulum tract, e.g. Figure 2(a)-(b), (loose thresholds) or (ii) terminate prematurely (conservative thresholds). In addition to this inherent trade-off, tractography suffers because it relies *solely* on the orientation of the current tensor and ignores the information in the tensors that were previously tracked. The proposed method—by optimally exploiting the information contained in *all* the tensor values, locations, and partial-volumed voxels in a unified framework—extracts the cingulum with significantly higher accuracy. Future work includes better quantification of the improvements obtained with the proposed method.

Acknowledgments

The authors gratefully acknowledge NIH support of this work via grants HD042974, HD046159, NS045839, and EB06266.

References

1. Lenglet, C., Rousson, M., Deriche, R., Faugeras, O., Lehericy, S., Ugurbil, K.: A Riemannian approach to diffusion tensor image segmentation. In: Proc. Info. Proc. Med. Imag, pp. 591–602 (2005)
2. Wang, Z., Vemuri, B.: DTI segmentation using an information theoretic tensor dissimilarity measure. IEEE Trans. Med. Imag. 24(10), 1267–1277 (2005)
3. Concha, L., Gross, D., Beulieu, C.: Diffusion tensor tractography of the limbic system. Amer. J. Neuroradiology 26, 2267–2274 (2005)
4. Jiang, G., Zang, Z., Xie, W., Guo, X.: Asymmetry analysis of cingulum based on scale-invariant parameterization by diffusion tensor imaging. Human Brain Map 24, 92–98 (2005)
5. Ziyan, U., Tuch, D., Westin, C.F.: Segmentation of thalamic nuclei from DTI using spectral clustering. In: Proc. Med. Image Comput. and Comp. Assisted Intervention, pp. 807–814 (2006)
6. Franklin, T., Acton, P., Maldjian, J., Gray, J., Croft, J., Dackis, C., O'Brien, C., Childress, A.: Decreased gray matter concentration in the insular, orbitofrontal, cingulate, and temporal cortices of cocaine patients. Biol. Psychiatry 51(2), 134–142 (2002)
7. Kinoshita, M., Yamada, K., Hashimoto, N., Kato, A., Izumoto, S., Baba, T., Maruno, M., Nishimura, T., Yoshimine, T.: Fiber tracking does not accurately estimate size of fiber bundles in pathological conditions: initial neurosurgical experience using neuronavigation and subcortical white matter stimulation. NeuroImage 25(2), 424–429 (2005)
8. Zhuang, X., Huang, Y., Palaniappan, K., Zhao, Y.: Gaussian mixture density modeling, decomposition, and applications. IEEE Trans. Image Proc. 5(9), 1293–1302 (1996)
9. Leemput, K.V., Maes, F., Vandermeulen, D., Seutens, P.: Automated model-based tissue classification of MR images of the brain. IEEE Tr. Med. Imaging 18, 897–908 (1999)
10. Pham, D., Prince, J.: An adaptive fuzzy segmentation algorithm for three-dimensional magnetic resonance images. In: Proc. Info. Proc. Med. Imag, 140–153 (1999)
11. Kim, J., Fisher, J.W., Yezzi, A.J., Cetin, M., Willsky, A.S.: A nonparametric statistical method for image segmentation using information theory and curve evolution. IEEE Trans. Image Processing 14(10), 1486–1502 (2005)
12. Awate, S.P., Tasdizen, T., Foster, N.L., Whitaker, R.T.: Adaptive, nonparametric Markov modeling for unsupervised, MRI brain-tissue classification. Medical Image Analysis 10(5), 726–739 (2006)
13. Fletcher, P.T., Joshi, S.C.: Principal geodesic analysis on symmetric spaces: Statistics of diffusion tensors. In: ECCV Workshops CVAMIA and MMBIA, pp. 87–98 (2004)
14. Arsigny, V., Fillard, P., Pennec, X., Ayache, N.: Geometric means in a novel vector space structure on symmetric positive-definite matrices. SIAM J. Matrix Analysis and Applications (in press)
15. Pennec, X., Fillard, P., Ayache, N.: A Riemannian framework for tensor computing. Int. J. Comput. Vision 66(1), 41–66 (2006)
16. Awate, S.P., Gee, J.C.: A fuzzy, nonparametric segmentation framework for DTI and MRI analysis. In: Proc. Info. Proc. in Med. Imag (IPMI) (to appear, 2007)
17. Chow, Y., Geman, S., Wu, L.: Consistant cross-validated density estimation. Annals of Statistics 11(1), 25–38 (1983)

Adaptive Metamorphs Model for 3D Medical Image Segmentation

Junzhou Huang[1], Xiaolei Huang[2], Dimitris Metaxas[1], and Leon Axel[3]

[1] Division of Computer and Information Sciences, Rutgers University, NJ, USA
[2] Department of Computer Science and Engineering, Lehigh University, PA, USA
[3] Department of Radiology, New York University, New York, USA

Abstract. In this paper, we introduce an adaptive model-based segmentation framework, in which edge and region information are integrated and used adaptively while a solid model deforms toward the object boundary. Our 3D segmentation method stems from Metamorphs deformable models [1]. The main novelty of our work is in that, instead of performing segmentation in an entire 3D volume, we propose model-based segmentation in an adaptively changing subvolume of interest. The subvolume is determined based on appearance statistics of the evolving object model, and within the subvolume, more accurate and object-specific edge and region information can be obtained. This local and adaptive scheme for computing edges and object region information makes our segmentation solution more efficient and more robust to image noise, artifacts and intensity inhomogeneity. External forces for model deformation are derived in a variational framework that consists of both edge-based and region-based energy terms, taking into account the adaptively changing environment. We demonstrate the performance of our method through extensive experiments using cardiac MR and liver CT images.

1 Introduction

Automated object boundary extraction is a fundamental problem in medical image analysis. It remains challenging to solve the problem robustly, however due to the common presence of cluttered objects, object texture, image noise, and various other artifacts in medical images. Efficiency is also often a concern, especially in 3D segmentation. Model-based methods have been extensively studied in recent years and achieved considerable success because of their ability to integrate high-level knowledge with low-level image processing [2,3,4,5]. The most commonly used models are either deformable models [2,3,1,4,5], or statistical models [6,7,8]. While both statistical shape [6] and appearance [7] models have been proposed to capture variations in an object in images, most deformable model frameworks [2,3,9] have been using primarily shape information, deriving external image forces from edge or gradient information. These shape-only deformable models often have difficulty in segmenting objects with texture patterns or in noisy images.

N. Ayache, S. Ourselin, A. Maeder (Eds.): MICCAI 2007, Part I, LNCS 4791, pp. 302–310, 2007.
© Springer-Verlag Berlin Heidelberg 2007

Some efforts have been made in the literature to integrate region information into shape-only deformable models. Geodesic Active Regions [4] deal with supervised texture segmentation in a frame partition framework. It assumes that the number of regions in an image is known and the region statistics are learned off-line using a mixture-of-Gaussian approximation. Region Competition [10] performs texture segmentation by combining region growing and active contours after applying a set of texture filters. The method assumes multivariate Gaussian distributions on the filter responses. In [11], an improved active contour deforms on a likelihood map instead of a heuristically-constructed edge map; however, the segmented objects are dilated versions of the truth objects, which is caused by artificial neighborhood operations. Metamorphs [1] is proposed as a new class of deformable models that integrate boundary information and nonparametric region statistics for segmentation. In Metamorphs, shape and appearance of a model are defined in a common pixel space and both edge- and region-based energy terms are differentiable with respect to the deformation parameters, so that boundary and region information are naturally integrated. Another key property of Metamorphs is that the object region statistics are adaptively learned from the evolving model-interior statistics, requiring no other *a priori* information. Good segmentation results are obtained using Metamorphs in 2D images. However, the original Metamorphs framework suffers from efficiency problems when being extended to 3D because it requires computation in the whole image volume. Furthermore, edges in the original framework were computed statically using the Canny edge detector with a global threshold and did not get updated adaptively as the object model deforms.

In this paper, we propose a new, efficient, 3D model-based segmentation method based on Metamorphs. Our main novelty is to propose a local and adaptive scheme that focuses computation on a subvolume and uses the model interior's gradient and intensity statistics for adaptive edge and region of interest (ROI) computation. During model evolution, on one hand, the online-learning aspect of the 3D Metamorphs model keeps up-to-date appearance statistics of the object and uses this information to constrain model deformation, and on the other hand, the adaptively changing statistics enable the model to better handle image noise and gradual changes in intensity. In addition, we develop a new ROI-based balloon energy term, from which one can derive anisotropic external forces that efficiently deform the model toward the ROI boundary.

In the remainder of the paper, we briefly review Metamorphs [1] in Section 2. We introduce the new 3D adaptive Metamorphs models in Section 3. In Section 4, experimental results are presented and we conclude in Section 5.

2   Metamorphs Deformable Models

Considering traditional deformable models as "active contours" or "evolving curve fronts", the deformable shape and appearance models, termed "Metamorphs" [1], are "deforming disks or volumes" that have not only boundary shape but interior appearance.

Model Shape and Appearance Representations. The object model shape in Metamorphs is represented implicitly as a distance function. In this way, model shape is defined by a distance map "image", in the common pixel space as image intensity. The intensity distribution of a Metamorphs model's interior region is represented using a nonparametric kernel-based method [12].

Model Dynamics. The deformations that a Metamorphs model can undergo are defined using a space warping technique, Free Form Deformations (FFD) [1]. FFD parameterizes warping deformations of the volumetric space in which the model is embedded, hence deforming both model boundary and interior simultaneously. When applied to segmentation, a Metamorphs model is initialized covering a seed region inside the object, and external image forces are derived in a variational framework consisting of both edge- and region-based energy terms. Both types of energy terms are differentiable with respect to the common set of FFD deformation parameters.

3   3D Adaptive Metamorphs Models

Shape Representation. The 3D extension of the Metamorphs implicit shape representation is straightforward. Let $\Phi : \Omega \to R^+$ be a Lipschitz function that refers to the distance transform for the model shape $\mathcal{M}$. By definition Ω is bounded since it refers to the image domain. The shape defines a partition of the domain: the region that is enclosed by $\mathcal{M}$, $[\mathcal{R}_{\mathcal{M}}]$, the background $[\Omega - \mathcal{R}_{\mathcal{M}}]$, and the boundary of the model, $[\partial \mathcal{R}_{\mathcal{M}}]$ (In practice, we consider a narrow band around the model $\mathcal{M}$ in the image domain as $\partial \mathcal{R}_{\mathcal{M}}$). Given these definitions, the following implicit shape representation is considered:

$$\Phi_{\mathcal{M}}(\mathbf{x}) = \begin{cases} 0, & \mathbf{x} \in \partial \mathcal{R}_{\mathcal{M}} \\ +D(\mathbf{x}, \mathcal{M}) > 0, & \mathbf{x} \in \mathcal{R}_{\mathcal{M}} \\ -D(\mathbf{x}, \mathcal{M}) < 0, & \mathbf{x} \in [\Omega - \mathcal{R}_{\mathcal{M}}] \end{cases}$$

where $D(\mathbf{x}, \mathcal{M})$ refers to the min Euclidean distance between the image pixel location $\mathbf{x} = (x, y, z)$ and the model $\mathcal{M}$. One example of shape representation is shown in Fig. 1 (2.e).

Appearance Representation. The nonparametric kernel-based method is used to represent the 3D model-interior intensity distribution [1]. Suppose the model is deforming on the image I, the image region $\mathcal{R}_{\mathcal{M}}$ is bounded by the current model $\Phi_{\mathcal{M}}$, then the nonparametric distribution over pixel intensity values i can be defined as:

$$\mathbf{P}(i|\Phi_{\mathcal{M}}) = \frac{1}{V(\mathcal{R}_{\mathcal{M}})} \iint_{\mathcal{R}_{\mathcal{M}}} \frac{1}{\sqrt{2\pi}\sigma} e^{\frac{-(i-I(\mathbf{y}))^2}{2\sigma^2}} d\mathbf{y} \tag{1}$$

where $V(\mathcal{R}_{\mathcal{M}})$ denotes the volume of $\mathcal{R}_{\mathcal{M}}$, and σ is a constant specifying the width of the Gaussian kernel. Using this nonparametric approximation, the intensity distribution of the model interior gets updated automatically while the model deforms. One example is shown in Fig. 1 (1.b).

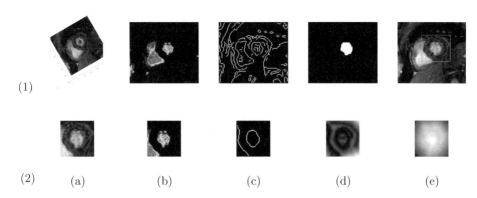

(1)

(2)   (a)   (b)   (c)   (d)   (e)

Fig. 1. An example of left ventricle segmentation in a 3D MR image. (1.a) Initial 3D sphere model; (1.b) Intensity probability map (only displaying one slice in a 3D image); (1.c) Edges based on global threshold; (1.d) ROI; (1.e) Localization of a subvolume of interest (IIV); (2.a) one slice from the 3D IIV; (2.b) updated Intensity probability map (2.c) updated edges based on local threshold in IIV; (2.d) distance map based on edges; (2.e) distance map based on ROI boundary.

Model Deformations. 3D Incremental Free Form Deformations (IFFD) is used to define model deformations. The essence of FFD is to deform the model by manipulating a regular control lattice F overlaid in its volumetric embedding space. Hence the model deformation parameters, $\mathbf{q}$, using FFD are deformations of control points in the lattice F:

$$\mathbf{q} = \{(\delta F^x_{h,w,s}, \delta F^y_{h,w,s}, \delta F^z_{h,w,s})\}; \ (h, w, s) \in [1, H] \times [1, W] \times [1, S]$$

The deformed position of a pixel $\mathbf{x} = (x, y, z)$ given the control lattice deformation from the initial regular configuration, F^0, to a new configuration, $F^0 + \delta F$, can be calculated through interpolation using cubic B-spline basis functions:

$$D(\mathbf{q}; \mathbf{x}) = \sum_{l=0}^{3} \sum_{m=0}^{3} \sum_{n=0}^{3} B_l(u) B_m(v) B_n(r) (F^0_{i+l,j+m,k+n} + \delta F_{i+l,j+m,k+n}) \quad (2)$$

- $\delta F_{i+l,j+m,k+n}$, $(l, m, n) \in [0, 3] \times [0, 3] \times [0, 3]$ are the deformations of pixel $\mathbf{x}$'s (sixty four) adjacent control points,
- (i, j, k) is the index (in global reference frame) of the control point located at the origin of a local reference frame defined by $\mathbf{x}$'s 64 adjacent control points.
- $B_l(u)$, $B_m(v)$ and $B_n(r)$ are the lth, m^{th} and n^{th} basis function of a Cubic B-spline respectively [1].

3.1 Adaptive Edge and Region Information

To efficiently find object boundary, our algorithm starts with a simple-shape object model that is initialized covering a seed region inside the object. Edge

306   J. Huang et al.

and region information are then extracted and integrated adaptively as the model
evolves over time. The overall model fitting process has the following steps.

- Step 1: Initialize a simple-shape (e.g. sphere, cylinder) 3D model centered
  around a seed point [Fig. 1(1.a)].
- Step 2: Compute nonparametric intensity statistics inside the model using
  Eqn. 1 [Fig. 1(1.b)]. The "Region Of Interest" (ROI) is determined as the
  largest possible region in the image that overlaps the model and has a consistent intensity distribution as the current model interior [1] (see [Fig. 1(1.d)]).
  Based on the ROI, we localize a subvolume of interest, which we call the "Interested Image Volume" (IIV) [Fig. 1(1.e)].
- Step 3: In IIV [Fig. 1(2.a)], compute the intensity probability map and update ROI based on a local probability threshold. Edges are also computed
  in IIV by performing 3D canny edge detection using a local gradient threshold. Comparing Fig. 1(2.b) and Fig. 1(2.c) with Fig. 1(1.b) and Fig. 1(1.c),
  one can see that the updated intensity probability map and edges are more
  accurate in our adaptive framework.
- Step 4: With edges and ROI computed in IIV, compute edge- and region-
  based energy terms(see section 3.2).
- Step 5: Evolve the deformable model, for a fixed number of iterations, toward
  object boundary based on model dynamics derived from the above energy
  terms. In [Fig. 2(b)], an intermediate model is shown.
- Step 6: Repeat steps 2-5 until convergence (e.g. when model deformation is
  sufficiently small). The converged model is shown in [Fig. 2(c)].

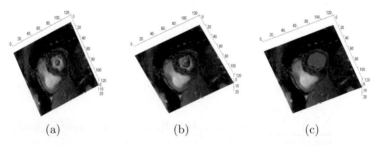

(a)   (b)   (c)

Fig. 2. Model evolution. (a) Initial model plus one slice in a 3D image; (b) Intermediate
model; (c) Converged model.

3.2   3D Model Dynamics

Two energy terms are defined to deform the model toward object boundary.

The ROI Based Balloon Term. The ROI-based balloon term is designed to
efficiently deform the model toward ROI boundary. After computing the intensity
probability map P_I within IIV (see Step 3 in section 3.1, [Fig. 1(2.b)]) based on
model-interior intensity statistics, a threshold (typically the mean probability
in IIV) is applied on P_I to produce a binary IIV P_B. Assuming the object to
be segmented is a solid without holes, we take the outer-most border of the

connected component on this binary image P_B that is overlapping the model as the current ROI boundary. We encode this ROI boundary by computing its "shape image", which is its signed distance transform [Fig. 1(2.e)]. Denote this "shape image" as Φ_r, the ROI-based balloon term is defined as:

$$E_B = \frac{1}{S(\partial\mathcal{R}_\mathcal{M})} \iint_{\partial\mathcal{R}_\mathcal{M}} \Phi_r(\mathbf{x})\big(\Phi_\mathcal{M}(D(\mathbf{q};\mathbf{x}))\big)d\mathbf{x} \qquad (3)$$

In the normalizing term, S means the surface normal. By the first component of this energy term $\Phi_\mathcal{M}(D(\mathbf{q};\mathbf{x}))$ alone, the model boundary affinity pixels $\mathbf{x}$ will be mapped outward to locations $D(\mathbf{q};\mathbf{x})$, where the model shape representation values $\Phi_\mathcal{M}(D(\mathbf{q};\mathbf{x}))$ are smaller. Hence the model would expand and grow like a balloon so as to minimize the value of the energy term. The second component in the energy term, Φ_r, is the ROI "shape image" and encodes the distance value of each pixel from the ROI region boundary. It serves as a weighting factor for the first component so that the speed of model evolution is proportional to the distance of the model from the ROI boundary. Then, the model moves fast when it is far away from the boundary and the underlying $\Phi_r(\mathbf{x})$ values are large; it slows down as it approaches the boundary, and stops at the boundary. This ROI-based balloon term is very effective in countering the effect of un-regularized or inhomogeneous region intensities such as that caused by speckle noise and spurious edges inside the object of interest. Moreover, the ROI term generates adaptively changing balloon forces that expedite model convergence and improve convergence accuracy, especially when the shape of the object is elongated, or has salient protrusions or concavities.

The Adaptive Shape Term. We encode the adaptive edge information using a "shape image" Φ, which is derived from the distance transform of the edge map computed within IIV. In the previous Metamorphs model [1], the edge map is computed with a global threshold applied to the whole image and stay unchanged during model evolution [Fig. 1(1.c)]. In our model, the edge map is computed in a ROI-related, adaptively-changing subvolume instead of in the whole image [Fig. 1(2.c)]. As the model evolves, the edge map is adaptively re-computed based on gradient statistics inside the new model. To evolve a 3D model toward edges, we define an edge-based data term E_E on pixels in a narrow band around the model boundary $\partial\mathcal{R}_\mathcal{M}$.

$$E_E = \frac{1}{V(\partial\mathcal{R}_\mathcal{M})} \iint_{\partial\mathcal{R}_\mathcal{M}} \big(\Phi(D(\mathbf{q};\mathbf{x}))\big)^2 d\mathbf{x} \qquad (4)$$

Intuitively, this term will encourage the deformation that maps the model boundary to edge locations where the underlying "shape image" distance values are as small (or as close to zero) as possible.

3.3   3D Model Evolution

A unified gradient-descent based parameter updating scheme can be derived using energy terms introduced above. The following evolution equation is derived for each element $\mathbf{q}_i$ in the model deformation parameters $\mathbf{q}$:

$$\frac{\partial E}{\partial \mathbf{q}_i} = \left(\frac{\partial E_E}{\partial \mathbf{q}_i} + a\frac{\partial E_B}{\partial \mathbf{q}_i}\right) \qquad (5)$$

– The motion due to the adaptive shape term is:

$$\frac{\partial E_E}{\partial \mathbf{q}_i} = \frac{1}{S(\partial \mathcal{R}_\mathcal{M})} \iint_{\partial \mathcal{R}_\mathcal{M}} 2\Phi(D(\mathbf{q};\mathbf{x})) \cdot \left(\nabla\Phi(D(\mathbf{q};\mathbf{x})) \cdot \frac{\partial}{\partial \mathbf{q}_i} D(\mathbf{q};\mathbf{x})\right)d\mathbf{x}$$

– The motion due to the ROI-based balloon term is:

$$\frac{\partial E_B}{\partial \mathbf{q}_i} = \frac{1}{S(\partial \mathcal{R}_\mathcal{M})} \iint_{\partial \mathcal{R}_\mathcal{M}} \Phi_r(\mathbf{x})\left(\nabla\Phi_\mathcal{M}(D(\mathbf{q};\mathbf{x})) \cdot \frac{\partial}{\partial \mathbf{q}_i} D(\mathbf{q};\mathbf{x})\right)d\mathbf{x}$$

where a is a constant balancing the contribution of the two parts and the partial derivatives with respect to the deformation (FFD) parameters, $\frac{\partial}{\partial \mathbf{q}_i}D(\mathbf{q};\mathbf{x})$, can be easily derived from the model deformation formula for $D(\mathbf{q};\mathbf{x})$ [Eqn. (2)].

4   Experiments

Heart. We applied our adaptive model to segmenting the endocardium of the left ventricle in tagged MRI images. The image data are 4D spatial-temporal short-axis cardiac tagged MR images. A 1.5T GE MR imaging system was used to acquire the images using an EGG-gated tagged gradient echo pulse sequence. Every 30ms, 2 sets of parallel short axis (SA) images were acquired: one with horizontal tags and one with vertical tags. Each set consists of 24 phases, with 16 slices (images) per phase. We collected 768 2D-images for testing. These 768 2D-images formed 48 3D images, each with the size of $192 \times 192 \times 16$. An expert was also asked to draw the left ventricle (LV) endocardium contours in these images for validation purposes.

Some example segmentation results are shown in Figure 3. Quantitative validation is performed by comparing the automated segmentation results with expert solutions. Denote the expert segmentation in the images as l_{true}, and the results from our method as l_{amm}. The True Positive Fraction (TPF) describes the fraction of the total amount of tissue in the true segmentation that is overlapped with the segmentation by our method: $FPF = \frac{|l_{amm} \cap l_{true}|}{l_{true}}$. On the entire test image set, the proposed method achieved an average 96.1% TPF. Our algorithm was implemented in MATLAB with embedded C code, and tested on a 2GHz Pentium 4 PC. The running time for LV endocardium segmentation in a 3D image of size $192 \times 192 \times 16$ is around 15 seconds.

Liver CT. Another application to which we applied our model-based method is segmenting tumors in liver CT images. These images were acquired using a LightSpeed Plus GE multi-slice CT scanner. The scans were reconstructed with a 38cm field of view. On average the CT system operated with an image acquisition time of 90 msec per slice. The scanner generated X-rays with a peak voltage of 120 kVp and a maximum current of 260 mA. The axial resolution was 7.5mm and the image resolution of each cross section slice is 512 by 512. We collected 28 3D CT scans of the liver with 392 2D image slices in total.

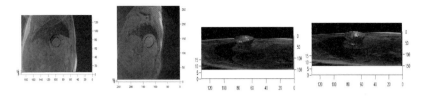

Fig. 3. Left ventricle endocardium segmentation example. Converged 3D model plus one slice in the 3D image from different views.

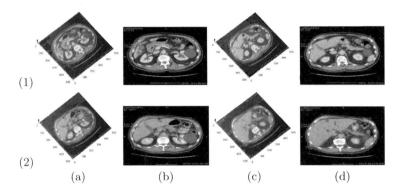

Fig. 4. Tumor segmentation examples. (1.a) The converged model representing the segmented tumor, plus one slice in a 3D CT image; (1.b) 2D view of the segmented contour in the same image slice; (1.c) The model plus another slice of the same 3D image; (1.d) The segmented contour in the same slice as in (1.c); (2) similar to (1) but for a different 3D image.

An expert was asked to draw the tumor contours in these test images. Some example segmentation results are shown in Figure 4. On the entire dataset, the proposed method achieved very encouraging segmentation results with an average of 91.7% TPF. The running time for tumor segmentation in these high-resolution CT images varied from 30 seconds to a few minutes, depending on the tumor size and the noise level.

5 Conclusions

We have presented a new 3D adaptive Metamorphs deformable model. It is a major extension of the 2D Metamorphs model [1]. Instead of computing edge and region information statically and in the whole image, we adaptively calculate a "focus of attention" subvolume, in which edges and region of interest (ROI) are extracted based on object-specific criterion. A new ROI-based balloon term is developed, which is effective in countering the effect of inhomogeneous region intensities, such as those caused by speckle noise and spurious edges inside the object. Compared to other works that integrate edge and region information for model-based segmentation, our model is novel in that it is an object model that has both boundary and interior. As the model evolves, its adaptively-changing appearance statistics will re-define its surrounding edges and ROI so that more reliable external image forces can be obtained. Focusing the computation on a subvolume containing the model also makes the framework more efficient.

Acknowledgement. This research has been partially funded by NSF funds ACI 0205671 and CNS-0428231 to Dr. Metaxas, NIH R21 AG27513-01 to Dr Metaxas and NIH R01 HL083309 to Dr Axel.

References

1. Huang, X., Metaxas, D., Chen, T.: Metamorphs: Deformable shape and texture models. In: IEEE Conf. on Computer Vision and Pattern Recognition, pp. 496–503 (2004)
2. Kass, M., Witkin, A., Terzopoulos, D.: Snakes: Active contour models. Int'l Journal of Computer Vision 1, 321–331 (1987)
3. Metaxas, D.: Physics-Based Deformable Models. Kluwer Academic Publishers, Dordrecht (1996)
4. Paragios, N., Deriche, R.: Geodesic active regions and level set methods for supervised texture segmentation. Int'l Journal of Computer Vision 46(3), 223–247 (2002)
5. Vese, L.A., Chan, T.F.: A multiphase level set framework for image segmentation using the Mumford and Shah model. Int'l Journal of Computer Vision 50(3), 271–293 (2002)
6. Cootes, T.F., Taylor, C.J., Cooper, D.H., Graham, J.: Active shape models - their training and application. Computer Vision and Image Understanding 61(1), 38–59 (1995)
7. Cootes, T.F., Edwards, G.J., Taylor, C.J.: Active appearance models. Proc. of European Conf. on Computer Vision 2, 484–498 (1998)
8. Leventon, M.E., Grimson, E.L., Faugeras, O.: Statistical shape influence in geodesic active contours. IEEE Conf. on Computer Vision and Pattern Recognition 1, 1316–1323 (2000)
9. Caselles, V., Kimmel, R., Sapiro, G.: Geodesic active contours. In: IEEE Int'l Conf. on Computer Vision, pp. 694–699 (1995)
10. Zhu, S., Yuille, A.: Region Competition: Unifying snakes, region growing, and Bayes/MDL for multi-band image segmentation. IEEE Trans. on Pattern Analysis and Machine Intelligence 18(9), 884–900 (1996)
11. Pujol, O., Radeva, P.: Texture segmentation by statistical deformable models. Intenational Journal of Image and Graphics 4(3), 433–452 (2004)
12. Comaniciu, D., Meer, P.: Mean shift: A robust approach toward feature space analysis. IEEE Trans. on Pattern Analysis and Machine Intelligence 24(5), 603–619 (2002)

Coronary Artery Segmentation and Skeletonization Based on Competing Fuzzy Connectedness Tree

Chunliang Wang and Örjan Smedby

CMIV, Linköping University Hospital
SE-58185 Linköping, Sweden
wcl_sd@hotmail.com, orjan.smedby@cmiv.liu.se

Abstract. We propose a new segmentation algorithm based on competing fuzzy connectedness theory, which is then used for visualizing coronary arteries in 3D CT angiography (CTA) images. The major difference compared to other fuzzy connectedness algorithms is that an additional data structure, the connectedness tree, is constructed at the same time as the seeds propagate. In preliminary evaluations, accurate result have been achieved with very limited user interaction. In addition to improving computational speed and segmentation results, the fuzzy connectedness tree algorithm also includes automated extraction of the vessel centerlines, which is a promising approach for creating curved plane reformat (CPR) images along arteries' long axes.

Keywords: segmentation, fuzzy connectedness tree, centerline extraction, skeletonization, coronary artery, CT angiography.

1 Introduction

In the past few years, noninvasive imaging of the coronary arteries has attracted growing interest. Thanks to the development of image acquisition techniques such as 64-slice scanners for CT angiography (CTA), the spatial and temporal resolution and image quality of the volumetric images have improved remarkably. Compared to the rapid development of the image capture technique, however, the visualization techniques used have not evolved correspondingly. Radiologists and cardiologists still largely depend on viewing original slices, oblique multiplanar reformatting (MPR) and curved plane reformatting (CPR) images, sometimes complemented by a slab maximum intensity projection (MIP) image. Panoramic MIP or volume rendering (VRT) images are less helpful for coronary artery disease diagnosis, due to the concealing effect of contrast medium in adjacent heart chambers and great vessels.

A key method to solve this problem is to segment the coronary arteries in the volumetric datasets. However, due to the close anatomic relationship between coronary arteries and heart chambers and resolution limitations in the images, many automated algorithms, which have been successfully utilized in peripheral vessel extraction, such as pattern reorganization techniques and model-based approaches [1], may fail with coronary artery datasets. Although several algorithms specifically designed for the coronaries have been published [2-4], they tend to have limited success with complicated cases, and important details of coronary artery system may

N. Ayache, S. Ourselin, A. Maeder (Eds.): MICCAI 2007, Part I, LNCS 4791, pp. 311–318, 2007.
© Springer-Verlag Berlin Heidelberg 2007

be lost during the segmentation. Interactive approaches may solve part of this problem but can be very time-consuming. The concept of fuzzy connectedness (greyscale connectedness), which has been proposed to separate arteries and veins in Magnetic resonance angiography (MRA) [5-7], shows great ability to separate two contrast-filled structures from each other. A previous feasibility study showed that this approach can be applied to 3D CTA data to separate the coronary arteries from other contrast-filled structures and thus permit coronary artery visualization in an angiographic mode similar to invasive X-ray angiography [8].

In this paper we propose a new algorithm based on competing fuzzy connectedness theory, which only requires limited interaction by the user. In addition to overcoming several problems of former algorithms [5-7], the new algorithm includes automated extraction of the vessel centerline, which is useful, e.g., for creating CPR images.

2 Method

In this section, we will first give a brief review of fuzzy connectedness theory, and then present the competing fuzzy connectedness tree algorithm. Finally, we will introduce how it can be extended into a skeletonization algorithm.

2.1 Fuzzy Connectedness and Relative Fuzzy Connectedness Theory

Just as the coronary arteries can be bluntly separated from the heart during surgery due to the varying connectivity of the wall structures, they can also be separated in 3D CTA images depending on the connectivity of the contrast agent in the vessel lumen.

In a 3D image, a path p joining two voxels, u and v, is a sequence of distinct points $u = w_0, w_1, \ldots w_{n-1}, w_n = v$, such that for each i, $0 \leq i \leq n$, w_{i+1} is a 26-neighbor of w_i. Let $g(w_i)$ be the strength that the voxel w_i can contribute to the path. The strength of connectedness of p is determined by the weakest point along the path:

$$S(p) = \min_{w_i \in p}(g(w_i)) \tag{1}$$

The connectedness between u and v is the strength of the strongest of all paths joining u and v:

$$C(u,v) = \max_{p(u,v)}(S(p)) \tag{2}$$

Although a more sophisticated strategy, such as the Fuzzy Affinity function developed by Udupa and collaborators [5] can be used to calculate the contribution function $g(w_i)$ of each voxel, we have chosen, for convenience and simplicity, to use the gray-scale function $f(w_i)$ directly, i.e. $g(w_i) = f(w_i)$, since our research does not focus on the evaluation of the "cost" function.

An example image (Fig. 1A) contains two seeds, $s1$ and $s2$ within objects $O1$ and $O2$, respectively. With the approach above, the degree of connectedness of a pixel u to each seed can be calculated. Then it can be easily decided to which object u should belong by comparing $C(u, s1)$ and $C(u, s2)$. Applying this strategy to all pixels in the image, a natural segmentation by "relative fuzzy connectedness" is achieved [5].

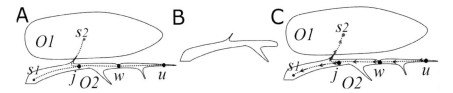

Fig. 1. A: p_{u-s1} and p_{u-s2} are the strongest paths from u to $s1$ and $s2$. **B**: segmentation result using relative fuzzy connectedness theory. **C**: competing fuzzy connectedness trees for p_{u-s1} and p_{u-s2}.

2.2 Shared Path Effect of Relative Fuzzy Connectedness

Although relative fuzzy connectedness can separate most parts of objects correctly, in some cases it will give wrong results. In Fig. 1A, we give an example of such a case. Suppose that p_{u-s1} and p_{u-s2} represent the strongest paths from u to $s1$ and $s2$ respectively. Both paths share a segment p_{u-j}, and a point w on p_{u-j} is the weakest point for both paths. Based on the theory above, all points between w and u will have the same strength of connectedness $g(w)$ to both seeds, and thus the membership of those points will depend on the strategy of the implementation of the algorithm. If $O1$ is the object of interest and $O2$ is the background, all points between u and w may belong to background ($O2$), even if the points on p_{j-w} belong to $O1$, as the segmentation result in Fig. 1B shows. With the "SeparaSeed" approach [6], which implemented fuzzy connectedness with a chamfer algorithm [10], the membership of points in p_{u-w} will depend on which seed will change the "color label" of those points first; i.e., the geometric distance between voxel and seeds will affect the result.

2.3 Competing Fuzzy Connectedness Algorithm Based on Connectedness Tree

To avoid the shared path effect, Udupa and collaborators proposed an Iterative Relative Fuzzy Connectedness algorithm which iteratively refines the competition rules for different objects depending upon the results of the previous iteration [5]. An obvious drawback of that algorithm is the computation time demands caused by the iteration. Here we propose a new algorithm which can avoid the "shared path effect" without adding extra iteration time. The basic idea is to calculate a connectedness tree at the same time as the seeds propagate. As a result, each voxel will point to the neighbor from which it is connected with its "strongest" seed. As shown in Fig. 1C, all points between w and u will be connected with $O1$ by pointing to the points on p_{j-w}; thus the potential mistake caused by the shared path will be avoided.

Our competing fuzzy connectedness tree (CFCT) algorithm is described in the following pseudo-code.

Input: A 3D Image $I = (C, f)$, and n seed regions S_j in C
Output: a fuzzy connectedness tree *pointer* and a 3D connectivity map $O=(C, g)$
Auxiliary Data Structures: a 3D array *marker* represents if current voxel should be checked, $N(v)$ denotes the set of neighbor points of v. $N^+(v)$ denotes the upper 13 neighbors of v, $N^-(v)$ denotes the lower 13 neighbors of v (details in [6])

```
1  for v∈ C, set g(v)=0, pointer(v)=nil, marker(v)=false
2  for v∈ S_j(1•j•n) set g(v)=f(v) and for w∈ N(v) set
```

```
    marker(w)=true
 3   for v∈ S_j(1•j•n) and S_j is stopping seeds, set g(v)=0
 4   repeat
 5      for v∈ S_j(1•j•n) from (0,0,0) to (x_max, y_max, z_max)
 6         if marker(v)=true
 7            find w_max in N'(v) such that g(w_max)= max(g(w))
 8            if g(w_max)>g(v)
 9               g(v) = min(f(v); g(w_max))
10               pointer(v)= w_max
11               for all w∈ N(v) set marker(w)=true
12            else
13               set marker(v)=false
14      for v∈ S_j(1•j•n) from(x_max, y_max, z_max) to (0,0,0)
15         if marker(v)=true
16            find w_max in N'(v) such that g(w_max)= max(g(w))
17            if g(w_max)>g(v)
18               g(v) = min(f(v); g(w_max))
19               pointer(v)= w_max
20               for all w∈ N(v) set marker(w)=true
21            else
22               set marker(v)=false
23  until no changes in O
```

The extra data structure *marker* limits the comparison within the 26-neighborhood to those voxels whose neighbors have a new optimized connectivity value. This strategy reduces the iteration time, as the number of changed points decreases roughly exponentially with each iteration in the main loop (rows 3-22).

By introducing the array *marker*, the CFCT algorithm has evolved into a variation of Dijkstra's shortest-path algorithm [9]. Here, *marker* is essentially equivalent to the queue Q, and setting *marker* (v) = true or false, equivalent to a push or pop operation on the queue Q. Using an array instead of a queue, multiple duplicated v existing in Q at the same time are avoided. Memory being allocated beforehand may prevent memory exhaustion during iteration. In practice, the marker array can be merged with the pointer array by using 1 bit of 1 byte, saving even more memory.

A bidirectional scan based on the location of voxels is carried out to decide which voxel should "pop out". This strategy, which was proposed to compute the distance transform [10], helps to accelerate the convergence. In addition, memory is read sequentially, which is faster than accessing memory randomly.

After the construction of the fuzzy connectedness tree, every voxel can get a property *color* by recursively asking its predecessor until a seed is reached. This color map can be used as a segmentation mask, defining a zone containing the anatomically interesting vessels, as well as part of the background

A new kind of seed, the stopping seed, has been introduced to separate the coronary artery from the root of the aorta. A stopping seed is defined as a seed with 0 as initial value (line 3). As it is a seed, its g will keep the initial value, so it will never propagate but terminate the propagation of other trees. To cut away the artery totally from the aorta, a stopping plane should be used instead of isolated points.

2.4 Centerline Extraction Algorithm Based on Fuzzy Connectedness Tree

Our centerline extraction algorithm is based on the following observation: if only one seed is included in a coronary artery segment, the CFCT algorithm can always, from any voxel u in this segment, find a path connecting $s1$ and u by searching upwards in the fuzzy connectedness tree (Fig. 2). As every voxel points to its strongest neighbor, this path always snaps onto the ridge of the fuzzy connectivity map. As long as the highest intensity is found in the center of the vessel, tracing from the distal end of a coronary artery to the root seed will actually follow the centerline of the vessel.

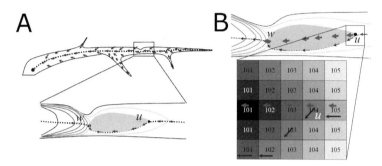

Fig. 2. A: Fuzzy connectedness path is distorted at a flat roof after a stenosis. **B**: Local optimization of the fuzzy connectedness tree, the grey-level represents the intensity in the input image, the number in the grid represents the *distance* to the root seed.

According to fuzzy connectedness theory, the peak intensities will be erased in certain areas of the fuzzy connectivity map. In cases such as Fig. 1, after a weak point w, a flat roof will appear (cf. Fig. 2A), because for any voxel u after w, $C_{u\text{-}s1}$ will be equal to $g(w)$ as long as $g(u) \geq g(w)$. In this area, the fuzzy connectedness path will prefer to follow one edge of the flat region as decided by the scan order.

To avoid distortion of the centerline in such cases, a refining step is added. First, a distance map $distance(v)$ is created to indicate the number of points on the path $p_{v\text{-}s}$ connecting the voxel v and the root seed s. Then local optimization of the fuzzy connectedness tree is carried out by searching from the distal end, based on the intensity scene of input image and steered by the distance map. Suppose voxel u is the point we have just found. To decide the next node, rather than using the *pointer(u)* directly, we search all neighbors having a distance less than $distance(u)$ (in Fig. 2B equal to 104), and choose the one with the maximum intensity value in the input image. To reduce noise in the input image, a Gaussian smoothing filter can be used.

In cases with more than one seed in the artery, the connectedness tree is rebuilt after deleting the extra seeds, and all voxels not belonging to a vessel segment are marked as stopping seeds. In the ensuing propagation, only the root seed will have the chance to grow in the coronary artery.

To find the distal endpoint of an artery, a possible strategy is to use the distance map to locate the farthest point, as in [11]. However, the result will be highly dependent on the accuracy of the geometric profile of the segmented artery. When using the strategy above, the distal end will sometimes be located in adjacent tissues with lower intensity. To avoid such mistakes, we use a weight function, when creating the distance map, to assign the step length of a voxel instead of using integer 1. The weight function is defined as: $weight(v) = g(v)/H$, where H is the highest intensity value of the entire input image.

After the longest centerline has been extracted, the centerline of any branch on the main trunk can be found by setting the former centerline as seed and recomputing the weighted distance map. The iteration can be terminated by defining the number of branches desired or by specifying a minimum length of branches (pruning).

3   Results

In 33 clinical coronary CTA datasets (240-450 slices of 0.75mm, 512×512 pixels), we tested both the CFCT algorithm and the older "SeparaSeed" algorithm implemented as plug-ins to Osirix on a Mac G5 (2.5GHz CPU and 2GB RAM). Fig. 3 compares the computation times for each iteration in the main loop for a dataset of 512×512×240 voxels. With the new algorithm, basic seed planting required 2–3 min for an experienced radiologist, the first round segmentation 3–5 min, and interactive seed modification 0–8 min. Using only basic seed planting (with one root seed placed in each coronary artery) resulted in all visible branches being completely segmented in

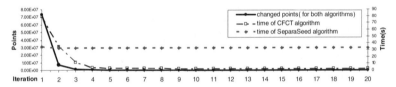

Fig. 3. Comparison of iteration time between "SeparaSeed" and CFCT algorithm

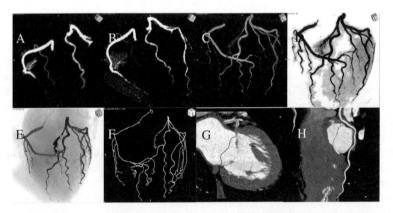

Fig. 4. A: Segmentation result with SeparaSeed. **B**: Result of CFCT algorithm using the same seeds. **C, D**: VRT and black-and white inverse MIP images mimicking coronary angiography. **E**: Different vessels shown with different opacity and different color. **F**: A complete skeleton of coronary artery system. **G, H**: Centerline extracted with CFCT algorithm and CPR along it.

18 cases, compared to 12 cases when using the same seeds with the "SeparaSeed" algorithm ($p<0.05$; McNemar's Test) (Fig. 4). In total, visually correct centerlines were obtained automatically in 95.3% (262/275) of the visible branches.

4 Discussion

As expected, the CFCT algorithm can run 7–8 times faster than the SeparaSeed algorithm. It can also yield more accurate segmentation results with limited user interaction by avoiding the "shared path effect", thus saving interaction time for planting more seeds. With a VOI definition tool, the whole procedure, including seed planting, segmentation and centerline extraction for the main coronary branches, can be completed within 10–15 min, which may be clinically acceptable. It should be noted that our goal is not an accurate estimation of arterial dimensions; for visualization, suppression of adjacent myocardium is achieved by the rendering algorithm.

The major difference between the CFCT algorithm and Udupa's Relative Fuzzy Connectedness or Iterative Relative Fuzzy Connectedness algorithm is that only one affinity scene is calculated during the whole procedure. By calculating a fuzzy connectedness tree, multiple iterative propagations are avoided. Another speed advantage of the connectedness tree is that previous iteration results can be reused after user modification to recalculate connectedness trees. When new seeds have been planted in the input seed regions, a new round propagation can start running with previous results directly from line 2 of the CFCT algorithm. New trees will grow from those seeds by "snatching voxels" from other trees. If seeds are deleted, the trees arising from those will be removed from the *pointer,* and the connectivity value g of relevant voxels will be reset to 0. After a few iterations, the empty region will be connected to branches extending from nearby trees, resulting in fast convergence. With further improvements, the user may be able to modify seeds at almost interactive speeds.

Compared to centerline extraction algorithms based on Minimum Cost Path Search, an advantage of the fuzzy connectedness tree is that the cost function will not be affected by the Euclidean distance of the "Minimum Cost Path". Since the coronary arteries surround the heart chambers, which may have equal or higher intensity than coronary arteries, the minimum cost path may prefer a short-cut across the narrow barrier (valley) between the heart chamber and arteries, if the cost function is based on intensity. With the fuzzy connectedness tree, this will never happen as long as the strength of the connectedness path between the root seed and distal end is somewhat higher than the lowest intensity of the barrier. Possibly, more accurate centerlines could be obtained by using Hessian-based filters instead of Gaussian filters to correct the distorted centerlines, but in coronary CTA, according to our experience, the latter is sufficient and probably more time-effective.

In summary, this study has shown that the CFCT algorithm is a promising segmentation and skeletonization tool for coronary CTA, requiring only limited interaction by the user. A clinical evaluation of this algorithm will be reported in a separate paper. Other future work includes applying the method to MRA datasets and extending 3D segmentation to 4D datasets for handling dynamic multiple phase CTA.

References

1. Kirbas, C., Quek, F.K.H.: Vessel Extraction Techniques and Algorithms: A Survey. In: Third IEEE Symposium on BioInformatics and BioEngineering, pp. 238–245 (2003)
2. Marquering, H., Dijkstra, J., Koning, P., de, S.B., Reiber, J.H.C.: Towards quantitative analysis of coronary CTA. Int. J. Cardiovasc. Imaging 21, 73–84 (2005)
3. Florin, C., Paragios, N., Williams, J.: Particle Filters. A Quasi-Monte Carlo Solution for Segmentation of Coronaries. In: Medical Image Computing and Computer-Assisted Intervention MICCAI, pp. 246–253 (2005)
4. Khan, M.F., Wesarg, S., Gurung, J., Dogan, S., Maataoui, A., Brehmer, B., Herzog, C., Ackermann, H., Aßmus, B., Vogl, T.: Facilitating coronary artery evaluation in MDCT using a 3D automatic vessel segmentation tool. Eur. Radiol. 16, 1789–1795 (2006)
5. Udupa, J.K., Saha, P.K.: Fuzzy connectedness and image segmentation. Proceedings of the IEEE 91, 1649–1669 (2003)
6. Tizon, X., Smedby, Ö.: Segmentation with gray-scale connectedness can separate arteries and veins in MRA. J. Magn. Reson. Imaging 15, 438–445 (2002)
7. Löfving, A., Tizon, X., Persson, A., Wiklund, G., Smedby, Ö.: Virtual contrast injection – a software tool for selective visualization of vessel structures. Eur. Radiol. 15, 425 (2005)
8. Löfving, A., Tizon, X., Persson, A., Smedby, Ö.: Angiographic visualization of the coronary arteries in computed tomography angiography with virtual contrast injection. The Internet Journal of Radiology 4 (2006)
9. Dijkstra, E.W.: A Note on Two Problems in Connexion with Graphs. Numer. Math. 1, 269–271 (1959)
10. Borgefors, G.: On digital distance transforms in three dimensions. Computer Vision and Image Understanding 64, 368–376 (1996)
11. Bitter, I., Kaufman, A.E., Sato, M.: Penalized-distance volumetric skeleton algorithm. IEEE Transactions on Visualization and Computer Graphics 7, 195–206 (2001)

Mixtures of Gaussians on Tensor Fields for DT-MRI Segmentation

Rodrigo de Luis-García and Carlos Alberola-López

ETSI Telecomunicación, University of Valladolid, Valladolid, Spain
{rodlui,caralb}@tel.uva.es

Abstract. In this paper, an original approach for the segmentation of tensor fields is proposed. Based on the modeling of the data by means of Gaussian mixtures directly in the tensor domain, this technique presents a wide range of applications in medical image processing, particularly for Diffusion Tensor Magnetic Resonance Imaging (DT-MRI). The performance of the segmentation method proposed is shown through the segmentation of the corpus callosum from a dataset of 32 DT-MRI volumes. Comparison with a recent and related segmentation approach is favorable to our method, showing its capability for the automatic extraction of anatomical structures in the white matter.

1   Introduction

DT-MRI is a medical imaging modality which provides, at each voxel, a symmetric second order tensor that describes the diffusion of water molecules [1]. The diffusion tensor can be thought of as the covariance matrix of a zero-mean trivariate Gaussian distribution that models the diffusion, and is represented by a symmetric and positive definite (SPD) 3×3 matrix. Brain imaging is the most common application of diffusion MRI, as it can be employed for the visualization of the fibre tracts in the white matter of the brain.

DT-MRI has proved to be particularly relevant in a wide range of neurological clinical pathologies, such as ischemia, multiple sclerosis or schizophrenia, among others. The interested reader is referred to [2,3] for a comprehensive introduction to the applications of DT-MRI to brain diseases.

The segmentation of anatomical structures from DT-MRI data is a relatively new topic in medical image processing. In the last years, several authors have addressed the issue of segmentation of white matter internal structures from DT-MRI data, such as the *corpus callosum* or the *corona radiata* [4,5,6,7,8,9,10,11].

Initially, most of the methods intended for the segmentation of tensor fields were based on scalar or vector values extracted from the tensors [4]. Later, segmentation methods have been proposed working directly in the tensor domain, using tensor dissimilarity measures. Feddern *et al.* first proposed a level set segmentation method that directly worked on tensor data [5]. In [6] a modified *k-means* algorithm was proposed by Wiegell *et al.* to segment the thalamic nuclei from DT-MRI, using a combination of the Mahalanobis voxel distance and the Frobenius tensor distance.

N. Ayache, S. Ourselin, A. Maeder (Eds.): MICCAI 2007, Part I, LNCS 4791, pp. 319–326, 2007.
© Springer-Verlag Berlin Heidelberg 2007

In [12], Wang and Vemuri proposed the use of a region-based active contour model for the segmentation of tensor fields, using the Frobenius norm of the difference of tensors as a tensor dissimilarity measure.

Jonasson *et al.*, in [11], faced the segmentation of DT-MRI data from a perspective somehow inspired on a fibre tracking approach. In a level set framework, the speed propagation of the front is proportional to the similarity between the tensors lying on the front and its neighbors, measured in terms of the *normalized tensor scalar product*.

Wang and Vemuri introduced in [7] a new tensor dissimilarity measure, the Kullback-Leibler (KL) divergence. Starting from the KL divergence, a level set is evolved minimizing an energy functional derived from the *Active Contours Without Edges* model [13]. This segmentation approach was successfully tested on real DT-MRI data. Its main drawback is, coherently with the Chan & Vese model on which it is grounded, its limitation to a piecewise constant model.

In [8], Lenglet *et al.* presented a segmentation approach that proposes the minimization of an energy functional based on the Gaussian modeling of the KL distances from the tensor at each voxel to the mean tensor over each region, thus improving the segmentation with the Chan & Vese model. A new tensor dissimilarity measure, the geodesic distance, was also introduced and applied in this segmentation approach.

Later, Lenglet *et al.* proposed a definition of Gaussian distributions between diffusion tensors [14,10], that are incorporated into the probabilistic setting of the *Geodesic Active Regions* (GAR) model [15]. This segmentation method has shown to be capable of successfully segmenting internal white matter anatomical structures such as the corpus callosum. However, its performance is limited by the Gaussian modeling of the data; problems can be encountered if the complexity of the data is high enough so as to render the model too simplistic, a fact that affects the robustness and accuracy of the segmentation.

In this paper, a novel segmentation method for tensor-valued data is presented based on the definition of mixtures of Gaussians (MoG) over tensor fields. The model introduced here is, consequently, a generalization of the former proposals, and it is aimed at providing more flexibility in the segmentation and the capability to deal with more complex distributions in the data. The segmentation is performed in a region-oriented level set framework, following the GAR model.

In order to illustrate the performance of the proposed segmentation method, the corpus callosum has been segmented out of a set of 32 DT-MRI volumes. The segmentation of this anatomical structure has been addressed in many of the tensor field segmentation approaches in the literature [4,8,9,10,11], and is therefore a good choice for benchmarking. However, the performance of the segmentation approaches in the literature has been customarily validated on a single or few volumes, and a study on a larger dataset has not been performed before.

The remainder of this paper is organized as follows: next section presents the proposed segmentation method, from the definition of MoG on tensors to the derivation of the level set evolution equation. In Section 3, experimental work is presented and discussed in order to validate the method proposed. Finally, a brief summary is presented.

2   Segmentation Method

2.1   Gaussian Mixtures on Tensors

In the work by Lenglet *et al.* [14,10], a Gaussian distribution between tensors belonging to the manifold $S^+(3, \mathbb{R})$ of the 3×3 real, SPD matrices was defined with the following probability density function (PDF):

$$p(\mathbf{T}_i|\bar{\mathbf{T}}, \mathbf{\Lambda}) = \frac{1}{\sqrt{(2\pi)^6|\mathbf{\Lambda}|}} \exp\left(-\frac{\varphi(\boldsymbol{\beta}_i)^T \mathbf{\Lambda}^{-1} \varphi(\boldsymbol{\beta}_i)}{2}\right) \tag{1}$$

The following elements need to be specified to complete the description of the Gaussian distribution:

- $\mathbf{T}_i$ is the 3×3 tensor located at voxel i in Ω.
- $\bar{\mathbf{T}}$ is the empirical mean tensor over a set of N diffusion tensors.
- $\mathbf{\Lambda}$ is the associated covariance matrix, whose size is 6×6 for a 3×3 tensor (that is, the number of free components).
- The symmetric matrix $\boldsymbol{\beta}_i$ is defined, for a given metric $\mathcal{D}_x$, by $\boldsymbol{\beta}_i = -\nabla_{\mathbf{T}_i}\mathcal{D}_x$ $(\mathbf{T}_i, \bar{\mathbf{T}})$.
- The map $\varphi : S^+(3, \mathbb{R}) \mapsto \mathbb{R}^6$ associates to each matrix $\boldsymbol{\beta}_i$ its 6 free components.

The definition of the Gaussian distribution is general in terms of the metric employed. In their work, Lenglet *et al.* considered three different choices: Euclidean metric, KL divergence and geodesic distance. As empirical evidence favours the geodesic distance [14,10], it will be employed in this work.

Starting from the definition of Gaussian PDF over tensor fields defined before, we now define a new PDF composed of a mixture of Gaussians. For a mixture of K Gaussians, the PDF for a tensor $\mathbf{T}_i$ will be:

$$p(\mathbf{T}_i|\mathbf{\Theta}) = \sum_{k=1}^{K} \alpha_k \frac{1}{\sqrt{(2\pi)^d|\mathbf{\Lambda}_k|}} \exp\left(-\frac{\varphi(\boldsymbol{\beta}_{i,k})^T \mathbf{\Lambda}_k^{-1} \varphi(\boldsymbol{\beta}_{i,k})}{2}\right) \tag{2}$$

where we denote by $\mathbf{\Theta}$ the set of parameters: $\alpha_k, k = 1, \ldots, K$ are the mixing probabilities of the different components of the mixture, and each Gaussian distribution is characterized by its mean tensor $\bar{\mathbf{T}}_k$ and its covariance matrix $\mathbf{\Lambda}_k$.

In order to estimate the parameter vector $\mathbf{\Theta}$, a *Maximum Likelihood* (ML) approach by means of the EM algorithm will be followed, as it is customary for Gaussian mixtures. Hereafter, and in order to simplify the notation, we will express the dependencies of φ_i simply as $\varphi_i(\bar{\mathbf{T}}_k)$ (note that $\varphi_i = \varphi(\boldsymbol{\beta}_i)$ and $\boldsymbol{\beta}_i = \boldsymbol{\beta}_i(\bar{\mathbf{T}}_k)$. The log-likelihood we seek to maximize will be given by

$$\log(\mathcal{L}) = \sum_{i=1}^{N} \log\left(p(\mathbf{T}_i|\mathbf{\Theta})\right) = \sum_{i=1}^{N} \log\left(\sum_{k=1}^{K} \alpha_k g_k(\mathbf{T}_i|\mathbf{\Theta}_k)\right) \tag{3}$$

where we have denoted by $g_k(\mathbf{T}_i|\boldsymbol{\Theta}_k)$ the PDF of each of the components of the mixture, with parameters $\boldsymbol{\Theta}_k = \{\alpha_k, \bar{\mathbf{T}}_k, \boldsymbol{\Lambda}_k\}$. We first derive the log-likelihood with respect to the mean tensor $\bar{\mathbf{T}}_k$:

$$\frac{\partial}{\partial \bar{\mathbf{T}}_k} \log(\mathcal{L}) = \sum_{i=1}^{N} \frac{1}{\sum_{k=1}^{K} \alpha_k g_k(\mathbf{T}_i|\boldsymbol{\Theta}_k)} \frac{\partial}{\partial \bar{\mathbf{T}}_k} \left(\sum_{k=1}^{K} \alpha_k g_k(\mathbf{T}_i|\boldsymbol{\Theta}_k) \right) \quad (4)$$

$$= \sum_{i=1}^{N} \frac{1}{\sum_{k=1}^{K} \alpha_k g_k(\mathbf{T}_i|\boldsymbol{\Theta}_k)} \alpha_k g_k(\mathbf{T}_i|\boldsymbol{\Theta}_k) \frac{\partial}{\partial \bar{\mathbf{T}}_k} \left[-\frac{1}{2} (\boldsymbol{\varphi}_i(\bar{\mathbf{T}}_k))^T \boldsymbol{\Lambda}_k^{-1} (\boldsymbol{\varphi}_i(\bar{\mathbf{T}}_k)) \right]$$

In order to provide a more compact expression, we can reformulate the Gaussian distributions on tensors as distributions on vectors, where tensor $\mathbf{T}_i$ is represented by its free components, $\mathbf{t}_i$. Using this representation, the derivative we need to compute can be rewritten:

$$\frac{\partial}{\partial \bar{\mathbf{t}}_k} \left[(\boldsymbol{\varphi}_i(\bar{\mathbf{t}}_k))^T \boldsymbol{\Lambda}^{-1} (\boldsymbol{\varphi}_i(\bar{\mathbf{t}}_k)) \right] = \frac{\partial}{\partial \boldsymbol{\varphi}_i} \left[(\boldsymbol{\varphi}_i(\bar{\mathbf{t}}_k))^T \boldsymbol{\Lambda}^{-1} (\boldsymbol{\varphi}_i(\bar{\mathbf{t}}_k)) \right] \frac{\partial \boldsymbol{\varphi}_i}{\partial \bar{\mathbf{t}}_k}$$

$$= (\boldsymbol{\varphi}_i(\bar{\mathbf{t}}_k))^T \boldsymbol{\Lambda}^{-1} \frac{\partial \boldsymbol{\varphi}_i}{\partial \bar{\mathbf{t}}_k} \quad (5)$$

Indeed, $\frac{\partial \boldsymbol{\varphi}_i}{\partial \bar{\mathbf{t}}_k}$ depends on the choice of the tensor distance, and therefore a closed-form expression for the mean tensor cannot be obtained in general. The mean tensor is obtained instead by means of a gradient-ascent evolution process:

$$\bar{\mathbf{t}}_k^{(t+1)} = \bar{\mathbf{t}}_k^{(t)} + \Delta t \frac{\partial}{\partial \bar{\mathbf{t}}_k^{(t)}} \log(\mathcal{L})$$

$$= \bar{\mathbf{t}}_k^{(t)} + \Delta t \sum_{i=1}^{N} \frac{\alpha_k g_k(\mathbf{t}_i|\boldsymbol{\Theta}_k)}{\sum_{k=1}^{K} \alpha_k g_k(\mathbf{t}_i|\boldsymbol{\Theta}_k)} (\boldsymbol{\varphi}_i(\bar{\mathbf{t}}_k^{(t)}))^T \boldsymbol{\Lambda}^{-1} \frac{\partial \boldsymbol{\varphi}_i(\bar{\mathbf{t}}_k^{(t)})}{\partial \bar{\mathbf{t}}_k^{(t)}} \quad (6)$$

If a random initialization is employed for the $\bar{\mathbf{t}}_k^{(0)}$, the iterative process is likely to get stuck in local maxima. Therefore, a k-means algorithm is performed previously to the gradient ascent, so as to obtain the initial mean tensors of each component of the mixture.

With regard to the estimation of the parameters $\boldsymbol{\Lambda}_k$ and α_k, their derivation does not change with respect to a vector-valued MoG:

$$\hat{\boldsymbol{\Lambda}}_k = \frac{\sum_{i=1}^{N} p(k|i)(\boldsymbol{\varphi}_i(\bar{\mathbf{T}}_k))(\boldsymbol{\varphi}_i(\bar{\mathbf{T}}_k))^T}{\sum_{i=1}^{N} p(k|i)} \qquad \hat{\alpha}_k = \frac{1}{N} \sum_{i=1}^{N} p(k|i)$$

$$p(k|i) = \frac{\alpha_k g_k(\mathbf{T}_i|\boldsymbol{\Theta}_k)}{\sum_{k=1}^{K} \alpha_k g_k(\mathbf{T}_i|\boldsymbol{\Theta}_k)} \quad (7)$$

For the estimation of the complexity of the MoG, we will follow the approach by Figueiredo et al. [16], based on the use of the MDL (*Minimum Description Length*) criterion and implemented by means of a modified EM algorithm that leads to an integrated model selection and estimation procedure. A maximum number of 5 components was set for each mixture to run the complexity selection algorithm. In practice, for most of the segmentation experiments 3 or 4 components were obtained. It was additionally verified that if the above mentioned maximum was increased (say 6,7), more than 5 components were never selected.

2.2   Level Set Evolution

Based on the well-known GAR model [15], the segmentation we seek to perform is formulated as the minimization of the following energy functional:

$$E(\mathcal{C}, \mathbf{\Theta_1}, \mathbf{\Theta_2}) = -\int_{\Omega_1} \log p(\mathbf{T(x)}|\mathbf{\Theta_1}) d\mathbf{x} - \int_{\Omega_2} \log p(\mathbf{T(x)}|\mathbf{\Theta_2}) d\mathbf{x} + \nu|\mathcal{C}| \quad (8)$$

where $p(\mathbf{T(x)}|\mathbf{\Theta_i})$ follows the MoG model introduced in the preceding section. In order to perform the segmentation, the energy functional must be minimized with respect to the statistical parameters $\mathbf{\Theta_i}$ and to the segmenting surface, that is represented by means of the level set function ϕ. This is done following the two-step *Expectation-Maximization* technique [17]. For a fixed level set, the statistical parameters are updated with their ML estimators. Next, the segmenting surface is evolved following the level set equation

$$\frac{\partial \phi}{\partial t}(\mathbf{x}) = \delta(\phi)\left[\nu\nabla \cdot (\frac{\nabla\phi}{|\nabla\phi|}) - \frac{p(\mathbf{T(x)}|\mathbf{\Theta_1})}{p(\mathbf{T(x)}|\mathbf{\Theta_2})}\right] \quad (9)$$

where $\delta(\phi)$ is the Dirac function. In the next section, we evaluate the performance of the method proposed through the experimentation on real DT-MRI data.

3   Experimental Results and Comparisons

Experiments were conducted on the extraction of the corpus callosum from a set of real DT-MRI data in order to validate the segmentation method proposed. Comparisons were also performed with a related recent approach in the literature.

Data acquisition: The employed dataset consists of DT-MRI volumes of 32 subjects, which were acquired on a 1.5 Tesla scanner. The acquisition parameters were: b value = 1000 sec$/mm^2$, TE=1000 msec, TR=89 msec, along six diffusion-sensitizing directions. The images were obtained on 79 planes with 128 x 128 pixels per slice [1]. An example of the resulting DT-MRI volumes is shown in Figure 1, where color coding of the main tensor orientation has been employed.

Experiments: As for initial contours, the body of the corpus callosum was roughly delineated for 3 central sagittal slices of the volume, upon the visualization of the *fractional anisotropy*, FA [18]. The delineation and the resulting initial surface are shown for a sample volume in Figure 1.

In order to illustrate the overall performance for all the volumes in the employed dataset, in Figure 2 we reproduce all the obtained segmentation results. A successful segmentation was achieved for all cases, proving MoG to be a robust

---

[1] This volume dataset was kindly made available by the Signal Processing Institute at the École Polytechnique Fédérale de Laussane, within a research collaboration under the scope of the 6th Framework Program Network of Excellence *SIMILAR*. This is thankfully acknowledged.

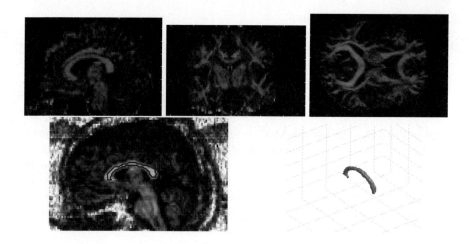

Fig. 1. Color coding of the main orientation in a sagittal, coronal and axial slice in a sample DT-MRI volume (top). Red means antero-posterior, green means left-right and blue inferior-superior. Delineation of the initial contour for the mid-sagittal slice, and initial level set surface (bottom).

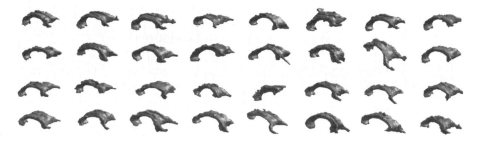

Fig. 2. Segmentation results for the corpus callosum of the 32 DT-MRI volumes using MoG on tensors proposed in this paper

model for the data. It can be also seen that the obtained segmentation is capable to capture both the genu and the splenium of the corpus callosum, which are the most difficult regions to segment.

For comparison purposes, we also show some segmentation results of our approach compared to those of the segmentation method in [14,10], based on the Gaussian modeling of the tensor probability density function (geodesic distance was also employed for this segmentation method, together with the same initial surfaces and identical segmentation parameters). Although this approach was able to obtain good segmentation results on the employed dataset, it encounters some problems in the region of the splenium in some cases when compared to the MoG approach, and it shows lower accuracy for some other subjects. In Figure 3, the segmentation results on a number of volumes show a better segmentation in the region of the splenium for the MoG model proposed in this paper. This

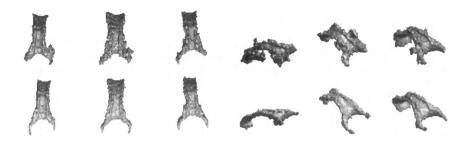

Fig. 3. Views of the segmentation results for the corpus callosum of different volumes using Gaussian model [14,10] (red) and MoG model proposed in this paper (green). Results show a better accuracy of our approach in the region of the splenium (three left cases), and a higher robustness to artifacts (three right cases).

increased performance is related to the ability of the MoG to capture a higher complexity in the data with respect to the single Gaussian model. In the same figure, some other segmentation results are shown where the MoG model shows a better accuracy than that of the Gaussian model, whose results present certain artifacts.

4   Summary

We have presented a novel technique for the segmentation of tensor fields applied to the extraction of anatomical structures from the brain white matter. The method is based on the definition of Gaussian mixtures on tensor-valued data, and experimental work on the segmentation of the corpus callosum from a large dataset of DT-MRI volumes shows a very good behaviour of the proposed model. Comparison with a recent and related approach based on a single Gaussian modeling is favorable in terms of the segmentation detail in specific areas such as the region of the splenium or robustness in the segmentation. We are currently working on the segmentation of other anatomical structures in the white matter and the shape analysis of the obtained structures.

Acknowledgments

The authors acknowledge the CICyT for research grant TEC2004-06647-C03-01, the FIS for grant PI-041483 and the European Commission for the funds associated to the NoE SIMILAR (FP6- 507609).

References

1. Bihan, D.L., Breton, E., Lallemand, D., Grenier, P., Cabanis, E., Laval-Jeantet, M.: MR imaging of intravoxel incoherent motions: Application to diffusion and perfusion in neurologic disorders. Radiology 161, 401–407 (1986)

2. Sundgren, P.C., Dong, Q., Gómez-Hassan, D., Mukherji, S.K., Maly, P., Welsh, R.: Diffusion tensor imaging of the brain: review of clinical applications. Neuroradiology 46, 339–350 (2004)
3. Horsfield, M., Jones, D.: Applications of diffusion-weighted and diffusion tensor MRI to white matter diseases-a review. NMR in Biomedicine 15, 570–577 (2002)
4. Zhukov, L., Museth, K., Breen, D., Whitaker, R., Barr, A.H.: Level set segmentation and modeling of DT-MRI human brain data. Journal of Electronic Imaging 12, 125–133 (2003)
5. Feddern, C., Weickert, J., Burgeth, B.: Level set methods for tensor-valued images. In: Proc. of the 9th IEEE Workshop on Variational, Geometric and Level Set Methods in Computer Vision, Nice, France, pp. 65–72 (2003)
6. Wiegell, M.R., Tuch, D.S., Larsson, H.B.W., Wedeen, V.J.: Automatic segmentation of thalamic nuclei from diffusion tensor magnetic resonance imaging. NeuroImage 19, 391–401 (2003)
7. Wang, Z., Vemuri, B.: An affine invariant tensor dissimilarity measure and its applications to tensor-valued image segmentation. In: Proc. of the IEEE Conference on CVPR, Washington DC, USA, pp. 228–233 (2004)
8. Lenglet, C., Rousson, M., Deriche, R.: Segmentation of 3d probability density fields by surface evolution: Application to diffusion MRI. In: Barillot, C., Haynor, D.R., Hellier, P. (eds.) MICCAI 2004. LNCS, vol. 3216, Springer, Heidelberg (2004)
9. Lenglet, C., Rousson, M., Deriche, R., Faugeras, O., Lehéricy, S., Ugurbil, K.: A Riemannian approach to diffusion tensor images segmentation. In: Proc. of Information Processing in Medical Imaging, Glenwood Springs, CO, USA (2005)
10. Lenglet, C., Rousson, M., Deriche, R.: DTI segmentation by statistical surface evolution. IEEE Transactions on Medical Imaging 25, 685–700 (2006)
11. Jonasson, L., Bresson, X., Hagmann, P., Cuisenaire, O., Meuli, R., Thiran, J.P.: White matter fiber tract segmentation in DT-MRI using geometric flows. Medical Image Analysis 9, 223–236 (2005)
12. Wang, Z., Vemuri, B.: Tensor field segmentation using region based active contour model. In: Proc. of the ECCV, Prague, Czech Republic, pp. 304–315 (2004)
13. Chan, T.F., Vese, L.A.: Active contours without edges. IEEE Trans. on Image Processing 10, 266–277 (2001)
14. Lenglet, C., Rousson, M., Deriche, R., Faugeras, O.: Statistics on the manifold of multivariate normal distributions: theory and application to diffusion tensor MRI processing. Journal of Mathematical Imaging and Vision 25, 423–444 (2006)
15. Paragios, N., Deriche, R.: Geodesic active regions: A new framework to deal with frame partition problems in computer vision. Journal of Visual Communication and Image Representation 13, 249–268 (2002)
16. Figueiredo, M., Leitao, J.M.N., Jain, A.K.: Unsupervised selection and estimation of finite mixture models. In: Proc. ICPR, Barcelona, Spain pp. 2087–2090 (2000)
17. Dempster, A., Laird, N., Rubin, D.: Maximum likelihood from incomplete data via the EM algorithm. Journal of the Royal Statistical Society 39, 1–38 (1977)
18. Basser, P., Pierpaoli, C.: Microstructural and physiological features of tissues elucidated by quantitative-diffusion tensor MRI. Journal of Magnetic Resonance B, 209–219 (1996)

Soft Level Set Coupling for LV Segmentation in Gated Perfusion SPECT

Timo Kohlberger, Gareth Funka-Lea, and Vladimir Desh

Siemens Corporate Research, Imaging and Visualization Department,
Princeton, NJ 08540, USA

Abstract. We present a new segmentation approach for the myocardium in gated and non-gated perfusion SPECT images. To this end, we represent the epi- and endocardium by separate signed distance functions and couple them by a soft constraint to give explicit control over the wall thickness. By an explicit modeling of the basal plane, the volume of the blood pool as well as the myocardium are determinable. Furthermore, prior shape information is incorporated by applying a kernel density estimation on a number of expert segmentations in a low-dimensional PCA subspace. Thereby, information along the time axis is fully taken into account by employing 4-dimensional embedding functions.

1   Introduction

Model-based imaging analysis of the left ventricle (LV) has gained an important role in diagnosis and treatment of heart diseases. Segmentation of the blood pool and myocardium has found to be a significant prerequisite of further quantitative analysis, such as the estimation of the ejection fraction within one cardiac cycle. The simultaneous assessment of myocardial perfusion and function with single photon emission computed tomography (SPECT) is a standard in clinical imaging practice [9].

In general, shape modeling has been done with either explicit representations by landmarks or binary images/volumes are employed, or implicit ones, describing the separating three-dimensional contour as the zero-level set of a four dimensional function [8]. In most cases, Principal Component Analysis (PCA) thereby is employed, which is, in case of explicit shape representations, either directly applied to the landmark coordinates or the components of deformations fields relative to a mean shape, or, for the implicit representations, to the components of the embedding level set functions. In addition, a prior shape probabilities are inferred from a number of representative training samples, in order to compensate for sparse image information.

On the other hand, prior information can also be incorporated in a non-statistical manner, such as the prior knowledge that the boundaries of an anatomical structure adhere to a certain geometrical relation. With the LV for example, it is known that the Euclidean distance (thickness) between the epi- and endocardium varies within a certain range. The same holds true for the cerebral

N. Ayache, S. Ourselin, A. Maeder (Eds.): MICCAI 2007, Part I, LNCS 4791, pp. 327–334, 2007.
© Springer-Verlag Berlin Heidelberg 2007

cortex as the outermost layer of the gray matter in the brain. Several work has been done exploiting this fact for either application scenario, either by highly heuristical, explicit approaches [4,2], or implicit ones [11,5,6,10,13]. With respect to the modeling of the thickness prior, all approaches being known to us thereby modify well-known edge-based or region-based data terms mostly on the basis of propagation equations, by adding more or less continuous scalar modulator functions measuring the Euclidean distance between the two surfaces. By this, the surface propagating 'forces' are adapted in order to keep the two surfaces at a certain distance in a more or less strict manner. Furthermore, with all approaches only closed surfaces are considered, which is not true for the epi- and endicardiac shape when excluding the basal plane.

As opposed to them, in Section 2, we present a new soft thickness term for the epi- and endocardium, which is separate from the existing data terms. This is realized via a formulation as an energy minimization, thereby giving a clear geometrical meaning without any heuristics involved. In addition, we address and give a solution to the problem of coupled open surfaces. In Section 3 we approximate the level sets description by a compact PCA subspace representation, which is followed by the introduction of a known prior shape probability term [12]. Subsequently, we extend the approach to spatio-temporal domain (4D) in application to gated SPECT data. After giving details on the energy minimization in Section 3.4, in Sec. 4 we present experimental results on 3D phantom data as well as expert annotated 4D data showing promising qualitative and quantitative results.

2   The Data Model

Let $I \in H^1(\Omega)$ denote a function of SPECT intensities on the closed rectangular volume $\Omega \in R^3$. We propose to model the epi- and endocardium implicitly as the zero level sets of the two singed distance functions $\phi_{ep}(\mathbf{x})$ and $\phi_{en}(\mathbf{x})$, [8], by which the bloodpool segment is described by $\{\mathbf{x} \mid \phi_{en}(\mathbf{x}) > 0\}$, the myocardium segment by $\{\mathbf{x} \mid \phi_{en}(\mathbf{x}) < 0 \land \phi_{ep}(\mathbf{x}) > 0\}$, and the background locations by $\{\mathbf{x} \mid \phi_{ep}(\mathbf{x}) < 0\}$.

Following the approach by Mumford and Shah, we then assume the SPECT intensities inside these three regions (bloodpool, myocardium, background) have similar values. While denoting the intensity means for each of the regions by μ_{bp}, μ_{my}, and μ_{bg}, we implicitly seek for those region boundaries which minimize the sum of deviations from each of the corresponding (empricial) means. We formulate this by minimizing the energy

$$E_{rn}(\phi_{ep}, \phi_{en}) = \int_{\Omega} |I - \mu_{bp}|^2 H_\epsilon(\phi_{en}) + |I - \mu_{my}|^2 \left(1 - H_\epsilon(\phi_{en})\right) H_\epsilon(\phi_{ep})$$

$$+ |I - \mu_{bg}|^2 \left(1 - H_\epsilon(\phi_{ep})\right) d\mathbf{x} \qquad (1)$$

with respect to ϕ_{ep} and ϕ_{en}, where H_ϵ refers to the approximate Heaviside step function, see [1]. However, E_{rn} obviously has many local minima with respect to ϕ_{ep} and ϕ_{en} and thus a minimization algorithm's result would highly depend on the initialization. In order to narrow down the number of local wrong minima, we suggest to introduce a soft constraint on the wall thickness of the myocardium. In terms of mathematical modeling, note that such a distance constraint can be easily realized here due to the implicit representation of the epi- and endocardium by signed distance functions. Excluding all locations beyond an infinite plane B, which is considered an approximation of the real basal plane section, a hard thickness constraint can be stated by $\phi_{ep}(\mathbf{x}) - d_{wall} - \phi_{en}(\mathbf{x}) = 0$, where d_{wall} denotes a given wall thickness. As a soft constraint, this can be realized by weighting and adding the energy term

$$E_{th}(\phi_{ep}, \phi_{en}) = \int_{\Omega} \Big(\phi_{en} - (\phi_{ep} - d_{wall})\Big)^2 d\mathbf{x} \qquad (2)$$

to (1). Unfortunately, (2) results in undesired solutions for ϕ_{ep} and ϕ_{en} for locations at or above the approximate basal plane B, since at B the zero level sets of both distance functions are assumed to coincide. As a remedy, we propose to limit the support of either distance function, such that the new support $\Omega_B \subset \Omega \in \mathbb{R}^3$ is bounded by B from above (excluding B), and replace every previous occurrence of ϕ_{ep} and ϕ_{en} by

$$\tilde{\phi}_{ep,B}(\mathbf{x}) := \begin{cases} \phi_{ep}(\mathbf{x}) & : \mathbf{x} \in \Omega_B \\ -d_{wall} & : \mathbf{x} \in \Omega \setminus \Omega_B \end{cases} \qquad \tilde{\phi}_{en,B}(\mathbf{x}) := \begin{cases} \phi_{en}(\mathbf{x}) & : \mathbf{x} \in \Omega_B \\ -2d_{wall} & : \mathbf{x} \in \Omega \setminus \Omega_B \end{cases} \qquad (3)$$

respectively[1]. By this, E_{th} has no effect at locations above and on B, whereas with E_{rn} they are considered as background, due to the substitutes $\tilde{\phi}_{ep,B}$ and $\tilde{\phi}_{ep,B}$ being negative there. Furthermore, because of $\tilde{\phi}_{ep}$ and $\tilde{\phi}_{en}$ being negative at locations at or above B, with the region model in (1), they are considered as background. Finally, the data model is crafted as a minimization of the weighted energies

$$E_{data}(\phi_{ep}, \phi_{en}, B) := E_{rn}(\tilde{\phi}_{ep,B}, \tilde{\phi}_{en,B}) + \omega_{th} E_{th}(\tilde{\phi}_{ep}, \tilde{\phi}_{ep}), \qquad (4)$$

with respect to ϕ_{ep} and ϕ_{en} on Ω_B, as well as the location and orientation of the basal plane B. Thereby, the scalar weight ω_{th} allows to adjust the extend of deviations from the given thickness.

3   The Shape Model

3.1   Parametrization in PCA Subspaces

Despite the additional thickness constraint, own experiments suggest that E_{data} still exhibits too many local minima of wrong segmentations, thus leaving the minimization highly dependent on the initialization. For that reason, we propose to incorporate prior shape knowledge derived from a shape model in addition.

---

[1] Note that $\tilde{\phi}_{ep,B}$ $\tilde{\phi}_{ep,B}$ are not signed distance functions and are possibly discontinuous at B.

In particular, given a set of N expert-segmented training shapes $\{\phi_i(\mathbf{x})\}_{i=1...N}$ of the epi- and endocardium, and the basal plane, we follow the approach by Rousson et al. [12] where a kernel density estimation is employed in a finite subspace spanned by the training shapes.

Each of the training shapes are first aligned with respect to translation and scale in R^3, which is implemented by minimizing the squared L^2-distance between ϕ_i and a chosen reference shape ϕ_{ref}:

$$\min_{\theta,\boldsymbol{t}} \int_\Omega \Big(\phi_i\big(\boldsymbol{R}(\theta)\mathbf{x} - \boldsymbol{t}, t\big) - \phi_{ref}(\mathbf{x}, t)\Big)^2 dx \ , \tag{5}$$

where $\boldsymbol{t} \in R^3$ denotes a translation vector and $\boldsymbol{R}(\theta) \in \mathbb{R}^{3\times3}$ a rotation matrix depending on orientation descriptors θ, e.g. a quaternion. Based on the aligned training shapes, the mean $\overline{\phi} = \frac{1}{N}\sum_{i=1}^N \phi_i$ is determined and a principal component analysis (PCA) employed in order to obtain the eigenmodes $\{\phi_i(\mathbf{x})\}_{i=1...N}\}$ which reflect the shape variations within the aligned training set, relative to $\overline{\phi}$. Subsequently, new distance functions, which lie in the linear subspace given by the training set, can be approximated as linear combinations of the first $n < N$ eigenmodes:

$$\phi_{\boldsymbol{\alpha}}(\mathbf{x}) = \overline{\phi}(\mathbf{x}) + \sum_{i=1}^n \alpha_i \psi_i(\mathbf{x}) \ , \tag{6}$$

cf. [8]. By this, a low-dimensional approximate representation of the distance functions is reached.

In our case, however, each of the training shape ϕ_i can have a different support, depending on the position and orientation of the basal plane. Extending the support as done in (3) obviously would not lead to a feasible training set to the PCA, because of possible strong discontinuities of $\tilde{\phi}_{ep}$ and $\tilde{\phi}_{en}$ at B. Alternatively we propose to align them in a way that all basal planes B_i to coincide. The common support then is given by the intersection of all aligned supports Ω_{B_i} based on which the PCA can be applied in a straightforward manner.

In terms of the implementation of this special alignment, a simple method is given by first choosing a reference shape ϕ_{ref} whose basal plane B_{ref} is colinear with one of the Euclidean coordinates planes, say the x/y-plane. Secondly, each training shape ϕ_i is first aligned to ϕ_{ref} with respect to a rigid transform. Thirdly, assuming the basal plane B_i of the ridigly aligned ϕ_i to be approximately colinear with B_{ref}, a subsequent translation along the normal vector of B_{ref} by the distance between B_{ref} and B_i is made.

Finally, such parametrized realizations of epi- and endocardium shapes, $\phi_{ep,\boldsymbol{\alpha}}$ and $\phi_{en,\boldsymbol{\alpha}}$, are bound to the position and orientation of the reference shapes $\phi_{ep,ref}$ and $\phi_{en,ref}$ they were aligned to. In aiming to represent shapes at any location and orientation, be make us of the common approach to replace $\phi_{\kappa,\boldsymbol{\alpha}}(\mathbf{x})$ ($\kappa \in \{ep, en\}$) by $\phi_{ep,\boldsymbol{\alpha}}\big(\mathcal{T}_{\theta,\boldsymbol{t}}(\mathbf{x})\big)$, with $\mathcal{T}_{\theta,\boldsymbol{t}}$ being the rigid transform: $\mathcal{T}_{\theta,\boldsymbol{t}} : \mathbf{x} \mapsto \boldsymbol{R}(\theta)\mathbf{x} - \boldsymbol{t}$.

3.2 Prior Shape Probabilities by Kernel Density Estimation

In aiming at introducing prior shape information, Rousson et al. [12] suggest inferring a prior probability by utilizing a Parzen-Rosenblatt kernel density estimator:

$$P(\boldsymbol{\alpha}) = \frac{1}{N\sigma^n} \sum_{i=1}^{N} \exp\left(-\frac{(\boldsymbol{\alpha} - \boldsymbol{\alpha}_i)^2}{2\sigma^2}\right). \tag{7}$$

Thereby it is assumed single Gaussian distributions of uniform width σ at each training function ϕ_i being projected to the linear subspace by $\boldsymbol{\alpha}_i = \int_{[1,T]}\int_{\Omega}\psi_i(\mathbf{x},t)$ $(\phi(\mathbf{x},t) - \bar{\phi}(\mathbf{x},t))\,d\mathbf{x}\,dt$. As proposed in [12], reasonable choices for σ are given by the average nearest neighbor distance $\sigma^2 = \frac{1}{N}\sum_{i=1}^{N}\min_{j\neq i}|\boldsymbol{\alpha}_i - \boldsymbol{\alpha}_j|$. As opposed to implying one multivariate Gaussian as deployed in [8] (while utilizing the covariance σ^{-1} matrix of the PCA), the Parzen estimator results both in a more flexible and more accurate shape model based on the training shapes.

In terms of computational costs, evaluating (7) obviously requires more operations than a single Gaussian distribution, since a Gaussian has to be calculated for each training shape. However, because of the much lower dimensionality of the linear subspace employed in (6), in comparison to discretizations of the $\{\phi_i\}$, this has emerged to have only a minor practical impact.

Different experiments employing the shape prior (7) to $\phi_{\boldsymbol{\alpha}_{ep}}(\mathbf{x})$ or $\phi_{\boldsymbol{\alpha}_{en}}(\mathbf{x})$, or both, suggest that a prior model with respect to the epicardium is empirically sufficient. Thereby, $\phi_{\boldsymbol{\alpha}_{en}}(\mathbf{x})$ is affected by the shape model only indirectly via the thickness constraint, which leaves it more sensitive to the image data, and thus presumably yielding blood volumes which are more independent from prior information. Hence, (4) is extended by prior energy term $\omega_{pr}E_{prior}(\cdot) = -\omega_{pr}\log P(\cdot)$, whose influence is adjusted by the scalar weight ω_{pr}.

3.3   Including the Temporal Dimension

In gated perfusion SPECT, several intensity volumes of a moving heart are available at different time points t within the heart cycle $[0,T]$. As detailed in [7], it is reasonable to take also the information along the temporal dimension into account. Therefore, we propose to extend the current approach which relies on a three-dimensional spatial support Ω to the four-dimensional spatio-temporal support $\Omega \times [0,T]$. Consequently, $I(\mathbf{x})$ in (1) is to be replaced by a sequence of intensity volumes $I(\mathbf{x},t)$, $(\mathbf{x},t) \in \Omega \times [0,T]$, and any distance function $\phi(\mathbf{x})$ by $\phi(\mathbf{x},t)$, which describes separate shapes for every time point t.

By this, temporal dependencies now come into play by carrying out a PCA on a set of rigidly aligned *sequences of training shapes* $\{\phi_i(\mathbf{x},t)\}_{i=1...N}$, which, by a straightforward extension of the three-dimensional parametrization approach, yields a linear parametrization of shape sequences:

$$\phi_{\boldsymbol{\alpha}}(\mathbf{x},t) = \bar{\phi}(\mathbf{x},t) + \sum_{i=1}^{n} \alpha_i \psi_i(\mathbf{x},t). \tag{8}$$

Note that a linear weight α_i associated with the subspace dimension i effects the shapes at all time points $t \in [0,T]$. Consequently, $P(\phi(\mathbf{x},t))$ in (7) now infers the probability the of a shape sequence implicitly represented by $\phi(\mathbf{x},t)$ to occur given N training shape sequences implicitly encoded by $\{\phi(\mathbf{x},t)\}_{1,...,N}$.

3.4 Minimization

In aiming at solving the energy

$$E_{rn}\big(\tilde{\phi}_{\boldsymbol{\alpha}_{ep},\boldsymbol{t},\theta,B},\tilde{\phi}_{\boldsymbol{\alpha}_{en},\boldsymbol{t},\theta,B}\big) + \omega_{th}E_{th}\big(\tilde{\phi}_{\boldsymbol{\alpha}_{ep},\boldsymbol{t},\theta,B},\tilde{\phi}_{\boldsymbol{\alpha}_{en},\boldsymbol{t},\theta,B}\big) + \omega_{pr}E_{prior}(\boldsymbol{\alpha}_{ep})$$

with respect to the epi- and endocardial shape parameters $\boldsymbol{\alpha}_{ep}$ and $\boldsymbol{\alpha}_{en}$, the rigid transform parameters $\boldsymbol{t}$ and θ, as well as the plane B, it is required the first variation of (3.4) w.r.t. to the first four entities to vanish. To this end, the gradients for each of the involved energy terms read:

$$\frac{\partial E_{rn}}{\partial \phi_{ep}} = 2\Big(|I-\mu_{my}|^2\big(1-H_\epsilon(\phi_{en})\big)\,\delta_\epsilon(\phi_{ep}) - |I-\mu_{bg}|^2\,\delta_\epsilon(\phi_{ep})\Big),\quad\text{and}$$

$$\frac{\partial E_{rn}}{\partial \phi_{en}} = 2\Big(|I-\mu_{bp}|^2\,\delta_\epsilon(\phi_{en}) - |I-\mu_{my}|^2\,\delta_\epsilon(\phi_{en})\,H_\epsilon(\phi_{ep})\Big),$$

$$\frac{\partial E_{th}}{\partial \phi_{en}} = 2\Big(\phi_{en} - (\phi_{ep} - d_{wall})\Big),\quad \frac{\partial E_{th}}{\partial \phi_{ep}} = -2\Big(\phi_{en} - (\phi_{ep} - d_{wall})\Big),\quad\text{where}$$

$$\frac{\partial E_\xi}{\partial \boldsymbol{\alpha}_\kappa} = 2\int_{[1,T]}\int_\Omega \frac{\partial E_\xi}{\partial \phi_\kappa}(\mathbf{x})\,\psi_i(\mathbf{x},t)\,d\mathbf{x}\,dt,\quad \xi\in\{\text{rn, th}\},\ \kappa\in\{\text{ep, en}\},\text{ as well as}$$

$$\frac{\partial E_{prior}}{\partial \boldsymbol{\alpha}_i} = \frac{1}{\sigma^2}\frac{\sum_{i=1}^N(\boldsymbol{\alpha}-\boldsymbol{\alpha}_i)\,K_i}{\sum_{i=1}^N K_i},\quad\text{with}\quad K_i = \frac{1}{(2\pi)^{\frac{3}{2}}}\exp\left(-\frac{(\boldsymbol{\alpha}-\boldsymbol{\alpha}_i)^2}{2\sigma^2}\right),$$

where $\delta_\epsilon(\cdot)$ refers to the regularized Dirac measure. Gradients with respect to the rigid transform parameters are of the form:

$$\frac{\partial E_\kappa}{\partial \boldsymbol{t}} = \frac{\partial E_\kappa}{\partial \phi_{ep}}\nabla\phi_{ep}\frac{d\mathcal{T}}{d\boldsymbol{t}} + \frac{\partial E_\kappa}{\partial \phi_{en}}\nabla\phi_{en}\frac{d\mathcal{T}}{d\boldsymbol{t}},\ \frac{\partial E_\kappa}{\partial \theta} = \frac{\partial E_\kappa}{\partial \phi_{ep}}\nabla\phi_{ep}\frac{d\mathcal{T}}{d\boldsymbol{t}} + \frac{\partial E_\kappa}{\partial \phi_{ep}}\nabla\phi_{en}\frac{d\mathcal{T}}{d\theta}$$

with $\frac{d\mathcal{T}}{d\boldsymbol{t}} = -(1\ 1\ 1)^\top$ and $\frac{d\mathcal{T}}{d\theta} = \frac{\partial\mathbf{R}}{\partial\theta}\mathbf{x}$. Minimization with respect to B can be implemented by a fitting to the upper rim of the myocardium intensities in I.

4 Experimental Results and Discussion

The proposed approach has been implemented and and tested at several gated studies (8 time phases each), followed by qualitative and quantitative comparison to expert annotations. Parameters were selected manually and the same for all experiments ($\omega_{th} = 0.04, \omega_{pr} = 500, \sigma = 200$). In particular, the soft thickness constraint parameter d_{wall} was set to 13 mm. PCA was conducted and subsequent Parzen estimation carried out on 30 expert-annotated SPECT sequences (also 8 phases). $\overline{\phi}$ served as initialization of the level set propagation.

Two representative results are depicted in Fig. 1 including their corresponding blood volume diagrams, both in comparison to the expert references. The MPR views show a high overlap between the automated results and reference segmentation. Furthermore, the influence of the new thickness constraint becomes apparent, which lets the distance between the epi- and endocardium vary in a certain range. With respect to the input data, the left study shows that the algorithm

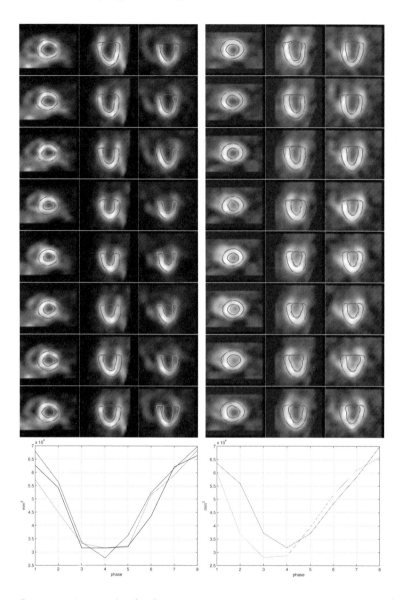

Fig. 1. Segmentation results (red) in comparison to an expert segmentations (green) for two different datasets. (a) and (b): Short axis and two long axis MPR views (left to right) for each of the eight heart phases (top to bottom, starting with ED). (c) and (d): Corresponding blood pool volume of the automated (red) and the expert segmentation(s) (green, and blue (if applicable)). Correlation factors: (c) automatic to green expert segmentation: 0.95, automatic to blue expert segm.: 0.97, green to blue expert segm.: 0.94 (inter-expert correlation), (d) automatic to expert segm.: 0.9. Ejection fractions: (c) automatic segm.: 60%, green expert segm. 52% expert, blue expert segm.: 53%, (d) automatic segm.: 52%, green expert segm. 54%.

is also able to detect the myocardial walls despite diminished image information (darker regions at the outer wall), which is compensated for by the prior shape model. In terms of the corresponding blood pool volumes, these and other experiments exhibit high correlation factors (0.95 and 0.9 here) which lie within the range of inter-expert variability, as well as close ejection fraction estimates.

We presented a segmentation approach for the bloodpool and myocardium in gated SPECT studies, which is based on a new thickness constraint between the epi- and endocardial shapes. By contrast to existing methods, this is realized on the basis of a sound energy minimization and kept separate from existing data-driven concepts, thereby giving explicit gradual control on its strength. First experiments yield good results with respect to expert annotations and suggest further studies on larger number of data sets.

References

1. Chan, T.F., Vese, L.A.: Active contours without edges. IEEE Trans. Image Processing 10(2), 266–277 (2001)
2. Faber, T., Cooke, C., Folks, R., Vansant, J., Nichols, K., De Puey, E., Pettigrew, R., Garcia, E.: Left ventricular function and perfusion from gated spect perfusion images: An integrated method. J. of Nuclear Medicine 40(4), 650–659 (1999)
3. Frangi, A.F., Rueckert, D., Schnabel, J.A., Niessen, W.J.: Automatic construction of multiple-object three-dimensional statistical shape models: Applications to cardiac modeling. IEEE Trans. Medical Imaging 21(9), 1151–1166 (2002)
4. Germano, G., Kavangh, P.B., Waechter, P., Areeda, J., Van Kriekinge, S., Sharir, T., Lewin, H.C., Berman, D.S.: A new algorithm for the quantitation of myocardial perfusion SPECT. I. J. of Nuclear Medicine 41(4), 712–719 (2000)
5. Goldenberg, R., Kimmel, R., Rivlin, E., Rudzsky, M.: Cortex segmentation: A fast variational geometric approach. IEEE T. Med. Im. 21(12), 1544–1551 (2002)
6. Gomes, J., Faugeras, O.: Reconciling distance functions and level sets. J. Visual Com. and Image Representation 11, 209–223 (2000)
7. Kohlberger, T., Cremers, D., Rousson, M., Ramaraj, R., Funka-Lea, G.: 4D shape priors for a level set segmentation of the left myocardium in SPECT sequences. In: Larsen, R., Nielsen, M., Sporring, J. (eds.) MICCAI 2006. LNCS, vol. 4190, pp. 92–100. Springer, Heidelberg (2006)
8. Leventon, M.E., Grimson, W.E., Faugeras, O.: Statistical shape influence in geodesic active contours. In: CVPR 2000, vol. 1, pp. 1316–1323. IEEE, Los Alamitos (2000)
9. Liu, Y., Sinusas, A., Khaimov, D., Gebuza, B., Wackers, F.: New hybrid count- and geometry-based method for quantification of left ventricular volumes and ejection fraction from ECG-gated SPECT. J. of Nuclear Cardiology 12, 55–65 (2005)
10. MacDonald, D., Avis, D., Evans, A.C.: Proximity constraints in deformable models for cortical surface identification. In: Wells, W.M., Colchester, A.C.F., Delp, S.L. (eds.) MICCAI 1998. LNCS, vol. 1496, pp. 650–659. Springer, Heidelberg (1998)
11. Paragios, N.: A variational approach for the segmentation of the left ventricle in cardiac image analysis. Int. J. Computer Vision 50(3), 345–362 (2002)
12. Rousson, M., Cremers, D.: Efficient kernel density estimation of shape and intensity priors for level set segmentation. In: Duncan, J.S., Gerig, G. (eds.) MICCAI 2005. LNCS, vol. 3750, pp. 757–764. Springer, Heidelberg (2005)
13. Zeng, X., Staib, L.H., Schultz, R.T., Duncan, J.S.: Segmentation and measurement of the cortex from 3-D MR images using coupled-surfaces propagation. IEEE Trans. Medical Imaging 18, 927–937 (1999)

Nonrigid Image Registration with Subdivision Lattices: Application to Cardiac MR Image Analysis

R. Chandrashekara[1], R. Mohiaddin[2], R. Razavi[3], and D. Rueckert[1]

[1] Department of Computing, Imperial College London, UK
[2] Royal Brompton Hospital, Imperial College London, UK
[3] Division of Imaging Sciences, King's College London, UK

Abstract. In this paper we present a new methodology for cardiac motion tracking in tagged MRI using nonrigid image registration based on subdivision surfaces and subdivision lattices. We use two sets of registrations to do the motion tracking. First, a set of surface registrations is used to create and initially align the subdivision model of the left ventricle with short-axis and long-axis MR images. Second, a series of volumetric registrations are used to perform the motion tracking and to reconstruct the 4D cardiac motion field from the tagged MR images. The motion of a point in the myocardium over time is calculated by registering the images taken during systole to the set of reference images taken at end-diastole. Registration is achieved by optimizing the positions of the vertices in the base lattice so that the mutual information of the images being registered is maximized. The presented method is validated using a cardiac motion simulator and we also present strain measurements obtained from a group of normal volunteers.

1 Introduction

Using magnetic resonance imaging (MRI) it is possible to obtain high resolution cine-images of cardiac motion noninvasively, enabling global functional parameters such as left ventricular volume, left ventricular mass, stroke volume, ejection fraction, and cardiac output to be measured once suitable pre-processing has been applied to the acquired images and the left ventricle (LV) has been segmented out. Although global measures of cardiac function are useful indicators of cardiac malfunction they do not reveal the regional wall motion abnormalities which are necessary for the early detection of cardiovascular diseases such as coronary heart disease. Tissue tagging ([18,2]) enables the measurement of the three-dimensional (3D) motion patterns within the walls of the heart. Radio-frequency (RF) pulses applied at the start of the cardiac cycle produce planes of saturated magnetization in the muscle walls which appear as dark stripes when imaged immediately afterwards, and can be tracked to reconstruct dense deformation fields within the myocardium. To do this multiple stacked short-axis (SA) and long-axis (LA) image sequences of the heart are acquired with tag planes in three mutually orthogonal directions so that the 3D motion of the heart over time can be measured.

N. Ayache, S. Ourselin, A. Maeder (Eds.): MICCAI 2007, Part I, LNCS 4791, pp. 335–342, 2007.
© Springer-Verlag Berlin Heidelberg 2007

Numerous methods have been developed for motion field extraction using tagged MR images. Among these methods optical flow ([14,7,6]), active contour models ([1,17,11]), and harmonic phase MRI (HARP) ([12]) have yielded moderately successful results although none have proved to meet all requirements in terms of accuracy and efficiency to come to dominate clinical practice. Among the main difficulties encountered is the need to estimate through-plane motion which is compounded by the effects of patient and respiratory motion. Recent work on image registration based techniques for tagged MR image analysis have yielded promising results for obtaining clinically meaningful information ([4,13,15]). The advantage of using image registration is that no assumptions are required about the nature of the tag pattern in the images. Moreover, the use of statistical measures of image similarity (e.g. mutual information) can account for the variation in tag intensity over time seen in tagged MR images. The approach in [4] uses free-form deformations (FFDs) to model the cardiac deformation. However, these models require the control points to be spaced on a regular grid covering the entire heart. A more natural approach is to adopt the control point mesh to the geometry of the LV using extended FFD models [8]. In this paper we present a new deformation model which is based on subdivision surfaces and subdivision lattices. The key advantage of this model is that the deformation of the LV can be controlled by a small number of control points and can therefore be efficiently optimized.

2   Method

One of the initial steps necessary for tagged MR image analysis is the segmentation of cardiac structures before subsequent motion tracking and deformation analysis. This is necessary to ensure that the blood flow patterns seen in the images do not interfere with the motion tracking of the heart muscle. One encounters a number of difficulties at this stage due to the nature of the images acquired. As there is no fully automated procedure for the accurate segmentation and fitting of surface and volumetric models to cardiac structures in tagged MR images our approach is to use a semi-automated method to construct the subdivision lattice used to model the deformation of the LV and do the motion tracking. We begin by first describing how the endocardial and epicardial surfaces of the LV are modeled using subdivision surfaces.

2.1   Modeling the Epicardium and Endocardium with Subdivision Surfaces

Subdivision surfaces were first proposed simultaneously by Catmull and Clark [3] and Doo and Sabin [5] in 1978 as a method for defining smooth surfaces by progressive refinement of a control polygon mesh. They are defined in terms of a base control polygon mesh and a set of geometric and topological rules which when applied to the mesh generate a sequence of polygon meshes which converge to a smooth surface. Subdivision surfaces combine the flexibility and ease of use of polygon meshes with arbitrary topology while retaining the smooth surface properties of spline-based surfaces.

We model the endocardial and epicardial surfaces using Catmull-Clark subdivision surfaces [3].

Generating Subject Specific Models of the Endocardium and Epicardium Using Surface Registration. To create surface models of the endocardium and epicardium we have adopted a semi-automatic approach in which the user places point markers defining the endocardium and epicardium of the LV to which template surfaces are then registered. To aid in the placement of the markers as well as making the initial alignment of the templates we have developed a graphical user interface (GUI) First, the user places point markers delineating the endocardium on the SA and LA images. The approximate positions of the apex, base, and septum are then specified to compute a transformation matrix which makes an initial alignment of a template surface (defined using a base polygon mesh consisting of 25 vertices) with the point markers.

After this, the template subdivision surface is then deformed so that it conforms as closely as possible to the endocardial point set by minimizing the distances between the point markers and the surface. This is done by optimizing the positions of the control vertices using a gradient descent optimization procedure. The registered endocardial surface is then duplicated and used as the input surface to register to the epicardial markers. From the endocardial and epicardial surfaces we now create the volumetric model of the LV which is described in the next section.

2.2   Construction of a Subject-Specific Model of the LV

The idea of subdivision surfaces was extended to volumes by MacCracken and Joy [9]. Starting with a base lattice, geometrical and topological rules of subdivision are applied to generate a sequence of lattices which converge to a volume of space.

The base lattice of the LV model is constructed simply from the base polygon meshes of the endocardium and epicardium by connecting their corresponding vertices as shown in figure 1. This approach ensures that the inner and outer surfaces of the subdivision lattice correspond to the surfaces computed in section 2.1 as the geometric rules of subdivision at the boundary faces of lattices are the same as the rules of subdivision for Catmull-Clark surfaces. The base lattice contains 50 vertices.

2.3   Motion Tracking by Image Registration

Once the subdivision lattice is aligned with the LV we are ready to do the motion tracking. Suppose that two sets of image sequences have been acquired, a SA sequence and a LA sequence. We denote by $I_{SA,t}(\mathbf{x})$ and $I_{LA,t}(\mathbf{x})$ the trilinearly interpolated values of the images at position $\mathbf{x}$ and time frame t in the SA and LA images respectively and we choose the images taken at the start of the cardiac

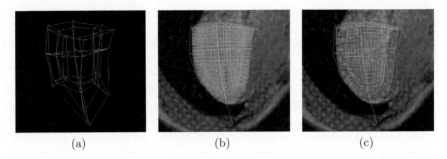

(a)   (b)   (c)

Fig. 1. This figure shows the volumetric model of the LV that is created from the surface models of the endocardium and epicardium. (a) The base lattice. (b) The model after 3 levels of subdivision. (c) The model after 3 levels of subdivision with only the boundary edges displayed.

cycle, $I_{\mathrm{SA},0}(\mathbf{x})$ and $I_{\mathrm{LA},0}(\mathbf{x})$, as the reference images (the target images). By registering the images taken during the cardiac cycle (the source images) to the target images we can determine the movement of points within the myocardium over time. Registration is being achieved by finding the displacements of the base vertices defining the subdivision lattice based transformation such that when the transformation is applied to the source images, the weighted sum of the mutual information of the images being registered is maximized ([4]).

Evaluation of Similarity Measure. Before we can evaluate the degree of similarity between the images being registered we need to transform the source images into the coordinate system of the target images. Given a set of displacements of the vertices, $\mathcal{U}^0 = \{\mathbf{u}_0^0, \mathbf{u}_1^0, \ldots, \mathbf{u}_{V_0-1}^0\}$, of the base lattice a source image is transformed into the coordinate system of the target image by finding for each voxel $\mathbf{x}_i$ within the subdivision lattice its transformed position, $T^L(\mathcal{U}^0, \mathbf{x}_i)$, in the source image. This is done by following the procedure given below,

1. We first find the cell, $\mathbf{c}_i^L$, in which the point resides. This can be done efficiently by partitioning the bounding boxes of the cells of the subdivision lattice using an octree data structure.
2. Then the local coordinates, $[u \ v \ w]^T$, of $\mathbf{x}_i$ within the cell $\mathbf{c}_i^L$ are calculated. To do this a numerical procedure based on Newton's method is used.
3. The vertices of the base lattice, $\mathcal{V}^0$, are now displaced by the vectors $\mathcal{U}^0$, and the positions of the vertices in the subdivided lattices are then updated according to the geometrical rules of subdivision given in the previous section.
4. Then, using the cell and local coordinates computed in step 2 we transform the $\mathbf{x}_i$ to their new positions in the deformed lattice.

The source image voxel values can now be interpolated at the transformed positions to obtain the image intensity values of the transformed source image $I_{\mathrm{SA},t}(T^L(\mathcal{U}^0, \mathbf{x}))$. This process is repeated for both the SA and LA images to obtain two transformed images, $I'_{\text{SA},t}$ and $I'_{\text{LA},t}$, which are then compared with their respective target images, $I_{\text{SA},0}$ and $I_{\text{LA},0}$. The similarity metric used is a weighted sum of the mutual information of the images being registered (note that only the image regions within the volume of the subdivision lattice are being registered). The weighting factors depend on the number of SA and LA image voxels which lie within the LV model.

Again, a gradient descent optimization procedure is used to find the optimal positions of the control points. However, other optimization methods such as the simplex method might also be suitable.

3   Results

3.1   Cardiac Motion Simulator

To validate our model we have used the cardiac motion simulator of Waks *et al.* [16]. The motion model used in the simulator is applied to a confocal prolate spherical shell and the simulator is capable of generating realistic tagged MR images of the motion of the heart. SA and LA image sequences were generated using k-parameter values sampled at ten equally spaced time points between end-diastole and end-systole from figure 4 of [16]. Using the method described in section 2 the motion field within the LV volume was estimated and compared with the true motion fields obtained from the simulator. The total time taken to do the motion tracking for a sequence of images with 10 time frames was 2800 s on an Intel Pentium IV 3.2 GHz PC with 2 GB of RAM. For each time instant and for all voxels within the myocardium the relative error, r, was calculated,

$$r = \frac{100}{N} \sum_{i=1}^{N} \frac{|\mathbf{t}_i - \mathbf{e}_i|}{|\mathbf{t}_i|} \tag{1}$$

where N is the number of voxels in the myocardium, $\mathbf{t}_i$ is the true displacement at voxel i, and $\mathbf{e}_i$ is the estimated displacement at voxel i. The relative error in the estimated displacement field was found to be 8.5%.

3.2   Normal Volunteers

A sequence of stacked SA and LA tagged MR image sequences were also acquired from nine normal volunteers and using the method described in section 2 we derived the motion fields within the myocardium for the cardiac cycle between end-diastole and end-systole. We also derived motion fields using the FFD-based motion tracking method described in [4] so that a comparison of the two methods could be made. The myocardium at $t = 0$ was then segmented along the length of the LA into three regions, the apical, mid-ventricular, and basal regions; and around the circumferential direction into the lateral, anterior, septal, and inferior regions. Figure 2 shows a comparison of the circumferential strain in the mid-ventricular region calculated using the subdivision lattice and free-form

340   R. Chandrashekara et al.

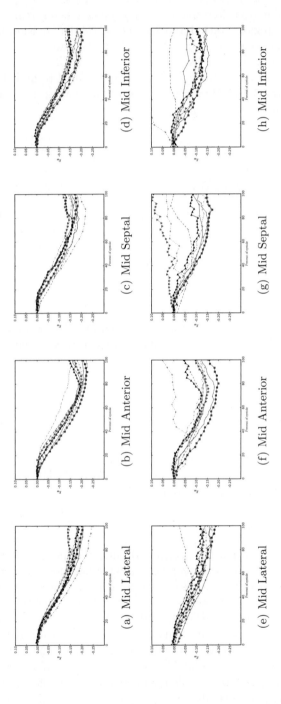

Fig. 2. Circumferential strain as a function of time expressed in terms of percentage of the cardiac cycle. The vertical axis represents strain and the horizontal axis represents time. The top and bottom rows show the strain computed using subdivision lattices and free-form deformations respectively.

deformation based motion tracking. In a normal healthy heart the circumeferential strain decreases during systole [10,15]. The figure indicates that the motion fields generated by the subdivision lattices are smoother than those generated by the FFDs and show less variability in the strain patterns seen across a group of normal volunteers.

4   Discussion and Conclusions

In this paper we have presented a method for cardiac motion tracking in tagged MR images based on nonrigid registration using subdivision lattices. We validated our method using a cardiac motion simulator and showed that accurate displacement and strain fields could be computed. The principal advantage of the method presented in this paper is the reduced number of degrees of freedom (the displacements of the base lattice vertices) which need to be optimized for. For the work presented in this paper to be of practical benefit one should build a large database of the strain distributions in normal volunteers so that comparisons could be made with the strain patterns seen in subsequent patient examinations.

References

1. Amini, A.A., Chen, Y., Elayyadi, M., Radeva, P.: Tag surface reconstruction and tracking of myocardial beads from SPAMM-MRI with parametric B-spline surfaces. IEEE Transactions on Medical Imaging 20(2), 94–103 (2001)
2. Axel, L., Dougherty, L.: Heart wall motion: Improved method of spatial modulation of magnetization for MR imaging. Radiology 172(2), 349–360 (1989)
3. Catmull, E., Clark, J.: Recursively generated B-spline surfaces on arbitrary topological meshes. Computer Aided Design 10(6), 350–355 (1978)
4. Chandrashekara, R., Mohiaddin, R.H., Rueckert, D.: Analysis of 3-D myocardial motion in tagged MR images using nonrigid image registration. IEEE Transactions on Medical Imaging 23(10), 1245–1250 (2004)
5. Doo, D., Sabin, M.A.: Behaviour of recursive subdivision surfaces near extraordinary points. Computer Aided Design 10(6), 356–360 (1978)
6. Dougherty, L., Asmuth, J.C., Blom, A.S., Axel, L., Kumar, R.: Validation of an optical flow method for tag displacement estimation. IEEE Transactions on Medical Imaging 18(4), 359–363 (1999)
7. Gupta, S.N., Prince, J.L.: On variable brightness optical flow for tagged MRI. In: Information Processing in Medical Imaging, pp. 323–334. Kluwer, Dordrecht (1995)
8. Lin, N., Duncan, J.S.: Generalized robust point matching using an extended free-form deformation model: application to cardiac images. In: Proceedings of the 2004 IEEE International Symposium on Biomedical Imaging: From Nano to Macro (2004)
9. MacCracken, R., Joy, K.I.: Free-form deformations with lattices of arbitrary topology. In: Proceedings of the 23rd Annual Conference on Computer Graphics and Interactive Techniques, pp. 181–188. ACM Press, New York (1996)
10. Moore, C.C., McVeigh, E.R., Zerhouni, E.A.: Quantitative tagged magnetic resonance imaging of the normal human left ventricle. Topics in Magnetic Resonance Imaging 11(6), 359–371 (2000)

11. O'Dell, W.G., Moore, C.C., Hunter, W.C., Zerhouni, E.A., McVeigh, E.R.: Three-dimensional myocardial deformations: Calculation with displacement field fitting to tagged MR images. Radiology 195(3), 829–835 (1995)
12. Osman, N.F., McVeigh, E.R., Prince, J.L.: Imaging heart motion using harmonic phase MRI. IEEE Transactions on Medical Imaging 19(3), 186–202 (2000)
13. Petitjean, C., Rougon, N., Preteux, F., Cluzel, P., Grenier, P.: Measuring myocardial deformation from MR data using information-theoretic nonrigid registration. In: FIMH, pp. 162–172 (2003)
14. Prince, J.L., McVeigh, E.R.: Optical flow for tagged MR images. In: Proceedings of the 1991 International Conference on Acoustics, Speech, and Signal Processing, pp. 2441–2444 (1991)
15. Tustison, N.J., Amini, A.A.: Biventricular myocardial strains via nonrigid registration of AnFigatomical NURBS models. IEEE Transactions on Medical Imaging 25(1), 94–112 (2006)
16. Waks, E., Prince, J.L., Douglas, A.S.: Cardiac motion simulator for tagged MRI. In: Proceedings of the IEEE Workshop on Mathematical Methods in Biomedical Image Analysis, pp. 182–191 (June 1996)
17. Young, A.A., Kraitchman, D.L., Dougherty, L., Axel, L.: Tracking and finite element analysis of stripe deformation in magnetic resonance tagging. IEEE Transactions on Medical Imaging 14(3), 413–421 (1995)
18. Zerhouni, E.A., Parish, D.M., Rogers, W.J., Yang, A., Shapiro, E.P.: Human heart: Tagging with MR imaging — a method for noninvasive assessment of myocardial motion. Radiology 169(1), 59–63 (1988)

Spatio-temporal Registration of Real Time 3D Ultrasound to Cardiovascular MR Sequences

Weiwei Zhang, J. Alison Noble, and J. Michael Brady

Wolfson Medical Vision Lab, Department of Engineering Science, University of
Oxford, Parks Road OX1 3PJ, Oxford, UK
{weiwei,noble,jmb}@robots.ox.ac.uk.

Abstract. We extend our static multimodal nonrigid registration [1] to
a spatio-temporal (2D+T) co-registration of a real-time 3D ultrasound
and a cardiovascular MR sequence. The motivation for our research is
to assist a clinician to automatically fuse the information from multiple
imaging modalities for the early diagnosis and therapy of cardiac disease.
The deformation field between both sequences is decoupled into spatial and temporal components. Temporal alignment is firstly performed
to re-slice both sequences using a differential registration method. Spatial alignment is then carried out between the frames corresponding to
the same temporal position. The spatial deformation is modeled by the
polyaffine transformation whose anchor points (or control points) are automatically detected and refined by calculating a local mis-match measure based on phase mutual information. The spatial alignment is built in
an adaptive multi-scale framework to maximize the phase-based similarity measure by optimizing the parameters of the polyaffine transformation. Results demonstrate that this novel method can yield an accurate
registration to particular cardiac regions.

1 Introduction

Cardiovascular disease is one of the world's leading causes of death. The comparison and fusion of information from multiple cardiac image modalities, e.g.
cardiovascular magnetic resonance imaging (CMR) and real-time 3D echocardiography (RT3DUS), is of increasing interest in the medical community for
physiological understanding and diagnostic purposes.

Most of the current cardiac image registration methods focus on establishing
the spatial correspondence between image sequences, while ignoring the temporal correspondence [2]. However, incorporating temporal information into the
alignment of multi-modal cardiovascular images can contribute to the study of
dynamic properties or motion patterns of the heart. For example, Huang et al.
have presented a method for rapid spatio-temporal registration of RT3DUS and
CMR images [3]. They first calibrate and synchronize both sequences by integrating electrocardiogram (ECG) and a spatial tracking system to a RT3US
machine. These augmented sequences are then manually co-registered to generate a temporal transformation matrix on which the real-time registration step is
based. But the dependence of temporal alignment on the ECG signal might be

N. Ayache, S. Ourselin, A. Maeder (Eds.): MICCAI 2007, Part I, LNCS 4791, pp. 343–350, 2007.
© Springer-Verlag Berlin Heidelberg 2007

error-prone due to the sampling errors in the ECG signal. In addition, the limited number of degree of freedoms (DOFs) assumed in that work can not be sufficient to represent the heart as a deformable model in the real case. In other work, Perperidis et al. report two algorithms for spatio-temporal registration of CMR sequences [4]. The transformation model is separated into spatial and temporal components. The first algorithm optimizes the spatial and temporal components simultaneously while the second algorithm optimizes the temporal component before optimizing the spatial component. However, the first algorithm is computationally expensive and the second algorithm can only align limited temporal positions in the cardiac cycle. To our knowledge, spatio-temporal (2D+T) non-rigid registration of RT3DUS and CMR sequences has not been reported before.

In this paper, we extend our static (gated) multi-modal registration method to multi-frame RT3DUS and CMR registration to enable correlation of 3D information between these two modalities [1]. The novelty is to perform the temporal alignment by re-slicing both sequences to contain the same number of frames in order to make them correspond to the same temporal position by using a differential registration technique. The spatial alignment is achieved by a polyaffine transformation framework whose control points are automatically identified by a local mis-match measure using phase information. Therefore the optimization of the proposed method is computationally efficient.

2   Method

We describe the 2D+T version of the method, although it extends naturally to 3D+T. An image sequence $I(x, y, t)$ can be represented as a series of 2D images, where $(x, y) \in \Omega_I$ denotes a point in the 2D image domain and $t \in [0, T - 1]$ denotes the temporal position of a scene and T usually represents the total number of the frames recorded in a cardiac cycle. The goal of our image sequence registration is to find a deformation field that maps each point in the floating image sequence to its corresponding point in the reference image sequence. As in the work of Perperidis et al [4], the spatio-temporal registration problem is solved by decoupling the deformation field $\mathbf{D}$ into the spatial component and the temporal component respectively:

$$\mathbf{D}_{temporal}(t) = t'(t) \quad and \quad \mathbf{D}_{spatial} = (x'(x, y), y'(x, y)) \tag{1}$$

More precisely, the temporal alignment is performed before the spatial alignment to ensure that each temporal frame in the floating image sequence is registered with the corresponding temporal frame in the reference image sequence. This prevents different image scenes in the same sequence being deformed in different temporal directions. After temporal alignment is complete, the spatial alignment can be taken between both frames that correspond to the same position in the cardiac cycle.

One assumption of the proposed method is that both modality images are in the same spatial coordinate view, e.g. in the short axis (SA) or long axis (LA) view. We use the orientation information acquired during the CMR examination to bring the RT3D dataset into the same spatial coordinate system as the CMR dataset using commercial software. In the experimental section, every frame in the cardiac sequence is taken from the mid slice of the SA and LA views.

2.1 Spatial Alignment

The heart is undergoing a spatially varying motion during the cardiac cycle. Even at the same phase of the cardiac cycle, multi-modal cardiac images exhibit local differences due to the motion between the examinations and the different ways to acquire and slice the datasets, which are not easily modeled only by a global rigid transformation. We assume the deformation of the ventricles in multi-modal cardiac images is composed of a locally affine transformation. The polyaffine frame work is employed to obtain a globally non-rigid transformation to model the deformation that presents several local behaviours [5]. The idea behind the polyaffine transformation is to weight the sum of local displacements according to a weight function for each arbitrary image region:

$$\mathbf{D}_{spatial}(x,y) = \frac{\sum_i w_i(x,y)\mathbf{D}_i(x,y)}{\sum_i w_i(x,y)} \tag{2}$$

where w denotes the weight function for image region i within a cardiac scene and $\mathbf{D}$ denotes the local displacement in each image region. The weight function is modeled by a Gaussian function that acts as a pre-defined shape for each region and models its influence in the image space. The local displacement modeled by an affine transformation is obtained via an ODE to guarantee invertibility, since all transformations induced by an ODE are reversible [6]. Therefore it can avoid the 'folding' effect that a traditional spline-based transformation tends to produce at high image resolution [7,8].

A local mis-match measure is employed to automatically identify the anchor point (the centre of a local misaligned region) of a polyaffine transformation by removing superfluous degrees of freedom and avoiding the regular grid of control points that increases the computation. Therefore, the polyaffine transformation can effectively adjust these control points to align and correct the spatial difference using less transformation parameters. Adopting the local phase as the image descriptor has been shown to increase the accuracy of non-rigid registration in terms of the information theory based similarity measure [9,10]. Furthermore as the mutual information of local phase can avoid the intensity changes across multi-modalities and makes no assumption of a like-with-like correspondence, it is well-suited for cardiovascular image analysis [11,10]. A local mis-match measure based on the local mutual phase information in a small spatial neighbourhood is used to find the most misaligned region between the US and MR images [12].

2.2 Temporal Alignment - General Principles

Due to the variations in the temporal sampling rate, RT3DUS and CMR image sequences of the same subject are not generally synchronized. This implies that

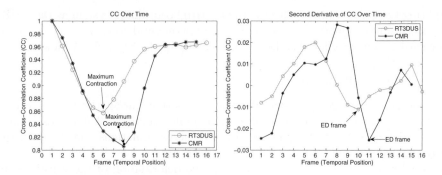

Fig. 1. Cross-correlation coefficient (CC) for MR and US sequences over time and their second derivatives. Left: CC of both MR and US sequences shown together. Right: Using the second derivative (central differences method) of CC to identify the end-diastole frame.

the spatial alignment of the corresponding frames between image sequences may lead to the comparison of frames at different positions in the cardiac cycle. One approach to accommodate this could combine spatial and temporal alignment in one optimization step. However, it has been reported that this combined optimization demands expensive computation and in practice, the floating image scene can be deformed in different temporal directions [4].

In our temporal alignment, we prefer to re-slice the multi-modal cardiac sequences in time to make each pair of frames correspond to the same time position. To this end, we identify key temporal positions in the cardiac cycle based on temporal cross-correlation. For each imaging modality sequence and for each identified segment (phase) of the cardiac cycle, we then estimate the total motion field by summation of the consecutive pairwise estimations of the motion between frames. Each sequence is then re-sliced to contain the same number of frames.

Detection of Key Cardiac Phases. Figure 1 shows how the cross-correlation coefficient (CC) is used to derive temporal information from a cardiac image sequence. This is achieved by calculating the cross-correlation coefficient of each subsequent frame with respect to the initial frame, which is proposed by Perperidis et al [4]. The initial frame is arbitrarily assumed to be the beginning of the cardiac cycle (end-diastole). The maximum contraction frame can be easily identified by finding the minimum value of the cross-correlation coefficient since it has the lowest degree of similarity with the initial frame (frames 6 and 8 respectively for RT3DUS and CMR). Similarly, the end-diastolic frame should have a high degree of similarity with the initial frame, which can be identified by finding the minimum value of the second derivative of the cross-correlation coefficient after the location of maximum contraction (frame 10 and 11 respectively for RT3DUS and CMR).

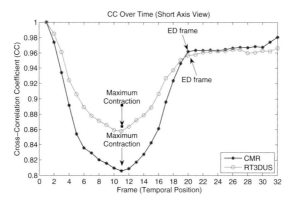

Fig. 2. The result of re-slicing multi-modal cardiac sequences to contain the same number of frames (32 frames) in a cardiac cycle

Re-slicing Cardiac Sequence. Using temporal cross-correlation, the cardiac cycle is now defined into four phases. But as observed in figure 1, the equivalent frame numbers are not aligned to the same point in the cardiac cycle. To align them, the dense estimated motion field is firstly re-sliced between these positions and the local transformation flow is then used to non-linearly interpolate and generate a new frame. Figure 2 shows the CC versus frame number curves of RT3D and CMR sequences sliced to 32 frames across the cardiac cycle.

Key to doing re-slicing is the estimation of the motion field. The differential local affine transformation is employed for estimating the motion field between two consecutive frames [13]. $I(x, y, t)$ and $I(x', y', t-1)$ are denoted as the consecutive frames. The motion field can be modeled by a local affine transformation, assuming the brightness and contrast between frames are constant:

$$I(x, y, t) = I(m_1 x + m_2 y + m_5, m_3 x + m_4 y + m_6, t - 1) \tag{3}$$

where m_1, m_2, m_3, m_4 are the linear affine parameters and m_5, m_6 are the translation parameters. A quadratic error function is minimized in order to estimate these transformation parameters. This error function can be approximated using a first order truncated Taylor series expansion. By differentiating with respect to the unknowns, setting the result to zero and solving for $\vec{m}$, the error function can be estimated analytically:

$$\vec{m} = \left[\sum_{x,y \in \Omega} \vec{c} \, \vec{c}^T \right]^{-1} \left[\sum_{x,y \in \Omega} \vec{c} \, k \right] \tag{4}$$

where $\vec{m} = (m_1 \cdots m_6)^T$ and Ω denotes a small spatial neighborhood; and the scalar k and vector $\vec{c}^T$ are given as: $k = I_t + x I_x + y I_y$ and $\vec{c}^T = (x I_x, y I_x, x I_y, \cdots y I_y, I_x, I_y)$.[1]

---

[1] For notational convenience, the dependencies/parameters of $I_x(\cdot), I_y(\cdot)$ and $I_t(\cdot)$ with respect to t are dropped.

The invertibility of the matrix $\overline{m}$ can be guaranteed by integrating a large enough spatial neighborhood. Moreover, to account for intensity changes and to ensure that model parameters vary smoothly across space, additional parameters that capture a change in contrast and brightness and a smoothness constraint term can be added to equation 3 and the quadratic error function respectively. The algorithm is built in a coarse-to-fine scheme to speed up the computation. Finally, the motion field between the ultrasound frames is estimated by applying the differential technique to the phase image rather than intensity [9]. It should be noted that the registered (or newly-generated) frame is produced by warping the intensity image instead.

When estimating the motion field across the whole cardiac cycle, the total motion field is obtained from the contribution of the partial motion fields of the consecutive pairs over the cardiac phases [14]. Both forward and backward consecutive registrations are performed to reduce registration errors. The total motion field is given by the maximum likelihood of the accumulated motion field from the consecutive pairs, assuming the error distribution of the consecutive registration is identically distributed:

$$\mathbf{M}_{0,t} = \omega_t \mathbf{M}_{0,t}^{forward} + (1 - \omega_t)\mathbf{M}_{0,t}^{backward} \ (\omega_t = \frac{T-t}{T}) \tag{5}$$

where $\mathbf{M}_{0,t}^{forward} = \mathbf{M}_{0,t-1}^{forward} + \mathbf{M}_{t-1,t}^{forward}$ denotes the accumulated motion field from the forward consecutive pairs and $\mathbf{M}_{0,t}^{backward} = \mathbf{M}_{T,t+1}^{backward} + \mathbf{M}_{t+1,t}^{backward}$ denotes the accumulated motion field from the backward consecutive pairs. For further implementation details see [9].

3   Results

Figure 3 shows the results of the proposed spatio-temporal registration of multimodal cardiac sequences. Due to space constraints, we show the results at two temporal positions in two different views. Alternatively, the results can be viewed as a movie (http://www.robots.ox.ac.uk/robots/people/WeiweiZhang.html).

4   Validation

We follow our previous work to validate the method using expert-identified landmarks. For each pair of the corresponding frames, the anatomical landmarks such as the conjoint of the anterior and anterior septum, the conjoint of the septum and inferior PPM, and the APM, were carefully identified by an experienced clinical expert. The RT3DUS slice identified anatomical landmarks were registered to the CMR image as the reference standard. The measure of the registration accuracy is defined as the root mean square error (RMS) distance of the identified anatomical landmarks between the nonrigidly registered RT3D slice and the reference standard. In this experiment, the registration accuracy were $4.35 \pm 1.25mm$ and $5.23 \pm 1.65mm$ for the SA and LA sequences respectively.

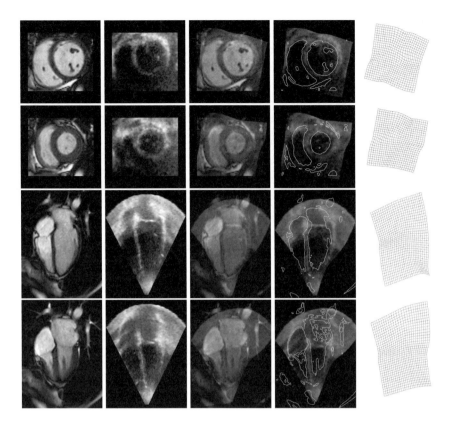

Fig. 3. The result of spatio-temporal registration of RT3DUS and CMR sequences (top two rows in SA view and bottom two rows in LA view). From left to right column: CMR image frames at two temporal positions (the beginning of the cardiac cycle, the peak contraction of the left ventricle); the corresponding RT3DUS frames; the registered RT3DUS frames superimposed to the CMR frame with iso contours; the spatial transformation grids generated by the polyaffine transformation.

5   Discussion

In this paper, a novel method has been presented to solve the problem of non-rigidly registering RT3DUS and MR sequences. The deformation field between both cardiac sequences has been decoupled into spatial and temporal components and each component is optimized separately. The temporal alignment is an important part of our method and is solved by re-slicing both sequences using a differential registration technique. After the temporal alignment, each sequence has the same number of frames and each frame is ensured to correspond to the same temporal position. Therefore our previous static registration method can be extended to multi-frame registration. Since the algorithm only uses the image information, it can reduce the dependence on ECG signal and spatial tracking system which might be a source of error. A visual comparison from several key cardiac phases has shown that the polyaffine transformation can correct spatial differences in small regions like the myocardium and papillary muscles. In the future, we will investigate the application of RT3DUS/CMR in clinical practice.

Acknowledgements. We thank the Oxford Centre for Clinical MR Research (Dr Matthew Robson) and the Oxford John Radcliffe Hospital Cardiology Department (Dr Harold Becher) for providing the clinical motivation and data.

References

1. Zhang, W.W., Noble, J.A., Brady, J.M.: Adaptive non-rigid registration of real time 3d ultrasound to cardiovascular mr images. In: IPMI 2007. LNCS, vol. 4584, pp. 50–61 (2007)
2. Makela, T.J., et al.: A review of caridac image registration methods. IEEE Trans. Med. Imag 21, 1001–1021 (2002)
3. Huang, X.S., et al.: Dynamic 3d ultrasound and mr image registration of beating heart. In: Duncan, J.S., Gerig, G. (eds.) MICCAI 2005. LNCS, vol. 3750, pp. 171–178. Springer, Heidelberg (2005)
4. Perperidis, D., Mohiaddin, R.H., Rueckert, D.: Spatio-temporal free-form registration of cardiac mr image sequences. Med. Imag. Anal 9, 441–456 (2005)
5. Arsigny, V., Pennec, X., Ayache, N.: Polyrigid and polyaffine transformations: A novel geometrical tool to deal with non-rigid deformations - application to the registration of histological slices. Med. Imag. Anal. 9, 507–523 (2005)
6. Tenebaum, M., Pollard, H.: Ordinary differential equations. Dover (1985)
7. Rueckert, D., et al.: Non-rigid registration using free-form deformation: Application to breast mr images. IEEE Trans. Med. Imag. 18, 712–721 (1999)
8. Meyer, C.R., et al.: Demonstration of accuracy and clinical versatility of mutual information for automatic multimodality image fusion using affine and thin plate spline warped geometric deformations. Med. Imag. Anal. 1, 195–206 (1997)
9. Zhang, W.W.: Multimodal Cardiovascular Image Analysis Using Phase Information. PhD thesis, University of Oxford, PhD Thesis forthcoming (2007)
10. Mellor, M., Brady, J.M.: Phase mutual information as a similarity measure for registration. Med. Imag. Anal. 9, 330–343 (2005)
11. Felsberg, M., Sommer, G.: A new extension of linear signal processing for estimating local properties and detecting features. In: Proc. DAGM, 195–202 (2000)
12. Park, H., Bland, P.H., Brock, K.K., Meyer, C.R.: Adaptive registration using local information measures. Med. Imag. Anal. 8, 465–473 (2004)
13. Periaswamy, S., Farid, H.: Elastic registration in the presence of intensity variations. IEEE Trans. Med. Imag. 7, 865–874 (2003)
14. Ledesma-Carbayo, M., et al.: Cardiac motion analysis from ultrasound sequences using nonrigid registration. In: Niessen, W.J., Viergever, M.A. (eds.) MICCAI 2001. LNCS, vol. 2208, pp. 889–896. Springer, Heidelberg (2001)

Nonlinear Registration of Diffusion MR Images Based on Fiber Bundles*

Ulas Ziyan[1], Mert R. Sabuncu[1], Lauren J. O'Donnell[2,3],
and Carl-Fredrik Westin[1,3]

[1] MIT Computer Science and Artificial Intelligence Lab, Cambridge MA, USA
ulas@mit.edu
[2] Department of Neurosurgery, Brigham and Women's Hospital, Harvard Medical
School, Boston MA, USA
[3] Laboratory of Mathematics in Imaging, Brigham and Women's Hospital,
Harvard Medical School, Boston MA, USA

Abstract. In this paper, we explore the use of fiber bundles extracted
from diffusion MR images for a nonlinear registration algorithm. We
employ a white matter atlas to automatically label major fiber bundles and to establish correspondence between subjects. We propose a
polyaffine framework to calculate a smooth and invertible nonlinear warp
field based on these correspondences, and derive an analytical solution
for the reorientation of the tensor fields under the polyaffine transformation. We demonstrate our algorithm on a group of subjects and show
that it performs comparable to a higher dimensional nonrigid registration
algorithm.

1   Introduction

Diffusion tensor imaging (DTI) measures the molecular diffusion, i.e., Brownian
motion, of the endogenous water in tissue. This water diffusion is anisotropic in
fibrous biological tissues such as cerebral white matter. Quantification of water
diffusion in tissue through DTI provides a unique way to look into white matter
organization of the brain [1].

Tractography is a common post-processing technique for DTI which aims at
reconstructing fibers from the tensor field [2]. The method works by tracing the
principal diffusion direction in small steps. The resulting tracts can be grouped
together into bundles. Even though the resolution of DTI is too low to measure
any individual axons, these bundles show similarity to anatomical structures and
suggest that at the bundle level we are able to capture structural information [3, 4].

A popular technique to investigate white matter anatomy is to manually select
regions of interest (ROIs) that are thought to correspond to a particular anatomical white matter tract, and to analyze scalar measures derived from the diffusion

* This work was supported by NIH NIBIB NAMIC U54-EB005149, NIH NCRR NAC
P41-RR13218, R01-MH074794 and the Athinoula A. Martinos Foundation. We are
grateful to Susumu Mori at JHU for the diffusion MRI data (R01-AG20012 / P41-
RR15241) and Serdar Balci for the ITK help.

N. Ayache, S. Ourselin, A. Maeder (Eds.): MICCAI 2007, Part I, LNCS 4791, pp. 351–358, 2007.
© Springer-Verlag Berlin Heidelberg 2007

tensors within the ROI. ROI based methods could be subject to user bias if the ROIs are manually traced. Therefore several methods have been proposed to identify anatomically meaningful regions from the DTI data. One class of methods uses tractography results and groups them into regions either interactively or automatically, e.g. [3, 4]. A recent study reported that tractography-based definitions of a pyramidal tract ROI are more reproducible than manual ROI drawing [5].

An alternative to ROI-based studies is to perform spatial normalization for the whole data set followed by voxel based morphometry in the white matter. There are many registration techniques designed for aligning scalar MR images such as structural T1 weighted images. Some of these linear and non-linear methods have been applied to scalar images derived from the diffusion tensor data [6, 7, 8, 9, 10].

However, DTI is by nature a non-scalar image and potentially offers rich information that can be used to determine voxel-wise correspondence across subjects. This has been observed in some studies and resulted in: 1) multi-channel scalar registration techniques that aim to account for orientational information, and 2) correspondence validation techniques that are not not only based on voxel-wise similarities but also on fiber tracts generated from the DTI data sets.

The contributions of this paper are multi-fold. Firstly, we propose a novel algorithm to non-linearly register DTI data sets (of multiple subjects) based on fiber bundles that have been automatically segmented. We employ a polyaffine framework [11] to fuse the bundle-based transformations. This yields a global, one-to-one nonlinear deformation. Secondly, we derive an analytical solution for the reorientation of the tensor fields after the application of the polyaffine deformation. Finally, we propose a new measure (of fiber-tensor fit, FiT) to quantify the quality of the match between a deformed fiber tract and underlying diffusion tensor field.

2   Methods

2.1   Fiber Bundles

Organization of tract fibers into bundles, in the entire white matter, reveals anatomical connections such as the corpus callosum and corona radiata. By simultaneously clustering fibers of multiple subjects into bundles, major white matter structures can be discovered in an automatic way [12]. The results of such a clustering can then saved as bundle models along with expert anatomical labels to form a white matter atlas, which can later be used to label tractography results of new subjects [12].

In this work, we use such an atlas to automatically label tractography results of a group of subjects. Since the labeling is consistent among multiple subjects, the use of such an atlas not only provides individual's label maps but also correspondence between subjects. As described in the following Section, we employ this correspondence determined by the label maps to perform nonlinear inter-subject registration.

2.2   Registration of Fiber Bundles

Inter-subject registration using fiber tracts is not a well studied problem. To our knowledge, the only study that deals with this question performs registration on a tract by tract basis utilizing a rigid invariant tract parametrization [13]. The drawback of this framework is that it only allows for rigid transformations (with 6 independent variables) and is computationally very expensive due to the need to process fibers individually.

Instead of registering tracts individually, we propose to register corresponding bundles. To align the bundles from two subjects, we compute 3 dimensional spatial probability maps for each fiber tract bundle in each subject. The goal of our registration is to maximize the correlation between two corresponding bundles' probability maps. A fiber bundle b_i consists of a set of tracts $\{t_j\}$, where t_j is represented by a set of points $\{x_k\}$. Given a fiber bundle we define b_i's spatial probability map as:

$$P_{b_i}(x) = \frac{1}{Z} \sum_{t_j \in b_i} \sum_{x_k \in t_j} \kappa(x - x_k),$$

where Z is the appropriate normalization for a valid probability density (calculated by summing the estimated spatial probability map), and $\kappa(x - x_k)$ is a (Gaussian) kernel centered around x_k, the kth sample from the tract t_j.

Next, we discretize these probability maps to obtain a 3D scalar image for each tract bundle in each subject. We employ a sequential quadratic programming method [14] to find the 9 affine parameters that maximize the correlation coefficient between corresponding probability maps in different subjects. For a pair of subjects, this yields a set of affine transformations that relate each corresponding bundle pair. The last step of our algorithm is to fuse these affine transformations to achieve a global, invertible nonlinear deformation. There are several ways to achieve this. In this study, we employed the log-Eucledian polyaffine framework [11] which guarantees invertibility.

2.3   Polyaffine Framework

The log-Euclidean polyaffine framework offers a fast method to calculate an invertible and smooth nonlinear warp field with a small number of parameters [11]. matrices that define three dimensional affine transformations in homogeneous coordinates. Abusing notation, we denote the affine transformation defined by the matrix A as a vector valued function $A(x) \in \mathbb{R}^3$ for $x \in \mathbb{R}^3$. Our goal is to obtain a global deformation field, $\Phi(x)$, that is computed by a weighted fusion of these affine transformations (A_i's). The most obvious way to combine these transformations is through a weighted sum, but that does not in general yield a smooth and invertible deformation [11]. One way of achieving a well behaved deformation is to use the following stationary ordinary differential equation:

$$\frac{d}{dt}x(t) = \sum_{i=1}^{S} w_i(x(t)) \log(A_i)(x(t)), \tag{1}$$

with $\boldsymbol{x}(0) = \boldsymbol{x}_0$ and $\log(\boldsymbol{A}_i) \in \mathbb{R}^{4\times4}$ is the principal logarithm of $\boldsymbol{A}_i$. Note $\log(\boldsymbol{A}_i)(\boldsymbol{x})$ is an affine transformation. The fused transformation is defined as: $\Phi(\boldsymbol{x}_0) = \boldsymbol{x}(1)$. A numerical solution to (1) is computed in the following manner. Define:

$$T_N(\boldsymbol{x}) = \sum_{i=1}^{S} w_i(\boldsymbol{x}) A_i^{2^{-N}}(\boldsymbol{x}) \ , \tag{2}$$

where N is a small positive integer (typically 4 or 5), $\boldsymbol{A}_i^{2^{-N}}$ denotes the Nth square root of $\boldsymbol{A}_i$ and the weights sum up to one, i.e., $\sum_i w_i(\boldsymbol{x}) = 1$ for all $\boldsymbol{x}$. Note that $A_i^{2^{-N}}(\boldsymbol{x})$ is also an affine transformation. The global transformation Φ is then obtained in N steps:

$$\Phi(\boldsymbol{x}) = \underbrace{[T_1 \circ T_2 \circ \cdots \circ T_N]}_{N \ times} \circ T_N(\boldsymbol{x}) \ , \tag{3}$$

where $T_n = T_{n+1} \circ T_{n+1}$, for $n \in \{1, \dots, N-1\}$, and $\circ$ denotes concatenation. The inverse of $\Phi(\boldsymbol{x})$ is also calculated using the same formulation by replacing each A_i with A_i^{-1} in Equation 2 [11].

2.4   Diffusion Tensor Rotation

Deforming a tensor field is not as easy as interpolating the tensors at their new locations. Since they carry directional information, diffusion tensors need to be rotated when they undergo a spatial transformation [6]. Given the rotational component $\boldsymbol{R}$ of the transformation, the tensors $\boldsymbol{D}$ should be reoriented to $\boldsymbol{R}^T \boldsymbol{D} \boldsymbol{R}$. This rotational component is readily available in an affine transformation. However, it needs to be estimated for a nonlinear deformation field. One way to do so is to calculate the deformation gradient tensor (i.e., Jacobian matrix) $\boldsymbol{J}_\Phi(\boldsymbol{x}) \in \mathbb{R}^{3\times3}$ of the deformation Φ. This captures the locally linear component of the deformation and can be employed via the finite strain method [6] to estimate the rotational component: $\boldsymbol{R} = (\boldsymbol{J}\boldsymbol{J}^T)^{-1/2}\boldsymbol{J}$. For an arbitrary deformation field the Jacobian can be approximated with finite differences. We used this method for the nonlinear benchmark algorithm in Section 3.

An interesting property of the polyaffine framework is that an analytic expression for the Jacobian can be derived. Let's re-write $A_i^{2^{-N}}$ from (2) as $A_i^{2^{-N}}(\boldsymbol{x}) = \boldsymbol{M}_i\boldsymbol{x} + \boldsymbol{t}_i$. Notice that $T_N(\boldsymbol{x}) = \sum_{i=1}^{S} w_i(\boldsymbol{x})\boldsymbol{M}_i\boldsymbol{x} + w_i(\boldsymbol{x})\boldsymbol{t}_i$. Then the Jacobian of T_N is:

$$\boldsymbol{J}_{T_N}(\boldsymbol{x}) = \sum_{i=1}^{S} w_i(\boldsymbol{x})\boldsymbol{M}_i + (\boldsymbol{M}_i\boldsymbol{x} + \boldsymbol{t}) \left(\nabla w_i(\boldsymbol{x})\right)^T$$

$$= \sum_{i=1}^{S} w_i(\boldsymbol{x})\boldsymbol{M}_i + T(\boldsymbol{x}) \left(\nabla w_i(\boldsymbol{x})\right)^T \ , \tag{4}$$

where $.^T$ denotes transpose. Given $\boldsymbol{J}_{T_N}(\boldsymbol{x})$ and using (3), the Jacobian of Φ is computed with the chain rule in N steps:

$$\boldsymbol{J}_{\phi(\boldsymbol{x})} = \underbrace{[\boldsymbol{J}_{T_1}(T_2(\boldsymbol{x})) \cdots \boldsymbol{J}_{T_{N-1}}(T_N(\boldsymbol{x})) \cdot \boldsymbol{J}_{T_N}(T_N(\boldsymbol{x}))]}_{N \ times} \cdot \boldsymbol{J}_{T_N}(\boldsymbol{x}) \ ,$$

where $\boldsymbol{J}_{T_n} = \boldsymbol{J}_{T_{n+1}}(T_{n+1}(\boldsymbol{x})) \cdot \boldsymbol{J}_{T_{n+1}}(\boldsymbol{x})$, for $n \in \{1, \dots, N-1\}$, $\boldsymbol{J}_{T_N}(.)$ is defined in (4) and $\cdot$ is matrix multiplication.

2.5   Measure for Registration Quality: FiT

Two diffusion tensor images can be considered well registered if the tracts generated from one data set match well with the other data set's tensor field after deformation. To quantify this, we propose a measure we name Fiber-Tensor Fit (FiT).

Given a three dimensional probability density $p(\boldsymbol{x})$, its orientation distribution function (ODF) is defined as [15]:

$$\psi(\boldsymbol{u}) = \int_0^\infty p(\boldsymbol{u}r)dr \ ,$$

where $\boldsymbol{u} \in \mathbb{R}^3$ is a unit vector and r is a scalar parameter (the radius in polar coordinates).

In diffusion imaging, water diffusion is commonly modeled with a Gaussian distribution. $\boldsymbol{D}(\boldsymbol{x})$ be the diffusion tensor at that location. The ODF at $\boldsymbol{x}$ can be written as:

$$\psi(\boldsymbol{u}(\boldsymbol{x})) = \int_0^\infty \frac{1}{\sqrt{(2\pi)^3|\boldsymbol{D}(\boldsymbol{x})|}} \exp(-\frac{1}{2}r\boldsymbol{u}(\boldsymbol{x})^T\boldsymbol{D}^{-1}(\boldsymbol{x})\boldsymbol{u}(\boldsymbol{x})r)dr$$

$$= \frac{1}{\sqrt{(4\pi)^2|\boldsymbol{D}(\boldsymbol{x})|}} \frac{1}{\sqrt{\boldsymbol{u}(\boldsymbol{x})^T\boldsymbol{D}^{-1}(\boldsymbol{x})\boldsymbol{u}(\boldsymbol{x})}} \ ,$$

Note that for a given a diffusion tensor $\boldsymbol{D}(\boldsymbol{x})$, the ODF is upper bounded: $\psi(\boldsymbol{u}(\boldsymbol{x})) \leq \sqrt{\lambda_1(\boldsymbol{x})}/\sqrt{(4\pi)^2|\boldsymbol{D}(\boldsymbol{x})|}$, where $\lambda_1(\boldsymbol{x})$ denotes the maximum eigenvalue of $\boldsymbol{D}(\boldsymbol{x})$. The tract ODF value at $\boldsymbol{x}$ is defined as $\psi(\boldsymbol{t}_i(\boldsymbol{x}))$, where $\boldsymbol{t}_i(\boldsymbol{x})$ denote the tangent vector to a fiber tract t_i at $\boldsymbol{x}$. We define FiT as the sum of the log ratios of the tract ODF values to the maximum ODF values. Thus, ignoring constants, the FiT of a fiber tract t_i on a tensor field $\boldsymbol{D}$ is defined as:

$$\varphi(t_i; \boldsymbol{D}) = -(\sum_{\boldsymbol{x} \in t_i} \log(\boldsymbol{t}_i(\boldsymbol{x})^T\boldsymbol{D}^{-1}(\boldsymbol{x})\boldsymbol{t}_i(\boldsymbol{x})) + \log(\lambda_1(\boldsymbol{x}))).$$

Notice that $\varphi(t_i; \boldsymbol{D})$ is not sensitive to an arbitrary ordering of eigenvectors that have very close eigenvalues. Also, the value of FiT is maximized for the first-order streamline tractography solution, since that would mean a perfect alignment between the tract tangent vector and the principle eigenvector at every sample along the tract. Even though FiT is well suited for quantifying the fiber-tensor alignment, a direct optimization of this measure may not be feasible since the algorithmic complexity of each iteration would be the same as running a full brain tractography.

3   Experiments

We analyzed 15 full brain Diffusion Tensor MR images of resolution 2.5 x 2.5 x 2.5 mm. Tractography was performed in each subject using Runge-Kutta order two integration. As a benchmark, we employed an ITK implementation [16] of an FA-based non-linear registration method (known as the demons algorithm) that has been successfully applied to DTI data [7]. This method performs a dense matching on the intensity images using a diffusion process. Regularization is achieved through Gaussian smoothing.

Selecting the first subject as the template, we provide results for 14 pairwise registrations using: 1) an FA-based global affine registration algorithm [17], 2) the demons algorithm, and 3) the proposed bundle-based polyaffine algorithm. Figure 1 includes 3D renderings of the registered tracts from a subject (in green)

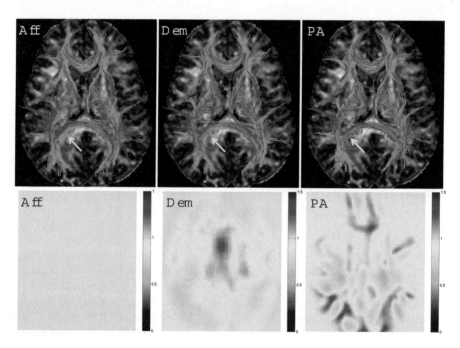

Fig. 1. Top Row: 3D renderings of the registered tracts of a subject (in green) and the template (in red) within ±5mm of the central axial slice overlayed on the central FA slice of the template. "Aff" (left) stands for the FA based global affine, "Dem" (middle) for the demons algorithm and "PA" (right) for the polyaffine framework as proposed in this work. Arrows point to an area of differing qualities of registration. Overlapping of the red and green fibers is indicative of better registration. Bottom Row: Jacobian determinant images from the central slice of the volume: Yellow represents areas with small changes in size, and the shades of red and blue represent enlargement and shrinking, respectively. The Jacobian of the global affine registration is constant. The Jacobian of the demons algorithm is smooth due to the Gaussian regularization. The Jacobian of the polyaffine algorithm reflects the underlying anatomy because of the fiber bundle-based definition of the deformation.

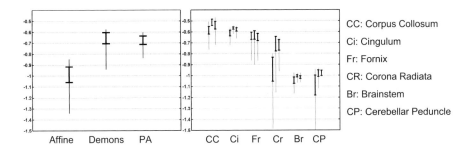

Fig. 2. Left: Mean FiT values from 14 subjects' DTI sets. Each subject's DTI data is aligned with the template and compared with the template's fiber tracts. Thin lines indicate the range of the FiT values, and the thick crossbars indicate the regions within one standard deviation from the mean. Right: Mean FiT values from 14 subjects' major fiber bundles. For each bundle, the left error bar is for affine; the middle one is for demons and the right one is polyaffine. Relative ranges of the fit values for major structures are similar to the averages from the whole data sets, however differ from each other in absolute terms.

and the template tracts (in red) overlayed on the central axial FA slice of the template. The second row shows the central slice of the Jacobian determinant volumes for the corresponding deformations computed by each registration algorithm. Note that certain anatomical structures are visible in the proposed algorithm's Jacobian image. This is due to the bundle-based definition of the underlying deformation field. The Jacobian image of the demons algorithm, however, demonstrates no clear relationship with the underlying anatomy. A close investigation of the fiber tract renderings in Figure 1 reveals that both non-linear algorithms, in general, achieve significantly better alignment of the tracts. There are some regions in this image, e.g. the corpus callosum, where the bundle-based algorithm yields more accurate matching than the demons algorithm. Figure 2 includes plots of average FiT values for the different algorithms and some major bundles of interest. The nonlinear algorithms achieve consistently better registrations than to the affine algorithm. The two nonlinear algorithms yield comparable results.

4   Discussion

This paper explores an inter-subject bundle-based nonlinear registration algorithm for DTI data sets. The algorithm performs comparable to a higher dimensional nonrigid registration algorithm, and it has certain advantages that many nonlinear algorithms lack, such as the ease of calculating the inverse transform. We also showed that there is an analytic expression for the Jacobian matrix of our deformation field, which was used for the reorientation of the deformed diffusion tensor field. Furthermore, the quality of the registration can be improved with higher degrees of freedom, such as multiple affine components per structure, without losing the cited advantages.

References

[1] Basser, P.J., Mattiello, J., Bihan, D.L.: MR diffusion tensor spectroscopy and imaging. Biophys. J. 66, 259–267 (1994)

[2] Basser, P., Pajevic, S., Pierpaoli, C., Duda, J., Aldroubi, A.: In vivo fiber tractography using DT–MRI data. Magnetic Resonance in Medicine 44, 625–632 (2000)

[3] O'Donnell, L., Westin, C.F.: White matter tract clustering and correspondence in populations. In: Duncan, J.S., Gerig, G. (eds.) MICCAI 2005. LNCS, vol. 3749, pp. 140–147. Springer, Heidelberg (2005)

[4] Maddah, M., Mewes, A., Haker, S., Grimson, W.E.L., Warfield, S.: Automated atlas-based clustering of white matter fiber tracts from DTMRI. In: Duncan, J.S., Gerig, G. (eds.) MICCAI 2005. LNCS, vol. 3749, pp. 188–195. Springer, Heidelberg (2005)

[5] Partridge, S.C., Mukherjee, P., Berman, J.I., Henry, R.G., Miller, S.P., Lu, Y., Glenn, O.A., Ferriero, D.M., Barkovich, A.J., Vigneron, D.B.: Tractography-based quantitation of diffusion tensor imaging parameters in white matter tracts of preterm newborns. Magnetic Resonance in Medicine 22(4), 467–474 (2005)

[6] Alexander, D.C., Pierpaoli, C., Basser, P.J., Gee, J.C.: Spatial transformations of diffusion tensor magnetic resonance images. IEEE TMI 20 (2001)

[7] Park, H.J., Kubicki, M., Shenton, M.E., Guimond, A., McCarley, R.W., Maier, S.E., Kikinis, R., Jolesz, F.A., Westin, C.-F.: Spatial normalization of diffusion tensor MRI using multiple channels. Neuroimage 20(4), 1995–2009 (2003)

[8] Jones, D.K., Griffin, L., Alexander, D., Catani, M., Horsfield, M., Howard, R., Williams, S.: Spatial normalization and averaging of diffusion tensor MRI data sets. Neuroimage 17(2), 592–617 (2002)

[9] Leemans, A., Sijbers, J., Backer, S.D., Vandervliet, E., Parizel, P.M.: Affine coregistration of diffusion tensor magnetic resonance images using mutual information. In: Blanc-Talon, J., Philips, W., Popescu, D.C., Scheunders, P. (eds.) ACIVS 2005. LNCS, vol. 3708, pp. 523–530. Springer, Heidelberg (2005)

[10] Xu, D., Mori, S., Shen, D., van Zijl, P.C., Davatzikos, C.: Spatial normalization of diffusion tensor fields. Magnetic Resonance in Medicine 50(1), 175–182 (2003)

[11] Arsigny, V., Commowick, O., Pennec, X., Ayache, N.: A fast and Log-Euclidean polyaffine framework for locally affine registration. Research report RR-5865, INRIA Sophia-Antipolis (2006)

[12] O'Donnell, L., Westin, C.F.: High-dimensional white matter atlas generation and group analysis. In: Larsen, R., Nielsen, M., Sporring, J. (eds.) MICCAI 2006. LNCS, vol. 4191, pp. 243–251. Springer, Heidelberg (2006)

[13] Leemans, A., Sijbers, J., Backer, S.D., Vandervliet, E., Parizel, P.M.: Multiscale white matter fiber tract coregistration: a new feature-based approach to align diffusion tensor data. Magnetic Resonance in Medicine 55(6), 1414–1423 (2006)

[14] Fletcher, R., Powell, M.: A rapidly convergent descent method for minimization. Computer Journal 6, 163–168 (1963)

[15] Tuch, D.S., Reese, T.G., Wiegell, M.R., Wedeen, V.J.: Diffusion MRI of complex neural architecture. Neuron 40, 885–895 (2003)

[16] Ibanez, L., Schroeder, W., Ng, L., Cates, J.: The ITK Software Guide. 1st edn. Kitware, Inc. ISBN 1-930934-10-6. (2003)

[17] Zollei, L., Learned-Miller, E., Grimson, W.E.L., Wells III, W.M.: Efficient population registration of 3D data. In: ICCV, Computer Vision for Biomedical Image Applications (2005)

Multivariate Normalization with Symmetric Diffeomorphisms for Multivariate Studies

B.B. Avants, J.T. Duda, H. Zhang, and J.C. Gee

Penn Image Computing and Science Laboratory
University of Pennsylvania
Philadelphia, PA 19104-6389
avants@grasp.cis.upenn.edu

Abstract. Current clinical and research neuroimaging protocols acquire images using multiple modalities, for instance, T1, T2, diffusion tensor and cerebral blood flow magnetic resonance images (MRI). These multivariate datasets provide unique and often complementary anatomical and physiological information about the subject of interest. We present a method that uses fused multiple modality (scalar and tensor) datasets to perform intersubject spatial normalization. Our multivariate approach has the potential to eliminate inconsistencies that occur when normalization is performed on each modality separately. Furthermore, the multivariate approach uses a much richer anatomical and physiological image signature to infer image correspondences and perform multivariate statistical tests. In this initial study, we develop the theory for Multivariate Symmetric Normalization (MVSyN), establish its feasibility and discuss preliminary results on a multivariate statistical study of 22q deletion syndrome.

1 Introduction

Emerging imaging modalities such as very high resolution MRI (sub-millimeter), diffusion tensor (DT) MRI and cerebral blood flow imaging provide a unique opportunity for computing anatomically and functionally meaningful mappings between subjects. Traditional high-resolution T1 structural images capture gray matter (computational structure) white matter (connective tissue) and cerebrospinal fluid borders. The diffusion tensor imaging modality [1] provides insight into directional white matter organization in the human brain. This information, captured in a tensor, provides a guide to normalization within white matter that is unavailable to T1 MRI. Arterial spin labeling (ASL) perfusion MRI is another emerging quantitative functional magnetic resonance imaging (fMRI) method which directly measures cerebral blood flow (CBF) by using water molecules in inflowing arteries as an endogenous contrast agent [2,3]. Each modality captures complementary attributes of the underlying subject being imaged. Taken together and in the same coordinate system, the set of these images obtained in a single imaging session on the same subject can be considered as a single multivariate (or multi-spectral) image.

N. Ayache, S. Ourselin, A. Maeder (Eds.): MICCAI 2007, Part I, LNCS 4791, pp. 359–366, 2007.
© Springer-Verlag Berlin Heidelberg 2007

No current image registration method systematically addresses the problem of consistently mapping between two multivariate (MV) datasets. For example, clinical research imaging protocols may acquire T1, DT and cerebral blood flow images. In this case, an individual's anatomical-functional system is represented by, at minimum, these three modalities. MV normalization will directly model this correspondence problem on the level of the individual and her associated set of images, as opposed to on single modality image pairs.

Consider an n-modality dataset, $\mathbf{I}_n = \{I_1, \cdots, I_n\}$ and a second dataset, $\mathbf{J}_n$, from a different individual or the same individual at a different time. A common approach to mapping between these individuals is to select one image modality as the reference, for example, I_1, typically a T1 structural image, and to find the image registration between it and J_1. However, this approach ignores modality dependent distortions and also does not take advantage of the additional information provided by the alternative pictures of the individuals' anatomical-functional systems in modalities $2 \rightarrow n$.

There is little related work, in medical image registration, on this topic. However, in 1993, Miller, et al. published likely the first multivariate deformable normalization method [4] and applied this method to map between a 2D patient and template dataset. Similarly, Park, et al [5] developed a multiple channel elastic DT registration method for simultaneously mapping T2 and fractional anisotropy (FA) images. FA is a scalar value that measures the degree of anisotropy in each tensor voxel and is aligned, inherently, with the T2 modality. The full tensor is not used in Park's normalization. Miller's recent work [6] is more typical of the approach currently used where individuals' datasets are normalized only according to T1 structural images. Alternatively, normalization may be done only on the DT images [7,8]. Our goal is to use as much information about an individual as possible to guide the subject to template matching while allowing (Bayesian) weights modelling the uncertainty between modalities to be incorporated into the normalization optimization. This integrative approach, ideal for setting up multivariate studies, is illustrated in figure 1.

Our MV normalization uses the full MV image object as the basis for finding correspondences. This novel model includes intrasubject transformations between the modalities, intersubject intramodality maps and the ability to spatially vary the weighting of the combined MV data. Our hypothesis is that combining information from, for example, DT and T1 will improve the quality of both gray and white matter mappings and improve statistics derived from multivariate population studies. The diffusion data in DT provides information in white matter areas that appear homogeneous in T1. CBF images, on the other hand, give information about the current state of functionally related blood flow throughout the brain and may also contribute to normalization.

We now extend the symmetric normalization method (SyN) [9] to deal properly with MV datasets, yielding MVSyN. We develop the MVSyN theory for three modalities, two scalar and one tensor. The resulting map may be applied consistently to all three modalities. In our associated study, we use the MV symmetric diffeomorphic transformation model to estimate intersubject correspondences from fused T1 and diffusion tensor (DT) structural images. We compare results from MVSyN with standard single modality symmetric normalization in terms of the statistical power for a population study. Our preliminary results suggest the novel finding that combining the DT and T1 pictures of neuroanatomy may indeed improve upon structural normalization usually based on T1 structural data alone.

2   Multivariate Symmetric Normalization

Symmetric Diffeomorphic Registration. We now summarize the approach to symmetric normalization, but leave major details to external references [9]. Recall that a diffeomorphism is a differentiable map with a differentiable inverse and may be generated by integrating regularized velocity fields, $\boldsymbol{v}(\mathbf{x}, t)$, through an ordinary differential equation, $d\phi(\mathbf{x}, t) = \boldsymbol{v}(\phi(\mathbf{x}, t), t)$. We denote such a map, indexed by a spatial coordinate $\mathbf{x} \in \Omega$ and a "time" t, as $\phi \colon \mathbf{x} \in \Omega \times t \in [0, 1] \to \Omega$. These diffeomorphic maps are constrained to equal the identity at the boundaries of the domain Ω. The usual approach in image registration is to find a map $\phi(\mathbf{x}, 1)$ such that $I(\phi_1(\mathbf{x}, 1)) \approx J$. This parameterization of the problem is asymmetrically optimized with respect to I. The symmetric diffeomorphic parameterization instead seeks solutions ϕ_1 and ϕ_2 such that $I(\phi_1(\mathbf{x}, 0.5)) \approx J(\phi_2(\mathbf{x}, 0.5))$ where the composition $\phi_2^{-1}(\phi_1(\mathbf{x}, 0.5), 0.5)$ gives $\phi_1(\mathbf{x}, 1)$. This approach eliminates bias towards either I or J. For easier reading we write, for instance, $\phi_1(0.5)$ for $\phi_1(\mathbf{x}, 0.5)$.

Symmetric Diffusion Tensor Diffeomorphic Registration. We extend the scalar SyN technique for image registration to normalize full tensor data. Diffusion tensor data requires special handling because a transformation of the underlying space should preserve the tensor orientation. To date, no symmetric diffeomorphic image registration method works with the full tensor. Few nonrigid DT normalization strategies incorporate reorientation. We will outline our MV and DT methods for both normalization and reorientation with symmetric diffeomorphisms.

   Miller, et al gave an algorithm that maps DT images based upon fiber orientation, which requires projecting each tensor (matrix) to a vector quantity, the principal eigenvector of the tensor [7]. We have recently developed a method in which we are able to estimate small deformation optimization of a DT similarity metric while taking into account the reorientation [8]. We detail our method for using this small deformation model to define velocity fields that may be integrated in time, through the MVSyN framework, to define large deformation diffeomorphisms.

   First, define a diffusion tensor as $\mathbf{D_i}$, a symmetric, positive definite 3×3 matrix. The Euclidean distance between tensors gives a similarity measure that takes advantage of the full tensor of information,

$$\|\mathbf{D}_1 - \mathbf{D}_2\|_{DT} = \sqrt{\mathrm{Tr}((\mathbf{D}_1 - \mathbf{D}_2)^2)}. \tag{1}$$

This similarity metric is the DT analogy of the intensity difference measure that may be used for T1 to T1 structural image registration.

The difficulty, traditionally, in optimizing this similarity measure with respect to a generic deformable transformation is that the deformation affects the tensor values themselves. An analytical method for parameterizing a deformation in terms of a local affine patch [8] allows one to compute analytical derivatives of the similarity measure above with respect to small deformations.

Now consider I_{DT} and J_{DT}, two DT images with pixel values $I_{DT}(\mathbf{x}) = \mathbf{D}_1$, $J_{DT}(\mathbf{x}) = \mathbf{D}_2$. Our goal is to compute the similarity between these two diffusion tensor images with respect to a diffeomorphism, ϕ_1 or ϕ_2,

$$\int_\Omega \|I_{DT}(\phi_1(0.5)) - J_{DT}(\phi_2(0.5))\|^2_{DT} d\Omega, \qquad (2)$$

where we assume tensor reorientation (discussed below) is always used when a transformation is composed with DT images. Consider that a diffeomorphism, $\phi(\mathbf{x})$, is, by definition, a locally affine transformation. Then, in a small neighborhood, N, about $\mathbf{x}$, we can approximate the diffeomorphism as an affine transformation, F, expressed as $QS(\mathbf{x})\mathbf{x} + \mathbf{T}(\mathbf{x})$, where $\mathbf{T}$ is the translation, Q is the rotation matrix and S is the pure deformation component of F. We are able to deform images I_{DT} and J_{DT} by using the preservation of principle directions (PPD) method, as given in [10]. Therefore, we may write $I_{DT}(\phi_1(\mathbf{x})) = \tilde{I_{DT}}$ and $J_{DT}(\phi_2(\mathbf{x})) = \tilde{J_{DT}}$, regardless of the size of the ϕ_i, as they are guaranteed diffeomorphic and thus locally affine.

Now assume a small deformation of $\tilde{I_{DT}}$ as $\boldsymbol{v}_1$ such that we have $\|\tilde{I_{DT}}(\mathbf{x} + \boldsymbol{v}_1) - \tilde{J_{DT}}\|_{DT}$. Locally, we estimate $\mathbf{x} + \boldsymbol{v}_1(\mathbf{x}) \approx (QS)\mathbf{x} + \mathbf{T}$. We may then compute, at position $\mathbf{x}$, the equation 2 above as,

$$\|\tilde{I_{DT}}((QS\mathbf{x} + \mathbf{T}) - Q\tilde{J_{DT}}Q^T\|^2_{DT}, \qquad (3)$$

where $Q\tilde{J_{DT}}Q^T$ accounts for reorientation and F is estimated in N, a local neighborhood of $\mathbf{x}$. Here, we use the finite strain model to parameterize the reorientation, while the more accurate PPD method has been used to deform the tensor images by the ϕ_i. *This parameterization of the similarity allows us to take derivatives of the objective function in the space of diffeomorphisms while taking into account the effect of reorientation on the tensor values.* Analytical derivatives of equation 3 are in the proper Eulerian reference frame needed for estimating derivatives of the DT similarity criterion in equation 2. This specialized method, along with PPD reorientation, enables us to extend the SyN method to function with both scalar and diffusion tensor data. Other similarity measures, described in [8], may be parameterized in a similar way. The same approach as above is used to estimate the similarity gradient with respect to $\tilde{J_{DT}}$.

MVSyN with T1, DT, CBF. The extension to MV data requires the use of modality-dependent similarity criterion as well as a strategy for sensibly weighting information from each modality in the registration optimization. Define $\mathbf{I}_3$ as consisting of $\{I_1 = T1,\ I_2 = CBF,\ I_3 = DT\}$ image modalities, assumed to exist in the same patient space and in the same rigid orientation. Furthermore, define $\Pi_3(\mathbf{I_3}, \mathbf{J_3})$ as the similarity criterion operating on a MV pair, $\mathbf{I_3}$ and $\mathbf{J_3}$.

We now extend scalar symmetric normalization to deal with MV datasets,

$$E_{MVSyN}(\mathbf{I_3}, \mathbf{J_3}) =$$

$$\inf_{\phi_1} \inf_{\phi_2} \int_{t=0}^{0.5} \{\, \|v_1(\mathbf{x}, t)\|_L^2 + \|v_2(\mathbf{x}, t)\|_L^2 \,\}\, dt +$$

$$\int_{\Omega} \omega \Pi_3(\mathbf{I_3}, \mathbf{J_3}, 0.5)\, d\Omega\,,$$

with each ϕ_i the solution of:

$$\phi_i / dt = v_i(\phi_i(\mathbf{x}, t), t) \text{ with } \phi_i(\mathbf{x}, 0) = \mathbf{Id}. \qquad (4)$$

Equation 4 retains the transformation models used in symmetric normalization, but also uses additional similarity metrics, contained in Π_3, for multiple modality image sets. We define Π_3 as,

$$\Pi_3(\mathbf{I_3}, \mathbf{J_3}, 0.5) = \omega_1(\mathbf{x})|I_1(\phi_1(0.5)) - J_1(\phi_2(0.5))|^2 +$$
$$\omega_2(\mathbf{x}) MI(I_2, (\phi_1(0.5)), J_2(\phi_2(0.5))) + \omega_3(\mathbf{x})\|I_3(\phi_1(0.5)) - J_3(\phi_2(0.5))\|_{DT}^2 \quad (5)$$

where MI is the mutual information (defined in the usual way) and the ω_i weights each similarity term as a function of the domain. If this term is optimized, we write $\mathbf{I_3}(\phi_1(0.5)) \approx \mathbf{J_3}(\phi_2(0.5))$. Our previous work in curve matching [11] showed that weights which vary across the spatial domain allow results that may be superior to results found with constant weighting terms. A reasonable choice for weighting functions will depend upon the relative signal of the input images; for T1 and CBF, levels that are above noise; for DT, the weight may be higher in regions where the fractional anisotropy is strong enough to indicate the presence of white matter. The sum of the weighting functions will be constrained to add to one. We will also normalize each similarity derivative such that its maximum displacement, before weighting, is on the order of a single voxel. This latter step aids in making a fair combination of the different gradients.

Note that the MVSyN registration algorithm involves, qualitatively, taking derivatives of the objective function Π_3 and then regularizing in both space and time. Our approach to regularization uses a finite horizon temporal discretization and the full voxel resolution in the spatial domain. Therefore, the critical gradients which we must compute are the derivatives of Π_3 with respect to the current position of the diffeomorphism. Regularizing this derivative gives an estimate of the velocity. The gradients of MI may be found in [12], for the DT norm in [8].

3   Results

We now study a MV dataset containing both DT and structural T1 pediatric neuroimages, as described in [13], and containing 11 controls and 16 age-matched

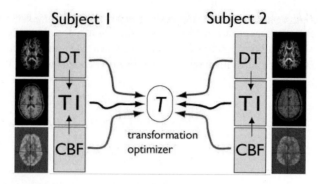

Fig. 1. Two integrative MV datasets of individual anatomical structure and function and the mapping between the MV datasets via transformation, T. Our methods are able to leverage all modalities (T1 structural, DT and cerebral blood flow) to guide the computation of T with maximal subject information. Therefore, in this case, there will be three intramodality inputs for determining T. The CBF and DT images are initially mapped into the structural coordinate system, as it is typically of highest resolution and has features shared by each modality. All mappings are diffeomorphic. Curved arrows indicate intersubject transformations while straight arrows indicate intrasubject transformations.

subjects suffering from 22q deletion syndrome. This genetic defect causes a variety of effects, the most prominent of which is brain matter loss and enlarged ventricles. We also chose this dataset because it has been analyzed previously with other methods [13] and contains a known population difference showing reductions in the gray matter of 22q subjects relative to controls.

Preprocessing, before normalization, involved mapping each subject's DT image into the T1 anatomical space by an affine registration. Affine registration was used to accommodate for modality-dependent distortion. The T1 structural images were also skull-stripped. We then select a control image as a template and normalize the full dataset to this template by optimizing equation 4. For this preliminary comparison, we choose constant weighting functions $\omega_1 = 0.5$, $\omega_2 = 0.0$ and $\omega_3 = 0.5$. The results of an example normalization, along with multivariate group difference statistics on the fractional anisotropy (FA) and Jacobian, are shown in figure 2. The statistics were assessed with Hotelling's T^2 distribution where the variables were, at each voxel, the value of the normalized FA and the log-Jacobian of the diffeomorphic map to the template space. The Jacobian estimates local structure sizes. The log-Jacobian is used as it has a symmetric distribution around zero. Therefore, our multivariate study assesses the probability of a control-patient difference in both FA and local structure sizes. For comparative purposes, we also performed the same study with SyN, using the T1 structural images alone to guide the mapping. This involved using MVSyN but with ω_2 and ω_3 set to zero. Both FA and Jacobian images were used for the MVSyN and SyN multivariate comparison.

The significance of our results were assessed with cluster-size based permutation tests. Permutation tests provide a non-parametric method for examining

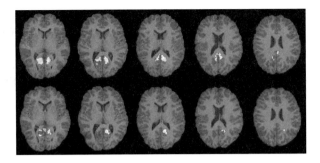

Fig. 2. The most significant cluster generated by MVSyN normalization is shown over-laid on the template in the top row. The cluster shows the areas where gray matter and FA are significantly larger in controls compared to subjects (non-parametric cluster level significance at $p < 0.005$). The bottom row shows the largest cluster generated by SyN normalization (1003 voxels, significant at $p < 0.025$. The MVSyN cluster is larger and also more bilateral. It is interesting that including DT information in the normalization increases the significance of a gray-matter focused result.

the random chance of finding results similar to those in one's true population. The procedure involves selecting a T or p-value threshold and then collecting the histogram of cluster sizes over hundreds or thousands of permutations of the dataset. We chose a threshold of $p < 0.001$ to generate clusters at each of 1000 permutations.

Our comparison found that MVSyN produced stronger MV statistics for this study. A cluster size of 938 voxels was significant at a level of $p < 0.05$ for MVSyN. A cluster size of 1113 voxels was significant for SyN at $p < 0.05$. These results, and the major cluster found by both methods, are shown in figure 2. The largest above threshold cluster, generated by MVSyN, was 1643 voxels. SyN's corresponding cluster was 1003 voxels in size. Both clusters show gray matter loss in 22q subjects relative to controls, as expected, as well as a difference in the FA. By examining the univariate statistics, we saw that the majority of this effect was due to volumetric, rather than FA, differences. Our finding, here, is consistent with previous studies [13], although our statistical threshold is more conservative.

4   Discussion

The most common approach for multiple modality studies is to perform normalization with respect to structural images alone. MVSyN absorbs this model while permitting much greater flexibility through parameter selection and using full MV datasets. We showed that the MVSyN model also improves the statistical significance of a MV statistical study on a known patient population. We also note that univariate statistics on the Jacobian values generated by SyN and MVSyN show the same trend as the multivariate statistics.

We believe that MVSyN provides an ideal complement to multivariate datasets currently being collected and will improve normalization-based studies. However, many issues remain, including parameter selection, similarity metric choice and evaluation. One pressing issue not explicitly dealt with here is the possibility of non-rigid deformation in the intrasubject T1 to DT or CBF to T1 mapping. Note that, if necessary, one may introduce explicit DT distortion correction models. Furthermore, development in parallel MR imaging are reducing the amount of distortion present in DT. For these reasons, and given our encouraging preliminary results, we believe MVSyN constitutes a valuable contribution to normalization methodology.

References

1. Basser, P J, Mattiello, J., Le Bihan, D.: MR diffusion tensor specstroscopy and imaging. Biophys. J. 66, 259–267 (1994)
2. Wang, J., Licht, D.J., Jahng, G.H., Liu, C.S., Rabin, J.T., Haselgrove, J.C.: Pediatric perfusion imaging using pulsed arterial spin labeling. J. Mag. Reson. Imag. 18, 404–413 (2003)
3. Wang, J., Aguirre, G., Kimberg, D., Roc, A.C., Li, L., Detre, J.: Arterial spin labeling perfusion fmri with very low task frequency. Magn. Reson. Med. 49, 796–802 (2003)
4. Miller, M.I., Christensen, G.E., Amit, Y., Grenander, U.: Mathematical textbook of deformable neuroanatomies. Proc. Natl. Acad. Sci (USA) 90, 11944–11948 (1993)
5. Park, H.-J., Kubicki, M., Shenton, M E, et al.: Spatial normalization of diffusion tensor MRI using multiple channels. Neuroimage 20, 1995–2009 (2003)
6. Miller, M.I., Beg, M.F., Ceritoglu, C., Stark, C.: Increasing the power of functional maps of the medial temporal lobe by using large deformation diffeomorphic metric mapping. PNAS 102, 9685–9690 (2005)
7. Yan, C., Miller, M.I., Winslow, R.L., Younes, L.: Large deformation diffeomorphic metric mapping of vector fields. tmi 24, 1216–1230 (2005)
8. Zhang, H., Yushkevich, P.A., Alexander, D.C., Gee, J.C.: Deformable registration of diffusion tensor MR images with explicit orientation optimization. In: Duncan, J.S., Gerig, G. (eds.) MICCAI 2005. LNCS, vol. 3749, Springer, Heidelberg (2005)
9. Avants, B., Grossman, M., Gee, J.C.: Symmetric diffeomorphic image registration: Evaluating automated labeling of elderly and neurodegenerative cortex. Medical Image Analysis (in press online, 2007)
10. Alexander, D.C., Pierpaoli, C., Basser, P.J., Gee, J.C.: Spatial transformations of diffusion tensor magnetic resonance images. IEEE Trans. Med. Imaging 20, 1131–1139 (2001)
11. Avants, B., Gee, J.C.: Formulation and evaluation of variational curve matching with prior constraints. In: Gee, J.C., Maintz, J.B.A., Vannier, M.W. (eds.) Biomedical Image Registration, pp. 21–30. Springer, Heidelberg (2003)
12. Hermosillo, G., Chefd'Hotel, C., Faugeras, O.: A variational approach to multimodal image matching. Intl. J. Comp. Vis. 50, 329–343 (2002)
13. Simon, T., Ding, L., Bish, J., McDonald-McGinn, D., Zackai, E., Gee, J.C.: Volumetric, connective, and morphologic changes in the brains of children with chromosome 22q11.2 deletion syndrome: an integrative study. Neuroimage 25, 169–180 (2005)

Non-rigid Surface Registration Using Spherical Thin-Plate Splines

Guangyu Zou[1], Jing Hua[1], and Otto Muzik[2]

[1] Department of Computer Science, Wayne State University, USA
[2] PET Center, School of Medicine, Wayne State University, USA

Abstract. Accurate registration of cortical structures plays a fundamental role in statistical analysis of brain images across population. This paper presents a novel framework for the non-rigid intersubject brain surface registration, using conformal structure and spherical thin-plate splines. By resorting to the conformal structure, complete characteristics regarding the intrinsic cortical geometry can be retained as a mean curvature function and a conformal factor function defined on a canonical, spherical domain. In this transformed space, spherical thin-plate splines are firstly used to explicitly match a few prominent homologous landmarks, and in the meanwhile, interpolate a global deformation field. A post-optimization procedure is then employed to further refine the alignment of minor cortical features based on the geometric parameters preserved on the domain. Our experiments demonstrate that the proposed framework is highly competitive with others for brain surface registration and population-based statistical analysis. We have applied our method in the identification of cortical abnormalities in PET imaging of patients with neurological disorders and accurate results are obtained.

1 Introduction

In order to better characterize the symptoms of various neuro-diseases from large datasets, automatic population-based comparisons and statistical analyses of integrative brain imaging data at homologous cortical regions are highly desirable in noninvasive pathophysiologic studies and disease diagnoses [1]. As a recent comparative study pointed out, intensity-based approaches may not effectively address the huge variability of cortical patterns among individuals [2]. Surface-based methods, which explicitly capture the geometry of the cortical surface and directly drive registration by a set of geometric features, are generally thought to be more promising in bringing homologous brain areas into accurate registration. One reason leading to this consideration is that the folding patterns (gyri and sulci) are typically used to define anatomical structures and indicate the location of functional areas [3].

In essence, cortical surfaces can be regarded as 3D surfaces. In the context of cortical structural analysis, representations based on the Euclidean distance are problematic, as it is not consistent with the intrinsic geometry of a surface [3]. For this reason, we adopted the strategy to first parameterize brain surface on a

N. Ayache, S. Ourselin, A. Maeder (Eds.): MICCAI 2007, Part I, LNCS 4791, pp. 367–374, 2007.
© Springer-Verlag Berlin Heidelberg 2007

canonical spherical domain using conformal mapping [4]. After that, subsequent matching and averaging of cortical patterns can be performed in this canonical space with enhanced efficiency since all geometric characteristics of the cortex are retained in this space. The benefits of this framework are as follows: first, because surface registration is modeled as a smooth deformation on a sphere, many confounding factors originally existing in the Euclidean space are eliminated; second, this registration method is implicitly scale-invariant as shapes are normalized on the canonical domain via conformal mapping; third, by means of deforming shapes in a parametric space, a 3D shape registration is reduced into a 2D space, thus largely simplifying computational complexity.

Even so, one needs to note that conformal mapping itself can not wipe off the inherent variability of individual human brains. To account for this nonlinear variation, non-rigid registration techniques need be used to deform one surface onto another with consistent alignment of primary anatomies. Towards this end, the spherical thin-plate splines (STPS) is presented to provide a natural scheme for this purpose. Given a set of point constraints, a smooth deformation field can be efficiently estimated with C^∞ continuity everywhere except at the location of lankmarks where the continuity is C^1. Optimization techniques can then be further appended afterwards in this framework as a back-end refinement in order to compensate for the discrepancies between piecewise spline estimation and the actual confounding anatomical variance.

For the purpose of accurately aligning two brain surfaces, a novel framework is systematically introduced in this paper. We first propose to use the conformal structure on a spherical domain to completely represent the cortical surface for registration. Building on that, we systematically derive the analytical and numerical solutions regarding spherical thin-plate splines (STPS) deformation and compound optimization based on the conformal factor and mean curvature of brain surfaces, which naturally induces a non-rigid registration between two brain surfaces. The effectiveness and accuracy of this framework is validated in a real application that intends to automatically identify PET abnormalities of the human brain.

2   Conformal Brain Surface Model

Based on *Riemannian geometry*, conformal mapping provides a mathematically rigorous way to parameterize cortical surface on a unit sphere, of which many properties have been well studied and fully controlled. Let ϕ denote this conformal transformation and (u, v) denote the spherical coordinates, namely, the conformal parameter. The cortical surface can be represented as a vector-valued function $\boldsymbol{f} : S^2 \to \mathbf{R}^3, \boldsymbol{f}(u, v) = (f_1(u, v), f_2(u, v), f_3(u, v))$. Accordingly, the local isotropic stretching of ϕ (conformal factor $\lambda(u, v)$) and the mean curvature $H(u, v)$ of surface $\boldsymbol{f}$ can be treated as functions defined on S^2. Since $\lambda(u, v)$ and $H(u, v)$ can uniquely reconstruct surface $\boldsymbol{f}$ except for a rigid rotation [4], the two functions are sufficient for representing arbitrary closed shapes of genus zero topology. We term this representation the *Conformal Brain Surface Model*

(CBSM). The orientational freedom of CBSM can be removed by SVD methods, based on the landmark correspondences representing homologous cortical features. The CBSM is illustrated in Figure 1.

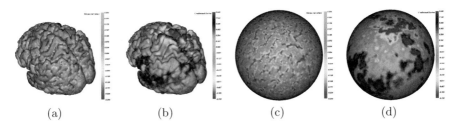

(a)   (b)   (c)   (d)

Fig. 1. Conformal Brain Surface Model. In (a) and (b), mean curvature and logarithmic conformal factor are color-encoded on the brain surface, respectively. (c) and (d) visualize the mean curvature function and the conformal factor function in accordance with the CBSM.

Suppose that M_1 and M_2 are two surfaces to be matched, and the parameterizations are $\varphi_1 : M_1 \to \mathbf{R}^2$ and $\varphi_2 : M_2 \to \mathbf{R}^2$, respectively. Then the transition map $\varphi_2 \circ \varphi_1^{-1} : M_1 \to M_2$ defines a bijection between M_1 and M_2. Given a matching criterion, the registration of 3D shapes can be consequently defined as an automorphism μ on the parameter domain, such that the transformation $\psi = \varphi_2 \circ \mu \circ \varphi_1^{-1}$ in 3D minimizes the studied matching error. In particular, given a conformal parameterization of brain surface S, a registration criterion can be losslessly defined using $(\lambda(x_1, x_2), H(x_1, x_2))$.

A few related ideas have been proposed in [4,5,6,7,8]. However, Gu et al. [4] only pursued solutions in the conformal space, which in most cases is over-constrained for an optimal registration in terms of anatomy alignment. In [6], the deformation for the brain surface was essentially computed in a rectangular plane. Since a topological change is required from a sphere to a disk, choices for the landmarks restricted by the large distortion at domain boundaries. The registration scheme employed in [7] is basically a variant of ICP (Iterated-Closest-Point) algorithm that is performed in the Euclidean space. As for the spherical deformation, diffeomorphic deformation maps constructed by the integration of velocity fields that minimize a quadratic smoothness energy under specified landmark constraints are presented in a recent paper [9]. When compared with STPS, its solution does not have closed-form.

3   Method

Generally, our method includes two main steps: First, the registration is initiated by a feature-based STPS warping. This explicit procedure largely circumvents local minimum and is more efficient when compared with using variational optimization directly. Second, a compound energy functional that represents a balanced measurement of shape matching and deformation regularity is minimized, which compensates for the potential improper localization of unmarked cortical features.

3.1 STPS Deformation

Thin-plate splines (TPS) are a class of widely used non-rigid interpolating functions. Because of its efficiency and robustness, intensive exploitation of TPS has been made for smooth data interpolation and geometric deformation.

The spherical analogue of the well-known thin-plate bending energy defined in Euclidean space was formulated in [10], which has the form

$$J_2(u) = \int_0^{2\pi} \int_0^{\pi} (\Delta u(\theta, \phi))^2 \sin \phi d\theta d\phi, \tag{1}$$

where $\theta \in [0, \pi]$ is latitude, $\phi \in [0, 2\pi]$ is longitude, Δ is the Laplace-Beltrami operator. Let

$$K(X, Y) = \frac{1}{4\pi} \int_0^1 \log h(1 - \frac{1}{h})(\frac{1}{\sqrt{1 - 2ha + h^2} - 1} - 1)dh, \tag{2}$$

where $a = \cos(\gamma(X, Y))$ and $\gamma(X, Y)$ is the angle between X and Y. With the interpolants

$$u(P_i) = z_i, \quad i = 1, 2, \ldots, n, \tag{3}$$

the solution is given by

$$u_n(P) = \sum_{i=1}^n c_i K(P, P_i) + d, \tag{4}$$

where

$$\mathbf{c} = \mathbf{K}_n^{-1}[\mathbf{I} - \mathbf{T}(\mathbf{T}^T \mathbf{K}_n^{-1} \mathbf{T})^{-1} \mathbf{T}^T (\mathbf{K}_n^{-1})]\mathbf{z},$$
$$d = (\mathbf{T}^T \mathbf{K}_n^{-1} \mathbf{T})^{-1} \mathbf{T}^T (\mathbf{K}_n^{-1})\mathbf{z},$$
$$(\mathbf{K}_n)_{ij} = K(P_i, P_j),$$
$$\mathbf{T} = (1, \ldots, 1)^T,$$
$$\mathbf{z} = (z_i, \ldots, z_n)^T,$$

in which $\mathbf{K}_n$ is the $n \times n$ matrix with its (i, j)th entry denoted as $(\mathbf{K}_n)_{ij}$.

Given the displacements $(\Delta\theta_i, \Delta\phi_i)$ of a set of points $\{P_i\}$ on the sphere in spherical coordinates, the STPS can be used to interpolate a deformation map $S^2 \to S^2$ that is consistent with the assigned displacements at $\{P_i\}$ and smooth everywhere, which minimizes J_2. Most anatomical features on brain surfaces, such as sulci and gyri, are most appropriate to be represented as geometric curves. The feature curves are automatically fitted using the cardinal splines, based on a set of sparse points selected by a neuroanatomist on the native brain surface. The framework also provides the automatic landmark tracking functions using the methods in [11]. In order to deal with curve landmarks on the sphere with STPS, we convert a curve to a dense set of ordered points, yielding precise control over curves. A global smooth deformation field $(u_\theta(P), u_\phi(P))$ can be consequently determined, which warps each landmark curve on the source CBSM into their counterpart on the target as shown in Figure 2 (a), (b) and (c). This deformation ensures the alignment of primary labeled features. However, other unlabeled cortical anatomies are not guaranteed to be perfectly matched to their counterparts. In the following, a global optimization scheme is proposed to address this issue.

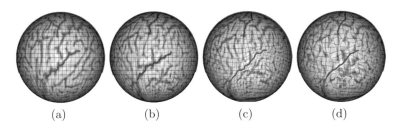

(a)   (b)   (c)   (d)

Fig. 2. The illustration of the CBSM deformations at each registration stage. (a) shows the target CBSM. (b) shows the source CBSM. (c) shows the effect of STPS deformation performed on (b). The result of a further refining optimization is shown in (d).

3.2   Compound Optimization

Since all the transformations applied so far are topology preserving, we generally consider that homologous anatomies have been laid very close to each other in the spherical space through the landmark-based STPS deformation. To further refine the alignment of anatomies besides the manually traced features, we define a global distance in the shape space via CBSM based on the conformal factor $\lambda(u, v)$ and the mean curvature $H(u, v)$:

$$d(S_1, S_2) = \int_{S^2} ((\log \lambda_1(u, v) - \log \lambda_2(u, v))^2 + (H_1(u, v) - H_2(u, v))^2) d\mu, \quad (5)$$

where the $d\mu$ is the area element of the unit sphere S^2. Here we compare the logarithm values of λ to eliminate the bias between the same extent of stretching and shrinking from conformal mapping. When this functional is minimized, two brain surfaces are registered. Additionally, we moderately smooth down the brain surface for mean curvature computation similar in spirit to [3], since we assume that the optimization should only be directed by large-scale geometric features while being relatively insensitive to those small folds that are typically unstable across subjects. Suppose the optimization procedure is performed by deforming S_2 to S_1. The optimal nonlinear transformation $\tilde{\phi}^*$ can be formulated as

$$\tilde{\phi}^* = \arg\min_{\phi}(d(S_1(u, v) - S_2(\phi(u, v)))). \quad (6)$$

In practice, simply minimizing the distance functional may cause undesirable folds or distortions in the local patch. To avoid this, we also add another term to the distance functional to maximize conformality while warping two spherical images into registration. This regularizing term is essentially a harmonic energy functional.

Note that the cortical surface, as well as the domain, are approximated by triangular meshes. We use the gradient descent method for the numerical optimization. Suppose $\boldsymbol{f}(\cdot)$ and $\boldsymbol{g}(\cdot)$ are the piecewise linear approximations of CBSM domains, p and q are neighbor vertices, and $\{p, q\}$ denotes the edge spanned between them. $\alpha_{p,q}$ and $\beta_{p,q}$ denote the two angles opposite to p, q in the two triangles sharing edge $\{p, q\}$. $A_{f(g)}(p)$ denotes the areal patch in $f(g)$ associated with p. Therefore, the gradient of this compound functional is given by

$$
\begin{aligned}
\frac{\partial E}{\partial \boldsymbol{f}(v)} = & \sum_{u \in N_1(v)} (\cot \alpha_{p,q} + \cot \beta_{p,q})(\boldsymbol{f}(v) - \boldsymbol{f}(u)) \\
& + \frac{\varphi A_f(v)}{\sum_{i \in K_f} A_f(i)} \lambda_{f-g}(v) \frac{\boldsymbol{f}(v) - \boldsymbol{f}(u^*)}{\|\boldsymbol{f}(v) - \boldsymbol{f}(u^*)\|} \nabla_{\overrightarrow{\{u^*, v\}}} \lambda_{f-g}(v) \\
& + \frac{\omega A_f(v)}{\sum_{i \in K_f} A_f(i)} H_{f-g}(v) \frac{\boldsymbol{f}(v) - \boldsymbol{f}(u^*)}{\|\boldsymbol{f}(v) - \boldsymbol{f}(u^*)\|} \nabla_{\overrightarrow{\{u^*, v\}}} H_{f-g}(v),
\end{aligned}
$$

$$(7)$$

where φ and ω are tunable weighting factors, $SF_{f-g}(\cdot) = SF_f(\cdot) - SF_g(\cdot)$, and u^* is defined as

$$
u^*(v) = \arg \max_{u \in N_1(v)} \nabla_{\overrightarrow{\{u, v\}}} (SF_f - SF_g)(v), \tag{8}
$$

in which the SF denotes either $\lambda(\cdot)$ or $H(\cdot)$, and $N_1(v)$ is the 1-ring neighbors of v. In practice, we also constrain the displacement of each vertex in the tangential space of the unit sphere. The optimized result after STPS deformation is shown in Figure 2 (d). Its improvement to brain surface registration will be further demonstrated in Section 4.

4   Experiments

We have tested our framework through automatic identification of Positron Emission Tomography (PET) abnormalities. In order to identify the functional abnormalities characterized by PET, the normal fusion approach [12] is used for MRI and PET integration as shown in Figure 3 (a) and (b). PET values are projected onto the high resolution brain surface extracted from MRI data. Then we apply the proposed framework to bring the studied subjects (high-resolution cortical surfaces) into registration and subdivide the cortical surfaces into registered, homotopic elements on the spherical domain. Similar to the element-based analysis of PET images in [13,14], we obtain the PET concentration for each of the cortical elements. A patient's data is compared with a set of normals to locate the abnormal areas in the patient brain based on the statistical histogram analysis of the PET concentration at the homotopic cortical elements. Figure 3 (c)

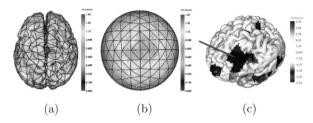

(a) (b) (c)

Fig. 3. Identification of PET abnormalities. (a) and (b) show the rendering of the PET concentration on the cortical surface and the spherical domain, respectively. The triangle-like elements are the defined homotopic cortical elements by the registration. (c) PET abnormalities are rendered on the cortical surface using a color map.

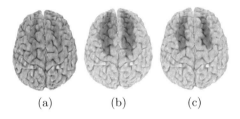

(a) (b) (c)

Fig. 4. Repetition Levels for Prominent Cortical Regions. (a) shows the regions of middle frontal gyri delineated by a neuroscientist; (b) shows the agreement using only STPS, while (c) gives the result when the compound optimization is enabled.

show the result of a pediatric patient with epilepsy. The blue color indicates decreased tracer concentration than normal. We use 8 normal pediatric datasets to establish the normal distribution for comparison. One of the normal dataset is treated as the template for registration. In our experiments, the detected abnormal spots well corresponds to the final clinical diagnoses because the high-quality inter-subject mapping and registration greatly improves cross-subject element matching for statistical analysis. This real application validates the registration capability of our framework from a practical perspective.

We also directly evaluated our methods on several prominent neuroanatomical regions in terms of group overlap using high-resolution MRI data. Since cortical regions have been well defined and indexed by elements, the overlap can be measured by area. The elements for a specific feature which agree on more than 85% cases are colored in red. Those that agree on 50%∼85% cases are colored in green. As an example, Figure 4 demonstrates the result on middle frontal gyri, delineated by a neuroscientist. It is evident that, after compound optimization, the features under study appear more consistent to the middle frontal gyrus regions on the template cortex because of the refined matching of geometric structures by compound optimization. The certainty with regard to the regional boundaries are increased. More comprehensive experiments indicate that significant agreements can be achieved via our method. The overall registration accuracy in terms of group overlap is about 80%.

5   Conclusion

We have presented a novel, effective non-rigid brain surface registration framework based on conformal structure and spherical thin-plate splines. To enable this procedure, we systematically derive the analytical and numerical solutions regarding STPS deformation and compound optimization based on the conformal factor and mean curvature of brain surfaces. Our experiments demonstrate that our method achieves high accuracy in terms of homologous region overlap. Our method is tested in a number of real neurological disorder cases, which consistently and accurately identify the cortical abnormalities.

References

1. Thompson, P., et al.: Mapping cortical change in alzheimer's disease, brain development and schizophrenia. NeuroImage 23(1), S2–S18 (2004)
2. Hellier, P., et al.: Retrospective evaluation of intersubject brain registration. IEEE TMI 22(9), 1120–1130 (2003)
3. Fischl, B., et al.: Cortical surface-based analysis II: Inflation, flattening, and a surface-based coordinate system. NeuroImage 9(2), 195–207 (1999)
4. Gu, X., et al.: Genus zero surface conformal mapping and its application to brain surface mapping. IEEE TMI 23(8), 949–958 (2004)
5. Fischl, B., et al.: High-resolution intersubject averaging and a coordinate system for the cortical surface. Human Brain Mapping 8(4), 272–284 (1999)
6. Wang, Y., et al.: Optimization of brain conformal mapping with landmarks. In: Duncan, J.S., Gerig, G. (eds.) MICCAI 2005. LNCS, vol. 3750, pp. 675–683. Springer, Heidelberg (2005)
7. Tosun, D., et al.: Mapping techniques for aligning sulci across multiple brains. Medical Image Analysis 8(3), 295–309 (2004)
8. Zou, G., et al.: An approach for intersubject analysis of 3D brain images based on conformal geometry. In: Proc. ICIP 2006 pp. 1193–1196 (2006)
9. Glaunès, J., et al.: Landmark matching via large deformation diffeomorphisms on the sphere. Journal of Mathematical Imaging and Vision 20, 179–200 (2004)
10. Wahba, G.: Spline interplolation and smooothing on the sphere. SIAM Journal of Scientific and Statistical Computing 2(1), 5–16 (1981)
11. Lui, L.M., et al.: Automatic landmark tracking and its application to the optimization of brain conformal mapping. In: Proc. CVPR 2006 pp. 1784–1792 (2006)
12. Stockhausen, H.V., et al.: 3D-tool - a software system for visualisation and analysis of coregistered multimodality volume datasets of individual subjects. NeuroImage 7(4), S799 (1998)
13. Ghias, S.A.: GETool: Software tool for geometric localization of cortical abnormalities in epileptic children. Master Thesis, Computer Science Department, Wayne State University (2006)
14. Muzik, O., et al.: Multimodality Data Integration in Epilepsy. International Journal of Biomedical Imaging 13963 (2007)

A Study of Hippocampal Shape Difference Between Genders by Efficient Hypothesis Test and Discriminative Deformation

Luping Zhou[1], Richard Hartley[1,2], Paulette Lieby[2], Nick Barnes[2],
Kaarin Anstey[3], Nicolas Cherbuin[3], and Perminder Sachdev[4]

[1] RSISE The Australian National University
[2] Vision Science and Technology Program, NICTA
[3] Centre for Mental Health Research, ANU
[4] Neuropsychiatric Institute, Prince of Wales Hospital, Sydney[*]

Abstract. Hypothesis testing is an important way to detect the statistical difference between two populations. In this paper, we use the Fisher permutation and bootstrap tests to differentiate hippocampal shape between genders. These methods are preferred to traditional hypothesis tests which impose assumptions on the distribution of the samples. An efficient algorithm is adopted to rapidly perform the *exact* tests. We extend this algorithm to multivariate data by projecting the original data onto an "informative direction" to generate a scalar test statistic. This "informative direction" is found to preserve the original discriminative information. This direction is further used in this paper to isolate the discriminative shape difference between classes from the individual variability, achieving a visualization of shape discrepancy.

1 Introduction

In this paper, we investigate methods of characterizing anatomical shapes as part of a clinical study. The purpose is to detect a statistically significant difference between two classes based on shape descriptors. In this paper we concentrate on classification for gender based on the hippocampus. Such analysis is typically used when attempting to discriminate between healthy and diseased populations, such as in the case of schizophrenia ([1]). We address two key problems in shape analysis: hypothesis testing and identifying the discriminative information.

The classification of the hippocampal shapes between genders is a difficult problem. Using common classifiers, such as kernel SVM and nonlinear discriminators, we could only generate a classification accuracy slightly better than chance. In this case, hypothesis testing becomes critical in answering whether the difference detected by the classifiers is a real difference or just random. Prevailing

---

[*] National ICT Australia is funded by the Australian Government's Backing Australia's Ability initiative, in part through the Australia Research Council. The authors thank the PATH research team at the Centre for Mental Health Research, ANU, Canberra, and the Neuroimaging Group (Neuropsychiatric Institute), Prince of Wales Hospital, Sydney, for providing the original MRI and segmented data sets.

N. Ayache, S. Ourselin, A. Maeder (Eds.): MICCAI 2007, Part I, LNCS 4791, pp. 375–383, 2007.
© Springer-Verlag Berlin Heidelberg 2007

methods for hypothesis testing in the existing medical applications make a distribution assumption for the test statistic, such as the t test or χ^2 test ([2,3,4,5]). A limitation of such methods is that a poor distribution model can result in unreliable testing results. For example, the Student's t test assumes a normal distribution of the population or a large sample size. However, this assumption is difficult to justify in many existing medical applications where the sample is small ([4,2,3]). Hence it is better to use hypothesis tests such as the Fisher permutation test and the bootstrap test, which make minimal assumptions about the sample distribution. However, the exact permutation and bootstrap tests are computationally intractable because of their formidably large test space. Generally practitioners only consider a small subset randomly drawn from the entire test space. This is known as the Monte-Carlo or the randomized permutation test.

Another issue to address is to identify the discriminative information between groups in order to understand the nature of the difference. One approach is to represent the shape as a Point Distribution Model (PDM) and analyze each landmark separately([3]). This method potentially ignores the correlations between the landmarks. Golland *et al.* in [2] recently proposed an approach introducing the concept of the "discriminative direction". This "direction" is a curved path with the property that when a shape deforms along its course, only the differences relevant for group discrimination appear.

This paper has two main contributions: (i) It applies the efficient permutation/bootstrap test proposed in [6] to the shape-determination problem; this involves adapting the method to multivariate data. The multivariate shape descriptors are "scalarized" by being projected onto a line. The projection direction is carefully selected using kernel Fisher discriminant analysis (KFDA) to preserve the discriminating information of the original data as much as possible. Compared with other approaches, our method is free of distribution assumptions and overcomes the problem of the overwhelmingly large search space involved in the exact permutation test. It searches the entire test space, resulting in a more accurate p-value estimation in trivial computational time. (ii) The "discriminative direction" is found by a different approach compared with [2]. In [2], the problem is formulated in terms of finding the movement direction in the original space that minimizes the movement in feature space parallel to a hyperplane determined using kernel SVM. Our method on the other hand formulates the problem from the perspective of movement in the feature space and links it to the inverse of the kernel problem ([7,8,9,10]) in machine learning. That is, when a shape descriptor moves along a direction found by KFDA in the feature space, the corresponding changes in the original space are computed as the preimages of the kernel mapping to form the course of the "discriminative direction". Thereby a more direct and conceptually simpler solution is achieved.

2   Method

In this paper, 3D hippocampal shapes are represented by the spherical harmonics expansion (SPHARM) [11,5,3]. A shape descriptor vector is composed of $3(l+1)^2$

spherical harmonic coefficients $(c_{x0}^0, c_{y0}^0, c_{z0}^0, \cdots, c_{xn}^{-m}, \cdots, c_{zn}^m)^\top$, where l is the degree, m the order and c the coefficient. Here hippocampal shape descriptors for two classes (men and women) are compared in order to determine if the shape vectors for the two classes are significantly different.

2.1   Review of the Efficient Permutation and Bootstrap Tests in [6]

Suppose we have m observations $x_1, x_2, \ldots, x_m$ belonging to class A (for instance males) and $n - m$ observations $x_{m+1}, \ldots, x_n$ belonging to class B (for instance females). A (scalar) statistic t_i (for instance height) is measured and the difference between the mean value of the statistic for classes A and B is found; thus

$$ t = \frac{1}{m} \sum_{i=1}^m t_i - \frac{1}{n-m} \sum_{i=m+1}^n t_i . $$

Suppose that this results in a higher value for class A than class B. The question is whether this difference is significant. Under the null-hypothesis, the value of this test statistic t should not be significantly different from zero.

For the Fisher permutation test, we randomly repartition the n samples into two classes A_r and B_r of sizes m and $n - m$, resulting in a test statistic t_r^* defined as before. The permutation test seeks the fraction p of times among all such partitions that the original statistic t is greater than t_r^*. The boostrap test differs from the permutation test in that the two classes A_r and B_r are drawn from the original observations with replacement.

The exact permutation/bootstrap test has an extremely large test space. The size of the entire test space, N, is C_n^m for the permutation test and n^n for the bootstrap test. Even when n is around 100, the exhaustive enumeration of all possible test statistic values is computationally intractable.

A more efficient method is proposed in [6] for the exact test. Instead of using the exhaustive enumeration, it expands p as an infinite Fourier series. The method is elaborated as follows. In [6], p is defined as $N^{-1} \sum_{r=1}^N H(t_r^* - t)$, where $H(x)$ is a step function: 0 if $x < 0$, $1/2$ if $x = 0$, and 1 otherwise. Assuming that H is a periodic function (with period exceeding the largest value of $t_r^* - t$), taking its infinite Fourier series and exchanging the order of the finite and infinite sums, p becomes a convergent series

$$ p = \frac{1}{2} + \frac{2}{\pi} \Im \left(\sum_{k=1}^\infty \frac{\Psi(2k-1) \exp(-i(2k-1)t)}{2k-1} \right) \tag{1} $$

where $\Im(z)$ is the imaginary part of z and $\Psi(2k-1) = N^{-1} \sum_{r=1}^N \exp(ikt_r^*)$. For details, refer to [6].

The advantage of this procedure is that the infinite sum converges rapidly when N is large. More significantly, when the test statistic is a linear combination of the observed data, the computation of $\Psi(k)$ may be carried out very efficiently, as shown in [6]. Note that this method converges to an exact p value without explicitly enumerating all the resamplings of the data.

2.2   Extension of the Method in [6] to Multivariate Data

The method in [6] is applicable to scalar data only. This can be clearly seen from the definition of p where the step function, $H(x)$, is only valid for scalars. We solve this problem by "scalarizing" the multivariate data. All data are projected onto an "informative" direction which can maximally preserve the discriminative information in the original data. The direction $\mathbf{w}$ is realized by maximizing the Fisher linear discriminant criterion (FLDA): $\mathcal{J}(\mathbf{w}) = (\mathbf{w}^{\top}\mathbf{S}_B\mathbf{w})/(\mathbf{w}^{\top}\mathbf{S}_W\mathbf{w})$ where $\mathbf{w}$ is the projection vector, $\mathbf{S}_B$ is the between-class scatter matrix, and $\mathbf{S}_W$ is the within-class scatter matrix. Hence the resulting projections are gathered compactly within classes, and separated between classes.

Actually we use a nonlinear version, known as kernel Fisher discriminant analysis (KFDA) [12], to seek the "informative" direction, because the real-world data is often not linearly separable. KFDA maps the data nonlinearly into another space of higher dimension, $\mathcal{F}$, and performs FLDA in $\mathcal{F}$ instead. Let $\mathbf{x}$ ($\mathbf{x} \in \mathcal{R}^d$) be a sample, and $\Phi : \mathcal{R}^d \to \mathcal{F}$ be the nonlinear mapping. In $\mathcal{F}$ we may write the discriminant criterion as $\mathcal{J}(\mathbf{w}) = (\mathbf{w}^{\top}\mathbf{S}_B^{\Phi}\mathbf{w})/(\mathbf{w}^{\top}\mathbf{S}_W^{\Phi}\mathbf{w})$ where $\mathbf{S}_B^{\Phi}$ and $\mathbf{S}_W^{\Phi}$ are defined in terms of values $\Phi(\mathbf{x})$ in $\mathcal{F}$.

The mapping Φ can be very complex. Hence KFDA uses the kernel trick to avoid computing it explicitly. Consider that $\mathbf{w}$ lies in a space spanned by the data samples: $\mathbf{w} = \sum_i \alpha_i \Phi(\mathbf{x}_i)$. The objective function $\mathcal{J}(\mathbf{w})$ may be written in terms of the coefficients α_i and the inner product $\langle \Phi(\mathbf{x}_i), \Phi(\mathbf{x}_j) \rangle$. Instead of explicitly computing Φ, we define a kernel function $k(\mathbf{x}_i, \mathbf{x}_j)$; the function Φ is then implicitly defined by the relationship $k(\mathbf{x}_i, \mathbf{x}_j) \equiv \langle \Phi(\mathbf{x}_i), \Phi(\mathbf{x}_j) \rangle$. The RBF (radial basis function) kernel $k(\mathbf{x}_i, \mathbf{x}_j) = \exp(-\|\mathbf{x}_i - \mathbf{x}_j\|^2/2\sigma^2)$ is used in this paper. With this kernel, the optimal values of α_i may be computed to maximize $\mathcal{J}(\mathbf{w})$. Then any data vector $\mathbf{x}$ may be scalarized by projection onto the discriminative direction $\mathbf{w}$ according to the formula $\mathbf{w}^{\top}\Phi(\mathbf{x}) = \sum_{i=1}^{l} \alpha_i k(\mathbf{x}_i, \mathbf{x})$.

Note that the projection direction $\mathbf{w}$ in KFDA is a non-linear discrimination axis in the original shape space. Moreover, the projection direction is a combination of the features in the shape space (linear in FLDA, and nonlinear in KFDA). The combination weights reveal the correlations of multiple variables with regard to the discrimination.

2.3   Discriminative Deformation

The shape difference needs to be located. We address this issue by deforming a particular male hippocampus to a female one and vice versa. This deformation reveals the discriminative differences between classes, excluding any differences due to the individual variability within a class. This is called a "discriminative deformation" in this paper, and is obtained by deforming a shape along the "discriminative direction" (see Section 1). This paper seeks the "discriminative direction" by utilizing the nonlinear mapping $\Phi : \mathcal{R}^d \to \mathcal{F}$ provided by KFDA and computing the inverse of the kernel mapping. In short, the "discriminative direction" is formed by simply computing the preimages of a movement parallel to the direction $\mathbf{w}$ (see Section 2.2) in $\mathcal{F}$ for a particular shape descriptor $\Phi(\mathbf{x})$. In this way, we avoid solving the complex optimization problem in [2].

In $\mathcal{F}$, if $\Phi(\mathbf{x})$ moves along the direction $\mathbf{w}$ for a step of λ, it arrives at a new position: $\Phi(\mathbf{x}) + \lambda\mathbf{w}$, where $\mathbf{w}$ is a unit vector. If the preimage of the new position in $\mathcal{R}$ is estimated as $\mathbf{z}$, the error $\rho = \|\Phi(\mathbf{x}) + \lambda\mathbf{w} - \Phi(\mathbf{z})\|^2$ should be minimized. This optimization problem is equivalent to maximizing $\langle\Phi(\mathbf{x}) + \lambda\mathbf{w}, \Phi(\mathbf{z})\rangle$ when a Gaussian RBF kernel is used. Notice that for an RBF kernel there is a relationship between the input space distance $d_{ij}^2 = \|\mathbf{x}_i - \mathbf{x}_j\|^2$ and the feature space distance $\tilde{d}_{ij}^2 = \|\Phi(\mathbf{x}_i) - \Phi(\mathbf{x}_j)\|^2$, namely $d_{ij}^2 = -2\sigma^2 \log((2 - \tilde{d}_{ij}^2)/2)$. Making a simplifying assumption that the preimage of $\Phi(\mathbf{x}) + \lambda\mathbf{w}$ does exist ($\rho = 0$), we obtain a closed form solution for $\mathbf{z}$, namely

$$\mathbf{z} = \frac{(2 - \tilde{d}^2(\phi(\mathbf{x}) + \lambda\mathbf{w}, \Phi(\mathbf{x})))\mathbf{x} + \lambda\sum_{i=1}^{l}\alpha_i(2 - \tilde{d}^2(\phi(\mathbf{x}) + \lambda\mathbf{w}, \Phi(\mathbf{x}_i)))\mathbf{x}_i}{2 - \tilde{d}^2(\phi(\mathbf{x}) + \lambda\mathbf{w}, \Phi(\mathbf{x})) + \lambda\sum_{i=1}^{l}\alpha_i(2 - \tilde{d}^2(\phi(\mathbf{x}) + \lambda\mathbf{w}, \Phi(\mathbf{x}_i)))},$$

(2)

where $\tilde{d}^2(\Phi(\mathbf{x}_i), \Phi(\mathbf{x}) + \lambda\mathbf{w})$ is $2 + \lambda^2\alpha^\top K\alpha + 2\lambda\alpha^\top K_x - 2k(x_i, x) - 2\lambda\alpha^\top K_{x_i}$. Given n training data, K is the $n \times n$ kernel matrix, $K_{ij} = k(x_i, x_j)$. Further, α denotes $(\alpha_1, \cdots, \alpha_n)^\top$, K_x denotes $(k(x, x_1), \cdots, k(x, x_n))^\top$, and K_{x_i} denotes $(k(x_i, x_1), \cdots, k(x_i, x_n))^\top$.

3 Results

A database of 353 left hippocampi of healthy individuals, including 180 males and 173 females, is used. The hippocampi have been hand-traced from MRI scans which are drawn from the 60-64 year old age cohort from the first wave of a longitudinal project, PATH through Life, from the Centre for Mental Health Research, the Australian National University. The whole data set is partitioned into a training data set of size 150 (used to train KFDA), and a test data set of size 203. All shapes are represented using SPHARM coefficients with degree 5.

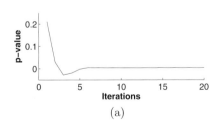
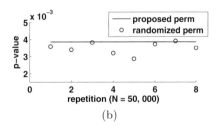

(a)   (b)

Fig. 1. (a) Convergence of the p-value calculated by the proposed permutation test. (b) In the randomized permutation test ($N = 50,000$), the p-value fluctuates around the value estimated by the proposed method when repeating the test with random resampling.

Hypothesis test. In our hypothesis test, the null hypothesis is defined by *a lack of significant statistical difference between the shapes of genders*. Two aspects are tested: the convergence speed and the discriminating ability. The convergence speed of our method is compared with the randomized permutation test. To facilitate a fair comparison, the convergence of the p-value is tested on the same KFDA projections in the randomized version. KFDA uses a RBF kernel. The parameters σ and μ for KFDA are tuned via a 5-fold cross validation. The results are obtained on a computer with a 3.0GHz CPU and 2.0GB RAM. In the randomized test, the p-value fluctuates around 0.0035 in eight repetitions of 50,000 random resamplings (Fig. 1 (b)). It takes 490 seconds for the randomized test to test only 10^{-57} of the entire test space. However, the p-value calculated by our methods takes only 10 iterations (2.28 seconds) in the permutation test and 36 iterations (0.05 seconds) in the bootstrap test to converge to 0.0039. Due to the large size of our test space, Fig. 1 (a) indicates that the p-value converges well without the "spike" effect mentioned in [6].

Table 1. Comparison of the p-value in different hypothesis tests

Test 1:	Test 2: FLDA		Test 3: KFDA	
Randomized	Permutation	Bootstrap	Permutation	Bootstrap
0.0339	0.0651	0.0645	0.0039	0.0039

The operation of projection may cause information loss. Hence we need to test the discriminating ability of our proposed methods. Three experiments have been conducted. Test 1 is independent of projection: a randomized permutation test is used whose test statistic is the Euclidean distance between the mean shape descriptors of two randomly selected groups. Test 2 and Test 3 seek the informative projection direction by FLDA and KFDA respectively. The p values in the hypothesis tests are summarized in Table 1. The smaller p value in Test 3 suggests that KFDA better preserves the discriminating information than both FLDA in Test 2 and the Euclidean distance in Test 1. Further experiments, not discussed here, show that KFDA achieves a better separation for the mean projections of the male and female groups.

The hypothesis test is conducted on normalized data, i.e. the hippocampi are normalized for volume. Indeed, it has often been reported that hippocampal volumes differ for the sexes ([13]). Our findings confirm other results that show male and female hippocampal shapes differ ([14]).

Discriminative shape deformation. A synthetic data set consisting of two concentric circles is used to test the discriminative direction method we derived (Fig 2). The circles are projected onto a direction $\mathbf{w}$ found by KFDA in the feature space (Fig 2 (a)). When a particular point p moves along $\mathbf{w}$ in the feature space, the corresponding moving trace, i.e. the discriminative direction at point p in the original space, is recovered in Fig 2 (b). It also can be seen that our method works consistently at different points. Our method is further applied

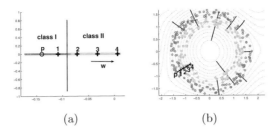

(a)   (b)

Fig. 2. Discriminative direction of two synthetic classes (dark and gray dots): (a) point p moving along $\mathbf{w}$ in the feature space; (b) the corresponding motion in the original space, i.e. the discriminative direction at p. Nine further examples are shown.

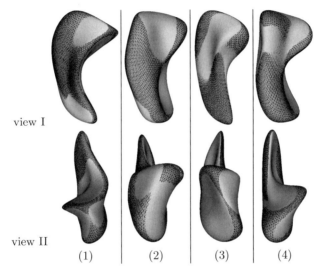

view I

view II

(1)   (2)   (3)   (4)

Fig. 3. Four left male hippocampi (each one in a column) are deformed to be female-like and viewed from two perspectives. The deformed female-like shape (in solid) and the original male shape (in mesh) are overlapped for comparison. The solid part is only visible when it protrudes the mesh, and vice versa. A female hippocampus is more likely to be thicker in the middle part of the hippocampal head than a male hippocampus.

on real hippocampi to expose the nature of shape changes between genders. Fig 3 gives four examples of left male hippocampi before and after the discriminative deformation. The original male shape and the deformed female-like shape are overlapped for comparison. It can be seen that a female hippocampus is more likely to be thicker in the middle part of the hippocampal head than a male hippocampus. This is supported by the findings in [14]. Note that each deformed hippocampus resembles its original shape since the deformation only changes the class features while maintaining the individual information.

4   Conclusions

Using the Fisher permutation and bootstrap tests applied to a KFDA projection of the shape vector, it was demonstrated that the difference between male and female hippocampal shapes is significant at the 99.6% level. The KFDA test outperforms a randomized test (Test 1) based on difference between shape-cluster distance (96.6%), and is very much faster.

The shape discrepancy revealed by our experiments is global for two reasons: (i) The shapes are represented by SPHARM coefficients, which are global features. (ii) Discriminative deformation is able to illustrate the localized shape changes as demonstrated in [2]. However, as our large data set is population representative, the significant inter-individual hippocampal shape variation renders localization of class difference difficult. Future work will be to investigate discrimination for pathology vs normal using local features like PDM.

References

1. Styner, M., Lieberman, J., Pantazis, D., Gerig, G.: Boundary and medial shape analysis of the hippocampus in schizophrenia. Medical Image Analysis 8(3), 197–2003 (2004)
2. Golland, P., Grimson, W.E., Shenton, M.E., Kikinis, R.: Detection and analysis of statistical differences in anatomical shape. Medical Image Analysis 9(1), 69–85 (2005)
3. Shen, L., Ford, J., Makedon, F., Saykin, A.: Hippocampal shape analysis surface-based representation and classification. In: Proceedings of SPIE-Medical Imaging, pp. 253–264 (2003)
4. Gerig, G., Styner, M., Shenton, M.E., Lieberman, J.: Shape versus size: Improved understanding of the morphology of brain structures. In: Niessen, W.J., Viergever, M.A. (eds.) MICCAI 2001. LNCS, vol. 2208, pp. 24–32. Springer, Heidelberg (2001)
5. Gerig, G., Styner, M., Jones, D., Weinberger, D., Lieberman, J.: Shape analysis of brain ventricles using spharm. In: Proceedings of Workshop on Mathematical Methods in Biomedical Image Analysis MMBIA, pp. 171–178 (2001)
6. Gill, P.M.: Efficient calculation of p-values in linear-statistic permutation significance tests. Journal of Statistical Computation and Simulation 77(1), 55–61 (2007)
7. Schoelkopf, B., Mika, S., Smola, A., Raetsch, G., Mueller, K-R.: Kernel PCA pattern reconstruction via approximate pre-images. In: Proceedings Eighth International Conference Artificial Neural Networks, pp. 147–152 (1998)
8. Mika, S., Schoelkopf, B., Smola, A.J., Mueller, K-R., Scholz, M., Raetsch, G.: Kernel PCA and de-noising in feature spaces. In: Proceedings of Advances in Neural Information Processing Systems, pp. 536–542 (1999)
9. Kwok, J.T., Tsang, I.W.: The pre-image problem in kernel methods. IEEE Transactions on Neural Networks 15(6), 1517–1525 (2004)
10. Rathi, Y., Dambreville, S., Tannenbaum, A.: Statistical shape analysis using kernel PCA. In: Proceedings of SPIE Electronic Imaging (2006) pp. 425–432 (2006)
11. Kelemen, A., Szekely, G., Gerig, G.: Elastic model-based segmentation of 3-D neuroradiological data sets. IEEE Transactions on Medical Imaging 18(10), 828–839 (1999)

12. Mika, S., Raetsch, G., Weston, J., Schoelkopf, B., Mueller, K-R.: Fisher discriminant analysis with kernels. In: Neural Networks for Signal Processing IX, 1999. Proceedings of the 1999 IEEE Signal Processing Society Workshop, pp. 41–48. IEEE Computer Society Press, Los Alamitos (1999)
13. Maller, J.J., Réglade-Meslin, C., Anstey, K.J., Sachdev, P.: Sex and symmetry differences in hippocampal volumetrics: Before and beyond the opening of the crus of the fornix. Hippocampus 16, 80–90 (2006)
14. Bouix, S., Pruessner, J.C., Collins, D.L., Siddiqi, K.: Hippocampal shape analysis using medial surfaces. NeuroImage 25, 1077–1089 (2005)

Graph Cuts Framework for Kidney Segmentation with Prior Shape Constraints

Asem M. Ali[1], Aly A. Farag[1], and Ayman S. El-Baz[2]

[1] CVIP Laboratory, University of Louisville, USA
asem,farag@cvip.uofl.edu
[2] Bioengineering Dept., University of Louisville, USA
aselba01@louisville.edu

Abstract. We propose a novel kidney segmentation approach based on the graph cuts technique. The proposed approach depends on both image appearance and shape information. Shape information is gathered from a set of training shapes. Then we estimate the shape variations using a new distance probabilistic model which approximates the marginal densities of the kidney and its background in the variability region using a Poisson distribution refined by positive and negative Gaussian components. To segment a kidney slice, we align it with the training slices so we can use the distance probabilistic model. Then its gray level is approximated with a LCG with sign-alternate components. The spatial interaction between the neighboring pixels is identified using a new analytical approach. Finally, we formulate a new energy function using both image appearance models and shape constraints. This function is globally minimized using s/t graph cuts to get the optimal segmentation. Experimental results show that the proposed technique gives promising results compared to others without shape constraints.

1 Introduction

Isolating the kidney from its surrounding anatomical structures is a crucial step in many unsupervised frameworks that assess the renal functions, such as frameworks that are proposed for automatic classification of normal kidneys and acute rejection transplants from Dynamic Contrast Enhanced Magnetic Resonance Imaging (DCE-MRI). Many techniques were developed for kidney segmentation, Priester et al. [1] subtracted the average of precontrast images from the average of early-enhancement images, and black-and-white kidney mask is generated by a threshold. This mask image is eroded and the kidney contour is obtained with help of manual interactions. Giele et al. [2] improved the previous technique by applying an erosion filter to the mask image to obtain a contour via a second subtraction stage. A hull function is used to close possible gaps in this contour, then via repeated erosions applied to this contour, several rings were obtained, which formed the basics of the segmentation of the cortex from the medulla structures. Boykov et al. [3] used graph cuts to get a globally

N. Ayache, S. Ourselin, A. Maeder (Eds.): MICCAI 2007, Part I, LNCS 4791, pp. 384–392, 2007.
© Springer-Verlag Berlin Heidelberg 2007

optimal object extraction method for dynamic N-data sets. They minimized cost function, which combined region and boundary properties of segments as well as topological constraints. Although the results looked promising, manual interaction was still required. Sun et al. introduced many computerized schemes for kidney segmentation and registration. In [4], after roughly alinement, they subtracted a high-contrast image from a pre-contrast image to obtain a kidney contour, which was propagated over the other frames searching for the rigid registration parameters. They used the level sets to segment the cortex and medulla. Most of these previous works, analyzed healthy transplants images. However, poor kidney function decreases the uptake of contrast agent, resulting in disjoined bright regions, so edge detection algorithms generally failed in giving connected contours.

The literature is rich with another segmentation approaches: simple techniques (e.g. region growing or thresholding), parametric deformable models and geometrical deformable models. However, all these methods tend to fail in the case of noise, gray level inhomogeneities, and diffused boundaries. In the area of medical imaging, organs have well-constrained forms within a family of shapes [5]. Therefore segmentation algorithms have to exploit the prior knowledge of shapes and other properties of the structures to be segmented. Leventon et al.[6] combine the shape and deformable model by attracting the level set function to the likely shapes from a training set specified by principal component analysis (PCA). To make the shape guides the segmentation process, Chen et al. [7] defined an energy functional which basically minimizes an Euclidean distance between a given point and its shape prior. Huang et. al. [8], combine registration with segmentation in an energy minimization problem. The evolving curve is registered iteratively with a shape model using the level sets. They minimized a certain function to estimate the transformation parameters. In Paragios's work[9], a shape prior and its variance obtained from training data are used to define a Gaussian distribution, which is then used in the external energy component of a level sets framework.

In this paper, we propose a new kidney segmentation approach that uses graph cuts to combine region and boundary properties of segments as well as shape constraints. We generate from a set of kidney aligned images an image consisting of three segments: common kidney, common background, and shape variability region. We model the shape variations using a new distance probabilistic model. This distance model approximates the distance marginal densities of the kidney and its background inside the variability region using a Poisson distribution refined by positive and negative Gaussian components. For each given kidney slice, to use the distance probabilistic model, we align the given image with the training images. Then its gray level is approximated with a linear combination of Gaussian distributions (LCG) with positive and negative components. Finally, we globally minimized a new energy function using s/t graph cuts to get the optimal segmentation. This function is formulated such that it combines region and boundary properties, and the shape information.

2 Proposed Segmentation Framework

Recently, graph cuts appeared as a powerful optimization technique to get the optimal segmentation because it optimizes energy functions that can integrate regions and boundary properties of segments. The weighted undirected graph is a set of vertices, and a set of edges connecting these vertices. Each edge is assigned a nonnegative weight. The set of vertices corresponds to the set of image pixels $\mathcal{P}$, and two specially terminal vertices s (source), and t (sink). An example for the graph that we used in kidney segmentation is shown in Fig. 4. Consider a neighborhood system in $\mathcal{P}$, which is represented by a set $\mathcal{N}$ of all unordered pairs $\{p, q\}$ of neighboring pixels in $\mathcal{P}$. Let $\mathcal{L}$ the set of labels $\{\text{"0"}, \text{"1"}\}$, correspond to kidney and background, respectively. Labelling is a mapping from $\mathcal{P}$ to $\mathcal{L}$, and we denote the set of labelling by $\mathbf{f} = \{f_p : p \in \mathcal{P}, f_p \in \mathcal{L}\}$. Now our goal is to find the optimal segmentation, best labelling $\mathbf{f}$, by minimizing a new energy function which combines region and boundary properties of segments as well as shape constraints. This function is defined as follows:

$$E(\mathbf{f}) = \sum_{p \in \mathcal{P}} S(f_p) + \sum_{p \in \mathcal{P}} D(f_p) + \sum_{\{p,q\} \in \mathcal{N}} V(f_p, f_q), \qquad (1)$$

where $S(f_p)$ measures how much assigning a label f_p to pixel p disagrees with the shape information, this will be explained in Sec. 2.1. $D(f_p)$ measures how much assigning a label f_p to pixel p disagrees with the pixel intensity I_p. $V(f_p, f_q)$ represents the penalty of the discontinuity between pixels p and q. The last two terms will be explained in Sec. 2.2.

2.1 Shape Model Construction

Kidney shape model is created from a training set of kidney DCE-MRI slices. Fig.1 illustrates the steps used to create the shape model. Fig.1(a) shows a sample of the DCE-MRI kidney slices. First, we manually segment the kidneys (by a radiologist), as shown in Fig.1(b). Then the segmented kidneys are aligned using 2D rigid registration [10], see Fig.1(c). The aligned images are converted to binary images, as shown in Fig.1(d). Finally, we generate a "shape image" $\mathcal{P}_s = \mathcal{K} \bigcup \mathcal{B} \bigcup \mathcal{V}$ as shown in Fig2(a). The white color represents $\mathcal{K}$ (kidney), black represents $\mathcal{B}$ (background), and gray is the variability region $\mathcal{V}$. To model the shape variations, variability region $\mathcal{V}$, we use a distance probabilistic model. The distance probabilistic model describes the object (and background) in the variability region as a function of the normal distance $d_p = \min_{c \in \mathbf{C}_{\mathcal{K}\mathcal{V}}} \|p - c\|$ from a pixel $p \in \mathcal{V}$ to the kidney/variability contour $\mathbf{C}_{\mathcal{K}\mathcal{V}}$. Each set of pixels located at equal distance d_p from $\mathbf{C}_{\mathcal{K}\mathcal{V}}$ constitutes an iso-contour $\mathbf{C}_{d_p}$ for $\mathbf{C}_{\mathcal{K}\mathcal{V}}$ as shown in Fig2(b) (To clarify the iso-contours, we enlarge the variability region without scale). To estimate the marginal density of the kidney, we assume that each iso-contour $\mathbf{C}_{d_p}$ is a normally propagated wave from $\mathbf{C}_{\mathcal{K}\mathcal{V}}$. The probability of an iso-contour to be object decays exponentially as the discrete index d_p increases. So we model the distance histogram by a Poisson distribution. We estimate the

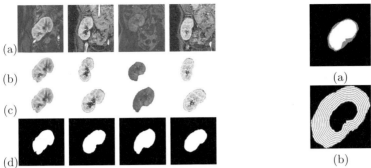

Fig. 1. Samples of kidney training data images: (a)Original , (b)Segmented , (c)Aligned (d)Binary

Fig. 2. (a) The labelled image, (b) The iso-contours

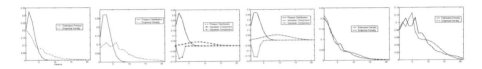

Fig. 3. [a,b]Empirical densities and the estimated Poisson distributions, [c,d] Components of distance probabilistic models, [e,f] Final estimated densities

kidney distance histogram as follows. The histogram entity at distance d_p is defined as

$$h_{dp} = \sum_{i=1}^{M} \sum_{p \in \mathbf{C}_{d_p}} \delta(p \in \mathcal{K}_i), \qquad (2)$$

where the indicator function $\delta(\boldsymbol{A})$ equals 1 when the condition $\boldsymbol{A}$ is true, and zero otherwise, M is the number of training images, and $\mathcal{K}_i$ is the kidney region in the training image i. We change the distance d_p until we cover the whole distance domain available in the variability region. Then we multiply the histogram with kidney prior value which is defined as follows:

$$\pi_{\mathcal{K}} = \frac{1}{M \mid \mathcal{V} \mid} \sum_{i=1}^{M} \sum_{p \in \mathcal{V}} \delta(p \in \mathcal{K}_i), \qquad (3)$$

We repeat the same scenario to get the marginal density of the background. The kidney and background distance empirical densities and the estimated Poisson distributions are shown in Fig.3 (a) and (b), respectively.

Distance Probabilistic Model: We define the shape penalty term $S(f_p)$ in Eq.1 as $S(f_p) = -ln \, P(d_p \mid f_p)$ where the distance marginal density of each class $P(d_p \mid f_p)$ is estimated as follow. Since each class f_p does not follow perfect Poisson distribution, there will be a deviation between the estimated and the empirical densities. We model this deviation by a linear combination of discrete

Gaussians with positive and negative components. So the distance marginal density of each class consists of a Poisson distribution and $K_{f_p}^+$ positive and $K_{f_p}^-$ negative discrete Gaussians components as follows:

$$P(d_p|f_p) = \vartheta(d_p|\lambda_{f_p}) + \sum_{r=1}^{K_{f_p}^+} w_{f_p,r}^+ \varphi(d_p|\theta_{f_p,r}^+) - \sum_{l=1}^{K_{f_p}^-} w_{f_p,l}^- \varphi(d_p|\theta_{f_p,l}^-), \quad (4)$$

where $\vartheta(d_p|\lambda_{f_p})$ is a Poisson density with rate λ, $\varphi(.|\theta)$ is a Gaussian density with parameter $\theta \equiv (\mu, \sigma^2)$ with mean μ and variance σ^2. $w_{f_p,r}^+$ means the rth positive weight in class f_p and $w_{f_p,l}^-$ means the lth negative weight in class f_p. This weights have a restriction $\sum_{r=1}^{K_{f_p}^+} w_{f_p,r}^+ - \sum_{l=1}^{K_{f_p}^-} w_{f_p,l}^- = 1$. We estimate the Poisson distribution parameter using the maximum likelihood estimator (MLE). To estimate the parameters of Gaussians components, we used the modified EM algorithm [11] to deal with the positive and negative components. Fig.3: (c) and (d) illustrate the probabilistic models components for kidney and background, respectively. The empirical and the final estimated densities are shown in Fig.3 (e) for the kidney and (f) for the background.

2.2   Image Appearance Models

Image appearance models are the gray level probabilistic model and the spatial interaction model.

A- Gray Level Probabilistic Model: To compute the data penalty term $D(f_p)$, we use the modified EM to approximate the gray level marginal density of each class f_p using a LCG with $C_{f_p}^+$ positive and $C_{f_p}^-$ negative components. Similar to distance probabilistic model the gray level probabilistic model is defined as follows:

$$P(I_p|f_p) = \sum_{r=1}^{C_{f_p}^+} w_{f_p,r}^+ \varphi(I_p|\theta_{f_p,r}^+) - \sum_{l=1}^{C_{f_p}^-} w_{f_p,l}^- \varphi(I_p|\theta_{f_p,l}^-). \quad (5)$$

B- Spatial Interaction Model: The pairwise interaction model which represents the penalty for the discontinuity between pixels p and q is defined as follows:

$$V(f_p, f_q) = \gamma \delta(f_p \neq f_q). \quad (6)$$

In this work we use a new analytical approach [11] to estimate the spatial interaction parameter γ. The simplest model of spatial interaction is the Markov Gibbs random field (MGRF) with the nearest 4-neighborhood. In the proposed approach, Gibbs potential is obtained analytically using MLE for a MGRF. The potential interaction is given by the following equation:

$$\gamma = \frac{K^2}{K-1} \left(f_{\text{neq}}(\mathbf{f}) - \frac{1}{K} \right), \quad (7)$$

where $K = 2$ is the number of classes in the image and $f_{\text{neq}}(\mathbf{f})$ denotes the relative frequency of the not equal labels in the pixel pairs.

2.3   Graph Cuts Optimal Segmentation

To segment a kidney, we construct a graph (e.g. Fig4) and define the weight of each edge as shown in table 1. Then we get the optimal segmentation boundary between the kidney and its background by finding the minimum cost cut on this graph. The minimum cost cut is computed exactly in polynomial time for two terminal graph cuts with positive edges weights via s/t Min-Cut/Max-Flow algorithm [12].

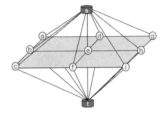

Fig. 4. Example of graph that used in image segmentation

Table 1. Graph Edges Weights

Edge	Weight	for
$\{p, q\}$	$V(f_p, f_q)$	$\{p, q\} \in \mathcal{N}$
$\{s, p\}$	$-ln[P(I_p \mid 1)P(d_p \mid 1)]$	$p \in \mathcal{V}$
	∞	$p \in \mathcal{K}$
	0	$p \in \mathcal{B}$
$\{p, t\}$	$-ln[P(I_p \mid 0)P(d_p \mid 0)]$	$p \in \mathcal{V}$
	0	$p \in \mathcal{K}$
	∞	$p \in \mathcal{B}$

3   Experiments

Our proposed kidney segmentation framework is tested on a data set of DCE-MRI of human kidney. To segment a kidney slice, we will follow the following scenario. The given image is aligned with the aligned training images. The gray level marginal densities of the kidney and its background are approximated using the proposed LCG model with positive and negative components. Fig.5(a) shows the original image, (b) shows the aligned image, (c) illustrates the empirical densities as well as the initial estimated density using dominant modes in the LCG model, (d) illustrates the LCG components, (e) shows the closeness of the final gray level estimated density and the empirical one. Finally, (f) shows the marginal gray level densities of the object and back ground with the best threshold. To illustrate the closeness of the gray level between the kidney and its background, (g) shows the segmentation using gray level threshold=72. To emphasize the accuracy of the proposed approach, (h) shows the segmentation using the graph cuts technique without using the shape constraints (all the t-links weights will be $-ln P(I_p \mid f_p)$), and (i) shows the results of the proposed approach.

Samples of the segmentation results for different subjects are shown in Fig.7, (a) illustrates the input images, (b) shows the results of graph cuts technique without shape constraints, and the results of the proposed approach are shown in (c).

Evaluation: to evaluate the results we calculate the percentage segmentation error from the ground truth (manual segmentation produced by an expert) as follows:

390   A.M. Ali, A.A. Farag, and A.S. El-Baz

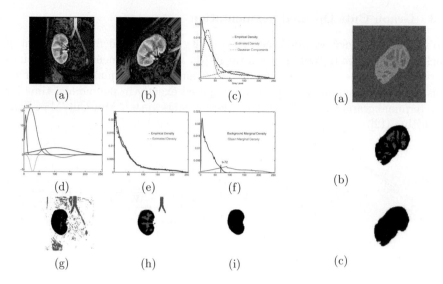

Fig. 5. Gray level probabilistic model for the given image (a) Original image (b) aligned image (c) Initial density estimation (d) LCG components (e) Final density estimation (f) Marginal densities. Segmented Kidney (g)Results of gray level threshold 102.6%(h) Results of Graph cuts without shape constraints 41.9% (i) Proposed approach results 2.5%

Fig. 6. Phantom Results (a) The phantom (b) Results of graph cuts without shape constraints 19.54% (c) Proposed approach results 0.76%.

$$error\% = \frac{100 * Number\ of\ misclassified\ pixels}{Number\ of\ Kidney\ pixels} \quad (8)$$

For each given image, the binary segmentation is shown as well as the percentage segmentation error. The misclassified pixels are shown in red color. The statistical analysis of 33 slices, which are different than the training data set and for which we have their ground truths, is shown in table 2. The unpaired t-test is used to show that the differences in the mean errors between the proposed segmentation, and graph cut without shape prior and the best threshold segmentation are statistically significant (the two-tailed value **P** is less than 0.0001).

4   Validation

Due to the hand shaking errors, it is difficult to get accurate ground truth from manual segmentation. Thus to evaluate our algorithm performance, we have created a phantom shown in Fig.6(a) with topology similar to the human kidney. Furthermore, the phantom mimics pyramids that exist in any kidney. The kidney, the pyramids and the background signals for the phantom are generated according to the distributions shown in Fig.5(f) using the inverse mapping

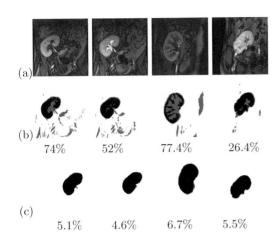

(a)

(b)

74%   52%   77.4%   26.4%

(c)

5.1%   4.6%   6.7%   5.5%

Fig. 7. More segmentation results (a)Original images (b) Results of Graph cuts without shape constraints (c) Proposed approach results.

Table 2. Accuracy of our segmentation on 33 slices in comparison to **G**raph **C**ut without shape and **TH**reshold technique

	Algorithm		
Error%	Our	GC	TH
Min.	**4.0**	20.9	38.4
Max.	**7.4**	108.5	231.2
Mean	**5.7**	49.8	128.1
Std.	**0.9**	24.3	55.3
Significance, **P**		< 0.0001	< 0.0001

methods. Fig.6(b,c) show our approach is almost 26 times more accurate than the graph cuts technique without shape constraints.

5   Conclusions

This paper proposed a new kidney segmentation approach that used graph cuts to combine region and boundary properties of segments as well as shape constraints. Shape variations were estimated using a new distance probabilistic model. The given image appearance models: image signal was approximated with a LCG with positive and negative components and the spatial interaction model was estimated using a new analytical approach. To get the optimal segmentation, we formulated a new energy function using the image appearance models and shape constraints and globally minimized this function using s/t graph cuts. Experimental results showed that the shape constraints overcame the gray level inhomogeneities problem and precisely guided the graph cuts to accurate segmentations (with mean error 5.7% and standard deviation 0.9%) compared to graph cuts without shape constraints (mean error 49.8% and standard deviation 24.3%).

Acknowledgement. This work is supported by the Kentucky Lung Cancer Program and the NSF Egypt program.

References

1. de Priester, J., Kessels, A., Giele, E., den Boer, J., Christiaans, M., Hasman, A., van Engelshoven, J.: MR renography by semiautomated image analysis: performance in renal transplant recipients. J. Magn. Reson Imaging 14(2), 134–140 (2001)

2. Giele, E.: Computer methods for semi-automatic MR renogram determination. PhD thesis, Eindhoven University of Technology, Eindhoven (2002)
3. Boykov, Y., Lee, V.S., Rusinek, H., Bansal, R.: Segmentation of dynamic N-D data sets via graph cuts using markov models. In: Niessen, W.J., Viergever, M.A. (eds.) MICCAI 2001. LNCS, vol. 2208, pp. 1058–1066. Springer, Heidelberg (2001)
4. Sun, Y., Jolly, M.P., Mourua, J.M.: Integrated registration of dynamic renal perfusion MR images. In: Proce. IEEE ICIP, pp. 1923–1926. IEEE Computer Society Press, Los Alamitos (2004)
5. Rousson, M., Paragios, N.: Shape priors for level set representations. In: Heyden, A., Sparr, G., Nielsen, M., Johansen, P. (eds.) ECCV 2002. LNCS, vol. 2351, pp. 78–92. Springer, Heidelberg (2002)
6. Leventon, M.E., Grimson, W.E.L., Faugeras, O.: Statistical shape influence in geodesic active contours. In: Proc. IEEE CVPR, p. 1316. IEEE Computer Society Press, Los Alamitos (2000)
7. Chen, Y., Thiruvenkadam, S., Huang, F., Wilson, D., Geiser, E.A., Tagare, H.D.: On the incorporation of shape priors into geometric active contours. In: IEEE VLSM, pp. 145–152. IEEE Computer Society Press, Los Alamitos (2001)
8. Huang, X., Metaxas, D., Chen, T.: Metamorphs:deformable shape and texture models. In: Proce. IEEE CVPR, pp. 496–503. IEEE Computer Society Press, Los Alamitos (2004)
9. Paragios, N.: A level set approach for shape-driven segmentation and tracking of the left ventricle. IEEE Trans. Medical Imaging 22, 773–776 (2003)
10. Viola, P.: Alignment by Maximization of Mutual Information. PhD thesis, Massachusetts Inst. of Technology, Cambridge, MA (1995)
11. Farag, A., El-Baz, A., Gimel'farb, G.: Pecise segmentation of multimodal images. IEEE Trans. Image Processing 15(4), 952 (2006)
12. Boykov, Y., Kolmogorov, V.: An experimental comparison of min-cut/max-flow algorithms for energy minimization in vision. IEEE Trans. PAMI 26(9), 1124 (2004)

Attenuation Resilient AIF Estimation Based on Hierarchical Bayesian Modelling for First Pass Myocardial Perfusion MRI

Volker J. Schmid[1], Peter D. Gatehouse[2], and Guang-Zhong Yang[1]

[1] Institute for Biomedical Engineering, Imperial College, South Kensington, London,
United Kingdom
{v.schmid,g.z.yang}@imperial.ac.uk
[2] Cardiovascular Magnetic Resonance Unit, Royal Brompton Hospital, London,
United Kingdom
p.gatehouse@rbht.nhs.uk

Abstract. Non-linear attenuation of the Arterial Input Function (AIF) is a major problem in first-pass MR perfusion imaging due to the high concentration of the contrast agent in the blood pool. This paper presents a technique to reconstruct the true AIF using signal intensities in the myocardium and the attenuated AIF based on a Hierarchical Bayesian Model (HBM). With the proposed method, both the AIF and the response function are modeled as smoothed functions by using Bayesian penalty splines (P-Splines). The derived AIF is then used to estimate the impulse response of the myocardium based on deconvolution analysis. The proposed technique is validated both with simulated data using the MMID4 model and ten *in vivo* data sets for estimating myocardial perfusion reserve rates. The results demonstrate the ability of the proposed technique in accurately reconstructing the desired AIF for myocardial perfusion quantification. The method does not involve any MRI pulse sequence modification, and thus is expected to have wider clinical impact.

1 Introduction

Early diagnosis and localization of myocardial perfusion defect is an important step in the treatment of Coronary Artery Disease (CAD). For prognostic evaluation and monitoring the efficacy of interventional measures of patients with CAD, myocardial perfusion imaging plays an important role in establishing the ischaemic burden and the viability of ischaemic myocardium. In recent years, the development of myocardial perfusion cardiovascular MRI has extended its role in the evaluation of ischaemic heart disease beyond the situations where there have already been gross myocardial changes such as acute infarction or scarring [1]. The ability to non-invasively evaluate cardiac perfusion abnormalities before pathologic effects occur, or as follow-up to therapy, is important to the management of patients with CAD. Differentiation of ischaemic but viable myocardium from infarcted regions requires detailed global quantitative assessment and modeling of myocardial perfusion characteristics. In MRI, quantitative results have been achieved in animal studies with intravascular agents

N. Ayache, S. Ourselin, A. Maeder (Eds.): MICCAI 2007, Part I, LNCS 4791, pp. 393–400, 2007.
© Springer-Verlag Berlin Heidelberg 2007

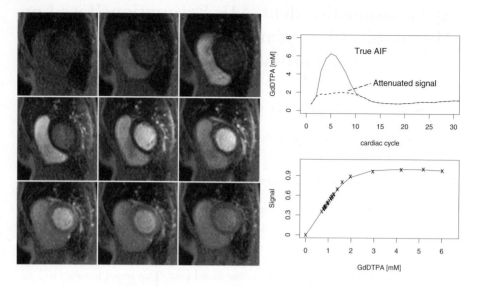

Fig. 1. Left: an example series of first pass myocardial perfusion MRI showing Gd-DTPA transit from the right ventricle, then to the left ventricle and finally entering into the myocardial tissue. Right top: attenuation of the AIF due to high Gd-DTPA concentration. Right bottom: Non-linear relationship between MR SI in the left ventricule (LV) and contrast concentration computed from a dual-imaging study [3].

(polylysine-Gd-DTPA) as a macromolecular blood pool marker and with conventional extracellular agents (Gd-DTPA) for human studies.

In general clinical practice, a high Gd-DTPA concentration is often required to achieve a good signal-to-noise ratio of the myocardium. However, the relationship between signal intensity (SI) and contrast concentration is linear only for low Gd-DTPA concentrations, typically up to about 2 mM (for long saturation time delay) [2]. Beyond this value, the overall SI and contrast concentration are not linearly related, thus leading to a non-linear attenuation of the SI time curve as shown in Fig. 1. Although this is usually not a problem for myocardium, as the perfused Gd-DTPA is relatively low, the SI of the Arterial Input Function (AIF), usually measured in the Left-ventricular (LV) blood pool, can be severely attenuated [3]. This non-linear attenuation of the AIF can lead to large errors in the estimation of myocardial perfusion reserve derived from the impulse response of the Gd-DTPA bolus.

Extensive research in MRI pulse sequence design has been conducted recently to tackle the problem of non-linear attenuation. The dual-bolus technique [4], for example, uses a low gadolinium dose to measure the AIF, followed by a high dose for the myocardial tissue signal. However, this protocol is complicated to implement for routine clinical use and extensive care must be taken to ensure the reproducibility of the boluses. An alternative approach of using T1-fast acquisition relaxation mapping (T1-FARM) [5] computes the T1 signal from two gradient-echo k-space data sets, but the signal-to-noise ratio (SNR) for this method is low. To overcome this problem, a dual-imaging approach has been proposed [3], which uses a shorter inversion recovery time to measure the AIF and a longer recovery time to assess the myocardial perfusion response.

Considering the potential pitfalls of using these elaborated perfusion pulse sequences in routine clinical practices, we propose in this paper an attenuation resilient AIF estimation method based on conventional perfusion imaging protocols with high-dosage gadolinium boluses. A recent study [6] has demonstrated the value of a Bayesian technique for estimating a parametric AIF in dynamic-contrast enhanced MRI (DCE-MRI) using a parametric prior model of the AIF. In this paper, we propose a Hierarchical Bayesian Model (HBM) for the reconstruction of the AIF, where the measured AIF is estimated simultaneously with the response function. Both the AIF and the response function are modelled as smoothed functions by using Bayesian penalty splines (P-Splines) [7]. Since the information from the myocardium is sparse, a relatively informative prior model is used for the response function in the reconstruction step. Subsequently, the derived AIF can be used in existing myocardial impulse response estimation techniques based on deconvolution analysis. The proposed technique is validated both with simulated data based on the MMID4 model [8] and ten *in vivo* data sets for estimating AIF, MBF and myocardial perfusion reserve (MPR) to demonstrate the potential clinical value of the technique.

2   Theory and Methods

Mathematically, HBM assumes the presence of latent variables, which are unknown and cannot be observed [9]. A HBM typically consists of three stages. The *data model* defines how the observed data — in this study the SI measurements in the myocardial tissue Y_{it} and in the blood pool Z_t — is generated from latent variables. The *process model* is a statistical description of the underlying physical process — in this study the flow of the contrast agent in blood and tissue, *i.e.* the (latent) response function in the myocardial tissue. In a third stage, *prior distributions* have to be specified to complete the HBM. Inference for the HBM is based on a Markov chain Monte Carlo (MCMC) algorithm.

2.1   Data Model

The observed signal intensities are realizations of stochastic processes, *i.e.* an observation consists of the signal and some noise. Let $S_i(t)$ be the true contrast concentration and Y_{it} be the observed signal intensity at time t in section i of the myocardium. Let $A(t)$ be the true AIF and Z_t the observed signal intensity in the LV blood pool at time t. We assume that the signal intensity both in the myocardium and in the LV blood pool is the true intensity plus white noise $Y_{it} \sim N(S_i(t), \sigma^2)$ for all i, t; $Z_t \sim N(A(t), \rho_t^2)$ for all t. The variance of the observation error σ^2 is estimated from the data with a flat inverse Gamma prior $\sigma^2 \sim IG(10^{-5}, 10^{-5})$. The variance ρ_t^2, however, is *a priori* fixed in this study depending on Z_t. This is because we know $A(t)$ is equal to Z_t for small values (up to observation error), so a small *a priori* variance of $\rho_t^2 = 10^{-5}$ is used. For higher values of Z_t (*i.e.* $Z_t > c \cdot \max(Z_t)$) the AIF is attenuated. So *a priori* we assume a high variance (*e.g.*, $\rho_t^2 = 10 \cdot \max(Z_t)^2$) for the AIF. So the prior information for the AIF is rather weak and the observed signal intensity in the myocardial tissue determines the AIF. The constant c can be chosen subject-specific, usual values are between 0.4 and 0.5.

2.2   Process Model

A general approach to modeling the blood flow in the myocardial tissue is to define the time curve of true signal in the myocardium $S_i(t)$ as a convolution of the arterial input function $A(t)$ and a response function f such that

$$S_i(t) = A(t) \otimes f_i(t) = \int_0^t A(t-u) f_i(u) \, du. \tag{1}$$

The signal intensity is measured at discrete time points $t_1, \ldots, t_n$, so Eqn. 1 can be discretized as

$$\tilde{S}_{it_k} = \sum_{l=1}^{T} A(t_k - t_l) f_i(t_l) \Delta t = \sum_{l=1}^{T} \tilde{A}_{kl} f(t_l), \tag{2}$$

where Δt represents the sampling interval [10]. The matrix $\tilde{A}$ may be interpreted as a convolution operator and is defined via

$$\tilde{A}_{kl} = \begin{cases} A(t_{k-l+1})\Delta t & \text{for } k \le l; \\ 0 & \text{else.} \end{cases} \tag{3}$$

Thus, the process model can be written as $\tilde{S}_i = \tilde{A} f_i$ for all i.

2.3   Prior Information

We assume that both the response function and the AIF are smooth functions and can be approximated by B-Splines, *i.e.*

$$f_i(t) = \sum_{j=1}^{p} \beta_{ij} B_{jt}, \qquad A(t) = \sum_j \gamma_j B_{jt}, \tag{4}$$

where B is the $n \times p$ design matrix of kth order B-splines with knots $s_1, \ldots, s_{p+k}$ [10]. In vector notation, $f_i = (f_i(t_1), \ldots, f_i(t_T))'$ and Eqn. 4 may be expressed via $f_i = B\beta_i$, $\tilde{A} = B\gamma$, where β_i and γ are regression parameters. We plug this representation of f into $\tilde{S}_i = \tilde{A} f_i$ and get

$$\tilde{S}_i = \tilde{A} f_i = \tilde{A} B\beta_i = D\beta_i, \tag{5}$$

where $D = \tilde{A}B$ is a $T \times p$ design matrix, which is the discrete convolution of the AIF with the B-Spline polynomials. However, in the HBM, D is dependent on A, *i.e.* D is unknown and is estimated along with the other parameters.

Following the theory of Bayesian P-Splines [7], a penalty function is used on the regression parameters $\boldsymbol{\beta_i}$ and $\boldsymbol{\gamma}$, respectively. Here a second order difference is used as stochastic restriction, known as "random walk of second order", where

$$\beta_{it} \sim N(2\beta_{i,t-1} - \beta_{i,t-2}, \phi_{it}) \text{ for } t > 2, \text{ for all } i \qquad (6)$$

and

$$\gamma_t \sim N(2\gamma_{t-1} - \gamma_{t-2}, \psi_t) \text{ for } t > 2. \qquad (7)$$

Due to the fast upslope at the beginning of the contrast uptake compared to the rest of the perfusion sequence, an adaptive prior has to be used for smoothing. That is, the variance parameters ϕ and ψ differ over time (and space) and are estimated from the data itself. To this end, flat inverse Gamma priors are used [7], where $\phi_{it} \sim IG(a,b), \psi_t \sim IG(a,b)$ with $a = 1, b = 10^{-5}$.

3   Simulation Study

To evaluate the proposed HBM AIF estimation method, simulated myocardial perfusion intensity curves were generated using the MMID4 model [8]. Data was simulated to represent healthy subjects and patients with different grades of stenoses both in rest and under stress. For each group and state, 12 sections of the myocardium with different MBF values were simulated 10 times (values for healthy subjects are MBF at rest 0.8-1.0, MBF under stress 1.5-2.0, MPR 1.88-2.30; for subjects with stenosis: MBF at rest 0.8-1.0, MBF under stress 0.9-1.5, MPR 1.13-1.50). The simulated concentration series were then attenuated following the measurements of [2], *i.e.* translated into normalized T1-weighted signal intensities. Random noise with a SNR of 6:1 was added to the signal intensities. The attenuated AIF was then reconstructed with the proposed HBM algorithm. Fig. 2 (left) depicts the true AIF used in the simulation, showing the simulated attenuated SI time intensity curve in the LV and the 10 reconstructions of the AIF from data representing healthy patients under stress. In

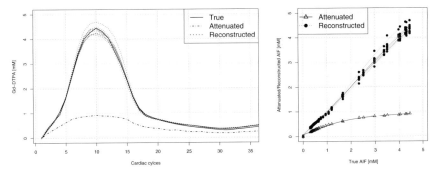

Fig. 2. Left: true AIF used in the simulation, attenuated AIF and the 10 reconstructions for a healthy patient under stress. Right: scatter plot of true AIF against attenuated and reconstructed AIF, respectively, with smoothing splines.

398 V.J. Schmid, P.D. Gatehouse, and G.-Z. Yang

Fig. 2 (right), the true AIF values are plotted against the attenuated AIF and the 10 reconstructions of the AIF. Cubic smoothing splines ($\lambda = 1$) are drawn for the reconstructions and the attenuated AIF, respectively.

The reconstructed AIF were then used in a semi-parametric analysis [11] to estimate the MBF at rest and under stress and the myocardial perfusion reserve (MPR), *i.e.* the ratio of hyperemic and baseline MBF. It can be deduced that with the reconstructed AIF, the mean overestimation of MBF is reduced from 118% to 28%. The mean squared error of MPR estimation was reduced by 60.6% with the proposed reconstruction of the AIF. For the analysis with the attenuated AIF the 95% confidence intervals (CI) of the estimated MPR values cover the true value in 33% of the sectors, whereas the 95% CI computed with reconstructed AIF always cover the true values.

4 In Vivo Study

To assess the clinical value of the proposed technique, the algorithm was applied to a study of 10 subjects. Results from the proposed technique were compared to results from a dual-imaging sequence [3]. The latter uses scanning protocol which includes an additional FLASH sequence with short saturaiton-recovery time delay to directly measure the input function in the LV.

For this study [3], images were acquired with a 0.1 mmol/kg injection of a Gadolinium-based contrast agent on a 1.5-T Siemens Sonata scanner with single-shot FLASH with 48×64 resolution with a short saturation recovery time (SSRT) of 3.4 msec, TE= 0.5msec, TR= 1msec. This was followed by measurement in the same cardiac cycles with a 108×256 resolution on the same FOV with a longer saturation recovery time (LSRT) of 63.4 msec, TE = 1.2 msec, TR = 1.86 msec. Each subject was scanned once under rest, followed by a scan after injection of 140 μg/minute/kg of adenosine for four minutes, *i.e.* under stress.

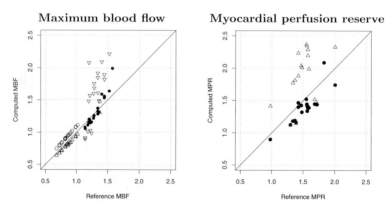

Fig. 3. Left: MBF computed with attenuated (Δ at rest, ∇ under stress) and reconstructed (o at rest, ● under stress) AIF plotted against reference values from the dual-imaging technique. Right: MPR computed with attenuated (Δ) and reconstructed (●) AIF against reference values from the dual-imaging technique.

Table 1. Mean squared difference between reference method and attenuated and re-constructed AIF for MBF at rest and under stress and MPR

	Subject 1		Subject 2		Subject 3		Subject 4		Subject 5	
	att.	rec.	att.	rec.	att.	rec.	att.	rec.	att.	rec.
MBF at rest	0.886	0.407	80.039	1.680	3.640	1.581	2.937	1.484	1.078	1.570
MBF under stress	1.658	0.945	1.269	0.281	2.489	0.678	3.096	0.929	1.163	0.962
MPR	1.878	0.827	0.141	0.122	0.684	0.450	1.053	0.627	1.093	0.613
	Subject 6		Subject 7		Subject 8		Subject 9		Subject 10	
	att.	rec.	att.	rec.	att.	rec.	att.	rec.	att.	rec.
MBF at rest	3.372	2.057	0.986	1.225	32.037	4.605	1.131	0.663	3.127	1.100
MBF under stress	3.356	0.629	1.195	0.944	0.937	0.033	0.864	0.438	2.614	1.035
MPR	1.029	0.306	1.206	0.771	0.029	0.007	0.765	0.659	0.836	0.941

Results from the analysis using three different input functions are used to illustrate the accuracy of the proposed technique:

a) the signal intensity measured in the LSRT scans, *i.e.* a conventional atten-uated AIF,
b) the signal intensity measured in the SSRT scans, *i.e.* an AIF from the dual-imaging technique, which is used as reference model here,
c) the AIF reconstructed with the proposed technique.

Maximum blood flow (MBF) and myocardial perfusion reserve (MPR) were computed from the data with the corresponding AIF. Fig. 3 (left) depicts the MBF at rest and under stress in the sectors of the myocardial tissue for subject 1. For the baseline scan, all three models agree reasonably well, *i.e.* non-linear attenuation does not represent a significant issue. However, for the hyperemic scan, MBF computed with the attenuated AIF is underestimated for small values and overestimated for larger values of MBF. MBF values computed from the reconstructed AIF however mostly agree with the reference method based on the dual-imaging sequence. Fig. 3 (right) depicts the MPR in different sections of the myocardium for subject 1. MPR estimates with the attenuated AIF show large differences compared to the reference method, whereas results from the reconstructed method correspond well with the reference data.

Tab.1 lists the mean squared difference of MBF and MPR between reference method and attenuated and reconstructed estimates, respectively, for the 10 sub-jects studied. The mean squared difference is noticeably reduced for all subjects.

5 Conclusion

In this paper, we have presented a technique for dealing with attenuated AIF in myocardial perfusion imaging based on HBM. The HBM uses information from the observed attenuated signal in the LV blood pool along with information from the signal in the myocardial tissue based on a smoothness constraint and Bayesian

P-splines [7]. Compared to recently proposed techniques such as dual-imaging, dual-bolus or T1-FARM, the proposed technique does not involve any MRI pulse sequence modification, and thus is more practical for routine clinical use. Although the proposed technique assumes a smooth AIF, the algorithm does allows for rapid changes. The cutoff parameter c has to be choosen patient-specifically; for all subjects in the *in vivo* study values of c between 0.4 and 0.5 were sufficient and changes to the c parameter of ± 0.1 did not change the results significantly.

Application of the proposed technique to simulated data and to *in vivo* scans clearly demonstrate the ability of the proposed technique to accurately reconstruct the desired AIF for myocardial perfusion quantification. The results illustrate the problems of correct estimation of MBF and MPR when using an attenuated AIF; especially for higher values of MBF (*e.g.*, for healthy patients under stress). By using the reconstructed AIF with HBM, estimates of MBF and MPR are similar to the ground truth data derived from the reference scans.

References

1. Panting, J., Gatehouse, P., Yang, G.-Z., Grothues, F., Firmin, D., Collins, P., Pennell, D.: Abnormal subendocardial perfusion in cardiac syndrome X detected by cardiovascular MRI. New Engl. J. of Med. 346, 1948–1953 (2002)
2. Kim, D., Axel, L.: Multislice, dual-imaging sequence for increasing the dynamic range of the contrast-enhanced blood signal and CNR of myocardial enhancement at 3T. J. of Mag. Res. Imag. 23, 81–86 (2006)
3. Gatehouse, P., Elkington, A., Ablitt, N., Yang, G., Pennell, D., Firmin, D.: Accurate assesment of the arterial input function during high-dose myocardial perfusion cardiovascular magnetic resonance. J. Mag. Res. Imag. 20, 39–45 (2004)
4. Christian, T.F., Rettmann, D.W., Aletras, A.H., Liao, S.L., Taylor, J.L., Balaban, R.S., Arai, A.E.: Absolute myocardial perfusion in canines measured by using dual-bolus first-pass MR imaging. Radiology 232, 677–684 (2004)
5. Bellamy, D.D., Pereira, R.S., McKenzie, C.A., Prato, F.S., Drost, D.J., Sykes, J., Wisenberg, G.: Gd-DTPA bolus tracking in the myocardium using T1 fast acquisition relaxation mapping (T1 FARM). Magn. Res. in Med. 46, 555–564 (2001)
6. Orton, M.R., Walker-Samuel, S., Collins, D.J., Leach, M.O.: A joint bayesian method for robust estimation of PK and AIF parameters for DCE-MR imaging. In: Proceedings of the 14th Annual Meeting of ISMRM, Seattle, p. 3490 (2006)
7. Lang, S., Brezger, A.: Bayesian P-splines. J. of Comp. and Graph Stat. 13, 183–212 (2004)
8. Kroll, K., Wilke, N., Jerosch-Herold, M., Wang, Y., Zhang, Y., Bache, R.J., Gassingthwaighte, J.B.: Modeling regional myocardial flows from residue functions of an intravascular indicator. Am. J. of Heart. Circ. Phys. 271, 1643–1655 (1996)
9. Gilks, W.R., Richardson, S., Spiegelhalter, D.J.: Markov Chain Monte Carlo in Practice. Chapman & Hall, London (1996)
10. Jerosch-Herold, M., Swingen, C., Seethamraju, R.: Myocardial blood flow quantification with MRI by model-independent deconvolution. Med. Phys. 29(5), 886–897 (2002)
11. Schmid, V.J, Whitcher, B., Yang, G.Z.: Semi-parametric analysis of dynamic contrast-enhanced MRI using Bayesian P-splines. In: Larsen, R., Nielsen, M., Sporring, J. (eds.) MICCAI 2006. LNCS, vol. 4190, pp. 679–686. Springer, Heidelberg (2006)

Real-Time Synthesis of Image Slices in Deformed Tissue from Nominal Volume Images

Orcun Goksel and Septimiu E. Salcudean

Department of Electrical and Computer Engineering
University of British Columbia, Vancouver, Canada
{orcung,tims}@ece.ubc.ca

Abstract. This paper presents a fast image synthesis procedure for elastic volumes under deformation. Given the node displacements of a mesh and the 3D image voxel data of an undeformed volume, the method maps the image plane pixels to be synthesized from the deformed configuration back to the nominal pre-deformed configuration, where the pixel intensities are obtained easily through interpolation in the regular-grid structure of the voxel volume. For smooth interpolation, this mapping requires the identification of the mesh element enclosing each image pixel. To accelerate this *point location* procedure, a fast method of marking the image pixels is employed by finding the intersection of the mesh and the image, and marking this intersection on the image pixels using *Bresenham's line drawing algorithm*. A deformable tissue phantom was constructed, it was modeled using the finite element method, and its 3D ultrasound volume was acquired in its undeformed state. Actual B-mode images of the phantom under deformation by the ultrasound probe were then compared with the corresponding synthesized images simulated for the same deformations. Results show that realistic images can be synthesized in real-time using the proposed technique.

1 Introduction

Medical simulators involving real-time imaging modalities, such as ultrasound, necessitate rapid and realistic image rendering of deformed tissue in response to probe or tool manipulation by a trainee. For real-time performance, tissue deformation, typically modeled by the finite element method (FEM), must be computed on a mesh having much coarser elements than the typical resolution of medical imaging modalities. Exploiting this fact, our work addresses the computational problems related to rapidly slicing a deformed 3D mesh. The need for real-time image synthesis in ultrasound simulation makes it our primary target application, although the techniques presented here are also applicable to other medical imaging modalities that need to slice deformed meshes.

Image generation inside deformed tissue has some concepts in common with the *elastic image registration* [1,2] and the *ultrasound volume reconstruction* [3,4,5] literature, where reconstruction refers to generating 3D voxel volume data from individual scans. However, compared to these fields that generally process

N. Ayache, S. Ourselin, A. Maeder (Eds.): MICCAI 2007, Part I, LNCS 4791, pp. 401–408, 2007.
© Springer-Verlag Berlin Heidelberg 2007

images offline, real-time medical image generation presents additional computational challenges, which have been studied for ultrasound B-mode image simulation in the literature. There exist two approaches for ultrasound image synthesis, *the generative approach* and *the interpolative approach*. The former models the ultrasonic wave propagation by using accurate representations of the probe, the tissue scatterers, and the wave interaction [6]. This complex and time-consuming approach is not suitable for real-time applications. The latter approach slices images from a pre-existing voxel volume data. UltraSim [7] and several others [8,9] follow this latter approach. However, these ultrasound simulators do not allow for tissue deformation.

In many medical procedures such as prostate brachytherapy, brain surgery, or breast biopsy, significant deformation is caused by medical tools or by the ultrasound probe. In certain applications, such as diagnosis of deep-vein thrombosis (DVT), deformation observed in ultrasound images during deliberate probe indentation contains essential diagnosis information. Fast synthesis of ultrasound images in soft tissues under deformation will facilitate the development of training simulators. With this goal, a DVT diagnosis simulator was proposed in [10,11]. It simulates the probe pressure by first slicing an image from the 3D ultrasound data set and then applying a 2D in-plane elastic deformation using quadtree-splines to this image. This 2D deformation applied is pre-computed offline by registering segmented anatomy from undeformed to deformed 3D models. However, an in-plane image deformation approach is not capable of simulating situations such as in Fig. 1(a-b), where anatomical structures enter or leave the imaging plane due to tissue deformation. In the example depicted, an inclusion which is nominally not in the ultrasound imaging plane later appears in it as a result of the depression by the probe. Real-time ultrasound image slicing using physically-valid 3D deformation models has not been addressed in the literature. Our work is motivated by this need for real-time realistic B-mode ultrasound simulation in medical training environments involving tissue deformation.

The paper is organized as follows. First, the overall interpolation approach of mapping image pixels back to the undeformed volume is introduced. Then, our acceleration technique for this approach is presented and it is applied to real-time ultrasound synthesis of a gelatin phantom while modeling deformation caused by the ultrasound probe, similarly to [12]. In this paper, deformed images of the phantom are acquired and compared with the simulated ones quantitatively. The change of the algorithm processing time with image size is also studied. Complementary detail on the specific numerical techniques presented below can be found in [12].

2   Methods

The techniques described below assume that a reconstructed voxel volume data of the region of interest is available *a priori*. Consider the deformed tissue configuration in Fig.1(c). To generate an image given the *reconstructed* voxel data, the intensity values (*gray-values*) at the planar locations shown need to be

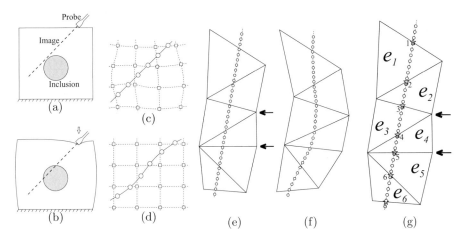

Fig. 1. A sample case where in-plane image deformation cannot capture the outcome of volume deformation from (a) nominal to (b) deformed configurations; Voxel data and image plane in (c) deformed and (d) undeformed states (the circles are the image pixels and the squares are the reconstructed data voxels); (e-f) mesh representation of an undeformation (reconstructed voxels are not depicted in here); and (g) flagging of pixels in a deformed 2D mesh

interpolated. Note that interpolating in the deformed data in the configuration given in Fig. 1(c) has two problems. First, the data is no longer in a regular-grid structure, requiring computationally-expensive scattered-data interpolation techniques. Second, although only a small subset of the nominal voxels are needed in the interpolation, it is time consuming to find which voxels are required. One can instead apply the inverse of the (deformation) displacement on image pixels in order to transform them back (*undeform*) into the regular-grid structure of the voxel volume as in Fig. 1(d). This latter approach is utilized in this paper.

Tissue tessellations for deformation models are generally much coarser than the imaging resolution due to computational constraints. Consider the situation in Fig. 1(e) where an image plane slices an object deformed under boundary constraints shown with the arrows as simulated by linear FEM using the given mesh. Mapping the mesh back to its nominal configuration (*undeforming*) as shown in Fig. 1(f) brings the image pixels to locations at which the given regular-grid data can be interpolated easily. Consequently, the simulation scheme for each pixel position P can be summarized as (*i*) finding its enclosing element e_i, (*ii*) computing the *undeforming* transformation T using e_i's shape functions, and (*iii*) interpolating the transformed position TP. Identifying the element enclosing a pixel in (*i*) is the bottleneck of this approach, since (*ii*) and (*iii*) are fast constant time $\mathcal{O}(1)$ operations. Note that this pixel-element mapping depends on both mesh deformation and the image position/orientation; therefore, it cannot be computed offline. This problem, called *point location* in computational geometry, has been extensively studied resulting in common techniques such as *slab decomposition* and *trapezoidal maps*. Nonetheless, execution time of any such method will not allow for real-time processing of conventional image resolutions. Indeed, the point location routine in QuickHull algorithm [13] locates the pixels of a single image presented in Section 3 in over 30 s. Instead of running point location individually for each pixel, in this paper, we exploit the fact that all the pixels lie on a planar image having finer resolution than the tissue tessellation.

Note that when pixels in an image are traversed in one direction, the elements that they belong to only alternate at the element edges. This fact can be utilized to rapidly identify the enclosing elements of pixels. For example, in a 2D mesh as in Fig. 1(g), if the pixels just below the upper-edge of each element are flagged by that element number, then a downwards traversal will reveal the elements enclosing the rest of the pixels in constant time. Similarly, in 3D this corresponds to flagging all the pixels along the entire surface cross-section of *sliced elements* (any element that is intersected by the image being generated), since these cross-sections are the borders where the assigned elements for consecutive pixels change. Accordingly, for each frame, a pre-computation of pixel flagging is introduced in order to reduce the step (i) above to negligible time.

Figure 2(a) demonstrates a sample flagging array slicing a geometrically-linear tetrahedral mesh. A plane can slice either 3 or 4 edges of a tetrahedron. Simple geometrical computations to find these intersections shown with stars require negligible $\mathcal{O}(1)$ time per sliced element. Then, a cross-section can be flagged by discretizing the lines connecting these intersections onto the flagging array. For this we use an optimized version of *Bresenham's line-drawing algorithm*. This only requires the assumption that the image pixels are equally-spaced in each individual axis. Assuming a top-down array traversal, only the top halves of triangles/quadrilaterals are flagged.

Let s be the number of sliced elements, then an average of $\sqrt{s}$ elements span one axis of the image, each causing $\sqrt{n}$ pixels to be flagged on average. This gives the cost $\mathcal{O}(\sqrt{ns})$ for preparing this flagging array prior to the generation of each frame. Since the frame interpolation still requires the traversal of $\mathcal{O}(n)$ pixels, the overall computational complexity is not reduced technically. Nonetheless, removing the significant hidden cost of point location from the $\mathcal{O}(n)$ loop practically achieves the anticipated speed gain.

3   Results

To obtain 3D ultrasound voxel data, a $60 \times 90 \times 90$ mm gelatin phantom was prepared. For contrast in ultrasound, a softer cylindrical inclusion of $\phi 25$ mm was made by varying the cellulose scatterer content. The phantom mesh, obtained using off-the-shelf meshing software, has 493 nodes and 1921 tetrahedra. For simulating deformation, considering the approximate values known for the materials, Young's modulus of the inclusion is set twice the substrate and a Poisson's ratio of 0.49 is used for both materials. Parallel slices of this volume were collected at 1 mm increments, paying attention to minimally deforming the phantom, using the Ultrasonix Sonix RP machine with a linear probe mounted on a precision

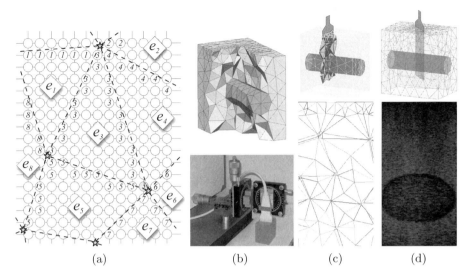

(a)   (b)   (c)   (d)

Fig. 2. (a) Flagging a sample 3D mesh projection on an array; (b) our phantom mesh and the image acquisition setup; (c) the cross-sections of the elements traversed and their boundaries; and (d) a synthesized image in tissue without any deformation

motion stage. The geometry and mesh of the phantom, and the setup for image acquisition can be seen in Fig. 2(b). Each image spans 37.5×70 mm and has a resolution of 220×410. This is the typical B-mode resolution on this ultrasound machine. This dense data is then used as the reconstructed voxel volume without any further interpolation. In this configuration, there is an average of 8750 voxels per element.

Figure 2(c) shows the cross-sections of traversed elements and the corresponding flagging array. A sample image without any phantom deformation (probe pressure) is shown in Fig. 2(d). To simulate deformation, the bottom layer of the phantom is fixed and the mesh nodes touching the probe on the top surface were displaced to conform to the probe. Two predetermined regions on the phantom had already been meshed with finer elements having nodes lying on the anticipated interfaces. In Fig. 3 the images were simulated as the probe indents $0, 5,$ and 10 mm into the phantom at two given positions/orientations. To measure the effect of n and s, the slice generation time of our implementation on a Pentium4 2.4 GHz computer was compared for various image *resolutions* and *widths* in Fig. 4(a). Note that the former only changes n, whereas the latter also affects s. The linearity and similarity of the lines show that generating flagging array takes negligible time and $\mathcal{O}(n)$ is the dominant factor. Thus, our approach of optimizing its hidden cost is an effective strategy for accelerating this scheme.

Simulated and acquired images at 1 mm indentation increments during the deformation in Fig. 3(top) were compared using their *mutual information* (MI) in Fig. 4(b). Plotted MI data were normalized with the average MI between each consecutive slice acquired for reconstruction throughout the volume. As

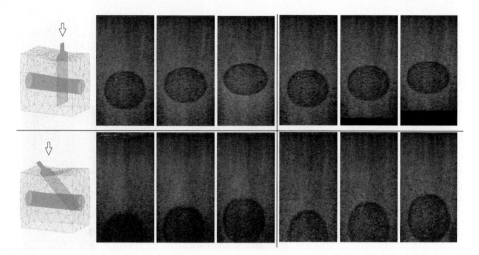

Fig. 3. Acquired (center) and simulated (right) images at 0, 5, and 10 mm indentation depths with vertical (top) and 45°-tilted (bottom) probe orientations (meshes (left) are depicted for 10 mm only)

expected, MI is the highest on the diagonal (i.e., each simulated image is most alike the acquired one at a similar indentation). A preliminary system for interactive ultrasound visualization with deformation has been developed using a SensAble Phantom interface as seen in Fig. 4(c). A simplified contact handling method of applying the deformation only to the closest node was implemented. A depth-dependent reaction force simulated with a spring from the nominal surface is applied on user's hand.

4   Discussion

In the literature, there have been image slicing implementations without taking deformation into account [5,7,8,9]. Also, there have been *in-plane image deformation* strategies for image registration, deformation correction for volume reconstruction [3,4], and a training simulation for DVT [10,11]. However, to the extent of our knowledge, our implementation is the first real-time image slicer inside 3D deformation models. Although only the probe indentation was presented here, the source of deformation can be also external such as needles or other medical instruments. In some procedures, e.g. prostate brachytherapy, the major tissue deformation is orthogonal to the imaging plane. In such cases, 2D in-plane deformation simply cannot be used and our method becomes essential.

Our acceleration techniques for this image synthesis method do not introduce any additional errors beyond the FEM simulation errors, i.e., we do not trade off accuracy with speed. As one will expect, for significantly large deformations, the acquired and the simulated images may not match exactly due to errors in the deformation model and differences between the estimated and the actual elasticity parameters.

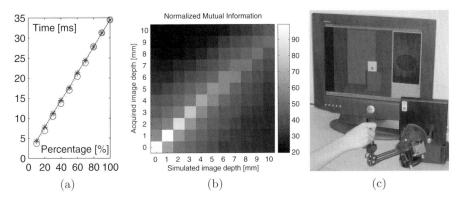

Fig. 4. (a) Slice generation time for various image resolutions (stars) and widths (circles) normalized to the full-scale size of the images presented above; (b) Mutual information in-between simulated and acquired images for vertical indentation at 1 mm increments; and (c) our real-time ultrasound examination simulator

We employ the linear FEM with tetrahedra for deformation due to its *shape functions* being simple, continuous, and easily invertible. Nonetheless, all presented methods also apply to the FEM with quadrilateral or other-geometry elements. Note that in flagging arrays, some pixels close to element corners/edges may be assigned to more than one element due to discretization. In order to successfully flag them, sliced polygons are first topologically sorted in linear time using their top-down partial ordering.

Due to speckle and other directional imaging artifacts, a deformed tissue does not necessarily generate the exact same nominal gray-values at its displaced position. Nevertheless, this assumption has been employed in many applications in the literature [3,4,5,7,8,9,10,11], with success. The speckle pattern (mainly its visual continuity) is also a major criterion in evaluating the realism of synthesized images. In this respect, the generated images were qualitatively found to be adequate for a training simulator.

5   Conclusions

We have presented a technique to synthesize planar images from the deformed mesh of a tissue model and the 3D image voxel data of the undeformed tissue. The deformation is assumed to be given by the node displacements of a mesh. A fast processing step was developed to identify the mesh element to which each pixel belongs by employing a plane enumeration technique. This allows the generation of image planes of considerable size at frame rates that are suitable for real-time applications. A phantom was constructed and its 3D B-mode ultrasound image was collected. The phantom was meshed and its deformation due to probe indentation was simulated using the FEM. Planar ultrasound images of the deformed phantom were synthesized and compared to the corresponding images acquired by deforming the phantom. The results show that the image synthesis method we developed produces realistic-looking images in real-time. In future work, we will target specific clinical applications in which we will carry out more extensive evaluation.

References

1. Krücker, J.F., LeCarpentier, G.L., Fowlkes, J.B., Carson, P.L.: Rapid elastic image registration for 3-D ultrasound. IEEE Trans. Med. Imag. 21(11), 1384–1394 (2002)
2. Zikic, D., Wein, W., Khamene, A., Clevert, D.A., Navab, N.: Fast deformable registration of 3D-ultrasound data using a variational approach. In: Larsen, R., Nielsen, M., Sporring, J. (eds.) MICCAI 2006. LNCS, vol. 4190, pp. 915–923. Springer, Heidelberg (2006)
3. Burcher, M.R., Han, L., Noble, J.A.: Deformation correction in ultrasound images using contact force measurements. In: IEEE Workshop Math Methods Bio Img Anal, Kauai, HI, USA, pp. 63–70 (2001)
4. Rohling, R.N., Gee, A.H., Berman, L.: A comparison of freehand three-dimensional ultrasound reconstruction techniques. Med. Image. Anal. 3(4), 339–359 (1999)
5. Gee, A., Prager, R., Treece, G., Cash, C., Berman, L.: Processing and visualizing three-dimensional ultrasound data. British J. Radiology 77, S186–S193 (2004)
6. Jensen, J.A., Nikolov, I.: Fast simulation of ultrasound images. In: IEEE Ultrasonics Symposium pp. 1721–1724 (2000)
7. Aiger, D., Cohen-Or, D.: Real-time ultrasound imaging simulation. Real-Time Imaging 4(4), 263–274 (1998)
8. Maul, H., Scharf, A., Baier, P., Wüstemann, M., Günter, H.H., Gebauer, G., Sohn, C.: Ultrasound simulators: Experience with sonotrainer and comperative review of other training systems. Ultrasound Obstet Gynecol 24, 581–585 (2004)
9. Tahmasebi, A.M., Abolmaesumi, P., Hashtrudi-Zaad, K.: A haptic-based ultrasound training/examination system (HUTES). In: IEEE ICRA, Roma, Italy, pp. 3130–3131 (2007)
10. Henry, D., Troccaz, J., Bosson, J.L., Pichot, O.: Ultrasound imaging simulation: Application to the diagnosis of deep venous thromboses of lower limbs. In: Wells, W.M., Colchester, A.C.F., Delp, S.L. (eds.) MICCAI 1998. LNCS, vol. 1496, pp. 1032–1040. Springer, Heidelberg (1998)
11. d'Aulignac, D., Laugier, C., Troccaz, J., Vieira, S.: Towards a realistic echographic simulator. Med. Image. Anal. 10, 71–81 (2005)
12. Goksel, O., Salcudean, S.E.: Fast B-mode ultrasound image simulation of deformed tissue. In: IEEE EMBC, Lyon, France (2007)
13. Barber, C.B., Dobkin, D.P., Huhdanpaa, H.T.: The Quickhull algorithm for convex hulls. ACM Trans. Math. Softw. 22(4), 469–483 (1996)

Quantitative Comparison of Two Cortical Surface Extraction Methods Using MRI Phantoms

Simon F. Eskildsen and Lasse R. Østergaard

Dept. of Health Science and Technology, Aalborg University, Denmark

Abstract. In the last decade several methods for extracting the human cerebral cortex from magnetic resonance images have been proposed. Studies comparing these methods have been few. In this study we compare a recent cortical extraction method with FreeSurfer, which has been widespread in the scientific community during recent years. The comparison is performed using realistic phantoms generated from surfaces extracted from original brain scans. The geometrical accuracy of the reconstructed surfaces is compared to the surfaces extracted from the original scan. We found that our method is comparable with FreeSurfer in terms of accuracy, and in some cases it performs better. In terms of speed our method is more than 25 times faster.

1 Introduction

Reconstruction of the human cerebral cortex from magnetic resonance (MR) images facilitates morphometric studies and brain mapping, and provides intuitive visualisation of the human brain for the use in e.g. surgical planning. Since the nineties a number of algorithms has been developed for extracting the boundaries of the cortex from MR images [1,2,3,4,5,6,7]. FreeSurfer has been around for more than seven years, and has, due to the fact that it is freely available, become widespread in the scientific community. We have recently published a method (henceforth designated Fast Accurate Cortex Extraction (FACE)), which resembles FreeSurfer in many aspects, but is significantly improved in terms of computational speed [8,9].

When performing morphometric studies the accuracy of the cortex reconstructions is very important. Therefore, it is of interest to investigate how well ACE performs in terms of accuracy compared to FreeSurfer. Quantification of the accuracy is difficult as the ground truth is rarely available. A means to measure the accuracy is using phantoms resembling real neuroanatomical data. Lee et al. [10] compared FreeSurfer [4], CLASP [7] and BrainVISA [2] using generated phantoms. They found that CLASP was more accurate than BrainVISA and FreeSurfer. However, CLASP is not publicly available, while the two other methods are. FreeSurfer performed second best in the study. In this study we compare our method, ACE, to FreeSurfer using realistic phantoms generated from real MR scans.

N. Ayache, S. Ourselin, A. Maeder (Eds.): MICCAI 2007, Part I, LNCS 4791, pp. 409–416, 2007.
© Springer-Verlag Berlin Heidelberg 2007

2   Methods

To evaluate the two cortex extraction methods, eight healthy young subjects (age: 32±7.4) and eight healthy middle-aged subjects (age: 54.3±6.0) were selected , and a comparison method similar to the method described by Lee et al. was used [10]. For each subject both methods were used to extract the cortical boundaries. The surfaces extracted by each method were used as reference for the generation of simulated MR scans as described below. The cortex of these customised phantoms were extracted by each method and the resulting surfaces were compared to the reference surfaces (see figure 1).

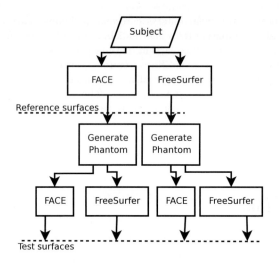

Fig. 1. Flow chart illustration of the comparison method

The following briefly describes the two cortex extraction methods, the generation of the test phantoms, and how the error between the reference surfaces and the test surfaces was quantified.

2.1   FreeSurfer Method

FreeSurfer [4,11] first registers the input MR volume to Talairach space[12]. Non-uniformities originating from inhomogeneities in the magnetic field are corrected, and the intensities are normalised. The resulting volume is skull stripped using an approach similar to BET [13]. The WM voxels inside the skull stripped volume is labelled using a two-step segmentation algorithm based on intensities and prior knowledge of the GM/WM interface. The ventricles and subcortical matter inside the WM component is filled, and the WM is separated into the two hemispheres by a sagittal cut through the corpus callosum and an axial cut through the pons. A connected component algorithm is used to isolate the main body of WM voxels, i.e. the cerebrum WM voxels.

From the WM voxels a surface mesh is constructed by generating connected triangles on the faces of the voxels. The resulting surface for each hemisphere is topology corrected to be isomorph to a sphere, and a deformation process smoothes the surface while maintaining it at the WM/GM interface. The pial, or GM surface is found by displacing the WM surface toward the GM/CSF interface using the local surface normals and intensity gradients.

2.2   Fast Accurate Cortex Extraction Method

FACE performs similar preprocessing steps as FreeSurfer. The registered, intensity corrected, and skull stripped volume is segmented into WM, GM, and CSF using a fuzzy clustering algorithm solely based on the intensities, and a WM labelling is performed by maximum membership classification. Cerebellum and the brain stem is removed using atlas information, and the hemispheres are separated by a sagittal cut through the corpus callosum. After a connected component analysis spherical topology of each hemisphere is obtained using a topology correction algorithm [14], and the WM hemispheres can be tessellated by an iso-surface algorithm yielding surfaces with Euler characteristics of a sphere (genus=0).

The iso-surface generated from the WM cerebrum voxels are deformed to fit the WM/GM interface under the influence of smoothing forces and forces derived from the surface normals, the fuzzy voxel classification, and gradient information of the original image.

The GM surface is found using the method described in [9]. The WM surface is displaced towards the GM/CSF interface using a combination of the local surface normals and a gradient vector field calculated from an edge map of the voxel segmentation. The influence of the two vector force fields on each vertex in the surface is weighted by the curvature of the surface, which enables different deformation behaviour according the position on the surface (sulcus or gyrus). The deformation is not minimising an objective function, which means that the complexity is low compared to the deformation process in FreeSurfer.

2.3   Phantom Generation

Membership volumes of WM, GM, and CSF were generated directly from the extracted surfaces. This was accomplished by labelling each voxel completely inside the WM surface as WM, and calculating the inside fraction of each voxel intersected by the surface. This was also done for the GM surface, and the memberships for the three tissue classes were calculated from the fuzzy labelled volumes (see figure 2). The three membership volumes were used as input to an MRI simulator [15] with the same acquisition parameters as the original MR scans (TR=18ms, TE=10ms, 1mm slices). The intensities of the resulting volume were normalised to the range of the original scan. Finally, subcortex, ventricles, cerebellum, brain stem, and extra-cerebral tissue were added from the original scan by superimposing the simulated brain scan onto the original (figure 3).

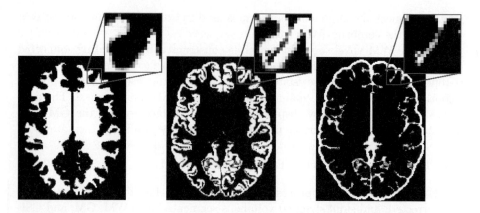

Fig. 2. Fuzzy membership volumes generated from the extracted surfaces. Left to right: WM, GM, and CSF.

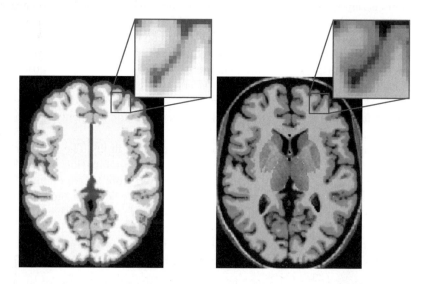

Fig. 3. Phantom produced by the MRI simulator (left), and final phantom after normalisation and added original tissue (right).

2.4   Accuracy Assessment

To test the accuracy of each method, reconstructions of the cortical boundaries were generated from the 32 phantoms. The reconstructions were then compared to the reconstructions of the original MR scans. Both methods ensures correct topology by volume- or surface-correction. Thus the comparison was based solely on geometrical factors. Four factors were considered, namely volume difference, surface area difference, over/under segmentation ratio, and the explicit geometrical error. Also the vertex density was taking into consideration in the comparison.

- **Volume Difference:** The enclosing volume of the surfaces was calculated and the difference (in percent) from the reference surfaces was measured.
- **Surface Area Difference:** Surface areas were calculated and the difference (in percent) from the reference surfaces was measured.
- **Over/under segmentation ratio:** Tissue membership volumes of WM, GM and CSF were created from the test surfaces similar to the procedure used in the phantom generation. The resulting fuzzy maps were compared to the maps generated from the reference surfaces, and the percentages of voxels respectively missing inside (false negatives) and added outside (false positives) the reference map were calculated.
- **Explicit Geometrical Error:** The Euclidean distance from each vertex in the reference surface to the closest face on the test surface was measured. The root mean square error of these distances was calculated for both the WM surface and the GM surface. Similarly, the distance was measured from the test surface to the reference surface. The latter was done to avoid that simply adding vertices to the surface did not necessarily reduce the error.

3   Results

The cortical extractions were performed on an AMD Opteron 2.6 GHz processor with 12 GB memory. The average extraction time from native scan to final surfaces for FreeSurfer was 20.1 hours, while it was 0.8 hours for FACE. The following presents the results on how well the methods reconstructed the original surfaces from the generated phantoms.

When comparing the reconstructed surfaces visually, only small differences can be discerned. Figure 4 shows the original GM surface along with the reconstructions by the two methods. The number of vertices in the surfaces generated by the two methods vary. FreeSurfer generates surfaces with almost twice the number of vertices compared to FACE (310,415±18,628 vs. 169,218±9,755).

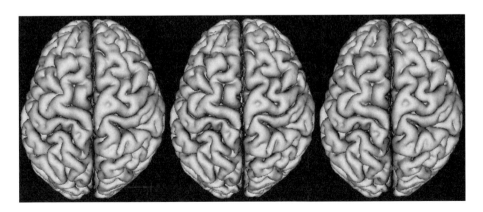

Fig. 4. Left: Surface extracted from original scan by FACE. Middle: Reconstruction from phantom by FreeSurfer. Right: Reconstruction from phantom by FACE.

Table 1. Errors measured by the four metrics on both WM and GM surfaces. Errors are deviation from the reference surfaces. For each metric the performance on both FreeSurfer and FACE phantoms is compared for the two methods (two-tailed paired t-test). Significant smaller errors are marked by bold font.

Metric	FreeSurfer Phantom			FACE Phantom		
	FreeSurfer	FACE	P-value	FreeSurfer	FACE	P-value
WM Δvol (%)	**1.2±1.1**	5.4±2.6	0.00	**1.7±1.9**	4.9±2.3	0.00
WM Δarea (%)	7.6±1.9	**3.1±1.5**	0.00	15.4±3.4	**9.4±1.9**	0.00
Brain Δvol (%)	4.4±1.2	4.0±1.0	0.36	5.5±2.0	**3.7±0.8**	0.01
GM Δarea (%)	5.4±1.4	5.0±3.1	0.54	2.5±2.4	1.6±1.5	0.22
WM FN (%)	8.5±1.3	**4.2±0.6**	0.00	10.0±2.1	**3.2±0.6**	0.00
WM FP (%)	**7.8±0.8**	9.1±2.3	0.01	8.7±0.8	**7.4±1.8**	0.00
GM FN (%)	23.4±1.3	**21.9±2.0**	0.01	26.4±3.7	**19.9±1.9**	0.00
GM FP (%)	15.7±1.4	**7.3±1.4**	0.00	17.6±3.1	**6.9±1.3**	0.00
WM ref2test (mm)	0.95±0.64	1.14±0.11	0.20	1.47±0.90	**0.63±0.07**	0.00
WM test2ref (mm)	0.75±0.14	0.84±0.17	0.13	1.28±0.17	**0.46±0.05**	0.00
GM ref2test (mm)	0.86±0.50	1.07±0.11	0.08	1.26±0.92	**0.64±0.08**	0.02
GM test2ref (mm)	0.83±0.14	**0.63±0.13**	0.00	1.39±0.19	**0.59±0.06**	0.00

Table 1 lists the results for each error metric averaged for the 16 subjects. The errors of the two methods for each metric was compared and tested by two-tailed paired t-test (the p-values are listed in the right hand column of each phantom). Significant smaller errors are marked by bold font. The volume and area errors are absolute percent change compared the to reference surfaces. The under/over segmentation error is measured by percent outside reference surface volume (false positives (FP)) and percent missing inside reference surface (false negatives (FN)). The explicit geometrical difference is measured by the RMS error in mm.

4   Discussion

From table 1 it can be observed that FACE has significantly fewer WM false negatives and GM false positives when testing on both groups of phantoms. The two metrics are related in that missing WM voxels most likely are classified as GM voxels. Generally, both methods seem to over-expand the surfaces when compared to the phantoms. This especially increases the GM false negatives percentage, as the GM tissue class is smaller than the WM tissue class.

The geometrical error rates show that the average distance between the test and reference surfaces is at subvoxel level when testing the accuracy of FACE. Reproducibility errors of FACE are consistently around half a voxel size, while FreeSurfer reproducibility errors are between 0.75 - 0.95 voxel size. For purposes of comparison the difference for the reference surfaces of the two methods was measured to 1.48±0.31 mm (average for both WM and GM surfaces).

When looking at the volume and area errors for the GM surfaces, i.e. cerebrum volume and area, there is little difference between the two methods, and the error is fairly small (1.6% - 5.5%). Also, the WM volume errors are low. However, higher error rates are found in the WM area. Looking at the area change per subject, it was found that all reconstructed WM surfaces had a smaller area than the reference, while the volume remained more or less the same. This could point to the fact that the WM voxels in the phantoms do not exactly resemble the original MR WM voxels leading to less deep sulci. Improvements of the phantoms could solve this bias. Also, visual inspection of the surfaces revealed significant differences in the surfaces at the base of the brain due to the different brain stem cutting strategies in the two methods. The inspection also revealed that FreeSurfer in a few surfaces missed part of the occipital lobe. This could be caused by registration errors which again could be caused by tissue voxels not resembling real MR data.

Generally, the tests show that the accuracy of FACE is comparable to Free-Surfer. In most cases FACE has a significantly better accuracy. FACE is on average more than 25 times faster than FreeSurfer. The longer extraction time in FreeSurfer can partly be explained by the high number of vertices in the surfaces. FreeSurfer generates surfaces with almost twice the number of vertices compared to FACE. Another reason for the speed difference is a very fast convergence of the deformation in FACE due to refraining from minimising an objective function.

Even though FACE in the comparison proved to be more accurate, results from some of the error metrics and visual inspections suggested that the phantoms could be improved to resemble real anatomical MR data. However, the results indicate that FACE is comparable to FreeSurfer in terms of accuracy.

The subjects used in this study were healthy without altered cortical morphology. Further studies must examine the accuracy of the two methods when analysing subjects with altered morphology (e.g. Alzheimer's patients), which is often the case in clinical trials.

Acknowledgements

Test data were provided courtesy of Dr. Peter Johannsen, Rigshospitalet, under grant number 22-04-0458 Danish Medical Research Counsil, and the International Consortium of Brain Mapping, McConnell Brain Imaging Centre, Montreal Neurological Institute, McGill University.

References

1. Cohen, L.D., Cohen, I.: Finite-element methods for active contour models and balloons for 2D and 3D images. IEEE Trans. Pattern Analysis and Machine Intelligence (1993)
2. Mangin, J.F., Frouin, V., Bloch, I., Régis, J., López-Krahe, J.: From 3d magnetic resonance images to structural representations of the cortex topography using topology preserving deformations. Journal of Mathematical Imaging and Vision 5(4), 297–318 (1995)
3. McInerney, T., Terzopoulos, D.: Topology adaptive deformable surfaces for medical image volume segmentation. IEEE Trans. Medical Imaging 18(10), 840–850 (1999)

4. Dale, A.M., Fischl, B., Sereno, M.I.: Cortical surface-based analysis i: Segmentation and surface reconstruction. NeuroImage 9(2), 179–194 (1999)
5. Zeng, X., Staib, L.H., Schultz, R.T., Duncan, J.S.: Segmentation and measurement of the cortex from 3-d mr images using coupled-surfaces propagation. IEEE Trans. Medical Imaging 18(10), 100–111 (1999)
6. Han, X., Pham, D., Tosun, D., Rettmann, M., Xu, C., Prince, J.: Cruise: Cortical reconstruction using implicit surface evolution. NeuroImage 23(3), 997–1012 (2004)
7. Kim, J.S., Singh, V., Lee, J.K., Lerch, J., Ad-Dab'bagh, Y., MacDonald, D., Lee, J.M., Kim, S.I., Evans, A.C.: Automated 3-d extraction and evaluation of the inner and outer cortical surfaces using a laplacian map and partial volume effect classification. NeuroImage 27(1), 210–221 (2005)
8. Eskildsen, S.F., Uldahl, M., Østergaard, L.R.: Extraction of the cerebral cortical boundaries from mri for measurement of cortical thickness. Progress in Biomedical Optics and Imaging - Proceedings of SPIE 5747(2), 1400–1410 (2005)
9. Eskildsen, S.F., Østergaard, L.R.: Active surface approach for extraction of the human cerebral cortex from mri. In: Larsen, R., Nielsen, M., Sporring, J. (eds.) MICCAI 2006. LNCS, vol. 4191, Springer, Heidelberg (2006)
10. Lee, J., Lee, J.M., Kim, J.S., Kim, I.Y., Evans, A.C., Kim, S.I.: A novel quantitative cross-validation of different cortical surface reconstruction algorithms using mri phantom. NeuroImage 31, 572–584 (2006)
11. Fischl, B., Sereno, M.I., Dale, A.M.: Cortical surface-based analysis ii: Inflation, flattening, and surface-based coordinate system. NeuroImage 9(2), 195–207 (1999)
12. Collins, D.L., Neelin, P., Peters, T.M., Evans, A.: Automatic 3d intersubject registration of mr volumetric data in standardized talairach space. Journal of Computer Assisted Tomography 18(2), 192–205 (1994)
13. Smith, S.M.: Fast robust automated brain extraction. Human Brain Mapping 17(3), 143–155 (2002)
14. Chen, L., Wagenknecht, G.: Automated topology correction for human brain segmentation. In: Larsen, R., Nielsen, M., Sporring, J. (eds.) MICCAI 2006. LNCS, vol. 4191, pp. 316–323. Springer, Heidelberg (2006)
15. Kwan, R.S., Evans, A., Pike, G.: MRI simulation-based evaluation of image-processing and classification methods. IEEE Transactions on Medical Imaging 18(11), 1085–1097 (1999)

Stabilization of Image Motion for Robotic Assisted Beating Heart Surgery

Danail Stoyanov and Guang-Zhong Yang

Institute of Biomedical Engineering,
Imperial College London, London SW7 2AZ, UK
{danail.stoyanov,g.z.yang}@imperial.ac.uk
http://vip.doc.ic.ac.uk

Abstract. The performance of robotic assisted minimally invasive beating heart surgery is a challenging task due to the rhythmic motion of the heart, which hampers delicate tasks such as small vessel anastomosis. In this paper, a virtual motion compensation scheme is proposed for stabilizing images from the surgical site. The method uses vision based 3D tracking to accurately infer cardiac surface deformation and augmented reality for rendering a motion stabilized view for improved surgical performance. The method forgoes the need of fiducial markers and can be integrated with the existing master-slave robotic consoles. The proposed technique is validated with both simulated surgical scenes with known ground truth and *in vivo* data acquired from a TECAB procedure. The experimental results demonstrate the potential of the proposed technique in performing microscale tasks in a moving frame of reference with improved precision and repeatability.

Keywords: Robotic Assisted Surgery, Beating Heart Surgery, Motion Compensation, Soft-Tissue Tracking.

1 Introduction

The use of master-slave robotic systems for minimally invasive surgery has made it possible to perform totally endoscopic beating heart surgery. This approach has a number of well documented patient benefits including reduced surgical trauma and avoidance of cardiopulmonary bypass. However, handling respiratory and cardiac motion under which these procedures must be performed is demanding even for skilled surgeons. Thus far, delicate tasks such as small vessel anastomosis during Totally Endoscopic Coronary Artery Bypass (TECAB) are normally performed under mechanical stabilization. Despite this, residual motion is still prominent, which is compounded by limited epicardial exposure and the complexity of instrument control. A potential solution to this is to introduce real-time *in situ* adaptive motion compensation.

Motion compensation involves synchronizing the movement of a robotic instrument with the deformation of the soft-tissue, hence allowing the surgeon to operate on a *virtually* stabilized operating field-of-view. Previous research has

N. Ayache, S. Ourselin, A. Maeder (Eds.): MICCAI 2007, Part I, LNCS 4791, pp. 417–424, 2007.
© Springer-Verlag Berlin Heidelberg 2007

demonstrated that by synchronizing instrument movement, it is possible to improve the accuracy of simulated surgical tasks [1]. Control requirements for a practical robotic device to operate in sync with the heart have also been investigated, illustrating the requirement for predictive control loops [2, 3, 4]. The pre-requisite of all motion stabilization techniques is accurate reconstruction of tissue deformation *in situ* and in real-time. Thus far, a number of approaches have been proposed to infer 2D deformation of the heart *in vivo* either by using projected fiducial markers [2] or by optical tracking techniques [3]. It has also been shown that the epicardial surface can be reconstructed in metric 3D space based on stereo-laparoscopes [5]. There is, however, limited investigation on the psychovisual and hand-eye coordination of the surgeon under such motion compensation schemes. The purpose of this paper is to present a vision based image stabilization scheme for motion compensation that combines real-time computational stereo tissue deformation recovery with 3D motion stabilization. Our study focuses on the visualization of the motion stabilized stereo-laparoscope images and does not describe a robotic tool synchronization system. The proposed technique forgoes the need of fiducial markers and can be integrated with an Augmented Reality (AR) scheme on a master-slave robotic console. The method is validated with both simulated surgical scenes with known ground truth and *in vivo* data acquired from a TECAB procedure.

2   Method

2.1   3D Tissue Deformation Recovery

For real-time motion compensation, accurate 3D tissue deformation recovery is essential. In order to compute 3D measurements using a stereo-laparoscope, the device is first calibrated using an existing planar object calibration algorithm [6]. This computes the intrinsic camera parameters and the spatial relationship between the stereo rig. The camera matrices and mapping between a world point $\mathbf{M} = [X \ \ Y \ \ Z]^{\mathsf{T}}$ and an image point $\mathbf{m} = [x \ \ y]^{\mathsf{T}}$ can be represented by the following equation:

$$\lambda \mathbf{m}_n = \mathbf{K}_n [\mathbf{R}_n \mid \mathbf{t}_n] \mathbf{M} \tag{1}$$

where $\mathbf{K}$ is the intrinsic parameter matrix, $\mathbf{R}$ and $\mathbf{t}$ are the extrinsic parameters, and λ is a scale factor. When these parameters are known, the 3D position of a landmark visible from both stereo-laparoscope views can be computed by finding the intersection of the rays back-projected from each camera. In practice, the true intersection point may not exist and a surrogate measure of identifying the mid-point of the shortest line segment between the rays is usually used.

For this purpose, the correspondence between image points in the two views must be established. To obtain stereo correspondence and subsequently track temporal tissue motion, we used a technique that extends previous work proposed in [7]. With this method, salient features are first selected on the epicardial surface based on the intensity gradient information [8]. They are then tracked in real-time using stereo-temporal constraints using the Lucas-Kanade (LK) algorithm. By denoting a warp function $\mathbf{W}_n(\mathbf{m}; \mathbf{p})$, which maps point $\mathbf{m}$ according to the parameter vector $\mathbf{p}$, the alignment of an image template $T_n(\mathbf{m})$ with an input image I_n in more than one camera can be formulated as the following minimization problem:

$$\sum_n \sum_{\mathbf{m}} [I_n(\mathbf{m} + \mathbf{P}_n(\mathbf{p})) - T_n(\mathbf{m})]^2 \qquad (2)$$

The selected parameterization of the warp function represents the 3D location of the target point $\mathbf{p} = \mathbf{M}$ and has an analytical *Jacobian* [9]. From a given starting solution, the LK parameter update term can be derived iteratively by approximating Eq. (2) with a first-order Taylor polynomial and obtaining the partial derivative with respect to $\Delta\mathbf{p}$. This leads to the following update equation:

$$\Delta\mathbf{p} = \mathbf{H}^{-1} \sum_n \sum_{\mathbf{m}} \left[\nabla I_n \frac{\partial \mathbf{W}_n}{\partial \mathbf{p}}\right]^{\mathsf{T}} [T_n(\mathbf{m}) - I_n(\mathbf{W}_n(\mathbf{m}; \mathbf{p}))]$$

$$\text{where} \quad \mathbf{H} = \sum_n \sum_{\mathbf{m}} \left[\nabla I_n \frac{\partial \mathbf{W}_n}{\partial \mathbf{p}}\right]^{\mathsf{T}} \left[\nabla I_n \frac{\partial \mathbf{W}_n}{\partial \mathbf{p}}\right] \qquad (3)$$

To obtain a starting solution, the same method as above was used but implemented in a pyramidal fashion to match across the stereo pair. This approach is effective as the hierarchical scheme allows for large disparity values. It is also particularly useful for improving the convergence of the algorithm for stereo-laparoscopes, where the cameras are arranged in a verged configuration. For feature detection, gradient based landmarks were used for improved computational performance suitable for real-time implementation [8]. To circumvent the effect of specular highlights, a threshold filter based on the intensity and saturation of the image was used to remove the associated outliers.

2.2 Motion Compensated Imaging

Once the motion of the target cardiac surface is reconstructed, virtual motion compensation is applied. To compensate for physiological motion, we use an AR scheme by creating a virtually moving camera, which renders the surgical field-of-view in a moving frame of reference.

For the calibrated stereo-laparoscope cameras, a ray $\mathbf{q}_n(\mathbf{m}_n)$ defining the line of sight for an image point $\mathbf{m}_n$ can be derived by using the camera matrix and the optical centre of the camera as:

$$\lambda \mathbf{q}_n(\mathbf{m}_n) = \mathbf{c}_n + \mathbf{P}_n^{\dagger} \mathbf{m}_n \qquad (4)$$

where $\mathbf{c}_n$ denotes the optical centre and $\mathbf{P}_n^{\dagger}$ the Moore-Penrose pseudo inverse of the projection matrix. A virtual surface rendered with a texture taken from the stereo-laparoscope will appear as the real scene in a virtual camera representing the stereo-laparoscope if all points on the surface satisfy Eq. (4). This effectively ensures the alignment of the virtual scene with the real images.

Compensating for the motion of a moving target on the cardiac surface can be achieved by directly moving the virtual camera with the respective motion of the target. Denoting the target motion as $\mathbf{J}^t = \mathbf{M}^t - \mathbf{M}^{t-1}$ and using Eq. (1), the position of the compensated camera must satisfy the following equation:

$$\mathbf{P}_n \mathbf{M}^t = \mathbf{P}_n' \left(\mathbf{M}^t + \mathbf{J}^t \right) \tag{5}$$

By using the decomposition of the camera matrix, it is clear that the intrinsic parameters remain constant and the above equation leads to an adjustment of the camera's extrinsic translation parameter as $\mathbf{t}_n^t = \mathbf{R}_n \mathbf{J}^t - \mathbf{R}_n \mathbf{c}_n^{t-1}$.

For an exact virtual scene representation from the new camera position, it is necessary to have the knowledge about the 3D geometry and photometric properties of the object. The scene geometry can be obtained with dense computational stereo techniques but this can be computationally demanding. In this study, an approximation of the cardiac surface was used instead in the vicinity of the compensated point by using a thin plate spline. The sparse set of landmarks around the compensated target was determined in §2.1 and their corresponding distance along rays defined in Eq. (4) was used as the control point to recreate the entire surface. The remainder of the surface was then interpolated back to a virtual plane satisfying Eq. (4). It should be noted that this interpolation does not necessarily represent the true perspective projection.

3   Experimental Setup and Results

In order to validate the proposed motion compensation approach, both simulated and *in vivo* data was used. In this study, the experimental environment consisted of a daVinci® console used for 3D visualization, a SenseAble Omni® haptic device for instrument manipulation, and a   3 GHz Pentium-D workstation with two NVIDIA GeForce 7600Gs graphics cards and 2 Gb of RAM for real-time processing. The proposed method was implemented using C++ and D3D for real-time 3D tissue-deformation recovery and motion compensated AR visualization. When motion compensation was applied the virtual instrument controlled by the haptic device was synchronized with the same motion signal as applied to the virtual camera.

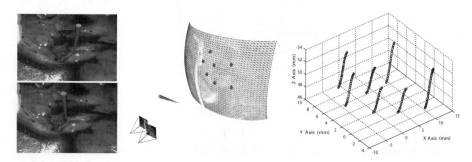

Fig. 1. The simulation environment used in this study, illustrating a stereo pair generated by the virtual camera (left), the corresponding virtual 3D scene and surface mesh (middle), and the 3D motion trajectories (right) of the highlighted control points used for validation

Ten volunteers (2 surgeons and 8 computer scientists) were asked to perform two separate tasks with and without motion compensation, respectively. *Task I* represents a simple targeting exercise and involves touching a sequence of markers on the moving surface as shown in Fig. 1. *Task II* simulates an incision required to expose an anastomosis site, which requires the user to follow a smooth path through a series of markers on the beating heart surface.

3.1 Validation with Simulated Data

For validation with simulated data, a 3D surface mesh textured with an *in vivo* image was used to represent the deforming cardiac surface. The dynamics of the motion were modeled by a sinusoidal Gaussian mixture function mimicking the respiratory and cardiac induced epicardial deformation. An example rendition of the virtual surface as observed from the stereo cameras is shown in Fig. 1.

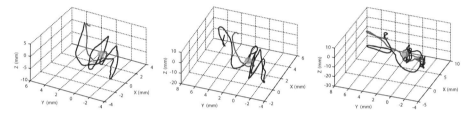

Fig. 2. Example trajectories in the moving frame of reference of a single target (green) for the instrument tip with (red) and without (blue) motion compensation for three of the subjects studied

The results obtained for the ten subjects performing *Task I* are summarized in Table 1 using the total path length (TPL) of the tooltip's motion, which is representative of the amount of movement required to reach the target. Example trajectories presented in the moving frame of reference of the target are shown in Fig. 2. It was found that with motion compensation, all subjects could reach the target with a faster and smoother trajectory compared to that without motion compensation.

For *Task II*, Table 1 summarizes the results for the ten subjects, where the mean path error (MPE) and its standard deviation (SPE) are used as performance measures. In this study, the path error was defined as the shortest Eucledian distance from the tooltip to the optimal path between the control points. It is evident that with motion compensation, there is a significant reduction in the MPE for most subjects along with a significant reduction in SPE. This indicates that subjects are much more confident and accurate in following the prescribed path along the cardiac surface, which is essential for exposing the anastomosis site.

To verify the statistical significance of the results presented in Table 1 we used a Kolmogorov-Smirnov test to find that the data did not adequately fit a Normal distribution. Therefore, we used the non-parametric Wilcoxon test for paired samples, which showed that the difference in results observed with and without motion compensation was significant for all performance metrics. The *p-value* given by the Wilcoxon test for TPL, MPE and SPE was 0.0273, 0.002 and 0.0098 respectively.

Table 1. Results obtained for the ten sujects performing *Tasks I* and *Task II*. The prefix (c) is used to distiguish the compensated version of the experiment and all measurements are in millimeters.

	S1	S2	S3	S4	S5	S6	S7	S8	S9	S10	Median [quartiles]
TPL	433.6	586.0	944.6	608.5	281.6	551.5	510.6	346.3	474.2	520.6	**515.6 [412, 592]**
cTPL	239.6	244.9	312.0	325.0	179.2	324.1	755.7	193.5	207.1	324.0	**278.4 [204, 324]**
MPE	2.43	2.79	2.45	2.20	1.80	2.48	3.41	1.85	1.48	1.95	**2.32 [1.84, 2.56]**
cMPE	1.48	1.67	1.72	0.97	1.07	1.42	3.04	1.13	0.82	1.59	**1.45 [1.04, 1.68]**
SPE	1.31	1.87	1.55	1.46	0.97	1.21	2.04	1.04	0.78	1.22	**1.27 [1.02, 1.63]**
cSPE	0.60	1.14	1.05	0.58	0.57	0.87	2.12	0.73	0.57	1.30	**0.8 [0.58, 1.18]**

3.2   Validation with *In Vivo* Data

For demonstrating the practical value of the proposed framework, an *in vivo* dataset from a TECAB surgery was used for further validation. In this experiment, the ground truth geometry was derived by tracking landmarks on the epicardial surface for the duration of the *in vivo* sequence (2100 frames) with the aforementioned 3D surface reconstruction technique. The reconstructed dense surface map and the corresponding 3D motion trajectory of an example tracked landmark are illustrated in Fig. 3. This result was then used as the ground truth 3D geometry as in previous experiments.

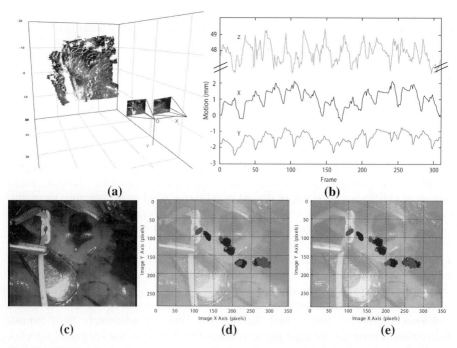

Fig. 3. (a-b) Dense cardiac surface reconstruction in 3D and the corresponding 3D motion components of the stabilization target along the *x*, *y*, and *z* axes **(c)** The reconstructed ground truth control points (blue circles) and the zero motion target (green). **(d-e)** Stereo pair from **(c)** showing the motion of each control point with (red) and without (blue) motion compensation.

Fig. 3 demonstrates the image motion of the control points back-projected to the camera view prior to (shown in blue) and after (shown in red) applying the proposed motion compensation scheme. It is apparent that the motion of the highlighted target point is close to zero, whereas the motion of the neighboring region is significantly reduced. The overall deformation of the surface is highly non-linear and thus there is residual motion.

Fig. 4 illustrates the results for the ten subjects performing *Task I* based on the *in vivo* data. It is evident that there is a marked improvement in performance for most of the subjects. This difference is statistically significant as demonstrated by a non-parametric Wilcoxon test for paired samples where the *p-value* was computed as 0.02 and 0.001 for the TPL and MPE metrics respectively.

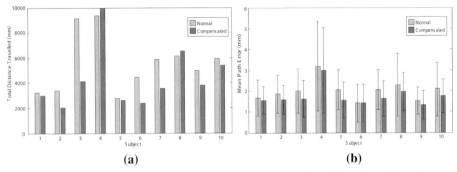

(a)   (b)

Fig. 4. (a) Bar chart illustrating the difference in the total path length in order to hit all targets during *Task I* with and without motion compensation. **(b)** The mean and standard deviation of the error between the tooltip and the ideal path for *Task II* for all the studied subjects.

4 Discussion and Conclusions

In conclusion, we have presented in this paper a method for motion compensation in robotic assisted beating heart surgery. The method uses vision based 3D tracking to accurately infer cardiac surface deformation and AR for rendering a motion stabilized view for improved performance of micro-scale surgical tasks such as vessel anastomosis. The experiments carried out in this study demonstrate the potential of the proposed technique in performing these delicate tasks in a moving frame of reference with greater precision and repeatability. An important area of future work is to develop methods that can adaptively select motion compensation target and seamlessly integrate the proposed motion compensation scheme into the current robotic assisted MIS workflows. Potential techniques include the use of tooltip tracking or to use real-time eye tracking to locate the surgeon's fixation point, thus leading to a gaze contingent adaptive motion compensation framework.

References

1. Trejos, A.L., Salcudean, S.C., Sassani, F., Lichtenstein, S.: On the Feasibility of a Moving Support for Surgery on the Beating Heart. In: Taylor, C., Colchester, A. (eds.) MICCAI 1999. LNCS, vol. 1679, pp. 1088–1097. Springer, Heidelberg (1999)

2. Ginhoux, R., Gangloff, J., De Mathelin, M., Soler, L., Sanchez, M.A., Marescaux, J.: Active Filtering of Physiological Motion in Robotized Surgery Using Predictive Control. IEEE Trans. Robotics 21(1), 67–79 (2005)
3. Ortmaier, T., Groger, M., Boehm, D.H., Falk, V., Hirzinger, G.: Motion Estimation in Beating Heart Surgery. IEEE Trans. Biomedical Engineering 52(10), 1729–1740 (2005)
4. Nakamura, Y., Kishi, K., Kawakami, H.: Heartbeat Synchronization for Robotic Cardiac Surgery. In: Proc. ICRA 2001, vol. 1, pp. 2014–2019 (2001)
5. Stoyanov, D., Darzi, A., Yang, G.-Z.: Dense 3D Depth Recovery for Soft Tissue Deformation During Robotically Assisted Laparoscopic Surgery. Computer Aided Surgery 10(4), 199–208 (2005)
6. Zhang, Z.: A flexible new technique for camera calibration. IEEE Trans. on Pattern Analysis and Machine Intelligence 22(11), 1330–1334 (2000)
7. Stoyanov, D., Mylonas, G., Deligianni, F., Yang, G.-Z.: Soft-Tisse Motion Tracking and Structure Estimation for Robotic Assisted MIS Procedures. In: Duncan, J.S., Gerig, G. (eds.) MICCAI 2005. LNCS, vol. 3750, pp. 139–146. Springer, Heidelberg (2005)
8. Shi, J., Tomasi, C.: Good Features to Track. In: CVPR 1994, vol. 1, pp. 593–600 (1994)
9. Devernay, F., Mateus, D., Guilbert, M.: Multi-Camera Scene Flow by Tracking 3D Points and Surfels. In: CVPR 2006, vol. 2, pp. 2203–2212 (2006)

Robotic Assistant for Transperineal Prostate Interventions in 3T Closed MRI

Gregory S. Fischer[1], Simon P. DiMaio[2],
Iulian I. Iordachita[1], and Gabor Fichtinger[1]

[1] Center for Computer Integrated Surgery, Johns Hopkins University, USA
[gfischer,iordachita,gaborf]@jhu.edu,
[2] Surgical Planning Lab, Harvard University, USA
simond@bwh.harvard.edu.

Abstract. Numerous studies have demonstrated the efficacy of image-guided needle-based therapy and biopsy in the management of prostate cancer. The accuracy of traditional prostate interventions performed using transrectal ultrasound (TRUS) is limited by image fidelity, needle template guides, needle deflection and tissue deformation. Magnetic Resonance Imaging (MRI) is an ideal modality for guiding and monitoring such interventions due to its excellent visualization of the prostate, its sub-structure and surrounding tissues. We have designed a comprehensive robotic assistant system that allows prostate biopsy and brachytherapy procedures to be performed entirely inside a 3T closed MRI scanner. We present a detailed design of the robotic manipulator and an evaluation of its usability and MR compatibility.

1 Introduction

Core needle biopsy is considered the definitive method of diagnosis for prostate cancer, and each year approximately 1.5M core needle biopsies are performed, yielding about 220,000 new prostate cancer cases in the U.S. [1]. When cancer is confined to the prostate, low-dose-rate permanent brachytherapy, where 50-150 radioactive pellets/seeds are placed into the prostate, is a common treatment option. A complex seed distribution pattern must be achieved, while minimizing radiation toxicity to adjacent healthy tissues. Transrectal Ultrasound (TRUS) is the current "gold standard" for guiding biopsy and brachytherapy. However, current TRUS-guided biopsy has a detection rate of 20-30% [2] and TRUS-guided brachytherapy cannot readily visualize seed placement in the US images. Further, the template in TRUS-guided procedures limits the placement precision and the ability to effectively guide oblique insertions. MRI has high sensitivity for detecting prostate tumors, high spatial resolution, excellent soft tissue contrast and multiplanar volumetric imaging capabilities, making it an ideal modality for guiding and monitoring such procedures.

The clinical efficacy of MRI-guided prostate biopsy and brachytherapy was demonstrated by D'Amico, Tempany, et al. using a 0.5T open-MRI scanner to plan and monitor transperineal needle placement [3]. Needles were manually

N. Ayache, S. Ourselin, A. Maeder (Eds.): MICCAI 2007, Part I, LNCS 4791, pp. 425–433, 2007.
© Springer-Verlag Berlin Heidelberg 2007

inserted using a plastic template, with the patient oriented in the lithotomy position, similarly to the TRUS-guided approach. Beyersdorff et al. performed targeted transrectal biopsy in 1.5T MRI with a passive articulated needle guide [4]. Krieger et al. present a 2-DOF passive, un-encoded and manually manipulated mechanical linkage to aim a needle guide for transrectal prostate biopsy with MRI guidance [5]. Robotic assistance has been investigated for guiding instrument placement in MRI, beginning with neurosurgery [6] and later percutaneous interventions [7]. Chinzei et al. developed a general-purpose robotic assistant for open MRI [8] that was subsequently adapted for transperineal intra-prostatic needle placement [9]. Stoianovici et al. has made developments in pneumatic stepper motors and applied them to robotic brachytherapy seed placement [10]. Other MRI-compatible mechanisms include pneumatic motors for a light puncture robot [11] and haptic interfaces for fMRI [12].

The patient is in the prone postion in [4] and [5], which make preoperative and intraoperative image fusion difficult; further, the transrectal approach precludes using commercially available endorectal imaging coils. The system presented in [10] is very complex and places the the patient in the fetal position, again preventing the pre- and intra-operative images from aligning and challenges traditional patient positioning for both MR imaging and and brachytherapy. The presented robotic system is of simpler design, lower cost, and above all, incorporates ergonomics suited for prostate biopsy and brachytherapy by allowing the patient to retain the supine (semi-lithotomy) pose used for preoperative imaging.

This work presents the design and development of a comprehensive robot-assisted system for transperineal prostate needle placement in 3T closed-bore MRI. The system integrates an image-based target planning interface, a robotic placement mechanism that allows for remote manipulation of the needle in the magnet bore without moving the patient out of the imaging space, as well as robot and needle tracking for navigation and control.

2   Methods

2.1   System Layout and Architecture

We have developed a comprehensive computer-integrated needle placement system to accurately target planned tissue sites by minimizing needle misplacement effects. The complete system comprises two main modules, integrated with high-field diagnostic MRI scanners. First is a visualization, planning and navigation system, and second is a robotic assistant for needle placement. The architecture of this system is outlined in Fig. 1.

In blocks **a** and **b**, 3D Slicer software (www.slicer.org) fuses multimodality pre-operative images with pre-procedural MR images for procedure planning. Kinematics of the needle trajectories are evaluated subject to anatomical constraints and constraints of the needle placement mechanism. Device and needle navigation are shown in blocks **c**, **d** and **e**, which are enclosed in a loop that represents device/needle positioning and sensing/localization. Blocks **d** and **e** guide the needle positioning device; an image-based servo loop tracks the needle

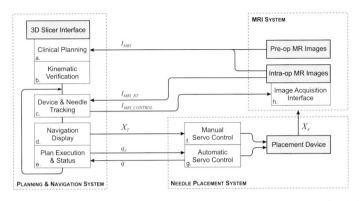

Fig. 1. System architecture (left) and component distribution (right)

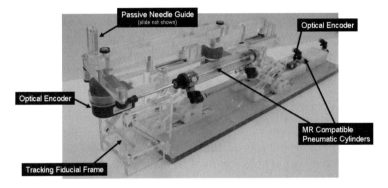

Fig. 2. Robot manipulator capable of two actuated DOFs with manual needle insertion. The tracking fiducial frame at the front of the robot is used for locating the robot in the scanner coordinate system.

and provides real-time images along it's axis to help detect and limit needle and tissue deflection effects. Blocks **f** and **g** are the robotic mechanism that provides remote operation of the needle while the patient is within the magnet bore.

2.2 Mechanical Design

The patient is positioned in the supine position such that their legs are placed on a leg support that provides a "tunnel" of access to the perineum. This creates a well defined workspace at the patient's perineum, while maintaining a compact profile to prevent interference with the patient, the scanner and adjacent equipment. The focus of the first phase is to bring MR guidance to the same degrees of freedom (DOF) available in traditional TRUS template-guided procedures. The kinematic requirements are $100mm$ in the vertical and horizontal directions and passive needle insertion guide with an encoded travel of $120mm$. To mimic the traditional TRUS procedure and also for increased safety, needle insertion is performed manually along the needle guide that is aligned by the robot. Already incorporated in the mechanical design, but not actuated in the present prototype system are two additional DOF; 15° of rotation in the vertical and horizontal planes will help avoid pubic arch interference that may typically be a contraindication using traditional techniques. This will be particularly important since space constraints of the MR scanner prevent positioning the patient in the full lithotomy position; thus, lowering the pubic arch and increasing the likelyhood of interference.

Vertical motion is generated by a modified scissor lift mechanism. Two such mechanisms actuated independently provide vertical motion and elevation angle. Horizontal motion is generated by a second planar bar mechanism that rests upon the vertical stage. Prismatic and rotational motions can be realized by coupling two such straight-line motion mechanisms. For both stages, actuation is provided by custom pneumatic cylinders described in Section 2.3. The actuators are oriented along the bore axis (B_0), thus reducing the overall width significantly. The complete assembly is shown in Fig. 2. Sterility is insured by making the top-most portion of the passive needle guide removable and draping the remainder of the robot. Further, the tissue contacting surface of the leg rest will be removable and sterilizable.

2.3   Actuation and Control

Pneumatic actuators were chosen because they offer relatively high speed and power for their weight and provide for compact means of actuation at the mechanism. They also do not require involved setup or allow the risk of fluid leakage, which is a sterility concern, associated with hydraulic systems. Servo control of the cylinders is provided by piezoelectrically actuated pressure regulator valves with switching times under $4ms$ (Hoerbiger-Origa Tecno Valve, Altenstadt, Germany). Custom MR compatible pneumatic cylinders are made with glass bores, graphite pistons, brass shafts and plastic housings (Made in collaboration with Airpel, Norwalk, CT). Pneumatic brakes are attached to each cylinder in order to lock and maintain needle position/orientation during needle insertion. They are unlocked by applying air pressure.

The robot uses linear strip optical encoders for the vertical motion stage and rotary encoders on the horizontal motion stage. Encoders were thoroughly tested in 3T MRI for functionality and imaging compatibility (US Digital EM1 with PC5 differential driver, Vancouver, Washington). Functionality was evaluated by confirming that no encoder counts were lost as the mechanism periodically oscillated in the bore of the scanner during imaging. Imaging compatibility was confirmed by monitoring the effect on the MR images under standard prostate imaging protocols as described later in Section 3.1.

A controller sitting in the MR scanner room near the foot of the bed provides low level control of the robot. Inside of the EMI shielded enclosure is an embedded computer with analog I/O for interfacing with valves and pressure sensors and an FPGA module for interfacing with joint encoders. Also in the enclosure are piezoelectric servo valves, piezoelectric brake valves and pressure sensors. The short distance between the servo valves and the robot is minimized, thus maximizing the bandwidth of the pneumatic actuators. The expected bandwidth is 100Hz. Control software on the embedded PC provides for low-level joint control and an interface to interactive scripting and higher-level trajectory planning. Communication with the planning and control workstation is through a fiberoptic ethernet connection.

Dynamic global registration between the robot and scanner is provided by passive tracking fiducials on the robot base and is described in detail in [13]. The rigid structure of the the fiducial frame is made up of seven rigid glass tubes with $3mm$ inner diameters that are filled with contrast extracted from MR Spot fiducials (Beekley, Bristol, CT). The rods are placed on three faces of a $60mm$ cube as shown in Fig. 2, and any arbitrary MR image slicing through all of the rods provides the full 6 DOF pose of the frame, and thus the robot, with respect to the scanner. Thus, by locating the fiducial attached to the robot, the transformation between patient coordinates (where planning is performed) and the robot's needle driver is known.

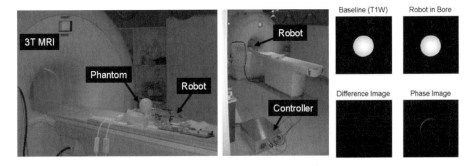

Fig. 3. Experimental setup for compatibility trials. The robot is placed on the bed alongside a spherical MR phantom (left) and the controller is placed in the scanner room near the foot of the bed(center). Images of the spherical phantom taken with the T1W sequence are shown with and without the robot present; the square at the center represents the field of view used for SNR calculations. Below them are the corresponding difference and phase images (right).

3   Results

3.1   MR Compatibility

MR Compatibility includes three main elements: 1) safety, 2) preserving image quality, and 3) maintaining functionality. Safety issues such as RF heating are minimized by isolating the robot from the patient, avoiding wire coils, and avoiding resonances in components of the robot; ferrous materials are completely avoided to prevent the chance of a projectile. Image quality is maintained by again avoiding ferromagnetic materials, limiting conductive materials near the imaging site, and avoiding RF sources. Pneumatic actuation and optical sensing, as described in Section 2.3, preserve full functionality of the robot in the scanner.

Evaluation and verification of the MR compatibility of the system was a primary goal of this work. Compatibility was evaluated on a 3T Philips Achieva scanner. A 10*cm* spherical MR phantom was placed at the isocenter and the robot placed such that the tip was at a distance of 120*mm* from the center of the phantom (a realistic depth from perineum to prostate) as shown in Fig. 3 (left). The phantom was imaged using three standard prostate imaging protocols: 1) **T2W TSE**: T2 weighted turbo spin echo (28cm FOV, 3mm slice, TE=90ms, TR=5600ms, 2) **T1W FFE**: T1 weighted fast field gradient echo (28cm FOV, 3mm slice, TE=2.3ms, TR=264ms) and 3) **TFE (FGRE)**: "Real time" turbo field gradient echo (28cm FOV, 3mm slice, TE=10ms, TR=26ms). A baseline scan with each sequence was taken of the phantom with no robot components using round flex coils similar to those often used in prostate imaging. The following imaging series were taken in each of the following configurations: 1) Phantom only, 2) Controller in room and powered, 3) Robot placed in scanner bore, 4) Robot electrically connected to controller and 5) Robot moving during imaging (only with T1W imaging). For each step, all three imaging sequences were performed and both magnitude and phase images were collected.

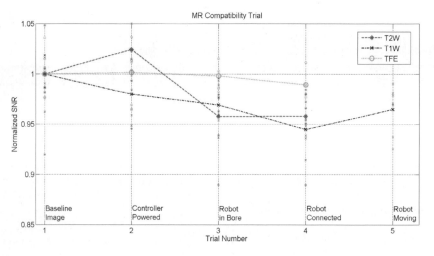

Fig. 4. Signal to noise ratio for three standard prostate imaging protocols with the system in different configurations. Lines represent mean SNR within 25mm cube at center of homogeneous phantom and discrete points represent SNR in the 25mm square on each of seven 3*mm* slices making up the cube.

The effect on image quality was judged by computing the signal to noise ratio (SNR). SNR of an MR image can be calculated with several techniques; we chose to define it as the mean signal in a 25*mm* square at the center of the homogeneous sphere divided by the standard deviation of the signal in that same region as shown in Fig. 3 (right). The SNR of the magnitude images was normalized by the value for the baseline image, thus limiting any bias in choice of calculation technique or location. SNR was evaluated at seven slices (representing 25mm width) at the center of the sphere for each of the three imaging sequences. The points in the graph in Fig. 4 show the SNR in the phantom for seven $3mm$ thick slices for each sequence at each configuration. The lines represent the average SNR in the $25mm$ cube at the center of the spherical phantom for each sequence at each configuration. When the robot was operational, the reduction in SNR of the $25mm$ cube at the phantom's center for these pulse sequences was 5.5% for **T1W FFE**, 4.2% for **T2W TSE** and 1.1% for **TFE (FGRE)**. Further qualitative means of evaluating the effect of the robot on image quality are obtained by examining prostate images taken both with and without the robot present. Fig. 5 (right) shows images of the prostate of a volunteer placed in the scanner bore on the leg rest.

3.2 System Integration

To evaluate the overall layout and workflow, the robot was placed in the bore inside of the leg rest with a volunteer as shown in Fig. 5 (left). Round flex receiver coils were used for this trial; endorectal coils can be used for clinical case to obtain optimal image quality. There was adequate room for a patient and the robot was able to maintain its necessary workspace.

Co-registration of the robot to the scanner was performed using the base tracking fiducial described in Section 2.3 that is shown in Fig. 2. Images of the robot's tracking fiducial provide the location of the robot base in the scanner's coordinate system with an RMS accuracy of $0.14mm$ and 0.37^o as described in [13]. Joint encoding provides end effector localization resolution of better that $0.01mm$ and $0.1mm$ for horizontal and vertical motions, respectively. In free space, the needle tip localization accuracy with respect to the MR images is expected to be better than $0.25mm$ and 0.5^o.

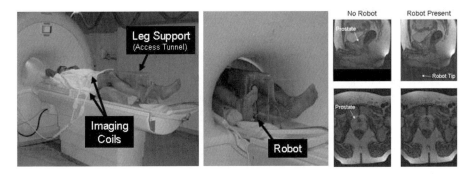

Fig. 5. Qualitative analysis of prostate image quality. Patient is placed on the leg support (left) and the robot sits inside of the support tunnel inside the scanner bore (center). T2 weighted sagittal and transverse images of the prostate taken when no robot components were present and when the robot was active in the scanner (right).

4   Discussion

MRI-guidance promises high quality, rapid, volumetric, multimodality imaging capabilities, but presents significant engineering challenges due to the harsh electromagnetic environment and tight spatial constraints in the scanner bore. We have developed a prototype robotic system for precisely targeting prostate tissue under realtime MR guidance. The current system provides the 2-DOF plus insertion of traditional TRUS-guided procedures with finer spatial resolution and image-based guidance. Needle placement accuracy can be improved from the $5mm$ grid that is standard today.

We have shown the system to be MR compatible under standard prostate imaging sequences, with sufficient accuracy for guiding prostate biopsy and brachytherapy procedures. Localization accuracy of the tracking fiducial that is attached to the robot and its application to visual servoing and dynamic scan plane control are described in our companion paper [13]. Detailed analysis of the true needle insertion error of the complete system in phantom studies, and ultimately animal and cadaver trials, is forthcoming. The next generation system will incorporate additional rotational DOFs such that pubic arch interference can be avoided, thus increasing the eligible population for these procedures. This work is also of relevance to the development of systems specialized for other organ systems and diseases that require targeted needle placement inside an MRI scanner.

This work was supported by NIH 1R01CA111288, CDMRP PCRP Fellowship W81XWH-07-1-0171, and NSF EEC-9731748.

References

1. Jemal, A., Siegel, R., Ward, E., Murray, T., Xu, J., Smigal, C., Thun, M.: Cancer statistics, 2006. CA Cancer J. Clin. 56(2), 106–130 (2004)
2. Terris, M.K., et al.: Comparison of mid-lobe versus lateral systematic sextant biopsies in detection of prostate cancer. Urol Int. 59, 239–242 (1997)
3. D'Amico, A.V., Tempany, C.M., Cormack, R., Hata, N., et al.: Transperineal magnetic resonance image guided prostate biopsy. J. Urol. 164(2), 385–387 (2000)
4. Beyersdorff, D., Winkel, A., Hamm, B., et al.: MRI-guided prostate biopsy with a closed MR unit at 1.5 T. Radiology 234, 576–581 (2005)
5. Krieger, A., Susil, R.C., Menard, C., Coleman, J.A., Fichtinger, G., Atalar, E., Whitcomb, L.L.: Design of a novel MRI compatible manipulator for image guided prostate interventions. IEEE TBME 52, 306–313 (2005)
6. Masamune, K., Kobayashi, E., Masutani, Y., Suzuki, M., Dohi, T., Iseki, H., Takakura, K.: Development of an MRI-compatible needle insertion manipulator for stereotactic neurosurgery. J. Image Guid. Surg. 1(4), 242–248 (1995)
7. Hempel, E., Fischer, H., Gumb, L., et al.: An MRI-compatible surgical robot for precise radiological interventions. In: CAS, pp. 180–191 (2003)
8. Chinzei, K., Hata, N., Jolesz, F.A., Kikinis, R.: MR compatible surgical assist robot: system integration and preliminary feasibility study. In: Delp, S.L., DiGoia, A.M., Jaramaz, B. (eds.) MICCAI 2000. LNCS, vol. 1935, pp. 921–933. Springer, Heidelberg (2000)

9. DiMaio, S.P., Pieper, S., Chinzei, K., Fichtinger, G., Tempany, C., Kikinis, R.: Robot assisted percutaneous intervention in open-MRI. In: MRI Symp. p. 155 (2004)
10. Muntener, M., Patriciu, A., Petrisor, D., Mazilu, D., Bagga, H., Kavoussi, L., Cleary, K., Stoianovici, D.: MRI compatible robotic system for fully automated brachytherapy seed placement. J. Urology 68, 1313–1317 (2006)
11. Taillant, E., Avila-Vilchis, J., Allegrini, C., Bricault, I., Cinquin, P.: CT and MR Compatible Light Puncture Robot: Architectural Design and First Experiments. In: Barillot, C., Haynor, D.R., Hellier, P. (eds.) MICCAI 2004. LNCS, vol. 3217, pp. 145–152. Springer, Heidelberg (2004)
12. Gassert, R., Moser, R., Burdet, E., Bleuler, H.: MRI/fMRI-Compatible Robotic System With Force Feedback for Interaction With Human Motion. T. Mech. 11(2), 216–224 (2006)
13. DiMaio, S., Samset, E., Fischer, G., Iordachita, I., Fichtinger, G., Jolesz, F., Tempany, C.: Dynamic MRI Scan Plane Control for Passive Tracking of Instruments and Devices. In: Ayache, N., Ourselin, S., Maeder, A. (eds.) MICCAI 2007. LNCS, vol. 4792, pp. 50–58. Springer, Heidelberg (2007)

Virtually Extended Surgical Drilling Device: Virtual Mirror for Navigated Spine Surgery

Christoph Bichlmeier[1], Sandro Michael Heining[2],
Mohammad Rustaee[1], and Nassir Navab[1]

[1] Computer Aided Medical Procedures (CAMP), TUM, Munich, Germany
{bichlmei,navab}@cs.tum.edu, {mohammad.rustaee}@gmail.com
[2] Trauma Surgery Department, Klinikum Innenstadt, LMU, Munich, Germany
{Sandro-Michael.Heining}@med.uni-muenchen.de

Abstract. This paper introduces a new method for navigated spine surgery using a stereoscopic video see-through head-mounted display (HMD) and an optical tracking system. Vertebrae are segmented from volumetric CT data and visualized in-situ. A surgical drilling device is virtually extended with a mirror for intuitive planning of the drill canal, control of drill direction and insertion depth. The first designated application for the virtually extended drilling device is the preparation of canals for pedicle screw implantation in spine surgery. The objective of surgery is to install an internal fixateur for stabilization of injured vertebrae. We invited five surgeons of our partner clinic to test the system with realistic replica of lumbar vertebrae and compared the new approach with the classical, monitor-based navigation system providing three orthogonal slice views on the operation site. We measured time of procedure and scanned the drilled vertebrae with CT to verify accuracy of drilling.

1 Introduction

Implantation of pedicle screws is a frequently performed procedure in spine surgery. The pedicle approach is not only used to perform minimally invasive spinal interventions like vertebroplasty and kyphoplasty in osteoporotic fracture conditions but also in most dorsal stabilization procedures. The region around an injured vertebra is stabilized with an internal fixateur attached to intact vertebrae with screws drilled into their pedicles. Drilling canals into intact pedicles around injured vertebrae is an essential, preparative procedure for implantation of pedicle screws. The surgical task of pedicle screw placement in the lumbar and thoracic spine remains interesting even after a decade of image-guided surgery in the spine, which has lead to a variety of computer-aided techniques using different imaging modalities [1]: Basic techniques developed from using anatomic descriptions of the entry points in different spinal levels and the typical directions for pedicle screws ("droit devant" [2]) and static x-ray control after instrumentation to intra-operative 2D-flouroscopic control; advanced techniques from CT-based surgical navigation to intra-operative Iso-C-3D-control.

N. Ayache, S. Ourselin, A. Maeder (Eds.): MICCAI 2007, Part I, LNCS 4791, pp. 434–441, 2007.
© Springer-Verlag Berlin Heidelberg 2007

Regarding this procedure, state-of-the-art navigation systems consist of an optical tracking system that locates surgical instruments and the patient at the operation site. Imaging data is presented with three orthogonal slice views on the operation site on an external monitor. Position of slices follows the drill, this means the intersection line is aligned with the drill axes. In addition some systems provide a 3D visualization of the region around the operation site using polygonal surfaces or direct volume rendering.

Augmented Reality (AR) for intra-operative visualization and navigation has been a subject of intensive research and development during the last decade [3,4]. Azar et al. presented a user performance analysis with four different navigation systems for needle placement. Results show that a HMD based system performs "better in avoiding the surrounding structures"' and needle procedures perform "in a shorter amount of time"[5]. Traub et al. presented a clinical evaluation of different visualization modes for surgical drilling [6]. Perceptive advantages of the virtual mirror were first described in [7]. Later the laparoscopic virtual mirror was introduced for liver resection [8]. Thanks to a virtual mirror using a stereoscopic video see-through head-mounted display (HMD) and an optical tracking system (see figure 1(b)), we introduce a new computer aided system for drilling in navigated spine surgery. Due to in-situ visualization (2.2) mental mapping of medical imagery, which is presented on radiographs or on a monitor within in the operating room (OR), to the patient is not necessary. The visualization can be directly registered with the real operation site for diagnoses, surgical planning, and intraoperative navigation. Perception of 3D in-situ visualization is intuitive, however interaction with such 3D data is not practical. In a laboratory setting one can move around the virtually augmented scene to perceive layout, size and its relative position to further objects. Although not every desired view on the object is possible. Regarding a typical scenario in the OR, the surgeon is surrounded by clinical staff, equipment and the patient. A point of view on the operation site for instance from beneath the operation table is impossible. Here, the virtual mirror assists to enable intuitively the desired perspectives.

2   Method

The following section provides a detailed description of the AR system, the setup of the clinical study and the integration of the virtual mirror.

2.1   AR System

For superior registration quality the system uses two synchronized tracking systems. The single camera inside-out tracking system allows for a high rotational precision [9] necessary for tracking the stereoscopic video see-through head mounted display (HMD)[10]. The optical outside-in tracking system from A.R.T GmbH (Weilheim, Germany) with four infrared cameras fixed to the ceiling covers a large working area ($3x3x2$ m). Once this system is calibrated, it provides stable tracking data for a long term unless cameras are moved. The system is capable of tracking the targets in our setup with an accuracy of $< 0.35[mm]$ RMS.

Both of the systems use the same kind of retro reflective fiducial markers offering a registration free transformation from one tracking system to the other. To recover the six degrees of freedom of a rigid body, the external optical tracking system requires at least four rigidly attached markers. Fiducial markers are attached to the surgical drill as well as to the phantom. The reference frame target has an exceptional function as it enables the transition between the inside-out and the outside-in tracking systems. Both tracking systems calculate the same coordinate system for the reference frame. All targets are shown in figure 1(a).Further details of the used hardware and the tracking system is described in [7,11].

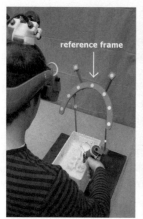 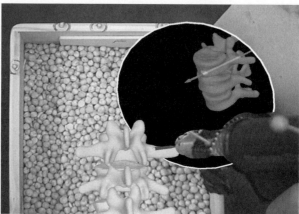

(a) View from outside.   (b) Surgeon's view through HMD.

Fig. 1. Virtual and real objects of the AR scene. Tracked targets are surgical drilling device, phantom and the reference frame with 9 fiducial markers.

2.2   In-Situ Visualization

All augmentations on targets, which are tracked by the optical outside-in tracking system, have to be positioned respective the reference frame of the inside-out tracking system. The transformation for in-situ visualization can be described by $^{CT}H_{ref}$.

$$^{CT}H_{ref} = ^{CT}H_{phantom} *^{phantom}H_{ext} * \left(^{ref}H_{ext}\right)^{-1} \tag{1}$$

Fiducial markers are attached to the boundaries of the wooden box. The optical outside-in tracking system provides the transformations $^{phantom}H_{ext}$ and $^{ref}H_{ext}$. Markers are segmented automatically from the volumetric imaging data. Correspondence of segmented positions and tracking data results in a registration matrix $^{CT}H_{phantom}$ that aligns the data volume with the tracked object.

Regarding a real surgical situation, data of an intraoperative CT scan with an optically tracked C-arm device can be registered with the patient and visualized [12].

2.3   Phantom

For primary tests and prospective evaluation, we built a phantom consisting of three vertebrae embedded in a silicone mold. The outer two vertebrae are replaceable. The use of the silicone mold avoids multiple scans for every new experiment. Therefore we created further silicone molds (see figure 2(a)) to reproduce the outer two vertebrae using synthetic two-component resin, which has similar physical properties as real vertebrae. According to the surgeons, material is slightly harder than real bone, which does not affect quality of drilling. Reproduced vertebrae fit precisely into the original silicon mold.

In a real scenario the surgeon only views a small area of vertebrae and therefore is able to roughly estimate the pose of the spinal column. Real pose of the spine can only be estimated. The silicone mold holding the three vertebrae was installed into a wooden box, which was filled with peas to simulate such restricted direct view in spine surgery (figure 2(b)).

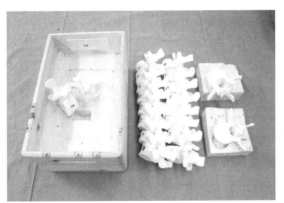 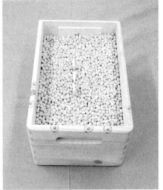

(a) Phantom, silicone mold and reproduced verte-   (b) Restricted view on vertebrae.   brae.

Fig. 2. Phantom for drilling experiments

2.4   Integration of the Virtual Mirror

We suggest dividing the procedure of drilling pedicles into two steps. First a drill canal is planed and defined, second the drilling itself is performed. Virtual components of the AR scene include a polygonal surface model of the vertebrae, a red arrow supporting the interactive planning of the drill canal, the virtual mirror and a blue cylinder representing the tracked drill. Depending on the position of objects, a virtual model of the drilling device is visible in the mirror image. Handling the problem of misleading depth perception is a major issue for AR systems. Virtual objects can only be presented superimposed on real objects. The model of the drilling device is used to create a depth mask with the stencil buffer[1] to provide occlusion, when the drilling device is positioned between the observer and visualization of segmented vertebrae or the virtual mirror.

Planning. The red arrow is initially orientated to the drill direction and positioned at its tip. The surgeon moves the drill to the visible entry point on the vertebrae and orientates the read arrow to the optimal drill canal. To ensure the correct position of the drill canal, the mirror is used to provide side views of the semi-transparent vertebrae. The mirror can be rotated on a circular path around the drill axes (radius=10cm) by rotating the drilling device around its axes. For ease of use the rotation angle of the drilling device is multiplied by an adjustable factor to change the position of the mirror. This enables the surgeon to move the mirror around the target while only rotating the drill by small angle. Thus only slight motion of the drilling device provides all desired side views (see figures 3,4). When the canal is positioned correctly, it can be locked. It will then remain at a fixed position inside the vertebrae during the following steps of the procedure.

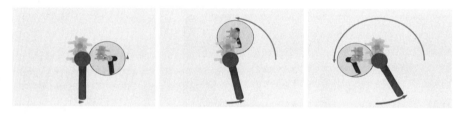

Fig. 3. Descriptive Illustration: Angle of mirror rotation around the drill tip(green/bright arrow) is the multiplied rotation angle of the drilling device around the drill axes (red/dark arrow)

Drilling. Once the canal is defined and locked the mirror automatically moves to a position in front of the drill, orthogonally to the drill direction. Now the surgeon moves the mirror to a desirable position that enables a view on the exit point on the bottom of the vertebrae but also allows for control of depth insertion. The mirror can be positioned automatically. However, we suggest to let the surgeon define its position according to the particular scenario, e.g. pose of the patient, position of equipment, surgeon and surgical staff during the operation and position of the operation site. When the ideal position for the mirror is found, it can be locked and remains respective the vertebrae.

A virtual spot light is attached to the drill tip and orientated to the drill direction. The non-realistic behavior of spot lights in OpenGL here turns into

---

[1] The stencil buffer is an additional buffer besides the color buffer and depth buffer found on modern computer graphics hardware. It can be used to limit the area of rendering.

an advantage. Spot lights are not blocked by surfaces. Even surfaces not visible for the light source are illuminated, if they are located inside the cone of the spot light. Therefore the spot light illuminates the entry point at the pedicle as well as the exit point on the opposite side of the vertebrae, which is visible only through the mirror (see figure 1(b)). Regarding the surgical task, the drill has to be aligned with the defined drill canal at the entry point using visual cues due to the spot light and intersection of drill, vertebrae and drill canal. Thereupon the drill has to be reoriented until the visible spot light is aligned with the exit point on the back of the vertebrae seen through the mirror.

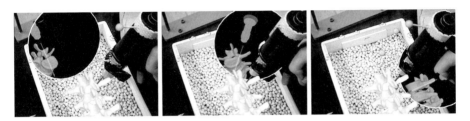

Fig. 4. Mirror is rotated around the operation site to check the position of the drill canal. Box was filled with peas to simulate the restricted view on the operation site.

3   Results

We asked five surgeons to drill preparative canals ($\varnothing_{drill} = 4mm$) for pedicle screw implantation into the two replaceable lumbar vertebrae described in section 2.3. We then compared a classical monitor based navigation system with the present method. Regarding navigated drilling for pedicle screw implantation, three of the surgeons were highly experienced, one had low experience and the last one had no experience. Furthermore all of them had been exposed to our system within the scope of a different evaluation study. In real surgery the surgeons prepare the pedicles to avoid gliding off and injuring anatomy before they start drilling. In this experiment, however the surgeons start drilling directly into bones. Each subject has to consecutively drill four canals using each method. Overall, we analyzed quality of 20 canals for each method and measured time of the procedure. Regarding the duration of drilling one canal, using the classical monitor based method is faster than the proposed method. This time lag is due to the fact that the present method requires a planning phase. This is not intended for the classical navigation system. However when comparing the quality of drill canals our method proves to be more accurate(see table 1).

Scale of accuracy was defined as 1=perfect, 2=acceptable and 3=perforation [13]. According to the surgeons the planning step enables a final check of canal position and allows for collaborative decision making before the vertebra is drilled.

Table 1. Tendency of measured data shows higher accuracy using the virtual mirror/HMD based method

method		mean	std. deviation	std. error mean
accuracy	virtual mirror	1,35	0,75	0,17
	monitor based	1,7	0,86	0,19
time	virtual mirror	173,75 sec	84,13 sec	18,81 sec
	monitor based	168,95 sec	103,59 sec	23,16 sec

4 Discussion

Regarding evaluation of the system, we know that experimenting with five surgeons, each drilling only 8 canals, is not enough for drawing statistically valid conclusions, however because of the limited accessibility of the surgeons such experiments need to be completed in the future. We also plan to test different materials for artificial vertebrae. In the current system the surgeon needs to wear the HMD, however we developed a HMD hanging from the ceiling, which removes the discomfort due to the weight.

5 Conclusion

This paper introduces a new method for navigated spine surgery using an augmented reality system. Medical imaging data is visualized and presented with a stereoscopic video see-through HMD. The virtual part of the AR scene is extended by a virtual mirror to support more intuitive visualization and more accurate navigation. Furthermore five trauma surgeons tested the method with an experimental setup. Analysis of measured data proves the system to be promising both in terms of accuracy and usability.

Acknowledgments

We would like to thank Frank Sauer, Ali Khamene from Siemens Corporate Research (SCR) for placing the HMD system at our disposal. Thanks to A.R.T. GmbH for providing the outside-in tracking system. We also want to thank the radiologists and surgeons of Klinikum Innenstadt München for their precious contribution in obtaining medical data and evaluating our system. Thanks also to Joerg Traub, Marco Feuerstein and Tobias Sielhorst for their support.

References

1. Hart, R.A., Hansen, B.L., Shea, M., Hsu, F., Anderson, G.J.: Pedicle screw placement in the thoracic spine: a comparison of image-guided and manual techniques in cadavers. spine 30, 326–331 (2005)
2. Roy-Camille, R., Saillant, G., Mazel, C.: Internal fixation of the lumbar spine with pedicle screw plating. Clin. Orthop. 203, 7–17 (1986)

3. Birkfellner, W., Figl, M., Huber, K., Watzinger, F., Wanschitz, F., Hummel, J., Hanel, R., Greimel, W., Homolka, P., Ewers, R., Bergmann, H.: A head-mounted operating binocular for augmented reality visualization in medicine - design and initial evaluation. TMI 21(8), 991–997 (2002)
4. King, A., Edwards, P., Maurer Jr., C., de Cunha, D., Gaston, R., Clarkson, M., Hill, D., Hawkes, D., Fenlon, M., Strong, A., Cox, T., Gleeson, M.: Stereo augmented reality in the surgical microscope. PresTVE 9(4), 360–368 (2000)
5. Azar, F.S., Perrin, N., Khamene, A., Vogt, S., Sauer, F.: User performance analysis of different image-based navigation systems for needle placement procedures. Proceedings of SPIE. 5367, 110–121 (2004)
6. Traub, J., Stefan, P., Heining, S.M.M., Tobias Sielhorst, C.R., Euler, E., Navab, N.: Hybrid navigation interface for orthopedic and trauma surgery. In: Larsen, R., Nielsen, M., Sporring, J. (eds.) MICCAI 2006. LNCS, vol. 4190, pp. 373–380. Springer, Heidelberg (2006)
7. Bichlmeier, C., Sielhorst, T., Navab, N.: The tangible virtual mirror: New visualization paradigm for navigated surgery. In: AMIARCS - The Tangible Virtual Mirror: New Visualization Paradigm for Navigated Surgery, Copenhagen, Denmark, MICCAI Society (2006)
8. Navab, N., Feuerstein, M., Bichlmeier, C.: Laparoscopic virtual mirror - new interaction paradigm for monitor based augmented reality. In: Virtual Reality, Charlotte, North Carolina, USA, March 2007, pp. 43–50 (2007)
9. Hoff, W.A., Vincent, T.L.: Analysis of head pose accuracy in augmented reality. IEEE Trans. Visualization and Computer Graphics 6 (2000)
10. Sauer, F., Schoepf, U.J., Khamene, A., Vogt, S., Das, M., Silverman, S.G.: Augmented reality system for ct-guided interventions: System description and initial phantom trials. Medical Imaging: Visualization, Image-Guided Procedures, and Display 5029, 384–394 (2003)
11. Sauer, F., Khamene, A., Bascle, B., Rubino, G.J.: A head-mounted display system for augmented reality image guidance: Towards clinical evaluation for imri-guided neurosurgery. In: MICCAI, London, UK, pp. 707–716. Springer, Heidelberg (2001)
12. Feuerstein, M., Mussack, T., Heining, S.M., Navab, N.: Registration-free laparoscope augmentation for intra-operative liver resection planning. In: SPIE Medical Imaging, San Diego, California, USA, vol. 203, pp. 7–17 (2007)
13. Arand, M., Schempf, M., Hebold, D., Teller, S., Kinzl, L., Gebhard, F.: Precision of navigation-assisted surgery of the thoracic and lumbar spine. Unfallchir. 106, 899–906 (2003)

Improved Statistical TRE Model When Using a Reference Frame

Andrew D. Wiles and Terry M. Peters

Dept. of Medical Biophysics, The University of Western Ontario and
Imaging Research Laboratories, Robarts Research Institute,
London, Ontario, Canada

Abstract. Target registration error (TRE) refers to the uncertainty in localizing a point of interest after a point-based registration is performed. Common in medical image registration, the metric is typically represented as a root-mean-square statistic. In the late 1990s, a statistical model was developed based on the rigid body definition of the fiducial markers and the localization error associated in measuring the fiducials. The statistical model assumed that the fiducial localizer error was isotropic, but recently the model was reworked to handle anisotropic fiducial localizer error (FLE).

In image guided surgery, the statistical model is used to predict the surgical tool tip tracking accuracy associated with optical spatial measurement systems for which anisotropic FLE models are required. However, optical tracking systems often track the surgical tools relative to a patient based reference tool. Here the formulation for modeling the TRE of a surgical probe relative to a reference frame is developed mathematically and evaluated using a Monte Carlo simulation. The effectiveness of the statistical model is directly related to the FLE model, the fiducial marker design and the distance from centroid to target.

1 Introduction

The statistical model for the target registration error (TRE) associated with a point-based registration, assuming an isotropic and uncorrelated fiducial localizer error (FLE) model, was developed by Fitzpatrick et al. [1] in 1998. Based on the registration technique that solves the "orthogonal procrustes" problem using singular value decomposition, this model is a function of (i) the FLE (zero mean and standard deviation σ on each cartesian axis), (ii) the fiducial marker rigid body definition ($\{x_i\}$ for $i = 1 \ldots N$) and (iii) the target location (r) in the rigid body space. The model was later extended to compute the independent variance components along the three orthogonal axes of the rigid body [2], and subsequently used to simulate the performance of optically tracked tools [3].

Recently, we extended this formulation to accept a generalized FLE model [4] that was (i) isotropic or anisotropic and (ii) correlated or uncorrelated. The anisotropic FLE model is particularly important for optical tracking systems where the error is typically three times larger along one axis than the other two orthogonal axes.

N. Ayache, S. Ourselin, A. Maeder (Eds.): MICCAI 2007, Part I, LNCS 4791, pp. 442–449, 2007.
© Springer-Verlag Berlin Heidelberg 2007

Registration algorithms exist that use the anisotropic FLE as a weighting factor in order to obtain a better estimate of the rigid transformation [5,6]. Moreover, algorithms using the extended Kalman filter have been developed to predict the noise parameters associated with a point-based registration [7,8]. However, in both cases the algorithms are iterative in nature and may not be suitable when algorithm speed is critical and estimates of the TRE are required[1]. Therefore, a closed-form estimate of the TRE statistics associated with the closed-form point-based registration method is still relevant.

In [1] and [3], the FLE model was originally defined as a normally distributed random variable with zero mean and root-mean-square (RMS) of $\text{RMS}_{\text{fle}} = 3\sigma^2$, or alternatively $\mathbf{fle} \sim \mathcal{N}_3\left(\mathbf{0}, \sigma^2 \boldsymbol{I}\right)$. In our improved model, the FLE was assumed to be a random variable with zero mean and specified covariance matrix, $\mathbf{fle} \sim \mathcal{N}_3\left(\mathbf{0}, \boldsymbol{\Sigma}\right)$. Using tensor notation, the FLE is defined by the covariance σ_{ij} in principal axes of the rigid body in a given orientation. The TRE mean goes to zero ($\mu_{\text{tre}} = 0$) while the covariance (Σ_{tre}) and root-mean-square (RMS_{tre}) at r are defined as

$$\left(\Sigma_{tre}\left(r\right)\right)_{ij} \approx$$

$$\epsilon^2 \left(\frac{\sigma_{ij}}{N} + \sum_{k \neq i}^{K} \sum_{m \neq j}^{K} \frac{r_k r_m \left(\Lambda_{kk}^2 \delta_{km} \sigma_{ij} - \Lambda_{kk}^2 \delta_{kj} \sigma_{im} - \Lambda_{ii}^2 \delta_{im} \sigma_{kj} + \Lambda_{ii}^2 \delta_{ij} \sigma_{km} \right)}{\left(\Lambda_{kk}^2 + \Lambda_{ii}^2 \right) \left(\Lambda_{mm}^2 + \Lambda_{jj}^2 \right)} \right)$$

$$(1)$$

$$\left\langle \left(\text{RMS}_{\text{tre}}\left(r\right) \right)^2 \right\rangle = \epsilon^2 \left(\sum_{i=1}^{K} \frac{\sigma_{ii}}{N} + \sum_{i=1}^{K} \sum_{j \neq i}^{K} \frac{r_j^2 \left(\Lambda_{jj}^2 \sigma_{ii} + \Lambda_{ii}^2 \sigma_{jj} \right)}{\left(\Lambda_{ii}^2 + \Lambda_{jj}^2 \right)^2} \right.$$

$$\left. + \sum_{i=1}^{K} \sum_{j \neq i}^{K} \sum_{\substack{k \neq i \\ k \neq j}}^{K} \frac{r_j r_k \Lambda_{ii}^2 \sigma_{jk}}{\left(\Lambda_{ii}^2 + \Lambda_{jj}^2 \right) \left(\Lambda_{kk}^2 + \Lambda_{ii}^2 \right)} \right) \quad (2)$$

where $\sigma_{ij}, \Sigma_{\text{tre}}$ are second order tensors in $\mathbb{R}^3$ and Λ_{aa} are the ath singular values of X which consists of the N demeaned fiducial marker positions in principal axes stacked in a $N \times K$ matrix ($K = 3$). ϵ is the smallness parameter used in perturbation theory and δ_{ij} is the Kronecker delta operator.

The new model formulation is limited to a single registration. In this paper, the model is extended to include the case where an optically tracked probe is measured relative to a reference tool. This was previously done by West and Maurer [3] for the TRE RMS statistic with the isotropic FLE model. Here, the TRE statistical model is extended to include the composition of transforms for the mean, covariance and RMS. Section 2 provides the mathematical derivation, while Section 3 provides details on the Monte Carlo simulation used to validate the model. The limitations of this model are discussed in Section 4 and Section 5 provides some concluding remarks.

---

[1] The algorithm speed criteria is highly dependent on the application.

2   Derivation of TRE by Composition of Transformations

West and Maurer [3] showed that the TRE RMS for an optical probe measured relative to a reference tool is the sum in quadrature of the TRE RMS for the tool tip location in probe space and reference space. The mean, covariance and RMS are similarly derived here for for our generalized TRE model presented in [4].

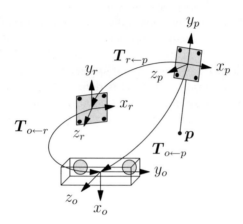

Fig. 1. Typical situation in image-guided surgery where probe p is tracked by the optical tracking system o relative to the reference tool r

Consider the case in Figure 1 where the tool tip of a probe is tracked by an optical tracking system relative to a reference tool. The tool tip is represented in probe, reference and optical tracker coordinate frames as $\boldsymbol{p}_p$, $\boldsymbol{p}_r$ and $\boldsymbol{p}_o$ respectively. In [4], the TRE is defined as the difference between the measured target location found via a point-based registration and the true (exact) target location. The definition is simplified by ignoring the gross transformations and only considering the erroneous portion of the transformation $\boldsymbol{T}_{e,p}$ (comprising rotation $\boldsymbol{R}_{e,p}$ and translation $\boldsymbol{t}_{e,p}$) in probe space[2]. The TRE at position $\boldsymbol{p}$ represented in probe space p and associated with the registration of the fiducial markers in p is given by

$$\mathbf{tre}_p\left(\boldsymbol{p}_p\right) = \boldsymbol{p}_p - \boldsymbol{p}_p^* = \boldsymbol{T}_{e,p}\boldsymbol{p}_p^* - \boldsymbol{p}_p^* = \boldsymbol{R}_{e,p}\boldsymbol{p}_p^* + \boldsymbol{t}_{e,p} - \boldsymbol{p}_p^*, \tag{3}$$

where $\boldsymbol{p}_p^*$ and $\boldsymbol{p}_p$ are the exact and measured tool tip positions respectively.

From [3], it was shown the TRE for a combination of transforms is given by

$$\mathbf{tre}_{\mathrm{comb}}\left(\boldsymbol{p}_r\right) = \boldsymbol{p}_r - \boldsymbol{p}_r^* \tag{4}$$

$$= \boldsymbol{T}_{r\leftarrow o}\boldsymbol{p}_o - \boldsymbol{T}_{r\leftarrow o}^*\left(\boldsymbol{p}_o - \mathbf{tre}_{o\leftarrow p}\left(\boldsymbol{p}_o\right)\right)$$

$$= \mathbf{tre}_r\left(\boldsymbol{p}_r\right) + \boldsymbol{R}_{r\leftarrow p}^*\mathbf{tre}_p\left(\boldsymbol{p}_p\right) \tag{5}$$

---

[2] Probe space is assumed to be in principal axes.

where equation (5) is the sum of reference TRE with the target at the "virtual tool tip" p_r and the probe TRE rotated into reference space. Both TRE values are computed in the principal axes and then transformed into the reference space. Since, the TRE represents a difference vector and not a spatial position, the transformation can be reduced to a rotation only.

In simulation, the exact transformations of the probe and reference tool are known, hence equation (5) can be used. However, if the formulation is used as a feedback mechanism during image-guided surgery then the exact transformations are no longer known but the TRE can be approximated using the measured transforms as shown in (6).

$$\mathbf{tre}_{\text{comb}}\left(\boldsymbol{p}_r\right) \approx \mathbf{tre}_r\left(\boldsymbol{p}_r\right) + \boldsymbol{R}_{r \leftarrow p}\mathbf{tre}_p\left(\boldsymbol{p}_p\right) \tag{6}$$

2.1   TRE Mean in a Reference Coordinate Frame

The mean of the target registration error for a point measured relative to the reference is zero since the expectation of the target registration error vector is zero for each tool.

$$\boldsymbol{\mu}_{\text{tre,comb}}\left(\boldsymbol{p}_r\right) = \left\langle\mathbf{tre}_r\left(\boldsymbol{p}_r\right)\right\rangle + \boldsymbol{R}^*_{r \leftarrow p}\left\langle\mathbf{tre}_p\left(\boldsymbol{p}_p\right)\right\rangle = 0 \tag{7}$$

2.2   TRE Covariance in a Reference Coordinate Frame

The covariance matrix is defined as:

$$\boldsymbol{\Sigma}_{\text{tre,comb}}\left(\boldsymbol{p}_r\right) = \left\langle\left(\mathbf{tre}_{\text{comb}}\left(\boldsymbol{p}_r\right)\right)\left(\mathbf{tre}_{\text{comb}}\left(\boldsymbol{p}_r\right)\right)^T\right\rangle. \tag{8}$$

Substitute (6) into (8) and expand to obtain

$$\boldsymbol{\Sigma}_{\text{tre,comb}}\left(\boldsymbol{p}_r\right) = \left\langle\left(\mathbf{tre}_r\left(\boldsymbol{p}_r\right)\right)\left(\mathbf{tre}_r\left(\boldsymbol{p}_r\right)\right)^T\right\rangle - 2\left\langle\left(\mathbf{tre}_r\left(\boldsymbol{p}_r\right)\right)\boldsymbol{R}^*_{r \leftarrow p}\mathbf{tre}_p\left(\boldsymbol{p}_p\right)^T\right\rangle$$
$$+ \boldsymbol{R}^*_{r \leftarrow p}\left\langle\left(\mathbf{tre}_p\left(\boldsymbol{p}_p\right)\right)\left(\mathbf{tre}_p\left(\boldsymbol{p}_p\right)\right)^T\right\rangle\boldsymbol{R}^{*T}_{r \leftarrow p}. \tag{9}$$

The expectations in the first and third terms reduce to the covariance matrix computed using equation (1)[3] for each respective rigid body registration with the target at $\boldsymbol{p}$. The expectation in the middle term goes to zero since the two TRE random variables are mutually independent resulting in a zero cross-covariance term.

$$\boldsymbol{\Sigma}_{\text{tre,comb}}\left(\boldsymbol{p}_r\right) = \boldsymbol{\Sigma}_{\text{tre},r}\left(\boldsymbol{p}_r\right) + \boldsymbol{R}_{r \leftarrow p}\boldsymbol{\Sigma}_{\text{tre},p}\left(\boldsymbol{p}_p\right)\boldsymbol{R}^T_{r \leftarrow p} \tag{10}$$

---

[3] Vector-matrix notation is used here for simplicity but the tensor notation used in (1) is needed for implementation within any simulation code.

2.3   TRE RMS in a Reference Coordinate Frame

The RMS for the combined TRE is

$$(\text{RMS}_{\text{tre,comb}}\,(\boldsymbol{p}_r))^2 = \left\langle (\textbf{tre}_{\text{comb}}\,(\boldsymbol{p}_r))^T\,(\textbf{tre}_{\text{comb}}\,(\boldsymbol{p}_r)) \right\rangle . \qquad (11)$$

Equation (6) is substituted into (11) where we expand the expression, use the mutual independence of the two TRE vectors to eliminate the middle term and obtain a similar expression as in [3].

$$(\text{RMS}_{\text{tre,comb}}\,(\boldsymbol{p}_r))^2 = (\text{RMS}_{\text{tre},r}\,(\boldsymbol{p}_r))^2 + \left(\text{RMS}_{\text{tre},p}\,(\boldsymbol{p}_p)\right)^2 \qquad (12)$$

Note that the rotation matrix disappears since the RMS is rotationally invariant.

3   Monte Carlo Simulations

Monte Carlo simulations were performed to validate the TRE model using combination of transformations. The simulations use the probe and reference tool designs in West and Maurer [3]. The probe fiducial markers were placed in a rectangular pattern where the height A and width B were set to 71mm and 54mm, respectively. The tool tip is 85mm away from the marker centroid on an axis that passes through the centroid and is parallel to the height dimension. The reference tool is a square geometry with a side length ℓ set to 32mm. Eight different simulations were defined whereby the FLE Model and the distance between the reference and tool tip were varied as shown in Table 1.

The isotropic and anisotropic FLE models were defined to have the same RMS statistic ($\text{RMS}_{\text{fle}} = 1/3$mm) but the standard deviation along the z axis was three times larger than the x and y axes in the anisotropic FLE model. The tool tip position was fixed at a specified location in the volume and the probe orientation was randomly selected under the restriction that the orientation was relevant in terms of an optical tracking situation. Similarly, the reference tool position and orientation were randomly selected so that the reference tool was at a distance d from the tool tip. After analyzing the results from the initial eight test cases, another four were simulated with the size of the reference tool increased from 32mm to 64mm.

In each case, $M = 1000$ random tool orientations were tested. For each random tool orientation, $N = 100,000$ sample measurements were simulated to obtain the TRE statistics. The predicted statistics were computed for each of the M random tool orientations using equations (7), (10) and (12) respectively.

Two forms of analysis were performed on the resulting data. First, hypothesis tests were used to determine whether the predicted mean and covariance matched the simulated statistics ($\alpha = 0.05$). The hypothesis tests were performed using the likelihood ratio function and the Wishart distribution (see [9,4]). Then the percent differences[4] between the predicted and simulated RMS results were examined. The summary of results are presented in Table 1.

---

[4] $\%\text{diff} = 100\,(\text{RMS}_{theory} - \text{RMS}_{sim})\,/\text{RMS}_{sim}$

Table 1. Monte Carlo simulation results for 12 cases where the FLE model, reference body size and the distance to the rigid body are varied. The hypothesis tests use the likelihood ratio and Wishart distribution [9]. Null Hypothesis for Test #1 is $H_0 : \Sigma_{sim} = \Sigma_{\text{tre}}$ and Test #2 is $H_0 : \mu = 0, \Sigma_{sim} = \Sigma_{\text{tre}}$.

Case	FLE Model	Ref. Size ℓ	Working Distance d	Hypothesis Test Percent Accepted #1	#2	RMS Percent Diff. Summary Statistics Mean	S.D.	Min	Max
1	Isotropic	32mm	100mm	94.8%	98.2%	-0.01%	0.15%	-0.47%	0.46%
2	Isotropic	32mm	200mm	94.6%	86.0%	0.00%	0.17%	-0.52%	0.60%
3	Isotropic	32mm	300mm	89.0%	39.2%	0.00%	0.17%	-0.52%	0.56%
4	Isotropic	32mm	400mm	79.2%	4.20%	0.00%	0.16%	-0.50%	0.54%
5	Anisotropic	32mm	100mm	95.3%	99.7%	0.00%	0.19%	-0.52%	0.62%
6	Anisotropic	32mm	200mm	71.4%	25.2%	-0.01%	0.20%	-0.56%	0.67%
7	Anisotropic	32mm	300mm	37.4%	3.8%	0.00%	0.19%	-0.82%	0.83%
8	Anisotropic	32mm	400mm	16.0%	0.0%	0.01%	0.20%	-0.75%	0.61%
9	Anisotropic	64mm	100mm	94.4%	98.3%	0.00%	0.19%	-0.61%	0.64%
10	Anisotropic	64mm	200mm	95.9%	98.9%	0.00%	0.19%	-0.71%	0.65%
11	Anisotropic	64mm	300mm	93.8%	91.4%	0.01%	0.19%	-0.61%	0.62%
12	Anisotropic	64mm	400mm	93.5%	80.7%	0.00%	0.20%	-0.76%	0.67%

4 Discussion

The results show two key findings. First, the acceptance of the hypothesis tests are significantly reduced as the distance d between the tool tip and the reference tool is increased. The hypothesis testing was expanded to include similar tests for the probe and reference tools separately. It was found that the probe maintained a high rate of acceptance of the null hypothesis (typically larger than 90%), but the reference tool exhibited a lower acceptance of the null hypothesis as the distance to the target increased. The predicted RMS percent differences agreed very well with the simulated results, but the percent differences may be misleading because the RMS results at $d = 400$mm (e.g., Case 8 RMS is 2.5mm to 4.4mm) will be significantly larger than the results at 100mm (e.g., Case 5 RMS is 0.7mm to 1.2mm). Hence a 1% difference in Case 8 is larger than a similar percentage in Case 5. Therefore, although the hypothesis tests and RMS look very different they may be exhibiting similar trends with varying degrees of sensitivity.

The second key finding was that if the rigid body size for the reference tool, i.e., ℓ increased to 64mm, the hypothesis tests accepted the null hypothesis at rates greater than 80% for all distances. By increasing the rigid body size, the moment of inertia of the rigid body is strengthened such that the rotational error is decreased given the same FLE model.

For both findings, it is suspected that the relationship between the target distance, rigid body size and the null hypothesis acceptance rate may be due to the rotational error in the registration. Recall from [1, 4] that a power series expansion was used to derive the TRE statistical model: $R = I + \epsilon R^{(1)} +$

$O\left(\epsilon^{2}\right)$. $\boldsymbol{R}^{(1)}$ is the erroneous portion of the transformation for the TRE, which is equivalent to $\boldsymbol{R}_{e,p}$ from equation (3). If we examine equations (1) and (2), it is clear that the TRE is normally distributed and formed by rotating, scaling and summing the contributions of the normally distributed FLE statistics. But if the error from (3) is separated into rotational and translational components, then we see that the portion of the error distribution attributed to the rotational error will lie on the surface of a sphere with a radius ρ equal to the distance from the target to the marker centroid. This distribution, suspected to be approximated by the von Mises-Fisher (spherical) distribution [10], is not normal. But if the rotational error is small then the von Mises distribution is approximated by a 2D projected normal distribution. The TRE becomes a 3D error distribution when the translational error component is taken into account. Consider a case restricted to 2D cartesian space, if the span (or 95% confidence interval) of the rotational error can be described by the angle θ that subtends from the mean to the error extents, then the path where the measured target may lie is related to the arc length $s = 2\rho\theta$. However, the span for the projected normal distribution is a chord for the arc s given by $w = 2\rho\sin\theta$. (This can be extended to 3D cartesian space by using a surface area subtended by a solid angle.) The ratio of the two spans becomes $b = \sin\theta/\theta$ which suggests that the rotational error given by the TRE model is underestimated by the factor b. Since θ is typically small, the underestimation is negligible for small ρ. For example, if $\theta = 2°$ then $b = 0.9998$ and the difference between s and w at $\rho = 100$mm is approximately 0.0014mm. As ρ increases, the underestimation becomes significant in terms of the Wishart based hypothesis tests but when used practically the difference between the simulated and predicted 95% confidence regions are not very different. In the future, an expression that defines the point at which the model significantly underestimates the true distribution would be useful.

In image registration applications, this is not a significant issue as the target is usually close to the centroid since it is typically contained within the convex hull formed by the fiducial markers. However, in image-guided surgery applications, such as those that track C-arms and fluoroscopes, it is common to track rigid bodies with targets that exist outside of the fiducial marker geometry at large distances such as 400mm and greater. Therefore, it is possible that when maintaining the same FLE and rigid body geometry while increasing the target distance, as done in this paper, the TRE model will underestimate the actual TRE error. However, as shown in the RMS percent differences, and by the example given, this underestimation is very small and hence the model is a very good approximation.

5   Conclusions

Overall, the proposed model performs well. However, this is only true for situations when the reference tool has an appropriate combination of rotational error and closeness to the target since the TRE model underestimates the TRE span as a function of target distance. This issue is not as significant in image registration applications where the target is often contained within the convex hull formed by the fiducial markers, but becomes significant when this formulation is used in the simulation of optically tracked tools for image-guided surgery.

Acknowledgements

This work was supported by CIHR, NSERC, ORDCF, CFI, UWO and NDI.

References

1. Fitzpatrick, J.M., West, J.B., Maurer Jr., C.R.: Predicting error in rigid-body point-based registration. IEEE Trans. Med. Imag. 17(5), 694–702 (1998)
2. Fitzpatrick, J.M., West, J.B.: The distribution of target registration error in rigid-body point-based registration. IEEE Trans. Med. Imag. 20(9), 917–927 (2001)
3. West, J.B., Maurer Jr., C.R.: Designing optically tracked instruments for image-guided surgery. IEEE Trans. Med. Imag. 23(5), 533–545 (2004)
4. Wiles, A.D., Likholyot, A., Frantz, D.D., Peters, T.M.: Derivation of TRE using anisotropic FLE. Technical Report NDI-TR-0421, Northern Digital, Inc. Waterloo, Ontario, Canada, Contact: support@ndigital.com (2007)
5. Chu, M.T., Trendafilov, N.T.: On a differential equation approach to the weighted orthogonal Procrustes problem. Statistics and Computing 8, 125–133 (1998)
6. Batchelor, P.G., Fitzpatrick, J.M.: A study of the anisotropically weighted Procrustes problem. In: Proceedings of IEEE Workshop on Mathematical Methods in Biomedical Image Analysis, Hilton Head, SC, USA, June 2000, pp. 212–218. IEEE Computer Society Press, Los Alamitos (2000)
7. Pennec, X., Thirion, J.-P.: A framework for uncertainty and validation of 3-d registration methods based on points and frames. International Journal of Computer Vision 25(3), 203–229 (1997)
8. Nicolau, S., Pennec, X., Soler, L., Ayache, N.: An accuracy certified augmented reality system for therapy guidance. In: Pajdla, T., Matas, J(G.) (eds.) ECCV 2004. LNCS, vol. 3023, pp. 79–91. Springer, Heidelberg (2004)
9. Anderson, T.W.: An Introduction to Multivariate Statistical Analysis. John Wiley & Sons, Toronto, Ontario (1984)
10. Mardia, K.V., Jupp, P.E.: Directional Statistics. John Wiley & Sons, Toronto (2000)

3D/2D Image Registration: The Impact of X-Ray Views and Their Number

Dejan Tomaževič, Boštjan Likar, and Franjo Pernuš

University of Ljubljana, Faculty of Electrical Engineering
Tržaška 25, 1000 Ljubljana, Slovenia
Tel.: +386 1 4768 248, Fax: +386 1 4768 279
{dejan.tomazevic,bostjan.likar,
franjo.pernus}@fe.uni-lj.si

Abstract. An important part of image-guided radiation therapy or surgery is registration of a three-dimensional (3D) preoperative image to two-dimensional (2D) images of the patient. It is expected that the accuracy and robustness of a 3D/2D image registration method do not depend solely on the registration method itself but also on the number and projections (views) of intraoperative images. In this study, we systematically investigate these factors by using registered image data, comprising of CT and X-ray images of a cadaveric lumbar spine phantom and the recently proposed 3D/2D registration method [1], [2]. The results indicate that the proportion of successful registrations (robustness) significantly increases when more X-ray images are used for registration.

Keywords: 3D/2D image registration, computed tomography, image-guided surgery, X-ray images.

1 Introduction

In radiation therapy and surgery, there is a constant demand to render the therapeutic procedures less and less invasive and to improve the accuracy with which a given procedure can be performed compared to conventional methods. Image guidance is the emerging technology that has the potential to decrease the invasiveness and increase the accuracy of procedures [3].The crucial part of image-guided systems that enable intra-therapy patient setup or provide intraoperative navigation guidance is registration of a patient in the treatment room to preoperative patient images or to models obtained from these images. A variety of rigid registration techniques have been proposed in the past that may be classified according to the data they use to compute the registration transformation [2], [4]. Geometry-based methods use points [5] or surfaces [6], [7], while intensity-based methods use contours of anatomical structures obtained by preoperative image segmentation [8] or image voxel intensity or gradient information [2], [4], [9]. Most of these techniques implement rigid registration of a 3D image to 2D images, while another set of methods exists, where a 3D anatomy model is non-rigidly registered to intraoperative 2D X-ray images [10,

N. Ayache, S. Ourselin, A. Maeder (Eds.): MICCAI 2007, Part I, LNCS 4791, pp. 450–457, 2007.
© Springer-Verlag Berlin Heidelberg 2007

11]. The methods that register preoperative 3D images/models to one or more intraoperative 2D images are commonly referred to as 3D/2D or 2D/3D registration methods. The accuracy and robustness of a 3D/2D registration method based on intraoperative X-ray images don't depend solely on the registration method but also on the specific anatomy, projections (views) and the number of X-ray images used for registration. To the best of our knowledge, we are not aware of any systematic study that would report on the impact of X-ray views and their number on the performance of a 3D/2D registration method. In the present study, we have therefore used image data, comprising of a CT and 18 X-ray images of a cadaveric lumbar spine phantom [1] and the validation protocol and validation metrics [2] to study the impact of the number of intraoperative X-ray images and selected projections (views) on the capture range and registration accuracy and robustness of our recently proposed 3D/2D registration method [2].

2 3D/2D Registration Method

Features that we use for rigid 3D/2D registration are normals $\mathbf{v}_A$ to surfaces of bony structures found in preoperative CT volumes and back-projected intensity gradients $\mathbf{v}_B$ of intraoperative X-ray images (Fig. 1) [2]. Let $\mathbf{r}_i^{S_v}$, a point on the surface of a 3D structure, be defined in the coordinate system S_v of a CT volume (Fig. 1). The position $\mathbf{r}_i$ of the same point in reference (patient) coordinate system S_{ref} is given by rigid transformation $\mathbf{T}$ defined by six parameters $\mathbf{q}=(t_x, t_y, t_z, \omega_x, \omega_y, \omega_z)^T$

$$\mathbf{r}_i^{S_{ref}} = \mathbf{r}_i = \mathbf{T}(\mathbf{r}_i^{S_v}) = \mathbf{R}\mathbf{r}_i^{S_v} + \mathbf{t} \tag{1}$$

where $\mathbf{R}$ and $\mathbf{t}$ describe, respectively, the rotation and translation of coordinate system S_v with respect to S_{ref}. Let $\mathbf{r}_s$ be the position of the X-ray source in the reference coordinate system S_{ref}. For a given position of a 3D image, defined by vector $\mathbf{q}$, the line which connects $\mathbf{r}_s$ and $\mathbf{r}_i$ and has direction defined by unit vector $\mathbf{e}_i$, intersects the X-ray image plane U at point $\mathbf{p}_i=\mathbf{p}(\mathbf{r}_i)$ (Fig. 1).

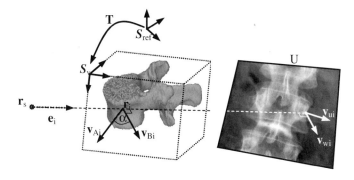

Fig. 1. 3D/2D registration geometrical setup

Rigid registration of a 3D preoperative image to M intraoperative 2D images is concerned with finding the set of parameters $\mathbf{q}$ that optimizes the criterion function CF

$$CF = \sum_{j=1}^{M} \frac{\sum_{i=1}^{N}\left|\mathbf{v}_{Ai}^{j}\right| \cdot \left|\mathbf{v}_{Bi}^{j}\right| \cdot f(\alpha)}{\sum_{i=1}^{N}\left|\mathbf{v}_{Ai}^{j}\right| \cdot \sum_{i=1}^{N}\left|\mathbf{v}_{Bi}^{j}\right|} \qquad (2)$$

where N is the number of surface points $\mathbf{r}_{i}^{Sv}$, $\mathbf{v}_{Ai}$ is the vector normal to the surface at point $\mathbf{r}_{i}^{Sv}$, $\mathbf{v}_{Bi}$ is the X-ray image gradient $\mathbf{v}_{Ui}$ back-projected to the $\mathbf{r}_{i}^{Sv}$, and $f(\alpha)$ is the weighting function depending on angle α between $\mathbf{v}_{Ai}$ and $\mathbf{v}_{Bi}$. The gradient $\mathbf{v}_{Bi}$ is obtained by back-projecting the gradient $\mathbf{v}_{Ui}(\mathbf{p}_{i})$, $\mathbf{v}_{Ui}(\mathbf{p}_{i})=\text{grad}_{U}I(\mathbf{p}_{i})$, of X-ray image intensity $I(\mathbf{p}_{i})$

$$\mathbf{v}_{Bi}(\mathbf{r}_{i}) = \frac{\left|\mathbf{p}_{i} - \mathbf{r}_{s}\right|}{\left|\mathbf{r}_{i} - \mathbf{r}_{s}\right|} \cdot \mathbf{v}_{w}(\mathbf{p}) = \frac{\left|\mathbf{p}_{i} - \mathbf{r}_{s}\right|}{\left|\mathbf{r}_{i} - \mathbf{r}_{s}\right|} \cdot \frac{\left(\mathbf{n} \times \mathbf{v}_{Ui}(\mathbf{p}_{i})\right) \times \mathbf{e}_{i}}{\mathbf{n} \cdot \mathbf{e}_{i}} \qquad (3)$$

where $|\mathbf{r}_{i}\text{-}\mathbf{r}_{s}|$ and $|\mathbf{p}_{i}\text{-}\mathbf{r}_{s}|$ are the distances from X-ray source $\mathbf{r}_{s}$ to points $\mathbf{r}_{i}$ and $\mathbf{p}_{i}$, respectively, $\mathbf{v}_{w}(\mathbf{p}_{i})$, $\mathbf{v}_{w}(\mathbf{p}_{i})=\text{grad}_{w}I(\mathbf{p}_{i})$, is the intensity gradient in the plane perpendicular to projection beam defined by $\mathbf{e}_{i}$, and $\mathbf{n}$ is the unit normal to projection plane U.

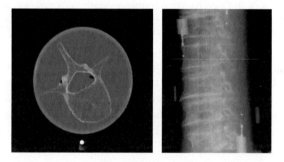

Fig. 2. Axial slice from a CT (*left*) and one of the 18 acquired X-ray images (*right*) of the spine phantom

3   Images and "Gold Standard" Registrations

Images used in the experiment were part of our 3D/2D registration "gold standard" lumbar spine phantom data set, which has been made publicly available [1]. A lumbar spine phantom had been constructed by placing a cadaveric lumbar spine, comprising vertebra L1-L5 with intervertebral disks and several millimeters of soft tissue, into a plastic tube filled with water. Six fiducial markers were rigidly attached to the surface of the tube. The CT image was obtained using a General Electric HiSpeed CT/i scanner. Axial slices were taken with intra-slice resolution of 0.27 x 0.27 mm and 1 mm inter-slice distance. X-ray images were obtained by PIXIUM 4600 (Trixell) digital X-ray detector with a 429 x 429 mm large active surface, 0.143 x 0.143 mm pixel size, and 14 bits of dynamic range. The X-ray source and detector-plane were fixed during image acquisition while the spine phantom was rotated on a turntable to simulate a setup with C-arm. By rotating (step=20°) the spine phantom around its long axis, 18 X-ray images were acquired. "Gold standard" registrations of CT to X-ray images were obtained by rigid registration of CT marker points to 3D marker points reconstructed from X-ray images, respectively. As such, the obtained "gold standard" registration defines the relative position of each of the X-ray images to CT volume and, consequently, relative positions between X-ray images. After registration, cubic sub-images of single vertebrae without markers, were defined manually in CT images. Each sub-volume was blurred using a Gaussian filter ($\sigma = 0.5$ mm) and isotropically re-sampled to the resolution of 1 mm. The Canny edge detector and a threshold were applied to automatically extract locations of points on surfaces of bony structures and to estimate surface normal directions at these points. The X-ray images were blurred with a Gaussian filter ($\sigma = 0.5$ mm) and the Roberts edge detector was applied to calculate intensity gradients $\text{grad}_U I(\mathbf{p})$.

4   Experiments

To test the impact of X-ray views and their number on the accuracy and robustness of the 3D/2D registration method, registrations were performed from a wide range of starting positions and orientations around the "gold standard" registration position using different projections and different numbers of X-ray images. Before registrations, the 6-dimensional parametrical space was normalized, so that a rotation of the volume containing a single vertebra of size 80 mm around its center for 0.1 radians (5.7°) was equivalent to mean translation of volume points for 2 mm. In this way, Euclidean metrics could be used to calculate the displacement (in parametrical space) of a starting position from the "gold standard" position [2]. Values of parameters defining a starting point were chosen randomly within 18mm (51.6°) around the "gold standard" position. Optimization of transformation parameters $\mathbf{q}=(t_x, t_y, t_z, \omega_x, \omega_y, \omega_z)^T$ was performed by Powel's method. To measure the registration error before and after registration, target registration error (TRE) [12] was calculated for eight target points (four on each pedicle) as the distance between target points in registered and "gold standard" position. Sixteen X-ray image sets, each containing 18 image subsets were formed (Table 1). The first set contained the 18 single images. Subsets in the next eight sets were comprised of image pairs taken at views, which differed by 20°, 40°,..., 160°, respectively. Subsets in the next four sets contained three images. The angles between the three images in a subset were 20°, 40°, 60°, or 80°. In the next two subsets of set 4 there were four images, the angles between them were 20° and 40°. In the 18 subsets of the last set there were eight images taken at views 20° apart. The 5 CT sub-volumes, each containing one of the vertebra L1-L5, were registered from 50 initial positions to each of the 18 subsets of X-ray images from all 16 image sets, which yielded 4500 (5x50x18) registrations for each set.

Table 1. The number and angle between two consecutive views in 16 sets of X-ray images registered to CT images

			X-ray images			
Set			**Subsets**			
No.	M	Δ	1	2	...	18
1	1		(0°)	(20°)	...	(340°)
2	2	20°	(0°,20°)	(20°,40°)	...	(340°,0°)
3		40°	(0°,40°)	(20°,60°)	...	(340°,20°)
4		60°	(0°,60°)	(20°,80°)	...	(340°,40°)
5		80°	(0°,80°)	(20°,100°)	...	(340°,60°)
6		100°	(0°,100°)	(20°,120°)	...	(340°,80°)
7		120°	(0°,120°)	(20°,140°)	...	(340°,100°)
8		140°	(0°,140°)	(20°,160°)	...	(340°,120°)
9		160°	(0°,160°)	(20°,180°)	...	(340°,140°)
10	3	20°	(0°,20°,40°)	(20°,40°,60°)	...	(340°,0°,20°)
11		40°	(0°,40°,80°)	(20°,60°,100°)	...	(340°,20°,60°)
12		60°	(0°,60°,120°)	(20°,80°,140°)	...	(340°,40°,100°)
13		80°	(0°,80°,160°)	(20°,100°,180°)	...	(340°,60°,140°)
14	4	20°	(0°,20°,40°,60°)	(20°,40°,60°,80°)	...	(340°,0°,20°,40°)
15		40°	(0°,40°,80°,120°)	(20°,60°,100°,140°)	...	(340°,20°,60°,100°)
16	8	20°	(0°,20°,...,140°)	(20°,40°,...,160°)	...	(340°,0°,...,120°)

M - number of images in a subset, Δ - angle between consecutive images in a subset .

5   Results

Table 2 shows means and standard deviations of TREs before and after successful (TRE of all 8 targets smaller than 2mm) registration and the proportion of successful registrations for three intervals of displacements. The results show that the registration errors fell with the higher number of images utilized for registration. The mean TRE achieved with one image was 0.9 mm, with 2 images between 0.32 and 0.41, and with 8 images 0.3 mm. The accuracy of registrations did not significantly depend on the projections. For instance, when registering image pairs to CT images, the best results were achieved with X-ray images being 80 or 100 degrees apart. However, the values for 80 and 100 degrees (0.32 mm) were not significantly smaller than the values for other angles between image pairs. The percentage of successful registrations increased with the higher number of images used for registration. It increased from 96% for two images to 99.5% for eight images if the initial displacements were between 0 and 6 mm. For the initial displacements between 6 and 12 mm the increase was much more dramatic. The proportion of successful registrations increased from 30% (one image), to 59% (two images), to 66% (three images), to 79% (four images) and, finally, to 80% for eight images. The same trend could be observed for displacements between 12 and 18 mm although, even with eight images the proportion of successful registrations was smaller than 40%.

Table 2. Registration errors and proportion of successful registrations for CT to X-ray registration using different X-ray projections and number of projections

Sets			Before registration	After registration	Successful registrations (%)		
No.	M	Δ	TRE [mm] Mean (Std)	TRE [mm] Mean (Std)	0÷6mm 0÷17.2°	6÷12mm 17.2÷34.4°	12÷18mm 34.4÷51.7°
1	1		3.3 (2.9)	0.90 (0.49)	61.8%	30.6%	13.5%
2	2	20°	5.2 (3.7)	0.41 (0.18)	96.4%	56.4%	13.7%
3		40°	5.1 (3.6)	0.34 (0.13)	95.6%	55.4%	13.1%
4		60°	5.0 (3.5)	0.33 (0.11)	95.2%	52.7%	11.3%
5		80°	4.9 (3.5)	0.32 (0.11)	94.7%	52.0%	10.5%
6		100°	4.9 (3.5)	0.32 (0.12)	94.2%	48.3%	11.2%
7		120°	5.0 (3.6)	0.34 (0.11)	93.8%	52.1%	12.3%
8		140°	5.1 (3.6)	0.34 (0.12)	95.8%	55.0%	13.6%
9		160°	5.3 (3.7)	0.40 (0.17)	95.3%	59.0%	15.1%
10	3	20°	5.5 (3.8)	0.34 (0.13)	98.4%	63.6%	18.6%
11		40°	5.4 (3.7)	0.31 (0.11)	98.6%	64.5%	16.4%
12		60°	5.5 (3.8)	0.31 (0.11)	97.9%	66.0%	19.4%
13		80°	5.4 (3.7)	0.31 (0.12)	97.7%	64.4%	18.2%
14	4	20°	5.8 (3.9)	0.32 (0.11)	98.9%	69.0%	23.8%
15		40°	5.7 (3.9)	0.30 (0.11)	99.2%	70.3%	23.1%
16	8	20°	6.3 (4.1)	0.30 (0.11)	99.5%	80.4%	36.7%

M - number of images in a subset, Δ - angle between consecutive images in a subset.

6 Discussion

The accuracy and robustness of registering a 3D preoperative image with 2D intraoperative images depends on the registration method and the anatomical structures that are to be registered. However, it is expected that the quality of 3D/2D registration also depends on the number of 2D intraoperative images and the projections under which these images are acquired. In the past, researchers have used one, two or more intra-operative images but have not systematically studied the impact of X-ray views and their number on the performance of an intensity-based 3D/2D registration method [13], [14]. To confirm the expectations that better registrations results can be achieved with more intraoperative images and with images taken at certain projections, we have conducted a study using the recently proposed 3D/2D intensity-based registration method and images and "gold standard" registration data.

As expected, the accuracy of successful CT/X-ray registrations for different initial displacements increased when more X-ray images had been used. Using two instead of one X-ray image, more than doubles registration accuracy, i.e. from 0.9 mm to 0.4 mm, which is more than enough for orthopedic procedures. The impact of the number of images used in registration accuracy could be explained with a fact that, when using a single X-ray image, the registration is well-defined for two in-plane translations and two in-plane rotations and ill-posed for one out-of-plane translation and one out-of-plane rotation [9, 13]. By adding an additional X-ray image, with significantly different angle of view, one out-of-plane translation becomes in-plane and thereby well-defined. Our experimental results on vertebra data suggested that a significantly different angle of view between two images would be 20 degrees, where sufficient accuracy of 0.41 mm was achieved, while the best accuracy of 0.32 mm was obtained for almost perpendicular views (80 and 100 degrees). The minimal angle between views can be useful information for those clinical applications that cannot afford time and space for acquiring X-rays with perpendicular views. Regardless of the angle of view, one out-of-plane rotation still remains, even if more than two X-ray views are employed in a single plane, which is the case when using C-arm with single rotation axis. However, even out-of-plane, the rotation could be well-defined, if the object of registration is not symmetric around one of its axis. This can explain our registration results, where adding additional X-ray images into the registration procedure has a small and clinically irrelevant impact on registration accuracy, since single vertebra body does not have symmetrical rotational axis. However, for other anatomy, for example for the shaft of the femur, which is close but not perfectly symmetric around one of the rotational axes, two X-ray images may not be sufficient to obtain the desired registration accuracy.

Similarly to registration accuracy, the percentage of successful registrations also increases where more X-ray images are used. The largest improvement is observed when deploying two, instead of one X-ray image, which can again be explained with ill-posed out-of-plane transformations. However, the percentage of successful registrations of 96% for initial displacement 0-6 mm (0÷17.2 degrees), when using two X-ray views, would probably be a border line for most spine clinical applications. Our results suggested that the percentage of registration increases significantly when more than two X-ray views were used. Adding more X-ray images into registration process increases the statistical power of criterion function calculation. Moreover, the information from additional images can also reduce the effect of outliers, e.g. occlusions, which can be present on one of X-ray images but not on the other images, while outliers can impose additional local optima into criterion function. Both, the increase of statistical power and the decreased effect of outliers, result in a smoother criterion function, which reduces the probability of optimization algorithm to converge to some local optimum.

This study justified the assumption that more X-ray image views improve registration accuracy and reliability. For the given imaged anatomy, e.g. for single vertebra object, and the given intensity based registration method [2], at least two X-ray images should be employed in the registration process to achieve desire registration accuracy, while for desired registration reliability, more X-ray images should be used. On the other hand, increasing the number of X-ray images to increase the reliability of registration result in increases radiation and acquisition times. Some care has to be taken when generalizing our registration results to clinical applications. Even though a real cadaver anatomy was used in our experiments, our gold standard images lack the presence of soft tissue and ribs that can occlude vertebra on X-ray images and can consequently harm the registration. Moreover, the calibration of our X-ray imaging system is almost ideal in comparison with the calibration of standard C-arm used in clinical procedures. By van Kraats et al. [13], it was reported that C-arm calibration errors have linear impact on registration errors. As a result, lower accuracy and reliability can be expected in real clinical use. However, we believe that our study provides general trends on how the number and the relative angle between X-ray image views affect the 3D/2D registration and gives some useful guidelines for further studies.

Acknowledgments. This work was supported by the Ministry of Higher Education, Science and Technology, Republic of Slovenia under Grant P2-0232.

References

1. Tomaževič, D., Likar, B., Pernuš, F.: Gold standard data for evaluation and comparison of 3D/2D registration methods. Comput. Aided Surg. 9, 137–144 (2004)
2. Tomaževič, D., Likar, B., Slivnik, T., Pernuš, F.: 3-D/2-D registration of CT and MR to X-ray images. IEEE Trans. Med. Imaging 22, 1407–1416 (2003)
3. Galloway, R.L.: The process and development of image-guided procedures. Annu. Rev. Biomed. Eng. 3, 83–108 (2001)
4. Livyatan, H., Yaniv, Z., Joskowicz, L.: Gradient-based 2-D/3-D rigid registration of fluoroscopic X-ray to CT. IEEE Trans. Med. Imaging 22, 1395–1406 (2003)
5. Maurer, C.R., Fitzpatrick Jr., J.M., Wang, M.Y., Galloway, R.L., Jr., M.R.J., Allen, G.S.: Registration of head volume images using implantable fiducial markers. IEEE Trans. Med. Imaging 16, 447–462 (1997)
6. Colchester, A.C.F., Zhao, J., Holton-Tainter, K.S., Henri, C.J., Maitland, N., Roberts, P.T.H., Harris, C.G., Evans, R.J.: Development and preliminary evaluation of VISLAN, a surgical planning and guidance system using intra-operative video imaging. Medical Image Analysis 1, 73–90 (1996)
7. Grimson, W.E.L., Ettinger, G.J., White, S.J., Lozano-Perez, T., Wells III, W.M., Kikinis, R.: Automatic registration method for frameless stereotaxy, image guided surgery, and enhanced reality visualization. IEEE Transactions on Medical Imaging 15, 129–140 (1996)
8. Gueziec, A., Kazanzides, P., Williamson, B., Taylor, R.H.: Anatomy-based registration of CT-scan and intraoperative X-ray images for guiding a surgical robot. IEEE Trans Med Imaging 17, 715–728 (1998)
9. Weese, J., Penney, G.P., Desmedt, P., Buzug, T.M., Hill, D.L., Hawkes, D.J.: Voxel-based 2-D/3-D registration of fluoroscopy images and CT scans for image-guided surgery. IEEE Trans. Inf. Technol. Biomed. 1, 284–293 (1997)
10. Zheng, G.Y., Ballester, M.A.G., Styner, M., Nolte, L.P.: Reconstruction of patient-specific 3D bone surface from 2D calibrated fluoroscopic images and point distribution model. In: Larsen, R., Nielsen, M., Sporring, J. (eds.) MICCAI 2006. LNCS, vol. 4190, pp. 25–32. Springer, Heidelberg (2006)
11. Fleute, M., Lavallee, S.: Nonrigid 3-D/2-D registration of images using statistical models. In: Taylor, C., Colchester, A. (eds.) MICCAI 1999. LNCS, vol. 1679, pp. 138–147. Springer, Heidelberg (1999)
12. Fitzpatrick, J.M., West, J.B., Maurer Jr., C.R.: Predicting error in rigid-body point-based registration. IEEE Trans. Med. Imaging 17, 694–702 (1998)
13. van de Kraats, E.B., Penney, G.P., Tomaževič, D., van Walsum, T., Niessen, W.J.: Standardized evaluation methodology for 2-D-3-D registration. IEEE Trans. Med. Imaging 24, 1177–1189 (2005)
14. McLaughlin, R.A., Hipwell, J., Hawkes, D.J., Noble, J.A., Byrne, J.V., Cox, T.C.: A comparison of a similarity-based and a feature-based 2-D-3-D registration method for neurointerventional use. IEEE Transactions on Medical Imaging 24, 1058–1066 (2005)

Magneto-Optic Tracking of a Flexible Laparoscopic Ultrasound Transducer for Laparoscope Augmentation

Marco Feuerstein[1], Tobias Reichl[1], Jakob Vogel[1], Armin Schneider[2], Hubertus Feussner[2], and Nassir Navab[1]

[1] Computer-Aided Medical Procedures (CAMP), TUM, Munich, Germany
[2] Department of Surgery, Klinikum rechts der Isar, TUM, Munich, Germany

Abstract. In abdominal surgery, a laparoscopic ultrasound transducer is commonly used to detect lesions such as metastases. The determination and visualization of position and orientation of its flexible tip in relation to the patient or other surgical instruments can be of much help to (novice) surgeons utilizing the transducer intraoperatively. This difficult subject has recently been paid attention to by the scientific community [1,2,3,4,5,6]. Electromagnetic tracking systems can be applied to track the flexible tip. However, the magnetic field can be distorted by ferromagnetic material. This paper presents a new method based on optical tracking of the laparoscope and magneto-optic tracking of the transducer, which is able to automatically detect field distortions. This is used for a smooth augmentation of the B-scan images of the transducer directly on the camera images in real time.

1 Introduction

Laparoscopic ultrasonography (LUS) nowadays plays an increasing role in abdominal surgery. Its main application areas include liver, biliary tract, and pancreas. Unfortunately LUS is often difficult to perform, especially for novice surgeons. Therefore, several groups tried to support surgeons by providing navigated LUS: The position and orientation ("pose") of the ultrasound transducer is estimated, so its body and B-scan images can be visualized in relation to the patient, other surgical instruments, or preoperative and intraoperative imaging data. This may greatly support surgeons utilizing LUS in cancer staging, radio frequency ablation, and other procedures.

To estimate the pose of a transducer with a rigid tip, a robot or optical tracking (OT) may be used [2]. In the latter case, a rigid body can be attached to the transducer handle to assure its continuous visibility. Several groups also try to localize rigid laparoscopic instruments in laparoscopic images by advanced image processing techniques, such as Voros et al. [7]. However, laparoscopic transducers most commonly used and preferred by surgeons feature a flexible tip providing rightward, leftward, forward, and backward steering. The tip also yields to external pressure from organ surfaces. Due to the missing line of sight to the flexible

N. Ayache, S. Ourselin, A. Maeder (Eds.): MICCAI 2007, Part I, LNCS 4791, pp. 458–466, 2007.
© Springer-Verlag Berlin Heidelberg 2007

transducer tip, an OT system cannot be used exclusively to localize this tip. A robot could only be utilized if the ultrasound probe was fully integrated into the end-effector. To the authors' knowledge no such system currently exists. Promising alternatives are the use of an electromagnetic tracking (EMT) sensor attached to the tip [4,5,6] or fully incorporated into the tip [1], or magneto-optic tracking, i.e. the combination of OT and EMT [3].

When clinically using EMT, a considerable problem is the distortion of the EMT field leading to erroneous tracking data. This distortion can be caused by metallic or electrically powered objects inside or in close vicinity to the working volume, for instance surgical instruments, an operating table, or imaging devices such as a C-arm or a computed tomography scanner. Depending on the operating room setup and instrumentation, tracking errors of several millimeters or even centimeters can occur [8,9]. To compensate for erroneous measurements caused by stationary objects, various calibration techniques were proposed [10]. They usually require the user to acquire a set of well distributed measurements within the EMT volume. This set is compared to a set of reference measurements to compute a field distortion function that is based on look-up tables or polynomials. Unfortunately, this function can only compensate static errors of non-moving distortion fields, so that the calibration process has to be repeated for every new operating room setup before an intervention. Dynamic changes of the field distortion, for example caused by the intraoperative relocation of the EMT transmitter or movement of instruments, cannot be compensated by the previously computed distortion functions. A first step towards the intraoperative detection of erroneous measurements caused by metallic objects distorting the field was presented by Birkfellner et al. [11]. They incorporate two sensors into a pointer, so redundant measurements can be obtained. Deviations of the fixed distance between the two sensors are used as a plausibility value.

This paper introduces a new method to detect field distortions online, i.e. intraoperatively without a pre-computed distortion function. It is applied to a flexible laparoscopic transducer whose pose is determined by a magneto-optic tracking system. The B-scan images of the transducer are overlaid on the live images of an optically tracked laparoscope in real time to provide surgeons with a better understanding of the spatial relationship between the two imaging modalities. Finally, a rigorous accuracy evaluation of both online field distortion estimation and laparoscope augmentation is presented.

2   System Setup

The hardware setup comprises following components: A flexible laparoscopic linear array transducer (LAP8-4, 5 MHz, 10 mm diameter) connected to a SONO-LINE Omnia US system by Siemens Medical Solutions, a laparoscopic camera with a forward-oblique 30° HOPKINS telescope by Storz, a standard workstation PC including two frame grabbers (for capturing the transducer and camera video in real time), and the magneto-optic tracking system. The OT system consists of 4 ARTtrack2 cameras and a book size PC running the DTrack tracking software. The EMT system in use is a 3D Guidance unit of Ascension equipped with a mid-range transmitter and insulated 1.3 mm sensors, which have a total diameter of 1.7 mm including the vinyl tubing. Time synchronization of all data streams and visualization is performed by CAMPAR [12].

3 Methods

In addition to an OT body, which is attached to the transducer handle (below referred to as "rigid body"), two EMT sensors are attached to the transducer shaft: One to the flexible tip ("flexible sensor"), the other one to the rigid part ("rigid sensor"), as close to each other as possible. Another OT body is mounted on the EMT transmitter ("transmitter body"). This setup allows us to co-calibrate EMT and OT and to obtain redundant tracking information of the rigid part of the transducer shaft, which is important to detect EMT errors. Finally, two OT bodies are attached to the laparoscopic camera, one to the head ("laparoscope body") and another one to the telescope to adjust for telescope rotations.

3.1 System Calibration

Spatial and temporal system calibration is performed offline in a distortion-free environment. All coordinate frames are visualized in figure 1.

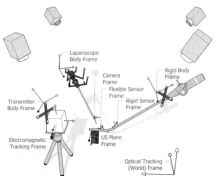
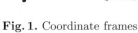
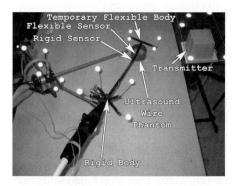

Fig. 1. Coordinate frames   **Fig. 2.** Setup for error evaluation

Hand-eye Calibration. To compute the Euclidean transformation $^{RigB}T_{RigS}$ between the rigid body and the rigid sensor frames, several poses with distinct rotation axes are recorded in both the OT and EMT coordinate frames. Stacked matrices A and B are generated from all movements between these poses. They are related to each other by the equation system $AX = XB$, which is solved by hand-eye calibration [13]. The same poses are used to estimate the rigid hand-eye transformation $^{EMT}T_{TransB}$ between the EMT transmitter coordinate frame and its OT body.

In a final optimization step, the two hand-eye calibration matrices $^{RigB}T_{RigS}$ and $^{EMT}T_{TransB}$ are optimized for all recorded poses by Levenberg-Marquardt. The matrix resulting from the transformation chain "rigid sensor to rigid body to OT to transmitter body to EMT to rigid sensor frame", which theoretically is an identity matrix, represents the accumulated transformation errors:

$$T_\delta = \begin{bmatrix} R_\delta & t_\delta \\ 0 & 1 \end{bmatrix} = {}^{RigS}T_{EMT} \cdot {}^{EMT}T_{TransB} \cdot {}^{TransB}T_{OT} \cdot {}^{OT}T_{RigB} \cdot {}^{RigB}T_{RigS} \quad (1)$$

We chose a cost function δ that weights translational to rotational errors 1:3, reflecting the root mean squared (RMS) error ratio provided independently by the two tracking system manufacturers: The RMS measurement errors of the OT system are stated as 0.4 mm (position) and 0.12° (orientation), the static RMS errors of the EMT system as 1.4 mm and 0.5°.[1]

$$\delta = \delta_{translational} + 3 \cdot \delta_{rotational} = \|t_\delta\| + 3 \cdot \frac{180}{\pi} \cdot \arccos\left(\frac{\text{trace}(R_\delta) - 1}{2}\right) \quad (2)$$

where the rotational error is the rotation angle of R_δ, decomposed into axis-angle parameters. The maximum error δ_{max} determined after optimization is chosen as a measure of distrust for the overall performance of the hand-eye calibration (cf. section 3.2).

Laparoscopic Camera. For laparoscopic camera calibration, the projection geometry including distortion coefficients and the transformation from laparoscope body coordinates to camera center coordinates are estimated, as described by Yamaguchi et al. [14].

Laparoscopic Ultrasound. For the determination of the pixel scaling of the ultrasound B-scan plane and its transformation to the flexible sensor frame, a single-wall calibration is performed [15]. Instead of scanning the planar bottom of a water bath, we scan a nylon membrane stretched over a planar frame, as proposed by Langø [16].

Temporal Calibration. In order to provide a smooth visualization without lag, all data is given a time stamp and brought into the same time frame. While the OT PC and our workstation are synchronized via the network time protocol (NTP) to the same reference time, the ultrasound and EMT systems require a more advanced synchronization. As these systems do not automatically provide reliable time stamps corresponding to the actual data acquisition time, a time stamp is generated when their data arrives at the workstation. Therefore, a fixed offset is subtracted from this time stamp to compensate for any lag introduced while traveling to the workstation. To determine this offset, the magneto-optically tracked transducer is moved up and down and the translation along the principal motion axes is compared, as proposed by Treece et al. [15].

---

[1] See also http://www.ar-tracking.de and http://www.ascension-tech.com

3.2   Online Error Estimation

Intraoperatively, every measured pose of the rigid sensor is transformed applying equation 1. If a corresponding error δ is determined, which is bigger than the distrust level δ_{max}, the surgical staff is automatically warned. Such errors are often caused by dynamic or static field distortions. Additionally, as the flexible sensor is in close proximity to the rigid one, its measurements will be most likely affected by these distortions as well.

In order to also approximate a correction of erroneous measurements of the flexible sensor, a simple approach is to apply the deviation between the previously hand-eye calibrated ("calib") and the measured ("meas") transformation of the rigid sensor to the measured flexible sensor transformation, all relatively to the fixed OT (world) reference frame:

$$^{OT}\boldsymbol{R}_{FlexS(corr)} = {^{OT}\boldsymbol{R}_{RigidS(meas)}}^{T} \cdot {^{OT}\boldsymbol{R}_{RigidS(calib)}} \cdot {^{OT}\boldsymbol{R}_{FlexS(meas)}} \quad (3)$$

$$^{OT}\boldsymbol{t}_{FlexS(corr)} = -{^{OT}\boldsymbol{t}_{RigidS(meas)}} + {^{OT}\boldsymbol{t}_{RigidS(calib)}} + {^{OT}\boldsymbol{t}_{FlexS(meas)}} \quad (4)$$

4   Experimental Evaluation Results

To avoid too many outliers, all EMT measurements were acquired in a restricted volume of 20–36 cm for x, and ±15 cm for y and z.

4.1   Ultrasound Calibration Error

After acquiring 40 flexible sensor poses and their corresponding lines that were automatically detected in the B-scan images, the calibration matrix was computed using the Levenberg-Marquardt optimizer. To determine the ultrasound calibration accuracy, a single EMT sensor with tip coordinates given in the EMT frame was submerged into the water bath. Its tip was segmented manually in 5 regions of the B-scan plane, which was repeated for 4 poses of the transducer differing from the ones used during calibration. The tip coordinates were transformed into the B-scan plane coordinates and compared to the segmented tip coordinates (scaled to mm). An RMS error of 1.69 mm with standard deviation of 0.51 mm and maximum error of 2.39 mm was obtained.

4.2   Laparoscope Augmentation Error

In order to estimate the laparoscope augmentation errors automatically, an additional OT body ("flexible body") was temporarily attached to the transducer tip and co-calibrated to the flexible sensor by another hand-eye calibration (cf. section 3.1 and figure 2). One marker of the flexible body was chosen as a reference and automatically segmented whenever visible in the laparoscopic video. We compared its center coordinates to the projection of its respective OT coordinates onto the image plane. Additionally, the corresponding EMT measurements as well as their approximated corrections were projected using the previously determined hand-eye calibration transformations.

Evaluation data was recorded using a laparoscope-to-marker distance of 5 to 10 cm, which is a typical intraoperative working distance. The current distance can be recovered from OT data and the camera calibration parameters. We also used this information to scale pixel units to mm.

For each of six evaluation series, the transducer was fixed at a different pose and the laparoscope

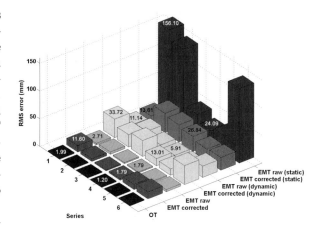

Fig. 3. RMS projection errors

was used to measure the projected distances from five differing poses, each in an undistorted and a distorted environment. To distort the EMT field, two alternatives were evaluated. A metal plate was placed on the table to simulate primarily static distortions caused for instance by an operating table. For dynamic distortions, a steel rod of 10 mm diameter was brought close to the transducer to simulate a surgical instrument, changing its proximity and angle to the transducer in five measurements.

The RMS errors are given in figure 3. For each of the six series, we plotted the errors of the three distortion cases (no distortion, static, and dynamic distortion), each scenario with our simple correction function enabled and disabled. While we have been able to predict and correct static interferences with high reliability, dynamic distortions yielded even worse results when attempting a correction.

In order to evaluate our distrust function statistically, we computed the distrust level (cf. equation 2) for each of the poses. An offset between the segmented marker and the EMT projections of more than 2 mm was regarded as erroneous measurement. In this case, we expect a distrust level δ of more than δ_{max} (during hand-eye calibration, δ_{max} was empirically determined to be 20). We defined the following cases for our evaluation:

– A *true positive* is a measurement, in which the EMT error was above 2 mm with a distrust level of above 20 – the detector rejected an erroneous reading correctly.
– A *true negative* is a measurement, in which the EMT error was below 2 mm with a distrust level below 20 – we correctly accepted the original EMT data.
– A *false positive* (type 1 error) is a measurement, in which the EMT error was below 2 mm, but the distrust level above 20 – we have not been able to detect a correct value and rejected it without necessity.

Table 1. Distortion detection rate by our distrust level

distortion		true	false
w/o:	positive	40.0%	10.0%
	negative	30.0%	20.0%
static:	positive	100.0%	0.0%
	negative	0.0%	0.0%
dynamic:	positive	73.8%	13.8%
	negative	12.4%	0.0%
avg:	positive	71.3%	7.9%
	negative	14.1%	6.7%

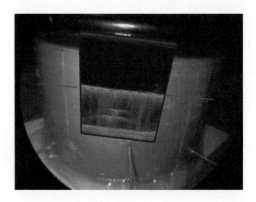

Fig. 4. Ultrasound plane augmented on the laparoscope video – Red line added manually to visualize the extension of the straight wire, which matches its ultrasound image

- A *false negative* (type 2 error) is a measurement, in which the EMT error was above 2 mm, but the distrust level below 20 – the record was accepted although the real error was large.

The results are listed in table 1. In about 85 % of all cases, we correctly detected the true situation (*true positives* and *true negatives*).

4.3 Ultrasound Augmentation

To visually inspect the overlay of the B-scan plane on the laparoscopic live video, we constructed a cylindric phantom containing straight wires, which extend through the walls of the phantom. It was filled with water of known temperature. Adjusting the pixel scaling factors to an adequate speed of sound, the B-scan plane was augmented, allowing the camera to view a wire on the augmented plane and its extension outside the phantom walls. A typical augmented laparoscope image can be seen in figure 4.

Whenever the occurrence of an error is determined, it is visualized by drawing a red frame around the ultrasound plane. Otherwise the frame is drawn in green. An attempt to correct the error can be visualized in yellow. The supplementary video demonstration[2] summarizes the results of all experiments and allows the observer to qualitatively evaluate the performance of automatic distortion estimation.

5 Discussion

The flat tablet transmitter recently presented by Ascension may be an alternative to overcome field distortions, e.g. caused by the operating table. However,

---

[2] http://campar.in.tum.de/files/publications/feuerste2007miccai.video.avi

due to its lower excitation, in the same setup it performed worse than the mid-range transmitter for ultrasound calibration, resulting in errors of about 4-8 mm. Bigger sensors could be used to improve the accuracy, but this would probably require bigger trocars. Using 1.3 mm sensors, the total diameter of the laparoscopic transducer is only 11.8 mm (including sterile cover), so it still fits a regular 12 mm trocar.

In gastrointestinal (laparoscopic) surgery conditions are different than in e.g. orthopedic surgery or neurosurgery. A discrimination of about 0.5 cm is usually sufficient for a number of reasons. Canalicular structures such as vessels, bile ducts, etc. play a critical role if they are equal to or thicker than 5 mm. Lymph nodes are considered to be inflicted by a tumor if the diameter is more than 10 mm and so on. Accordingly, an error of about 2-3 mm (as obtained for the distortion free environment) is certainly acceptable under clinical conditions.

While the error detection method is working well, the error correction method in the presented form turned out to be disappointing. This behavior may be explained by the facts, that (1) the accuracy of current electromagnetic tracking systems has still a lot of room for improvement, (2) during system calibration errors are accumulated, and (3), most importantly, field distortions at the flexible sensor differ a lot from those at the rigid sensor in terms of magnitude and direction, although both sensors are quite close to each other. To further improve the error correction and superimposition accuracy, the possible transducer tip movements can be modeled relatively to the rigid body and also the axis of the ultrasound tip can be segmented in the laparoscope images and backprojected into 3D to further correct the flexible sensor measurements. This is part of our current work and already gave very promising results by reducing dynamic errors of several centimeters to only around 5 mm, contrary to the here described simple correction approach, for which the corrected error grows proportionally to the original error. Additionally, a comparison to and integration of standard EMT calibration techniques is on its way. Our setup could even be used to generate a field distortion function online using the redundancy of the rigid sensor.

6   Conclusion

We presented a new method to detect EMT field distortions online by a magneto-optic tracking setup. We improve the state of art [2,3] for augmenting laparoscopic ultrasound images directly on the laparoscopic live images to give surgeons a better understanding of the spatial relationship between ultrasound and camera images. The laparoscopic ultrasound transducer tip is flexible. Therefore, our method could be applied to a larger set of applications. We are using two attached sensors and hence are able to additionally provide a distrust level of the current EMT measurements. Therefore, the system is able to automatically update and warn the surgical staff of possible inaccuracies.

References

1. Harms, J., et al.: Three-dimensional navigated laparoscopic ultrasonography. Surgical Endoscopy 15, 1459–1462 (2001)
2. Leven, J., et al.: Davinci canvas: A telerobotic surgical system with integrated, robot-assisted, laparoscopic ultrasound capability. In: Duncan, J.S., Gerig, G. (eds.) MICCAI 2005. LNCS, vol. 3749, Springer, Heidelberg (2005)
3. Nakamoto, M., et al.: 3d ultrasound system using a magneto-optic hybrid tracker for augmented reality visualization in laparoscopic liver surgery. In: Dohi, T., Kikinis, R. (eds.) MICCAI 2002. LNCS, vol. 2489, Springer, Heidelberg (2002)
4. Ellsmere, J., et al.: A new visualization technique for laparoscopic ultrasonography. Surgery 136, 84–92 (2004)
5. Krücker, J., et al.: An electro-magnetically tracked laparoscopic ultrasound for multi-modality minimally invasive surgery. In: CARS (2005)
6. Kleemann, M., et al.: Laparoscopic ultrasound navigation in liver surgery: technical aspects and accuracy. Surgical Endoscopy 20, 726–729 (2006)
7. Voros, S., Long, J.A., Cinquin, P.: Automatic localization of laparoscopic instruments for the visual servoing of an endoscopic camera holder. In: Larsen, R., Nielsen, M., Sporring, J. (eds.) MICCAI 2006. LNCS, vol. 4190, Springer, Heidelberg (2006)
8. Hummel, J.B., et al.: Design and application of an assessment protocol for electromagnetic tracking systems. Medical Physics 32, 2371–2379 (2005)
9. Nafis, C., Jensen, V., Beauregard, L., Anderson, P.: Method for estimating dynamic em tracking accuracy of surgical navigation tools. In: Medical Imaging 2006: Visualization, Image-Guided Procedures, and Display (2006)
10. Kindratenko, V.V.: A survey of electromagnetic position tracker calibration techniques. Virtual Reality: Research, Development, and Applications 5, 169–182 (2000)
11. Birkfellner, W., et al.: Concepts and results in the development of a hybrid tracking system for cas. In: Wells, W.M., Colchester, A.C.F., Delp, S.L. (eds.) MICCAI 1998. LNCS, vol. 1496, Springer, Heidelberg (1998)
12. Sielhorst, T., Feuerstein, M., Traub, J., Kutter, O., Navab, N.: Campar: A software framework guaranteeing quality for medical augmented reality. International Journal of Computer Assisted Radiology and Surgery 1, 29–30 (2006)
13. Daniilidis, K.: Hand-eye calibration using dual quaternions. International Journal of Robotics Research 18, 286–298 (1999)
14. Yamaguchi, T., et al.: Development of a camera model and calibration procedure for oblique-viewing endoscopes. Computer Aided Surgery 9, 203–214 (2004)
15. Treece, G.M., et al.: High-definition freehand 3-d ultrasound. Ultrasound in Medicine and Biology 29, 529–546 (2003)
16. Langø, T.: Ultrasound Guided Surgery: Image Processing and Navigation. PhD thesis, Norwegian University of Science and Technology (2000)

Evaluation of a Novel Calibration Technique for Optically Tracked Oblique Laparoscopes

Stijn De Buck[1], Frederik Maes[1], André D'Hoore[2], and Paul Suetens[1]

[1] Faculties of Medicine and Engineering, Medical Image Computing (ESAT and Radiology), K.U.Leuven, Herestraat 49, 3000 Leuven, Belgium
[2] Department of Abdominal Surgery, UZ Leuven, Herestraat 49, 3000 Leuven, Belgium
stijn.debuck@uz.kuleuven.ac.be*

Abstract. This paper proposes an evaluation of a novel calibration method for an optically tracked oblique laparoscope. We present the necessary tools to track an oblique scope and a camera model which includes changes to the intrinsic camera parameters thereby extending previously proposed methods. Because oblique scopes offer a wide 'virtual' view on the surgical field, the method is of great interest for augmented reality guidance of laparoscopic interventions using an oblique scope.

The model and an approximated version are evaluated in an extensive validation study. Using 5 sets of 40 calibration images, we compare both camera models (i.e. model and approximation) and 2 interpolation schemes. The selected model and interpolation scheme reaches an average accuracy of 2.60 pixel and an equivalent 3D error of 0.60 mm.

Finally, we present initial experience of the presented approach with an oblique scope and optical tracking in a clinical setup. During a laparoscopic rectum resection surgery the setup was used to augment the scene with a model of the pelvis. The method worked properly and the attached probes did not interfere with normal procedure.

1 Introduction

Laparoscopic techniques evolve very rapidly through a broad spectrum of enhancements [1] like the introduction of stereoscopic lenses, so called 'chip in the tip' lenses [1], etc. ... One of these enhancements is the use of scopes which have a viewing direction different from the mechanical rotation axis of the lens. Using such a scope holds the advantage of having a broader virtual field of view due to the easy rotation and the inclination. This property is considered a valuable asset in, for instance, laparoscopic rectum surgery and should thus be taken into account. In [2] Yamaguchi *et al.* introduced a camera model for an oblique (or tilted view angle) scope of which the angle is determined by a rotary encoder. The model tries to incorporate the physical behaviour of such a camera and introduces possible deviations from the ideal model. The resulting calibration

---

* We acknowledge the support of the IWT/OZM050811 project.

N. Ayache, S. Ourselin, A. Maeder (Eds.): MICCAI 2007, Part I, LNCS 4791, pp. 467–474, 2007.
© Springer-Verlag Berlin Heidelberg 2007

method is accurate but very specific to oblique scopes. It also does not incorporate changes to the camera intrinsic parameters.

In this paper we will present an accuracy evaluation of a novel calibration technique enabling the use of a tilted view angle laparoscope tracked only by an optical tracker. We extend the work of Yamaguchi *et al.* [2] by incorporating changes to the intrinsic camera parameters which renders the method more generic. Furthermore, we make use only of optical tracking for measuring the pose of the camera and lens thereby reducing hardware requirements as compared to the setup in [2]. This approach enlarges the application domain since it facilitates tracking of multiple bodies such as other instruments besides the laparoscopic camera (e.g. tracked ultrasound devices, ...). In fact, it provides a common reference frame in which multiple applications, with different requirements can be realized. The presented calibration approach can be applied when an oblique scope is used in such a generic setup. However, the use of an optical tracker will have an impact on the accuracy results. Therefore we conducted an extensive accuracy study of the proposed calibration approach.

2   Materials and Methods

The setup we use, consists of a CCD-camera, a 30° view angle laparoscope, an optical tracker (Flashpoint 5000, Image guided technologies) and an Octane workstation (SGI). Both the lens and the CCD-camera are equipped with IR-LEDs visible to the optical tracker (see Fig. 1) and can both be located accurately within the coordinate space of the optical tracker. In order to augment a laparoscope video with preoperative images we should know the parameters of the imaging system for each position and orientation of both lens and camera. Before we describe the computation of the parameters modeling the rotation of the oblique lens, we will present the camera model and its relation to the optical tracking device and explain how the angle θ between the CCD-camera and the lens can be determined.

2.1   Camera Model

A conventional straight laparoscope can be modeled sufficiently accurately by a pinhole model in conjunction with a radial distortion component [3]. The perspective model and radial distortion can be described by

$$\begin{bmatrix} \lambda p_i^{(u)} \\ \lambda \end{bmatrix} = KR(P_i - C) \quad \text{and} \quad \|p_i^{(u)} - c\| = (1 + \kappa)\|p_i^{(d)} - c\| \tag{1}$$

In these equations P_i is a point in world coordinates, $p_i^{(d)}, p_i^{(u)}$ are its corresponding image points, after and before distortion respectively. $c(C_x, C_y)$ is the center of distortion. The rotation matrix R and translation vector C relate the world coordinate system to the camera coordinate system. The projection matrix K projects the transformed point onto the undistorted image which is distorted using a radial distortion parameter κ.

Supposing that the tracker coordinate system coincides with the world co-ordinate system and we know C and R for one position ref of the scope, the projection in any other position l can be computed as:

$$\begin{bmatrix} \lambda p_i^{(u)} \\ \lambda \end{bmatrix} = K \begin{bmatrix} I_3 & 0 \end{bmatrix} T_{cam} T_{Tracker-LP}^{(l)} \begin{bmatrix} P_i \\ 1 \end{bmatrix} \tag{2}$$

in which $T_{Tracker-LP}$ is the matrix relating the tracker coordinate frame $O_{Tracker}$ to a local coordinate system of the camera IR-LEDs O_{LP}, I_3 is a unit matrix of size 3 and T_{cam} can be computed as follows

$$T_{cam} = \begin{bmatrix} R & -RC \\ 0 & 1 \end{bmatrix} {T_{Tracker-LP}^{(ref)}}^{-1} \tag{3}$$

and remains constant as long as the IR-LEDs are rigidly attached to the camera. This model applies to any orientation of an oblique scope as long as the camera head is not rotated about the lens axis.

Each orientation differs by the fact of having a different image plane. In an ideal oblique scope this difference is due to a rotation about the mechanical axis of the lens and, thus, the camera center C remains fixed. Because of lens imperfections both the center and the intrinsic parameters contained in K might change whenever the lens is rotated with respect to the camera head. Whereas others (e.g. [4]) use affine transformation to model variations in R and K, we propose a projective transformation or homography H. Changes in C can be modeled by a translation correction term. The projection of point P_i for an arbitrary orientation l of the lens w.r.t. the CCD-head about an angle θ can be written as follows:

$$\begin{bmatrix} \lambda p_i^{(u)} \\ \lambda \end{bmatrix} = K_{ref} H(\theta_l) \begin{bmatrix} I_3 & 0 \end{bmatrix} T_{cam}^{(ref)} T_{Tracker-LP}^{(l)} \left(\begin{bmatrix} P_i \\ 1 \end{bmatrix} + \begin{bmatrix} C_{corr}(\theta_l) \\ 1 \end{bmatrix} \right) \tag{4}$$

in which K_{ref} contains the parameters modeling a chosen reference orientation and $T_{cam}^{(ref)}$ is computed based on the same reference set. Since we have a pure rotation of the lens, one could omit $C_{corr}(\theta)$.

The intrinsic and extrinsic parameters of Eq. 1 for a straight lens or scope in a fixed position can be computed by means of a calibration jig (Fig. 1), that has a known geometry in the tracker reference frame. The centers of the discs are detected fully automatically and assigned to their proper 3D coordinates. After selection of a reference image, one can compute K_{ref}, R_{ref}, C_{ref} and thus $T_{cam}^{(ref)}$ based on the 2D-3D pairs [5,3].

2.2   Computation of Theta

The angle θ between the CCD-camera and the oblique lens can be computed on the basis of the relative pose of the IR-LEDs attached to the lens and the CCD-camera. In a first stage the invariant axis for a rotation of the camera head about the lens is computed. The second stage then determines the angle between measured poses about the invariant rotation axis.

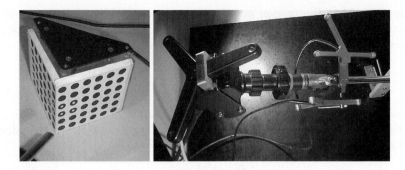

Fig. 1. Picture of the setup used for the calibration of an oblique scope. This includes the in house developed calibration jig with 3 attached IR-LEDs. An additional IR-LED probe was attached to the oblique lens, which is used to compute the angle between the lens and the CCD-camera.

2.3   Computation of the Center Correction Term and the Homography

Before computing the homography $H(\theta)$, we can compute the correction term $C_{corr}(\theta)$ by imposing that the camera center of a calibration image l should equal the reference camera center after applying the correction term. After constructing a set of $C_{corr}^{(l)}$ for each recorded pose of the oblique scope at θ_l, we can build a function $C_{corr}(\theta)$ by interpolation.

For the computation of H_l we acquire a set of images covering the range of orientations of camera and lens that is expected during the procedure. In order to keep the effect of measurement noise from the optical tracker minimal, the lens and jig remain fixed at one position while the CCD-head is rotated. The disc centers for all images are detected automatically and corresponding centers of the reference image are assigned. Subsequently, we can compute the homography H_l of each image l by finding the homography that maps

$$\begin{bmatrix} I_3 & 0 \end{bmatrix} T_{cam}^{(ref)} T_{Tracker-LP}^{(l)} \left(\begin{bmatrix} P_i \\ 1 \end{bmatrix} + C_{corr}(\theta) \right) \quad \text{onto} \quad K_{ref}^{-1} p_i^{(u)}$$

For the computation we use a method by Horaud $et\ al.$ [6].

Next, one can compute the parameters of a function $H(\theta)$ interpolating H_i which enables the computation of the homography for an arbitrary θ.

2.4   Interpolation of the Parameters

To be able to use the camera model of an oblique scope for arbitrary angles, we need to construct a function for both the homography $H(\theta)$ and the center correction $Ccorr(\theta)$. Two interpolation schemes were developed and tested: a truncated Fourier series

$$f(\theta) = \frac{a_0}{2} + \Sigma_{k=1}^{2} a_k \sin(k\theta) + b_k \cos(k\theta) \tag{5}$$

and a polynomial of an empirically determined fifth degree.

3   Experiments

3.1   Accuracy Assessment

In order to assess the accuracy of the approach and compare the two interpolation schemes, we performed a validation experiment on 4 sets of 40 images. The experiment was conducted as follows:

- First 5 times 40 images were acquired of the calibration jig with the lens in the same position and the camera head each time slightly rotated about the lens. Position and orientation of both lens and camera head were recorded by the optical tracker.
- Next, a calibration was computed for all (Sets A-E) of the 5 acquired sets while one set was used to validate (set A). Note that the reported results for set A depict a residue instead of a true validation.
- The image plane error ϵ_l was computed for each image l as

$$\epsilon_l = \frac{1}{n}\Sigma_{i=1}^{n}\|\widehat{p_{i,l}} - p_{i,l}\| \tag{6}$$

with

$$\begin{bmatrix} \lambda\widehat{p_{i,l}} \\ \lambda \end{bmatrix} = K_{ref}H(\theta_l)\begin{bmatrix} I_3 & 0 \end{bmatrix} T_{cam}^{(ref)}T_{Tracker-LP}^{(l)}(\begin{bmatrix} P_i \\ 1 \end{bmatrix} + \begin{bmatrix} C_{corr}(\theta_l) \\ 1 \end{bmatrix})$$

and $p_{i,l}$ equal to the image coordinate of the detected corresponding disc center and P_i the 3D coordinate of the disc center. n equals the number of detected disc centers for each image. Furthermore, a 3D equivalent error was computed as the distance between the back-projected ray through a disc center $p_{i,l}$ and the corresponding 3D point P_i.

This experiment was repeated for each calibration set altering both the interpolation scheme from a Fourier series to a polynomial interpolation and the camera model from the complete model including the center correction $C_{corr}(\theta)$ to the one neglecting this term.

A typical result from one set (set C) is plotted in Fig. 2 which visualizes the error as a function of θ. The resulting error function seems independent of θ.

The result of all experiments is summarized in Tab. 1 and 2. For each set (B-E) we show the mean and standard deviation of the error over all images of that set. The results are given for the 4 experiment types numbered as below:

1 no center correction & Fourier interpolation (NCC-FI)
2 no center correction & polynomial interpolation (NCC-PI).
3 center correction & Fourier interpolation (CC-FI).
4 center correction & polynomial interpolation (CC-PI).

Tab. 1 shows the image plane error in pixel while Tab. 2 shows the 3D error in mm. The latter is an objective way to represent the error as it is independent of the camera geometry. It does depend on the distance between the jig and the camera which we chose in the range expected in a real surgical setting.

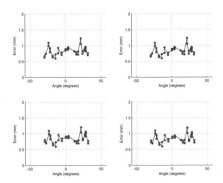

Fig. 2. A plot of the computed error in pixels where estimated projections of points are compared to detected ones. The 4 plots denote the result as a function of θ for the four types of modeling/interpolation. (top left = NCC-FI; top right = NCC-PI; bottom left = CC-FI; bottom right = CC-PI)

Table 1. Summary of the validation results for 5 sets. Each row represents the 2D image plane error in pixels computed on set A after calibration and interpolation using sets A-E and each considering a different combination of interpolating function and camera model (See Sec. 3). The average error over all experiments (sets B-E) is given in the last column.

	B	C	D	E	Average
NCC-FI	2.62 ± 0.96	3.58 ± 0.56	1.77 ± 0.79	2.41 ± 1.03	2.60 ± 0.84
NCC-PI	2.62 ± 0.96	3.58 ± 0.54	1.79 ± 0.82	2.44 ± 1.06	2.61 ± 0.85
CC-FI	2.54 ± 1.03	3.64 ± 0.57	1.78 ± 0.72	2.45 ± 0.89	2.60 ± 0.80
CC-PI	2.55 ± 1.03	3.60 ± 0.56	1.78 ± 0.74	2.62 ± 1.10	2.64 ± 0.86

From the results in Tab. 1 and 2, we can not deduce a significant difference between the polynomial and Fourier series interpolation. Because of its inherent periodicity and equally good performance, we chose to use the truncated Fourier interpolation.

As for the inclusion of C_{corr}, the experiment shows an increased error when adding this term to the model, although this difference is not significant. The increased error is probably due to the noise of the optical tracker measurement which leads to errors on the computed rotation angles θ. The use of a more complex model encompasses more degrees of freedom which, in the absence of a clear translation component, may merely model noise that is incorporated in the interpolation function. When evaluating a control set, the model will also render noisy estimates resulting in a higher error. This is confirmed by comparing the residue for set A shown in Tab. 3 before and after interpolation. Before interpolation the inclusion of C_{corr} results in a slightly higher accuracy. However, after interpolation, there is no significant difference noticeable.

Since the neglect of the term results in a model with fewer parameters which is less prone to noise and in a higher accuracy, we propose to use the approximation.

Table 2. Summary of the calibration results for the 5 sets (A-E) which were validated on set A. Each row represents the 3D error in mm computed on set A after calibration and interpolation and each considering a different combination of interpolating function and camera model (See Section 3). The average error over all experiments (sets B-E) is given in the last column.

	B	C	D	E	Average
NCC-FI	0.62 ± 0.22	0.83 ± 0.13	0.41 ± 0.18	0.56 ± 0.23	0.60 ± 0.19
NCC-PI	0.61 ± 0.22	0.83 ± 0.13	0.41 ± 0.18	0.57 ± 0.24	0.61 ± 0.19
CC-FI	0.59 ± 0.24	0.85 ± 0.14	0.41 ± 0.17	0.57 ± 0.21	0.61 ± 0.19
CC-PI	0.60 ± 0.24	0.84 ± 0.13	0.41 ± 0.17	0.61 ± 0.26	0.61 ± 0.20

Table 3. Residue of obtained by calibration of set A. Both the residue before and after interpolation are provided. The left column shows the 2D errors in pixel while the right column shows the 3D error in millimeter. This table shows that incorporating a center correction results in a more accurate model and that after interpolation the improvement is canceled out. This is probably due to measurement noise on the IR-LEDs.

	2D residue (pixel)	3D residue (mm)
No interpolation/no center corr	0.81 ± 0.11	0.19 ± 0.03
No interpolation/center corr	0.72 ± 0.03	0.17 ± 0.01
NCC-FI	1.48 ± 0.72	0.35 ± 0.17
NCC-PI	1.46 ± 0.64	0.34 ± 0.15
CC-FI	1.49 ± 0.73	0.35 ± 0.18
CC-PI	1.42 ± 0.59	0.33 ± 0.15

3.2   Clinical Usability

We also tested if the proposed method was usable in a clinical context. During a routine laparoscopic intervention in which an oblique scope is employed, we displayed a model of the pelvis on the acquired laparoscopic video stream. Calibration was performed as described above.

During the intervention, the sterilized lens was reattached to the CCD-head which was wrapped in sterile transparent plastic. The display of the virtual model on top of the real video stream worked well: under the used range of orientations, the model remained visibly stationary with respect to the patient. During the usage, the operator had to pay attention that the IR-LEDs were visible to the optical tracker, though once he found a comfortable position, this was easily asserted. Except for the wrapping of the CCD camera, which took slightly more time due to the size of the IR-LED probe, no significant delays in the surgical workflow were noted.

3.3   Discussion

By combining conventional calibration techniques, tracking of both lens and camera and a mapping technique based on homographies, we model the behaviour of a rotating oblique lens and can estimate the projection parameters for an arbitrary position of camera and lens. By providing a model for a lens based system that can cope with both changes to extrinsic and intrinsic parameters, we extend the work of Yamaguchi *et al.* [2]. Whereas they use a robotic device in their approach, we consider only optical tracking for obtaining pose data. That approach can be an advantage in the design of an (augmented reality) image-guided surgery system since it facilitates the tracking and representation of other devices (e.g. instruments) in a single reference frame.

Validation of this model and comparison with a simplified version on an extensive set of images, shows that for the application of oblique scopes we can neglect the center correction term C_{corr} without losing accuracy. This makes the model easier to update and less prone to noise. In our first clinical tests the calibration seems to work well and does not interrupt normal work flow.

The accuracy may be improved by reducing the influence of the IR-LED measurement noise on the computation of θ. This may be realized by the development of a dedicated circular IR-LED probe. This probe could consist of a circular array of IR-LEDs mounted around the mechanical rotation axis of the oblique lens such that it would present itself in a well conditioned way to the optical tracker, independent of the orientation of the probe.

References

1. Boppart, S.A., Deutsch, T.F., Rattner, D.W.: Optical imaging technology in minimally invasive surgery. Current status and future directions. Surgical Endoscopy 13(7); 718–722 (1999)
2. Yamaguchi, T., Nakamoto, M., Sato, Y., Nakajima, Y., Konishi, K., Hashizume, M., Nishii, T., Sugano, N., Yoshikawa, H., Yonenobu, K., Tamura1, S.: Camera model and calibration procedure for oblique-viewing endoscope. In: Ellis, R.E., Peters, T.M. (eds.) MICCAI 2003. LNCS, vol. 2879, pp. 373–381. Springer, Heidelberg (2003)
3. De Buck, S., Van Cleynenbreugel, J., Geys, I., Koninckx, T., Koninckx, P.R., Suetens, P.: A system to support laparoscopic surgery by augmented reality visualization. In: Niessen, W.J., Viergever, M.A. (eds.) MICCAI 2001. LNCS, vol. 2208, pp. 691–698. Springer, Heidelberg (2001)
4. Simon, G., Berger, M.O.: Registration with a zoom lens camera for augmented reality applications. In: IWAR 1999, p. 103. IEEE Computer Society, Washington, DC, USA (1999)
5. Tsai, R.: An efficient and accurate camera calibration technique for 3D machine vision. In: CVPR 1986, pp. 364–374 (1986)
6. Horaud, R., Csurka, G.: Self-calibration and euclidean reconstruction using motions of a stereo rig. In: ICCV 1998 pp. 96–103 (1998)

Fiducial-Free Registration Procedure for Navigated Bronchoscopy

Tassilo Klein[1], Joerg Traub[1], Hubert Hautmann[2], Alireza Ahmadian[3],
and Nassir Navab[1]

[1] Computer Aided Medical Procedures (CAMP), TUM, Munich, Germany,
[2] Pneumology Department, Klinikum rechts der Isar, TUM, Munich, Germany
[3] Tehran University of Medical Sciences, Iran

Abstract. Navigated bronchoscopy has been developed by various
groups within the last decades. Systems based on CT data and electromagnetic tracking enable the visualization of the position and orientation of the bronchoscope, forceps, and biopsy tools within CT data.
Therefore registration between the tracking space and the CT volume
is required. Standard procedures are based on point-based registration
methods that require selecting corresponding natural landmarks in both
coordinate systems by the examiner. We developed a novel algorithm
for a fully automatic registration procedure in navigated bronchoscopy
based on the trajectory recorded during routine examination of the airways at the beginning of an intervention. The proposed system provides
advantages in terms of an unchanged medical workflow and high accuracy. We compared the novel method with point-based and ICP-based
registration. Experiments demonstrate that the novel method transforms
up to 97% of tracking points inside the segmented airways, which was
the best performance compared to the other methods.

1   Introduction

Lung cancer is among the most common forms of cancer and by far the deadliest
of all types with a worldwide death toll of about one million annually [1]. In the
United States about 15% of all cancers are diagnosed in the lung, accounting to
31% of all cancer deaths in males and 26% in females [2]. According to this, modern computer-guided bronchoscopy has become an indispensable tool due to its
potential that enables doctors to examine and evaluate abnormalities for cancer
in the inside airways of patients even at remote spots. Especially in pulmonary diagnostics, biopsy specimens taken from lung lesions followed by histopathologic,
cytologic or microbiological assessments are a crucial procedure for the decision on an adequate therapy. The diagnostic success depends on various factors,
among others, skill of the examiner, nodule size and location. Especially when
it comes to accurately localizing peripheral solitary pulmonary nodules (SPN),
traditional image-guided bronchoscopy based on fluoroscopic images reaches its
limits. Inability or failure to reach designated targets and considering that many
SPNs are not visible under fluoroscopy, often more invasive approaches, e.g.,

N. Ayache, S. Ourselin, A. Maeder (Eds.): MICCAI 2007, Part I, LNCS 4791, pp. 475–482, 2007.
© Springer-Verlag Berlin Heidelberg 2007

CT-guided biopsy are facilitated, entailing an undesirable high exposure to radiation. Given the majority of SPNs situated in the lung periphery and the success rate using common techniques for biopsies typically between 18 and 62 percent, considerably depending on the lesion size and location [3], new procedures were facilitated. One possible solution to overcome the limits of traditional bronchoscopy is based on electromagnetic tracking (EMT) guided navigation as proposed by Hautmann et al. [4], Solomon et al. [5] as well as by Schwarz et al. [6], the latter using the commercial system by Superdimensions Inc.. All these studies showed good initial results. Their navigated bronchoscopy (NB) systems are based on tracking the tip of the bronchoscope by an electromagnetic (EM) sensor that is encapsulated in the tip of a flexible catheter pushed through the working channel of a bronchoscope or rigidly attached to its distal end. After a registration between tracking system and CT data, the sensor position can be visualized in the previously acquired CT images in real-time.

Recent attempts in registration and tracking for NB show considerable improvements. The approach of Wegner et al. [7,8] is to map the data from the EMT system to the closest point on a centerline of the segmented airways. Other approaches try to investigate more reliable and fully automatic registration procedures. Deguchi et al. [9] propose a method based on the iterative closest point (ICP) algorithm, to map the EM trajectory of the bronchoscope that is moved inside the airways to its segmented centerline from the CT data.

We propose a novel and fully automatic algorithm for the registration procedure in NB. Like the ICP approach we use the trajectory that is recorded during the routine examination of the airways at the beginning of the intervention. The algorithm is based on the assumption that the bronchoscope can be moved arbitrarily within the airways. In contrast to the ICP approach that enforces the trajectory to be close to the centerline, we try to create a more realistic model. We derived a new cost function for the registration that tests if a point, after applying the registration matrix, is inside or outside the segmented airways of the CT data. To make this approach fully automatic we developed an initialization procedure based on the main axes of both the segmented bronchial tree volume and the recorded trajectory. From experiments conducted on an airways phantom, we compared the results of different pneumologists using point-based, ICP-based and our newly developed registration method.

2   Method

Previously proposed and developed point and ICP-based registration techniques were integrated in our navigation system and compared with our fiducial-free approach.

2.1   Point-Based Registration

The simplest and most common method used to perform registration in NB is to find corresponding natural landmarks in the CT data and in the patient using the

EM sensor position data. Usually the anatomical landmarks inside the airways are chosen such that they are easy to recognize to avoid ambiguity and achieve better accuracy of the registration over external fiducials [5]. The localization procedure of the landmarks has to be performed meticulously since it directly affects the accuracy of the registration. Lacking accuracy and reproducibility, which are inherent to this method are among its main drawbacks.

The error associated with this matter is called Fiducial Localisation Error (FLE) [10]. However, for the evaluation of the registration accuracy the Target Registration Error (TRE) that is induced by FLE at a given target, is a more realistic error criteria. To determine the FLE an experiment was conducted. Experienced pneumologists were asked to identify five corresponding anatomical landmark sets: main carina, (RUL) right upper lobe carina, (ML) middle lobe carina, (LUL) left upper lobe carina, S6 carina. This procedure was carried out five times for each physician and the FLE determined subsequently. The results are listed in table 1. To visualize the TRE associated with point-based registration, error ellipsoids corresponding to SPN positions were computed in a Monte Carlo simulation based on the FLE determined in the experiment (see figure 1).

Table 1. Standard deviation for a selection of anatomical landmarks in CT and tracking space. In the CT half the element spacing $[0.47, 0.47, 2.0]$ was added.

	Main C.	RUL C.	ML C.	LUL C.	S6 C.	All
	STD Anatomical Landmarks CT Space (in mm)					
$\begin{pmatrix} x \\ y \\ z \end{pmatrix}$	$\begin{pmatrix} 0.924 \\ 0.987 \\ 1.720 \end{pmatrix}$	$\begin{pmatrix} 0.978 \\ 1.241 \\ 1.791 \end{pmatrix}$	$\begin{pmatrix} 1.033 \\ 5.465 \\ 8.235 \end{pmatrix}$	$\begin{pmatrix} 1.072 \\ 0.697 \\ 1.559 \end{pmatrix}$	$\begin{pmatrix} 0.777 \\ 0.812 \\ 1.562 \end{pmatrix}$	$\begin{pmatrix} 0.964 \\ 2.664 \\ 4.290 \end{pmatrix}$
	\multicolumn STD Anatomical Landmarks Tracking Space (in mm)					
$\begin{pmatrix} x \\ y \\ z \end{pmatrix}$	$\begin{pmatrix} 2.647 \\ 0.792 \\ 1.364 \end{pmatrix}$	$\begin{pmatrix} 0.741 \\ 0.499 \\ 0.737 \end{pmatrix}$	$\begin{pmatrix} 0.522 \\ 0.635 \\ 0.622 \end{pmatrix}$	$\begin{pmatrix} 0.355 \\ 0.399 \\ 0.354 \end{pmatrix}$	$\begin{pmatrix} 1.044 \\ 0.988 \\ 0.364 \end{pmatrix}$	$\begin{pmatrix} 1.345 \\ 0.695 \\ 0.781 \end{pmatrix}$

2.2 ICP-Based Registration

ICP was originally developed by Besl and McKay [11] to match two point clouds by iteratively minimizing the distances between point correspondences. The algorithm proceeds iteratively in two steps until convergence. At first establishing correspondences between spatial entities, in this specific case triangulated airways surface data or extracted centerlines from a CT and the trajectory, followed by estimation of a rigid transformation based on the correspondences that best maps one entity on the other. Subsequently, the transformation is applied to the trajectory points, aligning the respective entities closer. The underlying model for the approach assumes that the trajectory runs closely along the centerline or surface, respectively. However, this is not a realistic constraint, since the bronchoscope can move arbitrarily within the airways.

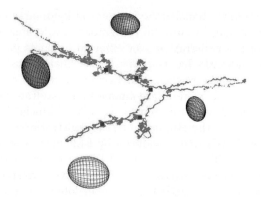

Fig. 1. TRE ellipsoids for exemplary SPNs. Squares indicate fiducial locations used

2.3   In-Volume Maximization Algorithm

During a pulmonary intervention the primary airways are initially examined using a bronchoscope. The covered path of the bronchoscope is tracked by an EMT system, which forms a three-dimensional trajectory. After the acquisition of the trajectory the in-volume maximization (IVM) algorithm optimally fits the trajectory into the segmented airways of the CT volume. Compared to the common approaches, IVM takes the most advantage of the current medical workflow and in contrast to ICP imposes no further constraints. The procedure consists of three steps: initialization, optimization and registration.

Initialization. Prior to optimization using non-linear techniques, the trajectory has to be roughly aligned with the CT data set. Therefore, we determine the approximate main carina location and spatial orientation of each entity (trajectory and CT). Given the natural constraint that the examination starts and ends within the trachea, its location can be recovered easily. Having estimated the trachea position, we approximate its direction by PCA regression. The main carina location coincides with one of the two ends of the trachea. A similar procedure is applied to the segmented CT data using PCA or the extracted centerline for recovering the orientation of trachea and the position of both main carina and RUL. The latter is identified by the anatomical property of the right main bronchus being wider, shorter and more vertical than the left one.

Let $R_{CT}, R_{trajectory} \in \mathbb{R}^{3x3}$ denote the matrices containing the orthogonal direction vectors in CT and recorded trajectory data, respectively. Further, let $t_{CT}, t_{trajectory} \in \mathbb{R}^3$ be the main carina position in the two data sets. We compute the initial transformation $T=\begin{pmatrix} R & t \\ \mathbf{0} & 1 \end{pmatrix} \in \mathbb{R}^{4x4}$ that maps the trajectory to the corresponding position in the CT, where $R = R_{CT}R_{trajectory}^t$ and $t = t_{CT} - R \cdot t_{trajectory}$.

Optimization. The IVM algorithm estimates the transformation that maximizes the number of trajectory points lying within the segmented airways volume after applying the transformation matrix. The accuracy of the EM sensor position measurements is influenced by many factors, among others, magnetic field distortion, sensor velocity and acceleration. Thus the permanent quality fluctuation should be accounted for in the cost function. Assuming that we can measure the degree of uncertainty at which a trajectory point is acquired, we weight each point within the cost function such that the target is biased favoring points fitted into the volume with low uncertainty.

Let $\mathcal{X} = \{x_i\}, x_i \in \mathbb{R}^3$ be the trajectory and x be an arbitrary point with measurement uncertainty ϵ_i, then we define a weight function $g : \mathbb{R}^3 \mapsto \mathbb{R}$ with $g(x_i) = \epsilon_i^{-1}$.

We determine the transformation T that maximizes the number of trajectory points located within the segmented airways volume. For measuring the quality of a registration step, we define a ratio-based cost function, penalizing trajectory points moving out of the airways of the registered CT data. This is, however, an assumption, which is valid only in the absence of noise and organ deformation.

Furthermore, let $M(\mathcal{X})_{in}$ denote the set of trajectory points after applying the transformation that are tested to be inside the airways. $M(\mathcal{X})_{out}$ are respectively the points tested to be outside the segmented volume. Additionally, let S be the ratio of trajectory points inside the segmented airways volume given the EM trajectory $\mathcal{X}$ and a transformation matrix T. Then the cost function $S(T, \mathcal{X}) : \mathbb{R}^{4 \times 4} \times \{\mathbb{R}^3\} \mapsto [0, 1]$ is defined as,

$$S(T, \mathcal{X}) = \frac{\sum_{x \in M(\mathcal{X})_{in}} g(x)}{\sum_{x \in M(\mathcal{X})_{in}} g(x) + \sum_{x \in M(\mathcal{X})_{out}} g(x)} \tag{1}$$

Let T^* be the transformation, which maximizes the number of trajectory points lying within the airways:

$$T^* = \max_T S(T, \mathcal{X}) \tag{2}$$

T^* is determined iteratively using an optimizer. Here we have a six-dimensional search space (3DOF translation, 3DOF rotation) and generally numerous local minima. To avoid convergence at a local minimum, a robust optimization algorithm is needed. Our first choice was the Simulated Annealing Simplex (SAS) algorithm, which is a modified version of the standard simplex in combination with simulated annealing. It is initiated with a virtual temperature of 10^6 that is lowered by 20% every two iterations. Occasionally the annealing procedure is restarted.

3   Navigation System Setup

For tracking of the bronchoscope (BF-1T180, Olympus) within the airways an EMT system was used (3D Guidance; Ascension Technology Corporation; Burlington, VT, USA). The setup contained a metal immune flat panel field generator and two minimized receiver sensors (diameter, 1.3 mm; length, 6.7 mm). Within the defined tracking volume of 400 x 400 x 460 mm, the 6DOF pose of each sensor is measured. One sensor is encapsulated in the tip of the

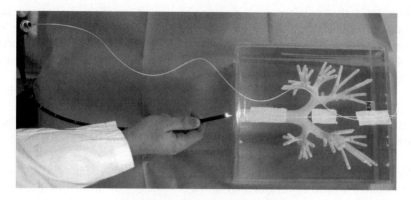

Fig. 2. The system setup for the bronchoscope navigation system. The flat panel field generator of the tracking system is positioned under the phantom. An EMT sensor is mounted on the tip of the bronchoscope.

bronchoscope. A second sensor is attached onto the surface of the phantom, approximately above the sternum. It is used as reference coordinate system. Thus, spontaneous transmitter and phantom patient motion can be compensated. We used a rubber lung dummy molded in silicone for our experiments.

4   Experiments and Results

In order to compare the registration performance of different algorithms we conducted a series of experiments. We acquired high resolution CT data of our phantom and segmented the airways up to the fourth bifurcation using a standard graph cuts algorithm. Subsequently, a centerline graph of the bronchial tree was extracted from the segmented airways. In the examination room experienced pneumologists performed a point-based registration (see section 2.1) selecting corresponding natural landmarks in the CT dataset and within the tracking space guided by the video of the bronchoscope. Furthermore, they performed a regular examination with the video bronchoscope throughout the entire visible bronchial tree with an attached EM sensor. The trajectory during this examination was recorded. In course of the experiments, we performed the initialization (see section 2.3), the ICP to the surface of the segmented model and its centerline (see section 2.2), and finally the IVM approach (see section 2.3).

The criterion to measure the quality of the registration is the percentage of recorded trajectory points inside the segmented bronchial tree after applying the transformation matrix. The point-based registration yields between 17 - 64%. With the initialization we achieve between 13 - 75%. The optimization using surface ICP achieves between 28 - 64%, using centerline ICP between 72 - 93%, and finally our IVM achieves between 75 - 97%. Table 2 shows the results of each trial of the experiments in detail. The computational time for both IVM and ICP registration took 2 to 5 minutes on a Intel Pentium M 1.73 GHz machine with 1 GByte of RAM.

Table 2. Registration performance for different registration algorithms. Indicated is the percentage of trajectory points inside the segmented airways volume after applying the various estimated registration transformations.

Experiment No.	Registration Method				
	Point-based	Initial	Surface ICP	Centerline ICP	In-Volume Max
1.	27	30	40	83	93
2.	64	20	52	72	75
3.	28	50	28	93	96
4.	18	59	62	88	97
5.	17	13	64	92	95
6.	31	30	58	85	86
7.	49	75	61	92	94
8.	37	28	64	89	96
9.	29	25	54	82	91
10.	31	35	55	86	92

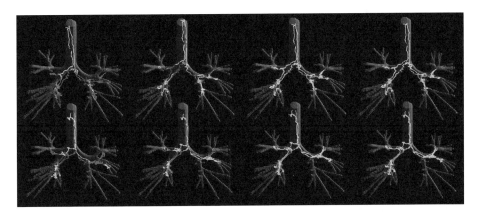

Fig. 3. Trajectories 4. and 8. from table 2 after registration. From left to right: point-based, surface ICP, centerline ICP and IVM. Bright spots are located inside the airways volume, gray ones outside.

5   Conclusion and Discussion

The low diagnostic success rate for SPNs without the support of navigation systems, especially crucial for peripheral SPNs with a diameter below $2cm$, facilitates the development of new methods. Various systems were proposed for navigation of a transbronchial biopsy needle within the previously acquired CT data by means of EMT. Standard procedures mainly employ point-based registration, which is often error prone and thus failing to provide the necessary accuracy. We showed in our experiments that registration can be based on the usage of an acquired EM trajectory data recorded during routine examination. Our developed IVM method smoothly integrates into the clinical workflow and improves the overall estimated accuracy. For the upcoming in-vivo tests, breathing and deformation will be an issue. A third sensor that is capable of tracking the respiratory state will allow to perform gated registration. The registration using the entire trajectory information is one further step towards a robust and non-rigid system for NB.

Acknowledgement. We thank Dr. K. Klingenbeck-Regn, Siemens Medical AX for the financial support and furthermore, Dr. F. Peltz for conducting experiments.

References

1. Parkin, D.M., Bray, F., Ferlay, J., Pisani, P.: Global Cancer Statistics, 2002. CA Cancer J. Clin. 55(2), 74–108 (2005)
2. Jemal, A., Siegel, R., Ward, E., Murray, T., Xu, J., Thun, M.J.: Cancer statistics, 2007. CA Cancer J. Clin. 57, 43–66 (2007)
3. Baaklini, W.A., Reinoso, M.A., Gorin, A.B.: Diagnostic yield of fiberoptic bronchoscopy in evaluating solitary pulmonary nodules. Chest 117, 1049–1054 (2000)
4. Hautmann, H., Schneider, A., Pinkau, T., Peltz, F., Feussner, H.: Electromagnetic catheter navigation during bronchoscopy: Validation of a novel method by conventional fluoroscopy. Chest 128, 382–387 (2005)
5. Solomon, S.B., White Jr., P., Wiener, C.M., Orens, J.B., Wang, K.P.: Three-dimensional ct-guided bronchoscopy with a real-time electromagnetic position sensor: A comparison of two image registration methods. Chest 118, 1783–1787 (2000)
6. Schwarz, Y., Greif, J., Becker, H.D., Ernst, A., Mehta, A.: Real-Time Electromagnetic Navigation Bronchoscopy to Peripheral Lung Lesions Using Overlaid CT Images: The First Human Study. Chest 129(4), 988–994 (2006)
7. Wegner, I., Biederer, J., Tetzlaff, R., Wolf, I., Meinzer, H.: Evaluation and extension of a navigation system for bronchoscopy inside human lungs. In: SPIE Medical Imaging (2007)
8. Wegner, I., Vetter, M., Schoebinger, M., Wolf, I., Meinzer, H.P.: Development of a navigation system for endoluminal brachytherapy in human lungs. SPIE Medical Imaging 6141, 23–30 (2006)
9. Deguchi, D., Ishitani, K., Kitasaka, T., Mori, K., Suenaga, Y., Takabatake, H., Mori, M., Natori, H.: A method for bronchoscope tracking using position sensor without fiducial markers. In: SPIE Medical Imaging (2007)
10. Fitzpatrick, J.M., West, J.B., Maurer, C.R.J.: Predicting error in rigid-body point-based registration. IEEE Trans. on Medical Imaging 14(5), 694–702 (1998)
11. Besl, P.J., McKay, N.D.: A method for registration of 3-d shapes. IEEE Trans. Pattern Anal. Machine Intell. 14(2), 239–256 (1992)

Automatic Target and Trajectory Identification for Deep Brain Stimulation (DBS) Procedures

Ting Guo[1,3], Andrew G. Parrent[2], and Terry M. Peters[1,3]

[1] Robarts Research Institute and University of Western Ontario
[2] The London Health Sciences Centre, Department of Neurosurgery
London, Ontario, Canada N6A 5K8
[3] Biomedical Engineering Graduate Program, University of Western Ontario
London, Ontario, Canada N6A 5B9
{tguo,tpeters}@imaging.robarts.ca

Abstract. This paper presents an automatic surgical target and trajectory identification technique for planning deep brain stimulation (DBS) procedures. The probabilistic functional maps, constructed from population-based actual stimulating field information and intra-operative electrophysiological activities, were integrated into a neurosurgical visualization and navigation system to facilitate the surgical planning and guidance. In our preliminary studies, we compared the actual surgical target locations and trajectories established by an experienced stereotactic neurosurgeon with those automatically planned using our probabilistic functional maps on 10 subthalamic nucleus (STN) DBS procedures. The average displacement between the surgical target locations in both groups was 1.82mm with a standard deviation of 0.77mm. The difference between the surgical trajectories was 3.1 ° and 2.3 ° in the lateral-to-medial and anterior-to-posterior orientations respectively.

1 Introduction

Deep brain stimulation (DBS) eliminates abnormally patterned activity from certain nuclei by implanting a multi-electrode stimulator into a specific midbrain structure where continuous high frequency electrical stimulation generated by a neuro-pacemaker is delivered [1]. Accurate implantation of the stimulator is critical to achieve the optimal surgical outcome, because small deviations in the electrode positioning may cause muscle contraction, speech and language disorders, ocular deviation, and visual defects [1,2]. In clinical practice, due to the inadequacy of the anatomical and functional information available pre-operatively, invasive electrophysiological measurements must be obtained intra-operatively with multiple exploratory electrodes to facilitate the mapping of functionally distinct deep brain structures and the identification of the optimal surgical target [1].

In addition to direct targeting on standard pre-operative medical images, rigid or non-rigid alignment of the digitized stereotactic atlases [3] with patient-specific pre-operative brain images is often utilized to assist the target identification. However the inherent limitations of current anatomical brain atlases may limit their applicability. Recently, Yelnik et al described a 3D deformable histological atlas of the human

N. Ayache, S. Ourselin, A. Maeder (Eds.): MICCAI 2007, Part I, LNCS 4791, pp. 483–490, 2007.
© Springer-Verlag Berlin Heidelberg 2007

basal ganglia [4] that contained functional information derived from immuno-histochemical studies. In addition, functional atlases [5,6] and databases [7] containing intra-operatively acquired subcortical electrophysiology from a number of patients have been implemented to complement the anatomical and histological atlases. Precise localization of the target is more likely to be achieved with the assistance of pre-operatively available electrophysiological information [7].

This paper focuses on constructing 3D probabilistic maps of functional data and integrating these maps into our neurosurgical system to accomplish automatic target and trajectory identification for DBS procedures. The optimal trajectory is identified with a probabilistic approach that maximizes the possibility of treatment efficacy while minimizing that of side effects. Preliminary studies were conducted to evaluate the effectiveness of this technique in surgical target and trajectory identification for subthalamic nucleus (STN) DBS procedures. Representing spatial distribution of population-based actual target stimulation information and deep-brain electro-physiological activities, novel probabilistic maps incorporated into our neurosurgical system, after non-rigidly aligned to a patient brain space prior to surgery, can provide robust and accurate automatic initialization of the surgical target and trajectory.

2   Materials and Methods

2.1   Image Registration

Frame-to-Image: The image-to-patient registration is achieved with a 0.5mm fiducial localization error (FLE) using an automatic frame-to-image registration procedure.

Post-operative-to-Pre-operative: The post- and pre-operative images are registered using a rigid registration that maximizes a cross-correlation metric to map the final DBS electrode placement information from the post- to the pre-operative image.

Functional Data Mapping: We employ a fast and completely unsupervised multi-resolution registration approach, AtamaiWarp [8], to generate the three-dimensional transformation matrix and warp grid describing the voxel to voxel mapping between each patient pre-operative image and a standard brain template.

2.2   Data Preparation

MR image acquisition: The pre- and post-operative MR images of 52 STN DBS procedures (26 left and 26 right) were acquired with a 3D SPGR sequence on a 1.5T GE Signa scanner (TR/TE 8.9/1.9ms, FA 20°, voxel size 1.17×1.17×1mm^3, in-slice resolution 256×256).

Electrode and stimulation field modeling: A B-spline based method allows a smooth contour of the DBS electrode (Medtronic 3389, Medtronic Inc., Minneapolis, MN, USA) on the post-operative image to be created with user defined control points. Theoretically, a patient specific electrical stimulation model [9] considering the tissue conductivity properties would describe the stimulation field distribution more accurately, however due to the unavailability of diffusion tensor imaging data for the patients recruited in this study it is not feasible for us to have such models. Assuming electrostatic, homogeneous, and isotropic tissue properties, we modeled the electrical stimulation field around the electrode as a Gaussian function (FWHM = 1mm). We discretized this function onto a 3D rectilinear grid ($6.3 \times 6.3 \times 1.5 \text{mm}^3$) with 0.1 mm isotropic cell size centered at the region of the electrode. The grid cells within and on the surface of the electrode were assigned a unit scalar value. Those surrounding cells representing the decreasing stimulation field have their values allocated as indicated by the calculated field strength.

Collection of intra-operative functional data: The intra-operative electrophysiological recording and stimulation data acquired during each procedure were coded in standard form and saved in patient MR image-space. Subsequently the annotated codes of intra-operative functional data were collected to the standard database using the resultant non-rigid transform from the third registration step. The inverse of the deformation grid was then used to map the data in the population-based database from the reference brain template back to an individual brain image.

2.3 Probabilistic Functional Map Construction

Two classes of probabilistic maps were generated to describe spatial distribution of population-based actual surgical target stimulation information and deep-brain intra-operative electrophysiological activities respectively.

The target and stimulation information map (**Fig. 1**) was computed based on the electrode and stimulation field models. First, the 3D grid file representing the electrode and stimulation field created on the post-operative image of each patient was rigidly registered to the pre-operative image-space of the same patient. Then a large rectilinear grid ($30 \times 30 \times 20 \text{mm}^3$) with the same cell size was created in the standard brain image-space and the cells were initialized to zero. When the discrete grid file of each patient is non-rigidly mapped to the standard coordinate system, it is superimposed over the large grid. Those grid cells overlapping non-rigid warped patient grid cells have their values incremented accordingly.

Adopting the collection of intra-operative stimulation measurements, we created two electrical stimulation maps ($50 \times 50 \times 50 \text{mm}^3$). One map incorporates the functional data relating to suppression of Parkinson's disease (PD) symptoms, while the other integrates data relating to side effects. The map grid cells overlapping the electrical stimulation data from the database have their values assigned and increased according to the stimulation parameters of the functional data. The assigned value is inversely proportional to the stimulation amplitude.

The intra-operative micro-recording data representing the characteristic signals of the STN were integrated into another functional map. A small grid ($10 \times 10 \times 10 \text{mm}^3$) covering the STN area of the standard brain template was generated. Since the micro-recording data have uniform parameters, the scalar value of each cell in the grid is determined only by the spatial frequency of the data presence.

We adopted Kriging interpolation [10] to generate the final probabilistic functional maps. Kriging, also called optimal spatial linear prediction, is capable of making inferences on unobserved values from data observed at known spatial locations. Kriging interpolation uses those grid cells with scalar values greater than a specified threshold to estimate the possible values for the rest grid cells. The minimum and maximum scalar values on each probabilistic functional map were set to zero and one respectively, and the remaining values within the range were normalized accordingly. Maximizing the use of the functional data available in our databases, the final three-dimensional probabilistic functional maps consisting of both the actual observed data and the optimal estimation values can be warped to a patient brain prior to surgery to predict the surgical target and trajectory.

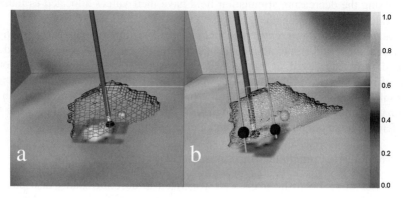

Fig. 1. The standard brain template (left) and a patient brain (right) are displayed by the neurosurgical system. The probabilistic map of surgical target and stimulation information is registered and fused with each image. The color map: probabilistic functional map on which the region in yellow indicates the optimal surgical target location. Dark line: central electrode whose tip is at the actual surgical target position; Bright lines: other four trajectories of "Ben-gun" electrode assembly; Mesh objects: segmented and registered STN in standard brain and a patient brain space; Bright yellow spheres: centroids of STN.

3   Clinical Application

The standard technique practiced by neurosurgeons at our institution for identifying the surgical target includes the combination of direct and indirect targeting strategies. In addition, the trajectory is determined based on the patient's cortical and subcortical anatomy as well as primary vasculature distribution on the pre-operative image to ensure reasonable trajectory entry point and procedure safety. Intra-operatively, the neurosurgeon employs a five-electrode assembly ("Ben-gun") to acquire deep brain electro-physiological information and refine target localization. On the other hand, our neurosurgical planning system [7] estimates the surgical target and trajectory automatically using the probabilistic functional maps described in the previous section. The surgical target location is initially defined as the grid cell with the greatest scalar value in the target and stimulation information map. The average scalar value of grid cells on a trajectory extending 10 mm above and below this target position at different orientation (lateral-medial: 0°-30° and anterior-posterior: 40°-90°) is computed. The trajectory with the highest value on the PD symptom relief map and the lowest on the side effect inducing map is considered the optimal trajectory (**Fig. 2**). Our trajectory identification approach is capable of eliminating any trajectory crossing the lateral ventricle and any sulcus by calculating the image intensity value of each voxel along and around the trajectory on the pre-operative patient brain image.

Therefore the appropriate entry point can be selected to ensure safety of the surgery. For each of the ten STN DBS cases (5 left and 5 right), we compared the automatically estimated target and trajectory with those identified by the neurosurgeon using standard clinical practice.

4 Results

4.1 Surgical Targeting Accuracy Analysis

As demonstrated in our previous work [7], stereotactic targeting of the STN using the registered actual surgical target data (centroid of the target cluster) provides less than 2.5mm localization error. Therefore we employed the probabilistic functional map containing population-based actual DBS electrode and stimulation field information to predict the surgical target positions. Because of the large sample size for Kriging interpolation, accurate predication of map values at locations where there are no previous patient data available can be accomplished. **Table 1** shows that the target locations estimated using this probabilistic map are on average 0.63 mm, 0.68 mm, and 0.75 mm away from the neurosurgeon-determined targets in x, y, and z directions respectively for the ten STN DBS procedures, indicating accurate initialization of the surgical target. As distinct from previous targeting techniques [7], this approach employing multiple population-based probabilistic functional maps containing a large number of stimulation field and functional activity data is completely unsupervised and yields higher reproducibility and less variance in target identification.

Table 1. Absolute differences between the probabilistic functional map-initialized and the real surgical targets (x: left-right; y: posterior-anterior, z: inferior-superior)

Difference	x	y	z	d(x,y,z)
Avg. (mm)	0.63	0.68	0.75	1.82
Max (mm)	1.76	1.51	1.39	3.15
Min (mm)	0.10	0.22	0.31	0.58
Sd (mm)	0.67	0.52	0.44	0.77

4.2 Surgical Trajectory Identification

A well-planned DBS trajectory ideally encounters stimulation responsive units that reduce tremor, rigidity, and bradykinesia, while avoiding units causing side effects. To identify the optimal surgical trajectory, our neurosurgical system searches the

Table 2. Absolute differences between the trajectory orientation angles estimated with probabilistic functional maps and those of real trajectories

Difference	Anterior-Posterior	Lateral-Medial
Avg. (°)	3.1	2.3
Max (°)	4.5	4
Min (°)	0	0
Sd (°)	1.8	1.5

functional map relating to PD symptom relief and that eliciting side effects. The final orientation of the trajectory is determined by the average scalar values of grid cells encountered by the tract (20 mm) centered at the established optimal surgical target on the two maps. High values on the first map and low values on the second are preferred. Most trajectories are 10° to 15° in a lateral-to-medial orientation and 45° to 70° anterior-to-posterior. **Table 2** reports the absolute difference in the two directions between the optimal trajectories predicted by the probabilistic electrophysiological maps and those identified by the neurosurgeon. In clinical practice, deep brain electrophysiological activity data, used to delineate functional borders and the surgical target, are obtained through only limited number of intra-operative trajectories. However the probabilistic functional maps can take advantage of the population based deep brain measurements. Hence the trajectory estimated with the maps is a result of more comprehensive analysis of electrophysiology.

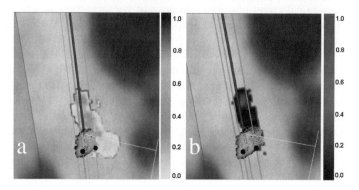

Fig. 2. Left: The functional map relating to PD symptom relief; Right: The functional map relating to side effects; Mesh objects: segmented STN

4.3 Micro-Recording Data Defined STN

Although the anterior portion of the STN can be seen on the T_2-weighted images, the distortion observed on T_2-weighted images and the lack of visibility of the posterior STN may limit their targeting efficacy. The probabilistic map, generated using the collection of characteristic signals of the STN observed during micro-recording processes, provides a functional representation of the STN. Grid cells with actual or predicted scalar values greater than 0.8 were considered to lie within the functional STN. We compared the centroid location of the functional STN and the real surgical target for each of the ten procedures. As the dorsolateral portion of STN is considered

Table 3. Absolute differences between the centroid locations of functional STN and the real surgical targets (x: left-right; y: posterior-anterior; z: inferior-superior)

Difference	x	y	z	d(x,y,z)
Avg. (mm)	1.32	1.81	0.80	2.63
Max (mm)	2.17	2.79	1.26	3.21
Min (mm)	0.15	0.08	0.10	0.96
Sd (mm)	0.71	1.06	0.32	0.75

the ideal surgical target position at our institution, average absolute difference of 2.63 mm between the surgical target and the STN centroid is reasonable (Table 3). Their spatial correlation is preserved for 80 percent of the cases.

5 Discussion

In this paper, we presented the construction of three-dimensional probabilistic maps of actual surgical target stimulation information and intra-operative functional data. Preliminary studies were conducted to assess the efficacy of target and trajectory prediction for ten STN DBS procedures. The results indicate that the probabilistic functional maps, integrated within our neurosurgical visualization and navigation system [7], facilitate completely automatic identification of surgical target and trajectory for individual patients prior to surgery. We also demonstrated the spatial correlation between the actual surgical target and the centroid of functional STN based on the probabilistic micro-recording data. Constructed with the spatial distribution data of stimulation and electrode contact, another probabilistic STN atlas contributed by Nowinski et al involves a great number of input data [11]. The part of this functional STN with medium and high probabilities correlates well with the anatomical STN derived from the Schaltenbrand-Wahren brain atlas [11]. Our probabilistic functional map for surgical target identification was calculated not only considering the DBS electrode, but also the probable electrical stimulation field. It is necessary to include the electrical stimulation information, since axons within 2.5 mm from the center of the electrode may be activated by monopolar stimulation [12]. Some studies demonstrated that brain shift and deformation caused by cerebrospinal fluid (CSF) leak occurring during DBS surgery around the functional target region is trivial (< 1mm) and does not affect the accuracy of target localization performed on pre-operative image space [13]. However, a more recent work by Pollo et al. [14] revealed displacement of the electrode in the distal direction that may be due to the patient position change, CSF leakage, and cannula and /or electrode insertion during image acquisition and surgical procedure. This issue should be further studied to quantify the influence of each contributive factor and eventually correct the possible brain shift. Three-dimensional probabilistic functional maps containing the actual intra-operatively obtained data at known locations and optimally predicted data generated by Kriging interpolation at the remaining areas enable comprehensive quantitative analysis of the surgical target and trajectory. The neurosurgical system saves target location, trajectory orientation, and the average scalar values of grid cells encountered by the trajectory centered at the optimal surgical target on the functional maps in a text file for additional evaluation. Although the system incorporating the probabilistic functional maps makes fully automatic surgical target and trajectory estimation feasible, thorough validation studies must nevertheless be carried out within a clinical context. In our ongoing studies we will obtain clinical information, analyze the correlation between the surgical target location and the surgical outcome, and re-present our previously conducted analysis with respect to the actual clinical evaluation data. Once this automatic surgical target and trajectory identification technique is clinically validated, the neurosurgeon at our institution would employ it for the planning and guidance of DBS procedures.

Acknowledgements. The authors acknowledge the financial support from CIHR, ORDCF, CFI, and OIT.

References

1. Machado, A., Rezai, A.R., Kopell, B.H., Gross, R.E., Sharan, A.D., Benabid, A.L.: Deep Brain Stimulation for Parkinson's Disease: Surgical Technique and Perioperative Management. Mov. Disord. 21(suppl. 14), S247–S258 (2006)
2. Halpern, C., Hurtig, H., Jaggi, J., Grossman, M., Won, M., Baltuch, G.: Deep brain stimulation in neurologic disorders. Parkinsonism Relat. Disord. 13, 1–16 (2007)
3. Ganser, K.A., Dickhaus, H., Metzner, R., Wirtz, C.R.: A deformable digital brain atlas system according to Talairach and Tournoux. Med. Imag. Analy. 8, 3–22 (2004)
4. Yelnik, J., Bardinet, E., Dormont, D., Malandain, G., Ourselin, S., Tande, D., Karachi, C., Ayache, N., Cornu, P., Agid, Y.: A three-dimensional, histological and deformable atlas of the human basal ganglia. I. Atlas construction based on immunohistochemical and MRI data. NeuroImage 34, 618–638 (2007)
5. D'Haese, P.F., Cetinkaya, E., Konrad, P.E., Kao, C., Dawant, B.M.: Computer-aided placement of deep brain stimulators: from planning to intraoperative guidance. IEEE Trans. Med. Imag. 24(11), 1469–1478 (2005)
6. Chakravarty, M.M., Sadikot, A.F., Mongia, S., Bertrand, G., Collins, D.L.: Towards a multi-modal atlas for neurosurgical planning. In: Larsen, R., Nielsen, M., Sporring, J. (eds.) MICCAI 2006. LNCS, vol. 4191, pp. 389–396. Springer, Heidelberg (2006)
7. Guo, T., Finnis, K.W., Deoni, S.C.L., Parrent, A.G., Peters, T.M.: Comparison of different targeting methods for subthalamic nucleus deep brain stimulation. In: Larsen, R., Nielsen, M., Sporring, J. (eds.) MICCAI 2006. LNCS, vol. 4190, pp. 768–775. Springer, Heidelberg (2006)
8. Guo, T., Starreveld, Y.P., Peters, T.M.: Evaluation and validation methods for intersubject non-rigid 3D image registration of the human brain. Proc. SPIE Medical Imaging 5744, 594–603 (2005)
9. Butson, C.R., Cooper, S.E., Henderson, J.M., McIntyre, C.C.: Patient-specific analysis of the volume of tissue activated during deep brain stimulation. NeuroImage 34, 661–670 (2007)
10. Cressie, N.A.C.: Statistics for Spatial Data. A Wiley-Interscience Publication, Chichester (1991)
11. Nowinski, W.L., Thirunavuukarasuu, A., Liu, J., Benabid, A.L.: Correlation between the anatomical and functional human subthalamic nucleus. Stereotact. Funct. Neurosurg. 85, 88–93 (2007)
12. Wu, Y.R., Levy, R., Ashby, P., Tasker, R.R., Dostrovsky, J.O.: Does stimulation of the GPi control dyskinesia by activating inhibitory axons. Mov. Disord. 16, 208–216 (2001)
13. Bardinet, É., Cathier, P., Roche, A., Ayache, N., Dormont, D.: A Posteriori Validation of Pre-operative Planning in Functional Neurosurgery by Quantification of Brain Pneumocephalus. In: Dohi, T., Kikinis, R. (eds.) MICCAI 2002. LNCS, vol. 2488, pp. 323–330. Springer, Heidelberg (2002)
14. Pollo, C., Vingerhoets, F., Pralong, E., Ghika, J., Makder, P., Meuli, R., Thiran, J.P., Villemure, J.G.: Localization of electrodes in the subthalamic nucleus on magnetic resonance imaging. J. Neurosurg. 106, 36–44 (2007)

Application of Open Source Image Guided Therapy Software in MR-guided Therapies

Nobuhiko Hata[1], Steve Piper[2], Ferenc A Jolesz[1], Clare MC Tempany[1],
Peter McL Black[2], Shigehiro Morikawa[3], Horoshi Iseki[4], Makoto Hashizume[5],
and Ron Kikinis[1]

[1] National Center for Image-guided Therapy, Department of Radiology,
Brigham and Women's Hospital and Harvard Medical School
hata@bwh.harvard.edu
[2] Department of Neurosurgery, Brigham and Women's Hospital
and Harvard Medical School
[3] Shiga Medical University
[4] Tokyo Women's Medical University
[5] Kyusyu University*

Abstract. We present software engineering methods to provide free open-source software for MR-guided therapy. We report that graphical representation of the surgical tools, interconnectively with the tracking device, patient-to-image registration, and MRI-based thermal mapping are crucial components of MR-guided therapy in sharing such software. Software process includes a network-based distribution mechanism by multi-platform compiling tool CMake, CVS, quality assurance software DART. We developed six procedures in four separate clinical sites using proposed software engineering and process, and found the proposed method is feasible to facilitate multicenter clinical trial of MR-guided therapies. Our future studies include use of the software in non-MR-guided therapies.

1 Introduction

Among image-guided therapy (IGT) tools, MR-guided therapy is a widely used option as evidenced by the more than 400 articles published in a literature database. We have even observed the acceleration of its prevalence since clinicians started to use diagnostic close-bore scanners in surgery.

However, the active development of new MR-guided therapy option is restricted in the scope of procedures, sites of implementation, and most importantly lack of flexibility in enabling software tools. The long-term goals of improving interventional and surgical procedures and attendant outcomes, reducing costs, and achieving broad utilization of software tools can be achieved by identifying the commonality of the enabling software and developing a software framework that can dynamically accommodate the specific needs of applications.

* Supporting grant: 5P41RR013218, 5P01CA067165,5U41RR019703, 5R01CA109246, 1R01CA111288, 5U54EB005149 from NIH, NSF 9731748, CIMIT, METI.

N. Ayache, S. Ourselin, A. Maeder (Eds.): MICCAI 2007, Part I, LNCS 4791, pp. 491–498, 2007.
© Springer-Verlag Berlin Heidelberg 2007

Such software should be open-source and proprietary free so that the openness lets programmers obtain, critique, use, and build upon the source code without licensing fees [1]. A similar model for sharing software has been actively developed in bioinformatics domain [2 , 3]. The open source software for bioinformatics has made it easier to create customized pipelines or analysis in gene expression study, or tailored medicine. There is no question that bioinformatics has embraced open source software and has been benefited from them in developing new methods.

Our objective in this paper is to present software engineering methods to share the commonality of software tools and provide robust testing, documenting, and version control mechanism in computer-enhanced MR-guided therapies. We refined these engineering methods over 2,000 cases of MR-guided brain, prostate, and liver therapies in four separate clinical centers by sharing the software platform but developing unique clinical applications in each centers. We used the 3D Slicer (www.slicer.org) originally developed for medical image processing, but modified to fit the needs of MR-guided therapy for this study. Our engineering challenge was to find the most commonality among the applications in different sites, while ensuring the flexibility to develop unique IGT application in those site with minimum overhead. The methods presented here contain summery of commonality we found over the course of clinical cases as well as unique enabling tools for each site's application.

2 Extending Medical Image Processing Software for MR-guided Therapy

We extended 3D Slicer [4] for MR-guided therapy to develop enabling software for MR-guided ablation therapy at four clinical sites. The 3D Slicer is freely available, open-source software for visualization, registration, segmentation, and quantification of medical data for diagnostic purposes. In addition to native tools originally developed for medical image processing, we developed tools and visualization methods useful for MR-guided therapies.

Fiducial/Locator. We prepared common graphical representation of tools specific to MR-guided therapy. Those models include fiducial points with arbitrarily changeable diameter and the locator representing the tracking wand. The locator model is mostly used to represent the digitally tracked wand; in-bore MR-guided surgery uses the optical tracking sensor placed over the area, and out-of-bore MR-guided surgery uses an optical tracking sensor placed outside the bore. In addition to mouse-controlled slice selection, the 3D Slicer provides slice selection using the locator, i.e. digital wand; this is the most common use of a digital wand in navigation software during surgery.

Users can define fiducial points in the three-dimensional space in both 2D image planes and 3D graphics scenes using a mouse pointer or digital wand. For instance, Morikawa et al. used fiducials to mark an ablated lesion in a liver during MR-guided microwave therapy [5]; in brain surgery at Brigham and Women's

Hospital, we used the fiducials for marking a cortical stimulation point on the cortex and compared them with the images.

Interconnectivity to Tracking Device. The 3D Slicer communicates with an external device in various formats. A relatively simple TCP/IP-based client/ server communication package has been in use in MR-guided interventions to retrieve updated images and the coordinates of digital wands[6]. A similar approach was used in linking the 3D Slicer to commercial navigation software, in which the coordinates of the tracker are shared between the two. In one study at Brigham and Women's Hospital, the optical tracking sensor is directly accessed from a module of the 3D Slicer, without client/server communication [6].

Patient-to-image Registration. The 3D Slicer provides patient-to-image registration using fiducial markers; a set of fiducials digitized by an external sensor is coupled with image-based digitization to estimate conversion matrix from physical (patient)-coordinate system to image coordinate system. The 3D Slicer provides digitization tools both for the external sensors and images using fiducial markers as the basis for user interaction.

Native image-to-image registration can also be used in MR-guided therapy by fusing a preoperative information-rich image to an intraoperative image, or by fusing the sequence of intraoperative images. Note that the users can bypass the fiducial placement if the optical tracking sensor is calibrated to the imager and confined in the image coordinate system.

Thermal Mapping. MRI can provide a thermal map for ablation therapy and monitor the extent of heat perfusion during microwave or laser-ablation therapy. The combination of stereotactic guidance using preoperative and preprocedural images and thermal mapping is useful to control the ablation therapy and maximize the coverage of an ablation lesion and lessen damage to surrounding critical tissue.

The 3D Slicer provides phase differential computation using a sequence of fast 2D spoiled gradient-recalled sequences as inputs. The magnitude, phase, real, and imaginary images can be transferred online in real time from the MRI scanner to the 3D Slicer workstation and presented to the physicians.

3 Software Process

Cross-platform Development. The 3D Slicer was developed using a cross-platform environment, CMake. CMake provides compilation management for Windows, Unix, and Mac OS platforms[7]. This multiplatform support was crucial to provide options for the IGT computer platform depending on the needs and requirements of the project. In our clinical applications, we used the Linux platform as well as Windows.

Software Distribution. We provided the software tools to facilitate their distribution to the collaborating institutions and researchers. Central to this effort were concurrent version systems (CVS), which records the history of sources files. A client/server version of CVS enables developers separated by geographic distance to function as a team. Documentation generation tools were Doxygen and LaTeX to produce online manual pages.

Quality Assurance. DART server was employed in the 3D Slicer for quality assurance in multiple projects. In addition, we enhanced DART to provide historical reporting, trending, and analysis of test results. DART currently supports results transmission using HTTP and FTP protocols. Regular testing is performed at scheduled intervals, often nightly, and it collects the overall software development activities for the past 24 hours. On-demand testing allows each developer to make local changes and immediately evaluate them against the established gold standard.

4   Results

The software we developed has been applied to multicenter clinical studies for MR-guided therapy at four different sites. Each center had one or two software engineers developing modules for clinical applications. Each center was also responsible for obtaining Institutional Review Boards' approval on human subject studies. The version of Slicer used in each site varies depending on the start of the clinical studies. In the following sections, we report the nature of the clinical application, number of cases, and unique function added. We found that average man-hours invested to develop new procedures were 286 man-hours and average number of codes per procedure was 2446.

4.1   MR-guided Brain Tumor Surgery

We used the 3D Slicer (version 2.0 - 2.6) to register serial intraoperative MRIs and for navigation [6]. The MRI scanner used was 0.5T vertical open magnet (Signa SP/i, GE Healthcare, London, UK). We performed 1,026 craniotomies, 336 biospies, 37 pituitary tumor cases, and 16 cyst drainage cases in MR-guided neurosurgery. Of these, 150 were performed using the 3D Slicer developed and controlled in the software engineering process discussed above. The estimated man-hours needed for this implementation was 160 man-hours and total number of lines in Tcl/Tk and shell script codes for on-line image transfer and tracker data control was 232.

Figure 1 highlights from the MR-guided brain tumor suregery.

4.2   In-Bore Prostate Biopsy

We used the 3D Slicer (version 2.6) for both MR-guided prostate brachytherapy in an open-bore MRI scanner as well as MR-guided prostate biopsy. We had 448 brachytherapy cases and 72 biopsy cases. The 3D Slicer has played a different role in each procedure. MRI scanner used was 0.5T vertical open magnet (Signa SP/i, GE Healthcare, London, UK).

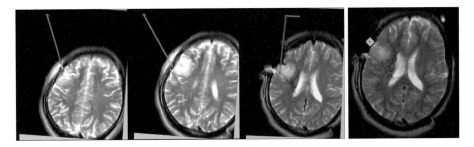

Fig. 1. 22-y-o male with approximately 3 cm x 3 cm left posterior frontal tumor. (Three images from far left) the 3D Slicer was helpful in confirming that tumor volume in the resection is not part of the active lesion in fMRI and DTI fused with intraoperative T2 MRI. Images are snapshots from physicians confirmation process using fMRI (shown as a red blob in the far left image), tumor-highlighted lesion (shown as a high-intensity lesion in second and the third images from left). The right image shows the craniotomy and the partially resected tumor. (Far right) The 3D Slicer was helpful in confirming the location of the Ojemann stimulator (blue dot) with respect to the lesion (in T2 image) and the margin.

The 3D Slicer is essential to the MR-guided prostate biopsy. The coordinates of suspicious tumor foci are specified in 3D Slicer and corresponding holes in the needle guiding template grid are computed, which effectively shortens surgery time and reduces the potential for computational errors. A key feature of the system is volumetric data fusion, allowing for target planning on high-resolution preoperative T2-weighted images mapped onto intraoperative 0.5T images. Patient-to-image registration methods was modified and used to calibrate the needle guiding template to MRI scanner's coordinate system. The template was calibrated to the MRI scanner using the optical tracking system; and 3D Slicer performed this operation by using both interconnectivity function to the tracker and the patient-to-image registration tool. The prostate biopsy module needed new development for real-time image transfer and scanner control, of which image transfer was already available from neurosurgical applications. Therefore, approximate man-hours invested was 320 man-hours and line of codes added was 3948 lines.

4.3   In-Bore Laser Ablation Therapy of Brain Tumor

The 3D Slicer (version 2.6) enabled software for monitoring laser-inducted interstitial therapy (LITT) of a brain tumor in intraoperative MRI. The 3D Slicer was useful to ablate the tumor with integrated tumor segmentation and thermal monitoring tools, processing the intraoperative MR imagery online and in real time. MRI scanner used was 0.5T vertical open magnet (Signa SP/i, GE Healthcare, London, UK).

The 3D Slicer, modified specifically for LITT, gave us options to objectively measure the extent of a tumor by image segmentation, mark the critical volume

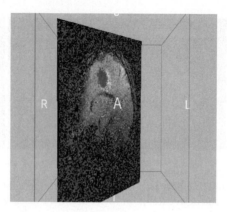

Fig. 2. A snap shot from In-bore laser ablation therapy of brain tumor showing the thermal image (in reddish color) overplayed on the T1-weighted MRI. The procedure uses shared tools of the thermal imaging, image transfer, image registration, and tracking and guidance using in-bore tracking system.

by thermal imaging, and update the treatment plan by comparing the original tumor lesion and treated lesion. Both the original tumor lesion and the ablated lesion were mapped onto the T1-weighted MRI. This overlapped mapping was then used to update the treatment plan, i.e., additional laser firing or repositioning of the fiber, to best cover the tumor with thermal ablation. Figure 2 demonstrates an highlights from the In-bore laser ablation therapy of brain tumor.

4.4   In-Bore Microwave Ablation Therapy of Liver Tumor

The team at Shiga Medical University, Shiga, Japan , used the 3D Slicer (version 2.2) in a similar manner as in the prostate biopsy above. The 3D Slicer could display an intraprocedural thermal MR image in combination with two reformatted images from preoperative high-resolution 3D volume data [7].

A unique innovation was the foot-printing, which recorded and displayed football-shaped coagulated areas of 20 mm in diameter and 30 mm in length along the electrode in the 3D space. The direction of the electrode was obtained from the optical tracking system information. The footprint was placed along the direction of the electrode to record the "coagulated area", was helpful to optimally cover the large tumor by placing electrode in multiple place inside the tumor. The number of man-hours spent on this development was 120 man-hours, and line of codes was 1659.

4.5   Slide-in-and-Out Ablation Therapy of Liver Tumor

In 11 Percutaneous Ethanol Injection Therapy (PEIT) and 3 Radiofrequency Ablation (RFA) interventions in Kyusyu University, Fukuoka, Japan, 3D Slicer (version 2.2) with intraoperative MR images provided useful information in determining the needle orientation and placement for the target tumors. MRI scanner used was low-field horizontal open magnet (Hitachi AIRIS-II, Tokyo, Japan).

By attaching the markers of optical position sensor to an ultrasound needle insertion adapter, a virtual needle path was intraoperatively displayed with tumor and vessel models constructed from segmentation. The reconstructed cross sectional MR images identical to ultrasound images including the needle positions were also provided after point-based MR registration with patient body using MRI visible markers. This MR based navigation provided physicians with strong confidence when the tumors were not clearly identified in conventional ultrasound guided procedures [8]. We observed deformation of liver which then led to discrepancy between MRI and ultrasound images. Approximately 480 man-hours were spent on this project.

4.6 Slide-in-and-Out Brain Tumor Surgery with Commercial Navigation Software

The team at Tokyo Women's Medical University, Tokyo, Japan have used the 3D Slicer, as navigation software in their MR-guided navigation therapy. The 3D Slicer was linked to a commercial neuro-navigation system (experimental product, Toshiba, Tokyo, Japan). MRI scanner used was low-field horizontal open magnet (Hitachi AIRIS-II, Tokyo, Japan).

Tumor segmentation method was developed and implemented in 3D Slicer. 3D Slicer's unique role in this study was transfer intraoperative images from the scanner and perform tumor segmentation followed by volume measurement. 3D slicer was set up next to the commercial neuro-navigation system and received tracker coordinates and patient-to-image registration using fiducial markers. The role of the 3D Slicer was complementary to the commercial navigation system, which doesnt provide interface to state-of-the-art segmentation, volume measurement, and visualization. Approximately 320 man-hours were spent on this project.

5 Discussion

We presented a software engineering methods to provide free open-source software for MR-guided therapy. We found that graphical representation of the surgical tools, interconnectively with the tracking device, patient-to-image registration, and MRI-based thermal mapping are crucial components of MR-guided therapy in sharing software. We developed six procedures in four separate clinical sites using proposed softare process, and found the method is feasible to facilitate multicenter clinical trial of MR-guided therapies.

There are surprisingly few efforts to share software resources in image-guided therapy; among them is Image Guided Surgery Toolkit (IGSTK) [9]. The toolkit contains the basic software components to construct an image-guided system, including a tracker and a default graphical user interface that includes a four-quadrant view with image overlay. Our solution is complementary to IGSTK; we have been trying to bridge medical image processing and image-guided surgery, yet requirements for the IGT-specific component are confined to target application. Our emphasis on bridging medical image computing (MIC) and computer assisted intervention (AI) was carried out in this stud. We found that registration and segmentation were the key enabling technology for new procedures.

Our future study include use of the software in non-MR-guided therapies, which should benefit from combined use of medical image processing and IGT-specific tools.

References

[1] McDonald, C.J., Schadow, G., Barnes, M., Dexter, P., Overhage, J.M., Mamlin, B., McCoy, J.M.: Open Source software in medical informatics–why, how and what. Int. J. Med. Inform. 69, 175–184 (2003)
[2] Marturano, A., Chadwick, R.: How the role of computing is driving new genetics' public policy. Ethics Inf. Technol. 6, 43–53 (2004)
[3] Stewart, J.E., Mangalam, H., Zhou, J.: Open Source Software meets gene expression. Brief Bioinform. 2, 319–328 (2001)
[4] Gering, D.T., Nabavi, A., Kikinis, R., Hata, N., O'Donnell, L.J., Grimson, W.E.L., Jolesz, F.A., Black, P.M., Wells, W.M.: An integrated visualization system for surgical planning and guidance using image fusion and an open MR. Journal of Magnetic Resonance Imaging 13, 967–975 (2001)
[5] Morikawa, S., Inubushi, T., Kurumi, Y., Naka, S., Sato, K., Demura, K., Tani, T., Haque, H.A., Tokuda, J., Hata, N.: Advanced computer assistance for magnetic resonance-guided microwave thermocoagulation of liver tumors. Academic Radiology 10, 1442–1449 (2003)
[6] Nabavi, A., Black, P.M., Gering, D.T., Westin, C.F., Mehta, V., Pergolizzi Jr., R.S., Ferrant, M., Warfield, S.K., Hata, N., Schwartz, R.B., Wells 3rd, W.M., Kikinis, R., Jolesz, F.A.: Serial intraoperative magnetic resonance imaging of brain shift. Neurosurgery 48, 797–798 (2001)
[7] Martin, K., Hoffman, B.: An open source approach to developing software in a small organization. IEEE Software 24, 46 (2007)
[8] Hong, J., Nakashima, H., Konishi, K., Ieiri, S., Tanoue, K., Nakamuta, M., Hashizume, M.: Interventional navigation for abdominal therapy based on simultaneous use of MRI and ultrasound. Med. Biol. Eng. Comput. (2006)
[9] Gary, K., Ibanez, L., Aylward, S., Gobbi, D., Blake, M.B., Cleary, K.: IGSTK: An open source software toolkit for image-guided surgery. Computer 39, 46 (2006)

Statistical Atlases of Bone Anatomy: Construction, Iterative Improvement and Validation

Gouthami Chintalapani[1], Lotta M. Ellingsen[2], Ofri Sadowsky[1],
Jerry L. Prince[2], and Russell H. Taylor[1]

Johns Hopkins University, Baltimore, USA
greddy@cs.jhu.edu

Abstract. We present an iterative bootstrapping framework to create and analyze statistical atlases of bony anatomy such as the human pelvis from a large collection of CT data sets. We create an initial tetrahedral mesh representation of the target anatomy and use deformable intensity-based registration to create an initial atlas. This atlas is used as prior information to assist in deformable registration/segmentation of our subject image data sets, and the process is iterated several times to remove any bias from the initial choice of template subject and to improve the stability and consistency of mean shape and variational modes. We also present a framework to validate the statistical models. Using this method, we have created a statistical atlas of full pelvis anatomy with 110 healthy patient CT scans. Our analysis shows that any given pelvis shape can be approximated up to an average accuracy of 1.5036 mm using the first 15 principal modes of variation. Although a particular intensity-based deformable registration algorithm was used to produce these results, we believe that the basic method may be adapted readily for use with any registration method with broadly similar characteristics.

1 Introduction

Statistical modeling and analysis of anatomical shape is an active subject of medical imaging research. Uses include image segmentation, analysis of anatomical variations within populations, identification of pathological anomalies, etc. Statistical characterization using principal component analysis (PCA) and point distribution models is presented in [1]. Following Cootes *et al.*, a number of authors (e.g., [2],[3],[4],[5]) have applied similar methods to construct statistical atlases of bony anatomy from CT scans of multiple individuals. The basic method used is to identify landmark points, establish point-based correspondences between subjects, and then perform statistical analysis to study shape variations. Typically, subject anatomical shapes are represented as surface meshes [4] or volumetric tetrahedral meshes [2],[5],[3]. Often, a template mesh representing an anatomical structure is created, deformably registered to each subject, and mesh vertex points are used as the corresponding landmark points. Wu *et al.* created a statistical model using surface triangular meshes and a non-rigid point matching

N. Ayache, S. Ourselin, A. Maeder (Eds.): MICCAI 2007, Part I, LNCS 4791, pp. 499–506, 2007.
© Springer-Verlag Berlin Heidelberg 2007

algorithm to register different shapes. Our atlas approach, originated by Yao *et al.* [2] and subsequently also adopted by others [5][3], represents the shape using tetrahedral meshes and registers the datasets using a grayscale deformable registration method. Bone density information is incorporated into the model using polynomials. Some drawbacks of these methods are that a bias is introduced in selecting a template shape and the sampling points on the surface are over determined when a deformable registration method is used. Bookstein *et al.* proposed an iterative ridge curve based algorithm to register each curve/shape to the average shape [6]. However, this approach poses difficulties when applied to volumetric data. Chui *et al.* presented an iterative process where multiple sample point sets are non rigidly deformed to the emerging mean shape [7]. Chui's method requires that each subject be separately segmented to identify the points. Although he suggests that the method can be useful in atlas construction, he does not address evolution of statistical modes. Rueckert *et al.* [8] constructed an intensity atlas by using deformable 3D-3D intensity image-to-image based registration to approximate the deformations between subjects and a template using B-spline polynomials, and then constructed a statistical atlas to the B-spline control points.

This paper proposes a systematic method for construction and iterative bootstrapping of a statistical mesh atlas from multiple CT data sets. Our approach most closely follows Yao's. It resembles Rueckert's by using image-to-image intensity-based registration to determine an initial set of deformations, but differs by applying them to our mesh data structure, in the use of PCA on the mesh to produce statistical modes, and in the use of 3D-3D atlas-to-image intensity-based registration in iterative bootstrapping. Although the method is potentially useful with any deformable mesh registration algorithm capable of incorporating prior statistical information, we demonstrate it with a new method that incorporates whatever prior information is available. We present validation results on a full pelvis atlas created from 110 datasets using this iterative process. We present the algorithm and results below.

2   Method

This section describes the iterative process of creating the statistical atlas. The statistical atlas consists of a tetrahedral mesh representing the average shape, Bernstein polynomials representing the CT intensities and the variational modes representing shape variations. A typical cross sectional view of the tetrahedral mesh skeleton is shown in Figure 1. Although our current atlas includes bone density parameters, for the purpose of this paper we are restricting ourselves to shape parameters. Our atlas construction method relies on the use of a deformable registration method developed by Ellingsen *et. al* [9] that has been modified to use prior statistical knowledge from our atlas in registering the volumetric datasets. Several authors (e.g., [2],[10],[11]), have proposed similar registration methods. Generally, these methods include the following steps: 1) similarity

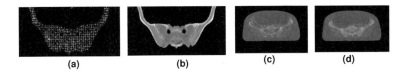

Fig. 1. (a) A cross-sectional view of tetrahedral mesh skeleton (b) mesh fitted with density polynomials (c) a CT slice of a typical subject with voxelized tetrahedral mesh (in blue) overlaid before registration (d) after registration

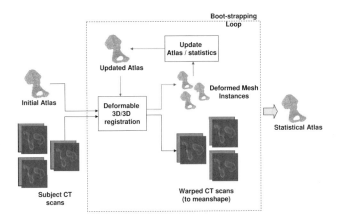

Fig. 2. Statistical atlas creation process using iterative bootstrapping technique

registration, 2) statistical mode matching, and 3) local deformation. In our current implementation, the gray scale deformable registration algorithm uses a continuously varying weighting parameter to smoothly vary from mode matching to purely image-driven local deformation, while preserving correct mesh topology.

A flowchart describing the iterative process is shown in Figure 2 and the algorithmic steps are shown below:

1. Select a template CT dataset C_{master} and manually label the voxels of the anatomy of interest, resulting in $C_{master}^{segmented}$. Create a tetrahedral mesh M_{master} from $C_{master}^{segmented}$. We have used the meshing application developed by [12].
2. Select n_{seed} CT datasets from the population, say C_i, where $i = 1, 2, 3, ..n_{seed}$. Deformably register each dataset to the template C_{master} using a 3D grayscale deformable registration. The output of this step would be a deformation field $Dmap_i$ and a warped subject CT, C_i^{warped}.
3. For each CT subject, create a mesh instance, M_i by interpolating the deformation field D_i at each vertex of the master mesh M_{master}.

4. Do a rigid registration between all the meshes and perform principal component analysis on the registered mesh instances. This results in meanshape M_0 and shape variational modes D_k, refered to as $Atlas_j$ where $j = 0$. Any given shape can be expressed as a linear combination of the anatomical modes of variation

$$S = M_0 + \Sigma_{k=1}^{n} \lambda_k D_k \qquad (1)$$

5. Create a CT-like volume $C_{meanshape}$ from the meanshape mesh M_0 and the mean density polynomial.
6. For each CT subject C_i, deformably register C_i to $C_{meanshape}$. This registration method uses prior knowledge (meanshape M_0 and modes D_i) to constrain the deformation process and to increase the registration accuracy. The resulting deformed mesh instance is M_i
7. Compute a new statistical model using principal component analysis on the mesh instances. The result of this step is a meanshape M_0^j and modes D_i^j, refered to as $Atlas_{j+1}$
8. Compare the two models, $\Delta = Compare(Atlas_j, Atlas_{j+1})$. Various tools for comparing any two given models are presented in the following section. If $\Delta > \epsilon$, then $j = j + 1$ and iterate steps 7 through 10. Stop otherwise.

With this bootstrapping process, the vertex correspondences are stabilized and the residual variance after principal component analysis is reduced after each iteration. Moreover, this iterative procedure removes the bias introduced in selecting the template subject and removes the artifacts introduced by the registration algorithms, thereby stabilizing the anatomical modes of variation. Our atlas creation process is modular and robust and we believe that the underlying concept can be readily adapted for use with any similar deformable registration method.

3   Results

We have created a statistical model of full pelvis anatomy from 110 CT scans of healthy patients using this new iterative method. The tetrahedral mesh model consists of 26875 vertices, 105767 tetrahedra, and 25026 outer surface triangles. This mesh was created from a 512x512x256 CT volume with a voxel size of 0.9375 cm^3. Results from four iterations of this boot-strapping method are presented. The zeroth iteration corresponds to basic atlas creation by registering all the subjects to a template subject without any prior knowledge. In later iterations, we use the statistical model from the previous iteration as a template. Figure 3 shows surface rendered mean shape and the first three modes of pelvis anatomy from the final iteration.

For validation purpose, we have randomly selected 20 datasets from our CT population and excluded all these 20 datasets from the atlas creation. The goal is to estimate these 20 left out subjects from atlases at different stages. Given a left-out shape instance, S^{true}, align this shape instance with the mean shape using similarity transformation. And then the shape can be estimated with deformable

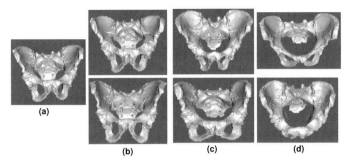

Fig. 3. Surface renderings of mean shape and first three principal modes. (a) mean shape; (b) top: mean+3σ1model, bottom: mean-3σ1 model; (c)top: mean+3σ2mode2, bottom: mean-3σ2mode2; (d) top: mean+3σ3 mode3, bottom: mean-3σ3mode3;

mode matching step as follows: Compute the mode weights using the mean shape ($overlineM$) and the modes of variation (Y)

$$\lambda = Y' * (S^{true} - \overline{M}) \qquad (2)$$

Use the dominant eigen modes to estimate the given shape

$$S^{est} = \overline{M} + \Sigma_{i=1}^{n} \lambda_i Y_i \qquad (3)$$

After estimating a given shape with the atlas, we define two types of metrics to measure the error between the estimated shape and the true shape: 1) vertex to vertex correspondence error assuming that the graphs of the meshes are similar and 2) surface to surface distance computed by measuring distances from the vertices of the model instance to the closest points on the subject surface [13]. We have performed four iterations of the boot-strapping algorithm and the residual error plots are shown below. The residual error as estimated from the leave-out validation tests in each iteration of the bootstrapping process is shown in Figure 4. For each iteration, we have created an atlas using 90 datasets and

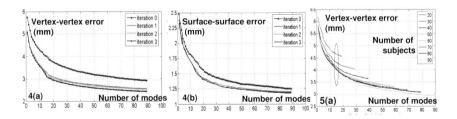

Fig. 4. Residual error plots from leave-out validation tests as a function of number of principal modes: (a) vertex to vertex correspondence error; (b) surface to surface distance; (c) Vertex to vertex correspondence error as a function of number of principal components used shown for different numbers of CT subjects used to form the atlas;

performed leave-out validation experiments using the remaining 20 datasets. Figure 4 shows that after first two iterations, the process more or less converged. There is a significant reduction in the vertex to vertex correspondence metric from iteration 0 to iteration 1 indicating that the vertex correspondences have improved. This process seems to have converged after iteration 2. A similar trend can be seen with surface to surface distance error metric. We have used our surface to surface distance metric to select the number of principal components to be used in the later experiments. Even though large number of eigen modes result in lower residual errors, it is computationally expensive to use a large set of principal modes. Typically, a threshold on the residual errors is used to determine the number of eigen modes. Here, we set the surface distance threshold to be approximately 1.5 mm and hence selected the first 15 shape modes in later experiments.

In order to analyze the size of the population and the number of principal modes needed to extract stable statistics, we performed the following experiment. We randomly selected n meshes, where $n = 20, 30, 40, ..80$ and created statistical models using these datasets. This process was repeated 20 times for each value of n. Figure 4(c) shows the average residual vertex correspondence error in the

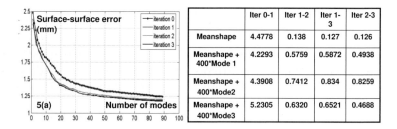

	Iter 0-1	Iter 1-2	Iter 1-3	Iter 2-3
Meanshape	4.4778	0.138	0.127	0.126
Meanshape + 400*Mode 1	4.2293	0.5759	0.5872	0.4938
Meanshape + 400*Mode2	4.3908	0.7412	0.834	0.8259
Meanshape + 400*Mode3	5.2305	0.6320	0.6521	0.4688

Fig. 5. (a) Residual surface to surface distance error from using iteration 3 as ground truth; (b) Surface to surface distance metric between mean shapes and modes from iterations 0-3

leave-out tests for different atlases as a function of number of modes used for various atlas population sizes. This graph shows that around 40 to 50 datasets are sufficient to capture the shape variations of a healthy pelvis anatomy using 15 modes. Adding more instances to this database results in a very small improvement, less than $0.1mm$, in terms of residual errors.

We analyzed the convergence in terms of the stability of the atlas. This analysis is shown in Table 1. The surface to surface distance between mean shapes from iterations 2 and 3 is around 0.126 mm and the volume overlap between the mean shape CT volumes is around 97%. Similarly, the average surface to surface distance betwen the shape modes for iterations 1, 2, and 3 is around 0.6 mm. After iteration 2, the mean shape and modes did not vary much. These values indicate that the atlas has become stable and the bootstrapping process has converged. As one of the reviewers mentioned, it could so happen that the process has converged to a consistent sub-optimal solution rather than the optimal solution. The intuition behind the iterative process is that after every iteration, residual errors are decreased by deforming/stretching the mesh vertices beyond the PCA mode matching step. To verify the convergence against ground truth, we selected mesh instances from the final iteration as our ground truth shapes. and performed leave-out validation analysis. The bootstrapping process has converged in iteration 3 as shown in Figure 5(b). However, we have measured the closest point distance between a few hand segmented meshes and the corresponding atlas instances from the final iteration. The average error is around 2.0153 mm. This number is roughly comparable to the 1.5036 mm accuracy achieved from using final iteration as ground truth. However, it is difficult to interpret these numbers in the absence of a firm consensus segmentation since manual segmentations are subject to random errors. We plan to do a thorough systematic evaluation of the algorithm against a consensus from multiple independent segmentations.

4   Conclusions and Future Work

This paper has presented an iterative bootstrapping technique to create statistical atlases of bony anatomy from collections of CT data sets, along with various error metrics to evaluate these atlases. Advantages of our approach include: 1) very minimal initial segmentation is required (once to create an initial mesh) and may be done manually or semi-automatically; 2) point correspondences are established automatically through intensity-based registration, avoiding landmark selection; 3) atlas bias/uncertainty is minimized through iterative refinement of an initial atlas; 4) the method requires little or no explicit prior anatomical information, although such information may be added in a separate annotation phase; and 5) the atlases produced are useful as prior information for assisting 3D/3D and 2D/3D (e.g., [5]) registration, as well as assisting in tomographic reconstruction from incomplete data [5].

Although we used a particular intensity-based registration method [9] to create this atlas, the technique can be adapted readily for use with other registration algorithms, although this must be demonstrated in actual experiments. Our method is modular and robust, thereby enabling us to build large population atlases fairly easily. As part of the validation framework, we have developed various tools and strategies to compare and analyze any given number of statistical models. In this paper, we have focused on shape statistics only and we are currently using mean density for our applications. An immediate extension would be to incorporate density statistics in to our atlas construction pipeline and combine the shape and density statistics to give us a better atlas.

We have demonstrated this approach by creating an atlas of the human male pelvis from 110 subjects. Our population analysis shows that up to 40-50 subjects are required to capture inherent shape variations of pelvic bone anatomy, although additional subjects further improve the results somewhat. The leave-out validation experiments indicate an accuracy of 1.5036 mm in approximating any given pelvis shape with the first 15 eigen modes of the 90 dataset atlas. Our next experiment will be to validate the bootstrapping process with a consensus multiple independent segmentations. In related ongoing work, we will shortly apply our boot-strapping approach to create male and female femur atlases.

Acknowledgments

We would like to thank Dr. Ted Deweese and Dr. Lee Myers for their assistance in providing us with the data. This work is supported by NSF ERC Grant EEC9731478 and NIH/NBIB Grant R21-EB003616. We would also like to thank Pauline Pelletier for helping us with data processing.

References

1. Cootes, T., Taylor, C., Cooper, D., Graham, J.: Active shape models - their training and application. Computer Vision Image Understanding 61(1), 38–59 (1995)
2. Yao, J., Taylor, R.H.: Non-rigid registration and correspondence finding in medical image analysis using multiple-layer flexible mesh template matching. IJPRAI 17(7), 1145–1165 (2003)
3. Querol, L., Buchler, P., Rueckert, D., Nolte, L.P., Ballester, M.: Statistical finite element model for bone shape and biomechanical properties. In: Larsen, R., Nielsen, M., Sporring, J. (eds.) MICCAI 2006. LNCS, vol. 4190, pp. 405–411. Springer, Heidelberg (2006)
4. Wu, C., Murtha, P.E., Mor, A.B., Jaramaz, B.: A two-level method for building a statistical shape atlas. In: CAOS (2005)
5. Sadowsky, O., Ramamurthi, K., Ellingsen, L., Chintalapani, G., Prince, J., Taylor, R.: Atlas-assisted tomography: registration of a deformable atlas to compensate for limited-angle cone-beam trajectory. In: IEEE International Symposium for Biomedical Imaging pp. 1244–1247 (2006)
6. Cutting, C.B., Bookstein, F.L., Haddad, B., Dean, D., Kim, D.: Spline-based approach for averaging three-dimensional curves and surfaces. Mathematical methods in medical imaging II, SPIE 2035, 29–44 (1993)
7. Chui, H., Zhang, J., Rangarajan, A.: Unsupervised learning of an atlas from unlabeled point-sets. IEEE Trans. Pattern Analysis and Machine Intelligence 26(2), 160–173 (2004)
8. Rueckert, D., Frangi, A., Schnabel, J.: Automatic construction of 3d statistical deformation models using non-rigid registration. In: Medical Image Computing and Computer Assisted Intervention, pp. 77–84 (2001)
9. Ellingsen, L., Prince, J.: Deformable registration of ct pelvis images using mjolnir. In: IEEE 7th Nordic Signal Processing Symposium (NORSIG) (2006)
10. Cootes, T., Beeston, C., Edwards, G., Taylor, C.: A unified framework for atlas matching using active appearance models. In: IPMI, pp. 322–333 (1999)
11. Shen, D., Davatzikos, C.: Adaptive-focus statistical shape model for segmentation of 3d mr structures. In: Delp, S.L., DiGoia, A.M., Jaramaz, B. (eds.) MICCAI 2000. LNCS, vol. 1935, pp. 206–215. Springer, Heidelberg (2000)
12. Mohamed, A., Davatzikos, C.: An approach to 3d finite element mesh generation from segmented medical images. In: IEEE International Symposium on Biomedical Imaging (ISBI) (2004)
13. Besl, P., McKay, N.: A method for registration of 3-d shapes. IEEE Trans. on Pattern Analysis and Machine Intelligence 14(2), 239–256 (1992)

A New Benchmark for Shape Correspondence Evaluation

Brent C. Munsell, Pahal Dalal, and Song Wang

Department of Computer Science and Engineering
University of South Carolina, Columbia, SC 29208, USA
{munsell,dalalpk,songwang}@engr.sc.edu

Abstract. This paper introduces a new benchmark study of evaluating landmark-based shape correspondence used for statistical shape analysis. Different from previous shape-correspondence evaluation methods, the proposed benchmark first generates a large set of synthetic shape instances by randomly sampling a specified ground-truth statistical shape model. We then run the test shape-correspondence algorithms on these synthetic shape instances to construct a new statistical shape model. We finally introduce a new measure to describe the difference between this newly constructed statistical shape model and the ground truth. This new measure is then used to evaluate the performance of the test shape-correspondence algorithm. By introducing the ground-truth statistical shape model, we believe the proposed benchmark allows for a more objective evaluation of the shape correspondence than those that do not specify any ground truth.

1 Introduction

Statistical shape models have been applied to address many important applications in medical image analysis, such as image segmentation for desirable anatomic structures [1,2] and accurately locating the subtle difference of the corpus-callosum shapes between the schizophrenia patients and normal controls [3]. Accurate and efficient shape-correspondence algorithms [4,5] to identify corresponded landmarks are essential to the accuracy of the constructed statistical shape models. However, how to objectively evaluate the results produced by these shape-correspondence algorithms is still a very difficult problem. One major reason is the unavailability of a ground-truth shape correspondence: given a set of real shape instances, say the kidney contours from a group of people, even the landmark points identified by different experts may show substantial difference from each other [6].

To address this problem, Davies and Styner [6] introduce three general measures to describe the compactness, specificity, and generality of the statistical shape model constructed from a shape-correspondence result and suggest the use of these three measures for evaluating shape-correspondence performance. However, without introducing the ground truth, these three measures may not be reliable in some cases [7]. For example, according to these measures, we prefer

N. Ayache, S. Ourselin, A. Maeder (Eds.): MICCAI 2007, Part I, LNCS 4791, pp. 507–514, 2007.
© Springer-Verlag Berlin Heidelberg 2007

a shape correspondence that leads to a statistical shape model with high compactness (or smaller shape variation space), which may not be true for certain structures.

In this paper, we present a new benchmark study with ground truth to more objectively evaluate the shape correspondence for statistical shape analysis. Specifically, the statistical shape analysis chosen for this paper is the widely used point distribution model (PDM) [1]. For simplicity, this paper focuses on the 2D case, where a point distribution model (PDM) is a $2m$-dimensional Gaussian distribution with m being the number of landmarks identified from each shape instance. In this benchmark, we start with a ground-truth PDM by specifying a $2m$-dimensional mean-shape vector and a $2m \times 2m$ covariance matrix. We then randomly sample this PDM to generate a set of synthetic continuous shape instances. A test shape-correspondence algorithm is then applied to correspond these shape instances by identifying a new set of landmarks. Finally we construct a new PDM from the corresponded landmarks and compare it with the ground truth PDM to evaluate the accuracy of the shape correspondence.

2   Problem Description

Given n sample shape instances (or continuous *shape contours* in the 2D case) S_i, $i = 1, 2, \ldots, n$, shape correspondence aims to identify corresponded landmarks from them. More specifically, after shape correspondence we obtain n corresponded landmark sets $\hat{V}_i$, $i = 1, 2, \ldots, n$ from S_i, $i = 1, 2, \ldots, n$, respectively. Here $\hat{V}_i = \{\hat{\mathbf{v}}_{i1}, \hat{\mathbf{v}}_{i2}, \ldots, \hat{\mathbf{v}}_{im}\}$ are m landmarks identified from shape contour S_i and $\hat{\mathbf{v}}_{ij} = (\hat{x}_{ij}, \hat{y}_{ij})$ is the jth landmark identified along S_i. Landmark correspondence means that $\hat{\mathbf{v}}_{ij}$, $i = 1, 2, \ldots, n$, i.e., the jth landmark in each shape contour, are corresponded, for any $j = 1, 2, \ldots, m$.

In practice, structural shape is usually assumed to be invariant to the transformations of any (uniform) scaling, rotation, and translations. Therefore, shape normalization is applied to $\hat{V}_i$, $i = 1, 2, \ldots, n$ to remove such transformations among the given n shape contours. Denote the resulting landmark sets to be $V_i = \{\mathbf{v}_{i1}, \mathbf{v}_{i2}, \ldots, \mathbf{v}_{im}\}$, $i = 1, 2, \ldots, n$, in which the absolute coordinates of the corresponded landmarks, e.g., $\mathbf{v}_{ij} = (x_{ij}, y_{ij})$, $i = 1, 2, \ldots, n$ are directly comparable.

Finally, we calculate the statistical shape model by fitting the normalized landmarks sets $V_i = \{\mathbf{v}_{i1}, \mathbf{v}_{i2}, \ldots, \mathbf{v}_{im}\}$, $i = 1, 2, \ldots, n$ to a multivariate Gaussian distribution. Specifically, we columnize m landmarks in V_i into a $2m$-dimensional vector $\mathbf{v}_i = (x_{i1}, y_{i1}, x_{i2}, y_{i2}, \ldots, x_{im}, y_{im})^T$ and call it a *(landmark-based) shape vector* of the shape contour $\hat{V}_i$. This way, the mean shape vector $\bar{\mathbf{v}}$ and the covariance matrix $\mathbf{D}$ can be calculated by

$$\bar{\mathbf{v}} = \frac{1}{n} \sum_{i=1}^{n} \mathbf{v}_i, \quad \mathbf{D} = \frac{1}{n-1} \sum_{i=1}^{n} (\mathbf{v}_i - \bar{\mathbf{v}})(\mathbf{v}_i - \bar{\mathbf{v}})^T. \tag{1}$$

The Gaussian distribution $\mathcal{N}(\bar{\mathbf{v}}, \mathbf{D})$ is the resulting PDM that attempts to model the deformable or probablistic shape space of the considered structure.

The accuracy of the PDM is largely dependent on the performance of shape correspondence, i.e., the accuracy in identifying the corresponded landmarks $\hat{V}_i$, $i = 1, 2, \ldots, n$. However, the performance of shape correspondence is not well defined because in practice, a ground-truth shape correspondence is usually not available and the landmarks manually labeled by different experts may be quite different from each other [6].

3   Proposed Method

The proposed benchmark starts from a specified ground-truth PDM, from which we can randomly generate a set of synthetic shape contours. A shape-correspondence algorithm should be able to identify corresponded landmarks from these shape contours and leads to a PDM that well describes the shape space defined by the ground-truth PDM. As shown in Fig. 1, the proposed benchmark consists of the following five components: (C1) specifying a PDM $\mathcal{N}(\bar{\mathbf{v}}^t, \mathbf{D}^t)$ as the ground truth, (C2) using this PDM to randomly generate a set of shape contours $S_1, S_2, \ldots, S_n$, (C3) running the test shape-correspondence algorithm on these shape contours to identify a set of corresponded landmark sets, (C4) deriving a PDM $\mathcal{N}(\bar{\mathbf{v}}, \mathbf{D})$ from the identified landmark sets using Eq. (1), and (C5) comparing the derived PDM $\mathcal{N}(\bar{\mathbf{v}}, \mathbf{D})$ to the ground truth PDM $\mathcal{N}(\bar{\mathbf{v}}^t, \mathbf{D}^t)$ and using their difference to measure the performance of the test shape-correspondence algorithm.

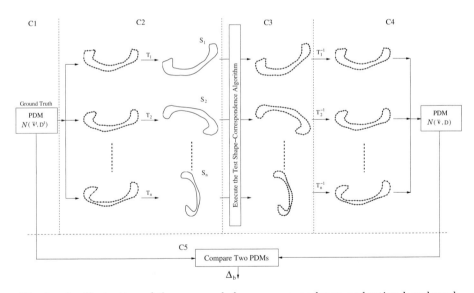

Fig. 1. An illustration of the proposed shape-correspondence evaluation benchmark

We can see that, in essence, this benchmark evaluates the shape-correspondence algorithm's capability to recover the underlying statistical shape model from a set of sampled shape instances. This reflects the role of the shape correspondence in statistical shape modeling. In these five components, (C3) and (C4) are for PDM construction and have been discussed in detail in Section 2. The task of Component (C1) is to specify a mean shape vector $\bar{\mathbf{v}}^t$ and a covariance matrix $\mathbf{D}^t$. Ideally, they can take any values only if $\mathbf{D}^t$ is positive definite. In practice, we can pick them to resemble some real structures as detailed in Section 4. In this section, we focus on developing algorithms for Components (C2) and (C5).

3.1   Generating Shape Instances

Given the ground-truth PDM $\mathcal{N}(\bar{\mathbf{v}}^t, \mathbf{D}^t)$ with k landmarks (k might be different from m, the number of landmarks identified by shape correspondence in Component (C3)), we can randomly generate as many sample shape vectors $\mathbf{v}_i^t$, $i = 1, 2, \ldots, n$ as possible. More specifically, with $\mathbf{p}_j^t$ and λ_j^t, $j = 1, 2, \ldots, 2k$ being the eigenvectors and eigenvalues of $\mathbf{D}^t$, we can generate shape instances in the form of

$$\mathbf{v}^t = \bar{\mathbf{v}}^t + \sum_{j=1}^{2k} b_j^t \mathbf{p}_j^t, \tag{2}$$

where b_j^t is independently and randomly sampled from the 1D Gaussian distribution $\mathcal{N}(0, \lambda_j^t)$, $j = 1, 2, \ldots, 2k$.

Each shape vector $\mathbf{v}_i^t$, $i = 1, 2, \ldots, n$ in fact defines k landmarks $\{\mathbf{v}_{i1}^t, \mathbf{v}_{i2}^t, \ldots, \mathbf{v}_{ik}^t\}$. By assuming that these k landmarks are sequentially sampled from a continuous shape contour, we can estimate this continuous contour S_i' by landmark interpolation. For constructing a closed shape contour, we interpolate the portion between the last landmark $\mathbf{v}_{ik}^t$ and the first landmark $\mathbf{v}_{i1}^t$. For constructing an open shape contour, we do not interpolate the portion between $\mathbf{v}_{ik}^t$ and $\mathbf{v}_{i1}^t$. While we can use any interpolation technique to connect these landmarks into contours, we use the Catmull-Rom cubic spline in this paper. If the ground-truth landmarks are sufficiently dense to represent the underlying shape contour (this is usually required for shape correspondence [8]), we expect that different interpolation techniques do not introduce much difference in the resulting shape contour.

For each synthetic shape contour S_i', we also apply a random affine transformation T_i, consisting of a random rotation, a random (uniform) scaling and a random translation. We define the resulting continuous contour to be the shape contour S_i. We record the affine transformation T_i, $i = 1, 2, \ldots, n$ and then pass $S_1, S_2, \ldots, S_n$ (in fact, their control points) to the test shape-correspondence algorithm. Note that the recorded affine transformations T_i, $i = 1, 2, \ldots, n$ are not passed to the test shape-correspondence algorithm (Component (C3)). This way, we test the capability of the shape-correspondence algorithm to handle affine transformations among the different shape contours. If the test shape-correspondence algorithm introduces further transformations, such as Procrustes analysis, in Component (C3), we record and undo these transformations before outputting the shape-correspondence result. This ensures the corresponded land-marks identified by the test shape-correspondence algorithm are placed directly back onto the input shape contours $S_1, S_2, \ldots, S_n$. Then in Component (C4), we directly apply the inverse transform T_i^{-1}, $i = 1, 2, \ldots, n$, to the landmarks identified on S_i. This guarantees the correct removal of the random affine trans-formation T_i before PDM construction in Component (C4).

3.2 Comparing a PDM Against the Ground Truth PDM

The goal of comparing the PDM $\mathcal{N}(\bar{\mathbf{v}}, \mathbf{D})$ derived in Component (C4) against the ground-truth PDM $\mathcal{N}(\bar{\mathbf{v}}^t, \mathbf{D}^t)$ is to quantify the difference of the deformable shape spaces that are represented by these two PDMs. However, directly com-puting the ℓ^2 norms (or any other vector or matrix-based norms) between $\bar{\mathbf{v}}$ and $\bar{\mathbf{v}}^t$, or $\mathbf{D}$ and $\mathbf{D}^t$ can not achieve this goal. In fact, in these two PDMs, the number of landmarks identified from each shape contour can be different, i.e., $\bar{\mathbf{v}} \in \mathbb{R}^{2m}$, $\bar{\mathbf{v}}^t \in \mathbb{R}^{2k}$ and $m \neq k$, where m and k are the number of landmarks along each shape contour in these two PDMs. The reason is that, when using different shape-correspondence algorithms, or the same shape-correspondence algorithm with different settings, we may get different number of corresponded landmarks along each shape contour.

Therefore, in this paper we compare two PDMs in the continuous shape space instead of using the sampled landmarks. For example, we can estimate the con-tinuous mean shape contours $\bar{S}^t$ and $\bar{S}$ by interpolating the landmarks in $\bar{\mathbf{v}}^t$ and $\bar{\mathbf{v}}$, respectively. In our experiments, we use the Catmull-Rom spline for this interpolation. After that, we measure the difference of two continuous shape con-tours using the widely used Jaccard's coefficient, which is landmark independent. More specifically, the mean-shape difference is defined as

$$\Delta(\bar{S}, \bar{S}^t) = 1 - \frac{|R(\bar{S}) \cap R(\bar{S}^t)|}{|R(\bar{S}) \cup R(\bar{S}^t)|}, \tag{3}$$

where $R(S)$ indicates the region enclosed by the contour S and $|R|$ computes the area of the region R. If S is an open contour, we connect its two endpoints by a straight line to form a closed contour for calculating $R(S)$ [8]. We can see that this difference measure takes value in the range of $[0, 1]$ with 0 indicating that $\bar{S}$ is exactly the same as $\bar{S}^t$.

However, $\Delta(\bar{S}, \bar{S}^t) = 0$ does not guarantee the shape spaces represented by the two PDMs are the same. To evaluate the difference between the two shape spaces, we use a random-simulation strategy: randomly generating a large set of N shape vectors from each PDM using Eq. (2), interpolating these landmarks defined by these shape vectors into continuous shape contours, and then measuring the similarity between these two sets of shape contours. We denote the N continuous shape contours generated from PDM $\mathcal{N}(\bar{\mathbf{v}}, \mathbf{D})$ to be $S_1^c, S_2^c, \ldots, S_N^c$ and the N continuous shape contours generated from the ground-truth PDM $\mathcal{N}(\bar{\mathbf{v}}^t, \mathbf{D}^t)$ to be $S_1^t, S_2^t, \ldots, S_N^t$. When N is sufficiently large, the difference between these two sets of continuous shape contours can well reflect the difference of the shape spaces underlying these two PDMs.

Given two continuous shape contours, we can measure their difference using Eq. (3). Therefore, the problem we need to solve is to measure the difference between shape-contour sets $\{S_i^c\}_{i=1}^N$ and $\{S_j^t\}_{j=1}^N$ with a given difference measure between a pair of shape contours, i.e., $\Delta(S_i^c, S_j^t)$, $i, j = 1, 2, \ldots, N$. In this paper, we suggest the use of the bipartite-matching algorithm to evaluate the difference between these two shape-contour sets. In the bipartite-matching algorithm, an optimal one-to-one matching is derived between two shape-contour sets so that the total matching cost, which is defined as the total difference between the matched shape contours, is minimal. Based on this, we define a difference measure between these two PDMs as

$$\Delta_b \triangleq \frac{\sum_{i=1}^N \Delta(S_i^c, S_{b(i)}^t)}{N}, \qquad (4)$$

where S_i^c and $S_{b(i)}^t$ are the matched pair of shape contours in the bipartite matching. In this difference measure, we introduce a normalization over N so that Δ_b takes values in the range of $[0, 1]$. Using the bipartite-matching algorithm, the measure Δ_b assesses not only whether the two shape spaces (defined by two PDMs) contain similar shape contours, but also whether a shape contour has the same or similar probability density in these two shape spaces.

4   Experiments

In this section, we use the proposed benchmark to evaluate five 2D shape-correspondence algorithms: Richardson and Wang's implementation of an algorithm that combines landmark sliding, insertion and deletion (SDI) [8], Thodberg's implementation of the minimum description length algorithm (T-MDL) [9], Ericsson and Karlsson's implementation of the MDL algorithm (E-MDL) [7], Ericsson and Karlsson's implementation of the MDL algorithm with curvature distance minimization (E-MDL+CUR) [7], and Ericsson and Karlsson's implementation of the reparameterisation algorithm by minimizing Euclidean distance (EUC) [7].

While, in principle, the ground truth PDM can be arbitrarily specified, we intentionally construct it to make it resemble some real anatomic structures. The basic idea is to collect real shape contours of a certain structure, apply any reasonable available shape-correspondence algorithm on them and then construct a PDM using Procrustes analysis and Eq. (1). In our experiment, this shape correspondence is achieved by manually labeling one corresponded landmark on each shape contour and then picking the others using a uniform sampling of the shape contour. For open shape contours, such as kidney and femur, we assume the endpoints are corresponded across all the shape contours and therefore manual labeling is not needed. We use these PDMs as ground truth for the proposed benchmark. Specifically, in our experiments we collect kidney, corpus callosum (callosum for short), and femur contours and construct three ground-truth PDMs, all with 64 landmarks.

From each ground-truth PDM, we randomly generate $n = 800$ sample shape contours that are passed to the shape-correspondence algorithm for testing. In the random simulation for Δ_b, we generate $N = 2,000$ sample shape contours from both the ground-truth PDM and the PDM constructed from the shape-correspondence result. In addition, in evaluating each shape-correspondence algorithm on each ground-truth PDM, 50 rounds of random simulations are conducted to analyze the stability of Δ_b. For all five test shape-correspondence algorithms, we set the expected number of corresponded landmarks to be 64 in Component (C3). For bipartite matching, we use the cost scaling push relabeling algorithm implemented by Goldberg and Kennedy [10] with a complexity of $O(\sqrt{VE}\log(CV))$, with V and E being the number of vertices and edges and C being the maximum edge weight when scaled and rounded to integers.

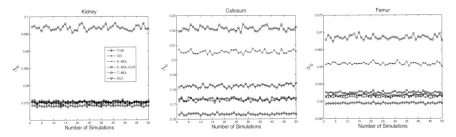

Fig. 2. Δ_b obtained from three ground-truth PDMs that resemble (a) kidney, (b) callosum, and (c) femur, respectively. The x-axis indicates the round of the random simulation. The curves with dimond show Δ_b between each ground-truth PDM and itself.

The evaluation results are shown in Fig. 2, from which we can see that the values of Δ_b do not significantly change over the 50 random simulations. It also shows that, in general, the performance of T-MDL is lower than the performance of SDI, E-MDL, E-MDL+CUR, and EUC on all three ground-truth PDMs. SDI has a similar performance to E-MDL, E-MDL+CUR, and EUC for the ground-truth PDM that resembles the kidney while has a lower performance than E-MDL, E-MDL+CUR, and EUC for the ground-truth PDMs that resemble the callosum and femur. In general, the performance of E-MDL, E-MDL+CUR, and EUC are all similar to each other. Note that, different shape-correspondence algorithms may be more suitable for different ground-truth PDMs. Also note that, the choices of n and N depend on the variance of the ground-truth PDM: if the ground-truth PDM has large eigenvalues along many principal directions, we may need to choose larger values for n and N. In this paper, the ground-truth PDMs resemble several real structures with limited variance. In fact, the stability of the Δ_b value over 50 rounds of random simulations may indicate that $N = 2,000$ is sufficiently large. In addition, if a shape-correspondence algorithm produces a Δ_b value that is close to the Δ_b value between the ground-truth PDM and itself, this may indicate that $n = 800$ is sufficiently large.

5   Conclusion

In this paper, we introduced a new benchmark for evaluating the landmark-based shape-correspondence algorithms. Different from previous evaluation methods, we started from a known ground-truth PDM and then evaluate shape correspondence by assessing whether the resulting PDM describes the shape space defined by the ground-truth PDM. We introduced a new measure to quantify this difference. We applied this benchmark to evaluate five available 2D shape correspondence algorithms.

Acknowledgements

This work was funded by NSF-EIA-0312861 and AFOSR FA9550-07-1-0250.

References

1. Cootes, T., Taylor, C., Cooper, D., Graham, J.: Active shape models - their training and application. Computer Vision and Image Understanding 61(1), 38–59 (1995)
2. Leventon, M., Grimson, E., Faugeras, O.: Statistical shape influence in geodesic active contours. In: IEEE Conference on Computer Vision and Pattern Recognition, pp. 316–323 (2000)
3. Bookstein, F.: Landmark methods for forms without landmarks: Morphometrics of group differences in outline shape. Medical Image Analysis 1(3), 225–243 (1997)
4. Davies, R., Twining, C., Cootes, T., Waterton, J., Taylor, C.: A minimum description length approach to statistical shape modeling. IEEE Transactions on Medical Imaging 21(5), 525–537 (2002)
5. Wang, S., Kubota, T., Richardson, T.: Shape correspondence through landmark sliding. In: IEEE Conference on Computer Vision and Pattern Recognition, pp. I–143–150 (2004)
6. Styner, M., Rajamani, K., Nolte, L.P., Zsemlye, G., Szekely, G., Taylor, C., Davies, R.: Evaluation of 3D correspondence methods for model building. In: Information Processing in Medical Imaging Conference (2003)
7. Ericsson, A., Karlsson, J.: Geodesic ground truth correspondence measure for benchmarking. In: Swedish Symposium in Image Analysis (2006)
8. Richardson, T., Wang, S.: Nonrigid shape correspondence using landmark sliding, insertion and deletion. In: International Conference on Medical Image Computing and Computer Assisted Intervention, pp. II–435–442 (2005)
9. Thodberg, H.: Minimum description length shape and appearance models. In: Information Processing in Medical Imaging Conference, pp. 51–62 (2003)
10. Goldberg, A., Kennedy, R.: An efficient cost scaling algorithm for the assignment problem. Mathematic Programming 71, 153–178 (1995)

Automatic Inference of Sulcus Patterns Using 3D Moment Invariants

Z.Y. Sun[1,2], D. Rivière[1,2], F. Poupon[1,2], J. Régis[3],
and J.-F. Mangin[1,2]

[1] Neurospin, I2BM, CEA, France
zysun@cea.fr
[2] IFR 49, France
[3] Service de Neurochirurgie Fonctionnelle, CHU La Timone,
Marseille, France

Abstract. The goal of this work is the automatic inference of frequent patterns of the cortical sulci, namely patterns that can be observed only for a subset of the population. The sulci are detected and identified using brainVISA open software. Then, each sulcus is represented by a set of shape descriptors called the 3D moment invariants. Unsupervised agglomerative clustering is performed to define the patterns. A ratio between compactness and contrast among clusters is used to select the best patterns. A pattern is considered significant when this ratio is statistically better than the ratios obtained for clouds of points following a Gaussian distribution. The patterns inferred for the left cingulate sulcus are consistent with the patterns described in the atlas of Ono.

1 Introduction

Human brain cortex folds to increase its surface area during development. It is intriguing to look at these folds. They are very complicated and variable, yet there is a certain consistency across brains [1]. Do they contain some information on the functional organization of the human brain? From the folds alone can we observe a pattern characteristic of a certain neurological disease? Thanks to recent advances in softwares dedicated to automatic recognition of cortical sulci [2,3,5,4], this kind of issues can now be tackled using large brain databases [6].

Each brain looks different and none of them looks exactly like the ones in the text books. Current studies of this variability focus on simple morphometric features like the length or the depth of the standard sulci or gyri. Unfortunately, the standard naming system cannot always account for the folding pattern variability. Hence some of the standard sulci can be difficult to define or to measure. This weakness of the nomenclature imposes difficulties on both morphometric studies and the pattern recognition softwares dedicated to automatic recognition of the sulci.

The most detailed description of the sulcus variability has been proposed in the atlas of Ono [7]. This atlas is not based on one single individual but on twenty different brains. For each sulcus, the authors propose a list of possible patterns and their frequencies. These patterns are defined for instance from the

N. Ayache, S. Ourselin, A. Maeder (Eds.): MICCAI 2007, Part I, LNCS 4791, pp. 515–522, 2007.
© Springer-Verlag Berlin Heidelberg 2007

variability of the sulcus interruptions. In a way, the goal of the method proposed in this paper is to automate the work performed by Ono. We want to discover folding patterns that can be observed only for a subset of the population. For this purpose, once a sulcus has been defined in a population of brains, a non supervised clustering method provides subsets of brains with a characteristic trait. Each of these subsets is supposed to represent one of the patterns of interest.

In the following, we use two datasets of brains provided by the designers of brainVISA, an open software suite including a package dedicated to the study of cortical folds (http://brainvisa.info). The folds have been detected first using BrainVISA, then the sulci have been labeled either manually or automatically. The first dataset is made up of 36 brains, where each sulcus has been reliably labeled manually by a neuroanatomist. This dataset is used to train BrainVISA's sulcus recognition system. We also use another set of 150 brains, with the sulci automatically labeled. This database was provided by the International Consortium for Brain Mapping (ICBM) and acquired in the Montreal Neurological Institute of McGill University. The automatic recognition of the folds is less reliable but still gives reasonably good results [5].

The clustering of the sulci is based on 3D shape descriptors called moment invariants [6]. The first part of the paper describes several studies proving that these descriptors are well adapted to our purpose. The second part of the paper proposes a sketch of the agglomerative algorithm used to select interesting brain clusters [8]. Finally some results are shown for the cingulate sulcus, which provided the strongest patterns according to our criterion.

2   Shape Space and 3D Moment Invariants

The 3D moment invariants have been proposed as an interesting set of descriptors for the study of the shape of cortical sulci because they can be computed for any topology [6]. Hence they allow the management of the various sulcus interruptions. The construction of these descriptors is filtering out the influence of localization, orientation and scale from the 3D coordinate moments in order to obtain pure shape descriptors. While their theoretical derivation is complex, they can be computed in a simple and robust way from a black and white image defining an object. In the following, we use only the 12 invariants derived from the coordinate moments up to the power three. These 12 invariants denoted by $I1, I2, ..., I12$ are calculated from the software brainVISA and used as input to our clustering program.

Some investigations are carried out to verify that the set of moment invariants is a reasonably good shape representation to study the fold patterns. In order to confirm that similar shapes lead to similar representations, we verified first that a small shape variation leads to a small variation of the invariants. This is mandatory for our clustering purpose. Our experiments consist in creating series of shapes sampling a continuous shape transformation. An example of the resulting behaviour of the invariants is shown in Fig. 1.left. It is impossible to claim from these simple investigations that the invariants vary smoothly whatever the

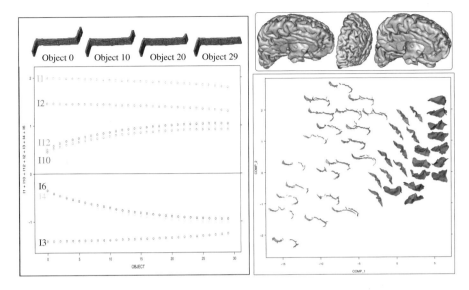

Fig. 1. Left: Variations of 7 moment invariants following continuous changes of a cylinder shape. **Right:** Two first axes of a PCA performed with 3 different sulci and 36 brains. Some of the sample points have been replaced by a snapshot of the corresponding sulcus in order to visualize the underlying shape. One can see gradual changes of the shapes, which shows that the invariant-based representation varies smoothly in the shape space.

underlying shape, and we will see further that we discovered some exceptions. Nevertheless, the behavior of these invariants seems to be continuous in general, except for two of them.

Studying the variability of the invariants across brains, we noticed that $I6$ and $I10$ were presenting bimodal distributions for some sulci. One mode was made up of positive values and the other one of negative values. There is no apparent correlation between the shape and the sign of $I6$ and $I10$. Furthermore, we managed to create slowly changing series of simulated shapes giving sign changes in $I6$ and $I10$. Such a series is illustrated in Fig. 2.left. This series evolves from a strong S cylinder towards a flat S by shortening both arms simultaneously. Notice that while most of the invariants behave smoothly all over the evolution, I6 and I10 fluctuate unexpectedly. They change sign three times very rapidly. To investigate this behavior further, we designed a new series using the finest-grain changes we could afford with our voxel-based representation (see Fig. 2.right). We discovered that adding only one single voxel could trigger the sign change. We do not know yet what kind of property would emerge if the shape space was sampled further with smaller voxels. The behaviour of the invariant could be continuous but very chaotic. Therefore, for further studies, we have chosen to discard $I6$ and $I10$ from our invariant-based representations.

It should be noted that our observation of the sign change of these two invariants has never been reported elsewhere. 3D moment invariants, indeed, have

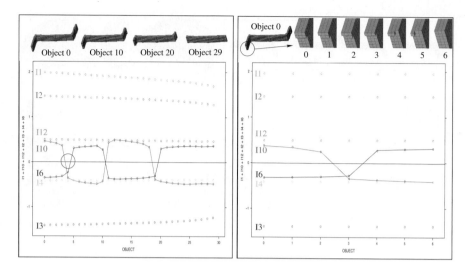

Fig. 2. Left: Variations of 7 moment invariants following continuous changes of a S-shaped cylinder. Note that I6 and I10 change signs abruptly several times. **Right:** A zoom on one of the sign change. Each step corresponds to the removal of one single voxel from the lower arm of the object.

mainly been considered as curiosities, because of the complexity of their derivation. Therefore, they were almost never used for actual applications. The invariants are made up of a sum of several hundreds of homogeneous polynomials of the central moments. This complexity is bound to hide some singularities. In fact we observed some sign change for a few other invariants, but for less than one percent of our total dataset. Therefore we decided to keep the ten remaining invariants as the basis of the representation used in this paper.

A second investigation aims at verifying that the information embedded in the invariants can distinguish the kind of patterns that characterize the cortical folds. For this purpose, we merge the datasets of several sulci, and we plot the resulting dataset using the two first axes of a principal component analysis. In most cases, the plot is made up of several clouds of points corresponding to the different sulci. An example is shown in Fig. 1.right. These clouds overlap more or less according to the shape of the sulci. The fact that each sulcus leads to a consistent cloud means that the invariant-based representations can be used to cluster groups of folds with similar shapes. To conclude, our different investigations have shown that the set of ten moment invariants can be considered as a good representation of the 3D shapes of the folds.

3 Clustering Sulci into Patterns

The cortical folding process can be considered as a chaotic phenomenon, in the sense that a slight difference among the factors that influence this process can lead to a large difference in the folding patterns. The folding patterns are the result of the competition between a large number of forces influencing brain geometry. Some of these forces are for instance the tensions induced by the long fiber bundles trying to pull two different parts of the cortex as close as possible [9]. In our opinion, the huge variability observed at the level of the folding patterns results from the large number of attractors embedded in the dynamics of this folding process. Modeling this dynamics globally is at the present time largely beyond reach. In this paper, however, we focus only on local aspects: we try to infer automatically, sulcus by sulcus, some of the alternative patterns resulting from this multiplicity of attractors. The goal is not yet to perform an exhaustive enumeration of all the possible patterns but to detect a few very contrasted patterns. If such patterns can be defined, we hypothesize that their relative frequencies could be different in some patient populations compared to control subjects. Developmental pathologies, indeed, could modify the folding dynamics and favor some specific folding patterns for some of the sulci. Hence, the folding patterns could provide some signatures useful for diagnosis.

With this goal in mind, we designed a method looking for such patterns on a sulcus by sulcus basis. For each sulcus, the method is looking for reasonably large groups of brains that exhibit a similarity in shape. Each such group is representing a pattern. At least two patterns are required and the detected patterns have to be as different as possible. It is important to emphasize that the goal here is not to assign each sulcus to a pattern. Reproducible patterns may only characterize a subset of the population.

We have chosen to address our goal using unsupervised agglomerative clustering methods. Such hierarchical approaches to clustering, indeed, fit completely our need for finding compact clusters and discarding numerous outliers. Among the variants of agglomerative clustering algorithms, we have chosen the average-linkage method for its robustness and space conserving properties [8]. In the following, the algorithm is applied to the n different instances of a given sulcus. Each instance comes from a different brain and is represented by a vector of ten moment invariants. The clustering algorithm is building a tree by successive agglomeration of the closest clusters of sulci. At the initial stage, each sulcus is a singleton cluster. The two closest sulci are joined first, leaving us with $n - 1$ clusters, one of which being the pair of joined sulci. In all succeeding steps, the two closest clusters are merged.

The complete agglomerative hierarchical tree has n levels. The lowest tree level corresponds to n singletons and the highest level to one single cluster gathering the whole set. To decide which level gives the best partition, we introduce a ratio defined as the average pairwise distance between cluster centers divided by the average cluster compactness. The compactness of a cluster is simply the average pairwise distance between the sulci. Note that the ratios are computed using only a subset of the sulci making up the kernel of each cluster. This kernel is defined as the t tightest sulci of the cluster, namely the t sulci that agglomerated the earliest in the hierarchy. Only these sulci will be considered as belonging to the putative patterns. Furthermore, only the clusters including at least t sulci will generate a putative pattern. A good set of patterns should provide a very high ratio of distance versus compactness.

The optimal kernel size t is defined as the size providing the most reliable set of patterns. The null hypothesis is that the sulcus set follows a Gaussian distribution. If the null hypothesis is true, our sulcus set should embed only one single pattern. Therefore, whatever the choice for t, the ratio should be low. In order to evaluate the distribution of the ratio for each value of t, 1000 different random sets are generated using a multivariate Gaussian distribution based on the covariance matrix of the sulcus of interest. The hierarchical tree is built up for each of these random sets and the best ratio is obtained for each value of t. From these ratio distributions, we can test the null hypothesis: for a given t, we compute the p-value as the percentage of random sets providing a better ratio than the best ratio obtained with the actual data. Then, the best t is simply the one providing the best p-value. Finally, this p-value is used to evaluate the quality of the set of patterns associated with this best t.

4   Results

The method has been applied to the ten largest sulci of the left and right hemi-spheres using the database of 36 manually labelled brains. Among the 20 sulci, 3 provided a set of patterns endowed with a p-value lower than 0.01 (the left cingulate sulcus, the left inferior precentral sulcus, and the superior frontal sulcus). The sulcus providing the best p-value (0.001 for $t = 4$) is the left cingulate sulcus (see Fig. 3). For this sulcus, a first pattern is made up of sulci presenting a large anterior interruption, a second pattern is made up of sulci presenting a smaller and more posterior interruption, and a third pattern is made up of sulci appearing continuous. It should be noted that these patterns can not be inferred just from the number of connected components. Indeed, the sulci of the third pattern are only apparently continuous: some of them are made up of several connected components overlapping each other when the sulcus is viewed from above. In fact, the moment invariants are blind to connectivity. Therefore, these three patterns would be interpreted more reliably in terms of shape than in terms of interruption. For instance, the first pattern corresponds to sulci much deeper in the posterior part than in the middle, while the last pattern corresponds to sulci with more homogeneous depth.

It is not an accident that the cingulate sulcus provides the best p-value. This sulcus is one of the sulci with very varied shapes and many interruptions. According to Ono's atlas, around 60% of the instances of this sulcus have no interruption, around 24% have two segments with a posterior interruption or an anterior interruption, and around 16% are divided into three segments [7]. It should be noted that the small size of the manually labelled database used here (36 brains) prevents the detection of rare patterns. Therefore, much larger databases will be required to achieve a more exhaustive pattern enumeration.

To illustrate possible applications of our pattern inference process, we use the three patterns obtained with this database to mine the left cingulate sulci of

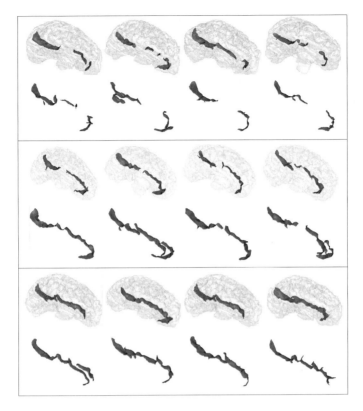

Fig. 3. The three patterns detected for the left cingulate sulcus. *Row 1,3,5:* the four tightest instances of each pattern in manually labelled database. *Row 2,4,6:* the four closest instances to the above pattern center in automatically labelled database.

another database, here the ICBM database. We selected in this database the closest samples to each of the three patterns. We observed that the shapes of these samples are consistent with the corresponding patterns (see Fig. 3). Note that when the anterior part of the sulcus is made up of two parallel folds (fourth row of Fig. 3), it is equivalent to a deeper sulcus for the moment invariants. To project the patterns from the first database onto the second database, we classify the sulci according to the closest distance to the pattern centers. This classification attributes 14 brains to the first pattern, 97 to the second and 35 to the third. It was found that the percentage of females increases gradually from 36% in the first class, to 41% in the second and to 49% in the third (global percentage of female is 42%).

5   Discussion

Compared with the traditional methods to characterize the folds by certain parameters such as the length, the number and position of interruptions, etc,

522   Z.Y. Sun et al.

the moment invariants that are used in this study provide a more comprehensive description of the 3D shapes. The drawback of using the moment invariants is that the clusters found do not necessarily provide an easy physical explanation that can be readily observed. This presents a difficulty in the description of the patterns found. Furthermore, even when we found an explanation of the possible groupings, that explanation is not necessarily the reason that groups the folds by the moment invariants. However, the final goal is not necessarily to characterize the patterns physically using words or a set of measurements such as the length or number of interruptions. These patterns, indeed, can be directly described by their moment invariants. A future direction of research could consists in mixing different kinds of features, for instance simple morphometric parameters like length and depth with 3D moment invariants. This approach, however, requires large databases to overcome problems induced by the curse of dimensionality.

In this paper, the search for patterns has been applied to folds already labeled, either manually or automatically. A more ambitious project, that will be addressed in the future, will be the design of methods looking for patterns without the knowledge of the traditional nomenclature. Such an approach applied to large databases could reveal patterns beyond the reach of the first anatomists.

One possible use of the patterns we found is to compare the frequency of occurrence among normal and patient datasets. Similar comparisons can be carried out on other datasets for pure neuroscience questions: musicians versus athletes, kids with an early development on language versus an early development on motor-skills, etc. The hypothesis is that a certain developmental event or a certain strong training would leave an observable imprint on the folding patterns.

References

1. Welker, W.: Why does cerebral cortex fissure and fold? In: Cerebral Cortex, vol. 8B, pp. 3–136. Plenum Press, New York (1988)
2. Le Goualher, G., Procyk, E., Collins, D.L., Venugopal, R., Barillot, C., Evans, A.C.: Automated extraction and variability analysis of sulcal neuroanatomy. IEEE Trans. on Medical Imaging 18(3), 206–217 (1999)
3. Lohmann, G., von Cramon, D.Y.: Automatic labelling of the human cortical surface using sulcal basins. Medical Image Analysis 4(3), 179–188 (2000)
4. Fillard, P., Arsigny, V., Pennec, X., Hayashi, K.M., Thompson, P.M., Ayache, N.: Measuring brain variability by extrapolating sparse tensor fields measured on sulcal lines. Neuroimage 34(2), 639–650 (2007)
5. Rivière, D., Mangin, J.F., Papadopoulos-Orfanos, D., Martinez, J.M., Frouin, V., Régis, J.: Automatic recognition of cortical sulci of the human brain using a congregation of neural networks. Medical Image Analysis 6(2), 77–92 (2002)
6. Mangin, J.F., Poupon, F., Duchesnay, E., Rivière, D., Cachia, A., Collins, D.L., Evans, A.C., Régis, J.: Brain morphometry using 3D moment invariants. Medical Image Analysis 8, 187–196 (2004)
7. Ono, M., Kubik, S., Abernathey, C.D.: Atlas of the cerebral sulci. Thieme (1990)
8. Kaufman, L., Rousseuw, P.J.: Finding groups in data. Wiley series in probability and statistics (1990)
9. Van Essen, D.C.: A tension-based theory of morphogenesis and compact wiring in the central nervous system. Nature 385, 313–318 (1997)

Classifier Selection Strategies for Label Fusion Using Large Atlas Databases

P. Aljabar[1], R. Heckemann[2], A. Hammers[3], J.V. Hajnal[2],
and D. Rueckert[1]

[1] Department of Computing, Imperial College London, UK
[2] Imaging Sciences Department, MRC Clinical Sciences Centre, Imperial College
London, UK
[3] Division of Neuroscience and Mental Health, MRC Clinical Sciences Centre,
Imperial College London, UK*

Abstract. Structural segmentations of brain MRI can be generated by propagating manually labelled atlas images from a repository to a query subject and combining them. This method has been shown to be robust, consistent and increasingly accurate with increasing numbers of classifiers. It outperforms standard atlas-based segmentation but suffers, however, from problems of scale when the number of atlases is large. For a large repository and a particular query subject, using a selection strategy to identify good classifiers is one way to address problems of scale. This work presents and compares different classifier selection strategies which are applied to a group of 275 subjects with manually labelled brain MR images. We approximate an upper limit for the accuracy or overlap that can be achieved for a particular structure in a given subject and compare this with the accuracy obtained using classifier selection. The accuracy of different classifier selection strategies are also rated against the distribution of overlaps generated by random groups of classifiers.

1 Introduction

As increasing numbers of MR images have become available over recent years, the creation and maintenance of repositories of atlases consisting of MR images with corresponding reliable structural segmentations (manual or otherwise) has become more feasible. It has been a natural consequence to use such expert annotations to assist in providing automatic segmentations of query or unseen images. A popular approach is atlas-based segmentation, where a segmented anatomical atlas is registered with a query subject and the atlas labelling is propagated to give an estimate for the segmentation in the query subject [1,2]. If multiple atlases are available, the labels from each atlas can be aligned with the query image and treated as classifiers. A rule can be applied to combine or fuse these classifiers to generate a segmentation estimate. This can be a simple

* We are grateful to David Kennedy at the Centre for Morphometric analysis for providing the data for this work and we are grateful to the EPSRC who funded this work under the IBIM project.

N. Ayache, S. Ourselin, A. Maeder (Eds.): MICCAI 2007, Part I, LNCS 4791, pp. 523–531, 2007.
© Springer-Verlag Berlin Heidelberg 2007

majority vote rule for each voxel [3] or a more sophisticated approach based on, for example assigning weights to classifiers [4].

Using a database of images of bee brains, Rohlfing et al. [3] showed that fusing the classifiers according to a simple vote or majority rule is robust and accurate compared with other methods. The vote rule has also been shown to outperform other classifier combination methods for more general applications [5]. In the context of the segmentation of human brain structures, Heckemann et al. [6] showed that this approach exceeds the accuracy of previous automatic methods and compares well with manual labelling. Using 30 expert labellings of human brains [7], a model was developed for the asymptotic level of accuracy achievable as the number of input classifiers increases. For classifier numbers beyond 15 to 20 atlases, the improvement in terms of segmentation accuracy tended to be very small.

If such an approach is applied to a repository consisting of a very large number of atlases, other factors become relevant. For example, the effort required to segment an unseen subject increases linearly according to the number of subjects if every atlas is registered to the query image. It is also likely that the population represented among the atlases is diverse with respect to factors such as age or pathology. This means that certain subjects in the database are more appropriate than others as potential classifiers for a query image. In the context of these considerations, and the diminishing returns from the use of increasing number classifiers, it is desirable to have a strategy for selecting atlases from among the population that are the most appropriate for the particular query subject and for the structure(s) which need to be segmented. Wu et al. investigated methods for optimal selection of a single template for atlas-based segmentation [8]. Our work contrasts with this in that we select multiple atlases for subsequent fusion.

In this work we present an investigation of practical selection strategies using a database consisting of 275 MR images and accompanying manual labels. We rate the performance of selections against an estimate of the 'best' possible segmentation accuracy and against the performance of random groups of classifiers. Finally we investigate the effect of selecting increasing numbers of classifiers from a ranked set of atlases.

2   Data and Methodology

The data used consisted of T1 weighted MR brain images of 275 male and female subjects with ages between 4 and 83 years acquired in multiple centres. Various structures in these images were manually delineated by the Centre for Morphometric Analysis (Massachusetts General Hospital, Charlestown, MA) following a single segmentation protocol. Manual delineations for 35 structures were present in all images. For our experiments, a number of subjects were randomly selected and used as test or query subjects and the remaining subjects' images and manual segmentations were treated as an atlas repository.

In this work, the term 'atlas' describes the pairing of an anatomical image and its corresponding manual labelling. If the anatomies of an atlas and a query subject are in alignment, the atlas labels can be considered to be a 'classifier', providing an estimate for a segmentation of the query. If multiple atlases are available as classifiers for a particular query, then these classifiers can be 'fused' or 'combined' to provide an improved segmentation estimate [3,6]. We describe as a fusion experiment the process of selecting a number of the repository subjects as classifiers and subsequently combining them with the majority vote rule to provide a fused segmentation estimate for a particular structure within a chosen query subject.

All subjects were registered to the MNI Brainweb single subject simulated T1 weighted MR image [9] to image avoid the computational burden that would be associated with registering every atlas to every query subject. The registrations consisted of an affine registration step followed by a non-rigid registration using a B-spline based free form deformation model [10] which was applied hierarchically with successive control point spacings of 20, 10 and 5mm. The metric used during registration was normalised mutual information (NMI) [11]. The resulting transformations were used to spatially normalise all anatomical images and their manual labels. After spatial normalisation, a region of interest (ROI) was defined for each structure studied as the minimum bounding box containing the structure for all repository subjects expanded by two voxels along each dimension.

The strategy for selecting atlases as classifiers is the main focus of this work, and this was carried out based on a set of ranks assigned to the repository images. The following describes the different methods used to select atlases from the repository:

- **Classifier selection based on segmentation similarity:** For a given query subject, the Dice overlaps [12] between the subject's manual label and all the repository subjects were found. The repository images were then ranked according to these values. Clearly, this method is not a realistic option in a practical setting as the manual segmentations for query subjects are generally unavailable (in fact, the segmentation of the query subjects is the overall goal). The accuracy of the resulting fused segmentation does, however, provide a reference value to compare against other selection methods.

- **Classifier selection based on image similarity:** For a given query subject, a number of different image similarity metrics can be calculated using the T1 weighted images of the query and of the repository atlases. The similarity ranking strategy breaks down into four methods based on the metrics used: sum of squared differences (SSD), cross correlation (CC), mutual information (MI) and normalised mutual information (NMI). The metric was calculated using voxels in the ROI defined for the chosen structure. The repository atlases were then ranked according to the resulting similarity metric values.

- **Classifier selection based on demographics:** In general, it is possible to select classifiers based on non-image information, e.g. age, sex or pathology. We have selected from atlases that were ranked according to how close their ages were to the query subject's age. This ranking is therefore independent of the image data.

3   Experiments and Results

3.1   Experiments

Fifteen classifiers were used for each fusion experiment and the accuracy of each resulting segmentation was measured by its Dice overlap with the manual segmentation for the query subject, which was treated as the 'gold standard'. To assess the performance of a selection method, the overlap of the resulting segmentation with the gold standard label was calculated and compared with the distribution of overlaps obtained from multiple fusions of randomly selected classifiers ($N = 1000$, 15 classifiers per experiment). In this work, we present the results of experiments using the hippocampus, the lateral ventricles and the thalamus which were chosen as representative structures in terms, size, image intensity and of the segmentation accuracy achievable by automated methods. In previous work [6], average Dice coefficients for the accuracy of fusion based segmentations of these structures have been 0.90 for the lateral ventricles and the thalamus and 0.82 for the hippocampus. Each structure's left-right pair was treated as a single structure.

A number of subjects were used as a test set and classifiers were selected from the remaining subjects which were used as a repository. For selection based on segmentation or image similarity, 20 subjects were randomly selected as the test set. For selection based on age proximity, the test set consisted of 15 random subjects equally divided among each of three age intervals: $0 - 10$, $30 - 45$ and $70+$ years.

The effect of selecting different numbers of ranked classifiers was also investigated. For each of the 20 subjects in the test set used for similarity selection, the repository atlases were ranked by segmentation similarity. Subsequently, starting with the top-ranked atlas, successively larger numbers of *ordered* atlases were used as classifiers, i.e. each group of classifiers was formed from the previous group with the inclusion of one further classifier.

3.2   Selection Strategy Comparisons

After fusion of 1000 sets of 15 random classifiers for all 20 query subjects, the mean (SD) overlap values were: Hippocampus 0.79 (0.03), lateral ventricle 0.90 (0.02), thalamus 0.88 (0.02). The random overlap distributions obtained for the hippocampus and lateral ventricle are shown in Figure 1 as box-and-whisker plots. Each box shows the lower quartile, the median and the upper quartile (q_1, q_2 and q_3). The whisker lengths are set at 1.5 times the inter-quartile range (distributions for the thalamus are qualitatively similar but were omitted for reasons of space). A negligible number of overlap values fell outside the whisker ranges which were not plotted for readability: 0.2% gave values above the whiskers and 2% below. Figure 1 also shows the overlaps achieved after similarity based selection, these can be compared against the random overlap distributions.

To summarise the performance of the image similarity selection methods, their overlap measures with the gold standard were compared with the quartiles

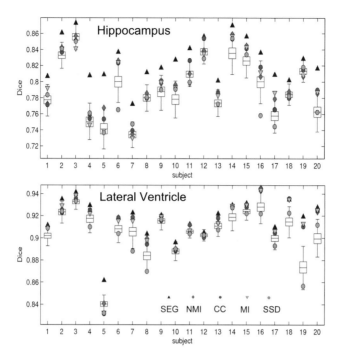

Fig. 1. Comparisons of performance for the segmentation similarity (SEG) and image similarity selection methods for 20 randomly selected test subjects. The similarity measures used were normalised mutual information (NMI), mutual information (MI), cross-correlation (CC), and sums of squared differences (SSD). For comparison, each box-and-whisker plot shows the Dice overlap distribution for 1000 random fusions of 15 classifiers.

Table 1. Performance ratings for image similarity selection using quartiles and z-scores. d represents the Dice overlap obtained by a particular metric, q_1, q_2, q_3: the quartiles for the random overlap distribution. Entries indicate the number of each case among the 20 query subjects. Bottom row: Mean z-scores for each combination of similarity metric and structure across all query subjects.

	Lateral Ventricle				Hippocampus				Thalamus			
	NMI	MI	CC	SSD	NMI	MI	CC	SSD	NMI	MI	CC	SSD
$q_3 \leq d \leq 1$	16	16	15	5	14	11	13	8	16	19	17	2
$q_2 \leq d < q_3$	2	3	2	4	4	1	3	2	4	0	2	5
$q_1 \leq d < q_2$	2	0	1	1	1	6	1	4	0	1	1	7
$0 \leq d < q_1$	0	1	2	10	1	2	3	6	0	0	0	6
Mean z	1.8	1.8	1.7	-0.4	1.2	0.8	1.2	-0.1	2.1	1.9	2.0	-0.5

of the random overlap distributions. The quartiles define four intervals $[0, q_1)$, $[q_1, q_2)$, $[q_2, q_3)$, $[q_3, 1]$ and the number of overlaps within each interval for each image similarity selection method and structure are shown in Table 1. With

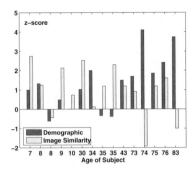

Fig. 2. A comparison of age based selection (green) with image similarity selection (NMI, yellow) using hippocampus overlap z-scores for subjects with different ages. The subjects' ages are on the horizontal axis.

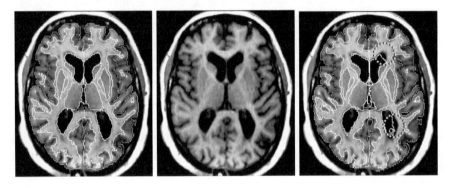

Fig. 3. Label fusion for the image of a 74 year old query subject. Left: Segmentation obtained by fusing the nearest 15 subjects in age. Centre: T1 weighted image. Right: A segmentation based on 15 randomly selected classifiers; dashed circles indicate regions of segmentation failure.

the exception of SSD, the image similarity selection methods all outperformed the median random overlap in 17 or more cases for the lateral ventricle. NMI selection exceeded the median in 18 of the 20 subjects for the hippocampus and lateral ventricle and in all cases for the thalamus.

The overlap values for each ranking method were also rated by converting them to z-scores using the mean and standard deviation of the random overlap distribution for the corresponding query subject and structure. The z-score expresses the signed difference between the measured value and the distribution mean as a multiple of standard deviations. The mean z-scores for the image similarity metrics are shown in Table 1, where it can be seen that the highest mean z-score was always achieved by image similarity selection using NMI. The mean z-scores after segmentation similarity selection were 3.2, 4.5 and 3.6 for the lateral ventricle, hippocampus and thalamus.

Using the test set for age based selection, classifiers were selected for each query subject according to age proximity and overlaps were calculated for the resulting

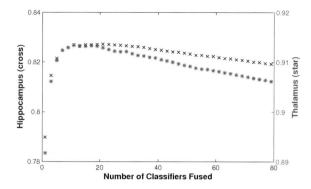

Fig. 4. Selecting increasing numbers of classifiers from the repository after after segmentation similarity ordering: The effect upon thalamus and hippocampus overlaps

fusions. Figure 2 shows these overlaps in the form of z-scores where the figures obtained after image similarity (NMI) selection for the same subjects are also shown for comparison. As an illustration, the image for a particular 74 year old subject is shown in Figure 3. This diagram also shows the labels produced by fusing the 15 age-selected classifiers along with a segmentation produced using 15 randomly selected classifiers. The fusion of randomly selected classifiers has, for example, overestimated the white matter on the right side of the brain and the segmentation of the right ventricle has failed in this case.

3.3   Varying the Number of Classifiers

In separate experiments, using the similarity selection test set, increasing numbers of classifiers were selected from an ordered set of atlases and fused. The atlases were ordered by segmentation similarity for each structure. The mean overlaps obtained across the test subjects for the hippocampus and thalamus are shown in Figure 4 (The data for the ventricles are similar but have been omitted for reasons of space). The main feature of these results is that the overlap values improve rapidly, reach their highest value for approximately 10–20 classifiers and subsequently decrease gradually as more classifiers are chosen from the ranked set.

4   Discussion

We have presented and tested strategies for classifier selection which can reduce the effects of scale when using large atlas repositories to segment structures in unseen images. The tested selection strategies are based on segmentation or image similarity and on age. Performance of the different methods was assessed in comparison with the distributions of overlap values obtained from a series of random classifier fusion experiments. In order to avoid the computational burden of registering every atlas with every query subject, the selection of classifiers and their fusion was carried out in a single reference space. We are currently adapting these methods to use reference space classifier selection in order to generate further improvements in segmentation accuracy in the query subject's native space. The high overlaps achieved by segmentation similarity based selection suggest they are good upper bound estimates for the accuracy possible with classifier fusion.

Using image similarity selection, the performance figures clearly show SSD as being the least reliable in identifying a good set of classifiers. The other metrics, NMI, MI and CC, vary more subtly; NMI selection generally performed best, being most likely to achieve an overlap value above the median of the random distribution and obtaining the highest z-scores throughout. This may be expected since NMI was used as the metric during registration.

How well a structure can be segmented for each query subject is estimated by the overlap distributions of randomly fused labels. Predictably, these show that the lateral ventricles are the easiest to segment. Additionally, the random overlap averages vary significantly between subjects showing a subject dependence for the segmentation accuracy. It is also noted that the quality of fused segmentations for one structure does not directly translate to another. For example subject 19 (Figure 1) has overlaps that are good for the hippocampus but poor for the lateral ventricle relative to the group. This provides some justification for the use of regional local metrics for selection.

Using age-based selection, the z-scores for NMI-based and age-based selection (Figure 2) suggest comparable performance for the young and middle aged groups. For the older group, however, selection by age significantly outperformed NMI selection in every case suggesting the potential demographic criteria have for increasing segmentation accuracy through classifier selection. The segmentations for the 74 year old subject shown in Figure 3 highlight how random classifiers can fail where age-based atlas selection provides a much better estimate. In our experience, such segmentation failures are possible for subjects with, for example, enlarged ventricles when using normal atlases. Selection strategies that combine image similarity and demographic data should provide an interesting area for further work.

The selection of increasing numbers of ranked classifiers after ordering the repository images ($N = 255$) showed that the highest overlap values were achieved for groups of 10–20 classifiers. This indicates that the choice of 15 subjects for the fusion experiments was reasonable. Moreover, the gradual decline in overlap values as more of the ordered classifiers are fused suggests that there is merit in avoiding the use of large numbers of classifiers when the repository is large and selection is applied. Clearly as the number of classifiers continues to increase, the resulting fused segmentations will approach the population mean and the overlaps will reach an asymptotic value. Heckemann et al. [6] showed that selecting increasing numbers of random sets of classifiers gave overlap values that monotonically increased to an asymptotic value, and they presented a model for convergence to this value. We feel that the limiting overlap value obtained by selecting from an ordered set of classifiers will be the same, and establishing this could prove an interesting task for further work.

In conclusion, we have presented and compared different strategies for classifier selection that should help towards reducing the computational burden associated with the use of large atlas databases. The results suggest that image and demographic based classifier selection can perform well in terms of segmentation accuracy and that there is merit in ranking and limiting the number of classifiers used when a large number are available.

References

1. Svarer, C., Madsen, K., Hasselbalch, S.G., Pinborg, L.H., Haugbol, S., Frokjaer, V.G., Holm, S., Paulson, O.B., Knudsen, G.M.: MR-based automatic delineation of volumes of interest in human brain PET images using probability maps. NeuroImage 24, 969–979 (2005)
2. Iosifescu, D., Shenton, M., Warfield, S., Kikinis, R., Dengler, J., Jolesz, F., Mccarley, R.: An automated registration algorithm for measuring MRI subcortical brain structures. Neuroimage 6, 13–25 (1997)
3. Rohlfing, T., Brandt, R., Menzel, R., Maurer Jr., C.R.: Evaluation of atlas selection strategies for atlas-based image segmentation with application to confocal microscopy images of bee brains. NeuroImage 21, 1428–1442 (2004)
4. Warfield, S., Zou, K., Wells, W.: Simultaneous truth and performance level estimation (STAPLE): an algorithm for the validation of image segmentation. IEEE Transactions on Medical Imaging 23, 903–921 (2004)
5. Kittler, J., Hatef, M., Duin, R., Matas, J.: On combining classifiers. IEEE Transactions on Pattern Analysis and Machine Intelligence 20, 226–239 (1998)
6. Heckemann, R.A., Hajnal, J.V., Aljabar, P., Rueckert, D., Hammers, A.: Automatic anatomical brain MRI segmentation combining label propagation and decision fusion. Neuroimage 33, 115–126 (2006)
7. Hammers, A., Allom, R., Koepp, M., Free, S., Myers, R., Lemieux, L., Mitchell, T., Brooks, D., Duncan, J.: Three-dimensional maximum probability atlas of the human brain, with particular reference to the temporal lobe. Human Brain Mapping 19, 224–247 (2003)
8. Wu, M., Rosano, C., Lopez-Garcia, P., Carter, C.S., Aizenstein, H.J.: Optimum template selection for atlas-based segmentation. NeuroImage 34, 1612–1618 (2007)
9. Cocosco, C., Kollokian, V., Kwan, R.S., Evans, A.: BrainWeb: Online interface to a 3D MRI simulated brain database. NeuroImage 5 (1997)
10. Rueckert, D., Sonoda, L., Hayes, C., Hill, D., Leach, M., Hawkes, D.: Non-rigid registration using free-form deformations: Application to breast MR images. IEEE Transactions on Medical Imaging 18, 712–721 (1999)
11. Studholme, C., Hill, D.L.G., Hawkes, D.J.: An overlap invariant entropy measure of 3D medical image alignment. Pattern Recognition 32, 71–86 (1998)
12. Dice, L.R.: Measures of the amount of ecologic association between species. Ecology 26, 297 (1945)

Groupwise Combined Segmentation and Registration for Atlas Construction

Kanwal K. Bhatia[1], Paul Aljabar[1], James P. Boardman[2], Latha Srinivasan[2],
Maria Murgasova[1], Serena J. Counsell[3], Mary A. Rutherford[2,3], Jo Hajnal[3],
A. David Edwards[2], and Daniel Rueckert[1]

[1] Visual Information Processing, Department of Computing, Imperial College London
[2] Department of Pediatrics, Faculty of Medicine, Hammersmith Hospital
[3] Imaging Sciences Department, MRC Clinical Sciences Centre, Hammersmith
Hospital, Imperial College London

Abstract. The creation of average anatomical atlases has been a growing area of research in recent years. It is of increased value to construct
representations of, not only intensity atlases, but also their segmentation
into required tissues or structures. This paper presents novel *groupwise
combined segmentation and registration* approaches, which aim to simultaneously improve both the alignment of intensity images to their average
shape, as well as the segmentations of structures in the average space.
An iterative EM framework is used to build average 3D MR atlases of
populations for which prior atlases do not currently exist: preterm infants at one- and two-years old. These have been used to quantify the
growth of tissues occurring between these ages.

1 Introduction

Anatomical atlases representative of populations are of tremendous value in
medical image analysis and have allowed the investigation of structural and
functional characteristics of the brain. There has been a recent increase in the
construction of atlases representing the *average anatomy* of a population [1]
[2] [3] [4] [5] [6] either through using pure groupwise registration techniques or
through the averaging of transformations from pairwise registrations, which are
less biased towards any single subject. In addition to average structure intensity atlases, it is also valuable to have segmentations of this average shape [7].
Segmentation allows for the quanitification of structural volumes, which can be
used to analyse morphological differences over time or between subjects [8] [9],
or for 3D visualisation and analysis [10].

Atlases representing segmented structures are useful in determining typical
anatomy in a given group. Additionally, they are often used in the segmentation
of new subjects of the same population [11] [12]. The construction of corresponding intensity and segmentation atlases can be achieved either through the
segmentation of images followed by the registration of these segmentations [6],
or through the alignment of intensity images and the propagation of individual
segmentations [11]. Clearly, in the first case, the registration is dependent on the

N. Ayache, S. Ourselin, A. Maeder (Eds.): MICCAI 2007, Part I, LNCS 4791, pp. 532–540, 2007.
© Springer-Verlag Berlin Heidelberg 2007

quality of the segmentation, and, in the second method, the final segmentation is dependent on the accuracy of the registration. Segmentation and registration would therefore appear to be complementary processes and an improvement in one is likely to lead to an improvement in the other.

Much previous work on supervised segmentation of brain MR images has used probabilisitic atlases (*priors*) to help classify voxels [13] [12] according to their location. However, problems may occur if the population from which the prior was created differs from that of the image to be segmented, for example, in the use of adult priors, such as the MNI305 priors, to segment child brain images [14]. It may not, however, be easy to obtain representative priors, as they themseleves are created from the segmentation of multiple subjects of the same population.

There has therefore been recent development in non-rigidly aligning priors to an image to be segmented [15]. The most recent work has shown that integrating the registration parameters into the Bayesian framework of maximum likelihood or maximum a-posterior estimation [16] [17] benefits the segmentation. However, no attempt is made to use segmentations to assist in the registration of images. This is done in [18], where a segmented target and a floating image are registered. The transformation between these images is used to improve the segmentation in the target space. The combined segmentation, registration and modelling of sets of images is considered in [19] which iteratively registers a current estimate of the transformed intensity image to a reconstruction of the image based on its current segmentation. However, it is not obvious in their work how the integration of these methods provides an improvement over sequential techniques.

In this paper, we introduce novel *groupwise combined segmentation and registration algorithms*. The aim is to concurrently align to, and segment a *population* of images in, the *average coordinate system* of the population. This is defined as the coordinate system which requires least deformation from itself to all subjects in the population [4]. To do this we combine methods which previously have been shown, individually, to perform well for their respective tasks - groupwise registration using the Kullback-Leibler divergence [6] and the Expectation-Maximisation (EM) algorithm for segmentation [13] [12] - and demonstrate the mutual benefit of their integration. Furthermore, we incorporate an iterative update into the segmentation process which uses the current probabilistic segmentations of the population to create representative prior models for the next iteration. The use of these dynamic models, created from the population concerned, reduces the bias as compared to priors based on standard atlases.

2   Methods

2.1   The EM Algorithm for Single-Subject Segmentation

For an image i, let $\mathbf{Y}$ be the collection of J voxels, each with intensity y_j, i.e. $\mathbf{Y} = \{y_j, j = 1, 2...J\}$. Assume we wish to segment this image into K tissue classes. Let the unknown tissue labelling $\mathbf{Z}$ be represented by a vector $\mathbf{z}$ of length K for each voxel. When a voxel is classified as being tissue class l, $z_l = 1$ and $z_{k \neq l} = 0$. Each tissue class, k, can be assumed to approximate a Gaussian distribution, with mean intensity μ_k and variance σ_k^2, forming the distribution parameters $\theta = \{\mu_k, \sigma_k^2, k = 1, 2...K\}$. The overall image can be considered to be a mixture of Gaussian distributions, with the mixing coefficients given by the prior probabilities of each of the labels, $p(z_{jk} = 1) = \pi_{jk}$, for each voxel j. The aim is to find the segmentation and Gaussian parameters which maximise the log-likelihood:

$$\sum_j \log \sum_k p(y_j|z_{jk} = 1, \theta) \cdot p(z_{jk} = 1) = \sum_j \log \sum_k G_{jk} \cdot p(z_{jk} = 1) \quad (1)$$

where $G_{jk} = p(y_j|z_{jk} = 1, \theta)$ gives the Gaussian probability density calculated from the distribution parameters. The EM algorithm solves this by iterating between two steps, details of the solution being given in [12]:

1. *Expectation step.* Calculate the posterior probability distribution, $w_{jl} = p(z_{jl} = 1|y_j, \theta)$, of a voxel j being labelled as tissue class l.
2. *Maximisation step.* Find the Gaussian parameters that maximise Eq. 1.

2.2 Groupwise Segmentation

The aim of our proposed groupwise segmentation method is to segment a group of n images, which have been non-rigidly aligned to their average coordinate system, using representative priors created from the current estimate of the segmentations of the individuals in the group. In order to create initial soft segmentations, $p(z_{ijk} = 1|y_{ij}, \theta)$, for each image, i, the EM algorithm is run for just a single iteration using MNI priors. The voxel-wise mean of these soft segmentations is then used to create a new prior model, $\pi_k^{(t+1)}$, of each class, k, to be used in the next iteration $t + 1$:

$$\pi_{jk}^{(t+1)} = \frac{\sum_i^n p(z_{ijk} = 1|y_{ij}, \theta)}{n} = \frac{\sum_i^n w_{ijk}}{n} \quad (2)$$

To avoid magnifying inaccuracies caused by bias of an initial prior model, the EM process continues with the model being updated at every iteration, using Eq. 2. However, although at each iteration the log-likelihood (and therefore the theoretical segmentation) is improved for the current model, constantly updating the model means that, overall, the log-likelihood will not converge. Instead, the algorithm is terminated when the complexity of the model converges. When the images are segmented with greatest confidence and perfectly aligned, the entropy of the model will always be at a minimum. We therefore instead aim to reduce the entropy of the model, and terminate the segmentation-registration process when this converges. The entropy of the prior model, M, at iteration t is given by:

$$H(M^{(t)}) = -\sum_j \sum_k \pi_{jk}^{(t)} \log \pi_{jk}^{(t)} \quad (3)$$

2.3   Groupwise Non-rigid Registration

In order to ensure the alignment of the priors to each of the images, the images need first to be aligned to a common, and preferably average, space. This could be done using a variety of either pairwise, or groupwise, non-rigid registration methods [4] [2] [1] [20] [3] [5] [6]. However, as the segmentation of each image gets more certain, this addtional knowledge can also be used to further improve the registration. The Kullback-Leibler divergence (KLD) is an additive metric for comparing distances between probability distributions. As individual segmentations become more accurate, the prior model becomes a more specific representation of the average shape. Reducing the distance between the model and each subject will therefore improve the alignment of the population to the average shape. The KLD similarity measure is given by the distance between the prior model π_{jk} and the classification of each subject w_{ijk}:

$$Minimise: \sum_i \sum_j \sum_k w_{ijk} \log \left(\frac{w_{ijk}}{\pi_{jk}} \right) \tag{4}$$

This aims to align each probability map with the current average probability map of the group. When they are all perfectly aligned, all distributions will be the same. This metric is particularly useful as a similarity measure for pure groupwise registration [6] as it reduces sensitivity to largely varying image intensities. The performance of the registration method is, however, dependent on the quality of the segmentations.

2.4   Integrated Segmentation-Registration

The groupwise registration method described in the previous section aims to align a group of subjects by using their segmentations. The quality of the registration is likely to be improved with improved segmentations. However, there is no requirement of the registration to provide an optimal solution to aid segmentation. The registration can instead be incorporated into a Bayesian maximum a-posteriori (MAP) framework for segmentation, as in [16]:

$$(\theta^{(t+1)}, R^{(t+1)}) = \arg\max_{\theta, R} \log \sum_{\mathbf{Z}} P(\theta, R, \mathbf{Z} | \mathbf{Y}) \tag{5}$$

This aims to maximise the probability of the Gaussian parameters, θ, the registration parameters, R, and the tissue labelling, $\mathbf{Z}$, given the image intensities, $\mathbf{Y}$. Extending the approach in [16] to include multiple deformable images gives:

$$(\theta^{(t+1)}, R^{(t+1)}) = \arg\max_{\theta, R} \sum_j \sum_k w_{ijk}^{(t)} \cdot \left[\log G_{jk} + \log \pi_{jk}^{(t)} \right] \tag{6}$$

This can be solved using the Expectation Conditional Maximisation (ECM) algorithm [21] by optimising Eq. 6 with respect to θ and R in turn. The term on the right-hand-side of Eq. 6 represents a cost function to be maximised. This can be rewritten by adding $(w_{ijk} \log w_{ijk} - w_{ijk} \log w_{ijk} = 0)$:

$$\arg\max_{\theta,R} \sum_{j} \sum_{k} w_{ijk} \log \left(G_{jk} \cdot w_{ijk}\right) - w_{ijk} \log \left(\frac{w_{ijk}}{\pi_{jk}}\right) \qquad (7)$$

The final term represents the KLD between the posteriors and the model, and thus the alignment of the image to the group average. However, the first term depends only on the image under consideration. Maximising these two terms concurrently, as in the integrated method, need not necessarily result in improved alignment.

2.5   Interleaved Segmentation-Registration

An alternative method is to interleave groupwise segmentation and groupwise registration such that each term of Eq. 7 is optimised individually. The groupwise registration algorithm in Section 2.3 maximises only the second term of Eq. 7. Any resulting reduction in the value of the first term can be compensated for by subsequently applying the groupwise segmentation algorithm of Section 2.2. This second stage finds the Gaussian parameters that maximise only the first term without affecting the registration result. The interleaved segmentation-registration algorithm therefore aims to improve both the segmentation and the registration by iterating between the two processes.

3   Results

3.1   Evaluation of Methods on Simulated Data

A population of 100 subjects was created by deforming the MNI Brainweb image by known deformation fields (generated using a free-form deformation model based on B-splines [22]), which were constrained to sum to zero deformation across the population. The MNI Brainweb image also has ground truth and probabilistic segmentations for WM, GM, CSF and background (BG) tissue classes. The transformations to the average space, as well as the segmentations of the individual images are therefore known. In addition, varying levels of Gaussian noise (with zero mean and standard deviation ranging from 0-5) were applied across the population. The proposed methods of interleaved (INLVD) and integrated (INTGD) segmentation-registration approaches have been tested on the simulated dataset. An initial estimate of the alignment is used, created using a groupwise registration approach based on B-splines [4] with a KLD similarity metric. The MNI305 priors are used as the initial prior probability maps. Additionally, the groupwise segmentation method alone has been applied, using the known, actual transformations to average space (GW).

Effect on segmentation. The segmentation of each subject using the described techniques is compared to that obtained using the standard EM algorithm on each individual, using affinely-aligned MNI priors. Average Dice overlaps between the known and obtained segmentations are computed for each structure and are shown in Table 1. It can be seen that the use of groupwise segmentation-registration improves the accuracy and consistency of the segmentation.

Table 1. Mean and standard deviation of dice similarity for each structure using each segmentation method

Method	BG	CSF	GM	WM
EM	0.976 ± 0.0044	0.779 ± 0.0247	0.871 ± 0.0067	0.922 ± 0.0066
INGTD	0.988 ± 0.0009	0.847 ± 0.0063	0.882 ± 0.0037	0.949 ± 0.0023
INTLV	0.988 ± 0.0009	0.850 ± 0.0060	0.884 ± 0.0038	0.950 ± 0.0023
GW	0.989 ± 0.0008	0.862 ± 0.0059	0.891 ± 0.0036	0.955 ± 0.0021

Effect on registration. Both integrated and interleaved methods used constrained groupwise registration [4], using the KLD similarity measure, to ensure the atlas represents average shape of the population. The average root-mean-squared (RMS) error of the final voxel deformations from the original shape were calculated. The average RMS deformation of the unregistered population was 2.92mm. The average error after only groupwise registration was found to be 1.93mm. This improved to 1.70mm when using the interleaved method of segmentation-registration. However, as predicted, no improvement was found from the integrated method which resulted in a final RMS error of 1.97mm.

3.2 Average Brain Atlases of Preterm Infants at One and Two Years

Populations of 22 preterm-born subjects imaged at one year and again at two years were initially aligned to their average shapes, by averaging pairwise transformations [2]. The pure groupwise segmentation algorithm was run on each of these aligned populations, using the MNI305 priors for the initial iteration. The prior atlases were recalculated after each iteration. Convergence of these atlases for the two-year-old population is shown in Fig. 1. Fig. 2 shows the final average intensity and tissue class probability atlases for the average shape of each population.

The model of priors has additionally been used to calculate volumes of the segmented tissue classes of each average shape. It was found that the mean volume of WM increases from 278 to $326cm^3$ (+17%) and the mean volume of GM increases from 536 to $612cm^3$ (+14%) between one and two years.

4   Discussion

The groupwise segmentation-registration methods developed have been used to create average intensity and probabilistic segmentations of populations, representing their average shape. Additionally, these techniques have been used to

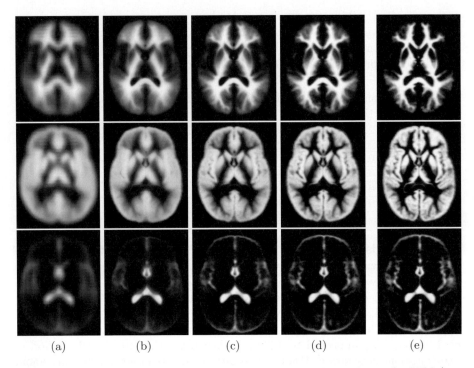

(a)   (b)   (c)   (d)   (e)

Fig. 1. The evolution of prior models for the two-year-old population for WM (top row), GM (middle row) and CSF (bottom row). (a) MNI 305 priors; (b)-(d) updated models at iterations 1-3; (e) convergence of model entropy at iteration 6.

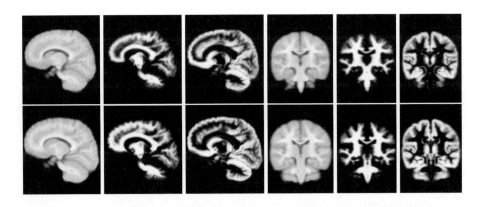

Fig. 2. Average shape atlases of 22 one- (top row) and two-year-olds (bottom row). L-R: sagittal intensity, WM and GM atlases, coronal intensity, WM and GM atlases.

segment the individual subjects of each population in their native space. On the simulated dataset, both combined segmentation-registration methods outperform the EM algorithm at segmentation of the original images. The best segmentation occurs when the images are perfectly aligned, as obtained when the known transformations to the average space are applied. However, only the interleaved method, which explicitly aims to maximise the registration, improves the alignment of the images over that obtained by pure groupwise registration.

The groupwise segmentation algorithm has also been used to create average shape and probabilistic segmentation atlases of populations of preterm infants at one- and two-years-old, as well as hard segmentations of the individual subjects in their native space. The atlases obtained have been used to quantify tissue growth between one and two years.

It is acknowledged that validation on a simulated dataset is limited as real populations contain differing brain topologies and imaging artifacts such as noise and inhomogeneity. Manual segmentations of the infant dataset are not available at time of writing, and it is intended to compare the results on real data to gold standard segmentations in the future.

References

1. Guimond, A., et al.: Average brain models: A convergence study. Computer Vision and Image Understanding 77(9), 192–210 (2000)
2. Rueckert, D., et al.: Automatic construction of 3-d statistical deformation models of the brain using nonrigid registration. IEEE TMI 22(8), 1014–1025 (2003)
3. Joshi, S., Davis, B., Jomier, M., Gerig, G.: Unbiased diffeomorphic atlas construction for computational anatomy. NeuroImage 23, S151–S160 (2004)
4. Bhatia, K.K., et al.: Consistent groupwise non-rigid registration for atlas construction. In: ISBI 2004, pp. 908–911 (2004)
5. Christensen, G.E., Johnson, H.J., Vannier, M.W.: Synthesizing average 3D anatomical shapes. NeuroImage 32(1), 146–158 (2006)
6. Lorenzen, P., et al.: Multi-modal image set registration and atlas formation. Medical Image Analysis 10(3), 440–451 (2006)
7. Xu, S., et al.: Group mean differences of voxel and surface objects via nonlinear averaging. In: ISBI 2004, pp. 758–761 (2006)
8. Aljabar, P., et al.: Analysis of growth in the developing brain using non-rigid registration. In: ISBI 2004, pp. 201–204 (2006)
9. Boardman, J.P., et al.: Abnormal deep grey matter development following preterm birth detected using deformation-based morphometry. NeuroImage 32 (2006)
10. Kikinis, R., et al.: A digital brain atlas for surgical planning, model-driven segmentation, and teaching. NeuroImage 2, 232–241 (1996)
11. Hammers, A., et al.: Three-dimensional maximum probability atlas of the human brain, with particular reference to the temporal lobe. HBM 19, 224–247 (2003)
12. van Leemput, K., et al.: Automated model-based bias field correction of MR images of the brain. IEEE TMI 18(10), 885–896 (1999)
13. Wells, W.M., et al.: Adaptive segmentation of MRI data. IEEE TMI 15(4), 429–442 (1996)
14. Murgasova, M., et al.: Segmentation of brain MRI in young children. In: Larsen, R., Nielsen, M., Sporring, J. (eds.) MICCAI 2006. LNCS, vol. 4190, pp. 687–694. Springer, Heidelberg (2006)

15. D'Agostino, E., et al.: Non-rigid atlas-to-image registration by minimization of class-conditional image entropy. In: Barillot, C., Haynor, D.R., Hellier, P. (eds.) MICCAI 2004. LNCS, vol. 3216, pp. 745–753. Springer, Heidelberg (2004)
16. Pohl, K., et al.: A Bayesian model for joint segmentation and registration. NeuroImage 31, 228–239 (2006)
17. Ashburner, J., Friston, K.: Unified segmentation. NeuroImage 26, 839–851 (2005)
18. Chen, X., et al.: Simultaneous segmentation and registration of medical image. In: Barillot, C., Haynor, D.R., Hellier, P. (eds.) MICCAI 2004. LNCS, vol. 3216, pp. 663–670. Springer, Heidelberg (2004)
19. Petrovic, V., et al.: Automatic framework for medical image registration, segmentation and modeling. In: MIUA 2006 (2006)
20. Twining, C., et al.: A a unified information-theoretic approach to groupwise non-rigid registration and model building. In: Christensen, G.E., Sonka, M. (eds.) IPMI 2005. LNCS, vol. 3565, pp. 1–14. Springer, Heidelberg (2005)
21. Meng, X.L., Rubin, D.B.: Maximum likelihood estimation via the ECM algorithm: A general framework. Biometrika 80(2), 267–278 (1993)
22. Rueckert, D., et al.: Non-rigid registration using free-form deformations: Application to breast MR images. IEEE TMI 18(8), 712–721 (1999)

Subject-Specific Biomechanical Simulation of Brain Indentation Using a Meshless Method

Ashley Horton, Adam Wittek, and Karol Miller

Intelligent Systems for Medicine Laboratory
School of Mechanical Engineering
The University of Western Australia
kmiller@mech.uwa.edu.au

Abstract. We develop a meshless method for simulating soft organ deformation. The method is motivated by simple, automatic model creation for real-time simulation. Our method is meshless in the sense that deformation is calculated at nodes that are not part of an element mesh. Node placement is almost arbitrary. Fully geometrically nonlinear total Lagrangian formulation is used. Geometric integration is performed over a regular background grid that does not conform to the simulation geometry. Explicit time integration is used via the central difference method. To validate the method we simulate indentation of a swine brain and compare the results to experimental data.

1 Introduction

Calculation of soft tissue deformation for surgical simulations have typically been based on Finite Element Analysis (FEA) [1,2,3,4,5]. The results from these FEA calculations have been promising, showing that near real-time simulations of surgical procedures, using nonlinear (both geometric and material) biomechanical models, can be achieved with a high level of precision [2,6,7]. Accuracy in FEA, relies heavily on the element mesh which discretises the geometry in question, and when dealing with incompressible continua such as soft tissue, we wish to use only hexahedral elements. When the geometry is highly irregular, an experienced analyst is required to manually create such a mesh which consumes valuable time. This is a major bottleneck; efficient generation of models to be used in real-time simulation of surgical procedures [8].

One solution to this bottleneck is to use a numerical method that does not have such strict discretisation requirements. For example, a meshless algorithm which uses a cloud of unconnected nodes to discretise the geometry instead of elements. Placement of these nodes can be done automatically since their arrangement is almost arbitrary.

Any algorithm to be used in surgical simulations must be capable of producing dynamic results in near real-time. Our algorithm uses Total Lagrangian (TL) formulation to calculate reaction forces. In TL, quantities are calculated with respect to the original configuration as detailed in [9,7]. Hence our method precomputes the constant strain-displacement matrices for each integration cell

N. Ayache, S. Ourselin, A. Maeder (Eds.): MICCAI 2007, Part I, LNCS 4791, pp. 541–548, 2007.
© Springer-Verlag Berlin Heidelberg 2007

and uses the deformation gradient to calculate the full matrix at each time step. For the sake of fast simulations, we also use explicit time integration based on the central difference method.

The purpose of this study is to evaluate the usefulness of our method for 3D surgical simulation. For this purpose, we perform simple indentation experiments on a swine brain and compare the results to those obtained with our method. While indentation is only a simple procedure, calculation of reaction forces on surgical instruments is an important field of study [10,11,12,13]. This is also a necessary validation to make before simulating more complicated procedures.

2   Meshless Method

The following is a brief description of the meshless algorithm we used to simulate indentation of brain tissue. The notation is based on that used in [9] where a left superscript indicates the time when a quantity occurs.

Preprocessing

1. Load simulation geometry in the form of two lists:
   - Node locations.
   - Integration point locations.
2. Load boundary conditions.
3. Loop through list of integration point locations[1]. For each integration point:
   - Identify n local nodes associated with the integration point.
   - Create and store the $3 \times n$ matrix $D\Phi(\mathbf{x})$ of moving least squares shape function derivatives $D\Phi_{k,i}(\mathbf{x}) = \frac{\partial \phi_i(\mathbf{x})}{\partial x_k}$ where $k = 1,2,3$ $i = 1,2 \cdots n$.
4. Loop through nodes and associate to each a suitable mass.
5. Initialise global nodal displacements $^{-\Delta t}\mathbf{U}$ and $^{0}\mathbf{U}$.

Solving
In every time step t:

1. Loop through integration points.
   - From precomputed list, load n local nodes and associated shape function derivatives $D\Phi(\mathbf{x})$ for the given integration point $\mathbf{x}$.
   - Find $n \times 3$ matrix of local nodal displacements ^{t}U.
   - Calculate deformation gradient ^{t}X.
   - Calculate full strain-displacement matrix $^{t}B_L$.
   - Calculate second Piola-Kirchoff stress vector $^{t}\hat{S}$.
   - Calculate and store local nodal reaction forces ^{t}f.
2. Put ^{t}f for each integration point into global nodal reaction forces vector $^{t}\mathbf{F}$.
3. Calculate the global nodal displacements for the next time step $^{t+\Delta t}\mathbf{U}$.

---

[1] Technically we should be looping through integration regions. We use single point integration so this is equivalent.

2.1   Support Domains and Moving Least Squares Shape Functions

Support domain and Moving Least Squares theory deals with the relationship between integration points and nodes. The theory was initially developed by [14] and used in meshless methods such as the Diffuse Element Method and Element Free Galerkin in [15,16]. We use it in this simulation for its simplicity and robustness.

For each integration point, we only require the $n \times 3$ first partial, spatial derivatives of the shape functions $\frac{\partial \phi_i(\mathbf{x})}{\partial x_k}$ for $k = 1, 2, 3$ and n the number of nodes in the support domain.

2.2   Force Calculation

In the total Lagrangian formulation, we calculate forces on nodes local to a given integration point with

$$^t f = \int_{^0V} {}^t B_L^T \, {}^t\hat{S} \, d \, {}^0V$$

which we integrate numerically.

The full strain-displacement matrix ${}^t B_L$ has the following construction

$$
{}^t B_L =
\begin{bmatrix}
\begin{pmatrix}
\frac{\partial \phi_1(\mathbf{x})}{\partial x_1} & 0 & 0 \\
0 & \frac{\partial \phi_1(\mathbf{x})}{\partial x_2} & 0 \\
0 & 0 & \frac{\partial \phi_1(\mathbf{x})}{\partial x_3} \\
\frac{\partial \phi_1(\mathbf{x})}{\partial x_2} & \frac{\partial \phi_1(\mathbf{x})}{\partial x_1} & 0 \\
0 & \frac{\partial \phi_1(\mathbf{x})}{\partial x_3} & \frac{\partial \phi_1(\mathbf{x})}{\partial x_2} \\
\frac{\partial \phi_1(\mathbf{x})}{\partial x_3} & 0 & \frac{\partial \phi_1(\mathbf{x})}{\partial x_1}
\end{pmatrix}
{}^t X^T, \; \cdots \; ,
\begin{pmatrix}
\frac{\partial \phi_n(\mathbf{x})}{\partial x_1} & 0 & 0 \\
0 & \frac{\partial \phi_n(\mathbf{x})}{\partial x_2} & 0 \\
0 & 0 & \frac{\partial \phi_n(\mathbf{x})}{\partial x_3} \\
\frac{\partial \phi_n(\mathbf{x})}{\partial x_2} & \frac{\partial \phi_n(\mathbf{x})}{\partial x_1} & 0 \\
0 & \frac{\partial \phi_n(\mathbf{x})}{\partial x_3} & \frac{\partial \phi_n(\mathbf{x})}{\partial x_2} \\
\frac{\partial \phi_n(\mathbf{x})}{\partial x_3} & 0 & \frac{\partial \phi_n(\mathbf{x})}{\partial x_1}
\end{pmatrix}
{}^t X^T
\end{bmatrix}
$$

where each partial derivative is taken from the precomputed $D\Phi(\mathbf{x})$. The deformation gradient ${}^t X^T$ is also calculated with the shape function derivatives and compares the current node locations to the original configuration. Calculation of the second Piola Kirchoff stress ${}^t\hat{S}$ is specific to the material used in the simulation and is discussed in section 3.3. The $3n$ nodal forces calculated at each integration point are combined to form the global force vector ${}^t\mathbf{F}$. These forces are the only data that is stored at each step of the integration point loop.

2.3   Explicit Time Integration

We use Newton's second law

$$\mathbf{M} \, {}^t\ddot{\mathbf{U}} = {}^t\mathbf{R} - {}^t\mathbf{F}$$

where the forces on the right hand side are the difference between applied (boundary) forces and the reaction forces calculated in section 2.2. Mass is constant, so we apply the finite difference method to acceleration to find the nodal displacements

$$^{t+\Delta t}\mathbf{U} \approx \Delta t^2 \mathbf{M}^{-1}({}^t\mathbf{R} - {}^t\mathbf{F}) + 2 \, {}^t\mathbf{U} - {}^{t-\Delta t}\mathbf{U}$$

All mass in the simulation is located at the nodes. The mass of a given node is determined by the number of support domains it is included in. The number of support domains a node is included in reveals how many integration points influence and are influenced by the node. Each integration point is allocated a mass according to its volume and this mass is distributed to the nodes in its support domain.

This concludes the description of one time step. If the simulation involves any enforced displacements or contacts, they are enforced here by adjusting $^{t+\Delta t}\mathbf{U}$ appropriately.

3   Simulation of Swine Brain Indentation

3.1   Geometry

From MRI images of the brain, we were able to construct the volume and discretise it with 4250 nodes. These nodes were evenly distributed throughout the volume and their placement was done by a computer with no manual adjustment. Similarly, 6371 integration points were placed in the volume, independent of node location. We performed a convergence analysis and confirmed that using more nodes would not increase accuracy. It is worth noting here that a tetrahedral mesh using similar node placement would involve around 18000 elements, consuming much more computation time than our method. Fig. 1 shows the cloud of nodes and integration points whilst Fig. 2 gives a surface visualisation.

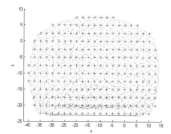
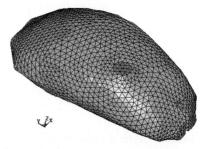

Fig. 1. Side view showing arbitrarily placed nodes (.) and regular integration grid (+)

Fig. 2. Surface visualisation. A circle can be seen, representing the nodes that are displaced during indentation. Note that the triangles shown are a visualisation aid rather than elements.

3.2   Boundary Conditions

The boundary conditions described here are chosen to simulate the indentation experiment detailed in section 4. To simulate a fixed base (Fig. 3), we constrain all nodes on the bottom surface of the brain. This is reasonable, given that the real swine brain was glued in place and the mould was significantly stiffer than the brain tissue.

Instead of simulating an indentor (which would require a contact algorithm) we enforce displacement on nodes contained withint a 10mm diameter circle on the brain surface. See Fig. 2 for the displaced nodes. The displacement is enforced vertically at a rate of 1mm s^{-1} for a period of 8.0s.

3.3 Material Properties

The purpose of this paper is to verify the algorithm rather than to conduct a complete simulation of actual surgery. It is therefore sufficient to model brain tissue constitutive behaviour with the Neo-Hookean hyperelastic model which has the strain-energy functional

$$W = \frac{\mu}{2}(\bar{I}_1 - 3) + \lambda(J - 1)^2$$

where μ, λ are Lamé parameters, $J = \det({}^t X)$ and $\bar{I}_1$ is the first strain invariant of the right Cauchy Green deformation tensor ${}^t C$. From this we calculate the second Piola-Kirchoff stress tensor

$$^t S = \lambda J(J - 1) \, {}^t C^{-1} + \mu J^{-\frac{2}{3}} \, I$$

and hence form the required vector ${}^t \hat{S}$. Our subject-specific shear modulus is $\mu = 210$Pa as was found for this particular brain in [3]. With Poisson's ratio of $\nu = 0.499$ we find $\lambda \approx 105$kPa. The mass density in our simulation is 10^3kg m^{-3}.

4 Brain Indentation Experiment

For our indentation experiment, the subject brain was that of a 6 month old swine (obtained as a by-product during a commercial slaughtering at Tokyo Shibaura Zooki, Tokyo, Japan) and can be seen in Fig. 3. This brain had a mass of 89.9g and was approximately 92.5mm, 62.5mm, 28.5mm in its major axis, minor axis and height respectively.

Throughout the experiment, the brain was constrained on its base by glue and a custom-made mould (see Fig. 3). To simulate in-vivo conditions, we submerged the brain and mould in a 37 °C saline solution.

The indentor was an aluminium cylinder of diameter 10mm and was attached to one end of a force sensor. The other end of the force sensor was attached to a linear motion table which moved vertically. See Fig. 4.

We lowered the indentor at a speed of 1mm s^{-1} so that the brain was indented by 8mm. Forces were recorded throughout the experiment at a sampling rate of 150 Hz. We performed 2 indentation experiments, one on the left and one on the right hemispheres. See section 5 for the recorded forces.

5 Results

At an indentation of 8mm, the swine brain experiments produced reaction forces of 0.181N and 0.125N for the left and right hemisphere respectively. Our simulation of 8mm indentation yielded a force of 0.131N. Looking at Fig. 5 we observe

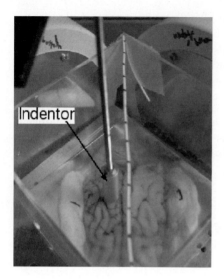

Fig. 3. Swine brain specimen glued onto mould, submerged in warm saline and positioned beneath the indentor

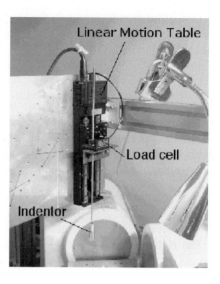

Fig. 4. Apparatus used to perform indentation

that our method is generating results that compare well with reality throughout the simulation.

The simulation was run on a standard desktop personal computer with a 3GHz Pentium 4 processor and 1Gb of internal memory. For this computer, the computation time was 55 seconds (The actual brain indentation took 8 seconds). As efficiency of parallel computing of biomechanical models models was reported to be as high as 90% [17], it can be expected that real-time computing of our model can be achieved with as few as 10 Pentium 4 processors.

6   Discussion

Given the results shown in section 5, we consider our simulated forces to be accurate in magnitude. However, we qualitatively notice that the simulation curve shown in Fig. 5 appears more linear than the experimental results which may call for a higher order hyperelastic material (such as Ogden's rubber formulation [18]) to be used in future work. We also note that no pia was included in our simulation which would lead us to expect lower reaction forces [3]. A more realistic future simulation may require simulation of the pia.

Ultimately we note that the simulation involved no tuning and gave results similar to reality. The simulation was performed with automatically positioned nodes and integration points. Future possibilities for our method include simulation of large deformation and topological changes which occur often in surgical procedures but cannot be easily dealt with using FEA.

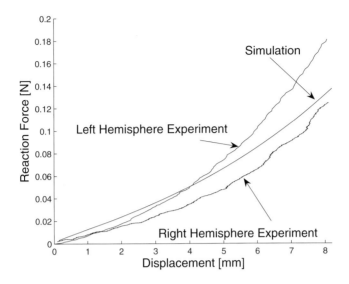

Fig. 5. Reaction force against displacement for our simulation and both swine brain experiments

Acknowledgments

The financial support of the Australian Research Council is gratefully acknowledged, Grant No. DP0664534.

References

1. Cotin, S., Delingette, H., Ayache, N.: Real-time elastic deformations of soft tissues for surgery simulation. In: Hagen, H. (ed.) IEEE Transactions on Visualization and Computer Graphics, pp. 62–73. IEEE Computer Society Press, Los Alamitos (1999)
2. Wittek, A., Miller, K., Kikinis, R., Warfield, S.: Patient-specific model of brain deformation: Application to medical image registration. Journal of Biomechanics (Accepted 2006)
3. Wittek, A., Dutta-Roy, T., Taylor, Z., Horton, A., Washio, T., Chinzei, K., Miller, K.: Analysis of needle insertion into the brain using non-linear biomechanical model. In: 7th International Symposium on Computer Methods in Biomechanics and Biomedical Engineering (2006)
4. Nienhuys, H.W.: Cutting in Deformable Objects. PhD thesis, University of Utrect, Utrect, The Netherlands (2003)
5. Szekely, G., Brechbuhler, C., Hutter, R., Rhomberg, A., Ironmonger, N., Schmid, P.: Modelling of soft tissue deformation for laparoscopic surgery simulation. Medical Image Analysis 4, 57–66 (2000)
6. Wittek, A., Kikinis, R., Warfield, S.K., Miller, K.: Brain shift computation using a fully nonlinear biomechanical model. In: Duncan, J.S., Gerig, G. (eds.) MICCAI 2005. LNCS, vol. 3750, Springer, Heidelberg (2005)

7. Miller, K., Joldes, G., Lance, D., Wittek, A.: Total lagrangian explicit dynamics finite element algorithm for computing soft tissue deformation. Communications in Numerical Methods in Engineering 23(2), 121–134 (2007)
8. Viceconti, M., Taddei, F.: Automatic generation of finite element meshes from computed tomography data. Critical Reviews in Biomedical Engineering 31, 27–72 (2003)
9. Bathe, K.J.: Finite Element Procedures. Prentice Hall, New Jersey (1996)
10. DiMaio, S., Salcudean, S.: Needle steering and motion planning in soft tissues. IEEE Transaction on Biomedical Engineering 52, 965–974 (2005)
11. Okamura, A.M., Simone, C., O'Leary, M.D.: Force modeling for needle insertion into soft tissue. IEEE Transactions on Biomedical Engineering. 51, 1707–1716 (2004)
12. Wittek, A., Laporte, J., Miller, K.: Computing Reaction Forces on Surgical Tools for Robotic Neurosurgery and Surgical Simulation. In: Proceedings of the Australasian Conference on Robotics and Automation 2004 (2004)
13. Brett, P.N., Parker, T.J., Harrison, A.J., Thomas, T.A., Carr, A.: Simulation of resistance forces acting on surgical needles. Proceedings of the Institution of Mechanical Engineers Part H: Journal of Engineering in Medicine 211, 335–347 (1997)
14. Lancaster, P., Salkauskas, K.: Surfaces generated by moving least squares methods. Mathematics of Computation 37(155), 141–158 (1981)
15. Nayroles, B., Touzot, G., Villon, P.: Generalizing the finite element method: Diffuse approximation and diffuse elements. Computational Mechanics 10(5), 307–318 (1992)
16. Belytschko, T., Lu, Y., Gu, L.: Element-free Galerkin methods. International Journal for Numerical Methods in Engineering 37(2), 229–256 (1994)
17. Koh, B.I., Reinbolt, J.A., Fregly, B.J., George, A.D.: Evaluation of parallel decomposition methods for biomechanical optimizations. Computer Methods in Biomechanics and Biomedical Engineering 7(4), 215–225 (2004)
18. Ogden, R.W.: Non-Linear Elastic Deformations. Ellis Horwood Ltd. Chichester, Great Britain (1984)

Towards an Identification of Tumor Growth Parameters from Time Series of Images[*]

Ender Konukoglu[1], Olivier Clatz[1,3], Pierre-Yves Bondiau[2],
Maxime Sermesant[1], Hervé Delingette[1], and Nicholas Ayache[1]

[1] Asclepios Research Project, INRIA Sophia Antipolis, France
ender.konukoglu@sophia.inria.fr
[2] Centre Antoine Lacassagne, Nice, France
[3] SPL Harvard, Boston, USA

Abstract. In cancer treatment, understanding the aggressiveness of the tumor is essential in therapy planning and patient follow-up. In this article, we present a novel method for quantifying the speed of invasion of gliomas in white and grey matter from time series of magnetic resonance (MR) images. The proposed approach is based on mathematical tumor growth models using the reaction-diffusion formalism. The quantification process is formulated by an inverse problem and solved using anisotropic fast marching method yielding an efficient algorithm. It is tested on a few images to get a first proof of concept with promising new results.

1 Introduction

Glial based tumors account for approximately 40-45% of all primary intracranial cancer, forming the largest class in this pathology [1]. Tumors within this group show a high variation extending from benign to fatal. Determining different characteristics of each specific case and following their change during the treatment is crucial in therapy planning and patient follow-up. Although medical imaging is not the sole source of information used for this, it plays an important role in understanding the pattern and speed of invasion of healthy tissue by cancerous cells. One of the most important hints that can be obtained from images is the progression of the Critical Target Volume (CTV) and Gross Tumor Volume (GTV), which are important in radiotherapy. For low grade gliomas, CTV corresponds to the enhanced region in the T2-weighted magnetic resonance images (MRI) and at its extent tumor cells are diffused into the brain tissue. In the case of high grade gliomas CTV corresponds to the extents of the tumor infiltrated edema [2]. GTV in both cases is taken as the image abnormality in T1 weighted images corresponding to the region where tumor cells are dense. As shown by Giese *et al.*, speed of invasion of tumor cells in grey and white matter are different, hence the speed of CTV progression [3]. Quantifying this progression of

[*] This work has been partly supported by the European Health-e-Child project (IST-2004-027749) and by the CompuTumor project (http://www-sop.inria.fr/asclepios/projects/boston/).

CTV in different tissues would be helpful in initial grading of the tumor and assessing the efficacy of the current treatment procedure.

Mathematical modeling of tumor growth dynamics gives us an insight on the physiology of the process by linking different types of observations under theoretical frameworks. There has been a large amount of models proposed to describe the growth dynamics of glial tumors. Different approaches can be coarsely classified into two groups, macroscopic and microscopic ones. Macroscopic models describe the evolution of local tumor cell densities and try to capture the dynamics by general equations [4,5,6]. Most of the macroscopic models are based on the reaction-diffusion formalism introduced by Murray in [7,4].

In this paper we are proposing a method for quantifying the progression of the CTV of glial based tumors. The formulation is based on the tumor growth model proposed by Clatz *et al.* in [5], which uses reaction-diffusion formalism. With the proposed method, we obtain quantitative estimates for the speed of invasion in white and grey matter by solving the patient specific parameter identification problem for this growth model using MR images taken at two different time instances from the same patient. The parameter identification problem is formulated using the front approximation of reaction-diffusion equations, which results in anisotropic Eikonal equations. The anisotropic fast marching method proposed in [8] is used for numerical solutions yielding an efficient algorithm.

2   Method

Quantitative measures for the speed of CTV progression can be obtained using reaction-diffusion based growth models, which explain the invasion through diffusion process. Clatz *et al.* proposed such a model in the form of a Fisher-Kolmogorov (F-KPP) equation in [5] based on the observation of Giese *et al.*:

$$\frac{\partial u}{\partial t} = \nabla \cdot (D(\mathbf{x})\nabla u) + \rho u(1 - u) \ , \ D(\mathbf{x})\nabla u \cdot \overrightarrow{n}_{\Sigma} = 0 \qquad (1)$$

where u can be seen as the normalized tumor cell density or the probability of finding a tumor at a given point, D is the diffusion tensor explaining the invasion of tumor cells, ρ is the proliferation rate and $\overrightarrow{n}_{\Sigma}$ corresponds to the normal vector of the brain surface. We focus in this article on the D matrix, which defines anisotropic diffusion on the white matter following the main fiber directions and isotropic diffusion on the grey matter, constructed as:

$$D(\mathbf{x}) = \begin{cases} d_g \mathbf{I} & \text{if } \mathbf{x} \text{ is in grey matter} \\ d_w D_w(\mathbf{x}) & \text{if } \mathbf{x} \text{ is in white matter} \end{cases} \qquad (2)$$

where D_w is the water diffusion tensor obtained from MR diffusion tensor imaging (MR-DTI) providing the fiber direction. Quantities explaining the speed of invasion are d_g and d_w, diffusion coefficients in grey and white matter respectively. Identification of these parameters for each patient using images taken at two different times corresponds to the identification process.

2.1 Front Approximation of Reaction-Diffusion Equations

The model given in Equation 1 requires tumor cell density u to be known at every point as an initial condition. However, this is not the case for medical images where only contours around GTV and CTV are available. The front motion approximation of reaction-diffusion equations offers a solution for this discrepancy between information needed and observations available [8]. These approximations formulate the motion of the tumor front (the visible contour) based on a reaction-diffusion equation such as the one given in Equation 1. Taking the contour around the CTV as the last visible tumor front we can use such an approximation to model its evolution.

The front motion approximation for reaction-diffusion equations is based on the fact that these PDEs have travelling wave solutions under certain conditions. This can be illustrated in the simple one dimensional F-KPP equation where D is scalar. In [9] it is shown that any initial condition with compact support will evolve and converge to a traveling wave of the form $u = u(x - ct)$ in time, where $c = 2\sqrt{D\rho}$ is the asymptotic speed of a point taken on the front. The convergence of the front and the speed of the point $u = 0.5$ can be seen in Figure 1. The convergence property is carried to higher dimensions for contours

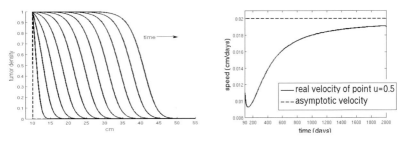

Fig. 1. Left: Front evolution starting from a step function. Steady wave-front is translating in time. Right: Speed of wave-front plotted versus time showing the convergence behavior and the asymptotic speed.

on the travelling wave with the asymptotic speed $c = 2\sqrt{\rho \mathbf{n}^t \mathbf{D} \mathbf{n}}$ under the condition that coefficients of the equation are constant and the front is planar, meaning the front has no curvature and its normal is given by $\mathbf{n}$. For more general fronts Γ like the tumor front mentioned where curvature exists and coefficients vary spatially we make the assumption that required conditions are satisfied within a voxel. Based on this assumption we can simply derive the travelling time formulation for Γ:

$$\sqrt{\nabla T^t \mathbf{D} \nabla T} = \frac{1}{2\sqrt{\rho}} \tag{3}$$

where $T(\mathbf{x})$ represents the time at which Γ passes from point $\mathbf{x}$ [10].

2.2   Numerical Method

The travelling time formulation given in Equation 3 is an anisotropic Eikonal equation. Very efficient methods for isotropic Eikonal equation $F|\nabla T| = 1$ have been proposed like fast marching (FM) methods [11]. These methods are based on the fact that characteristic directions of the equation are parallel to ∇T [12]. However, the anisotropic case poses extra difficulties for efficient numerical algorithms because this property is not satisfied [12]. The method we used to solve Equation 3 numerically is based on the original fast marching idea with the addition of a recursive correction phase to compensate the effects of anisotropy. In [8], it is demonstrated that this algorithm is fast and efficient in the case of high anisotropies and general meshes. Having an efficient numerical method for Equation 3 is essential in solving the parameter identification problem explained in the next section.

2.3   Parameter Identification Problem

The parameter identification process uses the front motion approximation given in Equation 3. In order to formulate this inverse problem we follow the modeling assumption as given in [5] and state $T(\Gamma_1) = 0$ and $T(\Gamma_2) = t_2 - t_1$, where Γ_1 and Γ_2 corresponds to contours around CTV regions observed in images taken at time t_1 and t_2 respectively. Parameter identification process tries to find parameters d_g and d_w that create a T function that would satisfy these conditions. Notice that ρ is a multiplicative factor in the travelling time formulation and it cannot be determined independently from the D matrix by just looking at the motion of the tumor front. To tackle this, we treat ρ as a known constant in the parameter identification problem. t_1 is not available in clinical circumstances hence we use $t_2 - t_1$. The formulation can be given as the minimization problem

$$C(d_w, d_g) = \frac{1}{2}(\text{dist}(\Gamma_2, \widehat{\Gamma_2}) + \text{dist}(\widehat{\Gamma_2}, \Gamma_2)) \;,\; d_w > 0 \text{ and } d_g > 0 \qquad (4)$$

$$\widehat{\Gamma_2} = \{\mathbf{x}|T(\mathbf{x}) = t_2 - t_1,\; \sqrt{\nabla T^t D \nabla T} = \frac{1}{2\sqrt{\rho}},\; T(\Gamma_1) = 0\}$$

where C is the objective function to minimize with respect to d_w and d_g, $\widehat{\Gamma_2}$ is the computed contour using the front approximation with the given parameters and $dist(A, B)$ is the distance between two isosurfaces taken as mean distance from voxels of A to the closest voxel of B.

The minimizing parameters d_w^* and d_g^* of the function C will create the closest contour $\widehat{\Gamma_2}^*$ to the observed contour Γ_2. This formulation poses a multidimensional minimization problem for which several methods have been proposed. One crucial observation is that explicit derivatives of C with respect to the variables are not available. Although we have constraints on d_w and d_g, these are not very restrictive so we choose to use the unconstrained minimization algorithm proposed by Powell in [13] and restrict the domain computation. The attractive feature of this algorithm is that it does not require derivatives of the objective function. Instead, local quadratic approximations of the objective functions are obtained and used in the minimization. The algorithm requires instances of the objective function to construct the quadratic approximation - which is computed using anisotropic fast marching - and updates it as the minimization proceeds. This minimization algorithm is prone to getting stuck at local minima. However, we observed in our experiments that the minimization surface is convex hence, this does not pose a problem.

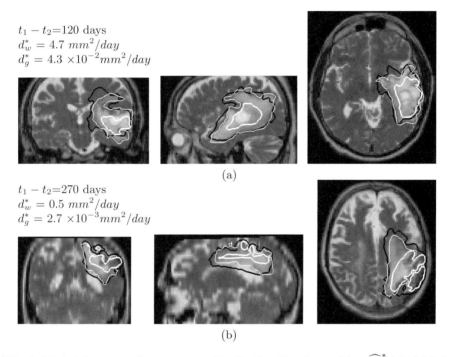

$t_1 - t_2 = 120$ days
$d_w^* = 4.7\ mm^2/day$
$d_g^* = 4.3 \times 10^{-2} mm^2/day$

(a)

$t_1 - t_2 = 270$ days
$d_w^* = 0.5\ mm^2/day$
$d_g^* = 2.7 \times 10^{-3} mm^2/day$

(b)

Fig. 2. Minimizing tumor front computed in the identification problem $\widehat{\Gamma_2}^*$ (thick black contours) is plotted with the initial and the final tumor fronts manually segmented from the images at taken at t_1 and t_2 respectively, (Γ_1 - thick white contours, Γ_2 - thin white contours). Underlying images are T2 weighted images taken at the second time instance. Estimated growth parameters (appearent diffusion coefficients) d_g^* and d_w^* for these patients are also given.

3   Results

We illustrate the use of the proposed algorithm on two different patient images both containing high grade gliomas, glioblastoma multiforme. In order to solve the parameter identification problem on patient images we need to construct tumor diffusion tensors as given in Equation 2, which requires MR-DTI and white matter segmentation of the patient. Diffusion images are not available for every patient and existence of the tumor and the low quality of patient images make it impossible to obtain an accurate white matter segmentation. Thus, in our experiments we used data acquired from a healthy subject, which consists of T1 and T2 weighted images alongside MR-DTI. This data is registered to the patient space using global affine transformation found using T1 weighted images. Tensors in the MR-DTI were re-oriented using finite strain strategy after applying the global affine transformation to take into account the effects of the transformation on the tensors [14]. To obtain the white matter segmentation, we use fractional anisotropy (FA) values of the DTI data and let points with FA > 0.3 form the white matter as an arbitrary value chosen for illustration of the method. This way we obtain perfect correspondence between diffusion tensors and the white matter segmentation. Lastly the ρ is set to 0.012/day as proposed in [4].

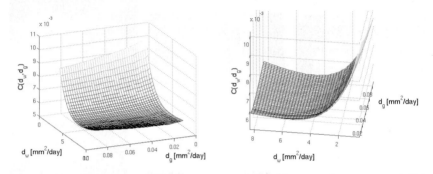

Fig. 3. The objective function $C(d_w, d_g)$ (minimization surface) for the patient whose image are given in Figure 2(a) is plotted from two different views

The minimization algorithm explained in Section 2.3 is applied to the patient images given in Figure 2(a) and Figure 2(b). Tumor segmentation at the initial time (thick white contour), tumor segmentation at the final time (thin white contour) the computed tumor front minimizing the objective function $\widehat{\Gamma}^*$ (thick black contour) are drawn on T2 weigthed images taken at the second time instance showing CTV at t_2. The minimizing parameters d_w^* and d_g^* for each patient are also given in these figures. In Figure 3 we plot the minimization surface (the function $C(d_w, d_g)$) computed for the patient image given in Figure 2(a). Notice the minimization surface has a wide valley which makes the optimization hard, on the other hand the surface is convex yielding only the global minimum. The minimizing criterion, which is the symmetric distance between the computed front and the delineated one, at this minimum reaches the value 0.05 mm for the first patient data and 0.078 mm for the second patient data demonstrating the similarity between the computed front and the real delineation.

4   Discussion

In this article, we proposed a novel method to quantify the speed of tumor invasion in white and grey matter for gliomas on MR images using mathematical growth models. This tool can be helpful in tumor grading and patient follow-up as it gives quantitative values about the growth of the tumor. Quantification process is formulated as a parameter identification problem and solved using the anisotropic fast marching method and multidimensional optimization. The speed estimates are given in terms of apparent diffusion coefficients d_g and d_w, which are used to construct tumor diffusion tensor as suggested by the growth model given in Equation 1.

Results given in Section 3 demonstrate the functioning of the proposed method. We observe that minimizing contours given in Figure 2 matches the actual Critical Target Volume delineation given in the image reasonably well. The discrepancies between these contours and the underlying CTVs are caused by different factors such as the use of registered DTI data instead of the one from the patient, lack of a good white matter segmentation of the patient, not taking into account the mass effect caused by the tumor and the fact that identification process assumes tumor growth is perfectly explained by the mathematical growth model used. The diffusion coefficients obtained, shows a big difference between the speed of the tumor in grey matter and in white matter coherent with the experimental results given in [3].

The method has been demonstrated on high grade gliomas where CTV corresponds to the edema region. However, the same tool can also be applied, and will be future work, to low grade gliomas since reaction-diffusion growth models have been proposed for these types of tumors as well [6]. Clinical values of the estimated diffusion coefficients should be assessed using a large database in order to understand their importance. Finally introducing different imaging modalities can give us the opportunity to find parameters more accurately and identify more parameters such as ρ.

References

1. Tovi, M.: Mr imaging in cerebral gliomas analysis of tumour tissue components. Acta Radiol. Suppl. (1993)
2. Kantor, G., Loiseau, H., Vital, A., Mazeron, J.: Descriptions of gtv and ctv for radiation therapy of adult glioma. Cancer Radiother (2001)
3. Giese, A., Kluwe, L., Laube, B., Meissner, H., Berens, M., Westphal, M.: Migration of human glioma cells on myelin. Neurosurgery 38(4) (1996)
4. Swanson, K., Alvord, E., Murray, J.: Virtual brain tumours (gliomas) enhance the reality of medical imaging and highlight inadequacies of current therapy. British Journal of Cancer 86 (2002)
5. Clatz, O., Sermesant, M., Bondiau, P., Delingette, H., Warfield, S., Malandain, G., Ayache, N.: Realistic simulation of the 3d growth of brain tumors in mr images coupling diffusion with biomechanical deformation. IEEE T.M.I. 24(10) (2005)
6. Jbabdi, S., Mandonnet, E., Duffau, H., Capelle, L., Swanson, K., Pélégrini-Issac, M., Guillevin, R., Benali, H.: Simulation of anisotropic growth of low-grade gliomas using diffusion tensor imaging. Magnetic Reson. in Med. 54 (2005)
7. Murray, J.: Mathematical Biology. Springer, Heidelberg (2002)

8. Konukoglu, E., Sermesant, M., Clatz, O., Peyrat, J.M., Delingette, H., Ayache, N.:
A recursive anisotropic fast marching approach to reaction diffusion equation: Application to tumor growth modeling. In: Karssemeijer, N., Lelieveldt, B. (eds.) IPMI
2007. LNCS, vol. 4584, Springer, Heidelberg (2007)
9. Aronson, D., Weinberger, H.: Multidimensional nonlinear diffusion arising in population genetics. Advances in Mathematics 30 (1978)
10. Keener, J., Sneyd, J.: Mathematical physiology. Springer, Heidelberg (1998)
11. Sethian, J.: Level set methods and fast marching methods: Evolving interfaces in
computational geometry, fluid mechanics, computer vision, and materials science.
Cambridge University Press, Cambridge (1999)
12. Sethian, J., Vladimirsky, A.: Ordered upwind methods for static hamilton-jacobi
equations: theory and algorithms. SIAM J. Numer. Anal. 41 (2003)
13. Powell, M.: Uobyqa: unconstrained optimization by quadratic approximation.
Math. Program. Ser. B 92 (2002)
14. Alexander, D., Pierpaoli, C., Basser, P., Gee, J.: Spatial transformations of diffusion
tensor magnetic resonance images. IEEE Trans. Med. Imag. 20 (2001)

Real-Time Modeling of Vascular Flow for Angiography Simulation

Xunlei Wu[1,2], Jérémie Allard[2], and Stéphane Cotin[1,3]

[1] Harvard Medical School, Boston, USA
wu.xunlei@mgh.harvard.edu
[2] SimGroup, CIMIT, Cambridge, USA
jeremie.allard@codrt.fr
[3] Alcove Project, LIFL/INRIA Futurs, Lille, France
stephane.cotin@lifl.fr

Abstract. Interventional neuroradiology is a growing field of minimally invasive therapies that includes embolization of aneurysms and arterio-venous malformations, carotid angioplasty and carotid stenting, and acute stroke therapy. Treatment is performed using image-guided instrument navigation through the patient's vasculature and requires intricate combination of visual and tactile coordination. In this paper we present a series of techniques for real-time high-fidelity simulation of angiographic studies. We focus in particular on the computation and visualization of blood flow and blood pressure distribution patterns, mixing of blood and contrast agent, and high-fidelity simulation of fluoroscopic images.

1 Introduction

Vascular diseases are the number one cause of death worldwide, with cardiovascular disease alone claiming an estimated 17.5 million deaths in 2005 [1]. An increasingly promising therapy for treating vascular diseases is interventional radiology procedures, where a guidewire-catheter combination is advanced under fluoroscopic guidance through the arterial system, thus allowing a minimally invasive therapy while reducing recovery time for the patient when compared to corresponding surgical procedures. However, the main difficulty in these therapies is navigating through the intricate human vascular system while relying on two-dimensional X-ray views of the patient. Yet, the best training method so far has been actual patients with a vascular pathology.

To reduce the risks due to training on patients, we have developed a real-time high-fidelity interventional neuroradiology simulator for physician training and procedure planning. The system relies on accurate patient-specific anatomical representations of the vascular anatomy [2] and uses new algorithms for fluoroscopic rendering and physics-based modeling of catheter-vessel interactions. The full body vascular model used in our simulator consists of over 4,000 arterial and venous vessels, and is optimized for real-time collision detection and visualization of angiograms.

In this paper, we aim to improve the vascular flow modeling accuracy over existing approaches [3,4] and yet maintain a real-time performance in order to

N. Ayache, S. Ourselin, A. Maeder (Eds.): MICCAI 2007, Part I, LNCS 4791, pp. 557–565, 2007.
© Springer-Verlag Berlin Heidelberg 2007

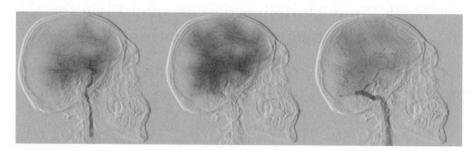

Fig. 1. High-fidelity real-time simulation of angiography in the brain, featuring contrast injection in arterial flow (*Left*); blush (*Middle*); and transition to venous side (*Right*)

improve training/planning immersiveness. We propose to simulate physiologic representations of arterial, parenchymal and venous phases of thoracic, cervical and intracranial vasculature. Synthetic fluoroscopy uses a volumetric approach which directly incorporates the same patient CT dataset as that used to reconstruct the vascular model. Laminar blood flow is modeled through a simplified version of the Navier-Stokes equations while contrast agent propagation is controlled by an advection-diffusion equation. The proposed method can handle very large anatomical dataset in real-time, and angiographic studies performed on our simulator closely approximate those on actual patients. This high level of fidelity is key to permit realistic simulation based training, and ultimately enables the planning and rehearsal of complex cases.

2   Real-Time Flow Computation in Large Vascular Networks

An angiogram is used to locate narrowing, occlusions, and other vascular abnormalities. By visualizing and measuring flow distributions in the vicinity of a lesion, angiographic studies play a vital role in the assessment of the pre- and post-operative physiological states of the patient. In this section we detail our real-time flow model, one of the three key elements of angiography simulation.

2.1   Flow Model

Aside from ventriculograms and some aortic angiograms, turbulent flow is rarely observed in interventional radiology procedures. In addition, flow distribution in the network is more relevant when identifying and quantifying vessel pathology than local fluid dynamic pattern. Hence, 1D laminar flow model is adequate under our application context.

Blood flow in each vessel is modeled as an incompressible viscous fluid flowing through a cylindrical pipe, and can be calculated from the Navier-Stokes equation. The resulting equation, called Poiseuille Law,

$$Q = \frac{\Delta P}{R} \quad with \quad R = \frac{8\eta L}{\pi r^4} \tag{1}$$

relates the vessel flow rate Q to the pressure drop ΔP, blood viscosity η, vessel radius r, and vessel length L. To compute such vascular flow, a set of algebraic equations are developed as follows. The arterial vasculature can be represented as a directed graph, with M edges and N nodes. If $M \neq N$, we form an augmented square matrix $\mathbf{K}$ by adding trivial equations, i.e. $\mathbf{P_s} = \mathbf{P_s}$ or $\mathbf{Q_s} = \mathbf{Q_s}$, to the set of Poiseuille equations. If $M < N$,

$$\mathbf{Q} = \mathbf{KP} \quad or \quad \begin{bmatrix} \vdots \\ Q_i \\ \vdots \\ \hline \mathbf{P_s} \end{bmatrix} = \begin{bmatrix} \vdots & \vdots & \vdots & \vdots & \vdots \\ 0 & \Omega_i & 0 & -\Omega_i & 0 \\ \vdots & \vdots & \vdots & \vdots & \vdots \\ \hline 0 \cdots & & \cdots & 0 & \mathbf{I} \end{bmatrix} \begin{bmatrix} \vdots \\ P_j \\ \vdots \\ P_k \\ \vdots \end{bmatrix} \tag{2}$$

where $\Omega_i = 1/R_i$ is the vessel i flow resistance. Boundary conditions are then added to the system as Lagrange Multipliers. There are two groups of constraints. The first set corresponds to the prescribed pressure values at the beginning and end nodes of the directed graph. These pressure values are defined as a function of time, the depth of the node, and ventricular pressure. The deeper an end node is in the graph, its pressure value is smaller and less variant in time. The second set of constraints relates to the conservation of flow, similar to Kirchhoff's circuit laws in electric circuits, such that for any internal node, the total flow flowing toward this node is equal to the total flow flowing away from this node. This is described by $0 \equiv \sum Q_{in} + \sum Q_{out} = \Psi^T \mathbf{P}$. The final system matrix of our 1D flow model is

$$\overline{\mathbf{Q}} \equiv \begin{bmatrix} \mathbf{Q} \\ \mathbf{P_e} \\ \mathbf{0} \end{bmatrix} = \overline{\mathbf{K}}\overline{\mathbf{P}} = \begin{bmatrix} \mathbf{K} & \Gamma & \Psi \\ \hline \Gamma^T & 0 & 0 \\ \hline \Psi^T & 0 & 0 \end{bmatrix} \begin{bmatrix} \mathbf{P} \\ \lambda_e \\ \lambda_f \end{bmatrix} \tag{3}$$

where λ_e and λ_f are vectors of Lagrange multipliers, and where Γ is a permutation matrix. Each row of Ψ^T is a summation of multiple rows from the first M rows of $\mathbf{K}$ in (2). $\mathbf{P_e}$ is the vector contains prescribed nodal pressure value.

Because the prescribed pressures $\mathbf{P_e}$ are varying in time, $\overline{\mathbf{Q}} = [\cdots 0 \cdots P_e^T 0]^T$ (containing both the initial conditions $\mathbf{Q} = 0$ and boundary conditions) needs to be updated at the beginning of each time step. So that $\overline{\mathbf{P}} = \overline{\mathbf{K}}^{-1} \overline{\mathbf{Q}}$. As a subset of $\overline{\mathbf{Q}}$, $\mathbf{Q} = [\mathbf{K}\ \Gamma\ \Psi]\overline{\mathbf{P}}$. Our model assumes that the vascular resistance is invariant in time, so that $\overline{\mathbf{K}}^{-1}$ can be precomputed. This permits real-time computation rates, even on very large vascular models. It costs 50 milliseconds to compute the flow distribution for an arterial vasculature with $2,337$ vessels on an Athlon 64 X2 2.4GHz processor.

2.2 Modeling Local Blood Flow Alterations

For the purpose of training, it is important to have access to a variety of scenarios. Each scenario does not necessarily need to be based on an existing patient dataset, but could be derived from a generic dataset that is altered to resemble a specific pathology. Our simulation system permits the creation of a stenosis or aneurysm at any location, as well as automatically accounting for the change in blood flow that it effects.

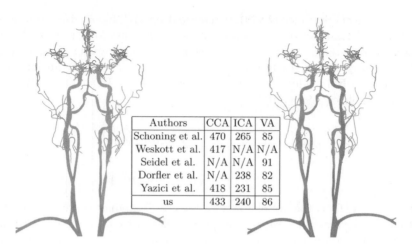

Authors	CCA	ICA	VA
Schoning et al.	470	265	85
Weskott et al.	417	N/A	N/A
Seidel et al.	N/A	N/A	91
Dorfler et al.	N/A	238	82
Yazici et al.	418	231	85
us	433	240	86

Fig. 2. *Left:* Blood pressure distribution due to a stenosis in the common carotid artery (CCA). *Right:* Restored blood pressure distribution after treatment. *Center:* Comparison of our computed blood flow (ml/min) in the CCA, internal carotid artery (ICA), and vertebral artery (VA) against the mean values measured by other authors [5].

Stenosis. During stenting or angioplasty simulation, a stent or balloon is deployed to expand the narrowed section of a vessel due to stenosis (as illustrated in the left of Figure 2). Therefore, the radius of the vessel is changed locally and its resistance is modified according to Equation (1). Assuming vessel i contains the stenosis, its initial resistance $R_i = R_1 + R_2 + R_s$ becomes $R'_i = R_i + (R'_s - R_s)$ after expanding the vessel's radius. This change in resistance requires $\overline{\mathbf{K}}'$ to be updated as $\overline{\mathbf{K}}'$ as well as its inverse of $\overline{\mathbf{K}}'$. To maintain the simulation interactivity, the computation of $\overline{\mathbf{K}}'^{-1}$ needs to be done in real-time. Notice that the local changes in $\overline{\mathbf{K}}$, namely row i in $\overline{\mathbf{K}}$ and two rows in Ψ^T, can be rewritten as $\overline{\mathbf{K}}' = \overline{\mathbf{K}} + \mathbf{U}\mathbf{V}^T$, where vector $\mathbf{U}^T = \begin{bmatrix} \cdots 1 \cdots 1 \cdots -1 \cdots \end{bmatrix}$, vector $\mathbf{V}^T = \begin{bmatrix} \cdots \Delta\Omega_i \cdots -\Delta\Omega_i \cdots \end{bmatrix}$, and $\Delta\Omega_i = R'_s - R_s$ represents the weight change of vessel i two nodes. Given $\overline{\mathbf{K}}^{-1}$, $\overline{\mathbf{K}}'^{-1}$ can be efficiently computed using Woodbury's formula [1].

The added fluid during injecting contrast agent, in particular, also changes the flow rate around the tip of catheter. In our vascular flow model, such influence is modeled as the whole vessel's flowrate being modulated by the injection rate. To correctly model the change of flow distribution due to injection, $\overline{\mathbf{K}}$ is augmented with one additional boundary condition $Q_{inj} = (P_{i,0} - P_{i,1})/R_i = \begin{bmatrix} \cdots \Omega_i \cdots -\Omega_i \cdots \end{bmatrix} \overline{\mathbf{P}} = \mathbf{U_{inj}}^T \overline{\mathbf{P}}$ such that

$$\overline{\mathbf{K}}_{\mathbf{inj}} = \begin{bmatrix} \overline{\mathbf{K}} & \mathbf{U_{inj}} \\ \mathbf{U_{inj}}^T & 0 \end{bmatrix} \tag{4}$$

---

[1] http://mathworld.wolfram.com/WoodburyFormula.html

To achieve real-time performance, $\overline{\mathbf{K}}_{\mathbf{inj}}^{-1}$ must be computed efficiently as well. Given $\overline{\mathbf{K}}^{-1}$, this objective is achieved by using block matrix decomposition [2].

3   Contrast Agent Propagation

3.1   Advection-Diffusion Model

An angiogram is done by taking a continuous series of X-rays while injecting a contrast agent into the vascular structure under examination. The contrast agent, usually an iodine solution, provides the density needed for detailed X-ray study of the blood vessels. Upon injection, the contrast agent is carried by blood stream and circulates through the vascular system (arterial, and venous) until it is eliminated in the kidneys and liver. We model the transportation of contrast agent by an advection-diffusion equation describing the distribution of contrast agent concentrations $\mathbf{C}(x, d, t)$ as a function of curvilinear coordinates $\mathbf{x}$ along the centerline of a vessel, the distance $\mathbf{d}$ to the centerline, and time $\mathbf{t}$,

$$\frac{\partial C(x,d,t)}{\partial t} + u(x,d,t)\frac{\partial C(x,d,t)}{\partial x} + \kappa_C \nabla \cdot \nabla C(x,d,t) = I(x,t) \tag{5}$$

where $I(x,t)$ is the injection rate of contrast agent, κ_C is the contrast agent diffusion factor and $u(x,d,t)$ is the laminar flow velocity along the axial direction of each vessel. From the vessel flow rate Q as computed by the vascular flow model (section 2), this velocity can be modeled as a parabolic profile:

$$u(x,d,t) = \frac{1}{4\eta}\frac{\Delta P}{\Delta x}(r^2 - d^2) = \frac{2}{\pi r^2}Q(1 - \frac{d^2}{r^2}) \tag{6}$$

Compared to only modeling concentration at the centerline, as in most previous works, this model provides two important flow features: the propagation front profile is not flat, and some contrast agent remains longer in vessels due to the low velocity near the borders. Since a precise variation depending on the radial position is not visually important, interpolation between the value at the border and at the center is sufficient, using the square of the radial distance to maintain a parabolic profile. We also apply the following simplifications:

- At the center due to high velocity, the advection term is stronger than the diffusion, which can be neglected. We solve this advection numerically using a unconditionally-stable semi-implicit scheme [6].
- At the border, only the diffusion is relevant as the velocity is zero. This diffusion can be computed numerically by combining the value from the previous timestep with the concentration at the center.

The resulting contrast propagation is visible in Figure 1.

3.2   Visualization

In this section we describe various techniques used for rendering a simulated angiogram with a high level of fidelity. While prior work [7] as well as commercial

---

[2] http://sepwww.stanford.edu/public/docs/sep121/paper_html/node93.html

products rely on polygon-based rendering techniques to simulate X-ray images, we propose a method based on volume rendering. Such a technique can provide a high level of realism yet can be optimized for real-time rendering on current consumer GPU, such as the NVIDIA GeForce 8800 GTX in our system.

Simulated fluoroscopy. Fluoroscopy is an imaging modality that uses a *continuous* beam of X-rays visualize the patient's internal anatomy. It follows the same principle as X-ray imaging, where the attenuation of a X-ray beam depends on the density and thickness of the tissue it traverses. The attenuation of an X-ray beam traversing a thin slice of homogeneous material is given as

$$I = I_0 e^{-\mu d} \approx I_0 e^{-\sum_j \mu_j d_j} \tag{7}$$

with I_0 the initial intensity, μ the attenuation coefficient of the material, and d the traversed material thickness. In order to simulate accurately the fluoroscopic process, we have developed a volume rendering approach which renders a CT scan dataset using a discrete transfer function to approximate the continuous beam attenuation equation (7), where d_j corresponds to the slice thickness along the ray and μ_j is the sampled attenuation coefficient of the anatomic structure at slice i. The value of μ_j can be derived from the intensity of each voxel in the CT scan. By computing the contribution of each slice of the CT scan image to the decrease of energy of the X-ray beam, then by summing all the contributions, we can derive a realistic synthetic X-ray image. Since the voxel intensity is directly related to Hounsfield Units, μ can be determined from Hounsfield Units [7]. Similarly, slice thickness and intra-slice distance of the CT scan allows us to measure d_j. What remains to be computed are $e^{-\mu_i d_i}$ and the sum of the contribution over each slice. A good approximation of (7) can be implemented in OpenGL by blending a texture element with the corresponding frame buffer element, taking advantage of recent programmable graphics boards.

Multi-scale voxel representation. Our contrast agent propagation model is based on 1D advection-diffusion as discussed in Section 3.1. To visualize the angiogram in 3D, our previous work [7] created a volumetric representation of the vessels' lumen by dividing this interior space into equal sized voxel elements which are then associated with a curvilinear location x along each vessel. The contrast agent concentration value of a sample point along a vessel is then mapped to the voxels in their vicinity. To deal with very detailed vascular models where the vessels radii vary from $0.5mm$ to $17mm$, more than 40 million equal sized voxels with size $0.25 \times 0.25 \times 0.25mm^3$ was generated, which can no longer be rendered in real-time.

To maintain both high-resolution visualization and real-time rendering, we developed a multi-scale approach based on subdivision. Similar to marching-cube, starting from a prescribed initial grid size, each voxel is tested and labelled as *internal*, *boundary*, and *external*. While the internal voxels are stored, the boundary voxels are subdivided into 8 equal sized sub-voxels. Each sub-voxel is examined against the set of surface polygons intersected by the parent voxel. If a sub-voxel does not intersect with surface and it is inside the surface, then that sub-voxel is labelled as internal and stored. Boundary sub-voxels are again subdivided. The iterative step continues until the predefined number of subdivisions is reached. As a result, starting from $2 \times 2 \times 2mm^3$ and 4 subdivision steps, i.e. the smallest particle is of $0.25 \times 0.25 \times 0.25mm^3$, we generate only 9.2 million multi-scale voxels.

Different sized particles have different amount of radiation attenuation under fluoroscopy. This is achieved by adjusting each particle's rendering size linearly and its intensity exponentially according to its dimensions. This approach is implemented using a programmable shader and runs at interactive frame rates.

Blush. As contrast agent propagates into invisible capillary vessels, it produces a blush that must be simulated, since it is an important visual cue for physicians. Unfortunately computing a volume-based diffusion would be time-prohibitive, so we instead use the GPU to compute an image-space diffusion. When the contrast agent propagates to small vessels in the blush area, we first render the multiscale particles, then use a two-pass (horizontal and vertical) convolution shader to compute a gaussian blur. The blur radius is tuned to achieve a high-level visual coherence with real angiogram. This image is then combined with the particles and x-ray volume to produces the final picture. The result, as shown in Figure 1, reproduces the visual effect with only a small impact on performance.

Cardiac and respiratory motion. Reproducing internal motions, mainly heart beating and respiratory motion, is required to produces realistic sequences. However, it is not possible to store and interactively render 4D scans, or animate by hand the vascular surface model. Instead, we rely on simple spatial affine transformations defined over a local volume of influence. Given a point p in 3D space, we compute its displaced position p' as follow :

$$p' = p + \sum\nolimits_i smoothstep\left(\frac{1-|(p-center_i)/radius_i|}{1-core_i}\right)(M_i - I)p \tag{8}$$
$$smoothstep(x) = 0 \ \text{ if } x < 0, \quad 1 \ \text{ if } x > 1, \quad 3x^2 - 2x^3 \ \text{ otherwise}$$

where the volume of influence is defined by $center_i$, $radius_i$ and $core_i$, while the motion is defined by a 4×4 matrix M_i. This transformation is animated over time using a cyclic profile curve. Equation 8 is simple enough to be implemented inside vertex shaders on the GPU, enabling real-time deformations of both surface and volumetric objects. Moreover, all parameters can be edited interactively using a simple visual editor, as visible in Figure 3. It provides enough controls to create simple but realistic motions. One important limitation is that it does not distinguish between bones and tissues, which are equally deformed. However, we can fine-tune visually the influence of each motion, so that the cardiac motions does not move the nearby ribs, while the respiratory motion do.

4   Results

We have applied our methods to different datasets, and performed both qualitative and quantitative validations. Blood flow and blood pressure distributions

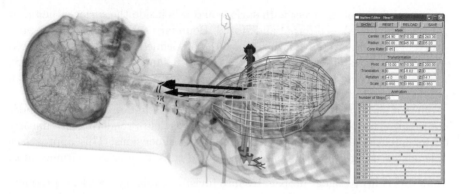

Fig. 3. *Left:* X-Ray rendering under deformation. *Right:* Interactive motion editor.

were computed on a dataset containing about 500 arterial vessels representing the cerebrovascular system, and on a dataset containing about 4,000 vessels (both arteries and veins) describing the full vascular circulation system with a higher level of detail in the brain. For both datasets the results were compared to results from Yazici *et al.* [5] as well as other studies referenced in [5]. The table in the center of Figure 2 compares various flow values in different main vessels of the cerebrovascular network. Our results match very closely these values, yet are computed in real-time. Changes in local flow patterns due to the treatment of a stenosis are also illustrated in the right of Figure 2. These results, as well as the real-time angiogram illustrated in Figure 1 are very similar to what can be observed during an actual procedure, and were qualitatively validated by a neuro-interventional radiologist.

5   Conclusion

We have proposed a series of methods for computing and rendering high-fidelity angiographic studies in real-time. These techniques can bring a new level of realism to simulation systems for interventional radiology, and increase the acceptance of such systems by the medical community.

References

1. Mackay, J., Mensah, G.: Atlas of Heart Disease and Stroke (2004)
2. Luboz, V., Wu, X., Krissian, K., Westin, C., Kikinis, R., Cotin, S., Dawson, S.: A segmentation and reconstruction technique for 3D vascular structures. In: Duncan, J.S., Gerig, G. (eds.) MICCAI 2005. LNCS, vol. 3749, pp. 43–50. Springer, Heidelberg (2005)
3. Alderliesten, T.: Simulation of Minimally-Invasive Vascular Interventions for Training Purposes. PhD dissertation, Utrecht University (2004)

4. Dawson, S., Cotin, S., Meglan, D., Shaffer, D., Ferrell, M.: Designing a computer-based simulator for interventional cardiology training. Catheterization and Cardiovascular Intervention 51(4), 522–527 (2000)
5. Yazici, B., Erdogmus, B., Tugay, A.: Cerebral blood flow measurements of the extracranial carotid and vertebral arteries with doppler ultrasonography in healthy adults. J. Diag. Interv. Radiol. 11, 195–198 (2005)
6. Stam, J.: Stable fluids. In: Proceedings of ACM SIGGRAPH 1999, pp. 121–128 (1999)
7. Manivannan, M., Cotin, S., Srinivasan, M., Dawson, S.: Real-time pc-based x-ray simulation for interventional radiology training. In: Proc. MMVR, pp. 233–239 (2003)

A Training System for Ultrasound-Guided Needle Insertion Procedures

Yanong Zhu[1], Derek Magee[1], Rish Ratnalingam[2], and David Kessel[3]

[1] School of Computing, University of Leeds, Leeds, UK
[2] Mid Yorkshire Hospitals NHS Trust, Wakefield, UK
[3] Leeds Teaching Hospitals NHS Trust, Leeds, UK

Abstract. Needle placement into a patient body under guidance of ultrasound is a frequently performed procedure in clinical practice. Safe and successful performance of such procedure requires a high level of spatial reasoning and hand-eye co-ordination skills, which must be developed through intensive practice. In this paper we present a training system designed to improve the skills of interventional radiology trainees in ultrasound-guided needle placement procedures. Key issues involved in the system include surface and volumetric registration, solid texture modelling, spatial calibration, and real-time synthesis and rendering of ultrasound images. Moreover, soft tissue deformation caused by the needle movement and needle cutting is realised using a mass-spring-model approach. These have led to a realistic ultrasound simulation system, which has been shown to be a useful tool for the training of needle insertion procedures. Preliminary results of a construct evaluation study indicate the effectiveness and usefulness of the developed training system.

1 Introduction

Needle placement into deep organs of a patient is a frequently performed interventional procedure, which may be carried out for a range of purposes, such as drainage of abscess, relief of blockages in the kidneys, radioactive seed implantation, and biopsy of deep tissues. Although usually guided by real-time ultrasound display, such procedures are still highly risky, and require a high level of spatial reasoning and hand-eye co-ordination skill, for successful performance and patient safety. The only reliable approach to acquisition of such professional skills is practicing in a specialised training regime. While practicing needle placement on human patients is dangerous and impractical, and the use of animals is inaccurate, an obvious solution is using simulation systems for the training of such interventional procedures.

Computerised surgical simulation is gaining extensive research interest among both medical and computing communities. Although major efforts have been devoted to simulation of minimally invasive surgery and open surgery involving large incisions, there is relatively limited development in the simulation of image-guided needle-based procedures [1]. Alterovitz et al [2] presented a program to simulate soft tissue deformation caused by needle movement. A single ultrasound image of the prostate is warped dynamically according to the deforming planar

N. Ayache, S. Ourselin, A. Maeder (Eds.): MICCAI 2007, Part I, LNCS 4791, pp. 566–574, 2007.
© Springer-Verlag Berlin Heidelberg 2007

mass-spring mesh. A key limitation of this study is that no 3D aspects of the procedure is implemented. Gorman *et al* [3] developed a system incorporating a mannequin and a haptic feedback device for the simulation of lumbar puncture procedure, which is based on offline CT data. This has no real-time visual feedback. Simulators for fluoroscopy (2D X-ray based imaging) guided procedures have also been reported [4,5]. Nonetheless, ultrasound is often preferable for the guidance of such procedures, as it is fully real-time and inherently safe, while exposure to X-ray should be minimised. Forest *et al* [6] presented an ultrasound simulator named HORUS. Some ultrasould artifacts, such as absorbtion and echos, were implemented, however the general appearance of the simulated ultrasound images was mainly based on CT images, which are essentially different from ultrasound. Moreover, although haptic devices may provide the feeling of "touching" and interacting with the virtual models to some degree, operating on a physical model is a more direct and realistic simulation of the real scenario.

Our target is to develop an ultrasound simulation system that reproduces the ultrasound-guided needle insertion procedure as closely as possible, such that the skills acquired on the simulator can be transported to practical operations with little effort. The hardware of our simulator consists of three components, a standard PC (Dual Intel® Xeon^{TM} CPU 3.20 GHz, 2.0 GB of RAM, running Microsoft® Windows® XP^{TM} Professional), a full scale penetrable model made of latex, plastic and foam, and a pair of Ascension PCIBirds magnetic 3D position/orientation sensors. One of the sensors is rigidly attached to a mock ultrasound probe, and the other attached to a standard biopsy needle. The system process flowchart is shown in Figure 1. For conciseness, in the following sections we will only briefly describe the offline processes in stage i, ii and iii, and focus on the real-time processes such as image synthesis and deformation modelling. Algorithmic details for data registration, sensor calibration, and construction of texture bank, may be found in [7] and [8].

2   Methods

2.1   Offline Processes

The synthesis of virtual ultrasound images requires the answer to three questions: where is the ultrasound scan plane w.r.t. the body, what is in the image, and what does it look like. The position and orientation of the scan plane are captured by the motion sensor that is rigidly attached to the ultrasound probe. A calibration function from the sensor to the calibration point at the centre of the end of the probe is estimated from multiple unique position samples using a standard Least Square Fitting method. Similar approach can be applied to the probe direction calibration, as well as the needle calibration [7]. A volumetric CT data set, acquired from a live patient, is first manually labelled, and then aligned to the physical model surface using a quadratic warping function estimated by a two-stage surface registration process [7]. Sampling this warped volume in the scan plane yields the tissue type of each pixel in the image. The basic appearance of ultrasound imaging is determined by a set of volumetric textures (one for

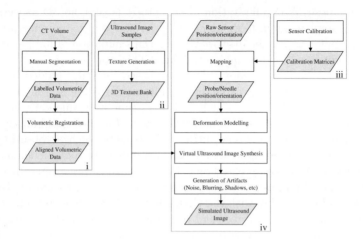

Fig. 1. Simulation process of ultrasound imaging

each visually distinct tissue type) that is synthesised from sets of selected 2D ultrasound examples [8].

2.2   Soft Tissue Deformation

Modelling of the deformation of soft tissue caused by the needle movement is essential for the simulation of ultrasound-guided needle placement as it increases the fidelity of the simulated process. More importantly, it provides immediate indication of needle location and orientation when the needle is invisible in the image but still reasonably close to the scan plane. On the other hand, however, we assume that a highly complex and accurate model for the deforming effect might be unnecessary in our case for two reasons, i) the deformation only needs to be accurate enough to indicate needle location and orientation, and ii) it must be simple enough to work in real-time.

Mass-spring and Finite Element methods are commonly applied methods in the domain of surgical simulation [9]. For the reason of computational efficiency and simplicity, we adopt a localised mass-spring model that is simplified to fit our problem. Firstly, all tissue types are assumed to have identical physical properties and interfaces between tissues are not considered. Although this would not allow the modelling of complex interactions, we have included some facilities that detect whether the needle hits bones or other crutial structures. Secondly, the needle is a thin and sharp device, and only causes deformation in the region local to the insertion path. Therefore, once the needle is detected to have broken the skin, a cylindrical deforming field centred at the predicted insertion path (i.e., the current direction of the needle) is created in the form of a tetrahedral mesh. Physical properties of the mesh elements, such as node mass, spring stiffness, and spring damping factor, are initialised using the methodology described in [10]. A reference mesh with identical topology, named $\hat{M}$, is created to represent the static locations of the vertices, while the deformed mesh, M, represents the dynamic vertex positions according to the mass-spring model. Although the mass-spring method is simple in concept, and has standard solutions, two key issues must be solved in our application, as discussed below.

Mesh Manipulation. In a mass-spring model, external forces can only be applied to its nodes. It is important that, during needle insertion, a mesh node is always constrained at the tip, and all penetrated nodes are constrained to only move along the needle shaft. We use a first-in-last-out stack, $\boldsymbol{v}_{shaft}$, to store the shaft nodes, and use v_{tip} to denote the current tip-node. When v_{tip} is penetrated, it is pushed into the stack, and a new tip-node is identified and assigned to v_{tip}. Figure 2 (a) shows the initial status of $\boldsymbol{v}_{shaft}$ and v_{tip} at a time point t, as well as the tetrahedron defined by $\{v_{j0}, v_{j1}, v_{j2}, v_{j3}\}$ that will enclose the needle tip at time $t + 1$. Let v_{j0} be the current tip-node ($v_{tip} = v_{j0}$), P_{tip} be the new tip position at time $t + 1$, and P_{inter} be the intersection point of the new needle direction with the triangle defined by $\{v_{j1}, v_{j2}, v_{j3}\}$. We consider v_{tip} as penetrated if $distance(P_{inter}, P_{tip}) \leq \lambda \cdot circumference(v_{j1}, v_{j2}, v_{j3})$, where λ is a constant that controls how much the tip node may be displaced before it is penetrated (empirically selected as 0.05 in our current model). The use of circumference ensures this criterion is invariant to the size of the enclosing tetrahedron. When the criterion is satisfied, the tip node is appended to $\boldsymbol{v}_{shaft}$, and v_{tip} is set to be empty. The mass-spring system is then advanced by one time step to $t + 1$ (see Figure 2 (b)). Subsequently, the closest of v_{j1}, v_{j2} and v_{j3} to P_{inter} is moved to P_{tip} and assigned as the new tip-node v_{tip} (v_{j3} in the example in Figure 2 (c)).

Moving a node to a new position in the mesh requires two sub-steps. Firstly, the corresponding node in the reference mesh must be moved accordingly. This is solved by using the Barycentric coordinates, which allow us to map an arbitrary point in the deformed mesh to its corresponding position in the reference mesh, or vice versa. Let $\boldsymbol{b} = \{b_0, b_1, b_2, b_3\}$ be the Barycentric coordinates of point P within the ith tetrahedron, T_i, i.e., $P = \boldsymbol{bv}'_i$, where $\boldsymbol{v}_i = \{v_{i0}, v_{i1}, v_{i2}, v_{i3}\}$ are the vertices of T_i. The corresponding position of P in $\hat{M}$, $\hat{P}$, is thus given by $\hat{P} = \boldsymbol{b}\hat{\boldsymbol{v}}'_i$. Secondly, physical properties of affected nodes/springs must be re-computed (see [10]). Since we maintain the lists of neighbouring nodes and connecting edges/tetrahedrons for all the mesh nodes, this can be done efficiently by iterating through the immediate neighbours of the moved node.

During needle retracking, there is no need to maintain a node at the needle tip. Hence we simply set v_{tip} to empty, and ordinally pop out the nodes in $\boldsymbol{v}_{shaft}$, as they come off the needle. To avoid oscillations after large movement of the needle, we linearly sub-sample the needle movements to ensure each step of movement is below a maximum length. This also ensures that the new tip node can be correctly identified even if the needle penetrates more than one tetrahedron in one time step.

Image Warping. Given the reference and deformed meshes at time t, the warped image can be produced by mapping each image pixel from the deformed

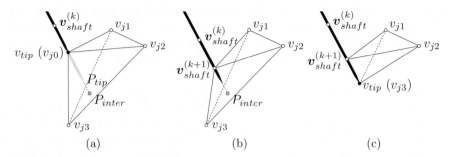

Fig. 2. Mesh manipulation for needle insertion in one step. The new position of the needle is shown in light grey, and current position in solid dark.

mesh to the reference mesh. It is safe to assume that, over a short period of time, most pixels will remain in the same tetrahedron as in the last frame, or appear in one of its neighbours due to mesh deformation. Thus we adopt a nearest-first strategy to perform efficient search of the appropriate tetrahedron for the computation of Barycentric coordinates. At the time when the mesh is first created, we search through the mesh to find the containing tetrahedron for every pixel. In later time steps, the search starts from the tetrahedron associated with the pixel in the previous frame, and propagates to its neighbours if necessary. This strategy greatly speeds up the mapping of coordinates between both meshes, which enables us to produce warped images in real-time.

2.3   Modelling the Needle

Apart from the deformation caused by the needle movement, the needle itself needs some specific handling. Since the motion sensor is fixed at the needle handle, the measured needle direction and tip position may be badly biased if the operator tries to adjust the needle direction by bending the needle. A bending constraining method is designed to minimise the measurement error, and approximate the location of the needle when it is bended within the body. Let $\mathbf{d_m}$ and $\mathbf{d_e}$ be the measured and entry direction of the needle, the constrained needle direction, $\mathbf{d_c}$, is given by $\mathbf{d_c} = w \cdot \mathbf{d_e} + (1 - w) \cdot \mathbf{d_m}$. The weight, w, is defined as $w = w_{max}/[1 + e^{-\alpha(l-\delta)}]$, where l is the inserted length of the needle shaft, w_{max} is the maximum value of weight, α defines the speed (smoothness) of transition from unconstrained to highly constrained bending as the needle is pushed forward, and δ controls the minimum needle length where the transition occurs (we currently use $w_{max} = 0.9$, $\alpha = 60$ and $\delta = 0.12$, based on extensive experiments and communication with our collaborating radiologists). To achieve realistic rendering of the needle, the ultrasound scan plane is assigned a thickness, t, and the brightness(visibility) of the needle shaft is determined by the intersection volume of the needle with the thickened scan plane. A value of t that is equal to the needle diameter appears to be appropriate in our simulator.

2.4   Simulation of Ultrasound-Specific Artifacts

Synthetic ultrasound images are generated by raster scanning through the pixels in the ultrasound portion of the scan plane. A number of imaging/graphic techniques are used to simulate ultrasound-specific artifacts and generate more realistic ultrasound images, as described in [8]. The speckle effect can be simply simulated by adding Gaussian distributed artificial noise to the image pixels. Shadows, caused by bones, air, and the needle shaft, are produced by a 2D ray-casting approach. The radial blur effect creates blurs around a specific point in an image, simulating the effects of a swirling camera. This is applied to simulate the radial scanning motion of a real ultrasound transducer.

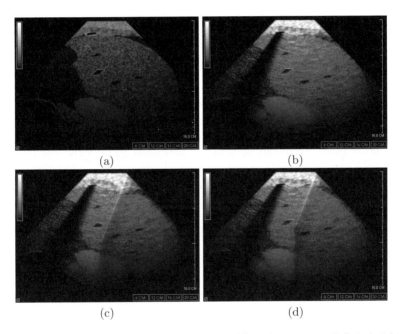

(a)   (b)

(c)   (d)

Fig. 3. Examples of synthetic ultrasound images. These images are slightly brightened for better display.

3   Results and Evaluation

Examples of simulated ultrasound images are shown in Figure 3. These include a "raw" synthetic ultrasound image constructed from the solid texture bank (Figure 3 (a)), and the final rendering results of the same image after artifact simulation (Figure 3 (b)). With the simulated features of speckle noise, blurring and shadowing, the improvement of realism is clear. The deformation due to needle movements may be better demonstrated dynamically. Figure 3 (c) and (d) illustrate the tissue deformation effect caused needle insertion and retracking, which is presented by the directional distortion of nearby structures.

Table 1. Definition of metrics

Principles	Metrics
The needle should not deviate from the optimal path (the straight line from entry point to the target).	m_1: Mean distance from needle tip to optimal path m_2: Mean angle from needle to optimal path
The needle should not deviate from the scan plane.	m_3: Mean distance from needle tip to scan plane m_4: Mean angle from needle to scan plane
The ultrasound probe should not move significantly after needle insertion	m_5: Mean angle from scan plane to entry plane
The needle should not be bended significantly	m_6: Mean distance from measured needle tip to constrained tip position. m_7: Mean angle from measured needle direction to constrained needle direction
The target should be visible in the image while the needle is inserted	m_8: Percentage of time when the target is visible m_9: Distance from target to scan plane
Needle tip should be close to the target.	m_{10}: Min distance from needle tip to target

A construct validation study of our simulation system as a training tool for ultrasound-guided needle insertion procedures is currently underway. The aim of the study is two-fold. On one hand, we hope to validate the realism of our system by showing that experienced experts are able to present superior performance on the simulator than novices as they are expected in real operation procedures. On the other hand, unskilled novices are predicted to perform less favourably due to the lack of practical experience, which may indicate the possibility to acquire and improve their skills through practicing on the simulation system.

We compare the performance of three groups of potential users of our system, including consultant radiologists, radiology registrars, and medical students. Each group consists of eight individuals. None of these twenty-four individuals has previous experience of our simulation system. The task for needle insertion is to find the target embedded in the liver, and hit it with a needle. Each individual is requested to perform three sessions with different target positions. Thus twenty-four sessions are recorded for each group.

Table 2. Performance comparison of three groups of users. All distances are in inches, and all angles are in radians. ($-^*$: $p < 0.05$, $-^{**}$: $p < 0.01$)

Metrics	Students	Registrars	Consultants	p-value (unpaired one-tail t-test)		
				Reg.vs.Stu	Con.vs.Stu	Con.vs.Reg
m_1	0.540 ± 0.122	0.541 ± 0.322	0.356 ± 0.045	0.5021	0.0160*	0.0702
m_2	0.258 ± 0.035	0.255 ± 0.040	0.170 ± 0.004	0.4826	0.0179*	0.0272*
m_3	0.282 ± 0.032	0.259 ± 0.086	0.221 ± 0.018	0.3717	0.0943	0.2827
m_4	0.152 ± 0.015	0.095 ± 0.007	0.070 ± 0.002	0.0344*	0.0015**	0.0999
m_5	0.066 ± 0.005	0.051 ± 0.002	0.054 ± 0.003	0.1906	0.2455	0.5756
m_6	0.088 ± 0.008	0.094 ± 0.003	0.055 ± 0.001	0.6093	0.0487*	0.0035**
m_7	0.041 ± 0.000	0.034 ± 0.000	0.025 ± 0.000	0.1256	0.0011**	0.0190*
m_8	0.927 ± 0.023	0.978 ± 0.005	0.999 ± 0.000	0.0726	0.0123*	0.0788
m_9	0.406 ± 0.049	0.388 ± 0.037	0.289 ± 0.023	0.3800	0.0194*	0.0281*
m_{10}	0.969 ± 0.967	0.635 ± 0.284	0.523 ± 0.102	0.0752	0.0200*	0.1909

A set of quantitive metrics, based on the essential principles for the procedure, are designed to quantify the performance of different groups. What we are most concerned in each session is the period from when the needle breaks the skin till it leaves the body. Therefore, all these metrics are defined over this period, as listed in Table 1. Comparison of the measured performance is presented in Table 2 for all three groups. The group of consultants, who have extensive practical experience in such procedures, performed significantly better than the medical students ($p < 0.05$ for 8 of 10 metrics). Also, though to a less significant level, the superiority of consultants over registrars can also be observed ($p < 0.05$ for 4 of 10 metrics). Registrars performed slightly better than medical students, but not significantly. During the experiments, we noticed that the consultants usually try to identify the optimal path by varying the needle direction when the needle just breaks the skin, then maintain a nice straight line once the path is determined. This is believed to account for the observation that, for some of the metrics (e.g., $m1$ and $m3$), although the consultants presented better performance than other groups, the absolute measurements are not optimal.

4   Discussion

We have presented a ultrasound simulation system for the training of ultrasound guided needle insertion procedures. A number of computational techniques are involved, covering data registration, solid texture modelling, mass-spring modelling, and image processing. All of these are devoted to the development of a useful training system based on realistic simulation of real-time ultrasound imaging. Apart from the visual appearance of simulated images, the fidelity and validity of the system are further demonstrated by the results of construct validation study. It is non-trivial to implement haptic feedback in the system, since a physical latex model is used. However, highly realistic modelling of haptic feedback is seen to be less essential given that the system is designed to improve spatial reasoning and hand-eye co-ordination abilities. Major focuses of future work will include a longitudinal evaluation study that traces the performance of a group of trainees during a structured training course, and the development of a virtual "self-deforming" model of the human body that simulates the motions of the internal anatomies (e.g., respiration).

References

1. Liu, A., Tendick, F., Cleary, K., Kaufmann, C.: A survey of surgical simulation: applications, technology, and education. Presence: Teleoper. Virtual Environ. 12, 599–614 (2003)
2. Alterovitz, R., Pouliot, J., Taschereau, R., Hsu, I., Goldberg, K.: Simulating needle insertion and radioactive seed implantation for prostate brachytherapy. In: Proc. of MMVR, pp. 19–25 (2003)
3. Gorman, P., Krummel, T., Webster, R., Smith, M., Hutchens, D.: A prototype haptic lumbar puncture simulator. In: Proc. MMVR, pp. 106–109 (2000)

4. Li, Z., Chui, C., Anderson, J., Chen, X., Ma, X., Huai, W., Peng, Q., Cai, Y., Wang, Y., Nowinski, W.: Computer environment for interventional neuroradiology procedures. Simulation and Gaming 32, 405–420 (2001)
5. Vidal, F.P., John, N.W., Cuillemot, R.M.: Interactive physically-based x-ray simulation: CPU or GPU? In: Proc. of MMVR, pp. 479–481 (2007)
6. Forest, C., Comas, O., Vaysière, C., Soler, L., Marescaux, J.: Ultrasound and needle insertion simulators built on real patient-based data. In: Proc. of MMVR, pp. 136–139 (2007)
7. Magee, D., Kessel, D.: A computer based simulator for ultrasound guided needle insertion procedures. In: Proc. IEE International Conference on Visual Information Engineering, pp. 301–308 (2005)
8. Zhu, Y., Magee, D., Ratnalingam, R., Kessel, D.: A virtual ultrasound imaging system for the simulation of ultrasound-guided needle insertion procedures. In: Proc. of Medical Image Understanding and Analysis (2006)
9. Delingette, H., Ayache, N.: Surgery simulation and soft tissue modeling. In: Ayache, N., Delingette, H. (eds.) IS4TM 2003. LNCS, vol. 2673, pp. 12–13. Springer, Heidelberg (2003)
10. Paloc, C., Bello, F., Kitney, R., Darzi, A.: Online multiresolution volumetric mass spring model for real time soft tissue deformation. In: Dohi, T., Kikinis, R. (eds.) MICCAI 2002. LNCS, vol. 2489, pp. 219–226. Springer, Heidelberg (2002)

Anisotropic Wave Propagation and Apparent Conductivity Estimation in a Fast Electrophysiological Model: Application to XMR Interventional Imaging

P.P. Chinchapatnam[1], K. S. Rhode[2], A. King[2], G. Gao[1],
Y. Ma[2], T. Schaeffter[2], D. Hawkes[1], R.S. Razavi[2],
D.L.G. Hill[1], S. Arridge[1], and M. Sermesant[2,3]

[1] University College London, Centre for Medical Image Computing, UK
[2] King's College London, Division of Imaging Sciences, UK
[3] INRIA Sophia Antipolis, Asclepios Team, France

Abstract. Cardiac arrhythmias are increasingly being treated using ablation procedures. Development of fast electrophysiological models and estimation of parameters related to conduction pathologies can aid in the investigation of better treatment strategies during Radio-frequency ablations. We present a fast electrophysiological model incorporating anisotropy of the cardiac tissue. A global-local estimation procedure is also outlined to estimate a hidden parameter (apparent electrical conductivity) present in the model. The proposed model is tested on synthetic and real data derived using XMR imaging. We demonstrate a qualitative match between the estimated conductivity parameter and possible pathology locations. This approach opens up possibilities to directly integrate modelling in the intervention room.

1 Introduction

Radio-frequency ablation (RFA) techniques are becoming increasingly preferred as an alternative to drug therapy for treatment of cardiac arrhythmias. These procedures are carried out under x-ray guidance, with specialised catheters for making invasive recordings of the electrical activity of the heart. Although RFA procedures can be highly effective with minimal side effects, they still have unsatisfactory success rates for some group of patients. There is still a need for substantial innovation in guiding these interventions. XMR suites are a new type of clinical facility combining in the same room a MR scanner and a mobile cardiac x-ray set. Registration of the two image spaces (MR and x-ray) makes it possible to combine patient anatomy with electrophysiology recordings [1].

The use of electrophysiology models simulating electrical propagation for various cardiac arrhythmias is a way forward in guiding the RFA procedures. Existing models however are computationally expensive and are presently not suitable for direct use in the intervention room. The aim of this research is to design

---

[1] Obtained from Ensite (St. Jude Medical) or Carto (Biosense).

N. Ayache, S. Ourselin, A. Maeder (Eds.): MICCAI 2007, Part I, LNCS 4791, pp. 575–583, 2007.
© Springer-Verlag Berlin Heidelberg 2007

electrophysiological models that are suited for clinical use and to propose methods to combine these models with interventional data in order to better estimate the patient cardiac function and aid in the guidance of RFA procedures.

Modelling the complete electrophysiology of the heart begins with the incorporation of electrical phenomena from the microscopic cellular level into the macroscopic set of partial differential equations (PDE) modelling a continuum. The resulting models are the bidomain and monodomain models [1]. The numerical solution of these models is computationally demanding due to a very small spatial scale associated with the electrical propagation in comparison to the size of the ventricles. Fortunately as the depolarisation occurs only in a narrow region, the depolarisation region can be considered as a propagating wavefront [2] and an Eikonal equation can be derived describing this activation phenomenon. Further, the solution of these models cannot be directly correlated with pathologies due to the complex interaction of various parameters present in the models. We believe that development of algorithms for identifying the hidden parameters in the electrophysiological models would help cardiologists in a quicker diagnosis and treatment of pathologies. For our interventional purpose and as parameter adjustment often requires several simulations, we propose to use the Eikonal equation to model the electrophysiology.

In this paper, we develop a Fast Marching Method (FMM) for the numerical solution of the anisotropic Eikonal-Curvature (EC) equation on surface triangulations and use it in an iterative algorithm to estimate the apparent conductivity parameter. This parameter is estimated first on a global basis and then local corrections are made. The developed model is validated on synthetic data and also applied to clinical data. We show that the proposed estimation procedure can potentially aid in the detection of scarred/infarcted regions in the myocardium using electrophysiological (Ensite) and geometrical (XMR) information.

2   Anisotropic Fast Marching Electrophysiology Model

Cardiac tissue is strongly anisotropic with wave speeds that differ substantially depending on their direction. For example, in human myocardium, propagation is about 0.5 m/s along fibres and about 0.17 m/s transverse to the fibres. In this section, we present a fast electrophysiological model for depolarisation wave propagation on anisotropic cardiac surfaces.

The static EC equation [3] for the depolarisation time (T) in the myocardium is given by

$$c\sqrt{kD}\{\sqrt{\nabla T^t \mathbf{M} \nabla T}\} - D\left[\{\sqrt{\nabla T^t \mathbf{M} \nabla T}\}\nabla \cdot \left(\frac{\mathbf{M}\nabla T}{\sqrt{\nabla T^t \mathbf{M} \nabla T}}\right)\right] = 1, \quad (1)$$

where c and k are constants related to the cell membrane. D is the volumetric electrical conductivity of the tissue and $\mathbf{M}$ [2] is a tensor quantity incorporating

---

[2] $\mathbf{M} = \mathbf{A}\bar{\mathbf{D}}\mathbf{A}^t$, where $\mathbf{A}$ is the matrix defining the fibre directions in the global coordinate system and $\bar{\mathbf{D}} = \text{diag}(1, \lambda^2, \lambda^2)$. λ is the anisotropic ratio of propagation speeds and is of the order 0.33 in human myocardium.

cardiac fibre directions. The term in square brackets in Eq. (1) is the anisotropic curvature flow term.

Sophisticated numerical techniques have already been developed to solve the Eikonal-Curvature equation to study propagation in normal myocardium [2,3,4]. These models generate accurate depolarisation times at the expense of high computational cost. However, the requirement for our electrophysiological model is that it should be fast. In accordance to this view, we propose an alternative fixed point iterative method combined with a very fast Eikonal solver based on a modified anisotropic Fast Marching Method (FMM) [5]. The fixed point iterative algorithm is presented in Algorithm 1. The curvature flow term in Step 2 is obtained by the anisotropic generalisation of the curvature term given in [6] and the Eikonal equations in Steps 1 and 3 are solved using the modified FMM.

Algorithm 1. Iterative Algorithm for Solving Eikonal Curvature Equation

---

1) Solve Eq. (1) without curvature term to get an initial estimate T_0. Set $T_{\text{curr}} = T_0$.
2) Compute anisotropic curvature flow term ($\widetilde{\kappa}(T)$) with the current estimate T_{curr}.
3) Solve $c\sqrt{kD}\left(\sqrt{\nabla T_{\text{new}}^t \mathbf{M} \nabla T_{\text{new}}}\right) = 1 + D\widetilde{\kappa}(T_{\text{curr}})$ to obtain new estimate of T.
4) **If** $\|T_{\text{new}} - T_{\text{curr}}\| < \varepsilon$, **Stop, Else** $T_{\text{curr}} = T_{\text{new}}$, **Goto** Step 2.

2.1 Validation of Algorithm

The algorithm presented to solve Eq. 1 is tested for its convergence and accuracy by performing numerical experiments. A square domain $[0,1] \times [0,1]$ is considered with the initialisation point being the origin. The parameter values used are $c = 3.89$ and $D = 0.005$. We tested the algorithm on a family of unstructured meshes ranging from $N = 121$ to $N = 5041$ mesh points. The myocardial tissue is simulated by requiring that the speed of propagation in the x-direction (along fibre direction) be three times the speed of propagation in the y-direction.

The results of numerical experiments conducted are presented in Fig. 1. The left sub figure (1.A) shows the convergence of the fixed point iterative algorithm for different mesh sizes. From this figure, it can be seen that the fixed point

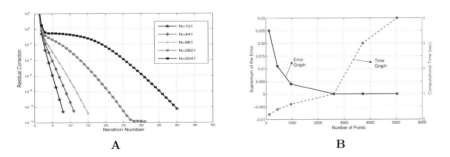

Fig. 1. A. Convergence of the fixed point algorithm for different meshes ($\|T_{k+1} - T_k\|_\infty$ vs k) **B.** Evolution of error (thick line) and Wall time (dashed) w.r.t mesh size.

algorithm converges to a pre-specified limit (say 10^{-10}) for different meshes and also that the convergence seems to be dependent on the number of mesh points N. For the densest mesh considered in the study (5000 nodes), the algorithm seems to converge in about 40 iterations which is very fast and hence may be suitable for faster computations in real time interventional cases.

Fig. 1.B shows the convergence of the solution to a fixed limit as $N \to \infty$ and also the wall time clocked by the FMM algorithm. As the exact solution of this problem is not available, we construct a reference solution by solving the problem on a fine mesh ($N = 5041$) and the convergence of the solution on coarser meshes is examined towards this limit. From the figure, it can clearly be seen that mesh convergence is achieved for this particular case. Note that in comparison to time taken by the sophisticated FEM method (about 4 minutes for 2300 nodes)[2], the FMM method obtains results on a 5000 node mesh in about 4 sec. Further, the stability of the FEM method depends on several terms (diffusion, boundary conditions etc.,) and is strongly dependent on the mesh size thus increasing the computational effort required. In contrast, we observe that the FMM method is quite stable even on coarser meshes and one can refine meshes with a correspondingly small increase in computational effort ($\mathcal{O}(n \log(n))$) and a reasonable first order accuracy [7].

3   Apparent Conductivity Estimation Procedure

Cardiologists generally base their analysis of electrophysiological data on the isochrones of depolarisation/repolarisation times of the epicardium and endocardium. However, these time variables are difficult to interpret due to the influence of the geometry and curvature of the propagating front and often need expert intervention. We hope that estimation of additional parameter maps related to conduction pathologies [3] would enable cardiologists to perform a quicker diagnosis. Additionally, a model based method has the advantage of allowing the use of the model in a predictive way, once adjusted to the data. This can be very useful to test therapies and plan interventions.

The idea in this section is to estimate these hidden parameters using the proposed anisotropic fast marching EC model and clinical measurements obtained during electrophysiology study. The two parameters that are present in the EC formulation are c (related to cell membrane) and the apparent conductivity D. As we have only one measure which is the depolarisation time, we can only chose to estimate one parameter. We aim to estimate the apparent conductivity D, which can be thought of as a good indicator in the case of pathologies. For example, in case of a scarred tissue, we expect that the apparent conductivity in the scarred region may be different (lower) than in the normal tissue.

The algorithm is based on matching the isochrones of measured depolarisation time T^m (from clinical data) to the simulated depolarisation time T^s (from model), in order to get an estimate of the conductivity value (D). To begin

---

[3] A similar goal of estimating myocardial conductivity from body surface potential measurements using a nonlinear system approach can be found in [8].

with, we assume that there is a nominal value of conductivity (D_{global}) on the entire cardiac surface and then you have local variations in conductivity (D_{local}) at each mesh point. We expect that these variations have a large magnitude at points near possible pathological locations.

The global conductivity is estimated by using a simple bisection method (Algorithm 2). As the FMM used in the estimation algorithm is very fast, the global estimation of apparent conductivity parameter is done in a very quick time. The obtained D_{global} after convergence is used as an initial guess for the local conductivity estimation algorithm.

Algorithm 2. Bisection Algorithm for Estimating Global Conductivity

---

1) Set $D = D_0$, where D_0 is the given user estimate for conductivity.
2) Evaluate the average value of measured depolarisation time $\overline{T^m}$
3) Solve Eq. (1) using FMM algorithm in Section 2 and calculate the average of simulated depolarisation time $\overline{T^s}$.
4a) **If** $|\overline{T^s} - \overline{T^m}| < \epsilon$, $D_{\text{global}} = D$, **Stop; Else,**
4b) **If** $\overline{T^s} < \overline{T^m}$, $D = D - 0.5D$; **Else,** $D = D + 0.5D$, and **Goto** Step 3.

The local correction of conductivity at each mesh point is obtained by minimisation of the quadratic error between the model and data. The algorithm works on minimising the cost function given by $J(\mathbf{D}) = \frac{1}{2} \sum_{i=1}^{N} (T_i(\mathbf{D}) - T_i^m)^2$, where T_i^m is the measured depolarisation time at vertex i and $T_i(\mathbf{D})$ is the solution of the Eikonal-Curvature equation with the given set of parameters $\mathbf{D}$. The minimisation is done using the method of steepest descent. The gradient vector is obtained using forward finite differences. i.e., $(\partial_D J)_i = [J(\mathbf{D} + \delta\tau_i) - J(\mathbf{D})]/\delta$, where τ_i is the unit vector in the ith dimension. We note that the algorithm (local estimation) can be expensive for a large number of points. However, this idea of gradient minimisation can be incorporated into a framework in which the conductivity is estimated on region by region basis, where the entire surface is divided into different regions. Further, we expect improved optimisation performance using more powerful descent algorithms such as conjugate gradients.

3.1   Propagation in a Slab of Tissue

We evaluate the performance of presented algorithms initially using synthetic data. A two dimensional slab of anisotropic cardiac tissue ($[0, 1] \times [0, 1]$) is considered for computations. The bottom surface represents the endocardium and the top represents the epicardium. The fibre directions are varied according to $\theta(y) = 2\pi y/3L$ where $L = 1.0$ represents the thickness of myocardium. The initial point of excitation is taken as the bottom leftmost corner of the slab. To simulate the myocardium propagation velocity of around 0.5 m/s, the value of the parameters taken was $c = 3.89$ and $D = 0.005$ along the fibre direction [3] and the anisotropy ratio is set to 0.33. The anisotropic Eikonal-Curvature equation was solved for a case where the conductivity distribution map is taken as shown in Fig. 2.A. Two regions were defined with a higher ($2D_0$) and lower

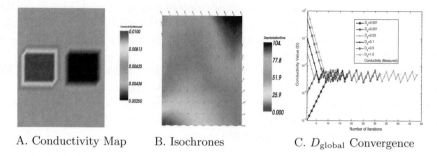

A. Conductivity Map   B. Isochrones   C. D_{global} Convergence

Fig. 2. A. Simulation of different conductivity zones with D twice the normal value (left square in red) and half the normal value (right square in blue); B. Resulting isochrones with the anisotropic Eikonal-Curvature equation (used as measured data for conductivity estimation); The arrows in the figure represent the fibre direction; C. Convergence of the global conductivity estimation procedure for different user values

$(0.5D_0)$ conductivities than the nominal conductivity $(D_0 = 0.005)$ over the entire domain. The resulting isochrones of depolarisation time obtained by using the fast electrophysiological model (shown in Fig. 2.B) are taken as the measured data for the conductivity estimation algorithm. Fig. 2.C shows the convergence of the global estimation procedure for different initial user values. From the figure, it can clearly be seen that the nominal conductivity values obtained by the bisection procedure are very near to the nominal conductivity value (D_0) used for obtaining measured data. Thus, the need for a good initial guess by the user is eliminated by this global conductivity estimation algorithm.

Next, we evaluate the performance of the estimation algorithm (global+local) for a case when the fibre directions are not known (Fig. 3.A) and when the fibre directions are given (Fig. 3.B). When the fibre directions are not known, we assume isotropic wave propagation. In the case of isotropic propagation, it can be seen that although the values of the estimated conductivities are not same as the measured values, a fair idea of the location of low conductivity region is obtained. The estimated low conductivity region is more diffused as compared to that in Fig. 2.A. A much sharper delineation of conductivity regions is obtained when the estimation algorithm is run with fibre data (Fig. 3.B). After convergence of the estimation procedure for the anisotropic case, we obtain a mean error of 2.8×10^{-2} on the depolarisation times which are between 0 and 104 ms. Further, we tested the estimation algorithm for the anisotropic case with noisy fibre data given by adding Gaussian noise to the fibre directions and the estimated conductivity map is shown in Fig. 3.C [4]. The estimated conductivity map with noisy fibre data corresponds more closely to the measured conductivity map (Fig. 2.A) than assuming isotropic wave propagation (Fig. 3.A). From these results,

---

[4] A zero mean Gaussian noise with a standard deviation of 10° was added to the fibre directions. We further note that the percentage change of the estimated conductivity w.r.t the added noise ranging from $0^o - 15^o$ standard deviations was less than 0.1%. This suggests that the algorithm is quite robust to Gaussian noise.

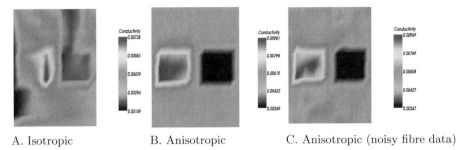

A. Isotropic   B. Anisotropic   C. Anisotropic (noisy fibre data)

Fig. 3. A. Estimated D with isotropic FMM ($\lambda = 1.0$); B. Estimated D with anisotropic FMM ($\lambda = 0.33$, $\theta(y) = 2\pi y/3L$); C. Estimated D with noisy fibre direction

it can be clearly seen that the global and local parameter estimation algorithm can successfully estimate different conductivity regions present in the domain. Further, in relation to clinical applications, as patient specific data on fibre orientations is difficult to obtain in-vivo, prior knowledge on these orientations has to be used. Statistical studies on these showed a variability of around 10 degrees [9], thus we tested the impact of such unknown (fibre orientations) on the estimation procedure.

4   Application to Clinical Data

In this section, we present some preliminary results of applying the conductivity estimation algorithm to clinical data obtained during an electrophysiology study in XMR environment. XMR registration makes it possible to incorporate the electrophysiology measurements and patient anatomy in the same coordinate space. This in turn enables to validate the conductivity estimation model developed by comparing the pathology location obtained from MR with estimated low conductivity regions.

The electrical measurements were obtained using the Ensite system, which is a non-contact invasive catheter based device for recording the electrical activity of the heart (reconstructed on 256 points). This data is from a patient with left bundle branch block, so the initialisation comes from the septum rather than the Purkinje network. The fibre orientation on the endocardium is taken as $+60^{o}$ to the circumferential axis $(\widehat{\xi})$ [5]. We assume that the 3D aspect of electrical propagation does not affect the endocardial surface recordings. The apparent conductivity is estimated on this case and is compared to scar locations estimated by segmentation of late enhancement MR image (see Fig. 4). We obtain a mean error of 6×10^{-2} on the depolarisation times which are between 0 and 66 ms.

---

[5] The circumferential direction at each mesh point is obtained by a cross product of the long axis vector $(\widehat{l})$ of the reconstructed geometry and the position vector of the considered point. Unit vectors in the radial $(\widehat{\eta} = \widehat{l} \times \widehat{\xi})$ and longitudinal $(\widehat{\zeta} = \widehat{\xi} \times \widehat{\eta})$ are obtained successively.

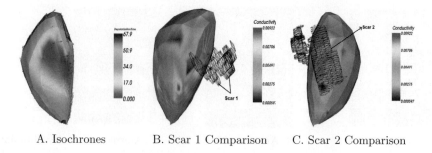

A. Isochrones   B. Scar 1 Comparison   C. Scar 2 Comparison

Fig. 4. A. Isochrones obtained using the anisotropic FMM algorithm; B, C. Matching between the estimated conductivity and scars segmented in a late enhancement MR image. Note that the scars do not lie on the ventricular surface as the late enhancement image was acquired one day before the procedure.

Visual inspection of Fig. 4 shows that the low conductivity areas and scars were co-localised to the accuracy of the MRI to Ensite registration.

5   Conclusion and Future Work

A novel anisotropic fast marching algorithm incorporating fibre data is presented to achieve fast simulations of electrophysiology, along with a parameter estimation procedure to adjust model parameters using interventional data. The apparent conductivity parameter present in the model is estimated on a global and local basis, to identify possible pathological locations (lower conductivity). The algorithm is used on both synthetic as well as real interventional data and the results obtained are very encouraging. Having such a model opens up possibilities for early detection of possible scar regions in the myocardium and also aid in treatment and planning of different strategies before the actual RFA procedure.

There can be several improvements made to the proposed model to enhance its estimation properties which will be the focus of our future research. In order to model re-entrant arrhythmias, we need to introduce the fast marching in a time-stepping fashion to enable nodes to become repolarised. Initial work demonstrating re-entrant wave behaviour using FMM applied to the classical Eikonal equation was presented in [10]. Further in this paper, the cardiac propagation is considered only on triangulated surfaces as relevant clinical data is present only on the endocardial surface. In order to build a more realistic model one should consider the propagation in the entire myocardial volume. A volumetric FMM has been developed for tetrahedral meshes and is currently under evaluation.

References

1. Sundness, J., Lines, G.T., Cai, X., Nielsen, B.F., Mardal, K.A., Tveito, A.: Computing the Electrical Activity in the Heart. Springer, Heidelberg (2006)
2. Tomlinson, K., Hunter, P., Pullan, A.: A FEM for an eikonal equation model of the myocardial excitation wavefront propagation. SIAM J. Appl. Math. (2002)

3. Keener, J.P.: An eikonal-curvature equation for action potential propagation in myocardium. J. Math. Biol. 29, 629–651 (1991)
4. Franzone, P.C., Guerri, L., Rovida, S.: Wavefront propagation in activation model of the anisotropic cardiac tissue. J. Math. Biol. (1990)
5. Konukoglu, E., Sermesant, M., Peyrat, J.M., Clatz, O., Delingette, H., Ayache, N.: A recursive anisotropic fast marching approach to reaction diffusion equation: Application to tumor growth modelling. In: Karssemeijer, N., Lelieveldt, B. (eds.) IPMI 2007. LNCS, vol. 4584, Springer, Heidelberg (2007)
6. Barth, T., Sethian, J.: Numerical schemes for the Hamilton-Jacobi and Level Set equations on triangulated domains. J. Comput. Phys. 145, 1–40 (1998)
7. Sethian, J.: Level Set Methods and Fast Marching Methods. CUP (1999)
8. Wang, L.W., Zhang, H.Y., Shi, P.C.: Simultaneous recovery of three-dimensional myocardial conductivity and electrophysiological dynamics: a nonlinear system approach. Computers in Cardiology 33, 45–48 (2006)
9. Peyrat, J.M., Sermesant, M., Delingette, H., Pennec, X., Xu, C., McVeigh, E., Ayache, N.: Towards a statistical atlas of cardiac fiber structure. In: Larsen, R., Nielsen, M., Sporring, J. (eds.) MICCAI 2006. LNCS, vol. 4190, pp. 297–304. Springer, Heidelberg (2006)
10. Sermesant, M., Konukoglu, E., Delingette, H., Coudiere, Y., Chinchapatnam, P., Rhode, K.S., Razavi, R., Ayache, N.: An anisotropic multi-front fast marching method for real-time simulation of cardiac electrophysiology. In: FIMH 2007 (2007)

Automatic Trajectory Planning for Deep Brain Stimulation: A Feasibility Study

Ellen J.L. Brunenberg[1], Anna Vilanova[1], Veerle Visser-Vandewalle[2],
Yasin Temel[2], Linda Ackermans[2], Bram Platel[3],
and Bart M. ter Haar Romeny[1]

[1] Department of Biomedical Engineering,
Eindhoven University of Technology, The Netherlands
e.j.l.brunenberg@tue.nl
[2] Department of Neurosurgery
[3] Department of Biomedical Engineering,
Maastricht University Hospital, The Netherlands

Abstract. DBS for Parkinson's disease involves an extensive planning to find a suitable electrode implantation path to the selected target. We have investigated the feasibility of improving the conventional planning with an automatic calculation of possible paths in 3D. This requires the segmentation of anatomical structures. Subsequently, the paths are calculated and visualized. After selection of a suitable path, the settings for the stereotactic frame are determined. A qualitative evaluation has shown that automatic avoidance of critical structures is feasible. The participating neurosurgeons estimate the time gain to be around 30 minutes.

1 Introduction

Parkinson's disease patients suffer from motor symptoms, caused by the loss of neurons and the subsequent subthalamic nucleus (STN) burst activity. In the early stage of the disease, patients are treated with dopamine. However, long-term drug taking usually results in severe side-effects. As a solution, deep brain stimulation (DBS) has been introduced [1]. This involves the implantation of electrodes, which, according to the general consensus, modulate STN activity.

Currently, the procedure can take more than eight hours. In our opinion, this could be shortened by refining the preoperative planning of the implantation trajectories. After indirect targeting of the STN, the conventional planning comprises manual selection of an entry point. The resulting path is examined slice by slice, to ensure that blood vessels, ventricles, and sulci are avoided. This is typically repeated a couple of times and can last more than one hour.

In previously developed planning systems for neurosurgery, often a great deal of user interaction is required. We would like to investigate the feasibility of automatically avoiding critical structures and shortening the path planning. After segmentation of the structures to be avoided, our contribution is the automatic calculation of possible paths to the STN in 3D. The resulting paths are then visualized, enabling the neurosurgeon to control their quality and select one.

N. Ayache, S. Ourselin, A. Maeder (Eds.): MICCAI 2007, Part I, LNCS 4791, pp. 584–592, 2007.
© Springer-Verlag Berlin Heidelberg 2007

Section 2 discusses previous research. Section 3 presents an overview of the algorithm, after which Section 4 focuses on segmentation. In Section 5, the path calculation is discussed, and the results are presented in Section 6. The validation can be found in Section 7, and finally some conclusions are given in Section 8.

2   Previous Work

Many of the existing planning algorithms require manual selection of entry points, for example those of Nowinski et al. [2] and Lee et al. [3]. Some only visualize the resulting path, others can also render target lesions and virtual tools. On the other hand, Bourbakis and Awad [4], Fujii et al. [5], and Vaillant et al. [6] describe elaborate path calculation algorithms. However, these require the manual assignment of tissue importance values, which is not very intuitive.

To our knowledge, there is no algorithm in literature that calculates safe paths automatically, without demanding manual setting of a complex cost function. We propose a possibility to select the costs easily by choosing two safety margins.

3   Method Overview

The proposal comprises anatomical segmentations, calculation of possible paths, and interactive visualization of the results. The desired pipeline is shown in Figure 1. The program separates MR and CT processing and is subdivided further to distinguish between user interaction and expensive calculations.

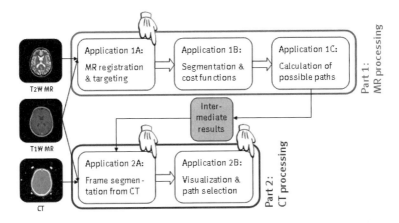

Fig. 1. Overview of the path planning algorithm with MR and CT processing parts. The hands indicate required interaction.

To find a safe path, the target and structures to be avoided, namely the blood vessels, ventricles, and sulci of the cortex, should be known. The corresponding calculations only need the MR images taken some days preoperatively. The developed MR processing part consists of three steps: registration and target selection, segmentation, and path calculation.

Contrast-enhanced T1- and T2-weighted MR and stereotactic CT have been collected for 4 patients. The MR images are registered manually and indirect atlas-based targeting of the STN is performed. Because these operations require user interaction, they are together in part 1A. In part 1B, the critical structures are segmented automatically. It is necessary to evade the blood vessels, also the small ones in the sulci of the cortex, in order to prevent hemorrhages. The ventricles should not be crossed to remain in control of the path, since the electrode is flexible. Subsequently, in part 1C, the target points and anatomical segmentations are used to calculate the possible paths for each side of the brain.

The CT processing is designed to be used on the operation day itself. It consists of two steps, both demanding interaction.

Part 2A involves manual registration of CT and MR. The frame is then segmented, and the parameters for the coordinate transformation from image space to frame space are calculated. The final part, 2B, visualizes the possible paths in 3D, together with the segmented structures. The security margins for the vessels and the ventricles can be changed interactively. Eventually, the most suitable paths can be chosen and inspected by the surgeon in probe's eye view.

For avoiding critical structures the blocks 1B, 1C, and 2B are of interest.

4   Segmentation of Anatomical Structures

To segment the blood vessels, ventricles and gyri, we use several existing methods which, to our knowledge, have not been used in this context before. In advance, the MR images are preprocessed using coherence-enhancing diffusion [7], in order to decrease the image noise while preserving edges.

For ventricle segmentation, we combine a method by Géraud, Bloch and Maître [8] that involves thresholding and mathematical morphology with a method from Schnack et al. [9], using region-growing. An ROI which definitely contains (part of) the ventricles is automatically defined on the MR. We segment the CSF using thresholding and eliminate noise by erosion followed by dilation to reconstruct the ventricle structure but stay inside its boundaries. Finally, the remaining points are used as seeds for gray value-based region-growing. The segmented ventricles can be seen in Figure 2 (left).

We have adapted Géraud's method [8] for brain tissue segmentation to our data. We use erosion and dilation, thresholding, connected components, and masking of T2- with results from T1-weighted MR. Afterwards, gyri and sulci are separated using the technique described by Lohmann [10]. The brain is closed and a depth level intersection with the original segmentation is calculated. The result can be seen in Figure 2 (middle). The gyri are then divided into two hemispheres and restricted to the frontal lobe, to avoid entering the motor cortex.

For the enhancement of blood vessels we use the vesselness measure by Frangi et al. [11]. After selecting the maximum response over 4 scales (0.75 - 3 mm), the image is thresholded to lose noise. To avoid false detection of vessels around

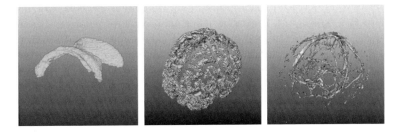

Fig. 2. Segmentations of anatomical structures. From left to right, the ventricles, gyri, and blood vessels can be seen.

the orbitae, the vessel image is masked with a slightly dilated segmentation of the brain tissue. The result can be seen in Figure 2 (right).

The segmentations are calculated fully automatically in MeVisLab. Due to the non-optimal implementation of the multi-scale vesselness, this takes around 60 minutes using a Pentium 4 3.06 GHz processor and 1 GB of working memory.

5 Path Planning

The automatic calculation of safe entry points is the most distinguishing part of this work. A safe path has to avoid blood vessels, ventricles, and sulci, should begin in front of the motor cortex (to avoid epilepsy or motor deficits) but behind the hairline (for cosmetic reasons), and should be safe up to a small distance below the target, to enable deeper insertion.

To a certain extent, it is valid that the further the path stays from the vessels and ventricles, the safer it is. Therefore, a Euclidean distance transform was calculated to obtain two cost functions. These distance maps were thresholded on the size of the set of electrodes that are implanted, in our case 3 mm, in order to have a value of 0 inside the segmented structure and the extra margin.

Existing studies on automatic planning applications require a lot of interaction for complex cost functions. We encountered basically two directions, one based on Dijkstra's path searching principle [12] and one on wave front propagation. However, these are not completely suitable for our application. First of all, they only find the minimum cost path, while we decided to determine every possibility and leave the choice to the surgeon. Furthermore, they need one proper cost function. We would have to add up the costs for the vessels and those for the ventricles in some artificial way, using extra normalization parameters. A linear cost accumulation also leads to the fact that almost hitting a vessel once gives the same cost as crossing the same vessel more often at a safer distance, which is not desirable. Finally, the paths proposed by the traditional methods are not restricted to straight lines, though necessary for our application. Therefore, we propose a very intuitive and easy-to-interact-with method.

Only pixels belonging to the frontal lobe gyri segmentation are considered to be possible entry points. For each of those, a straight line to the target position and 5 mm beyond is traced. Each point along this line is checked, calculating its distance to the vessels and ventricles using trilinear interpolation. If something is hit, e.g. if one of the distance maps is 0 at this point, the path is unsafe and therefore rejected. For all remaining paths, the minimum distance to a vessel and the minimum distance to a ventricle are stored. This enables the neurosurgeon to limit his options to safer paths.

Searching in a random list of entry points is of the order $\mathcal{O}(l)$, where l is the total number of possible paths and will probably not be interactive. A possible solution lies in using a 2D ordered array. Each entry point is then stored in a certain bin according to its minimum distance to a vessel and to the ventricles. For example, the entry point for a path with a minimum distance of 1.4 mm to a vessel and 3.2 mm to the ventricles is classified in the bin belonging to a vessel distance interval of [1.00, 1.50) mm and a ventricle distance of [3.00, 3.50) mm.

In this way, paths with distances higher than chosen thresholds can be proposed without further examination, while only the paths in bins at the margins have to be considered in detail. This is faster than a normal list search, accounting for an order of $\mathcal{O}(1+k)$, where k is the number of paths in a bin, which should be much smaller than the total number of possible paths l. For one of our patients, the mean l was 2852, while k was on average 61. Currently, each bin comprises an equal distance interval, namely 0.5 mm. The search is fastest when the size of the list per bin is balanced. Building the list of possible paths takes around 15 minutes.

6 Results

The user interface developed for visualization is shown in the top image of Figure 3. The desired safety margins to the ventricles and the blood vessels can be set on the right side. The remaining safe entry points and paths are then visualized together with the ventricles and blood vessels.

The bottom image in Figure 3 shows the user interface provided to inspect a selected path using a probe's eye view (MPR perpendicular to the path). Projections of the ventricle and blood vessel segmentations are shown on the reformatted data. The chosen safety margins are visualized as two circles and other distances can be measured by setting markers using the mouse. Meanwhile, the 3D context of the plane is shown to the right. The path's frame coordinates are presented in the bottom left corner.

In conclusion, the neurosurgeons now dispose of an automatic calculation of paths that avoid critical structures, of which the results are presented in 3D. Compared with the conventional path planning in 2D, this gives a more orderly overview of safe entrance regions and therefore speeds up the planning procedure.

7 Preliminary Validation

A qualitative validation has been performed to check whether the planning is indeed fastened by the developed algorithm. The procedure consisted of a

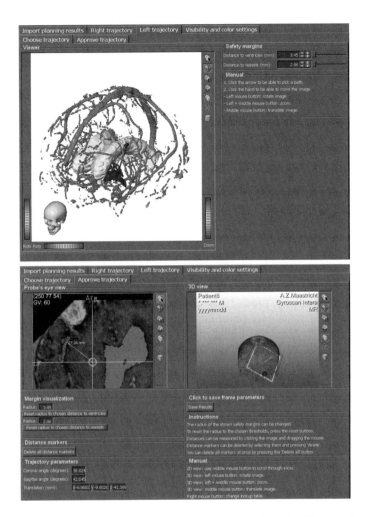

Fig. 3. User interfaces for visualization and inspection of paths. Top: paths together with ventricles and vessels. Bottom: inspection of selected path.

demonstration to one neurosurgeon and two resident neurosurgeons working in Maastricht University Hospital, with 10, 4, and 2 years experience with DBS, respectively. The neurosurgeons were not extensively trained on the new system. One resident attempted a planning himself after the demonstration. This took him about 25 minutes, while he needed on average about 45 minutes on the old system.

Subsequently, all three neurosurgeons were asked to fill out a questionnaire, containing questions about the functionality, appearance, and complexity of the system and its parts. A summary of their answers can be found in Table 1.

Evidently, the neurosurgeons have received the application with considerable enthusiasm. The average score (over 17 questions and 3 neurosurgeons) is 3.9,

E.J.L. Brunenberg et al.

Table 1. Average scores of questionnaire for qualitative validation. Scores were given on a scale of 1 to 5, where 1 means 'very poor' and 5 represents 'excellent'. Surgeon 1 has 10 years of experience, while surgeon 2 and 3 have 4 and 2 years, respectively.

	Surgeon 1	Surgeon 2	Surgeon 3	Mean
Path visualization (3 questions)	3.33	5.00	4.33	4.22
Path approval (2 questions)	4.50	4.00	3.50	4.00
General (4 questions)	4.00	4.00	3.75	3.92
Improvement compared to current system	yes	yes	yes	-
Amount of time to be gained (min)	40	20	30	30

and looking at the subapplication for path visualization and inspection, which was the main focus of this work, the mark increases to 4.1.

The neurosurgeons all think that automatic calculation and 3D visualization is an improvement compared to the currently used planning systems. They expect time gain of 30 minutes. Considering timing statistics for 380 procedures of STN DBS in 12 different centers, collected by the participating neurosurgeons [13], revealing a mean planning time of 1 hour and 3 minutes with a standard deviation of 29 minutes, the necessary planning time could be halved.

8   Discussion

In this study, the feasibility of a faster path calculation for STN DBS has been investigated. We use a combination of existing algorithms to segment the ventricles, blood vessels, and gyri. Cost functions are calculated from these segmentations and used to automatically determine the possible paths to the planned target, together with their distances to ventricles and vessels. Afterwards, the segmentations and paths are visualized in 3D, where the neurosurgeon has the possibility to change safety margins interactively. A suitable path can be selected and examined in a probe's eye view. Subsequently, the required frame parameters are calculated.

The participating neurosurgeons are enthusiastic, estimating the time gain to be 30 minutes, about half of the current procedure. They have many suggestions to improve the appearance and functionality of the current application. For example, they would like to optimize the visualization, using more anatomical information of the head and the basal ganglia, and would like to develop the path inspection further. Furthermore, an extensive quantitative validation has to be performed, to assess the accuracy and utility of the proposed system regarding the registration and segmentation steps.

Until now, we have performed a manual registration, because the inevitable inaccuracy was not important for a feasibility study. However, automating this step using 3D rigid registration based on for example mutual information, will be implemented and validated in the near future.

Validation of the segmentation of critical structures is not trivial, because a gold standard for the ventricles and blood vessels is not readily available.

Validation of the ventricles could be done using manual segmentations generated by collaborating physicians. For blood vessels a phantom could be used. However, the time-consuming generation of a ground truth and the subsequent validation were beyond the scope of this feasibility study.

For now, we projected the anatomical segmentations onto the probe's eye view visualization, as displayed in Figure 3 (bottom). This shows that the segmentation of the superior body of the ventricles is rather good. Nevertheless, looking at Figure 2 (left), it can be seen that the inferior horns of the ventricle are missing. The contrast between these horns and their surroundings is less and sometimes parts are invisible, probably due to partial volume effects. This causes gray value-based region-growing to miss these pieces. Therefore, it would be better to use model-based segmentation for this purpose. However, the inferior horns are not very important for STN DBS planning.

Regarding the blood vessels, the overlay in Figure 3 (bottom) and the segmentation in Figure 2 (right) are less convincing. The segmentation is noisy and the anterior part of superior sagittal sinus misses. However, we are aware of the fact that the used vesselness measure is not ideal, for example because it misses vessel junctions, and are planning to improve this in the near future.

In conclusion, every step in our prototype, from indirect targeting via rigid registration and vessel segmentation to the eventual visualization, can probably be replaced by a more sophisticated and better validated one. However, each of these steps constitutes in itself a field of research on which you can spend many years, while the presented work is just a feasibility study.

Apart from improvements on automatic avoidance of critical structures, another important subject for further research in this field is the STN targeting procedure. To save more time, the indirect atlas-based targeting should be replaced by an automatic segmentation of the target.

References

1. Benabid, A.: Deep brain stimulation for Parkinson's disease. Curr. Opin. Neurobiol. 13, 696–706 (2003)
2. Nowinski, W., Yang, G., Yeo, T.: Computer-aided stereotactic functional neurosurgery enhanced by the use of the multiple brain atlas database. IEEE Tr. Med. Im. 19(1), 62–69 (2000)
3. Lee, J., Huang, C., Lee, S.: Improving stereotactic surgery using 3-D reconstruction. IEEE Eng. Med. Biol. 21(6), 109–116 (2002)
4. Bourbakis, N.G., Awad, M.: A 3-D visualization method for image-guided brain surgery. IEEE Tr. Systems, Man, Cybernetics – Part B 33(5), 766–781 (2003)
5. Fujii, T., Emotoa, H., Sugoub, N., Mitob, T., Shibata, I.: Neuropath planner – automatic path searching for neurosurgery. CARS: ICS 1256(587), 596 (2003)
6. Vaillant, M., Davatzikos, C., Taylor, R.H., Bryan, R.N.: A path-planning algorithm for image-guided neurosurgery. In: Troccaz, J., Mösges, R., Grimson, W.E.L. (eds.) CVRMed-MRCAS 1997, CVRMed 1997, and MRCAS 1997. LNCS, vol. 1205, pp. 467–476. Springer, Heidelberg (1997)
7. Weickert, J.: Coherence-enhancing diffusion filtering. Int. J. Comp. Vis. 31(2/3), 111–127 (1999)

8. Géraud, T., Bloch, I., Maître, H.: 3D segmentation of brain structures from MR images using morphological approaches. Extract from 'Segmentation des structures internes du cerveau en imagerie par résonance magnétique'. PhD thesis, École Nationale Supérieure des Télécommunications, Paris, France (1998)
9. Schnack, H.G., Pol, H.E.H., Baaré, W.F.C., Viergever, M.A., Kahn, R.S.: Automatic segmentation of the ventricular system from MR images of the human brain. NeuroImage 14, 95–104 (2001)
10. Lohmann, G.: Extracting line representation of sulcal and gyral patterns in MR images of the human brain. IEEE Tr. Med. Im. 17(6), 1040–1048 (1998)
11. Frangi, A., Niessen, W., Vincken, K., Viergever, M.: Multiscale vessel enhancement filtering. In: Wells, W.M., Colchester, A.C.F., Delp, S.L. (eds.) MICCAI 1998. LNCS, vol. 1496, pp. 130–137. Springer, Heidelberg (1998)
12. Dijkstra, E.: A note on two problems in connexion with graphs. Numerische Mathematik 1, 269–271 (1959)
13. Coenen, V., Visser-Vandewalle, V.: Towards a standard of surgical care for Deep Brain Stimulation in Parkinson Disease: a 380 patients, multi center experience. Journal of Neurosurgery (submitted 2007)

Automatic Segmentation of Blood Vessels from Dynamic MRI Datasets

Olga Kubassova

School of Computing, University of Leeds, UK
olga@comp.leeds.ac.uk*

Abstract. In this paper we present an approach for blood vessel segmentation from dynamic contrast-enhanced MRI datasets of the hand joints acquired from patients with active rheumatoid arthritis. Exclusion of the blood vessels is needed for accurate visualisation of the activation events and objective evaluation of the degree of inflammation. The segmentation technique is based on statistical modelling motivated by the physiological properties of the individual tissues, such as speed of uptake and concentration of the contrast agent; it incorporates Markov random field probabilistic framework and principal component analysis. The algorithm was tested on 60 temporal slices and has shown promising results.

1 Introduction

In Dynamic Contrast-Enhanced Magnetic Resonance Imaging (DCE-MRI) sequences of images are acquired over time, during which a contrast agent (normally gadolinium diethylene triamine pentacetic acid (Gd-DTPA)) pre-injected into the patient enhances disease affected tissues [1]. Measurement of this enhancement, which is specific for voxels representing particular tissue types, allows assessment of the patient's condition [2,3].

The enhancement is reflected by the shape of signal intensity vs. time curves derived on the voxel-by-voxel basis from the temporal slices and can be measured by computing various heuristics such as maximum rate of enhancement (ME), initial rate of enhancement (IRE), and time of onset of enhancement (T_{onset}) [4,3,5]. Positioning of the imaging volume for acquisition of the data from the 2nd–5th metacarpophalangeal joints (MCPJs) and structure of the DCE-MRI experiment are shown in Fig. 1.

It was demonstrated [6] that signal intensity vs. time curves normalised over a baseline ($\hat{I}$) can be classified into one of the four categories based on their pattern of contrast agent uptake. The heuristics therefore can be extracted from these approximations rather than the raw data (Fig. 2), making their estimation more

* We gratefully acknowledge the advice and support of Dr. A. Radjenovic, Dr. S. F. Tanner [Medical Physics, University of Leeds] and Prof. R. D. Boyle, Dr. M. Everingham [School of Computing, University of Leeds]. Dr. Tanner is further thanked for providing medical data. O. Kubassova acknowledges with thanks the UK Research Councils for financial support via a Dorothy Hodgkin Award.

N. Ayache, S. Ourselin, A. Maeder (Eds.): MICCAI 2007, Part I, LNCS 4791, pp. 593–600, 2007.
© Springer-Verlag Berlin Heidelberg 2007

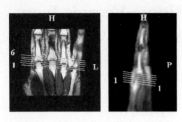 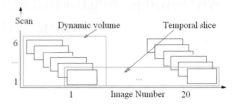

Fig. 1. Left: Positioning of imaging volume. Right: Structure of 4D DCE-MRI dataset with 6 temporal slices, 20 dynamic volumes.

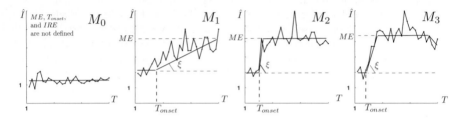

Fig. 2. Signal intensity vs. time curves normalised over a baseline ($\hat{I}$) approximated by M_0–M_3; ξ is a slope of the $\hat{I}$ that be taken as IRE; ME has not been reached for model M_1

robust to the noise effects and subjective opinion of the operator. Classification of $\hat{I}$ is based on the shape of the curve and the noise distribution presented in the temporal slice. The categories are:

M_0 – negligible enhancement, corresponding to the tissue allocated within cortical and trabecular bone, inactive joints, skin and disease unaffected areas.

M_1 – base/wash-in, corresponding to the curves in which by the end of the scanning procedure the maximal intensity has not been reached, indicating constant leakage into locally available extra-cellular space.

M_2 – base/wash-in/plateau. Full absorption of the contrast agent by the tissues.

M_3 – base/wash-in/plateau/wash-out. The wash-out phase is observed at the end of the scanning procedure.

To quantify the degree of RA, radiologists measure a number of voxels within a certain range of the heuristics ME and IRE. Due to the high vascularity that occurs in disease affected tissues, behaviour of the blood vessels and such tissues will be depicted in a very similar manner. This complicates visual analysis of the data and does not permit an objective assessment of the inflammation.

2   Related Work

A number of blood vessel segmentation techniques have been proposed [7,8,9]. Algorithms for static MRI and computer tomography (CT) data segmentation

[10,11] attempt to estimate the centre of the vessel paths and then employ various tracking techniques or prior knowledge about the imagery to determine vessel tree structure. In [7,12] explicit models (deformable models, parametric models, and template matching) were applied to extract the vasculature from DCE-MRI datasets. Such methods generally require manual or semi-automatic initialisation based on prior information about the diameter and location of the vessels.

Classification based methods are also popular for vessel segmentation from DCE-MRI data. Early methods [13] were based on the assumption that each voxel that enhances more than a certain threshold is vascular in origin. However, this approach can lead to the exclusion of up to 50% of the voxels from the image in enhancing tumours and other vascular tissues [5].

These methods have been enhanced by various modelling techniques. The Expectation Maximisation (EM) algorithm is widely used for tissues classification [14]. Commonly, classification is done based on intensity values [15] and whilst performance of these techniques is promising, intensity values of the tissues do not provide enough information for the data classification and the majority of the techniques require some post-processing in order to eliminate falsely detected regions.

We propose to perform blood vessel segmentation using heuristics ME, IRE, and a model number M as classification attributes rather than intensity values. These parameters utilise information about the tissues and should describe behaviour of the voxels better.

3   Segmentation Algorithm

Tissues with the most active perfusion and blood vessels normally exhibit a wash-out phase and assume model M_3, the rest of the disease-affected tissue is normally approximated with M_2, which indicates presence of the intensity plateau in $\hat{I}$ [6]. To isolate and locate tissues with the most significant temporal course variations we applied principal component analysis (PCA) to the temporal slices, where voxels, whose $\hat{I}$ curves were approximated by M_0 and M_1 were excluded.

Our experiments show that the first two principal components capture 97% of the variance in the data. It has also been illustrated that in DCE-MRI studies of the MCPJs, the first component shows temporal course compatible with inflammatory enhancement and the second – with blood vessels and areas with the most active perfusion [16]. Variation of the first two components around the mean and the projection of the data to the first and second components are shown in Fig. 3.

Global thresholding of the images, obtained as a projection of the original data to the second principal component with iterative thresholding [17] allows exclusion of the voxels with insignificant enhancement. Having excluded these, the task is to assign labels {vessel / non-vessel} to the remaining voxels.

Empirically it was observed that the distribution of the heuristics ME, IRE, and a model number M on the remaining voxels is bimodal, the heuristics exhibit

596   O. Kubassova

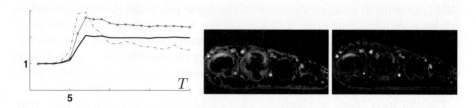

Fig. 3. From the feft: For a temporal slice: mean (bold), mean+2 first principal component($-\times-$), and mean+2 second principal component ($-\cdot-$); projection of the data on the first (middle) and second (right) princupal component

higher values on voxels corresponding to the vessels. We fit the mixture model of two Gaussians to the data using EM algorithm and assign a label {vessel / non-vessel} based on the assumption that the cluster with the higher mean corresponds to the vessel.

Let N be the number of voxels $\{x_i\}_{i=1...N}$ in the slice, each voxel characterised by three parameters $\mathbf{x} =< ME, IRE, M >$. Let Θ denotes the mixture parameters (the mean and standard deviation), and $l = \{l_1, l_2\}$ is vessel / non-vessel class, then:

$$p(\mathbf{x}|\Theta) = \sum_l p(\mathbf{x}|l,\Theta)\pi_l(l), \quad (1)$$

where π_l represents proportion of each class within the data and $p(\mathbf{x}|l,\Theta)$ – probability of a voxel to belong to the class l_1/l_2. We label each voxel with l_1/l_2, so that it gives the greater likelihood:

$$\Theta^*(\mathbf{x}) = \arg\max_\Theta \sum_{i=1}^N \log p(x_i|\Theta) \quad (2)$$

However, the noise presented in the data and imprecision in the model we used leave some error (see Fig. 5). Therefore, we exploit the fact that blood vessels have nonnegligible spatial support by assuming that neighbouring voxels are likely to have the same label in the absence of significant differences in the grey level between them.

Markov random field (MRF) [18] based filtering allows refining our initial labelling. Let Λ be a field of labels over the image, and C – a set of clicks, defined in 8-connected neighbourhood [19], then the energy function can be described by Eq. 3, where we omitted dependence on fixed parameters $\mathbf{x}$ and Θ for the sake of clarity.

$$E = \sum_{i=1}^N \log p(x_i|l_i) + \lambda \sum_{<i,j>\in C} \phi(f_i, f_j, l_i, l_j) \quad (3)$$

$\lambda \geq 0$ controls the relative importance of the terms. Based on the empirical observations, λ was set to 1, giving equal weight to both terms.

ϕ is 0 if $l_i = l_j$, and otherwise $\left(1 - \exp\{-|f_i - f_j|^2/(2\sigma^2)\}\right)$, where $\sigma = \sqrt{\frac{1}{C}|f_i - f_j|}$, C is a number of clicks, and f is pixel intensity in the post-contrast image. The assignment of the labels to the pixels which minimises the energy is found with the mincut maxflow algorithm, which is known to give the global minimum [19,20].

Given the assignment of vessel / non-vessel to each voxel, we can visualise the extent of inflammation via constructing parametric maps of the heuristics and excluding the voxels corresponding to the blood vessels (Fig. 4).

4   Experiments and Discussion

An algorithm for vessel segmentation from temporal DCE-MRI slices of the MCPJs was presented. In this section, we evaluate its performance in application to 60 temporal slices.

Imaging for this application was performed on a 1.5T MRI scanner (Gyroscan ACS NT, Phillips Medical Systems, Best, The Netherlands), using a 3D T1 weighted spoiled gradient echo sequence: repetition time/echo time/flip angle = $14/3.8/40°$; field of view = 100mm, slice thickness 3mm, imaging matrix is 128×256 [4].

The number of vessels seen in a slice varies from 8 to 17, and the diameter of a vessel ranges from 2 to 200 pixels. Firstly, we evaluate the algorithm's ability to detect the vessels in temporal slices by comparison of results with the ground truth (GT) provided by an experienced observer. Table 1 illustrates the results.

The algorithm did not deliver false positive results and no post-processing to remove over-segmented regions is needed. A small proportion of blood vessels of a small size (less than 5 pixels) has been classified as noise at the MRF step. However, analysing several corresponding slices, we can reconstruct the structure of the vessel tree using, for example, cubic interpolation on region locations. Fig.5 (right) illustrates the result for one of the studies. The reader gets a 'semi' 3D impression of the inflammatory distribution in the imaged area; moreover the location of under-segmented blood vessels can be recovered.

Table 1. Detection of blood vessels in temporal slices [Number of blood vessels delivered by the algorithm / Total number of vessel in the slice]; S – scan number; P – patient number

Patient / Slice	P_1	P_2	P_3	P_4	P_5	P_6	P_7	P_8	P_9	P_{10}
S_1	9/9	14/14	16/16	14/14	9/9	12/12	12/12	12/12	10/10	17/17
S_2	9/9	11/11	14/15	12/13	11/13	9/10	12/13	10/10	9/9	14/16
S_3	9/9	11/12	17/17	14/14	12/12	11/11	11/12	8/9	8/10	14/15
S_4	8/9	13/13	16/17	12/14	9/10	12/13	10/12	6/8	12/12	15/15
S_5	8/8	10/11	17/17	15/15	11/11	12/12	13/13	10/10	12/13	15/15
S_6	9/9	12/12	16/17	16/16	11/11	10/10	13/13	12/12	12/12	16/16

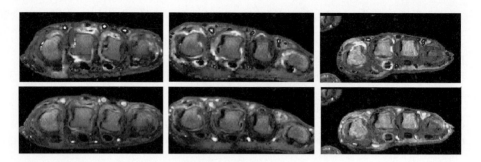

Fig. 4. Top: Parametric maps of ME corresponding to different DCE-MRI studies with segmented blood vessels (the contour is shown in blue). The lower values of the heuristic are plotted in red, then yellow and white as the values increase. Bottom: Corresponding post-contrast images.

The quality of the segmented boundaries of the vessels was evaluated using a mutual overlap based metric [21]. For 60 slices, at each step of the algorithm (PCA / PCA+EM / PCA+EM+MRF) we computed the number of erroneous voxels with respect to the overall number of voxels in the GT.

For comparison purposes we segmented BVs using the intensity of the voxels for probabilistic modelling rather than the heuristics (Alg.2 in Fig. 5).

The results obtained in this experiment indicate that the proposed algorithm generates accurate segmentation regardless of size and location of the vessels. At each step we observe an incremental increase in quality of results. On average the new algorithm detects 94% of vessels in dynamic MRI slices of the MCPJs, with mutual overlap between GT and obtained segmentations exceeding 90%.

Pixels identified as false negative are normally located around the border of segmented vessels. Their exclusion / inclusion might be due to observer mis-detection and could be improved by boundary refining algorithms.

An alternative approach, where intensity of the voxels was used for probabilistic modelling rather than the heuristics (Alg.2) failed to deliver reliable segmentation – often synovial tissue was classified as vessels and vice versa.

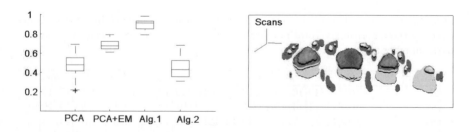

Fig. 5. Left: Mutual overlap between GT and segmented regions at each step of the proposed algorithm. Final results – Alg.1; results with an alternative segmentation technique (Alg.2). Right: Reconstructed vessels and bone interiors (3D view).

These results confirm that voxel intensity based modelling alone is not sufficient for accurate tissue classification.

5   Conclusion

The method presented in this paper delivers accurate segmentation of blood vessels from DCE-MRI datasets of the hand joints. Statistical mixture models motivated by the physiological properties of the individual tissues, such as speed of absorption and concentration of the contrast agent, have been employed to describe the behaviour of the vessels and synovitis. Spatial relationships between neighbouring pixels were incorporated through an MRF probabilistic framework. The combination of these methods provides promising results. The technique is fully automated, does not require any post-processing and can easily be adapted for other applications of the similar nature. Future work will focus on the testing of the method on datasets acquired from different joints and investigation of the algorithm's performance when other heuristics are included.

References

1. Taylor, P.C.: The value of sensitive imaging modalities in rheumatoid arthritis. Arthritis Research and Therapy 5(5), 210–213 (2003)
2. McQueen, F.M., Stewart, N., Crabbe, J., Robinson, E., Yeoman, S., Tan, P.L.J., McClean, L.: Magnetic resonance imaging of the wrist in early rheumatoid arthritis reveals a high prevalence of erosion at four months after symptom onset. Annals of the Rheumatic Diseases 57, 350–356 (1998)
3. Cimmino, M.A., Innocenti, S., Livrone, F., Magnaguagno, F., Silvesti, E., Garlaschi, G.: Dynamic gadolinium-enhanced MRI of the wrist in patients with rheumatoid arthritis. Arthritis and Rheumatism 48(5), 674–680 (2003)
4. Radjenovic, A.: Measurement of physiological variables by dynamic Gd-DTPA enhanced MRI. PhD thesis, School of Medicine, University of Leeds (2003)
5. Jackson, A.: Analysis of dynamic contrast enhanced MRI. Radiology 77(2), 154–166 (2004)
6. Kubassova, O., Boyle, R.D., Radjenovic, A.: Improved parameter extraction from dynamic contrast-enhanced MRI data in RA studies. In: Joint Disease Workshop, Medical Image Computing and Computer Assisted Intervention, vol. 1, pp. 64–71 (2006)
7. Kirbas, C., Quek, F.: A review of vessel extraction techniques and algorithms. ACM Computing Surveys 36(2), 81–121 (2004)
8. Suri, J.S., Liu, K., Reden, L., Laxminarayan, S.: A review on MR vascular image processing algorithms: acquisition and prefiltering: Part I. IEEE Transactions on Information Technology in Biomedicine 6(4), 324–337 (2002)
9. Sonka, M., Liang, W., Stefancik, R.M., Stolpen, A.: Vascular Imaging and Analysis. In: Sonka, M., Fitzpatrick, J.M. (eds.) Handbook of Medical Imaging. Medical Image Processing and Analysis, SPIE, pp. 808–914 (2000)
10. Bulpitt, A., Berry, E., Boyle, R., Scott, J., Kessel, D.A.: A deformable model, incorporating expected structure information, for automatic 3D segmentation of complex anatomical structures. Computer Assisted Radiology and Surgery 1, 572–577 (2000)

11. Magee, D., Bulpitt, A., Berry, E.: 3D automated segmentation and structural analysis of vascular trees using deformable models. IEEE Workshop on Variational and Level Set Methods in Computer Vision 1, 119–126 (2001)
12. McInerney, T., Terzopoulos, D.: Deformable models in medical image analysis: a survey. Medical Image Analysis 1(2), 91–108 (1996)
13. Tofts, P.S., Kermode, A.G.: Measurement of the blood-brain barrier permeability and leakage space using DEMRI. Magnetic Resonance in Medicine 17(2), 357–367 (1991)
14. Chung, A.C.S., Noble, J.A., Summers, P.: Vascular segmentation of phase contrast magnetic resonance angiograms based on statistical mixture modeling and local phase coherence. IEEE Transactions on Medical Imaging 23(12), 1490–1507 (2004)
15. Wilson, D.L., Noble, J.A.: An adaptive segmentation algorithm for time-of-flight MRA data. Medical Imaging 18, 938–945 (1999)
16. Klarlund, M., Østergaard, M., Rostrup, E., Skødt, H., Lorenzen, I.: Dynamic MRI and principal component analysis of finger joints in rheumatoid arthritis, polyarthritis, and healthy controls. International Society for MRI in Medicine (last access on 03.05.07) (1999), http://cds.ismrm.org/ismrm-1999/PDF2/409.pdf
17. Ridler, T.W., Calvard, S.: Picture thresholding using an iterative selection method. Man and Cybernetics 8(8), 630–632 (1978)
18. Geman, S., Geman, D.: Stochastic relaxation, Gibbs distributions, and the Bayesian restoration of images. IEEE Transactions on Pattern Analysis and Machine Intelligence 6, 721–741 (1984)
19. Boykov, Y., Lee, V.S., Rusinek, H., Bansal, R.: Segmentation of dynamic N-D data sets via graph cuts using Markov models. In: Niessen, W.J., Viergever, M.A. (eds.) MICCAI 2001. LNCS, vol. 2208, pp. 1058–1066. Springer, Heidelberg (2001)
20. Szeliski, R., Zabih, R., Scharstein, D., Veksler, O., Kolmogorov, V., Agarwala, A., Tappen, M., Rother, C.: Comparative study of energy minimization methods for markov random fields. European Conference on Computer Vision 2, 16–29 (2006)
21. Dice, L.R.: Measures of the amount of ecologic association between species. Ecology 26(3), 297–302 (1945)

Automated Planning of Scan Geometries in Spine MRI Scans

Vladimir Pekar[1,*], Daniel Bystrov[1], Harald S. Heese[1], Sebastian P. M. Dries[1],
Stefan Schmidt[1,2], Rüdiger Grewer[1], Chiel J. den Harder[3],
René C. Bergmans[3], Arjan W. Simonetti[3], and Arianne M. van Muiswinkel[3]

[1] Philips Research Europe – Hamburg, Germany
[2] University of Mannheim, Germany
[3] Philips Medical Systems, Best, The Netherlands
vladimir.pekar@philips.com

Abstract. Consistency of MR scan planning is very important for diagnosis, especially in multi-site trials and follow-up studies, where disease progress or response to treatment is evaluated. Accurate manual scan planning is tedious and requires skillful operators. On the other hand, automated scan planning is difficult due to relatively low quality of survey images ("scouts") and strict processing time constraints. This paper presents a novel method for automated planning of MRI scans of the spine. Lumbar and cervical examinations are considered, although the proposed method is extendible to other types of spine examinations, such as thoracic or total spine imaging. The automated scan planning (ASP) system consists of an anatomy recognition part, which is able to automatically detect and label the spine anatomy in the scout scan, and a planning part, which performs scan geometry planning based on recognized anatomical landmarks. A validation study demonstrates the robustness of the proposed method and its feasibility for clinical use.

1 Introduction

The diagnostic value of MRI scans greatly depends on the accuracy and consistency of scan planning. This procedure is typically carried out on a low resolution (often just a few orthogonal slices) survey dataset, the so-called "scout", in which scan geometries, such as off-center, angulation and field-of-view, are determined manually by the operator. The operators often need to plan several diagnostic scans with different parameters during one session, which requires high concentration and is potentially error-prone. Every operator has an individual planning style depending on his/her level of experience, training, etc. All these factors negatively influence the consistency and reproducibility in the resulting diagnostic scan geometries.

In order to improve the MR acquisition workflow, several research groups have proposed automated scan planning (ASP) methods for different anatomies, e.g. neurocranial [1,2], cardiac [3,4], and knee [5].

---

* V. Pekar is currently with Philips Medical Systems, Markham, ON, Canada.

N. Ayache, S. Ourselin, A. Maeder (Eds.): MICCAI 2007, Part I, LNCS 4791, pp. 601–608, 2007.
© Springer-Verlag Berlin Heidelberg 2007

Spine examinations represent one of the most important clinical applications of MRI. However, automated spine planning is a particularly difficult task, since several peculiarities have to be taken into consideration: i) Spine has a repetitive anatomical structure, so the correct order of visible vertebrae needs to be recognized and labeled. ii) The number of vertebrae may vary from one individual to another. iii) The appearance of vertebrae and intervertebral discs may be affected by different pathologies, e.g. deformity (scoliosis), fracture, neoplasm, degeneration, etc. iv) The ASP system has to be able to deal with partial spine acquisitions, for example, in examinations of the lower (lumbar) or upper (cervical) spine. The exact number of visible vertebrae in such examinations is not known in advance and the use of global registration or structural model-based methods for anatomy detection is difficult.

Robust anatomy recognition is a core requirement for an ASP system to be advantageous over manual planning in clinical routine. Automated spine detection and labeling is a technically challenging task even in diagnostic quality MRI. Peng et al. [6] aim at detecting the intervertebral discs in adjacent 2-D sagittal slices for segmentation of the whole spine column. A feature detector based on template matching is applied to detect candidates for disc centers followed by local post-processing. A semi-automated approach for labeling intervertebral discs in whole spine has been proposed by Weiss et al. [7]. After intensity correction step, the operator provides a seed point in the C2-C3 disc to start the search procedure based on intensity thresholds. Vrtovec et al. [8] detect the spine by searching for circular areas of homogeneous intensity in axial slices. The performance of the above mentioned approaches strongly depends on good image quality with reproducible contrasts. This may not be the case for scout data, of which the quality is usually limited by the clinically acceptable scanning time.

This paper develops a new approach for fast and robust automated spine detection and labeling in 3-D scout images. Analogously to earlier work [2,5], the detected anatomical landmarks are used to learn pre-defined geometries from a training set provided by the operator. In this way, the ASP system allows to consistently plan scan geometries tailored to individual needs and preferences of the radiologist. The focus of this paper is on planning lumbar and cervical partial examinations, although the approach can be extended to other types of examinations, e.g. thoracic or total spine.

The reliability of the proposed method is demonstrated by validating the anatomy detection on 60 spine scout images (30 cervical and 30 lumbar datasets). The experimental part of the paper also illustrates automated learning of scan plan geometries and their transfer from one area of the spine to another.

2   Method

Automated scan planning starts with the acquisition of a 3-D low-resolution scout scan. The scout image is analyzed by the anatomy recognition algorithm, which automatically detects the intervertebral discs and labels the corresponding vertebrae. In a clinical environment, the system would typically ask the operator to confirm (and, if needed, even adapt) the correctness of anatomy detection. After the labeling step, the positions and orientations of the intervertebral discs are used to generate a set of landmarks required for automated geometry planning.

2.1   Image Data

Scout protocols generally require a compromise between obtaining the image quality and resolution sufficient to successfully cope with the task of scan planning, and limited acquisition time, which should be kept as short as possible. The spine planning method in this work uses dedicated 3-D T1-weighted fast field echo (FFE) scans having sagittal slice orientation with $400 \times 400 \times 270$ mm field of view ($1.25 \times 1.25 \times 1.5$ mm voxel size) and acquisition time of 40 s. The datasets were acquired on a 1.5T Philips Achieva MR scanner.

2.2   Anatomy Recognition

The spine detection is implemented in the form of sequential application of three processing steps aiming at fast and reliable detection of the intervertebral discs.

Detection of disc candidates. As a pre-processing step, an interest point detector is applied to simplify the spine detection problem through analyzing a relatively small number of candidates. Since intervertebral discs appear as bright line-like structures in sagittal or coronal slices, our interest point detector is based on a special filter which detects approximately horizontal lines in sagittal 2-D slices of the scout image. This approach is computationally more efficient than searching for disc-like structures in 3-D. The filter response used is based on eigenanalysis of the image Hessian and is defined for image position $\mathbf{x}$ as: $V(\mathbf{x}, s) = \exp\left\{-\frac{\lambda_1^2/\lambda_2^2}{a^2}\right\}\left(1 - \exp\left\{-\frac{\lambda_1^2+\lambda_2^2}{b^2}\right\}\right)$, where λ_1 and λ_2 are the eigenvalues of the Hessian matrix at scale s with $|\lambda_1| \leq |\lambda_2|$, and a and b are sensitivity weights [9]. The value of a was set to 500 in this work, and the value of b was set to half of the maximum Hessian norm, as proposed in [9]. The first term suppresses blob-like structures while the second term suppresses the influence of the background noise. Admissible intensity range and principal Hessian eigenvector orientation are used to improve selectivity of the filter.

The filter is applied on a isotropically downsampled image with the voxel size of 3 mm^3, using the scale parameter $s = 1$. The filtered dataset is next converted to a binary image by applying the threshold $V > 10^{-4}$ and cleaned by morphological opening using a rectangular structural element. The centers of mass of the 3-D connected components in the filtered image are considered as candidates for the intervertebral disc centers. Additionally, the smallest principal component of each 3-D segment is computed to estimate the orientation vector orthogonal to the disc.

Spine detection. Unambiguous discrimination between true disc centers and false ones in the set of candidates is a very difficult task, even by exploiting the structural connectivity and vertical orientation of the spine column. We follow a different strategy and aim at reliably finding one single point belonging to the spine. Starting from that point, a progressive search is initiated which extracts the whole visible spine using prior structural knowledge.

Since the spine column can be considered as a tubular structure, most of the false candidates can be removed by applying an iterative procedure which removes candidates that form point triplets with angles in the range $[\pi/4, 3\pi/4]$. This is done to eliminate segments with unrealistically high curvature. In each pass, the candidate point responsible for the largest number of inadmissible triplets is eliminated from the set and the procedure is repeated until no such points are left. The topmost candidate point from the remaining set is marked as the first point belonging to the spine column in lumbar scouts. Analogously, the bottommost candidate point is used for cervical scouts.

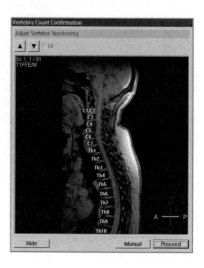

Fig. 1. GUI fragment with automatically labeled cervical scout

To improve the performance and robustness of the above method, a subset of 15 candidates mostly resembling intervertebral discs is taken instead of the whole set. This reflects the maximum number of visible discs in partial spine examinations. In order to select these candidates, the corresponding location in the image is evaluated for similarity with an intervertebral disc template represented by a triangulated surface mesh and positioned according to the disc orientation vector computed in the previous step. The similarity value for the k-th candidate is defined as: $S_k = \frac{1}{N}\sum_{i=1}^{N}\mathbf{n}_i^T\mathbf{g}_{i,k}$, where N is the number of triangles in the disc template mesh, $\mathbf{n}$ is the triangle normal unit vector and $\mathbf{g}$ is the normalized image gradient, computed at the triangle position.

Spine labeling. Starting at the first spine point, a progressive search is carried out upwards/downwards aiming at extracting the disc centers in the visible spine column from all candidates detected as interest points. The next spine point is selected as lying at a certain distance from the previously detected one, where the orientation of the corresponding intervertebral disc is used to define the search direction. If a candidate is missing at the expected position, e.g. due to pathology or image artifacts, an artificial disc candidate is inserted and searching continues using the same direction.

The search is terminated when several consecutive missing candidates are encountered. This criterion reliably identifies the C2-C3 disc in the cervical spine owing to the characteristic form of the C2 vertebra. In the lumbar spine, the L5-S1 disc can be found as being the one with the maximum forward angulation about the axis in right-left direction of the patient. After the entire set of visible discs are extracted, the vertebrae are labeled w.r.t. the disc found last, see Fig. 1.

2.3   Scan Geometry Planning

Analogously to previous work [2,5], the method uses a training set of manually planned geometries to propose a planning based on correlation with the
automatically detected anatomical landmarks. On the training samples, rigid
registration of the automatically detected landmarks is carried out. A robust
multi-variate median approach [10] has to be employed in the computation of
the "atlas" landmarks, since anatomical variability as well as variability in the
landmark extraction impede perfect alignment. The variance of the landmark
positions in the training samples w.r.t. the position of the corresponding "atlas"
landmark furthermore determines its contribution to the proposed planning. Finally, the planning algorithm performs rigid registration of the detected set of
landmarks from the current image with the "atlas" landmarks from the training
set based on these contributions.

Considerable contrast fluctuations in the scout protocol and possible presence
of severe pathologies, e.g. fractures, make accurate segmentation of structures
such as vertebrae or intervertebral discs for the purpose of landmark extraction
difficult. Instead, positions and orientations of the detected intervertebral discs
are used to define fixed extents around each disc, whose corner points are used as
landmarks. To account for the specific repetitive character of the spine anatomy,
the planning concept has been extended to transfer plans from one particular
area into another. For example, if the training set consists of lumbar anatomy
plans only, the system is still capable of planning on cervical scouts.

3   Results

Validation of the approach has been carried out using two criteria: i) robustness
of anatomy detection and ii) quality of automatically generated plans.

Validation of anatomy detection. Two cervical and two lumbar scout images
of 15 different volunteers were acquired. The volunteers were asked to change
their pose in-between, while the global positioning of each subject was kept
fairly consistent. Ground-truth information regarding the position of the visible
intervertebral discs was generated for all 60 datasets by a clinical expert.

In a first step, the performance of the disc candidate detection was evaluated,
showing a sensitivity of 95.6% for the interest point detector. As the interest
point detector responds on all horizontal line-like structures in the image, the
number of false disc candidate detections is rather high, especially in cervical
scouts owing to the smaller size of the intervertebral discs. The detailed statistics
discriminating between cervical and lumbar scouts are summarized in Table 1.

Secondly, the spine detection was evaluated. Fig. 2 illustrates the effect of
dramatically reducing the number of false candidates arising in disc candidate
detection by applying the spine detection procedure presented in Section 2.2.
The final candidate that was selected at the end of the procedure corresponded
in all 60 images to a valid detection of an intervertebral disc. In 28 out of 30
lumbar images, the detected point corresponded to the uppermost candidate, in

Table 1. Sensitivity results for detection of disc candidates in 60 datasets

	cervical	lumbar	all
visible discs (ground truth)	387	289	676
overall candidates	4480	841	5321
false candidates	4111	564	4675
true detections	369 (95.3%)	277 (95.8%)	646 (95.6%)
failed detections	18 (4.7%)	12 (4.2%)	30 (4.4%)

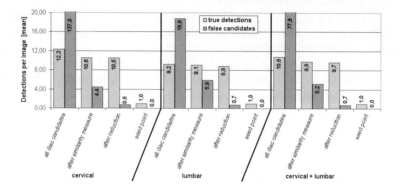

Fig. 2. Comparison of mean values per image for true detections and false candidates after different steps in the spine detection procedure

two images it was shifted downwards by one. Similarly, in 27 out of 30 cervical images the detected point corresponded to the lowermost candidate, in three images it was shifted upwards by one. These results imply that by performing the propagation process for the spine labeling, none of the intervertebral discs, that are within the clinically relevant area, are prone to be missed due to bad initialization.

Finally, the results of spine labeling were analyzed. In all 30 cervical images, the labeling was correct with the exception of one dataset, where one extra disc was erroneously detected. In particular, the progressive search was able to recover all relevant intervertebral discs for which disc candidate detection failed. Correspondingly, the labeling was correct in 25 out of 30 lumbar scouts. In the remaining 5 images L4-L5 was erroneously detected as the lowermost disc, however, in a clinical environment this error can be corrected by the operator.

Validation of automated planning. Qualitative assessment of consistency of the presented method with manual planning was carried out using 12 survey datasets. For the cervical and lumbar regions, manual plan sets were defined in six images each. Every plan set consisted of a mid-sagittal view of the total cervical or lumbar spine and two transverse views at different segmental levels: lower third of the vertebral body C6 or L4 and the disc below. Five plans were

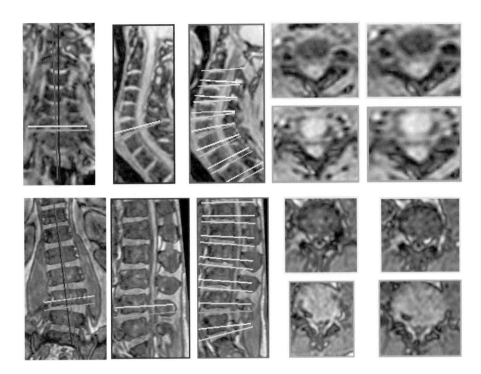

Fig. 3. Upper row: cervical, lower row: lumbar; left to right: manually planned frontal view, manually planned midsagittal view, automatically planned midsagittal view, manually planned vertebra/disc, automatically planned vertebra/disc. The blue and the red line in the frontal view correspond to the manually and automatically planned midsagittal planes. The yellow lines correspond to the planned vertebrae, the green lines correspond to the discs, the resulting transversal views are shown at the right.

based on the images of healthy volunteers from the anatomy detection validation study. These plans were used to train the ASP algorithm. For the sixth dataset, displaying a pathology, the corresponding plans were generated automatically and compared with the manual plans. The whole process including automated anatomy recognition and planning took about 6 seconds on a 2.4 GHz Linux PC.

The results were inspected visually as shown in Fig. 3, where the additional frontal view facilitates comparison of the automated and manual plans. The results reveal consistent planning of the requested segments. Furthermore, the 3rd column from the left in Fig. 3 shows the algorithm's successful extrapolation of the transverse plans to other segments.

A small in-plane rotation between the manually and automatically planned mid-sagittal views can be observed. Nevertheless, the automatically planned views have been rated as fully acceptable by a clinical expert. Note that the slight lumbar scoliosis and apparent cervical hyperlordosis were not present in the training data, which emphasizes the robustness of the method.

4   Conclusion

This paper has presented a novel method for automatically planning scan geometries in spine MRI scans. The approach makes use of automatically detected anatomical landmarks to learn and plan scan geometries for lumbar and cervical partial spine examinations. Since the number of visible vertebrae in such examinations is not known in advance, the proposed anatomy detection approach is based on analyzing locally extracted features aimed at determining the positions and orientations of intervertebral discs. The results of the validation study showed the anatomy labeling being correct in 54 out of 60 test datasets and shifted one level in the remaining 6 images. Based on a small number of training examples, automated planning showed consistent results for a clinical dataset with pathology, and in transferring plans to the areas of the spine other than those used for training. With the overall processing time of about 6 seconds, the proposed method is feasible for clinical use.

References

1. Itti, L., Chang, L., Ernst, T.: Automatic scan prescription for brain MRI. Magnetic Resonance in Medicine 45(3), 486–494 (2001)
2. Young, S., Bystrov, D., Netsch, T., Bergmans, R., van Muiswinkel, A., Visser, F., Springorum, R., Gieseke, J.: Automated planning of MRI neuro scans. In: Proc. of SPIE Medical Imaging, San Diego, CA, USA pp. 61441M–1–61441M–8 (2006)
3. Lelieveldt, R.P.F., van der Geest, R.J., Lamb, H.J., Kayser, H.W.M., Reiber, J.H.C.: Automated observer-independent acquisition of cardiac short-axis MR images: A pilot study. Radilogy 221, 537–542 (2001)
4. Jackson, C.E., Robson, M.D., Francis, J.M., Noble, J.A.: Computerized planning of the acquisition of cardiac MR images. Computerized Imaging and Graphics 28(7), 411–418 (2004)
5. Bystrov, D., Pekar, V., Young, S., Dries, S.P.M., Heese, H.S., van Muiswinkel, A.M.: Automated planning of MRI scans of knee joints. In: Proc. of SPIE Medical Imaging, San Diego, CA, USA pp. 65902Z–1–65902Z–9 (2007)
6. Peng, Z., Zhong, J., Wee, W., Lee, J.H.: Automated vertebra detection and segmentation from the whole spine MR images. In: Proc. of Engineering in Medicine and Biology, IEEE-EMBS, Shanghai, China, pp. 2527–2530 (2005)
7. Weiss, K.L., Storrs, J.M., Banto, R.B.: Automated spine survey iterative scan technique. Radiology 239(1), 255–262 (2006)
8. Vrtovec, T., Ourselin, S., Gomes, L., Likar, B., Pernus, F.: Generation of curved planar reformations from magnetic resonance images of the spine. In: Larsen, R., Nielsen, M., Sporring, J. (eds.) MICCAI 2006. LNCS, vol. 4191, pp. 135–143. Springer, Heidelberg (2006)
9. Frangi, A., Niessen, W., Hoogeveen, R., van Walsum, T., Viergever, M.: Multiscale vessel enhancement filtering. In: Wells, W., et al. (eds.) Proc. of MICCAI 1998, Cambridge, MA, USA, pp. 130–137 (1998)
10. Vardi, Y., Zhang, C.H.: The multivariate l1-median and associated data depth. Proc. National Academy of Sciences USA 97(4), 1423–1436 (2000)

Cardiac-Motion Compensated MR Imaging and Strain Analysis of Ventricular Trabeculae

Andrew W. Dowsey[1], Jennifer Keegan[2], and Guang-Zhong Yang[1]

[1] Institute of Biomedical Engineering, Imperial College London, SW7 2AZ, UK
{a.w.dowsey,g.z.yang}@imperial.ac.uk
[2] Cardiovascular Magnetic Resonance Unit, National Heart and Lung Institute,
Imperial College London, Royal Brompton and Harefield NHS Trust, SW3 6NP, UK
j.keegan@rbht.nhs.uk

Abstract. In conventional CMR, bulk cardiac motion causes target structures to move in and out of the static acquisition plane. Due to the partial volume effect, accurate localisation of subtle features through the cardiac cycle, such as the trabeculae and papillary muscles, is difficult. This problem is exacerbated by the short acquisition window necessary to avoid motion blur and ghosting, especially during early systole. This paper presents an adaptive imaging approach with COMB multi-tag tracking that follows true 3D motion of the myocardium so that the same tissue slice is imaged throughout the cine acquisition. The technique is demonstrated with motion-compensated multi-slice imaging of ventricles, which allows for tracked visualisation and analysis of the trabeculae and papillary muscles for the first time. This enables novel *in-vivo* measurement of circumferential and radial strain for trabeculation and papillary muscle contractility. These statistics will facilitate the evaluation of diseases such as mitral valve insufficiency and ischemic heart disease. The adaptive imaging technique will also have significant implications for CMR in general, including motion-compensated quantification of myocardial perfusion and blood flow, and motion-correction of sequences with long acquisition windows.

1 Introduction

Abnormality in the trabeculae carnae, a network of predominantly longitudinal muscular ridges that line the left and right ventricles, has been identified as a significant factor in a number of serious cardiomyopathies. Extensive non-compacted myocardium (isolated ventricular non-compaction) can lead to arrhythmia, thromboembolism and cardiac failure [1]. Similarly, the pathogenic replacement of trabeculae with fatty or fibrous tissue in arrythmogenic ventricular dysplasia can cause an electrical instability and is the primary cause of sudden cardiac arrest in young adults [2]. Amongst the trabeculae, at the base of both ventricles, reside the papillary muscles. The left ventricle contains two groups of papillary muscle that attach to the mitral valve leaflets through the chordae tendinae. They contract a fraction earlier in the cardiac cycle to ensure the mitral valve stays closed during systole. However, in patients with ischemic heart disease, displacement of the papillary muscles causes mitral insufficiency, both directly through ischemic dysfunction, and indirectly through dilation of

N. Ayache, S. Ourselin, A. Maeder (Eds.): MICCAI 2007, Part I, LNCS 4791, pp. 609–616, 2007.
© Springer-Verlag Berlin Heidelberg 2007

the left ventricle [3]. In basic haemodynamics, it is thought that the trabeculations reduce the turbulence of blood during systole. However, since detailed *in-vivo* measurement of trabecula and papillary muscle motion has not been possible due to their small structure and rapid systolic motion [4], the hypothesis remains unproved. Indeed, with advances in multi-detector CT, it was only discovered recently that the papillary muscles attach to the trabeculations rather than directly to the heart wall [5]. CT is now in common use for morphologic assessment of trabeculae in isolated ventricular non-compaction and arrythmogenic ventricular dysplasia. However, the required radiation dose involved limits its practical adoption. Furthermore, the temporal resolution is insufficient for accurate quantification of morphology and motion during the whole cardiac cycle.

Although recent developments in cardiovascular MR overcome many of these issues, cyclic through-plane motion causes structures to move in and out of the imaging plane, thus greatly affecting the depiction of trabecular morphology. To avoid this problem, it is necessary to adaptively track bulk movement of the heart during data acquisition so that the same structures remain localised throughout the cycle. The purpose of this paper is to present a prospective imaging scheme that tracks ventricular motion in real-time through a single breath-hold COMB multi-tag pre-scan. Our previous manually-seeded single tag tracking method [6] is extended through an objective and automatic real-time 4D multi-tag approach. This is performed whilst the subject remains in the scanner for subsequent motion-compensated multi-slice acquisition of the whole ventricle. Each *k*-space sample is corrected individually to ensure optimal motion compensation. Strain analysis of the trabeculae and papillary muscles was then quantified for the first time. Since traditional techniques such as MR tagging are too coarse to capture the fine detail and complex motion of the trabeculations [7], in this paper a method based on novel mass-invariant and bias-corrected free-form image registration of cylindrical and radial projections is presented.

2   Method

2.1   Adaptive Imaging with COMB Multi-tagging

The tagging technique implemented is an extension of that used by Kozerke *et al.* [8]. A cine gradient echo echo-planar sequence with a labelling pre-pulse (selective and non-selective 90° pulse pair) was implemented on a Siemens Avanto 1.5 Tesla scanner. With this method, the labelled images are generated by the complex subtraction of two datasets, with the phase of the selective component of the labelling pulse pair being reversed between the two. Interleaved horizontal (HLA) and vertical (VLA) long axis image planes were acquired during a single 18 cardiac cycle breath-hold, with labelling performed in the orthogonal short-axis plane. In this study, the selective 90° pre-pulse is a COMB radiofrequency pulse, which enables the simultaneous labelling of 4 parallel short axis planes (plane thickness = 7mm, plane separation = 20mm) centred in the middle of the left ventricle, as shown in Fig. 1(c-d). The parameters for the imaging sequence were as follows: slice thickness = 15mm, field of view = 400×260mm, matrix size = 128×71, echo-planar readout factor = 8 and temporal resolution (per interleaved cine pair) = 55ms.

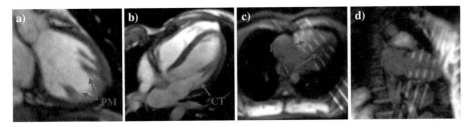

Fig. 1. (a) Mid-diastolic oblique view through the left ventricular papillary muscles (PM). (b) Perpendicular oblique view through lateral muscle showing connection of mitral valve to heads by chordae tendineae (CT). (c) Horizontal Long Axis (HLA) view showing 4 short-axis COMB tags through the left (LV) and right (RV) ventricles. (d) Perpendicular Vertical Long Axis (VLA) view showing the COMB tags placed through the left ventricle. (c) and (d) illustrate a systolic HLA/VLA pair in a single breath-hold COMB acquisition before complex subtraction.

In previous work, motion of a single COMB tag was tracked on HLA and VLA views using multi-resolution image registration with a hierarchical piece-wise bilinear transformation and BFGS optimization of the cross-correlation [6]. A single manual delineation on each of the two views was automatically propagated to the rest of the cardiac cycle, with the orthogonal distance regression plane calculated from the result.

To extend the tracking to multiple tagging of the whole ventricle, the regression plane was computed for each tag separately and Catmull-Rom interpolation used to derive the slice position and orientation for any slice offset between them. To delineate the tag objectively, a multi-resolution search was initiated along the tracked tag centerline in the set of acquired images, outwards from the tag centre, with the known tag location immediately after the ECG R-wave used as reference geometry. Gradient descent was used to minimize the sum of squared differences between the maximum observed intensity and the intensity of the tracked point through the cardiac cycle.

The result of the tracking is a list of the estimated sagittal, coronal and transverse components of the position and normal vectors of the COMB tags at all points in the cardiac cycle. A shared-phase cine TrueFISP sequence was adapted to read this output and to modify the orientation and offset (both through-plane and in-plane) for each k-space acquisition accordingly. Moving-slice breath-hold cine acquisitions were performed with a 300×300mm field of view (spatial resolution: 1.2×1.2mm) and a 6mm slice thickness. Twenty k-space samples (taking 60ms) were acquired per cardiac phase, with view-sharing enabling the reconstruction of data at 30ms intervals.

2.2 *In-vivo* Trabecular Strain Analysis

With slice-tracked coverage of the heart, it is now possible to visualize and quantify trabeculae and papillary muscle motion over the whole cardiac cycle. Furthermore, when the slices are arranged and visualised as a 4D volume, bulk cardiac motion is frozen. However, for accurate motion quantification in this coordinate space, it is essential to ensure mass conservation with the world coordinate space. Isotrophic mass-conserved volumes were derived by taking each longitudinal stack of voxels and deriving the change in sampling rate in world coordinates through the stack:

$$I = \left| \det\left(\beta'_x, \beta'_y, \beta'_z \right) \right| \beta_i \tag{1}$$

where $(\beta_x, \beta_y, \beta_z)$ is a uniform cubic B-spline curve fitted [9] to the world coordinates of each longitudinal stack of voxels, and β_i is a uniform cubic B-spline curve fitted to the intensity values. $I(z)$ therefore provides cubic B-spline interpolation weighted by the change in sampling rate at point z. The epicardial border and papillary muscles were then delineated with piecewise Catmull-Rom contours and the trabeculae segmented from the blood pool using a Gaussian Mixture Model (GMM) with expectation-maximization. Each output slice was then transformed into a one dimensional vector by summation of the densities along in-plane radial lines projected from the centre of the ventricle, so that each volume became a cylindrical manifold of radial density parameterised by in-plane angle and longitudinal slice location.

Circumferential motion could then be derived between volumes by performing free-form image registration [10] on the cylindrical manifolds generated in the previous step. To provide a realistic C2 continuous deformation field, a Haar multi-resolution pyramid and hierarchical uniform cubic B-spline tensor-product transformation model, periodic in the circumferential dimension, was employed, as previously demonstrated for smooth-wall myocardial strain analysis by MR tagging [7]. To avoid convergence to local optima, global motion was first derived using a single B-spline patch on heavily sub-sampled images (16×16 pixels). The B-spline patch was then iteratively sub-divided 5 times and the resolution increased so that motion was derived at different scales up to 16×16 B-spline patches on 512×512 pixel images.

Surface receiver coil signal intensity variations contaminate the MR images with a multiplicative bias-field. The bias-field affects the computation of the GMM, and therefore myocardial mass. An additive bias-field can also be observed due to errors in epicardial delineation regionally over or under-estimating radial density. Since the bias-fields are regionally continuous, in this study they are modelled as hierarchal tensor-product B-spline surfaces, which are optimized concurrently with the transformation model using the same multi-resolution schedule. The complete sampling function for the source image is therefore:

$$W_{s,C} = \left| \det\left(\beta'_\theta, \beta'_Z \right) \right| \cdot \left(I_s\left(\beta_\theta, \beta_Z \right) + \beta_V \right) \cdot e^{\beta_U} \tag{2}$$

where image I_s is under geometric transformation (β_θ, β_Z), multiplicative bias-field correction β_U, and additive bias-field correction β_V. Tissue incompressibility is preserved by weighting the deformed density projection by its change in volume $|\det(\beta'_\theta, \beta'_Z)|$. The total set of parameters for optimization is therefore $C=\{\theta, Z, U, V\}$. Since we deal with intensity correspondence between images explicitly with bias-field modeling, the similarity measure that drives the registration can be the sum of squared differences, defined as: $\text{sim}\left(W_{s,C}, I_r \right) = \sum_{(x,y) \in I_r} \left(W_{s,C}\left(x, y \right) - I_r\left(x, y \right) \right)^2$. For fast convergence with the quasi-Newtonian limited-memory BFGS optimizer [11], the first partial derivatives of the similarity measure with respect to the transformation parameters were derived in closed form, where each pixel $\mathbf{p}$ in the reference image I_r is compared to its corresponding pixel in the deformed sample image $W_{s,C}$:

$$\frac{\partial}{\partial \mathbf{C}} sim\left(W_{s,C}, I_r\right) = 2\sum_{\mathbf{p}\in I_r}\left[\left(W_{s,\mathbf{C}}\left(\mathbf{p}\right) - I_r\left(\mathbf{p}\right)\right)\cdot\frac{\partial W_{s,\mathbf{C}}\left(\mathbf{p}\right)}{\partial \mathbf{C}}\right] \tag{3}$$

Relative circumferential strain is then computed as the partial derivatives of β_θ in the derived transformation mesh.

Similarly, relative radial strain was computed by analysis of circumferential density projections, where density along in-plane concentric circles was summed to generate a manifold parameterised by in-plane radius and longitudinal slice location.

3 Results

Fig. 2 illustrates the effect of the adaptive slice-tracking in localization of the trabeculations. Motion-tracked left ventricles were acquired for 5 subjects and the right ventricle for one subject (ages 23 to 28, 1 female, 4 male), with an average study time of 50 minutes. 17 to 25 motion-tracked slices, spaced initially at 5mm intervals, were acquired for each dataset depending on ventricle length, resulting in full coverage.

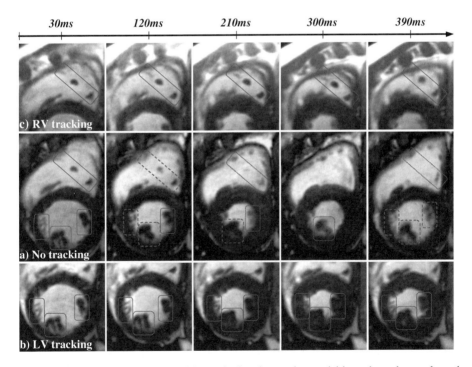

Fig. 2. Static and motion-tracked mid-ventricular short axis acquisitions through systole and early diastole for one of the subjects studied. (a) Conventional MR acquisition with a static imaging plane. The red boxes show localised trabeculae and papillary muscles that then start exhibiting motion blurring (dashed boxes) and begin to move out of the imaging plane (dotted boxes). With adaptive slice-tracking of the (b) left and (c) right ventricles, the trabeculae remain localized throughout the cardiac cycle.

Table 1. Mean, standard deviation and maximum error of slice position and orientation accuracy between an automatic and a manual tracking (*A vs M*), and two manual trackings (*M vs M*), for the left ventricle in 5 subjects and right ventricle (RV) in 1 subject

Data-set	Total Tags	Mis-tracked	*mean/stdev/max position error*		*mean/stdev/max orientation error*	
			A vs M (mm)	*M vs M (mm)*	*A vs M (°)*	*M vs M (°)*
1	88	2	0.68/0.37/2.28	0.94/0.60/3.10	1.38/0.77/4.08	1.45/0.78/3.62
2	96	0	1.03/0.44/2.13	0.86/0.35/1.74	1.39/0.56/3.41	1.50/0.79/3.69
3	88	1	0.58/0.26/1.38	0.63/0.31/1.56	1.30/0.83/3.44	1.66/0.85/3.85
4	80	0	0.93/0.45/3.23	0.94/0.52/2.80	1.85/0.96/4.95	1.88/0.94/4.56
5LV	88	3	0.93/0.45/2.74	0.88/0.72/2.95	1.33/0.74/3.82	1.80/0.88/3.82
5RV	88	11	1.78/1.34/8.94	2.22/1.77/8.27	2.73/1.66/6.95	2.78/1.99/8.48

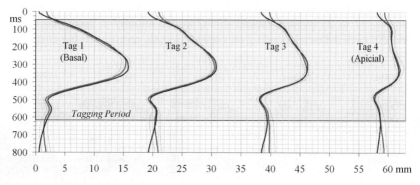

Fig. 3. Through-plane component of the centre of 4 moving slices through the cardiac cycle, derived from 4 left ventricular COMB tags imaged during the period shaded in turquoise. Two standard deviations from the mean of 10 expert manual delineations are shown in red. The automatic approach, including motion-correction for the known tag geometry immediately after the R-wave, is shown in blue.

For motion tracking, since the subject must remain static in the scanner during processing, real-time execution is necessary; the automatic approach takes 30 seconds including verification, as compared mean manual processing of 309 seconds. Validation of the tracking on the 6 datasets is presented in Table 1 and Fig. 3. Table 1 shows that slice position and orientation errors between the proposed automatic tracking and an expert manual delineation are equivalent. The right ventricle was more difficult to track due to the thinner wall and tagged blood remaining in the field of view. The relationship was then analysed further on one left ventricle dataset by obtaining manual delineations from 10 experts, and comparing the normal distribution (confirmed by Shapiro-Wilk tests) of position and orientation motion against the automatic approach. Fig. 3 illustrates tracked long-axis motion of the 4 tags. The automatic approach remained within the 95.5% confidence interval of the manual approach in 98.2% of samples. Variance in manual delineation increases at early systole and end diastole due to the issues of tagged blood and tag fade respectively. Furthermore, since the tags are only imaged after 40ms due to initialisation of the COMB pre-pulse, and before 620ms due to tag fade, motion interpolation is required for the other phases. It can be seen in the automatic approach that incorporating the known starting tag location at 2.5ms significantly aids tracking outside the tagging period.

An example cylindrical density projection with frozen bulk motion is shown in Fig. 4(b). It can be seen that from 420ms onwards, the papillary muscles rotates and shortens relative to the ventricle, as previously observed by invasive means [3]. Circumferential and radial components of the strain (Fig 4(b-c)) were then quantified with the proposed method and the derived strain maps reprojected onto the original volume (Fig. 4(a)). As expected, the radial strain of the myocardium can be seen compressing during systole and expanding during diastole. The circumferential strain is less deterministic, but more pronounced during diastolic relaxation of the muscle, as the trabeculations appear to swirl due to vortices in the filling blood pool. Note that the strain accuracy is affected by the partial volume effect caused by the 6mm slice thickness. This issue can be resolved through the use of super-resolution, but will require extension of our previous work [6] since the motion-tracked slices are no longer coplanar.

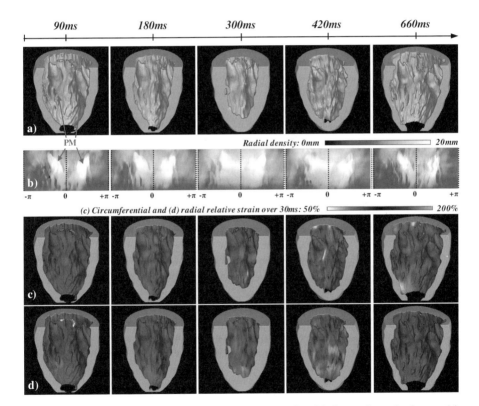

Fig. 4. Views of the left ventricle through the cardiac cycle with frozen through-plane and in-plane motion. (a) Volume rendering showing detailed trabeculations and papillary muscles (PM). (b) Unwrapped cylindrical density projection of the volume, with radial angle as *x*-axis and longitudinal depth as *y*-axis. Derived circumferential (c) and radial (d) relative strain of the myocardium, where 50% represents compression to half previous size over the last 30ms, and 200% is expansion by double. The scale is logarithmic *i.e.* black represents no strain (100%).

4 Conclusions

In this paper we have demonstrated a novel motion-tracked prospective imaging technique for revealing detailed ventricular trabeculation throughout the cardiac cycle. This is the first time that the motion of the trabeculae and papillary muscles are visualised and quantified in CMR. The morphologic and functional quantification achieved in this study will enhance our understanding and evaluation of cardiac diseases such as regional ischemia, isolated ventricular non-compaction, arrythmogenic ventricular dysplasia, and mitral insufficiency. Furthermore, the morphological structure revealed in this study will allow CFD analysis for elucidating the haemodynamic role of the trabeculations. The proposed multi-slice adaptive imaging technique will also have significant implications for CMR sequence design, including motion-compensated measurements of flow and myocardial perfusion, which are particularly sensitive to bulk cardiac motion. Furthermore, it is hoped that imaging sequences requiring long acquisition windows *e.g.* for small structures such as the coronary arteries, or T1 relaxation imaging, can now be utilized at any point in the cardiac cycle.

References

1. Petersen, S.E., Selvanayagram, J.B., Wiesmann, F., Robson, M.D., Francis, J.M., Anderson, R.H., Watkins, H., Neubauer, S.: Left Ventricular Non-Compaction. J. Am. Coll. Card 46, 101–105 (2005)
2. Kiumura, F., Sakai, F., Sakomura, Y., Fujimura, M., Ueno, E., Matsuda, N., Kasanuki, H., Mitsuhasi, N.: Helical CT Features of Arrhythmogenic Right Ventricular Cardiomyopathy. Radiographics 22, 1111–1124 (2002)
3. Levine, R.A., Vlahakes, G.J., Lefebvre, X., Guerrero, L., Cape, E.G., Yoganathan, A.P., Weyman, A.E.: Papillary Muscle Displacement Causes Systolic Anterior Motion of the Mitral Valve. Circulation 91, 1189–1195 (1995)
4. Karwatowski, S.P., Mohiaddin, R., Yang, G.-Z., Firmin, D.N, Sutton, M.S., Underwood, S.R., Longmore, D.B.: Assessment of regional left ventricular long-axis motion with MR velocity mapping in healthy subjects. J. Magn. Reson. Imaging 4, 151–155 (1994)
5. Axel, L.: Papillary Muscles Do Not Attach Directly to the Solid Heart Wall. Circulation 109, 3145–3148 (2004)
6. Dowsey, A.W., Lerotic, M., Keegan, J., Thom, S., Firmin, D., Yang, G.-Z.: Motion-Compensated MR Valve Imaging with COMB Tag Tracking and Super-Resolution Enhancement. In: Larsen, R., Nielsen, M., Sporring, J. (eds.) MICCAI 2006. LNCS, vol. 4191, pp. 364–371. Springer, Heidelberg (2006)
7. Tustison, N., Amini, A.A.: Biventricular Myocardial Strains via Non-Rigid Registration of Anatomical NURBS Models. IEEE Trans. Med. Imag. 25, 94–112 (2006)
8. Kozerke, S., Scheidegger, M.B., Pedersen, E.M., Boesiger, P.: Heart motion adapted cine phase-contrast flow measurements through the aortic valve. Magn. Reson. Med. 42, 970–978 (1999)
9. Thévenaz, P., Blu, T., Unser, M.: Interpolation Revisited. IEEE Trans. Med. Imag. 19, 739–758 (2000)
10. Dowsey, A.W., English, J., Pennington, K., Cotter, D., Stuehler, K., Marcus, K., Meyer, H.E., Dunn, M.J., Yang, G.-Z.: Examination of 2-DE in the Human Proteome Organisation Brain Proteome Project pilot studies with the new RAIN gel matching technique. Proteomics 6, 5030–5047 (2006)
11. Nocedal, J.: Updating quasi-Newton matrices with limited storage. Math. Comp. 35, 773–782 (1980)

High Throughput Analysis of Breast Cancer Specimens on the Grid

Lin Yang[1,2], Wenjin Chen[2], Peter Meer[1], Gratian Salaru[2],
Michael D. Feldman[3], and David J. Foran[2]

[1] Dept. of Electrical and Computer Eng., Rutgers Univ., Piscataway, NJ, 08544, USA
[2] Center of Biomedical Imaging and Informatics, The Cancer Institute of New Jersey,
UMDNJ-Robert Wood Johnson Medical School, Piscataway, NJ, 08854, USA
[3] Dept. of Surgical Pathology, Univ. of Pennsylvania, Philadelphia, PA, 19104, USA

Abstract. Breast cancer accounts for about 30% of all cancers and 15% of all cancer deaths in women in the United States. Advances in computer assisted diagnosis (CAD) holds promise for early detecting and staging disease progression. In this paper we introduce a Grid-enabled CAD to perform automatic analysis of imaged histopathology breast tissue specimens. More than 100,000 digitized samples (1200 × 1200 pixels) have already been processed on the Grid. We have analyzed results for 3744 breast tissue samples, which were originated from four different institutions using diaminobenzidine (DAB) and hematoxylin staining. Both linear and nonlinear dimension reduction techniques are compared, and the best one (ISOMAP) was applied to reduce the dimensionality of the features. The experimental results show that the Gentle Boosting using an eight node CART decision tree as the weak learner provides the best result for classification. The algorithm has an accuracy of 86.02% using only 20% of the specimens as the training set.

1 Introduction

Breast cancer is a malignant neoplasm that can affect both women and men. It is the leading cancer in both white and African American women, with more than 178,480 new cases for an estimated to be diagnosed in 2007 where 2030 cases are men, and will be responsible for estimated 40,460 deaths [1]. It is the second most common cause of cancer death in white, black, Asian/Pacific Islander and American Indian/Alaska Native women [1,2]. The incidence of breast cancer among women has increased gradually from one in 20 in 1960 to one in eight today. At this time there are slightly over 2 million breast cancer survivors in the United States. Women living in North America have the highest rate of breast cancer in the world [1].

In spite of the increase in the incidence of the disease, the death rates of breast cancer continue to decline. This decrease is believed to be the result of earlier detection through screening and analysis as well as improved treatment [1]. Some of the common methods screening of breast cancer include examination by a physician, self-performed routine examinations and routine mammograms. When suspicious lesions are detected by these methods, a fine needle aspirate or

N. Ayache, S. Ourselin, A. Maeder (Eds.): MICCAI 2007, Part I, LNCS 4791, pp. 617–625, 2007.
© Springer-Verlag Berlin Heidelberg 2007

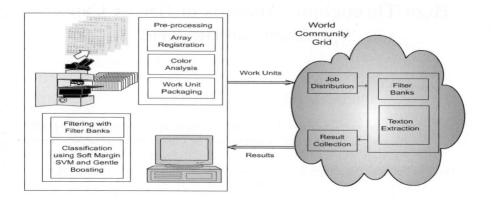

Fig. 1. The work-flow and logical units of the Grid-enabled tissue microarray

biopsy can be performed and the obtained tissue is examined [3]. The extracted tissue is mounted on glass slides and examined by a surgical pathologist to make decision of benign or cancer. Diaminobenzidine (DAB) and hematoxylin are standard staining methods used for breast cancer.

There has been increasing interest in investigating computer assisted diagnosis (CAD) system to help breast cancer diagnosis, e.g. [4]. However, to our knowledge, most of these studies were relatively limited in scale because the computation is often a bottleneck. In this paper, we report a Grid-enabled framework for analyzing imaged breast tissue specimens. We discriminate between benign and cancer breast tissues using the results obtained from the Grid. Without using the Grid, the filtering and generation of universal texture library would require 210 days of computation for 3744 samples because of the large image size and computational complexity of the process.

2   Grid Enabled Tissue Microarray and Features

Tissue Microarray (TMA) technology, e.g. [5], provides a platform to perform comparative cancer studies involving evaluation of protein expression. Several commercial products have been developed to automate the process of digitizing TMA specimens, e.g. T2 scanner, Aperio Technologies and MedMicro, Trestle Corporation. With the recent advance of the Grid technology [6,7], by now we can address the computational complexity of large-scale collaborative applications by leveraging aggregated bandwidth, computational power and secondary storage resources distributed across multiple sites. IBM has offered their World Community Grid to help research projects which require high levels of computation. Our Grid-enabled system was launched on the IBM World Community Grid in July, 2006. The work-flow and logical units are shown in Figure 1.

Textons are defined as repetitive local features that humans perceive as being discriminative between textures. We used the 49×49 LM filter bank [8] composed of 48 filters: eight LOG filter responses with $\sigma = 1, \sqrt{2}, 2, 2\sqrt{2}, 3, 3\sqrt{2}, 6, 6\sqrt{2}$, four Gaussian filtering responses with $\sigma = 1, \sqrt{2}, 2, 2\sqrt{2}$ and the bar and edge filtering response within six different directions, $\theta = 0, \pi/6, \pi/3, \pi/2, 2\pi/3, 5\pi/6$, $\sigma = 1, \sqrt{2}, 2$. All the σ-s are in pixel size. While textons are used to describe the appearance of breast cancer images, they are not specific for our applications.

The image filtering responses obtained from the Grid were collected together, and clustered using K-means, $K = 4000$ to capture a large enough code book. The texton library was constructed from the cluster centers. The appearance of each breast tissue image was modeled by a compact quantized description - texton histogram, where each pixel is assigned to its closest texton using

$$h(i) = \sum_{j \in I} count(T(j) = i) \tag{1}$$

and I denotes breast tissue image, i is the i-th element of the texton dictionary, $T(j)$ returns the texton assigned to pixel j. In this way, each breast tissue image is mapped to a point in the high dimension space R^d, where d is equal to the number of textons. Figure 2 shows the texton histograms of two imaged breast tissue specimens, one benign (top-left) and one cancer (bottom-left).

3   Dimension Reduction and Classification

Each breast cancer image is represented by a vector in the $d = 4000$ dimension space in which we have to consider the "curse of dimensionality". Traditionally, linear dimension reduction methods like multidimensional scaling (MDS) and principle component analysis (PCA) [9] have been used, which assume that the data can be represented by a lower dimensional linear subspace. In other cases, the data can be modeled by a low-dimensional nonlinear manifold, and nonlinear methods such as locally linear embedding (LLE) [10], isometric feature mapping (ISOMAP) [11] and local tangent space alignment (LTSA) [12] are more appropriate.

3.1   Dimension Reduction

Given a set of feature vector $Z = \{z_1, ...z_i, ..., z_n\}$ where $z_i \in R^d$. There exists a mapping T which can represent z_i in the low dimension as

$$z_i = T(x_i) + u_i \quad i = 1, 2, ..., n \tag{2}$$

where $u_i \in R^d$ is the sampling noise and $x_i \in R^{d'}$ denotes the representation of z_i in low-dimensional space.

PCA finds the mapping T which best represents the variance of data z_i in the original high-dimensional space. The low-dimensional space $R^{d'}$ is spanned by the d' largest eigenvectors of the covariance matrix of z_i. MDS finds the mapping T which preserves the pairwise distances between z_i-s in $R^{d'}$. If the data have certain geometric structure which can be modeled as a low-dimensional linear manifold, they are not expected to perform well.

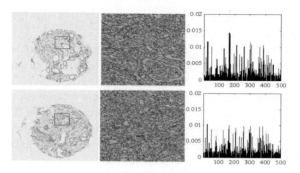

Fig. 2. Two breast tissue images on the left, benign (on the top) cancer (on the bottom). In order to keep the figure readable, only the texton maps of red rectangle regions were shown in the middle with different colors representing different textons. In practice the texton histograms of full images, shown on the right, were used for classification.

Although most of the geometric distances can not be used directly on the manifold, linear dimension reduction methods can be applied locally and Euclidean distances are valid on the local tangent space. The LLE preserves the geometry of the data points by representing points using their local neighbors. The ISOMAP approach applies a linear MDS on the local patch, but aim to preserve the geometric distance globally using the shortest path in the graph. The LTSA method maps each data point from the original space into the tangent space and align it to give a global coordinate.

If the data are approximately sampled from a low-dimensional manifold, the nonlinear methods generally perform better [10]. Otherwise the linear methods may be preferred because of their simplicity. In order to compare the performance of these methods, we used cross-validation (CV)

$$CV(\gamma) = \frac{1}{N} \sum_{i=1}^{N} \left| y_i - f^{-k(i)}(x_i, \gamma) \right| \tag{3}$$

where x_i is the feature vector in $R^{d'}$, $y_i = \{+1, -1\}$ represents the cancer and benign breast tissue labels. The $f^{-k}(x_i, \gamma)$ denotes the classification results using the γ-th dimension reduction method with the k-th part removed from the training data, and the number of partitioning $k = 5$ in our experiments. We tested the five different algorithms from 3 to 4000 dimensions and determined that ISOMAP is better (Figure 3). Good performance using ISOMAP was also reported in [13] for tissue characterization. Based upon these comparative results, ISOMAP with 500 dimensions are used for all subsequent operations.

3.2   Classification

In [14], KNN and $C4.5$ decision tree were integrated into a Bayesian classifier which provided good results for characterizing breast tissues. In [15], a cascade boosting classifier is used to detect prostate cancers. In our case, each breast

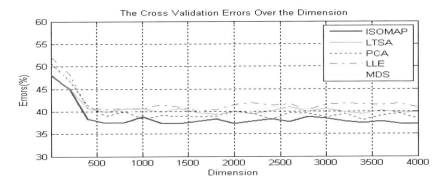

Fig. 3. The five different dimension reduction algorithms shown as five-fold cross-validation errors for different reduced dimensions

---

Input: Given n features $x_i \in R^{d'}$ and their corresponding labels $y_i = \{-1, 1\}$.

Training:

- Pick up 100 random pairs. Compute

  $\tau = \frac{1}{100} \sum_{i,j=1}^{100} \chi^2(x_i, x_j)$ where $\chi^2(x_i, x_j) = \frac{1}{2} \sum_{l=1}^{500} \frac{(x_i(l) - x_j(l))^2}{x_i(l) + x_j(l)}$.

- Build the Mercer kernel $\kappa(x_i, x_j) = \exp(-\frac{1}{\tau}\chi^2(x_i, x_j))$.
- Select the penalty parameter C and train the soft margin $SVM(\kappa, C)$. Record the model parameters.

Testing:

- Output the classification: $sign[SVM(x)] = sign\left[\sum_i y_i \alpha_i \kappa(x, x_i) + b\right]$

  where α_i and b are the learned weights and learned threshold.

Alg. 1. Soft Margin SVM using the Mercer kernel based on χ^2 distance

tissue image is represented by a feature vector in the reduced subspace $x_i \in R^{d'}$, where $d' = 500$. The maximum margin classifiers such as Support Vector Machine (SVM) [16] and Boosting [17] are more appropriate, especially when the number of training vectors are comparable with their dimensions.

Soft Margin Support Vector Machine. Because the training data are not linearly separable, we choose the Soft Margin SVM which allows training vectors to be on the wrong side of the support vector classifier with certain penalty. We use a nonlinear Mercer kernel [18] based on χ^2 distance. The detailed description is given in Algorithm 1.

The key parameters which affect the accuracy of soft margin SVM are the penalty and the kernel. The penalty parameter C can be selected according to cross validation (CV) errors. For the kernel selection, we tested linear, polynomial, Gaussian and the proposed Mercer kernel based on χ^2 distance, where the last one outperformed all the others.

Gentle Boosting on the Decision Tree. Boosting is one of the most important recent developments in machine learning. It works by sequentially applying

Input: Given n features $x_i \in R^{d'}$ and their corresponding labels $y_i = \{-1, 1\}$.
Training:
- Initialize the weights $w_i = 1/n, i = 1, ..., n$. Set $b(x) = 0$ and the number of nodes $M = 8$ in the CART decision tree.
- For $j = 1...J$
  - Each training sample is assigned its weight w_i. The weighted tree growing algorithm is applied to build the CART decision tree $T_j(x, M)$.
  - Update using $b(x) = b(x) + T_j(x, M)$.
  - Update the weights $w_i = w_i e^{-y_i T_j(x, M)}$ and renormalize w_i.
  - Save the j-th CART decision tree $T_j(x, M)$.
Testing:
- Output the classification: $sign\,[b(x)] = sign\left[\sum_{j=1}^{J} T_j(x, M)\right]$.

Alg. 2. Gentle Boosting using an eight nodes Classification And Regression Tree (CART) decision tree as weak learner

a classification algorithm on a reweighted version of the training data and the final label is decided by a weighted voting. Instead of using the most well-know Adaboost [17] with a simple linear classifier, as the weak classifier, we propose to apply Gentle Boosting [19] using an eight node CART decision tree as the weak learner, which experimentally provided higher accuracy than Adaboost. The detailed algorithm is provided in Algorithm 2.

The number of nodes of the CART decision tree can be selected using cross validation (CV). In our experiments, using eight nodes CART decision tree as weak learner provided the best results. The number of iterations J was chosen as 40 to achieve satisfactory accuracy and avoid overfitting as well.

4   Experiments

The tissue microarrays used in our experiments are prepared by different institutes: the Cancer Institute of New Jersey, Yale University, University of Pennsylvania and Imgenex Corporation, San Diego, CA. To date over 300 immunostained microscopic specimens, each containing hundreds of tissue image, were digitized at 40× volume scan using the Trestle MedMicro, a whole slide scanner system. The output images typically contain a few billions of pixels and are stored as a compressed tiled TIFF file sized at about two gigabytes. The registration protocol proposed by [20] was applied to automatically identify the rows and columns of the tissue arrays. Staining maps of the two dyes, diaminobenzidine (DAB) and hematoxylin, were generated from specimens and each of the two staining maps as well as the luminance of the original color image were submitted to the IBM World Community Grid for batch processing.

We have analyzed 3744 breast cancer tissues (674 hematoxylin and 3070 DAB staining) from the 100,000 images processed on the Grid. Without the Grid, it would require about 210 days of computation to generate the texton library even with an efficient C++ implementation on a PC with P3 1.5GHz processor and

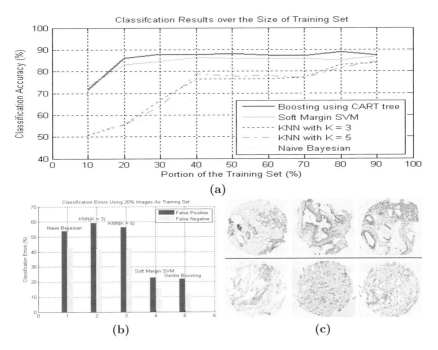

Fig. 4. The classification results. (a) Accuracy as the function of the size of training set using Gentle Boosting, Soft Margin SVM, KNN with $K = 3$ or 5 and naive Bayesian. (b) The false positive and false negative errors using 20% images as training set. (c) Some misclassified samples. The upper row is false positive and lower row is false negative.

1G RAM. However, we can build this universal texton library in less than 40 minutes in the largely distributed computing system [6].

The labels of all breast tissues from the hospitals and institutions are independently confirmed by certificated surgical pathologists. The dataset used in these experiments consisted of 611 benign and 3133 cancer samples. Each of the five algorithms was applied 10 times, using different parts of the training images drawn by random sampling. Figure 4 shows the average classification results. Because there were more positive samples than the negative samples, we obtained higher false positive errors but lower false negative errors (Figure 4b) than the average error (Figure 4a). It is clear that Gentle Boosting and Soft Margin SVM performed better, especially when the training set is small. The overall best one is the Gentle Boosting using an eight node CART decision tree as the weak learner, in which case the classification accuracy is 86.16% using only 20% of the dataset for training.

5   Conclusion

We have presented a Grid-enabled framework using texture features to perform high throughput analysis of imaged breast cancer specimens. A Gentle Boosting using an eight node CART decision tree as the weak learner provided the best results. In our experiments Atypical Duct Hyperplasia (ADH) gave highest false positive rates. In the future, we plan to subclassify the stages of breast cancer progression using the universal texton library, which were generated from the clustering results returned from the IBM World Community Grid.

Acknowledgements

This research was funded, in part, by grants from the NIH through contract 5R01LM007455-03 from the National Library of Medicine and 5R01EB003587-02 from the National Institute of Biomedical Imaging and Bioengineering. We would like to thank IBM's World Community Grid support team and our collaborators at The Cancer Institute of New Jersey and University of Pennsylvania.

References

1. American Cancer Society: Cancer Facts and Figures 2007. 2007 edn. American Cancer Society (2007)
2. U. S. Cancer Statistics Working Group: United states cancer statistics: 2003 incidence and mortality (preliminary data). National Vital Statistics 53(5) (2004)
3. Rosai, J.: Rosai and Ackerman's Surgical Pathology. 9th edn. Mosby (2004)
4. Suri, J.S., Rangayyan, R.M.: Recent Advances in Breast Imaging, Mammography, and Computer-Aided Diagnosis of Breast Cancer. 1st edn. SPIE (2006)
5. Hoos, A., Cordon-Cardo, C.: Tissue microarray profiling of cancer specimens and cell lines: Opportunities and limitations. Mod. Pathol. 81(10), 1331–1338 (2001)
6. Berman, F., Fox, G., Hey, A.J.G.: Grid Computing: Making the Global Infrastructure a Reality, 1st edn. Wiley, Chichester (2003)
7. Egan, G.F., Liu, W., Soh, W.S., Hang, D.: Australian neuroinformatics research - grid computing and e-research. ICNC 1, 1057–1064 (2005)
8. Leung, T., Malik, J.: Representing and recognizing the visual appearance of materials using three-dimensional textons. IJCV 43(1), 29–44 (2001)
9. Duda, R.O., Hart, P.E., Stork, D.G.: Pattern Classification. Wiley, Chichester (2000)
10. Rowels, S.T., Saul, L.K.: Nonlinear dimensionality reduction by locally linear embedding. Science 290(5500), 2323–2326 (2000)
11. Tenebaum, J., de Silva, V., Langford, J.: A global geometric framework for nonlinear dimensionality reduction. Science 290(5500), 2319–2323 (2000)
12. Zha, H., Zhang, Z.: Principal manifolds and nonlinear dimensionality reduction via tangent space alignment. SIAM J. on Sci. Comp. 26(1), 313–338 (2004)
13. Lekadir, K., Elson, D.S., Requejo-Isidro, J., Dunsby, C., McGinty, J., Galletly, N., Stamp, G., French, P.M., Yang, G.Z.: Tissue characterization using dimensionality reduction and fluorescence imaging. In: Larsen, R., Nielsen, M., Sporring, J. (eds.) MICCAI 2006. LNCS, vol. 4191, pp. 586–593. Springer, Heidelberg (2006)
14. Oliver, A., Freixenet, J., Marti, R., Zwiggelaar, R.: A comparison of breast tissue classification techniques. In: Larsen, R., Nielsen, M., Sporring, J. (eds.) MICCAI 2006. LNCS, vol. 4191, pp. 872–879. Springer, Heidelberg (2006)

15. Doyle, S., Madabhushi, A., Feldman, M., Tomaszeweski, J.: A boosting cascade for automated detection of prostate cancer from digitized histology. In: Larsen, R., Nielsen, M., Sporring, J. (eds.) MICCAI 2006. LNCS, vol. 4191, pp. 504–511. Springer, Heidelberg (2006)
16. Cortes, C., Vapnik, V.: Support vector networks. Mach. Learn. 20, 1–25 (1995)
17. Freund, Y., Schapire, R.E.: A decision-theoretic generalization of online learning and an application to boosting. J. Comp. and Sys. Sci. 55(1), 119–139 (1997)
18. Shawe-Taylor, J., Cristianini, N.: Kernel Mathods for Pattern Analysis, 1st edn. Cambridge University Press, Cambridge (2004)
19. Freund, Y., Schapire, R.E.: Experiments with a new boosting algorithm. Machine Learning, 148–156 (1996)
20. Chen, W., Reiss, M., Foran, D.J.: Unsupervised tissue microarray analysis for cancer research and diagnosis. IEEE Trans. Info. Tech. on Bio. 8(2), 89–96 (2004)

Thoracic CT-PET Registration Using a 3D Breathing Model

Antonio Moreno[1], Sylvie Chambon[1], Anand P. Santhanam[2,3],
Roberta Brocardo[1], Patrick Kupelian[3], Jannick P. Rolland[2], Elsa Angelini[1],
and Isabelle Bloch[1]

[1] Ecole Nationale Supérieure des Télécommunications (GET - Télécom Paris),
CNRS UMR 5141 LTCI - Signal and Image Processing Department, Paris, France
[2] Optical Diagnostics and Applications Laboratory, University of Central Florida,
USA
[3] Department of Radiation Oncology, MD Anderson Cancer Center Orlando, USA

Abstract. In the context of thoracic CT-PET volume registration, we
present a novel method to incorporate a breathing model in a non-linear
registration procedure, guaranteeing physiologically plausible deformations. The approach also accounts for the rigid motions of lung tumors
during breathing. We performed a set of registration experiments on one
healthy and four pathological data sets. Initial results demonstrate the
interest of this method to significantly improve the accuracy of multi-
modal volume registration for diagnosis and radiotherapy applications.

1 Introduction

Registration of multimodal medical images is a widely addressed topic in many
different domains, in particular for oncology and radiotherapy applications. We
consider Computed Tomography (CT) and Positron Emission Tomography
(PET) in thoracic regions, which provide complementary information about the
anatomy and the metabolism of the human body (Fig. 1). Their registration
has a significant impact on improving medical decisions for diagnosis and therapy [1,2,3]. Linear registration is not sufficient to cope with local deformations
produced by respiration. Even with combined PET/CT scanners which avoid
differences in patient orientation and provide linearly registered images, non-
linear registration remains necessary to compensate for cardiac and respiratory
motions [4].

Most of the existing non-linear registration methods are based on image information and do not take into account any knowledge of the physiology of
the human body. Landmark-based registration techniques do take physiology
into account by forcing homologous points to match. In this direction, several
breathing models were built for medical visualization, for correcting artefacts
in images or for estimating lung motion for radiotherapy applications, but few
papers exploit such models in a registration process (Section 2).

In this paper, we propose to integrate a physiologically driven breathing model
into a 3D non-linear registration (Sections 3 and 4). The registration problem is
defined between two CT volumes and one PET volume (Fig. 1).

N. Ayache, S. Ourselin, A. Maeder (Eds.): MICCAI 2007, Part I, LNCS 4791, pp. 626–633, 2007.
© Springer-Verlag Berlin Heidelberg 2007

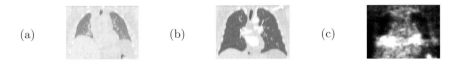

(a)   (b)   (c)

Fig. 1. CT images (a,b) corresponding to two different instants of the breathing cycle and PET image (c) of the same patient (coronal views)

2   Breathing Models

Breathing Models and Thoracic Imaging Registration – Currently, respiration-gated radiotherapies are being developed to improve the efficiency of radiations of lung or abdominal tumors [5]. Three techniques have been proposed so far: (i) *active techniques* controling the patient's breathing (airflow is blocked); (ii) *passive or empirical techniques* using external measurements in order to adapt radiation protocols to the tumor's motion [6,7,8]; (iii) *model-based techniques* employing a breathing model to evaluate lungs deformations during the breathing cycle [9]. Different bio-mathematical representations of the human respiratory mechanics have been developed [10]. Among *Mathematical tools*, the most popular technique is based on Non-Uniform Rational B-Spline (NURBS), surfaces which are bidirectional parametric representations of an object. In [11], NURBS surfaces were used to correct for respiratory artifacts of SPECT images, building NCAT (NURBS-based cardiac-torso) model. A multi-resolution registration approach for 4D Magnetic Resonance Imaging (MRI) was proposed in [12] with NCAT. In [13], a 4D NCAT phantom and an original CT image were used to generate 4D CT and to compute an elastic registration. *Physically-based models*, describing the important role of airflow inside the lungs, can be based on Active Breathing Coordinator (ABC allows clinicians to pause the patient's breathing at a precise lung volume) [9] or on volume preservation relations [14,15]. In [16], segmented MRI data were used to simulate PET volumes at different instants of the breathing cycle. These estimated PET volumes were used to evaluate different PET/MRI registration processes. Authors of [12,17] used pre-register MRI to estimate a breathing model. CT registration using a breathing model was presented in [9] but a specific equipement is needed. From a modeling and simulation point of view, physically-based deformation methods are better adapted for simulating lung dynamics and are easy to adapt to the patient, without the need for physical external adaptations.

Physics-Based Dynamic 3D Surface Lung Model – We employ an approach that was previously discussed in [15] and in which the two major components involved in the modeling efforts include: (1) Parameterization of PV (Pressure Volume) data from a human subject which acts as an ABC; (2) Estimation of the deformation operator from 4D CT lung data sets. In step (1) a parameterized PV curve, obtained from a normal human subject, is used as a driver for simulating the 3D lung shapes at different lung volumes. In step (2), the computation takes as inputs the nodal displacements of the 3D lung models and the estimated amount of force applied on the nodes of the meshes (which are on the surface of the lungs). Displacements are obtained from 4D CT data of a normal human subject. The direction and magnitude of the lung surface point's displacement are computed using the volume linearity constraint, i.e. the fact that the expansion of lung tissues is linearly related to the increase in lung volume. The amount of applied force on each node (that represents the air-flow inside lungs) is estimated based on a PV curve and the lungs's orientation with respect to the gravity, which controls the air flow. Given these inputs, a physics-based deformation approach based on Green's function (GF) formulation is estimated to deform the 3D lung surface models. Specifically the GF is defined in terms of a physiological factor, the regional alveolar expandability (elastic properties), and a structural factor, the inter-nodal distance of the 3D surface lung model. To compute the coefficients of these two factors, an iterative approach is employed and, at each step, the force applied on a node is shared with its neighboring nodes, based on local normalization of the alveolar expandability, coupled with inter-nodal distance. The process stops when this sharing of the applied force reaches equilibrium. For validation purposes, a 4D CT dataset of a normal human subject with four instances of deformation was considered [18]. The simulated lung deformations matched the 4D CT dataset with 2 mm average distance error.

3   Combining Breathing Model and Image Registration

We have conceived an original algorithm in order to incorporate the breathing model described above in our multimodal image registration procedure. Fig. 2 shows the complete computational workflow. The input consists of one PET volume and two CT volumes of the same patient, corresponding to two different instants of the breathing cycle (end-inspiration and end-expiration, for example, collected with breath-hold maneuver). The preliminary step consists in segmenting the lung surfaces (and, eventually, the tumors) on the PET data and on the two CT data sets, using a robust mathematical-morphology-based approach [19], and extracting meshes corresponding to the segmented objects.

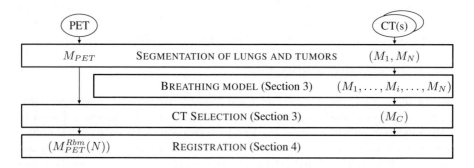

Fig. 2. Registration of CT and PET volumes using a breathing model

Computation of a Patient-Specific Breathing Model – For each patient, we only have two segmented CT datasets, therefore we first estimate intermediate 3D lung shapes between these two datasets and then, the displacements of lung surface points. *Directions* are given by the model (computed from a 4D CT normal data set of reference) while *magnitudes* are "patient-specific" (computed from the given 3D CT lung datasets). With known estimations of applied force and "subject-specific" displacements the coefficients of the GF can be estimated (Section 2). Then, the GF operator is used to compute the 3D lung shapes at different intermediate lung volumes.

CT Selection – Let us denote the CT simulated meshes M_1, M_2,..., M_N with M_1 corresponding to the CT in maximum exhalation and M_N to maximum inhalation. By using the breathing model, the transformation $\phi_{i,j}$ between two instants i and j of the breathing cycle can be computed as: $M_j = \phi_{i,j}(M_i)$. Our main assumption is that even if the PET volume represents an average volume throughout the respiratory cycle, using a breathing model, we can compute a CT volume that can be closer to the PET volume than the original CT volumes. By applying the continuous breathing model, we generate simulated CT meshes at different instants ("snapshots") of the breathing cycle. By comparing each CT mesh with the PET mesh (M_{PET}), we select the "closest" one (i. e. with the most similar shape). The mesh that minimizes a measure of similarity C (here the root mean square distance) is denoted as M_C: $M_C = \arg\min_i C(M_i, M_{PET})$.

Deformation of the PET – Once the appropriate CT (M_C) is selected, we compute the registration, f^r, between the M_{PET} mesh and the M_C mesh as:

$$M_{PET}^r(C) = f^r(M_{PET}, M_C), \tag{1}$$

where $M_{PET}^r(C)$ denotes the registered mesh. Then, the transformation due to the breathing is used to register the PET to the original CT (continuous line in Fig. 3) incorporating the known transformation between M_C and M_N:

$$\Phi_{C,N} = \phi_{N-1,N} \circ \ldots \circ \phi_{C+1,C+2} \circ \phi_{C,C+1}. \tag{2}$$

We apply $\Phi_{C,N}$ to $M_{PET}^r(C)$ in order to compute the registration with M_N:

$$M_{PET}^{Rbm}(N) = \Phi_{C,N}(M_{PET}^r) = \Phi_{C,N}(f^r(M_{PET}, M_C)), \tag{3}$$

where $M_{PET}^{Rbm}(N)$ denotes the PET registered mesh using the breathing model.

A *direct* registration, denoted f^{Rd}, can also be computed between M_{PET} and the original CT mesh M_N (dashed line in Fig. 3): $M_{PET}^{Rd}(N) = f^{Rd}(M_{PET}, M_N)$, where $M_{PET}^{Rd}(N)$ is the result of registering the PET directly to the CT mesh M_N (note that this could be done with another instant M_i). In the *direct* approach the deformation itself is not guided by any anatomical knowledge. In addition, if the PET and the original CT are very different, it is likely that this registration procedure will provide physically unrealistic results.

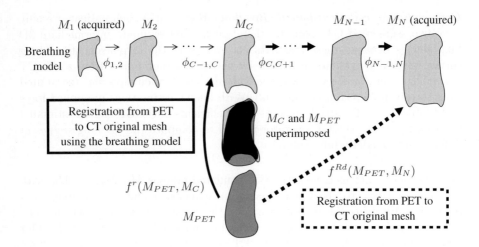

Fig. 3. Registration framework on PET (M_{PET}) and CT mesh (M_N) – The M_C mesh is the closest to the M_{PET} mesh. We can register M_{PET} to the M_N mesh (original CT) following one of the two paths.

4   Registration Method Adapted to Pathologies

The algorithm described in Section 3 can be applied with any type of registration method, to estimate f^{Rd} and f^r. These functions may be computed by any registration method adapted to the problem. We show here how the proposed approach can be adapted for registration of multi-modality images in pathological cases.

Registration with Rigidity Constraints – We have previously developed a registration algorithm for the thoracic region taking into account the presence of tumors, while preserving continuous smooth deformations [20]. We assume that the tumor is rigid and that a linear transformation is sufficient to cope with its displacements between CT and PET scanning. This hypothesis is relevant and in accordance with the clinicians' point of view, since tumors are often compact masses of pathological tissue. The registration algorithm relies on segmented structures (lungs and tumors). Landmark points are defined on both datasets to guide the deformation of the PET volume towards the CT volume. The deformation at each point is computed using an interpolation procedure where the specific type of deformation of each landmark point depends on the structure it belongs to, and is weighted by a distance function, which guarantees continuity of the transformation.

Registration with Rigidity Constraints and Breathing Model – Here, the following procedure is used to compute f^r (in our example M_N is the original CT):

1. Selection of landmark points on the CT mesh M_C (based on Gaussian and mean curvatures and uniformly distributed on the lung surface) [21];

2. Estimation of corresponding landmark points on the PET mesh M_{PET} (using the Iterative Closest Point (ICP) algorithm [22]);
3. Tracking of landmark points from M_C to the CT mesh M_N using the breathing model;
4. Registration of the PET and the original CT using the estimated correspondences with the method summarized in the previous paragraph.

The breathing model used in step (3) guarantees that the corresponding landmarks selected on the original CT are correct (and actually they represent the same anatomical point) and follow the deformations of the lungs during the respiratory cycle.

5   Results and Discussion

We have applied our algorithm on a normal case and on four pathological cases, exhibiting one tumor. In all cases, we have one PET (of size $144 \times 144 \times 230$ with resolution of $4 \times 4 \times 4$ mm^3 or $168 \times 168 \times 329$ with resolution of $4 \times 4 \times 3$ mm^3) and two CT volumes (of size $256 \times 256 \times 55$ with resolution of $1.42 \times 1.42 \times 5$ mm^3 to $512 \times 512 \times 138$ with resolution of $0.98 \times 0.98 \times 5$ mm^3), acquired during breathhold in maximum inspiration and in intermediate inspiration, from individual scanners. The breathing model was initialized using the lung meshes from the segmented CT. Ten meshes (corresponding to regularly distributed instants) are generated and compared with the PET. The computation time can reach two hours for the whole process (a few seconds for segmentation, a few minutes for landmark point selection and about ninety minutes for registration). Although this is not a constraint because we do not deal with an on-line process, this computation time will be optimized in the future.

As illustrated in Fig. 4 and 5 (one normal case and one pathological case), the correspondences between landmark points on the original CT and the PET are more realistic in the results obtained with the breathing model (images (e) and (f)) than without (images (b) and (c)). Using the model, it can be observed that the corresponding points represent the same anatomical points and that the uniqueness constraint is respected, leading to visually better looking PET registered images. In particular, the lower part of the two lungs is better registered using the model, the lung contour in the registered PET is closer to the lung contour in the original CT, cf. Fig. 4(g–i). In the illustrated pathological case, the tumor is well registered and not deformed. Moreover, the distance between the registered PET lungs and the original CT lungs is lower than using the direct approach.

In this paper, we consider the impact of the physiology on lung surface deformation, based on reference data of normal human subjects. Therefore the methodology presented in this paper will further benefit upon the inclusion of patho-physiology specific data once established. The use of normal lung physiology serves to demonstrate improvements in CT and PET registration using a physics-based 3D breathing lung model. Current work includes a quantitative comparison and evaluation on a larger database, in collaboration with clinicians.

632   A. Moreno et al.

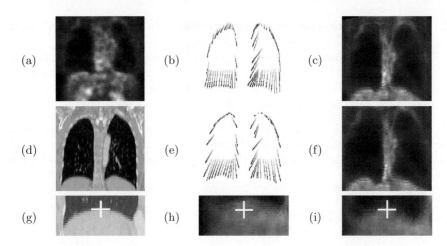

Fig. 4. (a) Original PET, (d) CT images in a normal case. Correspondences between selected points in the PET image and in the CT image are shown in (b) for the direct method and (e) for the method with the breathing model (corresponding points are linked). The registration result is shown in (c) for the direct method and in (f) for the method with the breathing model. Details of registration on the bottom part of right lung, (g) CT, (h) PET registered without breathing model, (c) with breathing model. The white crosses correspond to the same coordinates.

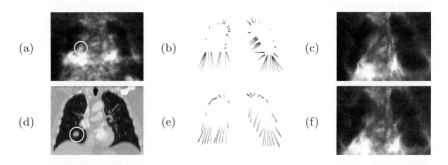

Fig. 5. Same as in Fig. 4(a–f) for a pathological case (the tumor is surrounded by a white circle)

References

1. Lavely, W., et al.: Phantom validation of coregistration of PET and CT for image-guided radiotherapy. Medical Physics 31(5), 1083–1092 (2004)
2. Rizzo, G., et al.: Automatic registration of PET and CT studies for clinical use in thoracic and abdominal conformal radiotherapy. Physics in Medecine and Biology 49(3), 267–279 (2005)
3. Vogel, W., et al.: Correction of an image size difference between positron emission tomography (PET) and computed tomography (CT) improves image fusion of dedicated PET and CT. Physics in Medecine and Biology 27(6), 515–519 (2006)

 4. Shekhar, R., et al.: Automated 3-Dimensional Elastic Registration of Whole-Body PET and CT from Separate or Combined Scanners. The Journal of Nuclear Medicine 46(9), 1488–1496 (2005)
 5. Sarrut, D.: Deformable registration for image-guided radiation therapy. Zeitschrift für Medizinische Physik 13, 285–297 (2006)
 6. McClelland, J., et al.: A Continuous 4D Motion Model from Multiple Respiratory Cycles for Use in Lung Radiotherapy. Medical Physics 33(9), 3348–3358 (2006)
 7. Nehmeh, S., et al.: Four-dimensional (4D) PET/CT imaging of the thorax. Physics in Medecine and Biology 31(12), 3179–3186 (2004)
 8. Wolthaus, J., et al.: Fusion of respiration-correlated PET and CT scans: correlated lung tumour motion in anatomical and functional scans. Physics in Medecine and Biology 50(7), 1569–1583 (2005)
 9. Sarrut, D., et al.: Non-rigid registration method to assess reproducibility of breath-holding with ABC in lung cancer. International Journal of Radiation Oncology–Biology–Physis 61(2), 594–607 (2005)
10. Mead, J.: Measurement of Inertia of the Lungs at Increased Ambient Pressure. Journal of Applied Physiology 2(1), 208–212 (1956)
11. Segars, W., et al.: Study of the Efficacy of Respiratory Gating in Myocardial SPECT Using the New 4-D NCAT Phantom. IEEE Transactions on Nuclear Science 49(3), 675–679 (2002)
12. Rohlfing, T., et al.: Modeling Liver Motion and Deformation During the Respiratory Cycle Using Intensity-Based Free-Form Registration of Gated MR Images. Medical Physics 31(3), 427–432 (2004)
13. Guerrero, T., et al.: Elastic image mapping for 4-D dose estimation in thoracic radiotherapy. Radiation Protection Dosimetry 115(1–4), 497–502 (2005)
14. Zordan, V., et al.: Breathe Easy: Model and Control of Human Respiration for Computer Animation. Graphical Models 68(2), 113–132 (2006)
15. Santhanam, A.: Modeling, Simulation, and Visualization of 3D Lung Dynamics. PhD thesis, University of Central Florida (2006)
16. Pollari, M., et al.: Evaluation of cardiac PET-MRI registration methods using a numerical breathing phantom. In: IEEE International Symposium on Biomedical Imaging, ISBI pp. 1447–1450 (2004)
17. Sundaram, T., Gee, J.: Towards a Model of Lung Biomechanics: Pulmonary Kinematics Via Registration of Serial Lung Images. Medical Image Analysis 9(6), 524–537 (2005)
18. Santhanam, A., et al.: Modeling Simulation and Visualization of Real-Time 3D Lung Dynamics. IEEE Transactions on Information Technology in Biomedicine. (in press, 2007)
19. Camara, O., et al.: Explicit Incorporation of Prior Anatomical Information into a Nonrigid Registration of Thoracic and Abdominal CT and 18-FDG Whole-Body Emision PET Images. IEEE Transactions on Medical Imaging 26(2), 164–178 (2007)
20. Moreno, A., et al.: Non-linear Registration Between 3D Images Including Rigid Objects: Application to CT and PET Lung Images With Tumors. In: Workshop on Image Registration in Deformable Environments (DEFORM), Edinburgh, UK, pp. 31–40 (2006)
21. Chambon, S., et al.: CT-PET Landmark-based Lung Registration Using a Dynamic Breathing Model. In: International Conference on Image Analysis and Processing, Modena, Italy (2007)
22. Besl, P., McKay, N.: A Method for Registration of 3-D Shapes. IEEE Transactions on Pattern Analysis and Machine Intelligence 14(2), 239–256 (1992)

Quantification of Blood Flow from Rotational Angiography

I. Waechter[1], J. Bredno[2], D.C. Barratt[1], J. Weese[2], and D.J. Hawkes[1]

[1] Centre for Medical Image Computing, Department of Medical Physics &
Bioengineering, University College London, UK
I.Waechter@cs.ucl.ac.uk
[2] Philips Research Aachen, Germany

Abstract. For assessment of cerebrovascular diseases, it is beneficial
to obtain three-dimensional (3D) information on vessel morphology and
hemodynamics. Rotational angiography is routinely used to determine
the 3D geometry and we propose a method to exploit the same acquisition to determine the blood flow waveform and the mean volumetric flow
rate. The method uses a model of contrast agent dispersion to determine
the flow parameters from the spatial and temporal development of the
contrast agent concentration, represented by a flow map. Furthermore,
it also overcomes artifacts due to the rotation of the c-arm using a newly
introduced reliability map. The method was validated on images from a
computer simulation and from a phantom experiment. With a mean error
of 11.0% for the mean volumetric flow rate and 15.3% for the blood flow
waveform from the phantom experiments, we conclude that the method
has the potential to give quantitative estimates of blood flow parameters
during cerebrovascular interventions.

1 Introduction

For diagnosis, treatment planning and outcome control of cerebrovascular diseases, such as atherosclerosis, aneurysms, or arteriovenous malformations (AVM),
it is beneficial to obtain three-dimensional (3D) information on vessel morphology
and hemodynamics. Rotational angiography (RA) allows 3D information on vessel morphology to be obtained during an intervention and is used routinely at the
beginning of aneurysm and AVM interventions. As it is possible to see how the
contrast agent moves with the blood, the sequence contains hemodynamic information as well. This information, however, is currently not exploited in clinical
systems. The goal of this work was to quantify the blood flow waveform and the
mean volumetric flow rate from rotational angiography data.

Several different approaches for the determination of blood flow information
from planar (not rotating) angiography have been reported previously. All existing approaches are based on analyzing changes in the x-ray image intensity
due to changes in the contrast agent concentration. Shpilfoygel et al. [1] give a
comprehensive review of established techniques, which include:

- techniques based on bolus tracking using time-intensity curves (TICs) at
different sites along a vessel

N. Ayache, S. Ourselin, A. Maeder (Eds.): MICCAI 2007, Part I, LNCS 4791, pp. 634–641, 2007.
© Springer-Verlag Berlin Heidelberg 2007

- techniques based on distance-intensity curves (DICs) at different points in time;
- and techniques based on optical flow.

Methods based on bolus tracking are known to give unreliable results in the case of pulsatile flow [1,2], and it is not possible to extract a time dependent waveform. Methods based on DICs and on optical flow enable a time-dependent waveform to be extracted. They, however, are sensitive to noise and the flow estimate depends on the distance to the injection site and the time from the start of the injection due to the effects of convective dispersion [2,3]. We propose a model-based flow estimation to overcome these problems by explicitly modeling convective dispersion.

To measure absolute flow parameters, it is necessary to know the 3D geometry of the vessel system, which cannot be obtained from a planar scan. As the 3D geometry can be obtained from RA, it is an advantage to extract the flow information from the same sequence. In this case only one contrast agent injection is required. Recently, there have been two approaches to achieve this: Chen at al. use a bolus tracking method [4], whereas Appaji and Noble use an optical flow method to reconstruct flow from RA [5]. However, both approaches do not address artifacts introduced by the rotation of the c-arm. In this paper, we propose a model-based flow estimation for RA, which addresses this problem.

2   Method

Our method first determines the so-called flow map and the newly introduced reliability map from the RA image sequence. The flow map is represented as an image, where the intensity is the concentration of contrast agent, the horizontal dimension is time and the vertical dimension is length along the vessel. Then a simulated flow map is fitted to the extracted flow map. The simulated flow map is generated using a model based on the physics of blood flow and contrast agent

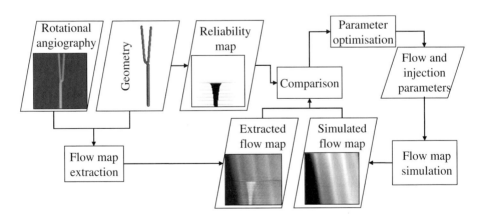

Fig. 1. Overview of the flow map fitting

transport. During the fitting, the optimal parameters for blood flow, including the flow waveform, and for the contrast agent injection are determined. An overview is given in Fig. 1 and all components are described in detail below.

2.1   Extraction of Flow Maps and Reliability Maps

At first the RA images are preprocessed to give quantitative information about the amount of iodine on the x-ray path. This can be done by digital subtraction of a mask scan and iodine calibration [6]. The RA sequence consists of M pre-processed images $I(x, y, t)$, acquired at the time steps $t \in [1, 2, \ldots, T]$ at different geometrical configurations $G(t)$ of the rotating c-arm.

Then, the 3D vessel centerline and radii are determined from the RA sequence as described in [7]. This method was tailored for RA sequences which show inflow and outflow of contrast agent. If $l \in [1, 2, \ldots, L]$ represents the length along the vessel, the centerline is given by a set of 3D points $(x, y, z) = P(l)$ and for each point the corresponding radius is given by $R(l)$. The projection function $\Pi(P(l), G(t))$ relates the positional co-ordinates of the 3D point $P(l)$ to the co-ordinates of the corresponding pixel within the x-ray image acquired at time t. A geometric calibration is used beforehand to determine the geometry parameters $G(t)$.

The uncorrected flow map $\mathbf{F}_U(l, t)$ is determined by projecting each 3D point of the centerline onto each image of the RA sequence and is given by

$$\mathbf{F}_U(l, t) = I(\Pi(P(l), G(t)), t). \tag{1}$$

Due to the rotation of the x-ray system, the flow map contains artifacts produced by two effects: Foreshortening and vessel overlap. In a projection image, vessels appear foreshortened if the direction of the x-ray is not perpendicular to the vessel. Vessels appear foreshortened frequently during a RA sequence. Vessel overlap occurs when more than one vessel segment lies on the x-ray beam path. The foreshortening error can be partially corrected: For every point $P(l)$ and every configuration of the c-arm $G(t)$, the length of the intersection of x-ray beam and current vessel is given by $\mathbf{L}(l, t)$ determined from the centerline and radii. This length is used for the correction of the flow map (referred to as extracted flow map) as given by

$$\mathbf{F}_E(l, t) = \frac{\mathbf{F}_U(l, t)}{\mathbf{L}(l, t)}. \tag{2}$$

As the amount of contrast agent is divided by $\mathbf{L}(l, t)$, $\mathbf{F}_E(l, t)$ represents the distribution and time course of the concentration of iodine. However, the information of foreshortened vessels is still less reliable and errors due to overlapping vessels cannot be corrected. The reliability map $\mathbf{R}_F(l, t)$ is used to overcome this problem. The reliability of each entry of the flow map is given by

$$\mathbf{R}_F(l, t) = \begin{cases} 0 & \text{, if vessel overlap is detected} \\ \cos \theta & \text{, otherwise,} \end{cases} \tag{3}$$

where vessel overlap is defined as the case when more than one vessel segments intersects with the x-ray beam and θ is the angle between the x-ray beam and the vessel centerline, which gives the degree of foreshortening.

2.2   Model-Based Flow Map Simulation

The model is used to predict a flow map, given the parameters of the blood flow and the injection. The blood flow is modeled by

$$Q_b(t) = \bar{Q}_b \cdot w(t), \tag{4}$$

where $\bar{Q}_b$ is the mean volumetric flow rate and $w(t)$ is the waveform

$$w(t) = \frac{\delta + cos(2\pi \cdot f_{\alpha,\beta,\gamma}(t/T))}{\int_0^1 \delta + cos(2\pi \cdot f_{\alpha,\beta,\gamma}(x))dx}, \tag{5}$$

where δ gives the baseline flow and $f_{\alpha,\beta,\gamma}(t) : [0,1] \rightarrow [0,1]$, with $f(\alpha) = a, f(\beta) = b, f(\gamma) = c$, $(a,b,c$ fixed), is a piecewise linear, monotonic function. α, β, γ specify the shape of the waveform. The injection flow $\widetilde{Q}_i(t)$ is assumed to be a rectangular function, defined by the maximum flow $\widetilde{Q}_i$, the start time T_s and duration T_d of the injection. The energy loss in the catheter is modeled by a lag element with characteristic time T_l. Mixing is assumed to be uniform. The concentration of iodine at the injection site is the given by

$$\mathbf{C}(r,0,t) = c \cdot \frac{m \cdot Q_i(t)}{Q_b(t) + m \cdot Q_i(t)}, \tag{6}$$

where $m \leq 1$ is a mixing factor and c is the concentration of iodine in the contrast agent. The flow is assumed to be laminar and axially symmetric. The vessel is divided in N laminae with average radius $r_n, n \in [1,2,\ldots,N]$. The velocity distribution in each laminae depends on the flow profile $p(r_n)$. A profile, given by

$$p(r_n) = 1 - (r_n/R)^k, 2 \leq k < \infty \tag{7}$$

can approximate a profile between plug flow $(k \rightarrow \infty)$ and parabolic flow $(k = 2)$. The velocity in laminae n is then given by

$$v(r_n,t) = v_0(t) \cdot p(r_n) = \frac{Q_b(t) + m \cdot Q_i(t)}{2\pi \sum_{n=1}^{N} p(r_n)r_n} \cdot p(r_n). \tag{8}$$

The transport of a soluble substance in a moving medium is determined by convection and diffusion [3]. Using the velocity of the laminae, the convection of iodine is then determined in 2D representation of the vessel tree, parameterized in terms of length l along and distance r from the vessel centerline [2]. Diffusion is modeled by applying a Gaussian low pass filter. The result is the time-dependent development of the concentration of iodine $\mathbf{C}(r,l,t)$. Finally, the simulated flow map is given by

$$\mathbf{F}_S(l,t) = \frac{1}{R} \sum_{n=1}^{N} \mathbf{C}(r_n,l,t). \tag{9}$$

2.3   Flow Map Fitting

For the flow map fitting, the simulated flow maps $\mathbf{F}_S$ are fitted to the extracted
flow map $\mathbf{F}_E$. The error between them is determined by

$$E(\mathbf{F}_S) = \sum_{l=1}^{L} \sum_{t=1}^{T} \left[(\mathbf{F}_S(l,t) - \mathbf{F}_E(l,t))^2 + (\nabla(\mathbf{F}_S(l,t)) - \nabla(\mathbf{F}_E(l,t)))^2 \right] \cdot \mathbf{R}_F(l,t),$$

(10)

where ∇ is the temporal gradient operator and the reliability map gives a weighting. A Gauss-Newton least-squares optimization is used to determine the injec-
tion and flow parameters, in particular, the waveform parameters $\alpha, \beta, \gamma,$ and δ
and the mean volumetric flow rate $\bar{Q}_b$ by minimizing $E(\mathbf{F}_S)$.

2.4   Validation

The proposed method for flow extraction was validated by computer simulations
and a phantom experiment. Three setups were used to determine the extracted
flow map as follows:

1. Simulated flow maps were corrupted by different levels of noise (Peak signal-
   to-noise ratio: 18, 22, 28) and used as extracted flow maps. The flow and
   injection parameters were varied according to Table 1. Three different waveforms (Fig. 2) were used. Overall 272 different flow maps were tested.
2. Flow maps were extracted from computer simulated RA. The contrast agent
   propagation was based on the model described above. The resulting concentrations $\mathbf{C}(r,l,t)$ were mapped to a voxel presentation of the vessel tree
   and converted to x-ray attenuation coefficients. The x-ray images were determined using a proprietary, analytical x-ray simulation software. Two example
   geometries were used: The first geometry was a curved tube with uniform
   radius, which produced a foreshortening artifact (see Fig. 3), and the second
   was a bifurcation, which produced an overlapping artifact(see Fig. 1). Flow
   and injection parameters were chosen as above.
3. Flow maps were extracted from the images from an experimental setup.
   The experimental setup consisted of a pulsatile flow circuit, a clinical contrast agent injector (MarkVProVis, Medrad) and a rotational x-ray system
   (Allura Xper with an FD20 detector, Philips Medical Systems). Seventeen
   image sequences were acquired following a contrast injection (Ultravist-370,
   Schering) into a straight tube. The tube was placed in an elliptical, water
   filled cylinder to generate realistic noise, beam hardening, and scatter. The
   ground truth flow was acquired by an electromagnetic flow meter (EMF).
   The flow parameters were estimated from a full length flow map (10 cm) and
   from a short flow map (1 cm).

The flow waveform was determined from each flow map using the flow map
fitting method described in Sec. 2.3 and compared with the ground truth waveform. The waveform was initialized to a cosine-function and the mean volumetric
flow rate was either initialized at half of the desired value or randomly chosen.

Table 1. Parameters of simulation

Parameters	Symbol	Unit	Values
Mean volumetric flow rate	$\bar{Q}_b$	[ml/min]	[100 - 300]
Flow profile	k	[]	[2, 5, 10]
Radius	R	[mm]	[2]
Max injection flow rate	$\tilde{Q}_i$	[ml/min]	[50 - 300]
Injection lag	T_l	[s]	[0.2 - 0.5]
Iodine concentration	c	[mg/ml]	[370]
Start injection	T_s	[s]	[0, 0.5, 1]
Injection duration	T_d	[s]	[3, 4]
Mixing factor	m	[]	[1]
Acquisition duration	T	[s]	[4]
Total number frames	M	[]	[120]
Number Laminae	N	[]	[10]

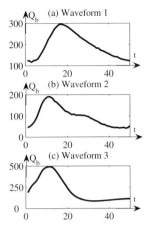

Fig. 2. Waveforms

The percentage error in the mean volumetric flow rate (mean flow) and waveform were calculated.

3   Results

The results of the three experiments were as follows:

1. For the first setup, the mean error of the mean flow and of the waveform were 0.7% and 7.3%, respectively. The accuracy of the waveform mainly depended on the shape of the wave form (Waveform 1: 4.5%, Waveform 2: 7.6%, Waveform 3: 9.8%; other flow and injection parameters had only

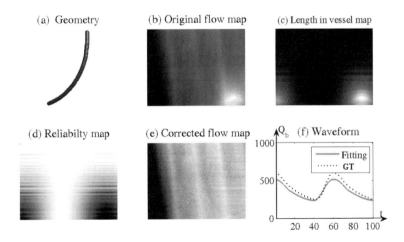

Fig. 3. Results from the computer simulation using the foreshortening phantom

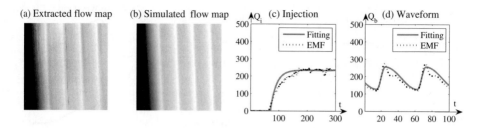

Fig. 4. Results from the experimental setup

minor influences. The influence of noise on the accuracy is relatively small (Waveform 1: No noise: 4.7%, low noise level: 4.5%, medium noise level: 4.6%, high noise level: 5.1%).

2. For the bifurcated geometry, the mean error of the mean flow and waveform were 11.8% and 16.4%, respectively. For the curved geometry, the mean error of the mean flow and waveform were 9.8% and 14.6%, respectively. Fig. 3 shows the uncorrected flow map, reliability map and corrected flow map for the curved geometry. Fig. 1 includes some results for the bifurcated geometry.

3. For the full length flow map from the experimental setup, the mean error of the mean flow and the waveform were 11.0% and 15.3%, respectively. For the short flow map, the error increased only to 13.0% and 17.3%. An example of a full length extracted flow map, the according fitted flowmap and estimated waveform together with the ground truth waveform are given in Fig. 4.

The optimization converged to an accurate solution, even when the start parameters were far away from the desired result parameters. It took 10 to 20 iterations for the convergence. The flow map fitting for the extraction of one waveform took about 5 min on a 3 GHz Xeon processor.

4   Discussion

In this paper, we have described a method for estimating a blood flow waveform and the mean volumetric flow rate from RA. Any method estimating blood flow from RA must be more robust than for planar angiography, because of image artifacts introduced by the rotation. To achieve this, we have introduced a novel approach, that utilizes a model-based flow estimation and the reliability map.

The reliability map is used to decrease the influence of artifacts on the flow estimation and to use as many segments of the vessel tree as possible. Existing methods use either only DICs (columns of the flow map) or TICs (rows of the flow map). Methods based on DICs in particular require a certain length of vessel to be unoccluded or foreshortened. In the case of rotational data and a non-trivial vessel geometry, it is not possible to determine sufficiently long, artifact-free DICs. However, even in complex geometries, enough segments should be not foreshortened and not overlapped at least in some parts of the RA sequence. The reliability map makes it possible to use this information.

The flow map fitting uses the flow map as a whole rather than single TICs or DICs. Therefore, it is more robust against noise and uncorrected artifacts compared with existing methods. The first experiment showed that even high levels of noise introduced only small errors into the waveform estimation.

A further advantage is that the proposed method incorporates a model of the underlying physics. Methods based on optical flow and DICs on the other hand have the disadvantage that the flow estimation changes with the distance from the injection site and time from the start of the injection. Our method models the convective dispersion and can therefore account for these different situations.

The last experiment showed that the flow model is able to explain real transport of contrast agent in a flowing medium. With a mean error of 11.0% for the mean volumetric flow rate and 15.3% for the blood flow waveform from the phantom experiments, we conclude that the method has the potential to give sufficiently accurate, quantitative estimates of blood flow parameters.

Such quantitative data can supplement the subjective information on flow currently obtained by visual interpretation during cerebrovascular interventions. For application of the method to clinical data, the frame rate of the RA sequence should be at least 30 fps. The distance between the injection site and the first observation should be known. Furthermore, a iodine calibration is beneficial. For the future, we plan experiments with more complex geometries and a comparison to a computational fluid dynamics simulations.

We thank the X-ray Pre-Development department at Philips Medical Systems Best for making the experiments possible.

References

1. Shpilfoygel, S.D., Close, R.A., Valentino, D.J., Duckwiler, G.R.: X-ray videodensitometric methods for blood flow and velocity measurement: A critical review of literature. Med. Phys. 27(9), 2008–2023 (2000)
2. Rhode, K.S., Lambrou, T., Hawkes, D.J., Seifalian, A.M.: Novel approaches to the measurement of arterial blood flow from dynamic digital X-ray images. IEEE Trans. Med. Imaging 24(4), 500–513 (2005)
3. Taylor, G.: Dispersion of soluble matter in solvent flowing slowly through a tube. In: Proceedings of the Royal Society of London. Series A-Mathematical an physical science, vol. 219(1137), pp. 186–203 (1953)
4. Chen, Z., Ning, R., Conover, D., Lu, X.: Blood flow measurement by cone-beam CT bolus imaging. In: Medical Imaging, Proceedings of the SPIE (2006)
5. Appaji, A., Noble, A.J.: Estimating cerebral blood flow from a rotational angiographic system. In: Biomedical Imaging: Macro to Nano, pp. 161–164 (April 6-9, 2006)
6. Molloi, S., Bednarz, G., Tang, J., Zhou, Y., Mathur, T.: Absolute volumetric coronary blood flow measurement with digital subtraction angiography. Int. J. Card Imaging 14(3), 137–145 (1998)
7. Waechter, I., Bredno, J., Weese, J., Hawkes, D.: Using flow information to support 3D vessel reconstruction from rotational angiography. Medical Physics 33, 1983 (2006)

Modeling Glioma Growth and Mass Effect in 3D MR Images of the Brain

Cosmina Hogea[1], Christos Davatzikos[1], and George Biros[2]

[1] Section of Biomedical Image Analysis, Department of Radiology, University of
Pennsylvania, Philadelphia PA 19104, USA
[2] Departments of Mechanical Engineering and Applied Mechanics, Bioengineering,
and Computer and Information Science, University of Pennsylvania, Philadelphia PA
19104, USA
hogeac@uphs.upenn.edu

Abstract. In this article, we propose a framework for modeling glioma
growth and the subsequent mechanical impact on the surrounding brain
tissue (mass-effect) in a medical imaging context. Glioma growth is modeled via nonlinear reaction-advection-diffusion, with a two-way coupling
with the underlying tissue elastic deformation. Tumor bulk and infiltration and subsequent mass-effects are not regarded separately, but
captured by the model itself in the course of its evolution. Our formulation is fully Eulerian and naturally allows for updating the tumor diffusion coefficient following structural displacements caused by
tumor growth/infiltration. We show that model parameters can be estimated via optimization based on imaging data, using efficient solution
algorithms on regular grids. We test the model and the automatic optimization framework on real brain tumor data sets, achieving significant
improvement in landmark prediction compared to a simplified purely
mechanical approach.

1 Introduction

Modeling brain tumor growth in conjunction with deformable registration algorithms can be used to construct brain tumor atlases and potentially assist
treatment planning [1, 2]. In order to improve registration between a normal
brain atlas and a tumor-bearing brain image, it is desirable to first construct
a brain atlas exhibiting tumor and mass-effect[1] similar to those of a patient at
study, thus reducing the problem to the (simpler) problem of registering two
relatively similar images.

Therefore, we need a way to simulate tumor growth and mass-effects for different brain anatomies. In [1,3,4], a purely mechanical 3D tumor growth model
targeted on simulations of tumor mass-effect was employed. The brain tissue was
modeled as an elastic material (linear or nonlinear) and the mechanical force
exerted by the growing tumor was approximated by a constant outward pressure P acting on the tumor boundary and controlling the tumor size and mass-
effect. This model was solved to obtain brain tissue displacements. Although this

---

[1] Deformation (compression) of the neighboring tissue induced by tumor growth is
commonly referred to as mass-effect.

N. Ayache, S. Ourselin, A. Maeder (Eds.): MICCAI 2007, Part I, LNCS 4791, pp. 642–650, 2007.
© Springer-Verlag Berlin Heidelberg 2007

approach was employed successfully for generating tumor-deformed brain atlases, it has two main limitations: (1) more irregularly shaped tumors are difficult to capture (the simulated tumors are generally quasi-spherical); and (2) it provides no information about the actual tumor evolution and infiltration into healthy tissue. In [2], the authors have used a relatively similar mechanical approach to model the mass-effect caused by the tumor bulk (GTV1) and added a separate reaction-diffusion model (similar to [5], [6], [7]) to account for the tumor infiltrative part only (GTV2, assumed to cause little mass-effect). In such an approach, the tumor reaction-diffusion equation is decoupled from the elasticity equations and the diffusion coefficient, which in reality is affected by tumor infiltration, is not updated [2].

Here, we propose a model that strongly couples glioma[2] growth with the subsequent deformation of the brain tissue. Using brain tumor MRI scans, model parameters can be estimated via a biophysically-constrained optimization formulation of a deformable image registration problem. In our approach, glioma growth is modeled via a nonlinear reaction-advection-diffusion equation, with a two-way coupling with the underlying tissue elasticity equations. Our formulation (fully Eulerian) naturally allows for updating the tumor diffusion coefficient following structural displacements caused by tumor growth/infiltration. The overall modeling framework results in a strongly coupled nonlinear system of partial differential equations, for which we use an efficient numerical solution procedure.

The main differences compared to the work in [2] are: (1) there is no sharp-interface separation between a tumor bulk and an infiltrative part; (2) the underlying tissue displacement (deformation) impacts the subsequent motion of the tumor cells in two ways: the diffusion coefficient changes (diffusion term in the tumor equation) and tumor cells are pushed around (advective term in the tumor equation); (3) the diffusion coefficient, affected by structural displacements following tumor growth and infiltration, is updated; (4) the numerical solution algorithm is based on fast hybrid finite element-finite difference solvers on fixed regular grids, coupled with an optimization algorithm for estimation of model parameters from patient imaging data.

2   Methods

The brain is regarded as a deformable solid occupying a bounded region ω in space. Let $U = \omega \times (0, T)$, where $(0, T)$ a specified time interval. Let $c = c(\mathbf{x}, t)$ be the tumor-cell density, normalized such that $0 \le c \le 1$. Using an Eulerian frame of reference, the tumor growth and the subsequent brain motion can be described by the following general set of equations:

$$\frac{\partial c}{\partial t} - \nabla \cdot (D\nabla c) + \nabla \cdot (c\mathbf{v}) - \rho c(1 - c) = 0 \qquad (1)$$

$$\nabla \cdot ((\lambda \nabla \cdot \mathbf{u})\mathbf{I} + \mu(\nabla \mathbf{u} + \nabla \mathbf{u}^T)) - p_1 e^{-\frac{p_2}{c^s}} e^{-\frac{p_2}{(2-c)^s}} \nabla c = 0 \qquad (2)$$

$$\mathbf{v} = \frac{\partial \mathbf{u}}{\partial t}, \qquad \frac{\partial \mathbf{m}}{\partial t} + (\nabla \mathbf{m})\mathbf{v} = 0, \qquad (3)$$

---

[2] Malignant gliomas are the most common primary brain tumors, originating in the glial cells; they are often resistant to treatment and carry a poor prognosis.

where $\mathbf{m} = (\lambda, \mu, D)$. In regions where $c \ll 1$ (infiltration), the customary proliferation term ρc corresponding to exponential growth at rate ρ is retrieved [5]. Proliferation is assumed to slow down in regions with c getting closer to 1 (tumor bulk), and it eventually becomes a death term if c becomes larger than 1[3]; D is the diffusion coefficient of tumor cells in brain tissue[4]. Here we consider the case of isotropic diffusion in both white and gray matter, with diffusion coefficients D_w and D_g, respectively [5]. $\mathbf{v}$ is the (Eulerian) velocity field[5], $\mathbf{u}$ is the displacement field.

We employ the linear elasticity theory and approximate the brain tissue as a linear elastic material, characterized by Lame's parameters λ and μ (related to Young's modulus E and Poisson's ratio ν). The elastic forces are pressure-like, directly proportional to the local gradient of the tumor cell density [9], [2]; the expression we use here, with p_1, p_2 and s positive constants, allows for flexibility in capturing both strong tumor mass-effect (generally caused by the tumor bulk) and milder mass-effects (generally caused by tumor infiltration), as illustrated in figure 1. The elastic material properties λ and μ and the tumor cell diffusivity D are assumed spatially varying (different in white matter, gray matter, ventricles, CSF). Boundary and initial conditions are specified to close the system of equations (1)-(3). We impose zero tumor cell flux and zero tissue displacement at the skull. The advection equations (3) are initial value problems, with the initial values assigned from the corresponding segmented MR image [3,4]. Equations (1)-(3) with prescribed boundary and initial conditions represent a mixed parabolic-elliptic-hyperbolic nonlinear system of PDEs. Next, we outline an efficient numerical algorithm for solving this system.

2.1   Numerical Methods

A significant challenge is posed by the fact that the underlying spatial domain ω occupied by the brain is a highly irregular one. Various techniques exist for solving PDEs on an irregular domain, from unstructured meshes that conform to the irregular domain boundary to immersed interface/ghost-fluid methods. Here, we employ a fictitious domain-like regular grid method. The target domain ω is embedded on a larger computational rectangular domain (box) Ω. The PDEs originally defined on ω, are appropriately extended to Ω, such that the true boundary conditions prescribed on $\partial\omega$ are approximated.

For simplicity, it is advantageous to split the problem into independent steps corresponding to the advection, diffusion, and reaction [10], [11]. Let $\mathbf{w} = (c, \mathbf{u}, \mathbf{v}, D, \lambda, \mu)$ denote the vector of unknowns. Let Δ, A_1, and R denote the diffusion, advection and reaction operators in the diffusion equation (1), and A_2 denote the advection operator in equations (3). Let $\mathbf{w}^n = (c^n, \mathbf{u}^n, \mathbf{v}^n, D^n, \lambda^n, \mu^n)$ is the solution at time $t = t_n$; to update the solution $\mathbf{w}^{n+1}$ at the next time step $t_{n+1} = t_n + \Delta t$ we use three steps.

---

[3] We do model tumor as a single species and we ignore heterogeneity.

[4] If tumor diffusion is assumed anisotropic, then D is a tensor.

[5] The velocity $\mathbf{v}$ in the tumor equation may well depend on tumor specific mechanisms (e.g., chemotaxis [8]). In our model the velocity accounts only for the tumor cells being displaced as a consequence of the underlying tissue mechanical deformation.

(I) We solve the advection equations (3) over time Δt to obtain $(D^{n+1}, \lambda^{n+1}, \mu^{n+1})$;

(II) We solve the diffusion equation (1) using a simple fractional step method [10]:   a) Solve $\frac{\partial c}{\partial t} = A_1(c, \mathbf{v})$ over time Δt with data $(c^n, \mathbf{v}^n)$ to obtain c^*;
b) Solve $\frac{\partial c}{\partial t} = \Delta(c, D)$ over time Δt with data (c^*, D^{n+1}) to obtain c^{**};
and c) Solve $\frac{\partial c}{\partial t} = R(c)$ over time Δt with data c^{**} to obtain c^{n+1}.

(III) Finally, we solve the elasticity equation (2) with data $(c^{n+1}, \lambda^{n+1}, \mu^{n+1})$ to obtain $\mathbf{u}^{n+1}$ and update the velocity $\mathbf{v}^{n+1}$.

Parameter estimation (optimization)

Consider the case of longitudinal data for a brain-tumor subject. We seek to compute the model parameters that generate images that 'best match' the patient data. This translates into a parameter-estimation problem for the model governing equations (1)-(3). Here we use an objective functional that defines a 'best match' by the Euclidean distance between model-generated landmarks and manually-placed landmarks in the target image(s). The results presented in the next section are obtained using the APPSPACK package [12], a derivative-free optimization library from Sandia National Laboratory. More efficient optimization algorithms, based on gradient estimation via the adjoints [13], are work in progress.

3   Results

Given the segmented image labels (generated from 3D MRI data), we assign piecewise constant material properties (white matter, gray matter, ventricles, and CSF). These values are used as initial condition in the transport equations (3). The 3D computational domain is the underlying domain of the image. It consists of the actual brain plus the surrounding fictitious material.

Synthetic brain tumor images

We first illustrate the capabilities of our proposed framework to simulate brain tumors with more complex patterns and mass-effect. For the simulations in Figure 1 we have used similar values for the elastic material properties as in [3, 4]. The tumor diffusivity in the white matter was set five times higher than in the gray matter [5], while the diffusivity in the ventricles (and eventually CSF) was set to zero. These simulations correspond to an aggressive physical tumor growth over T=365 days (one year), starting from the same small Gaussian seed located in the right frontal lobe. The numerical solution of our coupled system of PDEs (1)-(3) is obtained via the procedure described in section 2.1 using a hybrid finite element-finite difference method, with ten equal time steps and a spatial discretization of $65 \times 65 \times 65$ nodes[6]. The tumor growth illustrated in the second column (left to right) of figure 1 is less diffusive $(D_w = 7.5 \times 10^{-8} m^2/day; D_g = 1.5 \times 10^{-8} m^2/day)$ and more regularly shaped, while in the other two case scenarios depicted in the third and fourth

---

[6] By extensive numerical testing, we have found that such a discretization provides a reasonable trade-off between speed and accuracy.

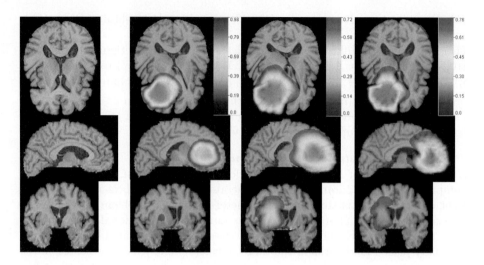

Fig. 1. Synthetic glioma growth, right frontal lobe: three different case scenarios starting from the same initial tumor seed. Left to right. The 1st column illustrates the 3D MRI of a normal brain image—axial, sagittal and coronal section respectively. The 2nd column shows the deformed image, with simulated tumor corresponding to low tumor diffusivity and long-range mass-effect ($p_2 = 0$). The 3rd column shows the deformed image, with simulated tumor corresponding to high tumor diffusivity (ten times higher) and long-range mass-effect ($p_2 = 0$). Finally, the 4th column shows the deformed image, with simulated tumor corresponding to high tumor diffusivity and short-range mass-effect ($p_2 = 0.1$). The tumor maps (here shown in RGB) are overlaid on the deformed template. The run time is about 500 seconds on an 2.2GHz AMD Opteron.

column (left to right) respectively, we increased the diffusivity by a factor of ten ($D_w = 7.5 \times 10^{-7} m^2/day; D_g = 1.5 \times 10^{-7} m^2/day$). For both simulations illustrated on the second and third columns (left to right) of figure 1, the parameter p_2 regulating the range of the mass-effect was set equal to zero, which is the minimum, corresponding to an extreme case scenario, with strong mass-effects propagating far away from the tumor core, which we refer to as 'long-range' mass-effects. This can be well observed by examining the ventricle deformation in the corresponding axial slices. If p_2 is increased, the mass-effects are more localized to areas close to the tumor core, which can be well observed on the fourth column of figure 1 and which we refer to as 'short-range' mass-effects. The rest of the model parameters are kept fixed to $\rho = 0.036/day, p_1 = 15kPa, s = 2$. More complex tumor patterns could be obtained by using more complicated initial tumor profiles and/or anisotropic diffusion (DTI-driven).

Optimization on real brain tumor data and comparison with simpler pressure-based mechanical model

In [3,4], the authors have investigated the ability of their proposed framework to realistically capture mass-effects caused by actual brain tumors in two dog cases with surgically transplanted glioma cells and a human case with progressive low-grade glioma. We use their data sets here for comparison purposes. For the two

Table 1. Landmark errors for the two dog cases (DC1, DC2) and for the human case
(HC) with the new model (optimized). The errors shown are with respect to landmarks
manually placed by an experienced human rater. Both the incremental pressure model
and the new model were numerically solved using a spatial discretization with 65^3
nodes; five equal pressure increments applied in the simple pressure model; four equal
time steps used in the new model for the two dog cases and five equal time steps for
the human case.

Landmark Error (mm)	Median	Min	Max	Run time (sec)
New model DC1	**0.89564**	0.0511	1.9377	200
Incremental pressure model	**1.6536**	0.3176	2.6491	300
Inter-rater variability DC1	**0.8484**	0.1304	2.8568	
New model DC2	**1.2980**	0.3803	2.6577	200
Incremental pressure model	**1.8912**	0.4795	3.7458	300
Inter-rater variability DC2	**1.3767**	0.1226	2.7555	
New model HC	**1.8457**	0.5415	4.1451	250
Incremental pressure model	**5.23**	1.15	8.9	300

dogs (DC1, DC2), a baseline scan was acquired before tumor growth, followed
by scans on the 6th and 10th day post-implantation. Gadolinium-enhanced T1
MR images were acquired. By the 10th day, tumors grew rapidly to a diameter
of 1-2 cm, and then the animals were sacrificed (prior to any neurological complications). For the human case (HC), two T1 MRI scans with approximately
2.5 years in-between were available. In all three cases, pairs of corresponding
landmark points were manually identified by human raters in the starting and
target images. For the dog cases, two human raters placed independent sets of
landmarks. All the results reported here are with respect to the most experienced
rater of the two; the inter-rater variability is included in table 1.

For the human case, only one human rater was available. We have fixed the
elastic material properties (stiffness and compressibility, respectively) to the values reported in [3, 4][7]. We consider a case-scenario with four optimization parameters: c_0, D_w, ρ, p_1 (p_2 fixed to zero). Here c_0 represents a scaling factor
(magnitude) of the initial tumor density, assumed again to be a Gaussian with
known center (here estimated from the serial scans). The landmark errors upon
optimization convergence are summarized in table 1; corresponding landmark
errors for the simplified purely mechanical approach in [3, 4] are included for
comparison. Relative landmark errors with respect to the maximum landmark
displacement for both the simplified incremental pressure approach [3, 4] and
the new model are shown for comparison in figure 2; the corresponding average
relative improvement achieved by the new (optimized) model are 17%, 20% and
51% for DC1,DC2 and HC, respectively. A visual illustration of simulations via
the two different approaches (new model vs. incremental pressure) is shown in
figure 3 (top row), highlighting the potential of the new model to capture more
information about the tumor compared to the pressure approach.

---

[7] In these three cases, the segmentation included only white matter and ventricles:
$E_{white} = 2100Pa, E_{ventricles} = 500Pa, \nu_{white} = 0.45, \nu_{ventricles} = 0.1$

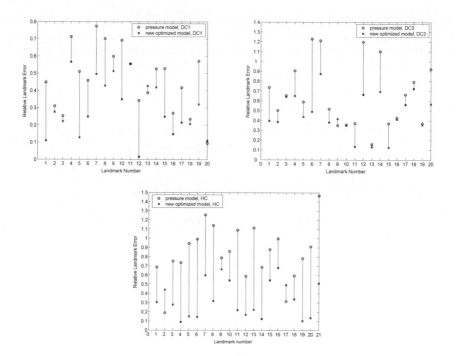

Fig. 2. Comparison of relative landmark errors (here with respect to the maximum landmark displacement) for the three cases DC1, DC2 and HC, via the the incremental pressure approach and the new model. The corresponding average relative improvements achieved by the new optimized model are 17%, 20% and 51% for DC1,DC2 and HC, respectively.

4 Conclusions and Further Research

In the present paper, we proposed a framework for modeling gliomas growth and the subsequent mass-effect on the surrounding brain tissue. Estimation of unknown model parameters is regarded as a constrained optimization problem. Although beyond the scope of the current paper, the long-term aims of this work are the following goals: to improve the deformable registration from a brain tumor patient image to a common stereotactic space (atlas) with the ultimate purpose of building statistical atlases of tumor-bearing brains; to investigate predictive features for glioma growth, after the model parameters are estimated from given patient scans. We illustrated the capabilities and flexibility of our new framework in capturing more complex/realistic tumor shapes and subsequent mass-effect, at reduced computational cost. We tested both the model and the optimization framework on real brain tumor data sets and showed significant improvement compared to a simplified purely mechanical approach [3, 4]. We are currently working on developing faster PDE-constrained optimization methods, with estimation of gradients via an adjoint-based formulation coupled to fast gradient-descent algorithms and general image similarity functionals.

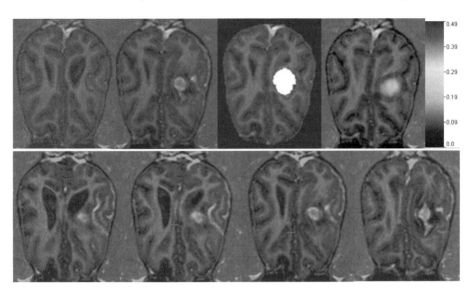

Fig. 3. Real brain tumor images, dog case DC1. **Top row**, from left to right: starting scan, T1 MR gadolinium-enhanced; target scan, T1 MR gadolinium-enhanced; our simulated tumor growth and mass-effect via the new optimized framework: tumor color maps overlaid on the model-deformed image, with corresponding color bar attached; simulated mass-effect via the simplified incremental pressure approach in [3], with tumor mask highlighted in white. The new tumor growth model shows potential to capture more information about the tumor compared to the pressure approach. **Bottom row**: illustration of a few of the target landmarks (marked with crosses) used for the model-constrained optimization in this case.

Finally, we are building non-uniform structured discretizations based on octree data structures to further reduce computational cost and allow more accurate approximations in regions of interest.

References

1. Mohamed, A., Davatzikos, C.: Finite element modeling of brain tumor mass-effect from 3d medical images. In: Proceedings of Medical Image Computing and Computer-Assisted Intervention, Palm Springs (2005)
2. Clatz, O., Sermesant, M., Bondiau, P.-Y., Delingette, H., Warfield, S.K., Malandain, G., Ayache, N.: Realistic simulation of the 3d growth of brain tumors in mr images coupling diffusion with mass effect. IEEE Trans on Med. Imaging 24, 1334–1346 (2005)
3. Hogea, C., Abraham, F., Biros, G., Davatzikos, C.: A framework for soft tissue simulations with applications to modeling brain tumor mass-effect in 3d images. In: Medical Image Computing and Computer-Assisted Intervention Workshop on Biomechanics, Copenhagen (2006)
4. Hogea, C., Abraham, F., Biros, G., Davatzikos, C.: Fast solvers for soft tissue simulation with application to construction of brain tumor atlases (Technical report) ms-cis-07-04, http://www.seas.upenn.edu/~biros/papers/brain06.pdf

5. Swanson, K.R., Alvord, E.C., Murray, J.D.: A quantitative model for differential motility of gliomas in grey and white matter. Cell Proliferation 33, 317–329 (2000)
6. Tracqui, P., Mendjeli, M.: Modelling three-dimensional growth of brain tumors from time series of scans. Mathematical Models and Methods in Applied Sciences 9, 581–598 (1999)
7. Habib, S., Molina-Paris, C., Deisboeck, T.: Complex dynamics of tumors: modling an emerging brain tumor system with coupled reaction-diffusion equations. Physica A: Statistical Mechanics and its Applications 327, 501–524 (2003)
8. Hogea, C.: Modeling Tumor Growth: a Computational Approach in a Continuum Framework. PhD thesis, Binghamton University (2005)
9. Wasserman, R.M., Acharya, R.S., Sibata, C., Shin, K.H.: Patient-specific tumor prognosis prediction via multimodality imaging. Proc. SPIE Int. Soc. Opt. Eng. 2709 (1996)
10. Tyson, R., Stern, L.G., LeVeque, R.J.: Fractional step methods applied to a chemotaxis model. J. Math. Biol. 41, 455–475 (2000)
11. Verwer, J., Hundsdorfer, W., Blom, J.: Numerical time integration for air pollution models. In: Report MAS-R9825, CWI Amsterdam (1991)
12. Kolda, T., et. al.: APPSPACK (2005), home page. http://software.sandia.gov/appspack/version5.0
13. Gunzburger, M.: Perspectives in Flow Control and Optimization. SIAM (2002)

Towards Tracking Breast Cancer Across Medical Images Using Subject-Specific Biomechanical Models

Vijay Rajagopal[1], Angela Lee[1], Jae-Hoon Chung[1], Ruth Warren[2],
Ralph P. Highnam[3], Poul M.F. Nielsen[1], and Martyn P. Nash[1]

[1] Bioengineering Institute, University of Auckland, NZ
v.rajagopal@auckland.ac.nz
[2] Department of Radiology, Addenbrooke's Hospital, Cambridge, UK
[3] Highnam Associates Limited, NZ

Abstract. Breast cancer detection, diagnosis and treatment increasingly involves images of the breast taken with different degrees of breast deformation. We introduce a new biomechanical modelling framework for predicting breast deformation and thus aiding the combination of information derived from the various images. In this paper, we focus on MR images of the breast under different loading conditions, and consider methods to map information between the images.

We generate subject-specific finite element models of the breast by semi-automatically fitting geometrical models to segmented data from breast MR images, and characterizing the subject-specific mechanical properties of the breast tissues. We identified the unloaded reference configuration of the breast by acquiring MR images of the breast under neutral buoyancy (immersed in water). Such imaging is clearly not practical in the clinical setting, however this previously unavailable data provides us with important data with which to validate models of breast biomechanics, and provides a common configuration with which to refer and interpret all breast images.

We demonstrate our modelling framework using a pilot study that was conducted to assess the mechanical performance of a subject-specific homogeneous biomechanical model in predicting deformations of the breast of a volunteer in a prone gravity-loaded configuration. The model captured the gross characteristics of the breast deformation with an RMS error of 4.2 mm in predicting the skin surface of the gravity-loaded shape, which included tissue displacements of over 20 mm. Internal tissue features identified from the MR images were tracked from the reference state to the prone gravity-loaded configuration with a mean error of 3.7 mm. We consider the modelling assumptions and discuss how the framework could be refined in order to further improve the tissue tracking accuracy.

1 Introduction

Breast cancer diagnosis and treatment typically involves the use of a number of imaging modalities and views of the breast. X-ray mammography is an effective screening tool for the detection of cancer at an early stage, and involves

N. Ayache, S. Ourselin, A. Maeder (Eds.): MICCAI 2007, Part I, LNCS 4791, pp. 651–658, 2007.
© Springer-Verlag Berlin Heidelberg 2007

compression of the breast between two plates in the cranio-caudal and medio-lateral oblique directions. MR images are taken for further characterization of suspicious lesions found in mammograms. Breast MRI is typically conducted with the subject lying in a prone position with the breasts hanging pendulously within a specialized MR coil.

During breast imaging and treatment procedures, significant shape changes can occur, whereby the internal tissues undergo large deformations between imaging orientations. Consequently, no two images of the breast show exactly the same tissues, thus tracking features between images is a difficult task. To this end, biomechanical models of the breast are being developed in order to constrain non-rigid image registration algorithms in order to provide transformations that are physically admissible [1,2].

We present a finite element modelling framework that we are developing to track features between medical images. We demonstrate our modelling approach by describing a pilot study based on MR images of one volunteer. In developing the model, we address two important issues that have not been previously reported: (i) the identification of the reference configuration of the breast when no load is applied (noting that images of the breast are almost always taken under gravity, and possibly compression loading conditions); and (ii) the estimation of subject-specific in-vivo mechanical properties of the breast tissues. Whilst the implications of the latter are somewhat intuitive, the importance of an accurate representation of the unloaded reference configuration of the breast has not been previously discussed. The large nonlinear deformations that the breast experiences can be modelled using the laws of physics, but this type of modelling depends on knowledge of a well-defined stress-free reference configuration. This unloaded state also serves as an ideal shape to which information and features from all images of the breast can be mapped and interpreted, since it is the configuration for which all loading and deformation effects imposed by the imaging procedures are removed. We have recently developed a computational technique to estimate this unloaded reference state [3], but this method remains to be validated for breast imaging in the clinical setting. For present purposes, we have experimentally estimated the reference configuration using neutral buoyancy imaging as explained in Section 2.2.

We first describe the methods that were employed to create the subject-specific biomechanical model for the pilot study. We then assess the performance of the model in predicting breast shape and tissue movement from the neutral buoyancy reference state to the prone gravity-loaded configuration.

2   Methods

We use a finite element implementation of large-deformation hyperelasticity theory to model breast biomechanics in our in-house software, CMISS [4]. This theory is more suitable to model the nonlinear deformations as opposed to small-strain linear elasticity techniques, which do not account for the large rotations that typical occur during finite deformations. The reader is directed to [5] and

[6] for further details on the theory of finite deformations and finite elements, respectively. The following sections outline the methods that were used to create a subject-specific finite element model of the breast under gravity loading conditions.

2.1 Subject-Specific Breast Geometry

We use smoothly continuous cubic-Hermite basis functions to represent breast geometry as they capture complex geometries with more realism than lower-order basis functions [7]. While a line represented with a 1D linear basis function has one degree of freedom per node (the x-coordinate, for instance), a representation with a 1D cubic-Hermite basis function consists of 2 degrees of freedom per node: the coordinate value and its arc-length derivative. The additional derivative information at the nodes implicitly enforces continuity of the spatial gradients at the interfaces between elements, thus requiring fewer elements to represent smoothly continuous anatomical surfaces compared to linear basis functions. Since cubic-Hermite functions use a greater number of degrees of freedom per node than linear basis functions, it follows that the use of fewer elements does not necessarily correspond to fewer geometric degrees of freedom. Indeed, for equal numbers of total geometric degrees of freedom, higher order basis functions are favoured because they provide better rates of solution convergence for finite elasticity problems [6].

Subject-specific finite element models are generated using a semi-automatic method that efficiently parameterizes the skin and muscle surface contours using geometric data that have been segmented from MR images (Fig. 1) [8]. The method uses a nonlinear least-squares approach to fit surfaces of volume elements to the segmented data sets [7].

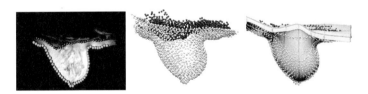

Fig. 1. Process of creating a subject-specific breast model. Left: Segmentation of tissue boundaries from an MR image. Grey points represent the skin surface, and black points represent muscle surface. Middle: Dataset of skin (grey points), and muscle (black points) after segmenting an entire MR image set. Right: Finite element model fitted to skin and muscle surface data.

This customization technique has been applied to MR datasets from six subjects with markedly different breast shapes. We found that geometric finite element models consisting of 24 tri-cubic Hermite elements (with 70 nodes and 1680 total geometric degrees of freedom) fitted the models with an average overall RMS error of 1.5 mm in representing the skin and muscle surfaces (see Fig. 2). For the mechanics study presented here, the breast was assumed to be

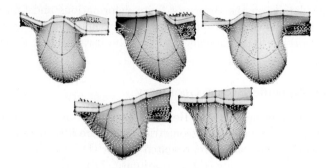

Fig. 2. Finite element model (surfaces) fitted to the skin surface data sets (spots) of 5 subjects lying prone in an MR scanner. The fitted model of subject 1 is shown in Fig. 1.

homogeneous after [2], thus the geometrical model did not need to account for any structural differences between the internal tissues.

2.2   Neutral Buoyancy Imaging and the Unloaded Configuration

Previous models have typically used the prone gravity-loaded configuration of the breast as the mechanical reference state. However, the effects of gravity loading mean that this is not the true stress-free reference configuration of the breast, hence this assumption may lead to large errors in mechanics predictions. In order to overcome this issue, we obtained MR images of the volunteer's breast when immersed in water and assumed that breast tissue density is close to that of water (see Fig. 4). Thus, we assume that neutral buoyancy offsets the effects of gravity, and more closely represents the unloaded configuration of the breast. These images are the first to capture the unloaded shape of the breast and will be used in future studies to investigate and quantify the importance of the representation of the reference configuration on the accuracy of breast mechanics modelling. For present purposes, neutral buoyancy images were used to create a finite element model of the volunteer's breast in the unloaded configuration. This neutral buoyancy model was used as the reference state for a mechanics simulation of the prone gravity-loaded configuration.

2.3   Loading and Boundary Conditions

Gravity loading was applied as a body force to the neutral buoyancy model. For the purposes of this study, it was assumed that the breast tissues and muscle were firmly attached to the rib cage, thus we applied fixed-displacment boundary conditions at the posterior surface of the model. Previous modelling studies have applied displacement boundary conditions to nodes across the entire skin surface to ensure that the outer shape of the breast in the deformed configuration was matched [1,2]. In contrast, the simulations in the present study are driven by the gravity loading condition alone and thus provide a more robust way of assessing the ability of the model to predict breast deformations.

2.4   Subject-Specific Mechanical Properties

The breast was assumed to be incompressible, homogeneous and isotropic as characterized by the neo-Hookean constitutive equation $W = c_1(I_1 - 3)$, where I_1 is the first principal invariant of the Lagrangian strain and c_1 is the material parameter that must be determined for the tissues [5]. Previous models have also used the neo-Hookean relationship, and they have typically used experimental data from the literature in order to characterize the mechanical behavior of breast tissues [1,2]. However, it is well known from experiments that breast tissue mechanical properties vary significantly between subjects [9]. Therefore, it is likely to be important to use a constitutive relationship that is customized to each individual. We used our existing material parameter optimization techniques [3,8] to estimate the value of c_1 using the model of the neutral buoyancy shape together with the segmented data from the images of the prone gravity-loaded configuration.

3   Results

The geometric finite element model of the neutrally buoyant breast had an RMS error of 0.78 mm for fitting the skin surface and 1.2 mm for fitting the muscle surface of the volunteer's breast. A displacement solution mesh convergence analysis was performed for the mechanics model by tracking eight material points located throughout the model and recording their displacements for successive refinements. The Euclidian displacements that each material point underwent during the deformation was calculated for each mesh resolution. The RMS errors between successive refinements were then recorded (see Fig 3) and the mesh corresponding to 112 tri-cubic Hermite elements, as illustrated in Fig. 4 (216 nodes; 5184 geometric degrees of freedom), was chosen as the most appropriate resolution for reliable model predictions. The material parameter optimization technique estimated a value of $c_1 = 0.08$ kPa for this model.

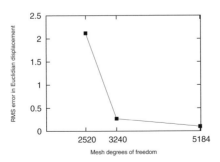

Fig. 3. Convergence of RMS error in Euclidean displacements of selected material points inside the fitted model with increasing mesh resolution

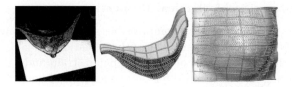

Fig. 4. MR image (Left) and refined finite element model (Right) of the right breast of a volunteer under neutral buoyancy. The bright region in the MR image represents the water bath.

3.1 Predicting the Prone Gravity-Loaded Configuration

Figure 5 illustrates the model's ability to predict the deformation of the breast in the prone gravity-loaded configuration. It shows that the homogeneous model provides a good match to the prone gravity-loaded configuration. The segmented surface data from the prone gravity-loaded shape was predicted with an RMS error of 4.2 mm. Four internal tissue regions were segmented from the neutral buoyancy images and tracked using the model to the prone gravity-loaded configuration. These segmented regions were not represented using finite elements, but were tracked as a set of embedded material points in the homogeneous model. Figure 5 illustrates the tracking process and Table 1 quantifies the accuracy with which the individual image features were tracked. On average, the homogeneous model tracked internal tissue deformations with an error of 3.7 mm.

Table 1. Total displacements of the four tissue regions tracked from the neutral buoyancy to the gravity-loaded configuration and the corresponding Euclidean errors between centroids of actual and predicted locations for the gravity-loaded configuration

Tissue region	1	2	3	4
Displacement (mm)	5.06	20.47	19.0	21.7
Euclidean Error (mm)	1.56	4.82	4.51	3.97

4   Discussion and Conclusions

This pilot study has shown that a homogeneous, subject-specific model is able to predict breast deformation from a neutral buoyancy state to a prone gravity-loaded configuration within a clinically acceptable localization accuracy (under 5 mm, after [2]). The gross surface characteristics are also reproduced by the model, tracking skin surface deformations with an RMS error of 4.2 mm. It is likely that incorporation of more structural detail, such as heterogeneities in breast tissue properties, will improve model predictions. As identified previously, a realistic representation of the boundary conditions at the chest wall may also improve accuracy [1,2]. Note however, that previous studies have enforced the surface of the model to match the skin surface configuration on the image using displacement boundary conditions. Our work predicts the entire deformation

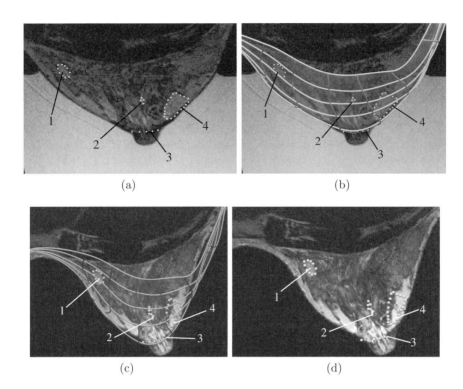

(a)   (b)

(c)   (d)

Fig. 5. Tracking surface and internal tissues from the neutral buoyancy reference configuration to the prone gravity-loaded deformed state. (a): Neutral buoyancy MR image with tissue features circled by white points and numbered sequentially. (b): Fitted finite element model of the unloaded state superimposed on the neutral buoyancy MR image and embedded with the same tissue features. (c): Predicted finite element model of the prone gravity-loaded configuration superimposed on prone gravity-loaded breast MR image. White points show predicted locations of the four tracked tissue features and the labelled points indicate actual locations of the features in the image. (d): Prone gravity-loaded breast MR image superimposed with the predicted locations of tracked tissue features in white, together with actual locations identified and labelled in white. See Table 1 for quantitative comparisons of tissue feature localization.

based only on the loading conditions, mechanical properties and fixed boundaries, thus providing a more robust validation of the model's predictability.

The framework presented in this paper incorporates the use of subject-specific mechanical properties and anatomically realistic geometry in modelling breast deformations. By acquiring neutral buoyancy images, we now have sufficient data to systematically assess the importance of each of the parameters (reference configuration, material properties, loading conditions and boundary conditions) of the biomechanical model. Results of these studies will help inform the modelling regarding the incorporation of biological detail that is necessary to perform reliable breast deformation predictions without compromising the speed of computations, which will be important for applications in the clinical setting such as image registration and biopsy procedures.

References

1. Tanner, C., Schnabel, J., Hill, D., Hawkes, D., Leach, M., Hose, D.: Factors influencing the accuracy of biomechanical breast models. Medical Physics Journal 33(6), 1758–1769 (2006)
2. Ruiter, N., Stotzka, R.: Model-based registration of x-ray mammograms and MR images of the female breast. IEEE Transactions on Nuclear Science 53(1), 204–211 (2006)
3. Rajagopal, V., Chung, J., Bullivant, D., Nielsen, P., Nash, M.: Finite elasticity: Determining the reference state from a loaded configuration. International Journal of Numerical Methods in Engineering (in press, 2007)
4. CMISS. software program (2007), http://www.cmiss.org
5. Fung, Y.: A First Course in Continuum Mechanics. Prentice-Hall, Englewood Cliffs (1977)
6. Zienkiewicz, O., Taylor, R.: The Finite Element Method: The Basis, 5th edn. vol. 1. Butterworth-Heinemann (2000)
7. Bradley, C., Pullan, A., Hunter, P.: Geometric modelling of the human torso using cubic Hermite elements. Annals of Biomedical Engineering 25(1), 96–111 (1997)
8. Rajagopal, V.: Modelling Breast Tissue Mechanics Under Gravity Loading. PhD thesis, University of Auckland (2007)
9. Sarvazyan, A., Skovoroda, A., Emelianov, S., Fowlkes, J., Pipe, J., Adler, R., Buxton, R., Carson, P.: Biophysical bases of elasticity imaging. Acoustic Imaging 21, 223–240 (1995)

Inter-subject Modelling of Liver Deformation During Radiation Therapy

M. von Siebenthal[1], G. Székely[1], A. Lomax[2], and Ph. Cattin[1]

[1] Computer Vision Laboratory, ETH Zurich, 8092 Zurich, Switzerland
{mvonsieb,szekely,cattin}@vision.ee.ethz.ch
[2] Paul Scherrer Institut, 5232 Villigen PSI, Switzerland

Abstract. This paper presents a statistical model of the liver deformation that occurs in addition to the quasi-periodic respiratory motion. Having an elastic but still compact model of this variability is an important step towards reliable targeting in radiation therapy. To build this model, the deformation of the liver at exhalation was determined for 12 volunteers over roughly one hour using 4DMRI and subsequent non-rigid registration. The correspondence between subjects was established based on mechanically relevant landmarks on the liver surface. Leave-one-out experiments were performed to evaluate the accuracy in predicting the liver deformation from partial information, such as a point tracked by ultrasound imaging. Already predictions from a single point strongly reduced the localisation errors, whilst the method is robust with respect to the exact choice of the measured predictor.

1 Introduction

The variability in shape and position of abdominal organs is an important issue in image acquisition, segmentation, patient setup and treatment. In the liver, the respiratory motion can lead to displacements of several centimetres [1]. Within a few minutes, a high reproducibility of the respiration was reported [2]. However, over larger intervals of 20 min or more, deformations of more than one centimetre were observed in addition to the quasi-periodic respiratory motion [3]. In radiation therapy such deformations lead to large uncertainties in target localisation.

One approach to improve targeting during treatment is to use deformation models as prior knowledge [4]. For the liver, models have been proposed that capture the subject specific quasi-periodic motion [5]. In contrast, we propose an inter-subject model, which is built from a training set of livers and can be applied to a previously unseen liver. Inter-subject models have been proposed for the cardiac shape and motion, which is close to periodic [6]. In the liver, the quasi-periodic component of motion can be handled to a large degree by breath-hold techniques or respiratory gating. Thus, the aim of this paper was to model the systematic motion and deformation of the liver, which occurs in addition to the quasi-periodic motion and can be considered as superimposed.

One direct application of this model is to predict the deformation of the entire liver from partial information. As a result, the displacement of a liver

N. Ayache, S. Ourselin, A. Maeder (Eds.): MICCAI 2007, Part I, LNCS 4791, pp. 659–666, 2007.
© Springer-Verlag Berlin Heidelberg 2007

tumour could be predicted from the displacement of vessel branchings that are tracked by ultrasound imaging, even though the tumour itself may not be visible in this modality. A deformable organ model offers the flexibility of non-rigid transformations between the planning and the treatment scene and should at the same time restrict the deformation to a tractable number of parameters.

2   Methods

2.1   Data Acquisition

To capture the intra-fraction deformation of the liver, 4DMRI sequences [3] were acquired from 12 healthy volunteers (6 female, 6 male, average age 31, range 17-75) after written consent was obtained. This produced time-resolved MR volumes consisting of 25-30 slices with a thickness of 4 mm and an in-plane resolution of 192×192 pixels and $1.8 \times 1.8 \, \text{mm}^2$. MR volumes with a temporal resolution of 290-410 ms were reconstructed, which produced 3300-6700 volumes during acquisition sessions of 40-75 min. In the following, we will only consider the variability of the liver at exhalation. Therefore, the volume with the most superior liver position was selected from each breathing cycle, yielding 220-850 exhalation volumes per volunteer.

The deformation of the liver at exhalation was determined for each volunteer by intensity-based non-rigid registration [3,7] between the reconstructed volumes. The resulting deformations describe the variability of the exhalation position at each point within the liver over time. Figure 1 illustrates how the exhalation position of discrete points varied over an acquisition session of 51 min. In addition to a small variation from cycle to cycle we observe large systematic displacements of more than 15 mm. Such deviations can be caused by drifts in the exhalation level, peristalsis, muscle distension or moving gases.

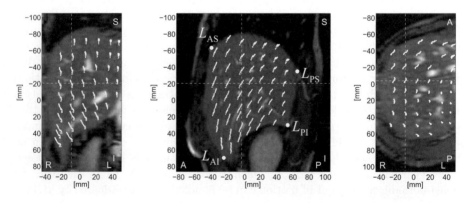

Fig. 1. Example point clouds in subject 1 showing a drift of the exhalation position in superior direction over 51 min

2.2 Inter-subject Correspondence

A key component for building a statistical model that covers different subjects is the inter-subject correspondence. This raises the question, with respect to which criterion two points should correspond. For example, in resective liver surgery correspondence should be based on the vascularisation. However, for modelling deformation in the abdomen, the goal is to find corresponding points that move comparably. We assume that for mechanical considerations the most relevant property of a point in the liver is its location relative to the liver surface, for example its distance from the diaphragm. We thus propose a scheme to establish correspondence based on landmarks on the liver surface.

In a preparatory step, the liver was segmented manually in one exhalation volume per subject. This produced fine triangular surface meshes with several thousand triangles but without correspondence between subjects. These surfaces were then remeshed with an approach similar to [8] in order to establish correspondence. For this purpose, mechanically relevant landmarks were identified. Figure 1 shows four landmarks $L_{AI}, L_{AS}, L_{PI}, L_{PS}$, where the indices indicate the location (anterior, posterior, superior, inferior). These points mark the delineations between the superior surface in contact with lung, the anterior and the posterior areas, which slide along the abdominal wall, and the inferior surface. The four landmarks were labelled manually in each sagittal slice from the inferior vena cava (IVC) to the inferior tip of the liver and were connected by B-splines. A prototype of the right liver lobe consisting of 46 triangles was then aligned to the fine mesh of each specific liver as illustrated in Fig. 2a, such that its four edges coincided with the marked delineations. In medio-lateral direction, the vertices of the prototype were regularly distributed along the landmark splines. The coarse prototype was then gradually refined to fit the fine surface mesh. In each refinement step, the triangles of the prototype were regularly subdivided into four smaller triangles and the newly generated points were projected onto the surface mesh. Figure 2b shows how a new point P'_{ab} was projected along the normal n.

Three refinement steps were performed for each of the 12 livers (Fig. 2c). Based on the resulting correspondences on the liver surface, a grid of corresponding points within the liver was defined. A regular grid of 290 points with 15 mm resolution was placed in the average liver shape and then transformed to each subject specific liver. Therefore, a Delaunay tetrahedrisation of the average liver was produced. The position of each point in the average liver is defined by the barycentric coordinates that give its position within a tetrahedron. Assuming the same tetrahedrisation in each subject specific liver, the grid point can be transformed to these livers by placing it at the same barycentric coordinates. The resulting points in each liver, which correspond to the regular grid of points in the average liver, will be further used for statistical modelling.

2.3 Statistical Modelling

We propose a model of the liver deformation that occurs during a treatment session in addition to the quasi-periodic breathing. The model captures the drift

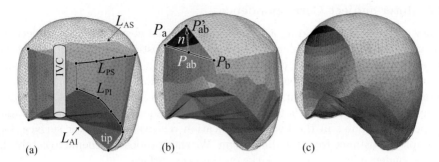

Fig. 2. (a) Coarse mesh prototype aligned with respect to manually identified delineations on the liver surface. (b) Refined mesh after correspondence preserving subdivision and projection. (c) Resulting mesh after three refinement steps.

of the exhalation position in each corresponding point. It should be noted that our aim was not to model the liver anatomy, which would describe the inter-subject variation of the position of the corresponding points. Instead, we describe the drift of each corresponding point in a point specific coordinate system, which is placed at the corresponding position in each subject. The axes of the point specific coordinate systems are chosen to reflect the orientation of the liver in the body. The left-right axis is perpendicular to the medial plane of the body and the superior-inferior axis points along the posterior abdominal wall.

To avoid a bias towards one specific dataset, an equal number of 200 sample exhalation positions was taken from each dataset, equally distributed over the duration of the acquisition session. From this data, a point distribution model was built, with $M = 290$ corresponding points and $N = 12 \times 200$ samples of each point. Each instance i of the liver was specified by a $3M$-dimensional vector p_i containing the position of each point. Principal component analysis was applied to determine the eigenvectors of the covariance matrix, i.e. the main modes of variation [9]. We assume that the matrix U is composed of the principal components as column vectors and that the diagonal matrix Λ contains the eigenvalues. With the mean shape vector $\bar{p}$, a specific instance can be defined as $p_i = \bar{p} + U b_i$, where b_i are the coefficients of the linear combination of eigenvectors.

2.4 Drift Prediction

The derived model can be used to predict the displacement of all considered points from a few measurements. Assuming that the displacement of a point j from its mean position is known, the most probable deformation that fulfils the constraint imposed by this fixed point is the one with minimum Mahalanobis distance from the mean shape. Based on the submatrix U_j, which contains only those rows of U that correspond to point j, we can calculate basis vectors $r_{x_j}, r_{y_j}, r_{z_j}$ that cause a unit translation of point j and have minimal Mahalanobis length [9]. With these basis vectors and the known point displacement $[\Delta x_j, \Delta y_j, \Delta z_j]^T$, the most probable instance $\check{p}$ is determined as

$$R_j = \begin{bmatrix} r_{x_j} r_{y_j} r_{z_j} \end{bmatrix} = \Lambda U_j^T \begin{bmatrix} U_j \Lambda U_j^T \end{bmatrix}^{-1}, \qquad \check{p} = \bar{p} + U R_j \begin{bmatrix} \Delta x_j \\ \Delta y_j \\ \Delta z_j \end{bmatrix}. \qquad (1)$$

If we assume that any point in the liver could be used as a predictor, we would choose the point P_{opt} that reduces the variance of the model as much as possible. As further elaborated in [9], the basis vectors R_j can be used to remove the variance of point j from the statistical model by subtracting R_j, weighted by the example specific displacements $[\Delta x_j, \Delta y_j, \Delta z_j]_i^T$, from the parametric representation b_i of each shape instance i.

$$\check{b}_i = b_i - R_j \begin{bmatrix} \Delta x_j \\ \Delta y_j \\ \Delta z_j \end{bmatrix}_i = b_i - R_j U_j b_i, \qquad \forall i \in \{1, ..., N\} \qquad (2)$$

To determine by how much the knowledge of point j has reduced the variability of the model, the variance of the coefficients $\check{b}_i$ after model reduction is compared to the variance of b_i before reduction. The point with maximum reduction potential, P_{opt}, is selected among all considered points and used as a predictor for the deformation of the entire liver.

To evaluate the predictive power of the model, leave-one-out experiments were performed. Models built from 11 of the 12 livers were used to predict the displacement of all points in the left-out liver following (1). In a practical setup it might not be possible to measure P_{opt}, for example due to the lack of trackable structures. For this reason, all 290 corresponding points were tested for their capability to predict the deformation of the left-out liver.

3   Results

The compactness of the derived model is characterised by the cumulative percentage of variance covered by the first few principal components. The cumulative variance was calculated from the eigenvalues Λ of a model containing all 12×200 sample exhalation positions.

components	1	2	3	4	5	6
cumulative variance [%]	78	88	91	94	96	97

Although the model describes the distribution of 290 points over 2400 sample deformations, it is compact and covers 91% of the full variance with 3 principal components. This shows that there are typical modes of deformation during treatment. Note that this model of intra-fraction deformation is not subject specific and has to be distinguished from a model of anatomical inter-subject variation, where with only 12 sample shapes a compact model would be less surprising.

Table 1 shows the extent of deformation observed in each subject over the acquisition sessions of 40-75 min. Whilst the mean displacement of all considered points is 5 mm or larger in 5 of 12 subjects, the maximum displacement is 5 mm or

Table 1. Euclidean displacements during complete acquisition sessions; average ± standard deviation and (maximum) over the right liver lobe. The prediction errors are given for three cases: (A) prediction from P_{opt} (B) worst prediction from one of the six neighbours of P_{opt} (C) prediction from the three points with maximum reduction potential according to the model.

subject	deformation [mm]	error A [mm] P_{opt} known	error B [mm] 1 point known	error C [mm] 3 points known
1	6.5±3.4 (18.8)	2.3±1.3 (7.7)	2.6±1.5 (8.7)	1.9±1.2 (5.8)
2	3.4±1.7 (7.1)	1.6±0.7 (3.2)	1.8±0.7 (3.5)	1.1±0.5 (2.7)
3	3.2±1.7 (8.4)	1.8±0.9 (5.1)	2.3±0.9 (6.5)	1.4±0.7 (4.0)
4	6.1±2.9 (14.8)	2.0±0.7 (3.3)	2.2±0.8 (3.9)	1.4±0.5 (2.6)
5	5.5±2.2 (10.2)	1.5±0.4 (3.2)	1.5±0.5 (3.8)	1.0±0.3 (2.2)
6	3.9±0.9 (5.7)	1.6±0.5 (3.0)	1.6±0.5 (3.1)	0.9±0.4 (1.9)
7	3.1±1.5 (7.0)	0.9±0.4 (2.0)	1.0±0.4 (2.0)	0.7±0.4 (1.8)
8	5.5±3.0 (12.1)	1.6±1.0 (5.0)	2.0±1.2 (5.8)	1.2±0.6 (3.1)
9	5.0±1.9 (10.1)	1.3±0.6 (3.8)	1.4±0.7 (4.0)	0.9±0.5 (2.7)
10	2.4±1.0 (5.0)	0.6±0.2 (1.4)	0.6±0.2 (1.5)	0.5±0.2 (1.5)
11	3.1±1.4 (6.0)	1.5±0.6 (3.0)	1.6±0.7 (3.3)	0.9±0.4 (2.4)
12	4.2±2.1 (9.4)	1.7±0.8 (4.2)	2.0±0.8 (4.4)	1.3±0.6 (3.0)

larger in all subjects and ranges up to 18.8 mm. This confirms that the considered deformations are an important source of localisation uncertainties.

Figure 3 depicts the results of the leave-one-out experiment for subject 1. The drift of each corresponding point over the acquisition session of 51 min, was predicted from a single point, for which we assume that the drift can be measured exactly. Each corresponding point was tested by using it as a predictor for the entire deformation. The resulting average error for each predictor is shown as the size of the marker at the respective position. Most points show a similar predictive power, which illustrates that the method is robust with respect to the choice of the predictor. However, we can identify two areas that are less suitable as predictors. First, this is the medial area toward the inferior vena cava, where the influence of the beating heart is largest, and second, points in the tip of the liver lobe show lower predictive power. These points are directly influenced by intestinal motion, which is in some cases poorly correlated to the deformation in the rest of the liver.

Table 1 shows the results for all 12 leave-one-out experiments and three different kinds of available partial information.

Case A: The prediction of the liver deformation based on the point P_{opt}, which has the maximum potential for variance reduction according to the model, leads to small average prediction errors ranging from 0.6 mm to 2.3 mm. Also the maximum prediction error is clearly smaller than the full deformation in all subjects. For subject 1, the location of P_{opt} is shown in Fig. 3. Not surprisingly, this point lies near the centre of the considered region. In subject 3, the deformation is successfully predicted with a mean residual error of 1.8 mm, but the maximum error is only reduced from 8.4 mm to 5.1 mm. This is possible because the

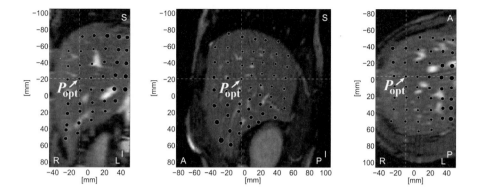

Fig. 3. Prediction errors when different points are used as predictors. The radius of the markers indicates the mean prediction error over the right liver lobe that results if this specific point can be measured. P_{opt} is the point with maximum potential for variance reduction according to the model.

prediction criterion, i.e. the Mahalanobis distance from the mean shape, takes the entire liver into account and may be not optimal for single points.

Case B: Table 1 further shows the prediction error if P_{opt} cannot be localised but one of its six direct neighbours. The small degradations again show the robustness with respect to the exact choice of the predictor.

Case C: To evaluate the further improvements in prediction accuracy with more available measurements, we applied (2) to find not only one but three points with maximum potential for variance reduction. In each leave-one-out model the triplet with maximum variance reduction was found by exhaustive search. These three points were then assumed to be measurable in the left-out liver and used as predictors. The quantitative results for three predictors in Table 1 show a clear reduction of the prediction error in all but one subject. Only subject 10 shows a slight increase from 1.4 mm to 1.5 mm in the maximum prediction error with 3 known points compared to the prediction based on P_{opt}. This is again possible, because the prediction criterion was defined over the entire liver lobe and may insufficiently reflect single point deviations. However, the mean prediction error of 0.5 mm in this subject is the smallest among all experiments.

4   Discussion and Conclusions

In the described experiments to evaluate the predictive power of the model we assumed accurately measurable predictors. An important further step will be to incorporate the uncertainty of measurements and to determine the achievable accuracy in practical setups. Moreover, the kind of partial information used for prediction may be adapted to a certain application. For example, if only the in-plane components of the predictor displacement are measurable, then the model and the prediction framework are not changed, but more measurements may be necessary for accurate predictions.

The mechanically motivated correspondences between subjects led to a compact model of liver deformation. However, a more complex scheme, which takes more mechanically relevant landmarks into account, such as the contact areas with the right kidney, the gall bladder or the portal vein, may further increase the predictive power of the model.

The presented model was built to specifically capture the deformation of the liver in addition to its quasi-periodic motion. A model of the full respiratory motion covering the complete respiratory cycle, changes in amplitude, and variations of the breathing speed would further broaden the spectrum of applications and is the subject of ongoing research.

Acknowledgments. This work has been supported by the CO-ME/NCCR research network of the Swiss National Science Foundation. The authors would like to thank Urs Gamper and Prof. Dr. Peter Boesiger (Institute for Biomedical Engineering, ETH Zurich) for their support in image acquisition.

References

1. Davies, S.C., Hill, A.L., Holmes, R.B., et al.: Ultrasound quantitation of respiratory organ motion in the upper abdomen. Br. J. Radiol. 67, 1096–1102 (1994)
2. Mageras, G.S., Yorke, E., Rosenzweig, K., et al.: Fluoroscopic evaluation of diaphragmatic motion reduction with a respiratory gated radiotherapy system. J. App. Clin. Med. Phys. 2, 191–200 (2001)
3. von Siebenthal, M., Székely, G., Gamper, U., et al.: 4D MR imaging of respiratory organ motion and its variability. Phys. Med. Biol. 52(6), 1547–1564 (2007)
4. Davatzikos, C., Shen, D., Mohamed, A., Kyriacou, S K: A framework for predictive modeling of anatomical deformations. IEEE T. Med. Imaging 20, 836–843 (2001)
5. Blackall, J.M., Penney, G.P., King, A.P., Hawkes, D.J.: Alignment of sparse freehand 3-D ultrasound with preoperative images of the liver using models of respiratory motion and deformation. IEEE T. Med. Imaging 24, 1405–1416 (2005)
6. Perperidis, D., et al.: Construction of a 4D statistical atlas of the cardiac anatomy and its use in classification. In: Duncan, J.S., Gerig, G. (eds.) MICCAI 2005. LNCS, vol. 3750, pp. 402–410. Springer, Heidelberg (2005)
7. Rueckert, D., Sonoda, L I, et al.: Nonrigid registration using free-form deformations: application to breast MR images. IEEE T. Med. Imaging 18, 712–721 (1999)
8. Styner, M., et al.: Evaluation of 3D correspondence methods for model building. In: Taylor, C.J., Noble, J.A. (eds.) IPMI 2003. LNCS, vol. 2732, pp. 63–75. Springer, Heidelberg (2003)
9. Hug, J., Brechbühler, C., Székely, G.: Model-based initialisation for segmentation. In: Vernon, D. (ed.) ECCV 2000. LNCS, vol. 1843, pp. 290–306. Springer, Heidelberg (2000)

Contributions to 3D Diffeomorphic Atlas Estimation: Application to Brain Images[*]

Matias Bossa, Monica Hernandez, and Salvador Olmos

GTC, Aragon Institute of Engineering Research (I3A), University of Zaragoza, Spain
{bossa,mhg,olmos}@unizar.es

Abstract. This paper focuses on the estimation of statistical atlases of 3D images by means of diffeomorphic transformations. Within a Log-Euclidean framework, the exponential and logarithm maps of diffeomorphisms need to be computed. In this framework, the Inverse Scaling and Squaring (ISS) method has been recently extended for the computation of the logarithm map, which is one of the most time demanding stages. In this work we propose to apply the Baker-Campbell-Hausdorff (BCH) formula instead. In a 3D simulation study, BCH formula and ISS method obtained similar accuracy but BCH formula was more than 100 times faster. This approach allowed us to estimate a 3D statistical brain atlas in a reasonable time, including the average and the modes of variation. Details for the computation of the modes of variation in the Sobolev tangent space of diffeomorphisms are also provided.

1 Introduction

The construction of brain atlases is central to the understanding of the anatomical variability. Currently there is a great interest in developing 3D atlases of the human brain. Most research in the framework of Computational Anatomy has been directed towards the development of 3D brain atlases using image mapping algorithms [1,2]. In this paradigm the atlas works as a deformable template and the nonlinear transformations encode the variability of the population.

As the anatomical variability is very large the non-rigid mappings between any two subjects must have a large number of degrees of freedom. Diffeomorphisms have been recently proposed to characterise such transformations. While there is no obvious reason to support the use of diffeomorphisms for inter-subject registration, the invertibility property is crucial for statistical analysis.

One problem that persists is that most current atlases have been based on arbitrarily chosen individuals. This introduces a bias into the analysis when comparing individual brains to the atlas and does not provide a meaningful baseline with which to measure individual anatomical variation.

Most recent work [3,4] of statistical atlas building avoids the bias introduced by template selection. These methods compute diffeomorphisms by solving a

---

[*] This work was partially funded by research grants TEC2006-13966-C03-02, FIS PI04/1795 from Spain. M. Bossa work was funded by DGA under the FPI grant B097/2004.

N. Ayache, S. Ourselin, A. Maeder (Eds.): MICCAI 2007, Part I, LNCS 4791, pp. 667–674, 2007.
© Springer-Verlag Berlin Heidelberg 2007

minimization of a functional energy over the set of non-stationary smooth vector fields. For stationary vector fields, a Log-Euclidean framework was recently proposed [5] to extend the computation of statistics from finite [6,7] to infinite dimensional manifolds.

In this work we tackle two issues that arise when trying to estimate statistical atlases (mean and modes of variation) of 3D brain anatomy. The first issue concerns about the logarithm map required to compute the mean diffeomorphism. Recently, the Inverse Scaling and Squaring (ISS) method has been proposed to estimate the logarithm map [5]. An alternative approach is proposed in this work that drastically reduces the computational time. The second issue concerns about the selection of the distance on the manifold of diffeomorphisms and its implication on the estimation of the mean and the modes of variation.

The article proceeds as follows. A review of the properties of the group of diffeomorphisms is given in Section 2. The methods for the computation of the logarithm map are described in Section 3. The details of the statistical analysis are given in Section 4. The results are given in Section 5. Finally, some concluding remarks are provided in Section 6.

2   The Group of Diffeomorphisms in $\mathbb{R}^n$

A diffeomorphism is an invertible function that maps a subset of points in $\mathbb{R}^n$ to another, such that both the function and its inverse are smooth. The composition operator provides a structure of group to the set of diffeomorphisms. A diffeomorphism can be obtained as the solution of the transport equation $\dot{\phi}(t) = v(t, \phi(t))$ with initial condition $\phi(0) = e$, where $v : [0, 1] \rightarrow V$ is a flow of smooth vector fields in a Hilbert space $(V, \langle \cdot, \cdot \rangle_V)$ [8,9], and e is the identity. The inner product in V is usually defined as $\langle v, w \rangle_V = \langle Lv, Lw \rangle_{L^2}$ where L is a linear invertible differential operator that guarantees the smoothness of v and therefore the smoothness and invertibility of $\phi(t)$. The metric obtained from this inner product endows the tangent space V with a topological structure of a Sobolev space and the group of diffeomorphisms with a Riemannian manifold structure. In Computational Anatomy L is usually chosen as $L = \gamma + \alpha \Delta$, where Δ is the Laplacian operator, because it is a simple way to guarantee the invertibility of φ [8].

In a recent work [5] a subgroup of diffeomorphisms was obtained by constraining v to be a *stationary* vector field $\dot{\varphi}(t) = v(\varphi(t))$. On one hand, these diffeomorphisms have fewer degrees of freedom than the general case, but they showed to be versatile enough to describe the anatomical variability within a dataset of human brains from normal subjects [5]. On the other hand, diffeomorphisms parameterized by stationary vector fields present some advantages: the exponential and logarithm maps can be more easily computed[1].

Although Lie groups are finite dimensional by definition, diffeomorphisms can be proven to fulfil the basic properties of Lie groups, except for being infinite

---

[1] To our knowledge there has not been proposed any formula to compute the logarithm map of diffeomorphisms from non-stationary vector fields.

dimensional. As in the case of finite dimensional Lie groups, the logarithm map is required in order to compute statistics of a sample of diffeomorphisms. Recently the ISS method for matrices was applied to compute the logarithm map for diffeomorphisms parameterized by stationary vector fields [5]. The Baker-Campbell-Hausdorff (BCH) formula can be applied to compute the logarithm of a composition of exponentials in finite dimension Lie groups as $\exp_G^{-1}(\exp_G(x) \exp_G(y))$ is analytic. Many infinite dimensional Lie groups share this property, they are the so-called BCH-Lie groups [10]. To our knowledge, it has not been theoretically shown whether the diffeomorphisms group is a BCH-Lie group or not. Similarly, the applicability of the ISS method has not been theoretically justified, neither. In this work, we assumed that both approaches may be used for our application, at least formally. A simulation study with controlled ground truth was designed for performance comparison.

3   Logarithm of Diffeomorphisms

3.1   Inverse Scaling and Squaring Method (ISS)

A popular method for computing the logarithm of matrices is the ISS method. In [5] this method was applied to diffeomorphisms making use of $\log(\varphi) = 2^N \log(\varphi^{2^{-N}})$. First the squared root of φ is computed N times recursively. Then, as the result is close to the identity, the logarithm can be approximated by $\log(\varphi^{2^{-N}}) \approx \varphi^{2^{-N}} - I$.

Although the approximation looks very simple, it involves the computation of $N \approx 10$ squared roots. In order to compute squared roots, it was proposed to perform a gradient descent on the functional

$$E_{SQRT}(T) = \frac{1}{2} \int \|T \circ T - \varphi\|^2 (x) dx, \tag{1}$$

that demands a large computation time[2].

3.2   Baker-Campbell-Hausdorff (BCH) Formula

In a Lie group, the BCH formula gives a solution of the expression $u = \log(\exp(v) \circ \exp(w))$ as a series in terms of the Lie bracket $[\cdot, \cdot]$[3]:

$$u = v + w + 1/2\,[v, w] + 1/12\,[v, [v, w]] + 1/12\,[[v, w], w] +$$
$$+1/48\,[[v, [v, w]], w] + 1/48\,[v, [[v, w], w]] + O((\|v\| + \|w\|)^5) \tag{2}$$

---

[2] Even though the original gradient proposed in [5] in order to minimize Equation (1) was $\nabla E_{SQRT}(T) = (DT^t) \circ T.(T \circ T - \varphi) + \|\det(D(T^{-1}))\|(T - \varphi \circ T^{-1})$, which involves the need to compute iteratively the inverse of T, we found that it is much more accurate and faster to use $\nabla E_{SQRT}(T) = (DT^t) \circ T.(T \circ T - \varphi)$ instead.

[3] A Lie bracket $[\cdot, \cdot]$ is a bilinear operation defined in the tangent space, such that $[x, y] = -[y, x]$ (and therefore $[x, x] = 0$), and fulfills the Jacob identity, i.e. $[x, [y, z]] + [y, [z, x]] + [z, [x, y]] = 0$.

In the group of diffeomorphisms the Lie bracket is defined as the Lie derivative $[v, w] = vw - wv$, where vw is the derivative of w in the direction of v, i.e. $vw = \frac{\partial w}{\partial v} = \sum_{j=1}^{3} v^j \frac{\partial w}{\partial x^j}$, where v^j are the components of vector field v and x^j are the Cartesian coordinates. Thus

$$[v, w] = \sum_j v_j \frac{\partial w}{\partial x_j} - w_j \frac{\partial v}{\partial x_j} \qquad (3)$$

Although the BCH formula does not provide a method for the computation of the logarithm map in a general case, in many practical applications the argument of the logarithm can be written as a composition of two exponentials of known vector fields. In practice the use of Equation (2) instead of the ISS method results in a tremendous reduction of computational complexity. Note that this formula could be straightforwardly applied to non-stationary vector fields.

4   Statistics on 3D Diffeomorphisms

4.1   Average Computation Using BCH

Several distances can be defined on a Riemannian manifold. For example, $d(\varphi_1, \varphi_2) = \| \log(\varphi_1) - \log(\varphi_2) \|$, which is inversion-invariant, was used in [5] for diffeomorphisms. This distance has the drawback that it is not invariant under the composition of diffeomorphisms, i.e. it is not translation invariant. The Riemannian or intrinsic distance is defined as the length of the geodesic connecting φ_1 and φ_2, and it is given by $D(\varphi_1, \varphi_2) = \| \log(\varphi_2 \circ \varphi_1^{-1}) \|_V$. This distance is inversion- and translation-invariant. The drawback now is that an iterative procedure is required to compute the mean of N instances:

$$\bar{\varphi}^{(k+1)} = \exp \left(\frac{1}{N} \sum_i \log \left(\varphi_i \circ (\bar{\varphi}^{(k)})^{-1} \right) \right) \circ \bar{\varphi}^{(k)}, \qquad (4)$$

which involves the computation of the logarithm map. Equation (4) is the generalization to infinite dimension of the algorithm given in [7] to obtain the Riemannian center of mass.

We propose to rewrite Equation (4) in terms of the tangent space representations:

$$\exp(\bar{v}^{(k+1)}) = \exp \left(\frac{1}{N} \sum_i \log \left(\exp(v_i) \circ \exp \left(-\bar{v}^{(k)} \right) \right) \right) \circ \exp \left(\bar{v}^{(k)} \right) \qquad (5)$$

The BCH formula (2) can be used to compute $\log \left(\exp(v_i) \circ \exp \left(-\bar{v}^{(k)} \right) \right)$ as well as $\bar{v}^{(k+1)}$ in Equation (5) as follows:

$$\bar{v}^{(k+1)} = r^{(k)} + \bar{v}^{(k)} + \frac{1}{2} [r^{(k)}, \bar{v}^{(k)}] + \cdots \qquad (6)$$

$$r^{(k)} = \frac{1}{N} \sum_i \left(v_i - \bar{v}^{(k)} - \frac{1}{2} [v_i, \bar{v}^{(k)}] + \cdots \right) \qquad (7)$$

where $r^{(k)}$ corresponds to $\frac{1}{N}\sum_i \log\left(\exp(v_i) \circ \exp\left(-\bar{v}^{(k)}\right)\right)$. With this approach neither exponentials nor logarithms need to be computed.

4.2 Principal Geodesic Analysis

Principal Geodesic Analysis is the generalization to non-linear spaces [6] of Principal Component Analysis defined on Euclidean vector spaces. In a Lie group, it consists on finding a set of ordered geodesics that pass through the Riemannian center of mass, orthogonal to each other and with maximum projected variance. Note that some computational schemes to compute PCA, such as SVD, are only valid when the norm is Euclidean. As vectors Lv_i belong to a Hilbert space with Euclidean norm SVD can be computed on them.

Let be $\mathbf{X} = [\text{vec}(Lv_1), \text{vec}(Lv_2), \ldots, \text{vec}(Lv_N)]$ the matrix associated to the N residuals and $\mathbf{WSU}^T$ the corresponding SVD decomposition. Let $\mathbf{w}_j$ be the j-th column of $\mathbf{W}$ and w_j the vector field such that $\text{vec}(w_j) = \mathbf{w}_j$. As L is a linear and invertible operator $v_i = \sum_j (L^{-1}w_j)s_j\mathbf{u}_{i,j}$. The vector fields $L^{-1}w_j$ form an orthonormal basis, with respect to $\|.\|_V$ norm, and are the principal components. The standard deviation of each mode is $s_j/\sqrt{N}$. The j-th principal geodesic is $\rho_j(\theta) = \exp(\theta(L^{-1}w_j))$, $\theta \in \mathbb{R}$.

5 Results

5.1 Logarithm of Diffeomorphisms

In the first experiment, we generated two 3D random diffeomorphisms $\varphi_1 = \exp(v_1)$ and $\varphi_2 = \exp(v_2)$, sampled on a $32 \times 32 \times 32$ regular grid. Then we measured the accuracy of the estimation of $v_3 = \log(\varphi_3)$, where $\varphi_3 = \varphi_1 \circ \varphi_2$. Two random fields v_1 and v_2 were generated from zero-mean unit variance Gaussian random displacements on a $8 \times 8 \times 8$ regular grid interpolated on the finner grid with cubic splines. Finally v_1 and v_2 were scaled in order to get a wide range of diffeomorphism energy.

Both methods, ISS and BCH formula, were used to estimate v_3. Several orders of accuracy (0,1, and 2) were used for the BCH formula. Left hand side of Fig. 1 shows root mean squared (RMS) difference between φ_3 and $\exp(v_3)$. The ISS method provided valid results only for energies lower than 0.08, which actually is a deformation energy larger than what one expect in registration between real brain images. The difference among ISS method and 1st-2nd-order BCH formula was small compared to the grid spacing (3×10^{-2}). However, the computational time spent by the ISS method was more than 100 times longer than the time spent by the 1st-order BCH formula.

The implementation of the BCH formula is straightforward while many parameters must be tuned in the optimization procedure used by the ISS method. Our implementation of the ISS method used the gradient estimation of Equation 1 avoiding the estimation of the inverse. While faster convergence and more accuracy is obtained for small deformations, it broke down at an energy value of 0.07 .

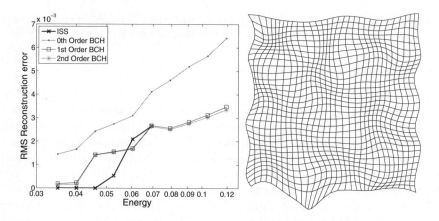

Fig. 1. Left: RMS difference between φ_3 and $\exp(v_3)$ vs. deformation energy. v_3 was estimated using ISS, 0th, 1st and 2nd Order BCH. Grid spacing is 3×10^{-2}. Right: 2D projection of a slice of φ_3 at energy 0.07.

5.2   Statistical Brain Atlas

A statistical brain atlas was built from a set of 19 T1-MRI images, acquired by a General Electric Signa Horizon CV 1.5 Tesla scan. As preprocessing steps, the images were resampled yielding a spatial resolution of $0.9 \times 0.9 \times 0.9$ mm, the skull was removed from the images using [11], the intensity images were normalised using a histogram matching algorithm, and aligned to a common coordinate system using a similarity transformation (7 dof).

Our scheme for unbiased atlas estimation is based on diffeomorphic registration with stationary vector fields, and was described in [12]. In this experimental section we make use of the benefit of the BCH formula.

The average brain atlas is shown in the bottom panels of Fig. 2. For comparison the linear average of brain images is also shown. Sharper details of anatomical structures can be seen in the atlas obtained with diffeomorphic transformations.

The first two modes of variation at ± 2 standard deviations are shown in Fig. 3 and 4. The modes of variation provide a nice and hierarchical illustration of the anatomical variability of the training set.

6   Conclusions

In this work the Baker-Campbell-Hausdorff formula was applied to the estimation of the logarithm map of 3D diffeomorphisms as well as to build a statistical atlas of brain images. We set up a simulation study for performance comparison in terms of accuracy and computational complexity of the ISS method and the BCH formula. Although the estimation error in both methods was similar, the computational time for BCH was more than 100 times shorter than for ISS. This reduction allowed us to estimate the mean and modes of variation from 19 3D brain images.

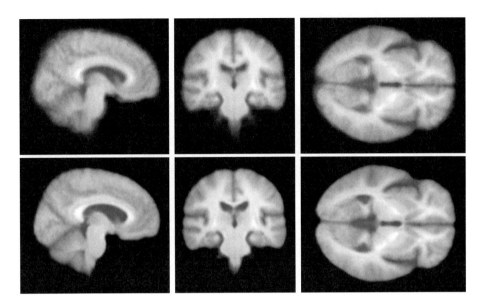

Fig. 2. Top: Linear average atlas. Bottom: Diffeomorphic atlas.

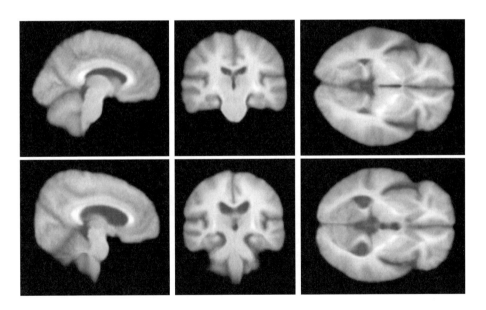

Fig. 3. First mode of variation at ±2 standard deviation

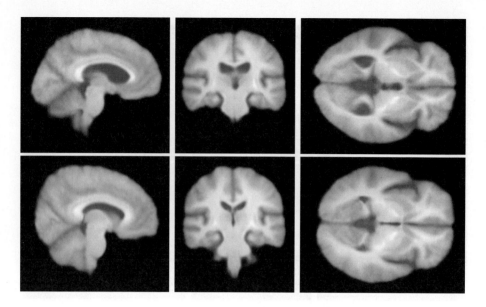

Fig. 4. Second mode of variation at ±2 standard deviation

References

1. Toga, A.W., Thompson, P.M.: A framework for computational anatomy. Computing and Visualization in Science 5, 13–34 (2002)
2. Grenander, U., Miller, M.I.: Computational Anatomy: an emerging discipline. Quaterly of Applied Mathematics 56, 617–694 (1998)
3. Avants, B., Gee, J.C.: Geodesic estimation for large deformation anatomical shape averaging and interpolation. Neuroimage 23(Supplement 1), S139–S150 (2004)
4. Joshi, S., Davis, B., Jomier, M., Gerig, G.: Unbiased diffeomorphic atlas construction for compuational anatomy. Neuroimage 23, 151–160 (2004)
5. Arsigny, V., Commonwick, O., Pennec, X., Ayache, N.: Statistics on diffeomorphisms in a Log-Euclidean framework. In: Larsen, R., Nielsen, M., Sporring, J. (eds.) MICCAI 2006. LNCS, vol. 4190, pp. 924–931. Springer, Heidelberg (2006)
6. Fletcher, P.T., Joshi, S., Lu, C., Pizer, S.M.: Principal geodesic analysis for the study of nonlinear statistics of shape. IEEE Trans. Med. Imaging 23(8), 994–1005 (2004)
7. Pennec, X.: Intrinsic statistics on Riemannian manifolds: Basic tools for geometric measurements. J. Math. Imag. Vis. 25(1), 127–154 (2006)
8. Arnold, V.: Mathematical methods of classical mechanics. Springer, Berlin, Germany (1989)
9. DoCarmo, M.P.: Riemannian geometry. Birkhäuser, Boston, USA (1992)
10. Glockner, H.: Fundamental problems in the theory of infinite-dimensional Lie groups. Journal of Geometry and Symmetry in Physics 5, 24–35 (2006)
11. Dodgas, B., Sattuck, D.W., Leahy, R.M.: Segmentation of skull and scalp in 3D human MRI using mathematical morphology. Hum. Brain Map (2005)
12. Hernandez, M., Bossa, M., Olmos, S.: Estimation of statistical atlases using groups of diffeomorphisms. Technical report, I3A, University of Zaragoza (2007), http://diec.unizar.es/intranet/articulos/uploads/I3ATR.pdf

Measuring Brain Variability Via Sulcal Lines Registration: A Diffeomorphic Approach

Stanley Durrleman[1,2], Xavier Pennec[1], Alain Trouvé[2], and Nicholas Ayache[1]

[1] INRIA - Asclepios Research Project, Sophia Antipolis, France
[2] Centre de Mathématiques et leurs applications, ENS de Cachan, Cachan, France

Abstract. In this paper we present a new way of measuring brain variability based on the registration of sulcal lines sets in the large deformation framework. Lines are modelled geometrically as currents, avoiding then matchings based on point correspondences. At the end we retrieve a globally consistent deformation of the underlying brain space that best matches the lines. Thanks to this framework the measured variability is defined everywhere whereas a previous method introduced by P. Fillard requires tensors extrapolation. Evaluating both methods on the same database, we show that our new approach enables to describe different details of the variability and to highlight the major trends of deformation in the database thanks to a Tangent-PCA analysis.

1 Introduction

Measuring brain variability among populations is a challenging issue. A very promising way as emphasized in [1,2] for instance is based on statistical analysis of brain deformations computed thanks to registrations of images or geometrical primitives like cortex surfaces, sulcal lines or landmarks. In the case of primitives, however, the registrations are rarely based on a consistent geometrical modelling of both primitives and deformations. We follow here the approach introduced in [3] and [4]: we model sulcal lines as currents. Such currents are then considered as 'geometrical landmarks' that guide a globally consistent deformation of the underlying biological material. After presenting this registration framework in section 2, we apply the method to a database of sulcal lines and deduce statistical measures of brain variability within the studied population in section 3. Eventually we show how the underlying geometrical modelling makes the measured variability different from this obtained in [5] on the same dataset but in a different framework (called here FAPA's), and how it enables to obtain new statistical results which may lead to new scientific findings.

2 Registering Lines Sets

Registering a lines set L_0 onto another L_1 consists in looking for the most regular deformation ϕ that acts on L_0 and best matches L_1. More precisely, we follow the approach proposed in [3]: the unknown deformation is searched in a subgroup of diffeomorphisms of the space $\mathbb{R}^3$ and the lines are modelled as currents. We find

N. Ayache, S. Ourselin, A. Maeder (Eds.): MICCAI 2007, Part I, LNCS 4791, pp. 675–682, 2007.
© Springer-Verlag Berlin Heidelberg 2007

the registrations thanks to the minimization of a cost function which makes a compromise between the regularity of the deformation and the fidelity to data.

2.1   Lines Modelled as Currents

The space of currents is a vector space which can be equipped with a norm that enables to measure geometrical similarity between lines. In this space, lines could be discrete or continuous and consists in several different parts. All these objects are handled in the same setting and inherit from many interesting mathematical properties: linear operations, convergence, etc.. Moreover, the distance between lines does not make any assumptions about point correspondences, even implicitly. This framework differs therefore from usual methods like in [6] where lines are considered as unstructured points set and "fuzzy" correspondences assumed.

We restrict now the discussion to what is needed in the following and we refer the reader to [7] and [3] for more details on the theory. We call here a line set L a finite collection of n continuously differentiable mappings $L_i : [i/n, (i+1)/n] \to \mathbb{R}^3$: $L = \cup_{i=0}^{n-1} L_i$. This formulation is compatible with discrete set of lines, each line L_i being given by n_i samples and $(n_i - 1)$ segments $[s_k^i, s_{k+1}^i]_{1 \leq k \leq n_i - 1}$.

A vector field ω is a differentiable mapping that associates to every points $x \in \mathbb{R}^3$ a vector $\omega(x) \in \mathbb{R}^3$. Let us denote W a linear space of vector fields. Our space of currents W^* is defined as the set of the continuous linear mappings from W to $\mathbb{R}$. A line set L can thus be seen as a current thanks to the formula:

$$\forall \omega \in W, \quad L : \omega \longrightarrow \int_0^1 <\omega(x_t), \tau(x_t)>_{\mathbb{R}^3} dt \qquad (2.1)$$

where τ is the unit tangent vector (defined almost everywhere) of the line set L at point x_t. For W we choose a reproducing kernel Hilbert space (r.k.h.s.) whose kernel K^W is isotropic and Gaussian (for more details on r.k.h.s, see [8]). This induces a norm on the space of currents that is computable in case of discrete lines. Indeed, when the line L is sampled, it can be approximated in W^* as the segments length tends to 0 by the sum of Dirac currents at the points (c_i) centers of the segments $[s_i, s_{i+1}]$: $L = \sum_k \delta_{c_k}^{\tau_k}$ where $\tau_k = s_{k+1} - s_k$. (for all vector field ω, $\delta_x^\alpha(\omega) = \langle \omega(x), \alpha \rangle_{\mathbb{R}^3}$: a Dirac current can be seen as a vector α concentrated at one point x). The Hilbertian inner product between $L = \sum_{i=1}^{n-1} \delta_{c_i}^{\tau_k}$ and $L' = \sum_{i=1}^{m-1} \delta_{c_i'}^{\tau_k'}$ where n *is not necessarily equal to* m is then given by: $\langle L, L' \rangle_{W^*} = \sum_{i=1}^{n-1} \sum_{j=1}^{m-1} \langle \tau_i, K^W(c_i, c_j')\tau_j' \rangle_{\mathbb{R}^3}$ where for all points x, y, $K^W(x, y) = g(x - y)\mathrm{Id}$ and g is a Gaussian function. The distance between two lines is then given by: $d^2(L, L') = \|L' - L\|_{W^*}^2 = \|L\|_{W^*}^2 + \|L'\|_{W^*}^2 - 2\langle L, L' \rangle_{W^*}$. This converges to the distance between two continuous lines when the segments lengths tend to zero. Eventually, this distance used as a fidelity to data term will prevent from systematically overfitted registrations.

2.2   Diffeomorphic Registration

We use here the large deformation framework founded in the paradigm of Grenander's group action approach for modelling objects (see [9,4,10,11]). This

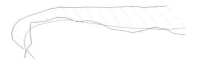

Fig. 1. Lines registration using an approach based on currents. Dark blue line is transported to the green line that matches the red line. The distance between red and green lines (i.e the precision of the matching) is computed although the sampling of each line is different, in particular no point to point correspondence is imposed.

framework enables to find a globally consistent deformation of the underlying space that best matches the lines sets. This differs from [5] where each line is registered individually without assuming spatial consistency of the displacement field. The global constraint as well as the introduction of a fidelity to data term lead to residual matching errors (the distance between red and green lines in figure 1) considered here as noise. In [5] denoising and matching are two separate processings.

The considered deformations are diffeomorphisms, solutions ϕ_1^v at time $t = 1$ of the flow equation: $\frac{\partial \phi_t}{\partial t} = v_t \circ \phi_t$ and $\phi_0 = \mathrm{id}_{\mathbb{R}^3}$. The tangent vector field v_t at each time t belongs to a r.k.h.s. V with kernel K^V that controls the regularity of the final diffeomorphisms. The induced norm defines in turn a distance between ϕ and the identity: $d_V^2(\mathrm{id}, \phi) = \inf \left\{ \int_0^1 \|v_t\|_V^2 \mid v \in L^2([0,1], V), \ \phi = \phi_1^v \right\}$.

In order to register a line onto another we define $\phi.L$ the action of a diffeomorphism ϕ on a current L by: $\phi.L(\omega) = L(\phi.\omega)$ and $\phi.\omega(x) = (d_x\phi)^t \omega(\phi(x))$ for all vector fields ω. This action coincides with the geometrical transportation of lines. In particular $\phi.\delta_x^\alpha = \delta_{\phi(x)}^{d_x\phi(\alpha)}$.

Our registration problem is to map a set of n labelled sulcal lines $L_0 = \cup_{i=1} L_{0,i}$ to another labelled set $L_1 = \cup_{i=1} L_{1,i}$. It is then reduced to the search of a family of vector fields $v : t \in [0,1] \longrightarrow v_t$ that minimizes the following cost function J: $J(v) = \gamma d_V^2(\mathrm{id}, \phi_1^v) + \sum_{i=1}^n \|\phi_1^v.L_{0,i} - L_{1,i}\|_{W^*}^2$ where γ controls the importance of the regularity against the fidelity to data.

It has been shown (in [4] for instance) that such an optimal diffeomorphism always exists, that its path defined by ϕ_t^v for the optimal v is geodesic with respect to the distance d_V and is an interpolation via the kernel K^V of the trajectories of the samples that numerically define the lines. Moreover we can show that one can recover the trajectory of any points of the space knowing only the initial speed at each lines samples. This means that a minimizing diffeomorphism is entirely determined by a finite set of parameters. This dramatic dimensionality reduction is of great importance to define statistics on deformations.

2.3 Experiments and Results

Through the Asclepios-LONI associated team **Brain-Atlas** we used the same dataset as in [5] of cortical sulcal landmarks (72 per brain) delineated in every subject scanned with 3D MRI (age: 51.8 +/- 6.2 years). In order to compare our measures of variability, we used the same set of 72 mean lines as in [5]. For 34 subjects in the database, we registered the mean lines set onto every subject's lines set. We computed the registrations thanks to J. Glaunès' algorithm detailed in [3]. We manually set $\gamma = 0.1$ and the standard deviation of K^V and K^W respectively to $\sigma_V = 25$mm and $\sigma_W = 5$mm. The diameter of the brains is about 120mm. For every subject deformations, we store the initial speed vectors of the mean lines samples that completely parametrize the deformation.

3   Statistics on Deformations

To do statistics, we take advantage of a tangent space representation like in [12] or [13] in case of finite dimensional manifolds. The deformations are indeed completely determined by their initial speed vector field that belongs to the linear space V provided by an Hilbertian norm $\|\|_V$. We recall that such a dense vector field is in turn parametrized by the finite set of initial speed vectors on the mean lines samples: $\{(v_{0,k}^s)\}$, $1 \le k \le N$ where N is the total number of mean lines samples, and that we stored these vectors for each of the 34 registrations. Statistics on deformations are then reduced to statistics in $\mathbb{R}^{3N}$ where the norm of the vector is the norm in V of its associated dense vector field. Our study is focused on variance which measures how locally the space is deforming and covariance which measures the correlations between different points trajectories.

Our results are then compared to those obtained by FAPA in [5] where the statistics are based on the mean lines samples displacement field computed from a point-to-point registration algorithm.

3.1   Variance of Deformations

At each mean lines sample k_0 we compute the empirical covariance matrix from the 34 initial speed vectors ($v_{0,k_0}^s \in \mathbb{R}^3$ for each subject s). These 3×3 matrices are represented as ellipsoids like in figure 2. They show how locally one point is varying among the studied population. On the other hand, thanks to the diffeomorphic approach, we can compute the tangent vector at each point of a 'mean brain surface' and hence the empirical covariance matrix of the deformations at those points. Figure 3 and 4 show such a surface where each point was coloured according to the 3D rms norm of the covariance matrix. In FAPA's method matrices computed on mean lines samples are downsampled and then extrapolated in the whole space thanks to a log-Euclidian framework ([13,14]). Comparing the results of both approaches highlights the different hypothesis made to model the lines, to remove noise and to extrapolate the variability to the brain surface.

Regularity of the Variability: The figure 2 shows that the point matching method of FAPA leads to irregular tensor fields at lines extremities and between lines whereas our global regularity constraint makes the retrieved variability spatially smoother. In our approach we leave aside the variability contained in the residual matching errors considered as noise. In FAPA's work the variability is denoised afterwards by removing extremal large tensors before the extrapolation.

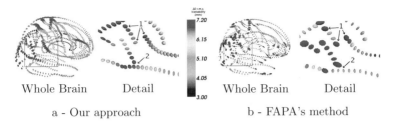

Fig. 2. At each sampling point, ellipsoids represent the square root of the empirical covariance matrix of the initial speed vectors (left hand side) or displacement field (right hand side). In FAPA's method, extremal points are supposed to be matched: this induces a high variability at lines extremities (area 1, right). This is avoided by the current approach (area 1, left). In FAPA's method each line is registered individually: the variance can vary dramatically at lines crossing (area 2, right). Our global regularity constraint leads to smoother results (area 2, left).

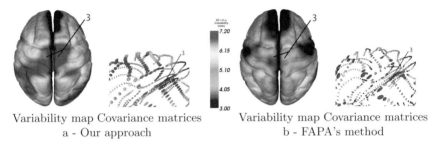

Fig. 3. On the variability maps, a tangential variability is retrieved in area 3 (extremities of central sulci) by our method and not by FAPA's one. The covariance matrices in this region show that the variability is mainly longitudinal. Since in FAPA's work large extremal tensors are removed before the extrapolation, the tangential variability is not captured and the total variability is small.

Tangential Variability: One major drawback of FAPA's method as underlined in [5] is the systematically under-estimated tangential variability. This aperture problem is particularly visible on the top of the brain as shown in figure 3. Our approach enables to find a larger part of this variability which is, as we will see, one of the major variation trends within the sample (cf fig. 6). Otherwise, the non-tangential part is in relative good agreement in most parts.

Distinction between correlated and anticorrelated motions: In our approach the deformation field is extrapolated before computing the covariance matrix. By contrast in FAPA's method the matrices are extrapolated without assuring that the extrapolated tensors derive from an underlying deformation. As shown figure 5 this difference theoretically enables in our case to distinguish between areas where samples are moving in a correlated or anti-correlated manner. This is a possible explanation of the different variability maps retrieved in

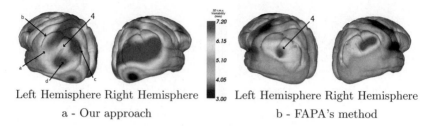

Left Hemisphere Right Hemisphere   Left Hemisphere Right Hemisphere

a - Our approach   b - FAPA's method

Fig. 4. Area 4 is surrounded by 4 major sulci: sylvius fissure (a), postcentral sulcus (b), intraparietal sulcus (c) and superior temporal sulcus (d). On the left hemisphere the first two move mostly in a decorrelated manner with respect to the last two sulci whereas their respective motions are much more correlated on the right hemisphere. Our approach tries to combine the motion of all lines and therefore leads to a small variability in area 4 on the left hemisphere and to a large one on the right hemisphere. With FAPA's method this asymmetry is not retrieved directly.

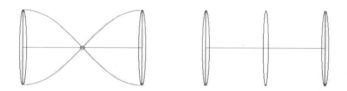

Fig. 5. Extrapolation schemes in the simple case of anti-correlated vectors. Right: In FAPA's framework the tensors are computed at the samples points and then extrapolated in the middle point: the tensor in the middle is similar to the two others. Left: In our approach we first extrapolate the vector field and then compute at each point the covariance matrix. Since the vectors are anti-correlated, the field is close to zero at the center and the variability measured at this point is negligible.

area 4 of figure 4. Note that the asymmetry we found between left and right hemispheres was also retrieved in other recent studies [15].

3.2   Principal Modes of Deformation

Let us see the field $\{v_{0,k}^s\}$ for each subject s as a unique vector in $\mathbb{R}^{3N}$ provided by the norm $\|\|_V$, (the norm of its associated dense vector field). We then carry out a Principal Component Analysis (PCA) on these vectors with respect to the given norm (e.g. the first principal mode is given by $\mathbf{argmax}_{v \neq 0} \frac{\sum_s \langle v_0^s, v \rangle_V^2}{\|v\|_V^2}$). This analysis enables to take into account the global correlations of all points motion together and synthesizes the main trends of deformation in the database.

Given a mode $\tilde{v} \in V$, we can compute the unique geodesic deformation process in the sense of the distance d_V whose initial tangent vector field is $\tilde{v}$. The eigenvectors $\tilde{v}$ were normalized ($\|\tilde{v}\|_V = 1$) so that the deformations are seen

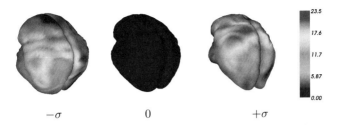

$$-\sigma \qquad\qquad 0 \qquad\qquad +\sigma$$

Fig. 6. First Mode of Deformation obtained by a PCA on initial vector speed fields. Original mean brain surface (Center) and its deformation at $-\sigma$ (Left) and $+\sigma$ (Right). Colours measure the displacement of each point along the deformation process (in mm).

between $[-\sigma, 0]$ for shooting the vector $-\tilde{v}$ and $[0, \sigma]$ for $\tilde{v}$. Results are shown figure 6. Movies of deformation are available at first author's webpage[1].

4   Conclusion and Perspectives

The framework presented here provides a consistent geometrical framework for measuring brain variability from sulcal lines registration. The lines are considered as *geometrical* objects and not as sets of landmarks, which means that we completely avoid computing point correspondences. A computable distance is defined on these lines that enables to include a noise model on lines within the framework. Although the optimal matching is parametrized with a finite set of parameters, the deformation field returned is dense, enabling to analyze the brain variability outside the data on the basis of an explicit deformation modelling. These three steps: denoising, lines matching and extrapolation are handled here consistlently in the same setting whereas they often lead to separate processings like in FAPA's work. This enables to give alternatives to some of the major drawbacks of other methods like the aperture problem for instance. The method is also generative: we can define an arbitrary deformation and hence generate deformed lines, illustrating thus the variability the method captured and highlighting the major trends of deformation within the database via a tangent-PCA analysis. Finally the approach is not limited to lines but could also be applied directly to register surface meshes (like in [16]) or images.

Besides such methodological advantages, the retrieved variability which differs from [5] are still to be validated by anatomical interpretations and by the model's predictive capability. At this stage, actually, the qualitative comparison mainly emphasizes the different hypothesis on which each model is based. Since our diffeomorphic constraint may be considered sometimes as too restrictive, one could define refinements that take into account possible local non diffeomorphic variations between subjects. Eventually, our new findings have to be confirmed by applying the method to other datasets of sulcal landmarks ([17]) or to other features that may be more relevant in an anatomical point of view. The integrative

---

[1] http://www-sop.inria.fr/asclepios/personnel/Stanley.Durrleman/

capability of the method could help actually to define a general model of brain variability based on multiple sources of input.

Acknowledgments We would like now to thank Paul Thompson (Lab of Neu-roImaging, UCLA School of Medicine) through the Asclepios-LONI associated team for providing the dataset of sulcal lines, Joan Glaunès (Lab. de Mathé-matiques Appliquées, Université Paris 5) whose code was used to compute the registrations and Pierre Fillard (INRIA-Asclepios) for giving access to his results. Images and movies were made using the software MedINRIA[2]. This work was partly supported by the European IP projet Health-e-Child (IST-2004-027749).

References

1. Ashburner, et al.: Identifying global anatomical differences: deformation-based morphometry. Human Brain Mapping 6(5-6), 348–357 (1998)
2. Chung, M., et al.: A unified statistical approach to deformation-based morphome-try. NeuroImage 18, 595–606 (2001)
3. Glaunès, J.: Transport par difféomorphismes de points, de mesures et de courants pour la comparaison de formes et l'anatomie numérique. PhD thesis, Université Paris 13 (2005), http://cis.jhu.edu/~joan/TheseGlaunes.pdf
4. Miller, M., Trouvé, A., Younes, L.: Geodesic shooting for computational anatomy. Journal of Mathematical Imaging and Vision (2006)
5. Fillard, P., Arsigny, V., Pennec, X., Hayashi, K., Thompson, P., Ayache, N.: Mea-suring brain variability by extrapolating sparse tensor fields measured on sulcal lines. NeuroImage 34(2), 639–650 (2007)
6. Chui, H., Rangarajan, A.: A new point matching algorithm for non-rigid registra-tion. Comput. Vis. Image Underst. 89(2-3) (2003)
7. Vaillant, M., Glaunès, J.: Surface matching via currents. In: Christensen, G.E., Sonka, M. (eds.) IPMI 2005. LNCS, vol. 3565, Springer, Heidelberg (2005)
8. Aronszajn, N.: Theory of reproducing kernels. Trans. Amer. Math. Soc. (68) (1950)
9. Grenander, U.: General pattern theory. Oxford Science Publications (1993)
10. Glaunès, J., Joshi, S.: Template estimation from unlabeled point set data and surfaces for computational anatomy. In: Proc. of Workshop MFCA (2006)
11. Marsland, S., Twining, C.: Constructing diffeomorphic representations for the groupwise analysis of non-rigid registrations of medical images. T.M.I (2004)
12. Vaillant, M., Miller, M., Younes, L., Trouvé, A.: Statistics on diffeomorphisms via tangent space representations. NeuroImage 23, 161–169 (2004)
13. Pennec, X., Fillard, P., Ayache, N.: A Riemannian framework for tensor computing. International Journal of Computer Vision 66(1), 41–66 (2006)
14. Arsigny, V., Fillard, P., Pennec, X., Ayache, N.: Log-Euclidean metrics for fast and simple calculus on diffusion tensors. M.R.M. 56(2), 411–421 (2006)
15. Fillard, P.: al: Evaluating brain anatomical correlations via canonical correlations analysis of sulcal lines (In: Stat. Registration and atlas formation)
16. Vaillant, M., Qiu, A., Glaunès, J., Miller, M.: Diffeomorphic metric surface mapping in subregion of the superior temporal gyrus. NeuroImage 34(3) (2007)
17. Mangin, J.F., et al: Object-based morphometry of the cerebral cortex. IEEE Trans. Med. Imag. (2004)

---

[2] http://www-sop.inria.fr/asclepios/software/MedINRIA/

Effects of Registration Regularization and Atlas Sharpness on Segmentation Accuracy

B.T. Thomas Yeo[1], Mert R. Sabuncu[1], Rahul Desikan[3], Bruce Fischl[2],
and Polina Golland[1]

[1] Computer Science and Artificial Intelligence Lab, MIT, USA
[2] Athinoula A. Martinos Center for Biomedical Imaging, MGH/MIT/HMS, USA
[3] Boston University School of Medicine

Abstract. In this paper, we propose a unified framework for computing atlases from manually labeled data at various degrees of "sharpness" and the joint registration-segmentation of a new brain with these atlases. In non-rigid registration, the tradeoff between warp regularization and image fidelity is typically set empirically. In segmentation, this leads to a probabilistic atlas of arbitrary "sharpness": weak regularization results in well-aligned training images and a "sharp" atlas; strong regularization yields a "blurry" atlas. We study the effects of this tradeoff in the context of cortical surface parcellation by comparing three special cases of our framework, namely: progressive registration-segmentation of a new brain to increasingly "sharp" atlases with increasingly flexible warps; secondly, progressive registration to a single atlas with increasingly flexible warps; and thirdly, registration to a single atlas with fixed constrained warps. The optimal parcellation in all three cases corresponds to a unique balance of atlas "sharpness" and warp regularization that yield statistically significant improvements over the previously demonstrated parcellation results.

Keywords: Registration, Segmentation, Parcellation, Multiple Atlases, Markov Random Field, Regularization.

1 Introduction

Automatic labeling of cortical brain surfaces is important for identifying regions of interests for clinical, functional and structural studies [3,14]. Recent efforts have ranged from the identification of sulcal/gyral ridge lines [15,17] to the segmentation of sulcal/gyral basins [3,5,8,9,11,13,14]. Similar to these prior studies, we are interested in parcellation of the entire cortical surface meshes, where each vertex is assigned a label, given a training set of manually-labeled cortical surfaces.

Probabilistic atlases are useful and prevalent in segmentation literature [3,5,12]. A typical initial step in atlas computation is the spatial normalization of the training images. Measures like the prior probability of a certain label at a location can then be computed. Spatial normalization can be achieved with different registration algorithms that can vary in the rigidity of warps, from affine [12] to fully nonrigid warps [5]. More restricted warps yield "blurrier" atlases that capture

N. Ayache, S. Ourselin, A. Maeder (Eds.): MICCAI 2007, Part I, LNCS 4791, pp. 683–691, 2007.
© Springer-Verlag Berlin Heidelberg 2007

inter-subject variability of structures, enlarging the basin of attraction for the registration of a new subject. However, the trade-off between robustness and accuracy, which is limited by the "sharpness" of the atlas, is typically ignored. Recent research [10] has shown that combining information about the warp rigidity and the residual image of the registration process can improve the classification accuracy of schizophrenic and normal subjects.

Finding the optimal warp regularization tradeoff has gathered attention in recent years. Twining *et al.* [2] and Van Leemput [7] propose frameworks to find the least complex models that explain the image intensity and segmentation labels respectively in the training images. This is useful if the goal is to analyze the training images. However, if the goal is new subject segmentation, then segmentation accuracy should drive the choice of warp regularization. An interesting question is whether outlier images require weaker regularization to warp closer to the population "average" and obtain better segmentation accuracy.

Joint registration-segmentation algorithms are generally more effective than sequential registration-segmentation as registration and segmentation benefit from additional knowledge of each other [1,12,18,19]. This paper proposes a joint registration-segmentation framework with Markov Random Field (MRF) priors on both segmentation labels and registration warps that incorporates multiple atlases. Our framework is an extension of Pohl *et al.* [12] and Fischl *et al.* [5].

Here we study the effect of atlas "sharpness" and warp regularization on segmentation accuracy. In particular, we compare 3 specific cases: (1) progressive registration of a new brain to increasingly "sharp" atlases using increasingly flexible warps, by initializing each registration stage with the optimal warps from a "blurrier" atlas; (2) progressive registration to a single atlas with increasingly flexible warps; (3) registration to a single atlas with fixed constrained warps.

Another contribution of this paper is the consistency of the co-registration of labeled images when computing the atlas and the normalization of an unlabeled test image to the atlas, i.e., we treat the atlas creation and new subject registration within the same framework. Finally, to the best of our knowledge, this is the first implementation of a joint registration-segmentation algorithm applied to the labeling of the cerebral cortex.

2   Theory and Implementation

2.1   Joint Registration and Segmentation

We define an atlas A_α to be an atlas trained from images aligned with warp smoothness parameter $S = \alpha$. We distinguish between α and S since one can use an atlas A_α for the registration of a subject with smoothness S where $\alpha \neq S$. Let R be the registration parameters, T be the image segmentation and Y be the observed image features. We obtain the joint registration-segmentation of a new image given a set of atlases A_α and smoothness S by maximizing the Maximum-A-Posteriori (MAP) objective function:

$$(R^*, T^*, S^*, A_\alpha^*) = \underset{R,S,A_\alpha,T}{\arg\max} \, p(R,T,S,A_\alpha|Y) = \underset{R,S,A_\alpha,T}{\arg\max} \, p(R,T,S,A_\alpha,Y) \quad (1)$$

where $p(\cdot)$ denotes probability. We can optimize Eq. (1) with coordinate ascent by iteratively optimizing one of the variables while fixing the remaining variables. Unfortunately, each iteration only finds the posterior mode of a random variable while disregarding its entire posterior distribution. Instead, we consider a variant of Eq. (1) where we marginalize over the segmentation T. Furthermore, for simplicity, we assume a uniform prior on S and A_α or equivalently treat them as non-random parameters, leading to the following formulation of the problem:

$$(R^*, S^*, A_\alpha^*) = \underset{R,S,A_\alpha}{\arg\max} \sum_T p(R,T,Y;S,A_\alpha) = \underset{R,S,A_\alpha}{\arg\max} \log \sum_T p(R,T,Y;S,A_\alpha). \quad (2)$$

This optimization can be solved by the Expectation-Maximization algorithm with the segmentation T as a hidden variable. To reduce computation time, instead of working with the continuous parameters α and S, we discretize S and A_α into a finite set $\{S, A_\alpha\} = \{S_1 > S_2 > \cdots > S_N, A_{S_1}, A_{S_2} \cdots A_{S_N}\}$, where larger values of α and S correspond to "blurrier" atlases and more restricted warps, respectively. The optimization criterion then becomes

$$\max_{S,A_\alpha} \left\{ \max_R \log \sum_T p(R,T,Y;S,A_\alpha) \right\} \quad (3)$$

With enough samples, the finite set $\{S, A_\alpha\}$ should sufficiently represent the underlying continuous space of atlases and warps. Given an unlabeled brain with image features Y, we consider the following schemes:

1. Multiple Atlas, Multiple Warp Scales (MAMS): multiscale approach where we optimize Eq. (3) w.r.t. R with "blurry" atlas A_{S_1} and warp regularization S_1, and use that to initialize the registration with sharper atlas A_{S_2} and warp regularization S_2, and so on.
2. Single Atlas, Multiple Warp Scales (SAMS): multiscale approach where we optimize Eq. (3) w.r.t. R with a fixed atlas A_{S_k} and warp regularization S_1, and use that to initialize the registration with the fixed atlas A_{S_k} and warp regularization S_2, and so on.
3. Single Atlas, Single Warp Scale (SASS): Optimize Eq. (3) w.r.t. R with a fixed atlas A_{S_k} and warp regularization S_m, where k might not be equal to m. This is most common in practice, especially when mixing and matching publicly available atlases and in-house registration algorithms.

Note that for each scheme, we do not search over values of S or α, but instead optimize the term within the curly brackets in Eq. (3), which we denote the mixed Maximum-Likelihood Maximum-A-Posteriori (ML-MAP) function:

$$\log \sum_T p(R,T,Y;S,A_\alpha) = \log p(R;S,A_\alpha) + \log \sum_T p(T,Y|R;S,A_\alpha) \quad (4)$$

$$= \log p(R;S) + \log \sum_T p(T,Y|R;A_\alpha) \quad (5)$$

where we have modeled the registration parameters R to be conditionally independent of the atlas A_α given the scale S. We also assume that both the segmentation T and the observation Y are independent of the scale S conditioned on the atlas A_α and registration R. Eq. (5) corresponds to the standard setup of the EM algorithm. In the E-step, we compute

$$Q(R; R^{(n)}) = \log p(R; S) + \sum_T p(T|Y, R^{(n)}; A_\alpha) \log p(T, Y|R; A_\alpha) \qquad (6)$$

where registration $R^{(n)}$ is obtained from the previous M-step. In the M-step we optimize $Q(R, R^{(n)})$ with respect to registration R:

$$R^{(n+1)} = \arg\max_R Q(R; R^{(n)}) \qquad (7)$$

So far, the derivations have been general without any assumptions about the atlases A_α, the prior $p(R; S)$ or the image-segmentation fidelity $p(T, Y|R; A_\alpha)$.

2.2   Model Instantiation

We now apply the above framework to the joint registration-parcellation of cortical brain surfaces, represented by triangular meshes with a spherical coordinate system that minimizes metric distortion [4]. The aim is to register an unlabeled cortical surface to a set of manually labeled surfaces and classify each vertex of the triangular mesh into anatomical units.

We model the warp regularization with a MRF parameterized by S:

$$p(R; S) = \frac{F(R)}{Z_1(S)} \exp\left\{ -S\left[\sum_i \sum_{j \in \mathcal{N}_i} \left(\frac{d_{ij}^R - d_{ij}^0}{d_{ij}^0} \right)^2 \right] \right\} \qquad (8)$$

where d_{ij}^R is the distance between vertices i and j under registration R, d_{ij}^0 is the original distance, $\mathcal{N}_i$ is a neighborhood of vertex i and $Z_1(S)$ is the partition function. Our regularization penalizes metric distortion weighted by a scalar S that reflects the amount of smoothness (rigidity) of the final warp. Function $F(\cdot)$ ensures invertibility and is zero if any triangle is folded by warp R and one otherwise.   Similarly, we impose a MRF prior on the parcellation labels:

$$p(T, Y|R; A_\alpha) = p(T|R; A_\alpha)p(Y|T, R; A_\alpha)$$
$$= \frac{1}{Z_2(A_\alpha)} \exp\left\{ \sum_i U_i(T_i; A_\alpha) + \sum_i \sum_{j \in \mathcal{N}_i} V(T_i, T_j; A_\alpha) \right\} \prod_i p(Y_i|T_i, R; A_\alpha) \,(9)$$

where T_i and Y_i are vertex i's parcellation label and observation respectively. The local potential $U_i(T_i; A_\alpha)$ captures the frequency of label T_i at vertex i. The compatibility function $V(T_i, T_j; A_\alpha)$ reflects the likelihood of labels T_i and T_j being neighbors. $Z_2(A_\alpha)$ is the partition function dependent on the atlas A_α.

Incorporating Eq. (8, 9) into $Q(R; R^{(n)})$ of Eq. (6) and discarding all terms independent of R yields (with some work!)

$$Q(R; R^{(n)}) = \log F(R) - S\sum_i \sum_{j \in \mathcal{N}_i} \left(\frac{d_{ij}^R - d_{ij}^0}{d_{ij}^0} \right)^2 + \sum_i \sum_{T_i} \left\{ p(T_i|Y, R^{(n)}; A_\alpha)U_i(T_i; A_\alpha) \right.$$
$$\left. + \left[\sum_{j \in \mathcal{N}_i} p(T_i, T_j|Y, R^{(n)}; A_\alpha)V(T_i, T_j; A_\alpha) \right] + p(T_i|Y, R^{(n)}; A_\alpha) \log p(Y_i|T_i, R; A_\alpha) \right\} \,(10)$$

where the first term prevents folding triangles, the second term penalizes metric distortion, the third and four terms are the Markov prior on the labels and the last term is the likelihood of the surface geometries given the segmentation.

2.3 Atlas Building

In our framework, the atlas construction is consistent with the registration of a new brain. Consider registering a training subject to the atlas A_{S_k} under the smoothness S_k. Using the same objective function from before, the E-step is trivial since we know the ground truth segmentation T^*, and hence $p(T|Y, R^{(n)}; A_\alpha)$ is the delta function $\delta(T^* - T)$. Simplifying the M-step gives (for each subject):

$$R^* = \arg\max_R \log p(R; S_k) + \log p(T^*, Y|R; A_{S_k}). \tag{11}$$

We can then warp each subject to a common coordinate system via registration R^*, and create atlas A_{S_k}. However, since A_{S_k} is unknown and yet appears on the right hand side of Eq. (11), we solve Eq. (11) using a fixed-point iterative method, where we initialize A_{S_k}, solve for the best R^*, create a new atlas A_{S_k} with R^* and repeat until convergence. In practice, we first create an atlas A_∞ after simple rigid-body registration and use it to initialize the creation of atlas A_{S_1}, where S_1 corresponds to an almost rigid warp. We then use atlas A_{S_1} to initialize the creation of atlas A_{S_2} where $S_1 > S_2$, and so on.

2.4 Implementation

The atlas A_S is defined by the local potential U, compatibility potential V and observation model $p(Y_i|T_i, R; A_\alpha)$. Features Y (sulcal depth and mean curvature) for the MRF and training follow that of Fischl et al. [5], except for simplicity, we set V to be spatially stationary and isotropic.

Computing $p(T_i|Y, R'; A_\alpha)$ and $p(T_i, T_j|Y, R'; A_\alpha)$ is NP-hard. Mean field approximation [6,16] yields the following fixed-point iterative solution:

$$b_i(k) \propto e^{U_i(k)+\log p(Y_i|T_i=k,R;A_\alpha)+\sum_{j\in\mathcal{N}_i}\sum_{T_j} b_j(T_j)[V_{ij}(k,T_j)+V_{ji}(T_j,k)]} \tag{12}$$

where $b_i(k)$ approximates the true belief $p(T_i = k|Y, R'; A_\alpha)$ and must be normalized at the end of each step. Estimating $p(T_i, T_j|Y, R'; A_\alpha)$ requires a variation of mean field [16]. To maximize over registration R in Eq. (10, 11), we warp each vertex of the mesh individually, and use conjugate gradient ascent with parabolic line search on a coarse to fine grid pyramid. The final segmentation is obtained by selecting the label with the highest posterior probability $p(T_i|Y, R^*; A_\alpha)$ for each vertex i and given atlas A_α.

3 Experiments

We consider 39 left hemispheres manually parcellated by a neuroanatomical expert, consisting of 35 labels (see Fig. 1). We use dice measure to evaluate

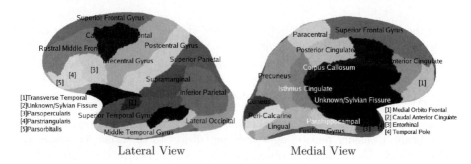

Lateral View   Medial View

Fig. 1. Example of manual parcellation shown on a partially inflated cortical surface. Note that our neuroanatomist prefer gyri labels to sulci labels. There are also regions where sulci and gyri are grouped together as one label, such as the superior and inferior parietal complexes. Some labels in the images are of different colors for contrast.

segmentation quality and compare our results to the algorithm demonstrated by Fischl et al. [5] and extensively validated by Desikan et al. [3]. The benchmark algorithm is essentially "Single Atlas, Single Warp Scale" (SASS), but with sequential registration-segmentation and a more complex MRF model.

We perform cross-validation 4 times by leaving out subjects 1 to 10 in the atlas construction, followed by joint registration-segmentation of subjects 1 to 10. We repeat with subjects 11 to 20, 21 to 30 and finally 31 to 39. We select S to be the set $\{100, 50, 25, 12.5, 8, 5, 2.5, 1, 0.5, 0.25, 0.1, 0.05, 0.01\}$, where we find that in practice, $S = 100$ corresponds to allowing minimal metric distortion and $S = 0.01$ corresponds to allowing almost any distortion.

Fig. 2(a) shows a plot of average dice (defined as the ratio of cortical surface area with correct labels to the total surface area averaged over the test set) for SAMS ($A_\alpha = A_1$) and MAMS as we vary S. The average dice peaks at $S = 1$ for all cross-validation trials, although individual variation exists (not shown). Smaller values of regularization parameter S allow larger warps for the outlier subjects because the tradeoff in the cost function is skewed towards data-fidelity over regularization. However, it is surprising to find that the optimal S is mostly constant across subjects.

In general, the mixed ML-MAP objective function of Eq. (3, 4) is not a good measure of the optimal (S, α): the ML-MAP function continues to improve as S decreases due to overfitting. Instead, we use dice as an independent measure of selecting the optimal (S, α). Empirically, finding the best S for each individual subject only improves the average dice minimally and hence, we are contented with choosing $S = 1$.

Fig. 2(b) shows a plot of dice averaged over all 39 subjects. SAMS performs the best for $\alpha = 1$. For illustration, we see that $SAMS$ with $\alpha = 0.01$ starts off well, but eventually overfits with a worse peak at $S = 1$ ($p < 10^{-5}$ for one-sided paired-sampled t-test). Similarly for SASS, the best α and S are both 1. We also show SASS with $\alpha = 0.01$ and $S = 1$ in Fig. 2(b). The differences among MAMS, SAMS or SASS at their optimum, $\alpha = 1$, $S = 1$, are not statistically significant.

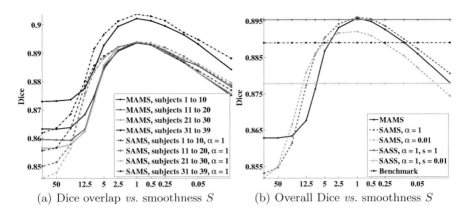

(a) Dice overlap *vs.* smoothness S (b) Overall Dice *vs.* smoothness S

Fig. 2. Summary of registration-segmentation results. S is plotted on a log scale.

On the other hand, their optimal performance is statistically significantly better than the benchmark, with all p-values less than 10^{-4}.

Because dice computed over the entire surface can be deceiving by suppressing small structures, we show in Fig. 3a the dice for each individual structure averaged over 39 subjects for MAMS ($S = 1$). The structures with the worst dice are the frontal pole and corpus callosum. Fig. 3a also shows the difference in dice between MAMS and the benchmark for each structure. For each structure, we perform the one-sided paired-sampled t-test between MAMS and the benchmark, where each subject is considered a sample. Results are shown in Fig. 3(b). Structures with p-values less than 0.05 are shown in dark blue. MAMS achieves statistically significant improvement over the benchmark for 16 structures. For the remaining 19 structures, the differences between the two segmentations are not statistically significant.

The optimal SAMS and SASS perform similarly to optimal MAMS, which is the unfortunate result of the local nature of gradient ascent. This is especially problematic on cortical surfaces where two adjacent sulci might appear quite similar locally. Incorporating multiscale features with multiple warp scales should therefore be more effective. Ultimately, however, a major hindrance is the accuracy of the manual segmentation. In well-defined regions such as pre- and post-central gyri, accuracy is already as high as 95% and within the range of inter-rater variability. In ambiguous regions, such as the frontal pole, inconsistent manual segmentation leads to poor atlas and less accurate segmentation validation.

Further work involves the application of our framework to other data sets and experiment with other models of data fidelity and regularization. We expect the optimal smoothness would change but it would be interesting to verify if the optimal smoothness for a given experimental condition stays almost constant for all subjects.

To conclude, we proposed a joint registration-segmentation framework that incorporates consistent atlas construction, multiple atlases and MRF priors on

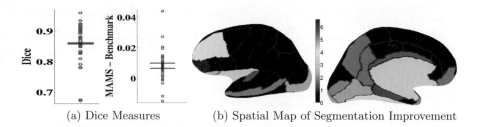

(a) Dice Measures   (b) Spatial Map of Segmentation Improvement

Fig. 3. (a) Dice of MAMS ($S = 1$) for individual structures (left) and improvement over the benchmark (right). (b) Spatial distribution of $-\log_{10}(p)$, where p is the p-value of the one-sided paired-sampled t-test between MAMS and the benchmark algorithm for each structure. Structures with p-values below 0.05 are colored dark blue.

both registration warps and segmentation labels. We showed that atlas "sharpness" and warp regularization are important factors in segmentation. With the proper choice of atlas "sharpness" and warp regularization, even with a less complex MRF model, the joint registration-segmentation framework has better segmentation accuracy than the state-of-the-art benchmark algorithm.

Acknowledgments. Support for this research was provided in part by the NIH NCRR (P41-RR14075, P41-RR13218, R01 RR16594-01A1 and the NCRR BIRN Morphometric Project BIRN002, U24 RR021382), the NIH NIBIB (R01 EB001550), the NIH NINDS (R01 NS052585-01 and R01 NS051826) the Mental Illness and Neuroscience Discovery (MIND) Institute, the National Alliance for Medical Image Computing (NAMIC, Grant U54 EB005149), and the NSF CAREER Award 0642971. Thomas Yeo is funded by the Agency for Science, Technology and Research, Singapore.

References

1. Ashburner, Friston: Unified Segmentation. NeuroImage 26, 839–851 (2005)
2. Twining, et al.: A unified information theoretic approach to groupwise non-rigid registration and model building. IPMI 9, 1–14 (2005)
3. Desikan, et al.: An auto. labeling system for subdividing the human cerebral cortex on MRI scans into gyral based regions of interest. NeuroImage 31, 968–980 (2006)
4. Fischl, B., et al.: Cortical Surface-Based Analysis II: Inflation, Flattening, and a Surface-Based Coordinate System. NeuroImage 9(2), 195–207 (1999)
5. Fischl, B., et al.: Automatically Parcellating the Human cerebral Cortex. Cerebral Cortex 14, 11–22 (2004)
6. Kapur, T., et al.: Enhanced Spatial Priors for Segmentation of Magnetic Resonance Imagery. In: Wells, W.M., Colchester, A.C.F., Delp, S.L. (eds.) MICCAI 1998. LNCS, vol. 1496, pp. 457–468. Springer, Heidelberg (1998)
7. Van Leemput, K.: Probabilistic Brain Atlas Encoding Using Bayesian Inference. In: Larsen, R., Nielsen, M., Sporring, J. (eds.) MICCAI 2006. LNCS, vol. 4190, pp. 704–711. Springer, Heidelberg (2006)
8. Klein, A., Hirsch, J.: Mindboggle: a scatterbrained approach to automate brain labeling. NeuroImage (24), 261–280 (2005)

9. Lohman, G., von Cramon, D.Y.: Automatic labelling of the human cortical surface using sulcal basins. Medical Image Analysis 4, 179–188 (2000)
10. Makrogiannis, S., et al.: A Joint Transformation and Residual Image Descriptor for Morphometric Image Analy. using an Equiv. Class Formulation. MMBIA (2006)
11. Mangin, et al.: Auto. construction of an attributed relational graph representing the cortex topography using homotopic trans. Proc. SPIE 2299, 110–121 (1994)
12. Pohl, K.M., et al.: A Bayesian model for joint segmentation and registration. NeuroImage, 31–228 (2006)
13. Rettmann, M.E., et al.: Automated Sulcal Segmentation Using Watersheds on the Cortical Surface. NeuroImage 15, 329–344 (2002)
14. Riviere, D., et al.: Automatic recognition of cortical sulci of the human brain using a congregation of neural networks. Medical Image Analysis 6, 77–92 (2002)
15. Tao, X., et al.: Using a Statistical Shape Model to Extract Sulcal Curves on the Outer Cortex of the Human Brain. Trans. Medical Imaging 21, 513–524 (2002)
16. Zhang, J.: The Mean Field Theory in EM Procedures for Markov Random Fields. IEEE Transactions on signal Processing 40(10), 2570–2583 (1992)
17. Zheng, S., et al.: A Learning Based Algorithm for Automatic Extraction of the Cortical Sulci. In: Larsen, R., Nielsen, M., Sporring, J. (eds.) MICCAI 2006. LNCS, vol. 4190, pp. 695–703. Springer, Heidelberg (2006)
18. Wyatt, P., Noble, J.: MAP MRF Joint Segmentation and Registration. In: MICCAI, pp. 580–587 (2002)
19. Yezzi, A., et al.: A variational Framework for Joint Segmentation and Registration. IEEE MMBIA (2001)

Generalized Surface Flows
for Deformable Registration and Cortical Matching

I. Eckstein[1], A. A. Joshi[2], C.-C. J. Kuo[2], R. Leahy[2], and M. Desbrun[3]

[1] Department of Computer Science, University of Southern California, USA
[2] Signal and Image Processing Institute, University of Southern California, USA
[3] Department of Computer Science, Caltech, USA

Abstract. Despite being routinely required in medical applications, deformable surface registration is notoriously difficult due to large intersubject variability and complex geometry of most medical datasets. We present a general and flexible deformable matching framework based on generalized surface flows that efficiently tackles these issues through tailored deformation priors and multiresolution computations. The value of our approach over existing methods is demonstrated for automatic and user-guided cortical registration.

1 Introduction

Matching (or registration) of deformable surfaces is a fundamental problem in medical image analysis and computational anatomy. One particularly challenging instance of the problem arises in the field of human brain mapping, where deformable registration of two cortical surfaces is required for intersubject comparisons and intrasubject analysis of neuroanatomical surface data. Related studies include progression of disorders such as Alzheimer's disease, brain growth patterns, genetic influences [1] and the effects of drug abuse on the structure and function of the brain [2]. The challenge in registering two cortices lies in the wide inter-subject variability and the convoluted geometry of the cortical surface, representing a real "stress test" for any general deformable registration technique. Various landmark-based and landmark-free methods have been developed [3,4,5,6,7,8]. Parameterization-based techniques first find a mapping between the cortical surface and a plane or a sphere, then align in the parameter domain cortical features such as mean curvature [2,5,6] or sulcal landmarks [8,9]. The often large change in metric due to the mapping needs to be accounted for while performing the alignment process in the parameter domain [9,10], adding to the computational costs. Another class of techniques operates directly in the ambient space by finding a 3D warping field that aligns the cortical features. Most of these methods are volume-based, aiming to align image features such as intensities [11] or invariant geometric moments [12], rather than surfaces. As a result, their matching of the cortices often exhibits inaccuracies.

In this paper we present a new, general, and flexible computational framework for deformable surface matching, based on the notion of *generalized* flows of discrete surfaces. Generalized flows were introduced recently in [13] and [14] in the Eulerian setting (i.e., for implicit surface representations), and extended to the Lagrangian (mesh-based) case in [15]. The proposed method iteratively deforms a 3D template

N. Ayache, S. Ourselin, A. Maeder (Eds.): MICCAI 2007, Part I, LNCS 4791, pp. 692–700, 2007.
© Springer-Verlag Berlin Heidelberg 2007

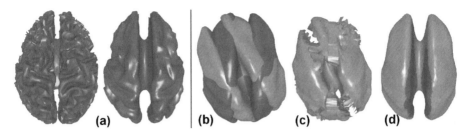

Fig. 1. A white matter cortex and its corresponding Partially Flattened Surface (**a**), where the major sulci are still clearly present. A basic Hausdorff gradient flow applied on a rotated, smoother version (**b**) creates spurious deformations (**c**) due to lack of coherence and local minima, while with a quasi-rigid deformation prior (**d**), it successfully recovers the transformation.

surface to match the target, until convergence criteria are met. As a result, the whole deformation trajectory is available as a by-product for evaluation and determination of the best fit.

The use of geometric flows in medical image analysis is not new: for instance, active contours (or snakes) and deformable models have been widely applied to reconstruct surfaces from volumetric images (*e.g.*, [16]). The main drawback of these methods is their sensitivity to local minima, which can become particularly severe when matching of geometrically complex objects is sought. Here we show a way to systematically deal with this issue using problem-specific prior knowledge. The contributions of this paper are as follows:

- We present a computational framework for surface matching based on *generalized* discrete geometric flows. By allowing custom *deformation priors*, the generalized approach significantly helps avoiding local minima and provides additional flexibility and control over the registration process, as well as robustness to noise.
- The proposed framework uses a triangle mesh (Lagrangian) representation for surface matching. Compared to the Eulerian methodology, this approach is both topology-preserving by definition and efficient by nature, confining computations strictly to the object boundary. Moreover, this representation can provide point correspondences between two surfaces at any chosen resolution.
- We formulate the alignment problem as a minimization process of a pseudo-Hausdorff distance and show a practical application of the method to cortical matching.
- The basic algorithm is optimized using a surface multiresolution representation, allowing efficient handling of complex models and faster convergence.

2 Method

A typical shape matching problem considers two 3D models—a *template* and an *instance*—assumed to have some "meaningful" but unknown mapping between them. The matching problem is thus to find such a valid mapping between the two shapes, generally involving a non-rigid mapping in medical applications. We start with a brief overview of our approach to the problem of deformable shape matching, before proceeding to the specific (and challenging) case of cortical surface matching.

2.1   Object Alignment as a Geometric Optimization

The task of aligning two objects is often cast as a geometric distance minimization problem: a common approach to registration is to deform one of the shapes (typically, the template) so as to minimize its "distance" to the other shape. Since an L^2-type distance measure is known to be too forgiving in comparing two shapes, we opt instead for the symmetric Hausdorff distance which, for two surfaces $\mathcal{S}$ and $\mathcal{T}$, is given by

$$d(\mathcal{S}, \mathcal{T}) = \max \left[\max_{p \in \mathcal{S}} \min_{q \in \mathcal{T}} \|p - q\| , \max_{q \in \mathcal{T}} \min_{p \in \mathcal{S}} \|p - q\| \right].$$

Since this expression is not differentiable, we adopt a pseudo-Hausdorff distance $d_H(\mathbf{X}, \mathbf{Y})$ between two distinct meshes $\mathbf{X} = \{\mathbf{x}_i\}_{i=1..P}$ and $\mathbf{Y} = \{\mathbf{y}_j\}_{j=1..Q}$, based on a method introduced in [17] in the context of Level Sets, and adapted in [15] to handle irregularly shaped polygonal meshes. This allows us to formulate distance minimization as an iterative gradient descent procedure, where the template mesh $\mathbf{X}$ is evolved (or flowed) at each step in the direction of the negative gradient of $d_H(\mathbf{X}, \mathbf{Y})$, with $\mathbf{Y}$ being the instance mesh. This process is known as *gradient flow*, and can be written as the following PDE:

$$\frac{d\mathbf{X}}{dt} = -\mathbf{M}^{-1} \frac{\partial d_H}{\partial \mathbf{X}}(\mathbf{X}, \mathbf{Y}), \tag{1}$$

where $\mathbf{M}$ is a finite element lumped (diagonal) *mass matrix* [18] associated with the mesh $\mathbf{X}$ to account for non-uniform sampling, and $\frac{\partial d_H(\mathbf{X}, \mathbf{Y})}{\partial \mathbf{X}}$ is given by

$$\frac{\partial d_H(\mathbf{X}, \mathbf{Y})}{\partial \mathbf{x}_i} = \frac{(d_H(\mathbf{X}, \mathbf{Y}) + \varepsilon)^{1-2\alpha}}{P \cdot Q} M_{ii}^x \sum_j \frac{\mathbf{x}_i - \mathbf{y}_j}{d_{ij}^{\alpha+1}} M_{jj}^y (f_i^{-2} + g_j^{-2}), \tag{2}$$

$$\text{where } d_H(\mathbf{X}, \mathbf{Y}) = \left[\frac{1}{P} \sum_i M_{ii}^x f_i^{-1} + \frac{1}{Q} \sum_j M_{jj}^y g_j^{-1} \right]^{\frac{1}{2\alpha}} - \varepsilon,$$

$$\text{and } f_i = \frac{1}{Q} \sum_j M_{jj}^y d_{ij}^{-\alpha}, \quad g_j = \frac{1}{P} \sum_i M_{ii}^x d_{ij}^{-\alpha}, \quad d_{ij} = |\mathbf{x}_i - \mathbf{y}_j|^2 + \varepsilon^2,$$

with M_{ii}^x and M_{jj}^y are elements of the mass matrices of $\mathbf{X}$ and $\mathbf{Y}$, respectively, and $\varepsilon > 0$, $\alpha \geq 0$ are parameters [15]. However, as illustrated by Figure 1 (right) such a naïve minimization is unlikely to yield relevant correspondences between two dissimilar shapes, as the energy landscape is too complex and non-linear to avoid getting stuck in one of the numerous local minima.

2.2   Generalized Hausdorff Flow

One important detail is that the definition of the gradient in Eq. 1 is implicitly based on the L^2 inner product on the deformation space [13], which in fact can be replaced by any valid inner product. In particular, given the L^2 inner product and *any self-adjoint positive-definite linear operator* $\mathbf{L} : U \rightarrow U$ (U being the deformation space), a *new* inner product can be defined by

$$\langle \mathbf{u}, \mathbf{v} \rangle_{\mathbf{L}} = \langle \mathbf{u}, \mathbf{L}\mathbf{v} \rangle_{L^2} = \langle \mathbf{L}\mathbf{u}, \mathbf{v} \rangle_{L^2}. \tag{3}$$

This is a special type of inner product, as it is defined with respect to the L^2 norm. The advantage is that, given the L^2-gradient ∇_{L^2} of any surface energy functional $\mathcal{E}$, the *generalized gradient* [13] of $\mathcal{E}$ can be defined by

$$\nabla_{\mathbf{L}}\mathcal{E}(\mathbf{X}) = \mathbf{L}^{-1}\nabla_{L^2}\mathcal{E}(\mathbf{X}) . \qquad (4)$$

This leads to the definition of a *generalized Hausdorff flow*:

$$\frac{d\mathbf{X}}{dt} = -(\mathbf{ML})^{-1}\frac{\partial\, d_H}{\partial\mathbf{X}}(\mathbf{X},\mathbf{Y}) .$$

The operator $\mathbf{L}$ should be chosen so as to reflect prior knowledge about the nature of a problem-specific deformation, and is therefore called a *deformation prior* (not to be confused with probabilistic priors used in Bayesian estimation). Thus, this procedure is of practical interest because it allows us to *modify any existing L^2 gradient flow*. Note that the energy itself is never altered by a prior—it is only the optimization *path* that is. We will now show two particular priors useful in many deformable registration contexts.

2.3   Deformation Priors

Sobolev Deformation Prior. As most conventional gradient flows are based on the L^2 norm of vector fields which disregards the spatial coherence of a deformation, they can produce highly irregular motion and are susceptible to noise and local minima. To address these flaws, Sundaramoorthi *et al.* [14] proposed a regularizing inner product, namely, a Sobolev norm, in the context of Eulerian (Level Sets) active contours. For meshes, the Sobolev norm H^1 derives from the following inner product:

$$\langle\mathbf{u},\mathbf{v}\rangle_{H^1} = \int_S \mathbf{u}(\mathbf{x})\cdot\mathbf{v}(\mathbf{x})d\mathbf{x} + \lambda\int_S \nabla\mathbf{u}(\mathbf{x})\cdot\nabla\mathbf{v}(\mathbf{x})d\mathbf{x} .$$

Using Eq. 3 and integration by parts, we can show that this inner product corresponds to the linear operator $\mathbf{L}_{H^1}(\mathbf{u}) = \mathbf{u} - \lambda\Delta\mathbf{u}$, where Δ is the discrete Laplace-Beltrami operator [19], and λ is an arbitrary weighting factor. Equipped with this deformation prior, we can define the H^1-gradient of the pseudo-Hausdorff distance (or any other surface energy $\mathcal{E}$), and perform an explicit integration of the corresponding gradient flow. This yields:

$$\mathbf{X}_{t+dt} = \mathbf{X}_t - dt\,(\mathrm{Id} - \lambda\Delta)^{-1}\frac{\partial\mathcal{E}}{\partial\mathbf{X}}(\mathbf{X}_t).$$

Thus, a step of Sobolev gradient flow is computed by solving the following linear system:

$$(\mathrm{Id} - \lambda\Delta)\mathbf{X}_{t+dt} = (\mathrm{Id} - \lambda\Delta - dt\,\frac{\partial\mathcal{E}}{\partial\mathbf{X}})\mathbf{X}_t. \qquad (5)$$

Consequently, the solution of this sparse and symmetric linear system couples the motion of each vertex to the motion of the other vertices. This exemplifies the regularization effect: vertices that move independently in an L^2 flow will now move in concord.

For a stronger regularization effect, we can extend to above scheme to higher order Sobolev-type norms. For instance, we can define a higher-order prior $\mathbf{L}(\mathbf{u}) = \mathbf{u} + \mu\Delta^2\mathbf{u}$,

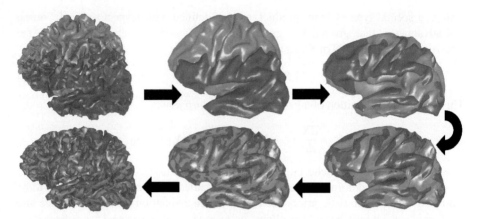

Fig. 2. Automatically matching a template (grey) to the subject cortex (blue). Partially flattened representations of both surfaces are iteratively aligned using a Hausdorff flow with a smoothing prior. The obtained alignment yields a correspondence between the original surfaces. The final color mix is due the fact that the surfaces lie on each other.

where $\Delta^2 = \Delta \circ \Delta$. With a slightly higher computational cost, the resulting scheme is equivalent to regularizing the instantaneous deformation with a thin-plate spline energy term (see e.g. [20]). In practice, we stick to the H^1 prior in this work.

Quasi-rigid Deformation Prior. Since the two input shapes are generally given in separate coordinate frames, it is often desired to first bring them into a rigid alignment. For that purpose we can use the quasi-rigid deformation prior $\mathbf{L}_R$ (see [13,15] for the Eulerian and Lagrangian derivations, respectively). Due to space constraints, we will not reproduce its formulation here. In essence, it can be seen as a linear filter that boosts the rigid component of a given motion field by a user-specified factor. As a result, an arbitrarily-rigid surface flow can be obtained. Figure 1 shows a successful quasi-rigid alignment of two cortices with this prior.

Note that since each of prior is given by a linear operator, we can also design a combined $\mathbf{L}_{R,H^1}$ prior which is a weighted combination of the two above operators, such that the rigid motion is prioritized and the non-rigid residual is smoothed. The result is a single prior that covers both phases of the registration process.

2.4 Matching Cortical Surfaces

Basic Algorithm We are now ready to apply the Hausdorff flow approach to match a template cortical surface (e.g., a digital atlas of the cortex) to an instance surface, e.g., segmented from a MRI scan. One naïve solution would be to perform the minimization directly on the input surfaces, combined with the H^1 deformation prior for regularization. This process is still likely to get stuck in a local minimum due to the highly convoluted geometry of the cortex. Even if we managed to get the two surfaces into a complete alignment, the result would hardly be adequate, as intercortex correspondence is in general not well-defined due to extreme variability of the cortical structures. In practice, quality of match is measured by the alignment of the major sulcal patterns that can be consistently identified in all brains. Thus, minimum intersurface distance alone is not a sufficient condition for an acceptable solution. In view if this problem, the use of Partially Inflated Surfaces (PFS) has been advocated for cortical matching [6]. The idea is to smooth out excessive surface detail through, e.g., Mean Curvature Smoothing [21]); a limited amount of smoothing is performed in order to facilitate matching while preserving the principal sulcal patterns—see Figure 1(a) for an illustration. We adopt this approach, with one important difference. While correspondence between two PFSs is typically computed by matching their maps in a common parameter domain, we eliminate these intermediate mappings by aligning the PFSs directly. Our strategy is summarized below, and illustrated in Figure 2:

ALGORITHM:

1. Partially flatten S and T, obtaining S' and T', respectively.
2. Apply Generalized Hausdorff Flow to achieve an arbitrarily close alignment of S' with T', yielding a correspondence map φ between the two.
3. Return $S \to S' \xrightarrow{\varphi} T' \to T$ as a bijective map between S and T.

The first step can be done rapidly using Mean Curvature Smoothing (MSC), with implicit time integration allowing an arbitrarily large time step. Note that MSC is a classical example of gradient flow, so our whole approach fits nicely into the flow-based methodology. The crux of the algorithm lies in the second step, where the template PFS S' (which can be precomputed for repeated use) is iteratively deformed to match T'. To regularize the flow, we use the $\mathbf{L}_{R,H^1}$ operator from Section 2.3. In practice, once the rigid component of the motion vanishes, $\mathbf{L}_{R,H^1}$ can be replaced with a simpler H^1 prior for efficiency. As the surfaces get closer, we switch to implicit time integration (Eq. 5) to avoid oscillations and accelerate convergence.

Finally, to make the process even more efficient for high-resolution models, the basic minimization algorithm is cast in a multiresolution framework, yielding a speedup of several orders of magnitude. A coarse match is first computed for simplified versions [22] of both PFSs, before refining them back to the original resolution (using *pyramid coordinates* [23]) for final alignment. Thus, our approach applies multiscale strategies to reduce both geometric and computational complexities: geometrically—using partial flattening to find a mapping, and computationally—employing coarser meshes to optimize performance.

Adding Constraints. As shown in Figure 3, the above procedure manages to automatically align most sulci, but cannot guarantee a correct match when a strong sulcal variability is present. A common remedy is to incorporate constraints, i.e., expert-specified sulcal curves, to control the mapping. In our case, adding constraints to the pseudo-Hausdorff energy is quite straightforward. Indeed, matching of two curves on opposite surfaces is just another distance minimization problem—this time, between sets of surface points that lie on the two curves. Thus, we can reuse the same Hausdorff distance approach, applying a separate, similar energy term to those mesh vertices that are incident on the curves (instead of the global Hausdorff potential). Adding point constraints, if needed, is even simpler. Note also that the constrained deformation is still kept smooth due to the use of the H^1 prior.

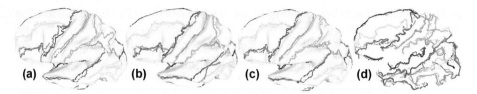

Fig. 3. a. Automatic matching of PFSs yields a close alignment for most sulcal curves. **b.** Constraining only 7 out of the 23 available curves reduces most misalignments, further improved by using the full set of constraints (**c**). **d.** Corresponding sulcal alignment for the original cortical surfaces. For clarity, a single cerebral hemisphere is shown.

3   Results

The proposed cortical matching algorithm was tested with a dataset of six subject brains, segmented from MRI scans using the BrainSuite tool [24], each supplemented with a set of sulcal curves marked by an expert according to the LONI Sulcal Tracing Protocol [1]. As illustrated by Figure 2, the algorithm automatically computes a near zero-distance alignment for two partially inflated cortical surfaces, effectively yielding an intercortex correspondence. It results in a reasonably close alignment for most sulcal curves, further improved through the addition of constraints. Figure 3 shows that most sulci could be matched automatically, and constraining only a subset of the sulcal curves is sufficient, thus significantly reducing the amount of manual effort required.

Table 1 summarizes a limited evaluation of our algorithm (GHF), compared to HAMMER [12], based on six pairs of subject brain images. Although the two methods operate on different modalities, distances between corresponding subject and deformed template sulcal curves can be measured in both cases. Even without resorting to constraints (to make a fair comparison to the landmark-free HAMMER), our method demonstrates a comparable quality of match, with clearly superior computation times: under 5 min on a standard PC, as opposed to several hours. Note also that for PFS sulci, registration error is even lower, which illustrates the quality of the core deformable matching procedure.

Table 1. Quality of match between deformed template and subject brains as average L^2 distances between corresponding sulcal curves

Method / Data	Mean L^2 Distance Per Case (mm)						Total Average
HAMMER / Original Sulci	4.67	4.62	4.79	5.05	5.13	4.90	4.87
GHF / Original Sulci	5.49	5.02	4.56	5.16	4.97	4.53	4.96
GHF / PFS Sulci	4.13	3.87	3.54	4.12	4.07	3.32	3.84

4   Discussion and Future Work

We have presented a practical and flexible multiresolution framework for deformable surface registration, based on generalized geometric flows. In the case of cortical matching, initial evaluation indicated quality comparable to state of the art methods, with near-interactive computation times. The presented solution is not without limitations: for instance, self-intersections may occur during the deformation, e.g., in presence of constraints (in fact, one can design constrained configurations not having any intersection-free solution). This shortcoming can be addressed through a special deformation prior added to the constraint energy term, e.g., a prior that prioritizes tangential motion. We are also investigating ways to generalize the definition of geometric distance and design new priors to improve automatic matching of sulcal features. Using generalized flows to compute continuous morphs that follow geodesics in shape spaces [25,26] is another exciting avenue of future work.

Acknowledgements. This work was partially funded by NSF (CAREER CCR-0133983, and ITR DMS-0453145), and DOE (DE-FG02-04ER25657).

References

1. Thompson, P.M., Mega, M.S., Vidal, C., Rapoport, J., Toga, A.W.: Detecting disease-specific patterns of brain structure using cortical pattern matching and a population-based probabilistic brain atlas. In: Insana, M.F., Leahy, R.M. (eds.) IPMI 2001. LNCS, vol. 2082, pp. 488–501. Springer, Heidelberg (2001)
2. Nahas, G.G., Burks, T.F. (eds.): Drug Abuse in the Decade of the Brain. IOS Press, Amsterdam (1997)
3. Hurdal, M.K., Stephenson, K., Bowers, P.L., Sumners, D.W.L., Rottenberg, D.A.: Coordinate system for conformal cerebellar flat maps. NeuroImage 11, S467 (2000)
4. Bakircioglu, M., Grenander, U., Khaneja, N., Miller, M.I.: Curve matching on brain surfaces using frenet distances. Human Brain Mapping 6, 329–333 (1998)
5. Fischl, B., Sereno, M.I., Tootell, R.B.H., Dale, A.M.: High-resolution inter-subject averaging and a coordinate system for the cortical surface. Human Brain Mapping 8, 272–284 (1998)
6. Tosun, D., Rettmann, M.E., Prince, J.L.: Mapping techniques for aligning sulci across multiple brains. Medical Image Analysis 8(3), 295–309 (2005)
7. Wang, Y., Gu, X., Hayashi, K., Chan, T., Thompson, P., Yau, S.: Brain surface parameterization using riemann surface structure. In: Duncan, J.S., Gerig, G. (eds.) MICCAI 2005. LNCS, vol. 3749, pp. 657–665. Springer, Heidelberg (2005)
8. Joshi, A., Shattuck, D., Thompson, P., Leahy, R.: A framework for registration, characterization and classification of cortically constrained functional imaging data. In: Christensen, G.E., Sonka, M. (eds.) IPMI 2005. LNCS, vol. 3565, Springer, Heidelberg (2005)
9. Thompson, P., Toga, A.: A framework for computational anatomy. Computing and Visualization in Science 5, 1–12 (2002)
10. Litke, N., Droske, M., Rumpf, M., Schröder, P.: An image processing approach to surface matching. In: Proceedings of the Symposium on Geometry Processing (2005)
11. Woods, R.P., Grafton, S.T., Holmes, C.J., Cherry, S.R., Mazziotta, J.C.: Automated image registration: I. J. Comp. Assist. Tomogr. 22, 139–152 (1998)
12. Shen, D., Davatzikos, C.: Hammer: Hierarchical attribute matching mechanism for elastic registration. IEEE Trans. Med. Imaging 21(8) (2002)
13. Charpiat, G., Keriven, R., Pons, J.P., Faugeras, O.: Designing spatially coherent minimizing flows for variational problems based on active contours. In: ICCV (2) pp. 1403–1408 (2005)
14. Sundaramoorthi, G., Yezzi, A., Mennucci, A.C.G.: Sobolev active contours. Int. J. of Comp. Vision (to appear)

15. Eckstein, I., Pons, J.P., Tong, Y., Kuo, C.C., Desbrun, M.: Generalized surface flows for mesh processing. In: Symposium on Geometry Processing (2007)
16. Xu, C., Prince, J.L.: Snakes, shapes, and gradient vector flow. IEEE TIP 7(3), 359–369 (1998)
17. Charpiat, G., Faugeras, O., Keriven, R.: Approximations of shape metrics and application to shape warping and empirical shape statistics. FoCM 5(1), 1–58 (2005)
18. Meyer, M., Desbrun, M., Schröder, P., Barr, A.: Discrete differential-geometry operators for triangulated 2-manifolds. In: Proc. of the Int. Workshop on Vis. and Math. (2002)
19. Pinkall, U., Polthier, K.: Computing discrete minimal surfaces and their conjugates. Experimental Mathematics 2(1), 15–36 (1993)
20. Chui, H., Rangarajan, A.: A new point matching algorithm for non-rigid registration. Computer Vision and Image Understanding 89(2-3), 114–141 (2003)
21. Desbrun, M., Meyer, M., Schröder, P., Barr, A.: Implicit fairing of irregular meshes using diffusion and curvature flow. ACM SIGGRAPH, 317–324 (1999)
22. Garland, M., Heckbert, P.: Surface simplification using quadric error metrics. In: Proceedings of ACM SIGGRAPH, pp. 209–216 (1997)
23. Sheffer, A., Kraevoy, V.: Pyramid coordinates for morphing. 3DPVT, 68–75 (2004)
24. Shattuck, D.W., Leahy, R.M.: BrainSuite: an automated cortical surface identification tool. Med. Image Anal 6(2), 129–142 (2002)
25. Beg, M., Miller, M., Trouvé, A., Younes, L.: Computing Large Deformation Metric Mappings via Geodesic Flows of Diffeomorphisms. IJCV 61(2), 139–157 (2005)
26. Kilian, M., Mitra, N.J., Pottmann, H.: Geometric modeling in shape space. In: ACM Transactions on Graphics (SIGGRAPH), ACM Press, New York (2007)

Real-Time Nonlinear Finite Element Analysis for Surgical Simulation Using Graphics Processing Units*

Zeike A. Taylor[1,2], Mario Cheng[1], and Sébastien Ourselin[1]

[1] BioMedIA Lab, e-Health Research Centre, CSIRO ICT Centre, Level 20, 300
Adelaide St, Brisbane, QLD, 4000, Australia
[2] Centre for Medical Image Computing, University College London, Gower St,
London, WC1E 6BT, UK
z.taylor@cs.ucl.ac.uk, {Mario.Cheng, Sebastien.Ourselin}@csiro.au

Abstract. Clinical employment of biomechanical modelling techniques
in areas of medical image analysis and surgical simulation is often
hindered by conflicting requirements for high fidelity in the modelling approach and high solution speeds. We report the development of
techniques for high-speed nonlinear finite element (FE) analysis for surgical simulation. We employ a previously developed nonlinear total Lagrangian explicit FE formulation which offers significant computational
advantages for soft tissue simulation. However, the key contribution of
the work is the presentation of a fast graphics processing unit (GPU)
solution scheme for the FE equations. To the best of our knowledge this
represents the first GPU implementation of a nonlinear FE solver. We
show that the present explicit FE scheme is well-suited to solution via
highly parallel graphics hardware, and that even a midrange GPU allows
significant solution speed gains (up to 16.4×) compared with equivalent
CPU implementations. For the models tested the scheme allows real-
time solution of models with up to 16000 tetrahedral elements. The use
of GPUs for such purposes offers a cost-effective high-performance alternative to expensive multi-CPU machines, and may have important
applications in medical image analysis and surgical simulation.

1 Introduction

The accurate simulation of tissue deformations arising during surgical procedures presents a formidable modelling challenge [1]. The constitutive behaviour
of soft tissues is well known to be nonlinear and time-dependent [2], and the
ability of these tissues to undergo large deformations without damage means
that linear small strain kinematic formulations are not strictly valid. In many
applications, notably surgical simulation [3,4] and intraoperative non-rigid medical image registration [5,6,7], there is a requirement for rigorous modelling of
nonlinear deformation. The most physically consistent procedure for estimating such deformations is to use differential equations of continuum mechanics,

---

* This work was performed while the first author was with the BioMedIA Lab.

N. Ayache, S. Ourselin, A. Maeder (Eds.): MICCAI 2007, Part I, LNCS 4791, pp. 701–708, 2007.
© Springer-Verlag Berlin Heidelberg 2007

solved using a numerical technique such as the finite element (FE) method [8]. However a major drawback of such procedures, especially nonlinear ones, is the significant computation times that may be required to solve large models. In many cases successful employment of simulation results depends crucially on the speed with which the results can be obtained. In the case of intraoperative image registration, extended delays while a patient is in the operating position are unacceptable, while interactive surgical simulations require solution at haptic feedback rates (>500Hz).

An efficient total Lagrangian explicit dynamic (TLED) FE algorithm was recently proposed for this purpose [9]. The main advantage of the formulation was that spatial derivatives were referred to the initial configuration of the body under analysis, and could therefore be precomputed. The use of explicit time integration also allowed calculations to be performed in an element-wise fashion, and so avoided the need for solution of large systems of algebraic equations, and allowed for easy incorporation of elaborate constitutive models. As will be seen, it is precisely this feature which renders the algorithm highly suitable for parallel execution.

In recent years there has been a growing body of work concerned with use of graphics processing units (GPUs) for general purpose computations [10]. By appropriately abstracting the graphics computational pipeline and the data upon which it operates, GPUs may be viewed as highly parallel computational engines. As a result GPU implementations of a range of non-graphics algorithms have been presented, for example including linear algebraic applications, ordinary and partial differential equation solvers, image analysis applications, and others (see review by Owens et al. [10]).

In this paper we present an efficient GPU implementation of the nonlinear TLED algorithm, suitable for simulation of soft tissues. The algorithm accounts for all geometric nonlinearities associated with the large deformations which occur in a surgical scenario. Importantly, we achieve significant improvements in solution speed compared with an equivalent CPU implementation, meaning that models of a useful size may be solved in real-time[1]. The significance of the results for purposes of surgical simulation and non-rigid image registration are discussed.

2   Total Lagrangian Explicit Dynamic Framework

Our implementation is based on the TLED algorithm described in [9]. Further details may be obtained from [8] also. The essential steps (from the point of view of GPU implementation) of the algorithm are as follows.

1. Precompute element shape function derivatives $\partial\mathbf{h}$ and mass matrix $\mathbf{M}$.
2. During each time step, n:
   - Apply loads (displacements) and boundary conditions to relevant nodal degrees of freedom.

---

[1] In which solutions for a time step are obtained in less time the size of the step itself.

- Loop over elements and compute the deformation gradient $\mathbf{X}^n$, strain-displacement matrix $\mathbf{B}_L^n$, 2nd Piola-Kirchhoff stresses $\mathbf{S}^n$, and element nodal forces $\hat{\mathbf{F}}^n$, and add these forces to the total nodal forces $\mathbf{F}^n$.
- Loop over nodes and compute new displacements $\mathbf{U}^{n+1}$ using the central difference method.

A detailed discussion of the formulation and computation of element matrices for various element topologies is presented in [8].

3 GPU Implementation of the TLED Algorithm

As is apparent from Section 2 the TLED algorithm consists of a precomputation phase and a time-loop phase. Since the precomputation phase is performed off-line and only once, our approach was to precompute relevant variables using standard CPU execution, load these variables into textures, and perform all time-loop computations using the GPU. Textures are arrays of values stored in GPU memory which are accessible by the fragment processors during a render pass. Individual texture elements are referred to as *texels*. Each texel may store up to four floating point values, representing red, blue, and green pixel colour values, plus a transparency value (RGBA). By maintaining all simulation variables (displacements, forces, etc) on the GPU itself, we minimise the amount of (time-consuming) CPU-GPU communication that takes place during the simulation.

The time-loop is executed as two render passes (RP1 and RP2), corresponding to the element- and node-loops described in Section 2. Computations are performed on the GPU's *fragment processors*. Loading is applied by prescribing displacements of loaded nodes.

We use a linear tetrahedral element formulation [8]. While these elements are known to produce inferior results when used for simulation of nearly incompressible materials [11], from a data structure point of view they provide significant advantages for GPU implementation. Since each element comprises four nodes, and each node posseses three degrees of freedom, all element matrices have dimensions which are multiples of these values, and are therefore very convenient for storage in four channel (RGBA) texels. Other element topologies such as hexahedra could be implemented in the same way, but all element matrices would be doubled in size and require twice as many texture reads. Additionally, recent efforts have produced 4-node tetrahedron formulations which overcome the locking phenomenon to a large extent [12]. For these reasons we do not feel that use of linear tetrahedra significantly diminishes the contributions of this first GPU development.

Material constitutive response is modelled using a Neo-Hookean model [8].

3.1 Render Pass 1: Element Loop

The purpose of RP1 is to compute element nodal force contributions $\hat{\mathbf{F}}^n$. All precomputed element data are stored in 2D textures on the GPU prior to commencement. The dimensions of the textures are calculated such that the number of texels equals the number of elements. At each time step, prior to execution of RP1, the GPU viewport is reset to these dimensions also to ensure the correct number of pixels are rendered. As the GPU renders the viewport the coordinates for each pixel are generated by the rasterizer and passed to the fragment processors [13]. By maintaining the same scale for rendered pixels and element-associated textures the coordinates of a pixel can be directly used to reference any data relevant to the corresponding element. This is known as 1:1 mapping and is commonly used in general purpose GPU applications.

Computation of element nodal forces requires the element nodal displacements, shape function derivatives, and volume. The latter two may be accessed from textures directly using the generated pixel coordinates. Displacements are accessed via a lookup texture, in which each texel contains the four node indices (from which displacement texture coordinates may be computed) for the current element. With these data retrieved the element nodal forces may be computed using the procedure decribed in [9].

For each element 12 force values are produced at each time step. The force contributions from each element must be summed to obtain the total forces on each node. Ideally, the computed forces would be added to a global nodal force vector as they are computed, but this would involve random texture writes (so-called *scatter operations*) which are currently prohibited. Therefore, force values computed in RP1 are written to textures, which are subsequently read and summed during the second render pass (node loop). The scatter operation is therefore reformulated as a *gather*. Four force textures are attached to the frame buffer to accommodate the four nodal force vectors produced by each element.

3.2   Render Pass 2: Node Loop

In RP2 the element nodal forces computed in RP1 are summed and used to compute new nodal displacements $\mathbf{U}^{n+1}$. The next set of imposed displacements on contacted nodes are also applied. The viewport is reformatted to dimensions equivalent to the number of nodes in the system in order to achieve a 1:1 mapping with the node-associated textures attached during this pass. Additionally, the four force textures rendered during RP1 are reattached as an array of input textures for RP2.

The major task of the fragment program for RP2 is the gathering of the element nodal force contributions for the current node. The locations and numbers of the relevant force values in the four force textures are determined via two lookup textures, labelled NodeElCrds and FCrds. The latter contains lists of force texture coordinates for each node in the system. Since node valencies are not constant, it is not possible (or is very inefficient) to structure this texture with a fixed mapping to the viewport dimensions. Therefore texture NodeElCrds (which does have the dimensions of the viewport), is used to provide the location of the first force texture coordinate in FCrds for the current node, and also the valence of this node. The fragment program then fetches and sums the required number of force values from the force textures using a dynamic loop structure. It then remains to compute $\mathbf{U}^{n+1}$, as mentioned.

4   Performance of the Algorithm

In order to assess the performance of the GPU implementation, we analysed two configurations: a cube model undergoing stretching and a brain model subject to indentation (see Fig. 1). The first served to illustrate the relative speed improvement achieved with the GPU, while the second constituted an example of relevance to both interactive surgical simulation and non-rigid image registration. In both cases we compared the solution times per time step for the GPU implementation with that of an equivalent CPU implementation. The GPU version was coded using Cg [14] and OpenGL [13], while the CPU version was written using C++. The test machine included a single 3.2GHz Intel P4 CPU and 2GB of RAM. An NVIDIA GeForce 7900GT GPU (550MHz clock speed, 512MB RAM) was used. Solution times were obtained for a range of mesh densities for each model. In each case five simulations were run, and the mean solution times are reported.

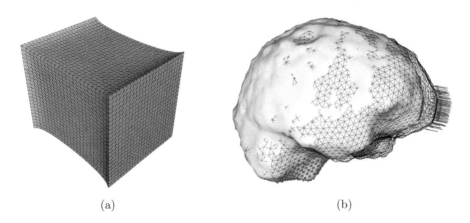

(a)   (b)

Fig. 1. (a) Cube model (82944 elements) after stretching by 20%. (b) Overlaid images of the undeformed (wire-frame) and deformed (surface) brain model (46655 elements). Anchor nodes near the brain stem are identified by spheres. Locations of displaced nodes and their displacement directions are indicated by arrows. Computation times for these mesh densities were 4.88ms/time step and 3.46ms/time step, respectively.

4.1   Stretching of a Cube Model

A series of cube models with edge lengths of 0.1m were constructed. Meshes with from 6000 to 82944 elements were used. The models were used to simulate stretching (by 20%) of a cube in which the displaced face and its opposing face were assumed to be fixed to loading platens. Lamé parameters were $\lambda = 49329$Pa and $\mu = 1007$Pa, chosen to correspond to a generally accepted stiffness value for brain tissue of $E = 3000$Pa, with a Poisson ratio of $\nu = 0.49$ (approximating incompressibility) [9]. Mass density was assumed to be that of water, i.e. $\rho = 1000$kg/m^3. It should be noted that the critical time step size for explicit analyses such as these is dependent on the material parameters used and the minimum characteristic element length in the mesh [8]. For this reason we report the solution times *per time step*, which are independent of these.

The GPU-computed deformed shape is shown in Fig. 1(a). The CPU and GPU solution results were identical in all respects. The mean solution times and ratios of solution times for each model size are plotted in Figs. 2(a) and (b), respectively. The solution times scaled approximately linearly with model size for both CPU and GPU implementations, which may be expected since the main computational effort of the algorithm is the *element-wise* computation of nodal forces $\hat{\mathbf{F}}^n$. A decisive speed improvement (up to approximately 16.4×) was achieved with the GPU implementation, as shown in Fig. 2(b).

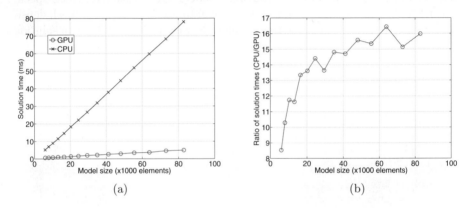

(a)   (b)

Fig. 2. (a) Mean solution times, and (b) ratios of CPU to GPU solution times for a single time step for stretching of a cube model, plotted against model size

4.2   Indentation of a Brain Model

The next set of tests involved simulation of the indentation of a brain model. The brain geometry was obtained from segmented magnetic resonance images used in the study by Clatz et al. [15]. Three meshes were generated from these data, with 11168, 25017, and 46655 elements, respectively. Material parameters were as used in the cube models. Anchor nodes (with all finite element degrees of freedom fixed) were selected from near the brain stem, while displaced nodes were selected from around the frontal lobes (see Fig. 1(b)). Displacements of 0.01m were applied. This configuration was not intended to represent any particular surgical scenario, but was presented as a generic example of "neurosurgical-type" deformations.

The undeformed (wire-frame) and GPU-computed deformed (surface) shapes are superimposed in Fig. 1(b). Again, CPU and GPU results were identical. The solution times, and ratios of solution times are plotted in Figs. 3(a) and (b), respectively. Again, significant speed improvements were observed (though somewhat less than for equivalent sized cube models), with a peak value of approximately 14×.

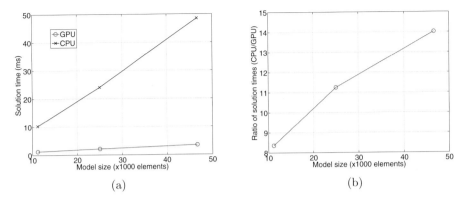

Fig. 3. (a) Mean solution times, and (b) ratios of CPU to GPU solution times for a single time step for indentation of a brain model, plotted against model size

5 Discussion and Conclusions

A novel GPU implementation of an efficient nonlinear FE algorithm suitable for soft tissue deformation simulation has been presented. It was shown that the algorithm employed was well suited to parallel execution, meaning solution speed improvements compared with an equivalent CPU implementation of greater than an order of magnitude were achieved. The largest achieved speed improvement was 16.4×, and we were able to achieve real-time solution of models of up to approximately 16000 tetrahedral elements. To the best of our knowledge this represents the first attempt to port a fully nonlinear FE algorithm to the GPU. Since the algorithm includes both kinematic and constitutive nonlinearities it is suitable for simulation of soft tissue deformation, for example in applications such as interactive surgical simulation and intra-operative non-rigid medical image registration. In view of the substantial speed gains achieved with this first GPU implementation we feel the present development is of great significance to such time-critical applications as these.

Use of biomechanical modelling in surgical simulation and image-guided therapy applications is becoming increasingly widespread. The large body of knowledge and techniques developed by the biomechanics community over many decades provide a powerful basis for addressing many problems in these areas. In many such applications there is a fundamental difficulty in reconciling conflicting requirements for modelling fidelity and expeditious solution. The rapid development of GPU technology has raised the possibility of an entirely new paradigm in high performance computing. The present contribution of a nonlinear FE algorithm implemented for GPU execution shows that this computing model provides a low cost means for performing realistic biomechanical simulations at speeds at or near real-time. We feel that this development has many applications in the areas mentioned.

Acknowledgements

The authors thank P. Raniga for helpful discussions and assistance with GPU programming, and B. Joshi for providing brain meshes. They also thank K. Miller and G. Joldes for much assistance with details of the TLED algorithm.

References

1. Miller, K., Taylor, Z., Nowinski, W.L.: Towards computing brain deformations for diagnosis, prognosis and neurosurgical simulation. Journal of Mechanics in Medicine and Biology 5(1), 105–121 (2005)
2. Taylor, Z.A., Miller, K.: Constitutive modelling of cartilaginous tissues: A review. Journal of Applied Biomechanics 22(3), 212–229 (2006)
3. Szekely, G., Brechbühler, C., Hutter, R., Rhomberg, A., Ironmonger, N., Schmid, P.: Modelling of soft tissue simulation for laparscopic surgery simulation. Medical Image Analysis 4, 57–66 (2000)
4. Picinbono, G., Delingette, H., Ayache, N.: Non-linear anisotropic elasticity for real-time surgery simulation. Graphical Models 65, 305–321 (2003)
5. Carter, T.J., Sermesant, M., Cash, D.M., Barratt, D.C., Tanner, C., Hawkes, D.J.: Application of soft tissue modelling to image-guided surgery. Medical Engineering & Physics 27(10), 893–909 (2005)
6. Wittek, A., Miller, K., Kikinis, R., Warfield, S.K.: Patient-specific model of brain deformation: Application to medical image registration. Journal of Biomechanics 40(4), 919–929 (2007)
7. Tanner, C., Schnabel, J.A., Hill, D.L.G., Hawkes, D.J., Leach, M.O., Hose, D.R.: Factors influencing the accuracy of biomechanical breast models. Medical Physics 33(6), 1758–1769 (2006)
8. Bathe, K.J.: Finite Element Procedures. Prentice Hall, Upper Saddle River, N.J (1996)
9. Miller, K., Joldes, G., Lance, D., Wittek, A.: Total lagrangian explicit dynamics finite element algorithm for computing soft tissue deformation. Communications in Numerical Methods in Engineering 23(2), 121–134 (2007)
10. Owens, J.D., Luebke, D., Govindaraju, N., Harris, M., Krüger, J., Lefohn, A.E., Purcell, T.J.: A survey of general-purpose computation on graphics hardware. Computer Graphics Forum 26(1), 80–113 (2007)
11. Hughes, T.J.R.: The Finite Element Method: Linear Static and Dynamic Finite Element Analyses. Prentice-Hall, Inc. Englewood Cliffs, NJ (1987)
12. Bonet, J., Marriott, H., Hassan, O.: An averaged nodal deformation gradient linear tetrahedral element for large strain explicit dynamic applications. Communications in Numerical Methods in Engineering 17(8), 551–561 (2001)
13. Shreiner, D., Woo, M., Neider, J., Davis, T.: OpenGL Programming Guide: The Official Guide to Learning OpenGL, Version 2, 5th edn. Addison-Wesley, Upper Saddle River, NJ (2006)
14. Fernando, R., Kilgard, M.J.: The Cg Tutorial: The Definitive Guide to Programmable Real-Time Graphics. Addison-Wesley Professional, Castleton, New York (2003)
15. Clatz, O., Delingette, H., Bardinet, E., Dormont, D., Ayache, N.: Patient-specific biomechanical model of the brain: application to parkinson's disease procedure. In: Ayache, N., Delingette, H. (eds.) IS4TM 2003. LNCS, vol. 2673, pp. 321–331. Springer, Heidelberg (2003)

Modeling of Needle-Tissue Interaction Using Ultrasound-Based Motion Estimation

Ehsan Dehghan[1], Xu Wen[1], Reza Zahiri-Azar[1], Maud Marchal[1,2], and Septimiu E. Salcudean[1]

[1] Department of Electrical and Computer Engineering,
University of British Columbia, Vancouver, Canada
tims@ece.ubc.ca

[2] TIMC-GMCAO Laboratory, Grenoble, France

Abstract. A needle-tissue interaction model is an essential part of every needle insertion simulator. In this paper, a new experimental method for the modeling of needle-tissue interaction is presented. The method consists of measuring needle and tissue displacements with ultrasound, measuring needle base forces, and using a deformation simulation model to identify the parameters of a needle-tissue interaction model. The feasibility of this non-invasive approach was demonstrated in an experiment in which a brachytherapy needle was inserted into a prostate phantom. Ultrasound radio-frequency data and the time-domain cross-correlation method, often used in ultrasound elastography, were used to generate the tissue displacement field during needle insertion. A three-parameter force density model was assumed for the needle-tissue interaction. With the needle displacement, tissue displacement and needle base forces as input data, finite element simulations were carried out to adjust the model parameters to achieve a good fit between simulated and measured data.

1 Introduction

During prostate brachytherapy, radioactive capsules are implanted inside the prostate and the surrounding tissue using a long needle with visual guidance from trans-rectal ultrasound (TRUS) and real-time X-ray fluoroscopy. The success of brachytherapy relies on the accuracy of the needle placement inside the tissue. However, due to prostate deformation and rotation [1], targeting errors are still common in brachytherapy [2] and can result in under-dosed and over-dosed regions that can lead to repeated treatments or complications, such as impotence or urinary incontinence. Since visual feedback is limited, significant skill is required to compensate for tissue deformation and decrease targeting errors. Brachytherapy simulators [3,4] and path planners represent new alternatives to train physicians and provide pre-operative planning.

There has been extensive research to model the needle-tissue interactions during needle insertion [5,6,7,8,9,10]. Okamura et al. [5] inserted a needle into bovine liver and divided the force applied by the tissue to the needle into three parts: 1) capsule stiffness; 2) friction and 3) cutting forces occurring at the needle

N. Ayache, S. Ourselin, A. Maeder (Eds.): MICCAI 2007, Part I, LNCS 4791, pp. 709–716, 2007.
© Springer-Verlag Berlin Heidelberg 2007

tip. The authors did not track tissue displacements in their work. Kataoka et al. [6] reported the tip and friction forces applied by a needle during penetration into a canine prostate. Podder et al. [7] reported the needle forces measured during brachytherapy of 25 patients and developed a patient-specific and procedure-specific statistical model to estimate the maximum force that the needle will experience during insertion into the prostate and the perineum. DiMaio and Salcudean [8] identified the force profile along the needle during penetration into a slab of PVC by tracking the motion of superficial markers using a camera. They identified a force model with a peak at the needle tip, following a constant shaft force density. Hing et al. [9] tracked the displacements of several implanted fiducial beads during needle insertion using a dual C-arm fluoroscope setup. They identified a local effective modulus during puncture and an approximate cutting force for soft tissue samples. Crouch et al. [10] introduced a velocity-dependent needle shaft force density. This model has a constant shaft force density followed by a dip and a peak at the tip. The force-displacement data were acquired from insertion of a needle into a transparent, homogeneous silicone gel phantom in which several layers of fiducial markers were implanted. Two digital cameras were used to track the movement of fiducial markers in 3-D.

In this paper, a new experimental method is proposed in order to model needle insertion into soft tissues. The method consists of measuring tissue displacements with ultrasound radio-frequency (RF) data, measuring needle base forces, and using a deformation simulation model to identify the parameters of a needle-tissue interaction model. The use of ultrasound imaging for tissue deformation measurement has several advantages: it is non-invasive and safe, it is the main imaging modality during many image-guided procedures such as prostate brachytherapy, and it does not require fiducial markers. The feasibility of this non-invasive approach was demonstrated in an experiment in which a brachytherapy needle was inserted into a non-homogeneous phantom composed of a harder inclusion mimicking the prostate and a softer surrounding tissue. The Time-Domain Cross-Correlation with Prior Estimates (TDPE) [11,12] was used to estimate the tissue displacements from ultrasound RF signals. This method has the ability to estimate the displacements in real-time. The RF correlation approach has demonstrated high resolution in elastography, hence high accuracy can be expected.

The paper is divided into five sections. In Sect. 2, the experiment design is detailed. Section 3 presents the measurements obtained. Section 4 proposes the modeling method. Section 5 draws conclusions and discusses future work.

2   Experiment Setup

An experiment was conducted to measure both the forces applied on a needle during its insertion into soft tissue and the resulting tissue displacements. The apparatus consists of a needle insertion device, allowing controlled insertion of a needle into a phantom, and an ultrasound machine used to track the tissue displacements.

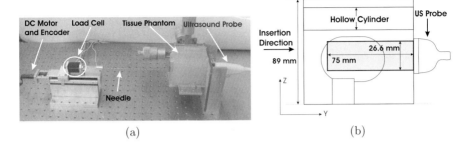

(a)   (b)

Fig. 1. (a) The experiment setup and (b) Side view of the phantom, showing the inclusion, hollow cylinder and the US field of view

2.1   Needle Insertion Device

An 18 gauge brachytherapy needle (Bard, NJ, USA) was mounted on a translational lead-screw stage powered by a Maxon DC motor with an optical encoder. A proportional controller was used to control the speed of the heavily geared drive motor. The needle was mounted on a load cell (MBD-2.5 Transducer Techniques, CA, USA) to measure the insertion and retraction forces applied on it. A computer was used to control the needle speed and to record the needle position and the feedback force at 20 Hz. The experiment setup is shown in Fig. 1(a).

2.2   Phantom Construction

A non-homogeneous phantom composed of a harder inclusion surrounded by a softer tissue has been constructed for the experiments. Fig. 1(b) shows its schematic diagram. The harder inclusion of the phantom – designed to mimic the prostate – is a cylinder with two hemispheres at the two ends. This inclusion was made from polyvinyl chloride (PVC) plasticizer (M-F Manufacturing Co., Inc. Fort Worth, TX, USA). The outside substrate was made from 66.7% PVC plasticizer and 33.3% plastic softener (M-F Manufacturing Co., Inc. Fort Worth). The inclusion was connected to the base with a cylinder of the same material to mimic the rotation of the prostate around the pubic bone. Cellulose (Sigma-Aldrich Inc., St. Louis, MO, USA) was added to the two parts as scattering particles. A cylindrical hole through the phantom represents the rectum. A stiff cylinder made of hard plastic was inserted into this hole to simulate the rectal probe and its effects on the motion of the prostate.

2.3   Tissue Deformation Tracking

A Sonix RP PC-based ultrasound machine and an L12-5 38-mm linear probe (Ultrasonix Medical Corp., Burnaby, BC, Canada) were used in the experiments.

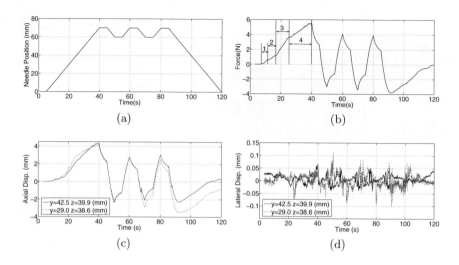

Fig. 2. (a) Needle tip position, (b) Measured insertion force, (c) Axial and (d) Lateral displacements of two sample nodes located in the ultrasound field of view. The legends show the initial location of the nodes. The needle was partially retracted and inserted again after the main insertion. Since in the second and third insertions the needle was inserted in the same path as the first insertion, no cutting occurred. Therefore, the second and third peak forces (t=60 and 80 s) are smaller than the first one (t =40 s).

Both B-mode ultrasound images and digitized radio-frequency (RF) signals were acquired simultaneously with this machine. The machine was synchronized with the computer, which controlled the insertion device and recorded the force data. The phantom was imaged to a depth of 75 mm using a linear array of 128 elements with 1.6 lines per millimeter in the lateral direction (70% sector). The centroid frequency was 5 MHz. RF frames were captured in real-time at 20 frames per second. The position of the ultrasound probe with respect to the tissue and the US field of view inside the tissue are shown in Fig. 1(b).

TDPE [11,12] was used to process the data off-line. Each RF-line was divided into 120 overlapping windows (1 mm window length and 60% window overlap). The axial [11] and lateral [12] components of the displacement (along y and z axes as shown in Fig. 1(b)) were estimated from RF frames. In this method, absolute motions are estimated by integration of relative motions. To increase the accuracy of the estimation, the following dynamic reference frame updating algorithm was used. For every RF frame, the displacements were estimated with respect to the reference frame which was originally set as the first frame. To compensate for RF de-correlation resulting from large displacements, the reference frame was moved to the latest estimated displacement, as soon as the average correlation coefficient corresponding to the latest simulated displacement dropped below 0.95. At each step, the absolute displacements for every spatial location were reported as the estimated motions at that location added to the accumulated displacement value in the integrator.

3   Force and Displacement Measurements

The needle was inserted along the y axis with a controlled position as shown in Fig. 2(a). The insertion line was 5 mm out of the ultrasound field of view to avoid the deteriorating effects of a metallic object on the US images and to increase the accuracy of the tracking algorithm. The tissue phantom was meshed using tetrahedral elements to be used in a model based on the finite element method (FEM) as described in Sect. 4. Some of the mesh nodes were located in the ultrasound field of view. The axial and lateral displacements of these nodes were measured during the experiment (see Figs. 2(c) and 2(d)). Due to the higher accuracy and resolution in the axial direction, only axial displacement estimations were used for modeling. The needle was fully retracted at t=118.5 s, since the measured force is zero after this time (see Fig. 2(b)). However, the measured nodal displacements in Fig. 2(c) show non-zero displacements after this time, which is due to the accumulation of residuals caused by integration of relative motions and the topological change caused by the needle insertion. The characterization of this drift and its effect on the identified model is the subject of future research. The measured force is shown in Fig. 2(b). The decrease in force noted when the needle stops moving is due to tissue relaxation.

4   Needle Shaft Force Distribution

A force distribution as shown in Fig. 3(b) was adopted to model the needle-tissue interaction. This force distribution has three parameters, a constant shaft force density f_s that can simulate friction, a peak force density f_p over the area close to the tip, which contributes to the cutting force, and the width of the peak force density, w. This choice was inspired by the measured force in Fig. 2(b), which shows four parts during insertion into two different tissue types and by the model presented in [8]. To identify the parameter values of this model, only the data from the first insertion portion ($0 \leq t \leq 40$ s) are used. Therefore, the tissue relaxation is not considered in the modeling part. In addition, the overall drift error is less than 1 mm over 120 seconds, while the maximum displacement, of the order of 4 mm, takes place in the first 40 seconds of the experiment. Therefore, the drift error is assumed to be negligible during the first insertion portion.

The tissue phantom was meshed using 991 nodes and 4453 linear tetrahedral elements to be used in a finite element analysis. The needle insertion process was simulated using the FEM. Since the tissue is confined in this experiment and is not allowed to rotate easily, a linear FEM model can be used as opposed to a non-linear one [13]. Due to the slow speed of insertion, the velocity dependent properties of tissue were neglected and the simulation was performed in a quasi-static mode. The force profile shown in Fig. 3(b) was implemented in the simulator and the corresponding displacements for nodes in the US field of view were simulated. In the simulation program, the shaft force density was integrated

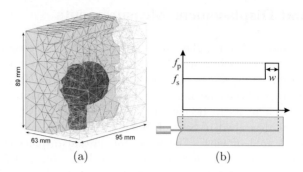

(a)   (b)

Fig. 3. (a) Tissue phantom meshed with tetrahedral elements and (b) The needle shaft force distribution

Table 1. Needle shaft force distribution and elastic parameters

	f_s(N/m)	f_p(N/m)	w(mm)	Young's Modulus(kPa)
Inclusion	72	320	7.0	10
Surrounding tissue	60	140	4.0	7

over the part of the needle which was inside the deformed tissue. This force was distributed over the nodes in contact with the needle. The nodes located on the bottom and back surfaces of the phantom and the nodes in contact with the stiff cylinder were fixed. The force distribution parameters were adjusted to fit the simulated force to the measured force. Since the tissue elastic parameters were unknown prior to the experiment, they were adjusted in the simulation program to fit the simulated axial displacements to the measured axial displacements. The Poisson's ratio was assumed to be equal to 0.49 to simulate the near incompressibility of tissue. The tissue force distribution and material elastic parameters are shown in Table 1 for the given phantom.

The simulated and measured forces are shown in Fig. 4(a). This figure shows the ability of the proposed force distribution model to simulate the needle force with high accuracy. The maximum error between simulated and measured forces is 0.33 N. The minor discontinuity in the simulated force around $t = 20$s is caused by the node repositioning method [4] used in the simulation program to increase the accuracy. Figure 4(b) shows the average simulated and measured axial displacements for the nodes in the ultrasound field of view. The simulated axial displacement has a maximum average error of 0.1 mm and standard deviation of 1.2 mm. Fig. 4(c) shows the position of the nodes in the US field of view in the deformed and undeformed configurations.

In the work presented, the elastic and force model parameters of two tissue types were identified. However, if the elastic parameters are identified using other methods prior to the modeling, the force model parameters can be identified for several layers of tissue. If the elastic parameters are unknown, the identification process for several tissue layers will be complicated, due to mutual effects of one layer of tissue on the displacement of the other ones.

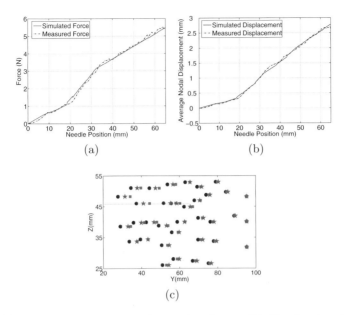

Fig. 4. (a) Simulated and measured insertion forces, (b) Simulated and measured average of nodal displacements in the axial direction, and (c) Position of the nodes in the US field of view. Only axial displacements are shown and were considered in identifying the model parameters. Circles denote the original positions, squares simulated positions and stars the positions measured with TDPE. The dotted line shows the projection of the needle on the US plane.

5   Conclusion and Future Work

A new experimental method has been presented to study and model the needle-tissue interactions. The method is based on measuring the tissue displacement from ultrasound RF data and measuring needle forces and needle base position during the insertion process. A three parameter force distribution model for the needle-tissue interactions has been presented. The model parameters were adjusted using the measurements of force-displacement data recorded during insertion of a needle into a non-homogeneous PVC phantom. The tissue phantom was composed of a harder inclusion to simulate the prostate and a softer surrounding tissue. It was not transparent and had no fiducial beads implanted in. An FEM based simulation was used to adjust the parameters and fit the simulated and measured forces. In addition, the Young's moduli of the tissues were adjusted to fit the simulated axial displacements to the measured axial displacements. The identified force profile and the elastic properties can be used to construct an FEM simulator to simulate the needle insertion process. Such a simulator can be helpful for path planning and for physician training.

In the future, the elastic parameters of the tissue will be identified with higher accuracy using a finer mesh. The dependency of the force model parameters to the insertion speed and the viscoelastic properties of the tissue will be investigated. Statistical analysis will be carried out by acquiring more insertion data from the phantom. In addition, the tracking algorithm will be validated by implanting beads in the tissue and by comparing TDPE results with other imaging modalities and tracking algorithms. During brachytherapy, images are acquired using TRUS. Therefore, the needle motion and major tissue displacements are in the lateral direction of the sagittal/parasagittal images. However, lateral displacement estimation has resolution that is one order of magnitude lower than the resolution in the axial direction. The effect of this discrepancy of resolution on the model depends on the tissue homogeneity and isotropy and will be the subject of further research.

References

1. Lagerburg, V., Moerland, M.A., Lagendijk, J.J., Battermann, J.J.: Measurement of prostate rotation during insertion of needles for brachytherapy. Radiotherapy and Oncology 77, 318–323 (2005)
2. Teschereau, R., Pouliot, J., Roy, J., Tremblay, D.: Seed misplacement and stabilizing needles in transperineal permanent prostate implants. Radiotherapy and Oncology 55, 59–63 (2000)
3. Alterovitz, R., Pouliot, J., Taschereau, R., Hsu, I.C., Goldberg, K.: Needle insertion and radioactive seed implantation in human tissue: Simulation and sensitivity analysis. In: Proc. IEEE ICRA pp. 1793–1799 (2003)
4. Goksel, O., Salcudean, S.E., DiMaio, S.P.: 3D simulation of needle-tissue interaction with application to prostate brachytherapy. Computer Aided Surgery 11(6), 279–288 (2006)
5. Okamura, A., Simone, C., O'Leary, M.: Force modeling for needle insertion into soft tissue. IEEE Trans. Biomed. Eng. 51, 1707–1716 (2004)
6. Kataoka, H., Washio, T., Chinzei, K., Mizuhara, K., Simone, C., Okamura, A.: Measurement of tip and friction force acting on a needle during penetration. In: Dohi, T., Kikinis, R. (eds.) MICCAI 2002. LNCS, vol. 2488, pp. 216–223. Springer, Heidelberg (2002)
7. Podder, T., Sherman, J., Messing, E., Rubens, D., Fuller, D., Strang, J., Brasacchio, R., Yu, Y.: Needle insertion force estimation model using procedure-specific and patient-specific criteria. In: Proc. IEEE EMBS Int. Conf, pp. 555–558 (2006)
8. DiMaio, S.P., Salcudean, S.E.: Needle insertion modeling and simulation. IEEE Trans. on Robot. Autom.: Special Issue on Medical Robotics 19, 864–875 (2003)
9. Hing, J.T., Brooks, A.D., Desai, J.P.: Reality-based needle insertion simulation for haptic feedback in prostate brachytherapy. In: Proc. IEEE ICRA, pp. 619–624 (2006)
10. Crouch, J.R., Schneider, C.M., Wainer, J., Okamura, A.M.: A velocity-dependent model for needle insertion in soft tissue. In: Duncan, J.S., Gerig, G. (eds.) MICCAI 2005. LNCS, vol. 3750, pp. 624–632. Springer, Heidelberg (2005)
11. Zahiri-Azar, R., Salcudean, S.E.: Motion estimation in ultrasound images using time domain cross correlation with prior estimates. IEEE Trans. Biomed. Eng. 53(10), 1990–2000 (2006)
12. Zahiri-Azar, R., Salcudean, S.E.: Real-time estimation of lateral motion using time domain cross correlation with prior estimates. In: Proc. IEEE Ultrasonics Symposium, pp. 1209–1212 (2006)
13. Dehghan, E., Salcudean, S.E.: Comparison of linear and non-linear models in 2D needle insertion simulation. In: Proc. Workshop on Computational Biomechanics for Medicine (In conjunction with MICCAI 2006), pp. 117–124 (2006)

Modelling Intravasation of Liquid Distension Media in Surgical Simulators

S. Tuchschmid[1], M. Bajka[2], D. Szczerba[1], B. Lloyd[1], G. Székely[1],
and M.Harders[1]

[1] Computer Vision Laboratory, ETH Zurich, Switzerland
{tuchschmid,domi,blloyd,szekely,mharders}@vision.ee.ethz.ch
[2] Clinic of Gynecology, University Hospital Zurich, Switzerland
michael.bajka@hin.ch

Abstract. We simulate the intravasation of liquid distension media into the systemic circulation as it occurs during hysteroscopy and transurethral resection of the prostate. A linear network flow model is extended with a correction for non-newtonian blood behaviour in small vessels and an appropriate handling of vessel compliance. We then integrate a fast lookup scheme in order to allow for real-time simulation. Cutting of tissue is accounted for by adjusting pressure boundary conditions for all cut vessels. We investigate the influence of changing distention fluid pressure settings and of the position of tissue cuts. Our simulation predicts significant intravasation only on the venous side, and just in cases when larger veins are cut. The implemented methods allow the realistic control of bleeding for short-term and the total resulting intravasation volume for long-term complication scenarios. While the simulation is fast enough to support real-time training, it is also adequate for explaining intravasation effects which were previously observed on a phenomenological level only.

1 Introduction

In both transurethral resection of the prostate and operative hysteroscopy, excess absorption of the distention fluid is one of the most serious complications [1,2]. During the intervention, the organ cavity is filled with a non-electrolytic distention fluid in order to allow for monopolar electrosurgery and to improve overall visibility. Fluid overload occurs when too much distention fluid is pressed through openly cut vessels into the patient's body, a process called intravasation. The amount of intravasation is influenced by the intrauterine pressure, the number and size of vascular openings and the duration of the procedure. Patients suffering from hyponatremia resulting from intravasation are at risk for pulmonary edema, cerebral edema, and cardiovascular collapse. Therefore, intrauterine pressure must be controlled to maintain a balance between too much pressure, increasing intravasation and too little pressure, decreasing visibility. In order to provide a means for learning the associated skills, we have extended our recently developed surgical simulator for hysteroscopy with a model of the intravasation process.

N. Ayache, S. Ourselin, A. Maeder (Eds.): MICCAI 2007, Part I, LNCS 4791, pp. 717–724, 2007.
© Springer-Verlag Berlin Heidelberg 2007

2   Methods

In order to model the intravasation process, we calculate the blood flow in an interconnected vascular system in dependence of changing boundary conditions. A fully interconnected network flow model was first used by Fatt [3] for petrochemical research of oil and water flow through reservoir rock. Since then, the model has also often been employed to estimate pressure and flow distribution in blood vessel networks (see [4,5] for an overview).

The vascularisation of the virtual surgical scene [6] is generated according to [7] relying on a postulated oxygen consumption of the tissue. This scheme was extended to ensure that the length and number of vessels are following Horton's law [8] which originates from the observation of river branching and states that the number and length of vessels of a particular order follows a geometric sequence. Although Horton's formulae only represent an approximation, they have been proven valid in various morphometric studies [5]. In our current growth framework, arterial and venous sections are grown as separate trees. To ensure that the flow at the arterial inlet (Q_{inlet}) is equal to the flow at the venous outlet (Q_{outlet}), all diameters of the latter system are adjusted with a factor equal to $\sqrt[4]{Q_{inlet}/Q_{outlet}}$.

Linear Intravasation Model. In the linear model, the network is simulated as a number of vessel segments which are formed as straight pipes connecting vessel nodes [5]. For all bifurcation nodes, conservation of mass requires that $\sum_{i=1}^{k} Q_{ij} = 0$, with Q_{ij} being the flow between vessel nodes i and j, and k the number of segments merging at node j. For laminar, steady flow in stiff, straight and uniform tubes, the flow can be calculated according to Poiseuille's law and depends on the vessel conductance G_{ij}

$$Q_{ij} = (P_i - P_j)\, G_{ij} \,, \quad with \ \ G_{ij} = \frac{\pi}{128} \cdot \frac{D_{ij}^4}{\mu_{ij} L_{ij}} \tag{1}$$

where D_{ij}, L_{ij} and μ_{ij} are the diameter, length and viscosity between nodes i and j.

While the viscosity is approximately constant for larger vessels, the Fahraeus-Lindquist effect causes non-Newtonian behaviour for vessels with small diameters often found in microcirculation. Therefore, we use in this case the modified blood viscosity relationship proposed in [9], which depends on tube diameter and hematocrit. For a hematocrit of 0.45, the apparent relative viscosity in dependence of the tube diameter $D[\mu m]$ is given by

$$\mu = 220 \cdot e^{-1.3D} + 3.2 - 2.44 \cdot e^{-0.06D^{0.645}} \tag{2}$$

The set of node equations can be reduced to a set of linear equations for the nodal pressures once the conductances have been evaluated for the given vessel geometry. Pressure boundary conditions have to be set for the arterial inlet node, the venous outlet node, and all arteriole/venule end nodes. In matrix form the set of equations is

$$\mathbf{G} \cdot \mathbf{P} = \mathbf{G}_B \mathbf{P}_B \tag{3}$$

with $\mathbf{G}$ the matrix of conductances, $\mathbf{P}$ the column vector of the unknown pressures, and $\mathbf{G}_B\mathbf{P}_B$ the column vector of the conductances times the boundary pressures of their attached vessel segments. This sparse system of equations is solved by a specialized solver [10]. When cutting through tissue, we simply remove the vessel segments that are cut and set the pressure boundary conditions of the neighboring nodes equal to the pressure of the distension fluid. We then solve (3) with the changed boundary conditions. The updated Q_{inlet} and Q_{outlet} indicate the value for intravasation into the arterial and venous system.

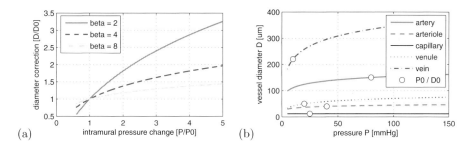

(a)   (b)

Fig. 1. Vessel diameter correction in dependence of changing pressure conditions for different stiffness indices (a) and different vessel types (b)

Compliant Intravasation Model. When vessels are cut, they are exposed to the differing pressure of the distension fluid, which causes a change in vessel diameter. Because of thinner walls and less connective tissue, the compliance of veins is considerably higher than for arteries [11]. Therefore, the integration of a compliance model is especially important for the intravasation into the venous tree. We use the phenomenological description discussed in [12] for the pressure-diameter relationship

$$ln(\frac{P}{P_0}) = \beta_{a/v}(\frac{D}{D_0} - 1) \qquad (4)$$

where P and D are the updated pressure and diameter, and P_0 and D_0 are reference values and correspond to the pressure and diameter of the given vessel at a given operation point. The parameters β_a and β_v are the stiffness indices for arterial and venous vessels and are fitted to experimental data (e.g. [13]). In contrast to a linear compliance model, the stiffness index provides a better approximation for a larger range of pressures. Figure 1(a) shows the resulting diameter correction for different stiffness indices in dependence of the relative intramural pressure change. Figure 1(b) shows examples for vessels with various operating points (P_0/D_0), with $\beta_a = 8$ for arterial and $\beta_v = 4$ for venous vessels. The dependence of the vessel conductance G on the diameter D (and therefore P) changes (3) to a non-linear system for the unknown pressures

$$\mathbf{G(P)} \cdot \mathbf{P} = \mathbf{G(P)}_B \mathbf{P}_B \qquad (5)$$

which we solve numerically by seeding the pressure variables with the linear solution, continue updating the diameters and conductances and iteratively solving the linear system until we reach steady-state conditions. Note that in the uncut model all vessel segments are at their respective operating points ($P=P_0/D=D_0$), diameter corrections are all equal to one and the compliant model therefore identical to the linear model.

Real-time Simulation. The full non-linear flow system consists of 19'144 vessel segments with diameters ranging from $220\mu m$ for the venous outlet to $16\mu m$ for the capillaries. Solving the full reference system for flow and pressure takes around 2 seconds on a dual-core 3GHz PC. To speed up computation, we first calculate pressure values for all vessel nodes in the reference system. We then select a threshold for the minimal simulated vessel diameter. Next, we crop all smaller vessel segments and set the pressure boundary condition of the new end nodes to the precomputed values. Therefore, we only have to solve the reduced vessel system during run-time simulation. This scheme allows a balance between level of detail and computation time when real-time capability is more important than accuracy.

3   Results

Figure 4 depicts the vessel system used in all experiments. In Fig. 4(a), the initial pressure distribution is shown. Figure 4(b) shows the resulting pressure distribution after a horizontal cut. The nomenclature and default values for all used variables are shown in Table 1. Reference values for all pressure boundary conditions are taken from literature data [11].

Table 1. Used variables and default values

	description	default value
$P_{inlet/outlet}$	pressure at arterial inlet/venous outlet	80/10 mmHg
$D_{inlet/outlet}$	diameter at arterial inlet/venous outlet	150/221 μm
$P_{art/ven}$	pressure at arteriole/venule	40/20 mmHg
$D_{art/ven}$	diameter of arteriole/venule	16 μm
$P_{distention}$	pressure of distention fluid	100 mmHg
$\beta_{a/v}$	stiffness index arteries/veins	8.0/4.0

The maximum pressure of the distention media $P_{distention}$ is set by the surgeon. While the recommended pressure range is between 60 and 100 mmHg [14], we have experienced cases where necessary settings for clear view were up to 150 mmHg. The influence of changing distention fluid pressure from 10 to 150 mmHg for the cut shown in Fig. 4(b) is depicted in Fig. 2. For the approximation (3), the intravasation is a linear function of $P_{distention}$ as expected. Q_{inlet} is negative for small pressure values, thus indicating bleeding. While the differences between the compliant and the linear model are small for Q_{inlet} due to the high β-value for arteries, the intravasation into the venous system Q_{outlet} is up to four times higher for the compliant model. For $P_{distention} = 100$ mmHg, the amount of

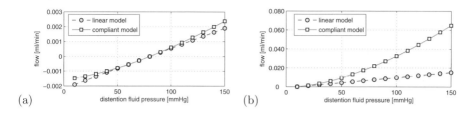

Fig. 2. Intravasation depending on distention fluid pressure for arterial inlet (a) and venous outlet (b)

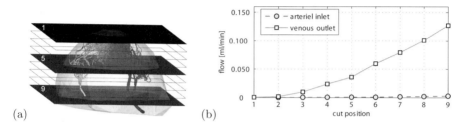

Fig. 3. Intravasation with compliant model (b) depending on cut position indicated by figure (a)

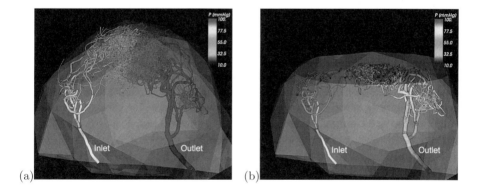

Fig. 4. Pressure distribution in myoma vascularisation before (a) and after (b) cut

intravasation into the venous system (Q_{outlet}) is about 50 times larger than the flow into the arterial system (Q_{inlet}).

According to medical literature, the amount of intravasation depends mainly on the size of cut vessels [14]. By changing the position of the horizontal cut, we investigated the influence of superficial vs. deep cuts on Q_{outlet} and Q_{inlet}. The cut positions are depicted in Fig. 3(a), while the resulting intravasation is displayed in Fig. 3(b). It can be clearly seen that significant intravasation only occurs into the venous system and only if larger vessels are cut.

We also investigated the necessary level of detail for the real-time simulation. With a minimal diameter for individually simulated vessel of 35 μm and setting

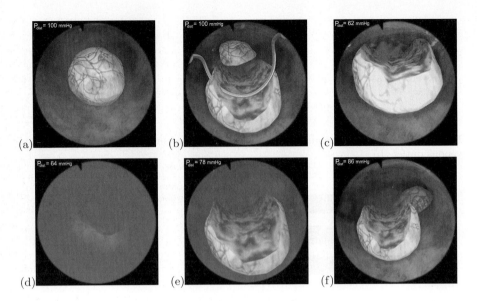

Fig. 5. Intravasation and bleeding simulation in the hysteroscopy simulator. The original situs with a myoma (a) has been cut (b) leading to bleeding (c) aggravated by the reduced distention fluid pressure ($P_{distention}$ top left corner). The completely obscured view (d) is then cleared by rinsing (e) leading to good visibility of the operation site (f).

the pressure boundary conditions to the initially computed values, the number of vessel segments was reduced from 19144 to 3839. This results in a computation speedup of 4.9 with a resulting error in Q_{outlet} of just 1.6%. Since we only have to update the simulation after a cut or when the distention fluid pressure has changed, the calculation time of 0.36 seconds is fast enough for real-time simulation in the training simulator. Figure 5 shows screenshots from an example intervention.

4   Discussion

A few of the assumptions of and possible extensions to our proposed model will be discussed in the following. Since the pressure of the distention fluid is in the same order of magnitude as the mean arterial pressure, the integration of a pulsatile flow model might be beneficial. However, we have not experienced any pulsating bleeding after cutting into a myoma. We also calculated Womersley and Reynolds numbers for all vessel segments and found them low enough to support the laminar flow model. In order to model flow behavior which departs from the parabolic velocity profile mandated by Poiseuille's law, a full three-dimensional finite element model would be necessary. However, the size of the full system with over 19'000 vessels prohibits the numerical solution with commercially available fluid solvers. While it would be possible to extend our model with correction factors based on a three-dimensional models for junctions and bended vessels, the literature shows that the expected effects are small for laminar flow and large length-diameter ratios [15].

Another open point is the effect of cutting into the vessel network. Due to the nature of electro-surgery, a thin layer of tissue is coagulated after a cut, effectively closing small vessels. In addition, small structures might buckle under the sudden pressure load. Also, vessels may deform after cutting because of residual wall stress. Since the discussed effects influence mainly the smallest vessel structures, their contribution to the overall intravasation might be even smaller than predicted by our model. The absolute value of the intravasation is highly dependent on the radii and overall morphometry of the vessel system (see Equation 1). A first visual comparison with data from a corrosion cast under electron microscopy [16] showed good agreement, yet no statistical analysis has been carried out. Unfortunately, there are no specific data available for the compliance in the vascular system of a myoma. However, while the absolute values for the resulting intravasation depend on diameter and compliance, the relative effects in changing cut position and distention fluid pressure are not affected.

5   Conclusion and Future Work

The presented framework enables the static analysis of pressure and flow distribution in large vessel networks. Based on the resulting flow, we control the bleeding for short-term complication scenarios in real-time. The intravasation volume and the resulting sodium serum level based on the performed surgery provide information on the long-term morbidity of the performed virtual surgery. According to our simulations, significant intravasation only occurs into the venous side, and only if larger veins are cut. While the simulation is fast enough to support real-time training, it is also adequate for explaining intravasation effects which were previously observed on a phenomenological level only.

Validation with real data is not meaningful without precise morphometric vessel data of the uterine cavity, since we could simply tune the base vessel's diameter until we get a good agreement. With the availability of such data, we will extend our model to cover intravasation through the endometrium into the lymphatic system by diffusion as well as fluid uptake through the tubal ostia. Together this will then allow the quantitative comparison of the total intravasation volume with data from real surgery. Screenshots, movies of sample interventions and detailed descriptions of all simulator modules can be found on our project web (http://www.hystsim.ethz.ch).

Acknowledgment. This work has been performed within the NCCR Co-Me supported by the Swiss National Science Foundation.

References

1. Rassweiler, J., Teber, D., Kuntz, R., Hofmann, R.: Complications of transurethral resection of the prostate (TURP)–incidence, management, and prevention. Eur. Urol. 50(5), 969–979 (2006)

2. Pasini, A., Belloni, C.: Intraoperative complications of 697 consecutive operative hysteroscopies. Minerva. Ginecol. 53(1), 13–20 (2001)
3. Fatt, I.: The network model of porous media: The dynamic properties of networks with tube radius distribution. Trans. AIME Petrol. Div. 207, 164–177 (1956)
4. Mayer, S.: On the pressure and flow-rate distributions in tree-like and arterial-venous networks. Bull. Math. Biol. 58(4), 753–785 (1996)
5. Kassab, G.S.: The coronary vasculature and its reconstruction. Ann. Biomed. Eng. 28(8), 903–915 (2000)
6. Sierra, R., Zsemlye, G., Székely, G., Bajka, M.: Generation of variable anatomical models for surgical training simulators. Med. Image. Anal. 10(2), 275–285 (2006)
7. Szczerba, D., Székely, G.: Simulating vascular systems in arbitrary anatomies. In: Duncan, J.S., Gerig, G. (eds.) MICCAI 2005. LNCS, vol. 3750, pp. 641–648. Springer, Heidelberg (2005)
8. Horton, R.: Erosional development of streams and their drainage basins: hydrophysical approach to quantitative morphology. Bull. Geol. Soc. Amer. 56, 275–370 (1945)
9. Pries, A.R., Neuhaus, D., Gaehtgens, P.: Blood viscosity in tube flow: dependence on diameter and hematocrit. Am. J. Physiol. 263(6 Pt 2), H1770–H1778 (1992)
10. Davis, T.A.: Algorithm 832: Umfpack v4.3—an unsymmetric-pattern multifrontal method. ACM Trans. Math. Softw. 30(2), 196–199 (2004)
11. Rooke, T.W., Sparks, H.V.: The Systemic Circulation, Medical Physiology, 2nd edn. ISBN: 0-7817-1936-4. Lippincott Williams & Wilkins (2003)
12. Hayashi, K., Handa, H., Nagasawa, S., Okumura, A., Moritake, K.: Stiffness and elastic behavior of human intracranial and extracranial arteries. J. Biomech. 13(2), 175–184 (1980)
13. Kassab, G.S., Molloi, S.: Cross-sectional area and volume compliance of porcine left coronary arteries. Am. J. Physiol. Heart. Circ. Physiol. 281(2), H623–H628 (2001)
14. Menacaglia, L., Hamou, J.: Manual of Gynecological Hysteroscopy. Endo-Press, Tuttlingen (2001)
15. Perry, R., Green, D. (eds.): Perry's chemical engineers' handbook, 7th edn. McGraw-Hill, New York (1997)
16. Walocha, J.A., Litwin, J.A., Miodonski, A.J.: Vascular system of intramural leiomyomata revealed by corrosion casting and scanning electron microscopy. Hum. Reprod. 18(5), 1088–1093 (2003)

Registration of Cardiac SPECT/CT Data Through Weighted Intensity Co-occurrence Priors

Christoph Guetter[1,2], Matthias Wacker[1], Chenyang Xu[1],
and Joachim Hornegger[2]

[1] Imaging & Visualization Department, Siemens Corporate Research, Princeton, USA
[2] Institute of Computer Science, Universität Erlangen-Nürnberg, Erlangen, Germany
christoph.guetter@siemens.com

Abstract. The introduction of hybrid scanners has greatly increased the popularity of molecular imaging techniques. Many clinical applications benefit from combining complementary information based on the precise alignment of the two modalities. In case the alignment is inaccurate, then this crucial assumption often made for subsequent processing steps will be violated. However, this violation may not be apparent to the physician. In CT-based attenuation correction (AC) for cardiac SPECT/CT data, critical misalignments between SPECT and CT can lead to spurious perfusion defects. In this work, we focus on increasing the accuracy of rigid volume registration of cardiac SPECT/CT data by using prior knowledge. A new weighting scheme for an intensity co-occurrence prior is introduced to assure accurate and robust alignment in the local heart region. Experimental results demonstrate that the proposed method outperforms mutual information registration and shows robustness across a selection of learned distributions acquired from 15 different patients.

1 Introduction

The use of multi-modality imaging, especially PET/CT and SPECT/CT, in clinical practice has become more popular. Common hybrid scanners combine low resolution molecular images with anatomical context from high-resolution CT by placing both, e.g. SPECT and CT, scanners next to each other. This setup allows for a good registration between the two modalities when the imaged anatomical structures are undergoing no or little motion such as structures in the head. However, in the imaging of other body parts, critical misalignments, as shown in Fig.1, still occur significantly often due to breathing, patient motion, or motion caused by acquisition protocol restrictions [1]. An accurate registration between the two modalities is imperative to ensure the diagnostic confidence of physicians. It has been reported, for example, in the application of quantitative cardiac SPECT/CT analysis that spurious perfusion defect artifacts are introduced in the CT-based attenuation correction (AC) images of the SPECT acquisition due to misalignments. The misalignments falsify the uptake values that are utilized for diagnosis [2,3]. Registration as preprocessing step to CT-based AC SPECT cannot involve user interaction or correction. These demands

N. Ayache, S. Ourselin, A. Maeder (Eds.): MICCAI 2007, Part I, LNCS 4791, pp. 725–733, 2007.
© Springer-Verlag Berlin Heidelberg 2007

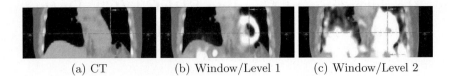

(a) CT   (b) Window/Level 1   (c) Window/Level 2

Fig. 1. Three anterior views of a misaligned cardiac SPECT/CT data set, the CT (a), and the SPECT overlayed on CT with two different window level settings 1, (b) and (c). The figure visualizes the challenging multi-modal registration problem.

may be somewhat addressed through a stringent acquisition protocol that, nevertheless, is both prone to errors and complicated to use in clinical practice. A better way of ensuring alignment is to utilize an automatic registration technique that is highly accurate and robust. In this paper, we propose a rigid registration method that is designed to address the above mentioned demands of cardiac SPECT/CT. The accuracy is achieved by incorporating weighted intensity co-occurrence priors about an accurate alignment of cardiac data. Using the joint probability distribution function (pdf) of previously registered image data as an intensity prior has been previously reported supporting for the accuracy of rigid as well as non-rigid multi-modal image registration by several research groups [4,5,6,7,8,9]. Hereby, an interesting energy minimization scheme of incorporating statistical priors was proposed as follows [7,8,9]:

$$E = \alpha\, E_{\mathrm{MI}} + (1 - \alpha)\, E_{\mathrm{prior}}, \tag{1}$$

where E_{MI} is the MI energy and E_{prior} denotes a dissimilarity measure towards the prior information. The factor α controls the influence of the prior. Two aspects are essential for this application: The usage of a data-driven as well as a prior model-driven term to ensure robust and accurate alignment in general, and in particular the requirement of an accurate heart alignment. In the following, we are deriving a new registration method considering those aspects. The achieved accuracy of the proposed approach, that exploits prior information from cardiac SPECT/CT acquisitions, is compared to the accuracy of standard mutual information (MI) [10,11] and a general learning-based approach [7]. This work extends previous works with the focus of applicability. Achieving higher accuracy and robustness than MI, the presented approach is not limited to the application of cardiac SPECT/CT imaging.

2   Description of Method

In order to achieve the registration accuracy and robustness needed in CT-based AC for SPECT reconstruction, several open issues need to be resolved. How does the choice of α influence the registration result and how should it be selected for this application? Secondly, is the Kullback-Leibler (KL) divergence a sufficient distance measure for joint pdfs? And the most intriguing open question: how well does the proposed scheme (1) generalize over a large pool of patients? We address those questions by deriving a new registration method that employs weigthed co-occurrence priors.

2.1 Image Registration Using Prior Knowledge

The α-influence is studied by investigating the energy behaviour, Eq.(5), while manually translating a cardiac SPECT/CT data set away from ground truth alignment. See Fig. 2(a) for results of using different α values. We note that a smaller α, i.e. more prior influence, has a smoothing effect on the overall cost function. Hereby, $\alpha = 0.2$ is observed to be a good trade-off between data driven and prior term. Decreasing the influence of MI allows to smooth out its local optima while still keeping the feature of maximizing the mutual information that both images share.

In previous work [4,6,7,8] the KL divergence is used to measure the dissimilarity of two distributions. In a discrete formulation, this can be written as:

$$E_{\text{prior}} = E_{\text{KL}}(p^{T_S}, p_{\text{prior}}) = \sum_{i,j} p^{T_S}(i,j) \log \left(\frac{p^{T_S}(i,j)}{p_{\text{prior}}(i,j)} \right), \tag{2}$$

where p^{T_S} is a joint pdf of two volumes related to each other by transformation T_S, and p_{prior} is a joint pdf learned from two previously aligned volumes. Fig. 2(b) illustrates the drawbacks of KL's asymmetry using two artificial distributions. We can observe that equal dissimilarities between the distributions create differently signed contributions to KL dependent on the variables' order of comparison. A more appropriate statistical measure is provided by the Jensen-Shannon (JS) divergence. The definition for the prior energy becomes:

$$E_{\text{prior}} = E_{\text{JS}}(p^{T_S}, p_{\text{prior}}) = \frac{1}{2} \left(E_{\text{KL}} \left(p^{T_S}, \bar{p} \right) + E_{\text{KL}} \left(p_{\text{prior}}, \bar{p} \right) \right), \tag{3}$$

where $\bar{p} = \frac{p^{T_S} + p_{\text{prior}}}{2}$. Fig. 2(c) shows the properties of JS divergence. These properties are of importance when we want to emphasize organ specific contributions in the joint pdf.

Misalignments of the SPECT heart image into the lung region of CT attenuation map introduce artifacts that can lead to false diagnosis. Prior knowledge about the correct mapping within this area is important to ensure such a mapping in future registrations. A problem of the general approach in [7] is that information stored in the learned joint pdf is global and influenced by the size of the background in both volumes. Local alignments are driven by the global matching especially if the transformation model is also global. Thus, we propose a new formulation that utilizes local information stored in the learned joint pdf. The new prior energy is written as:

$$\begin{aligned} E_{\text{prior}} = \; & E_{\omega,\text{JS}}(p^{T_S}, \; p_{\text{prior}}) = \omega \star E_{\text{JS}}(p^{T_S}, p_{\text{prior}}), \\ = \; & \tfrac{1}{2} \sum_{\Omega} \omega(i,j) \left[p^{T_S}(i,j) \log \left(\frac{p^{T_S}(i,j)}{\bar{p}(i,j)} \right) \right. \\ & \left. + p_{\text{prior}}(i,j) \log \left(\frac{p_{\text{prior}}(i,j)}{\bar{p}(i,j)} \right) \right] \end{aligned} \tag{4}$$

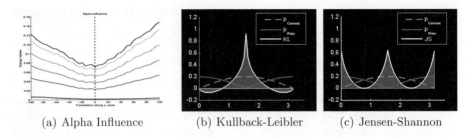

(a) Alpha Influence   (b) Kullback-Leibler   (c) Jensen-Shannon

Fig. 2. (a) Cost function influence of α values ranging from $\alpha = 0.6$ (top curve) to $\alpha = 0.1$ (bottom curve). (b) Plot of contributions (white curve) to KL divergence between two artificial distributions (green and magenta curve). The filled area denotes the KL value. (c) Plot of contributions to JS divergence. Distribution dissimilarities have positive, limited, and comparable contributions to JS.

where $\omega \in [0,1]^{N \times N}$, and $\star$ denotes the element-wise multiplication in the discrete case. The term ω will be chosen such that it penalizes organ specific intensity matchings that are inconsistent with a learned distribution. Hence, this penalty term introduces, to some extent, spatial information to intensity-based registration. Organ specific appearances in the joint intensity distribution can be estimated by either a segmentation or a manual outline of the organ of interest, see Section 2.2 for details on the choice of ω. A crucial assumption of ω is that penalties need to be assigned comparably for differences between prior and joint pdf, see discussion KL vs. JS. This requires a symmetric and strictly positive similarity measure on distributions. The transformation between the two data sets is obtained by solving the following equation:

$$\hat{T} = \underset{T=\{T_S, T_I\}}{\arg\min} \left[\alpha \cdot E_{\text{MI}}^*(p^T) + (1-\alpha) \cdot E_{\omega,\text{JS}}(p^T, p_{\text{prior}}^T) \right] \qquad (5)$$

where $E_{\text{MI}}^* = -\beta\, E_{\text{MI}}$, and $T = \{T_S, T_I\}$ is composed of a spatial rigid transformation T_S that aligns SPECT and CT volume and an intensity transformation T_I that warps p_{prior} to p^{T_S} to compensate for patient specific intensity variations. T_I is a 1-dimensional affine transformation between the prior SPECT intensities and the intensity range of the SPECT volume to be registered. We use the sum-squared-differences criterion for the matching. In our implementation, the two transformations are estimated sequentially but the framework above also allows for concurrent estimation.

2.2   Weighted Jensen-Shannon Divergence for Statistical Priors

The weighted Jensen-Shannon (WJS) divergence, defined in Eq. (4), is introduced to ensure an organ specific intensity co-occurrence. In order to derive a suitable ω for cardiac SPECT/CT registration, we segmented the heart in the SPECT volume using the method in [12]. The penalty area of ω, i.e. white area in Fig. 3(d), is then generated by studying the joint pdfs for different alignments

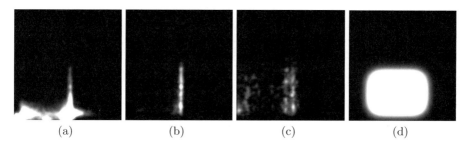

$$\text{(a)} \qquad\qquad \text{(b)} \qquad\qquad \text{(c)} \qquad\qquad \text{(d)}$$

Fig. 3. Observed joint pdfs of cardiac SPECT/CT data. The distributions are displayed for (a) the full volume overlap, (b) the heart overlap, and (c) the heart overlap at misalignment. Image (d) presents the penalty term ω of Eq. (4) that is generated from the observations made in (b) and (c).

of the segmented heart with the CT, see Figs. 3(b) and 3(c). In Fig. 3, the coordinate system is defined as follows: The origin is located in the lower left corner of each image, the horizontal and vertical axis refer to CT and SPECT volume intensities, respectively. Several interesting aspects are observed:

1. The joint intensity mappings corresponding to a segmented object in both modalities occur in a limited region within the joint pdf space. This is true for all possible spatial alignments of the two volumes (Fig. 3(c)).
2. In order to ensure consistency with a learned distribution, the penalty term needs to cover all intensity pairs that the object may generate in the joint pdf. The reason is that a learned pdf not only states which intensities do match but also provides knowledge about which intensities do not match.
3. Evaluating a similarity measure on a subset of the joint pdfs eliminates unwanted influences from the unweighted learned distribution, e.g. background size dependency, global structure dependencies.

Using the defined ω, Fig. 3(d), we applied the proposed approach to a pool of cardiac SPECT/CT patients.

3   Experiments

We applied the proposed approach (WJS), MI, and a general learning-based method (JS), i.e. using eq. (3) in eq. (5), to 15 different cardiac SPECT/CT acquisitions. The data sets were acquired by a Siemens Symbia T6 scanner. The field-of-view (FOV) for SPECT data ($128 \times 128 \times 128$, $4.79 \times 4.79 \times 4.79$mm) includes the lungs, heart, and abdomen, whereas the FOV for CT data ($512 \times 512 \times 25$, $0.97 \times 0.97 \times 5$mm) includes only heart and lungs. All volumes have been manually aligned for a precise match of the heart region. From this ground truth, priors are generated and several validation studies are executed. A validation study is defined as follows: For all data sets, multiple registrations are done per data set with different initial transformations away from ground truth alignment. For each registration, the error is computed as the distance from the obtained

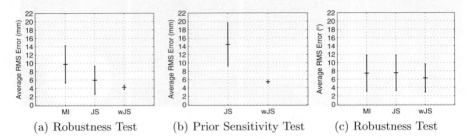

(a) Robustness Test   (b) Prior Sensitivity Test   (c) Robustness Test

Fig. 4. Comparison of error distributions for normalized MI, JS, and WJS over validation runs for translation (a) and (b), and rotation parameters(c). Using a mixture of prior and data driven model in combination with the newly weighted scheme, WJS, not only yields the best results but also generalizes well over multiple patients.

alignment to the ground truth alignment. Error mean and standard deviation of all registrations are then compared between the three methods.

Co-occurrence priors validation. In order to validate how sensitiv the proposed approach is towards the chosen prior, 15 different priors were generated. We then performed two validation studies, i.e. multiple data/single prior and single data/multiple prior validation. In the first one, all patient data sets are registered using one randomly chosen prior, i.e. robustness test. In the second study, one data set is randomly chosen among all patients and registered multiple times using the available priors respectively, i.e. prior sensitivity test. Note that the learning-based approaches utilize only one prior. The results of the two studies are presented in Figs. 4(a) and 4(b).

The proposed approach is by definition not bound to any specific transformation model. Here, we apply a rigid transformation model. The initializations range from -60mm to $+60$mm in steps of 30mm in x-/z- or in y-/z- direction for translation and from $-30°$ to $+30°$ in steps of $5°$ around the z-axis for rotation. We evaluated translation and rotation initializations separately. The chosen α value for all experiments is fixed to 0.2 for WJS and to 0.75 for JS.

Correcting for intensity variations between patients and studies. In Eq. (5), transformation T_I is also estimated during optimization. All 15 data sets showed minimal differences in the scaling parameter, i.e. it varied between 0.95 and 1.014, and no translational component was observed.

Validation results. Figures 4(a) and 4(b) show the mean registration error for the robustness and prior sensitivity validation results w.r.t. translation parameters. Figure 4(c) displays the mean angular registration errors for the robustness test. It can be observed that both JS and WJS are more accurate on average than MI, and WJS additionally shows a small standard deviation. The proposed approach, WJS, outperforms MI and the general learning-based method, JS, with a mean translation error of 4.19 ± 0.5mm. Note that the error is smaller than a SPECT voxel. Normalized MI and JS show a mean error of more than 2

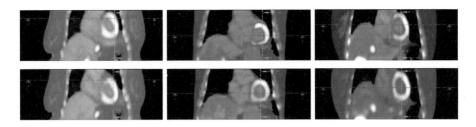

Fig. 5. Registration results for 3 out of 15 patients. The top row shows the MI result and the bottom row denotes the WJS results. The images illustrate the deviations from the optimum for MI registration and high accuracy achieved by WJS approach.

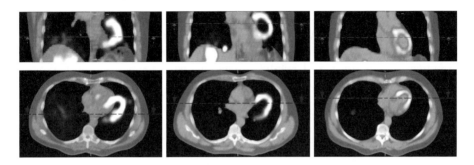

Fig. 6. Registration of a misaligned cardiac SPECT/CT scan. Two views are shown for misalignment after acquisition (left column), MI registration result (middle column), and weighted JS result using prior knowledge from a different scan(right column). The images show that the crucial alignment is only achieved by our proposed method.

[9.74±4.49mm] and more than 1 [5.9±3.36mm] voxel(s), respectively. We further noticed that optimization of MI is attracted to local optima and that the global optimum for MI deviates from the correct alignment if bright artifacts occur in CT data.[1] The learning-based methods do not get disturbed in those data sets. The rotation results also confirm the superiority of WJS over MI, see Fig. 4(c). The generally high observed mean angular error for WJS (6.2°), JS (7.5°) and for MI (7.4°) is probably due to the little structural information apparent in SPECT. The angular error is an accumulation of errors in all three axis. In addition, Fig. 6 shows a clinical scenario for registration where the scanned data is strongly mis-aligned. We were only able to register this data set using weighted intensity co-occurence priors.

The preliminary studies show that the proposed approach fullfills the clinical demands for registration accuracy of maximum 1 voxel mis-alignment in CT-based AC for cardiac SPECT, as mentioned in [2,3], and suggest the feasibility to use the approach for automated registration in hybrid scanners.

---

[1] The observation was made while investigating those data sets where the registration validation studies resulted in high errors.

4 Discussion and Conclusion

We have presented a robust registration approach for the application of CT-based AC of cardiac SPECT data. The achieved registration error of the proposed method (4.2 ± 0.5mm) is significantly lower than for MI (9.7 ± 4.49mm) and for a general learning-based method (5.9 ± 3.36mm). Clinical accuracy requirements are met for this application. The proposed approach can be easily extended to other applications where high accuracy in an organ specific region-of-interest is sought. Future work include validating this approach on a larger number of data sets and applying it to other modalities and applications.

Acknowledgements. The authors would like to thank Dr. Ponraj Chinnadurai for his valuable clinical input about SPECT and CT imaging, Christophe Chefd'Hotel for valuable research discussions, and Frank Sauer for his continued support of this research. We would like to particularly thank Jerome Declerck, Xavier Battle, Xinhong Ding, and Hans Vija at Siemens Medical Solutions for providing imaging data and helpful discussions with regards to the CT-based AC for cardiac SPECT problem.

References

1. Goetze, S., et al.: Prevalence of misregistration between SPECT and CT for attenuation-corrected myocardial perfusion SPECT. J. Nucl. Cardiol. 14, 200–206 (2007)
2. Fricke, H., et al.: A method to remove artifacts in attenuation-corrected myocardial perfusion SPECT introduced by misalignment between emission scan and CT-derived attenuation maps. J. Nucl. Med. 45, 1619–1625 (2004)
3. Kritzman, J., et al.: Changes in normal cardiac intensity distribution due to translation differences between CT and SPECT for a hybrid imaging system. J. Nucl. Cardiol. 12, 122–123 (2005)
4. Chung, A.C.S., et al.: Multi-modal image registration by minimising Kullback-Leibler distance. In: Dohi, T., Kikinis, R. (eds.) MICCAI 2002. LNCS, vol. 2489, pp. 525–532. Springer, Heidelberg (2002)
5. Zöllei, L., Fisher, J.W., Wells, W.M.: A unified statistical and information theoretic framework for multi-modal image registration. In: Proc. IPMI, pp. 366–377 (2003)
6. Soman, S., et al.: Rigid registration of echoplanar and conventional magnetic resonance images by minimizing the Kullback-Leibler distance. In: Gee, J.C., Maintz, J.B.A., Vannier, M.W. (eds.) WBIR 2003. LNCS, vol. 2717, pp. 181–190. Springer, Heidelberg (2003)
7. Guetter, C., et al.: Learning based non-rigid multi-modal image registration using Kullback-Leibler divergence. In: Duncan, J.S., Gerig, G. (eds.) MICCAI 2005. LNCS, vol. 3750, pp. 255–262. Springer, Heidelberg (2005)
8. Cremers, D., Guetter, C., Xu, C.: Nonparametric priors on the space of joint intensity distributions for non-rigid multi-modal image registration. In: Proc. CVPR pp. 1777–1783 (2006)
9. Zöllei, L., Wells, W.M.: Multi-modal image registration using Dirichlet-encoded prior information. In: Pluim, J.P.W., Likar, B., Gerritsen, F.A. (eds.) WBIR 2006. LNCS, vol. 4057, pp. 34–42. Springer, Heidelberg (2006)

10. Wells, W.M., et al.: Multi-modal volume registration by maximization of mutual information. Med. Image Anal. 1, 35–51 (1996)
11. Maes, F., et al.: Multimodality image registration by maximization of mutual information. IEEE T. Med. Imaging 16, 187–198 (1997)
12. Kohlberger, T., et al.: 4D shape priors for a level set segmentation of the left myocardium in SPECT sequences. In: Larsen, R., Nielsen, M., Sporring, J. (eds.) MICCAI 2006. LNCS, vol. 4190, pp. 92–100. Springer, Heidelberg (2006)

Prostate Implant Reconstruction with Discrete Tomography

Xiaofeng Liu[1], Ameet K. Jain[1,2], and Gabor Fichtinger[1]

[1] Department of Computer Science, Johns Hopkins University, Baltimore, MD, USA
[2] Philips Research North America, Briarcliff, NY, USA

Abstract. We developed a discrete tomography method for prostate implant reconstructions using only a limited number of X-ray projection images. A 3D voxel volume is reconstructed by back-projection and using distance maps generated from the projection images. The true seed locations are extracted from the voxel volume while false positive seeds are eliminated using a novel optimal geometry coverage model. The attractive feature of our method is that it does not require exact seed segmentation of the X-ray images and it yields near 100% correct reconstruction from only six images with an average reconstruction accuracy of 0.86 mm (std=0.46mm).

1 Introduction

Brachytherapy is a definitive treatment for low risk prostate cancer that represents the vast majority of new cases diagnosed nowadays. The brachytherapy procedure entails permanently implanting small radioactive seeds into the prostate. The main limitation of contemporary brachytherapy is faulty seed placement that may result in insufficient dose to the cancer and/or inadvertent radiation to the rectum, urethra, and bladder. Intra-operative implant optimization promises a major clinical breakthrough, but for this technique to succeed the implanted seeds must be reconstructed and registered with the anatomy [1]. This work concentrates on the first problem, reconstruction.

C-arm X-ray fluoroscopy is the gold standard in observing brachytherapy seeds and therefore is a natural candidate for implant localization. The 3D coordinates of the seeds can be calculated from multiple X-ray images upon solving the corres-pondence problem [2-6]. These methods uniformly require that seeds are accurately segmented in the X-ray images. Significant research has been dedicated to this problem, still without clinically robust and practical solution. To make the problem worse, typically 7%, but often as much as 43% of the seeds can be hidden in the X-ray images [7], and the recovery of these seeds is an exigent task that often leaves seeds undetected. Su *et al.* [7] proposed a solution to the hidden seed problem by resolving seed clusters and extending previously published approach [3], but it still required perfectly localizing all visible seeds all projection images.

Classic tomosynthesis might seem a suitable reconstruction, but unfortunately, it is impractical in brachytherapy because (1) the swing space of the C-arm is limited due to collision hazards and (2) the number of X-ray images is strictly limited in order to

N. Ayache, S. Ourselin, A. Maeder (Eds.): MICCAI 2007, Part I, LNCS 4791, pp. 734–742, 2007.
© Springer-Verlag Berlin Heidelberg 2007

save the patient and the OR crew from excessive toxic radiation. Tutar *et al.* [8] has proposed a variant of tomosynthesis denoted as selective back projection. However this method demands a large number of images (≥ 7) and wide C-arm angle ($\geq 25°$) to succeed. It is also prone to introducing false positive (FP) seeds, which from a dosimetric point of view are more troublesome than hidden seeds, because they act toward underdosing the cancer. Tutar *et al.* use a heuristic rule to recognize FP seeds by their sizes, but since C-arm pose estimation and calibration errors affect the size of objects, this may result in faulty separation of the true and false seeds.

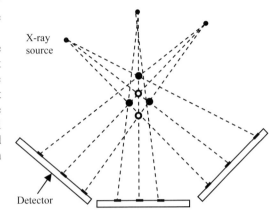

Our approach using discrete tomography is different in that after generating a 3D volume using back-projection we detect and remove the false positive seeds by solving an optimal coverage problem. We achieved high reconstruction rate with fewer images.

Fig. 1. Two false positive seeds are introduced by three legitimate seeds when their projectiles inter-sect the same voxels

2   Method

In the example in Figure 1, three X-ray images are used. Three seeds project in each image and leave a "mark" in the image, typically a dark blotch in fluoroscopy. After reconstructing a 3D voxel volume with common back-projection, five candidate seeds are found in the volume and all appear to be legitimate seeds in each image. The question is how to separate the true seeds from the false positives. In this simplistic example, it is very easy to identify the legitimate seeds (solid circles) because any other choice will lead to an inconsistency: there will be "seed marks" in one or more X-ray images to which no seed in the volume projects. Therefore, the intuition behind the reasoning is that each "seed mark" in each image must be "covered" by at least one seed in the voxel volume. To support this intuition, we develop a theoretical framework based on optimal geometry coverage.

Tomosynthesis with Distance Map and Seed Localization. Tomosynthesis [10] is the technique to reconstruct a 3D volume from multiple 2D projection images within a limited angle. The most commonly used approach is the back projection method, which was first introduced for CT reconstruction. In this method, each voxel in a 3D volume is projected onto all the images. The value assigned to this voxel is calculated as the average of the intensity values of its projected locations in the images.

A local coordinate system must be defined for the C-arm. For any arbitrary 3D point in the space, after C-arm calibration, its projected coordinates on the 2D image plane can be calculated by the rules of perspective projection.

In practice, the C-arm's pose is estimated with some error. Since the size of the seeds is small relative to the focal length, the reconstruction is quite sensitive to pose error. To make the reconstruction more robust to pose error, in the reconstruction of the 3D voxel volume we use distance maps rather than the projection image itself.

As preprocessing, in each image we first extract the so called 2D seed regions-- areas that contain seeds' projections--using adaptive thresholding and morphological operators and call the resulting images "seed-only" image. Then for each seed-only image, a distance map is calculated using a distance transform: the value at each pixel is the Euclidean distance to its nearest 2D seed region. (Pixels inside a 2D seed region all take a value of zero.) In reconstructing the 3D volume, the value of a voxel is the average of the distance values at all of its projected locations.

After the 3D voxel volume is reconstructed, candidate 3D seed regions are extracted by thresholding. The threshold value is based on estimated pose error. For example, in case of small pose error of less than 1 degree rotation, such as in Jain *et al.* [6], the threshold is set to ½ pixel. Upon thresholding, connected 3D seed regions are considered as candidate seeds. The candidate seeds are then labeled using the standard 3D "connected component labeling" method, i.e. any two neighboring voxels in the 3D seed regions are assigned the same label and considered as parts of the same seed. After that, the centroids of all the candidate seeds are calculated by averaging the 3D coordinates of all voxels wearing the same label. Each candidate seed is then represented by the location of its centroid, in addition to its label.

As we mentioned earlier, a decisive advantage of tomosynthesis over the three-film technique and its derivatives [6] is that, in addition to not requiring precise seed segmentation, it can reconstruct all hidden seeds. But the disadvantage is that tomosynthesis introduces false positive seeds, often as much as 20%. Next, we propose a theoretical framework for separating the true seeds from the false ones.

Theoretical Framework for Separating True Seeds. The problem is formulated as an optimal geometric coverage problem [11]. The general optimal coverage problem arises, for example, in wireless network design. From a given set of "server" points, we must select the minimum subset that can cover a given set of "client" points. The goal is formulated as to minimize a total cost function, which is the sum of the cost functions defined on all the selected server points.

In our problem, based on the intuition mentioned earlier, we want to find the M true seeds from the set of N candidates, such that all the 2D seed regions are "covered" in all projection images, i.e. every 2D seed region must have at least one true seed projected in it. In constructing the appropriate cost function, we can use the observation that a false positive (FP) seed, owing to its very nature, is projected close to some true seed in every image. While a true seed may be projected close to some other true seeds in some images, it usually is not the case for every image. (While it is common that a true seed can be hidden in some projection images, we have never encountered a situation where a true seed was hidden in all images. We also note that no existing method can recover such a seed.)

Hence for the server model, we define the cost function of a given seed (potential server point) as the sum of the closest distances between the projections of this seed and the projections of all other true seeds, in all images. We formulate the problem as such a general optimal coverage problem: Given the N candidate seeds, we want to find M seeds ($x_1, x_2, ..., x_M$) from them such that all 2D seed regions in the seed-only images are covered, and the below cost function is minimized

$$C = -\sum_{m=1 i=1}^{M} \sum_{i=1}^{n} \hat{d}_i(x_m) \tag{2}$$

where $\hat{d}_i(x_n) = \min_m \| P^j x_m - P^j x_n \|, \quad \forall n \in [1,2,\cdots,M], \text{and } n \neq m \tag{3}$

and P^j is the projection operator that projects a 3D point onto the jth image.

Unfortunately, the optimal coverage problem is NP-hard [12] and its computational complexity is $O(C_M^N)$, where C_M^N means N choose M. Thus for a large set of seeds, it is not possible to find its global optimal solution. We, however, managed to reduce the size of the problem by using the 2D seed-only images for regularization. To further reduce the problem, we also used greedy search to minimize local costs rather than the global cost function in Eq. (2).

Seed Clustering. To ensure that the projections of selected true seeds cover all the 2D seed regions in all seed-only images, the candidate seeds are clustered based on their projections in each image. For this purpose, we label all 2D seed regions in all seed-only images, in the similar way as 3D labeling described, e.g. the separated seed regions are assigned different labels and pixels in the same connected region wear the same label. The projections of seeds can then be clustered based on these labels. An example is shown in Fig. 2. Unlike Su *et al.* [7], the purpose of seed clustering is not to segment the 2D seed projections from 2D seed clusters in the images, or to identify the number of true seeds in each cluster. Instead, we use the seed clustering as a way to relating the 3D seeds, and the relationship is used in the coverage function that is to be minimized.

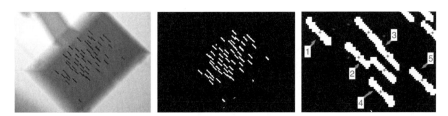

Fig. 2. (Left) X-ray image on phantom data; (Middle) the seed-only image resulted after preprocessing; (Right) Example of seed region labeling and seed grouping

On a projection image, the projections of all candidate seeds are first computed using Eq. (1). We denote a 3D candidate seed as x_n, and its 2D projection on the jth image is $P^j x_n$. For each $P^j x_n$, we find its nearest seed region, which is labeled as $L^j(P^j x_n)$. The distance from $P^j x_n$ to its closest seed region is also calculated and denoted as d_n^j ($d_n^j = 0$ if $P^j x_n$ is inside a seed region). The seed projections are then clustered based on $L^j(P^j x_n)$. Let there be K^j seed regions on the jth seed-only image, and they are labeled as $1, 2, ..., K^j$. The projections of the N candidate seeds on the jth image are then clustered into K^j sets Ω_k^j, such that

$$\forall p_1, p_2 \in \Omega_k^j, \; L^j(p_1) = L^j(p_1), \qquad j = 1, 2, ..., N_p, \; k = 1, 2, ..., K^j \qquad (4)$$

Let $\| \Omega_k^j \|$ be the cardinal of set Ω_k^j, we say the seed region with label k in j^{th} image is covered by $\| \Omega_k^j \|$ seeds. $\| \Omega_k^j \| \geq 1$. The clustering is repeated on all images.

In the example in Fig. 2(c), the seed regions are labeled from 1 to 5 and red asterisks mark the 2D projections of the candidate seeds. The three regions labeled with 1, 4 and 5 contain one true seed each. The two regions labeled with 2 and 3contain two (or more) true seeds each. Since the seeds in region 2 (and 3) are connected, it is considered as a single seed region. The candidate seeds include both true seeds and a few false seeds. In this example, upon clustering, the sets with label from 1 to 5 have 2, 3, 4, 1, and 1 element(s) individually

Local Coverage and Greedy Search. The seed clustering according to each projection can help reduce the size of our optimization problem. If a seed region is covered only by one seed, this seed must be a true one, because otherwise this region is not covered. The set of such seeds can be expressed as:

$$G = \bigcup_j \{ x_n : L^j(P^j x_n) = k \text{ and} \| \Omega_k^j \| = 1, \; k = 1,2,...,K^j \}, \quad j = 1,2,...,N_p \qquad (5)$$

where N_p is the number of projection images. These seeds are always chosen as true seeds. Hence the optimization problem is reduced to choose $(M-\|G\|)$ true seeds from $(N-\|G\|)$ candidate seeds. This can also be seen in the example in Fig. 2(c). The two regions labeled with 4 and 5 contain only one seed each. Therefore these two seeds are considered as true seeds and are always chosen.

Besides, instead of finding the global optimization of the cost function in (2), we use greedy search to find an approximate optimal solution. We also redefine the local coverage cost function as

$$C = \sum_n c(x_n), \quad c(x_n) = -\sum_{j=1}^{N_p} \frac{1 + D^j(x_n)}{1 + d_n^j}, \quad \text{for all } x_n \notin G \qquad (6)$$

where

$$D^j(x_n) = \min_{m \neq n} \| P^j x_n - P^j x_m \|, \quad \forall x_m \in S - G, \text{ and } L^j(P^j x_n) = L^j(P^j x_m) \qquad (7)$$

is the minimum distance between the projection of x_n and the projections of other seeds in the cluster in the jth image that includes x_n, and d_n^j is the distance from $P^j x_n$ to the nearest seed region. d_n^j is added in the cost function to include the effect of imperfect X-ray pose estimation.

The minimization problem in (6) is solved using greedy search iteratively. During each cycle of iteration, the seed that has the largest cost value $c(x_n)$ is considered as a false seed and is removed from the candidate seed set. G is updated at the beginning of each cycle of iteration, for after the removal of one seed, there may be additional seeds that cover some region alone (i.e. no other seed covers this region.) These seeds need to be extracted and added to **G**. The algorithm is summarized as below.

Algorithm 1. find M good seeds from N candidate seeds using greedy search
1. Initialize **S** be the set of candidate seeds.
2. For $i = 1:N\text{-}M$
3. Calculate **G** using (5).
4. Calculate local cost function $c(x)$ of all seeds x in **S - G** using (6).
5. Find $x_k \in \mathbf{S} - \mathbf{G}$, such that $x_k = \arg_x \min c(x)$.
6. Remove x_k from **S**: $\mathbf{S} = \mathbf{S} - \{x_k\}$.

3 Experiments and Results

Simulations. Synthetic C-arm images were used to verify our method. The images simulated a 50 cc prostate with a seed density of 2.0 seed/cc. The C-arm's focal length was 1000 mm, and the pixel size was 0.25 mm. Six images were generated on a $20°$ cone around the AP axis with evenly distributed angles. The seeds were represented by cylinders with a radius of 0.4 mm and a length of 1.45 mm. A typical synthetic image is shown in Fig. 3(a). No pose estimation error was assumed.

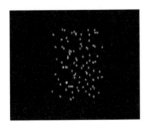 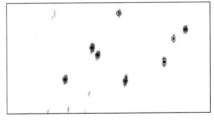

Fig. 3. (Left) Part of a synthetic C-arm image; (Right) One slice of the reconstructed 3D volume. The red circles mark the true seeds, and the green squares represent the FP seeds.

Table 1. Seed reconstruction results using different number of synthetic images

Number of images used	Number of true seeds implanted	Number of candidate seeds before FP removal	Correctly reconstructed seeds after FP removal (%)	Mean reconstruction error (mm)	Reconstructio n error STD (mm)
3	96	105.6	99.4	0.19	0.19
4	96	97.7	100	0.12	0.09

We reconstructed the seeds using 3, 4 and 6 images. For 3 images, 20 experiments were performed by using all the 20 combinations of selecting 3 images from the 6 available images. For 4 images, four experiments were performed using different image combinations. The results are shown in Table 1. In each experiment, the number of implanted seeds was assumed known. After FP removal, a set of candidate seeds that equal to the number of implanted seeds were chose. These chosen seeds were then compared with the known 3D locations of implanted seeds. When using 3 images, there were about 10% FP seeds reconstructed initially and then almost all were successfully removed, indicated by the near 100% correct final reconstruction rate. This means that when there is no pose estimation error, the seeds can be reconstructed accurately even from as few as 3 images using our method.

Phantom Studies. Experiments were performed on a seed phantom constructed from acetol. The FTRAC fiducial was used to track the C-arm (with accuracy of 0.56 mm translation and $0.33°$ rotation). It was attached to the seed phantom, as shown in Fig. 4. The seed phantom is comprised of twelve slabs with 5mm thickness each. Each slab has more than 100 holes with 5 mm spacing, into which the seed can be inserted. By precise manufacturing, the seed phantom was attached in a known position to a radiographic C-arm tracking fiducial, replicated after Jain *et al.* [13]. In this way, the exact location of each implanted seed was known relative to the tracking fiducial, serving as ground truth. Because some rotation error got introduced during assembly, the ground absolute seed positions had about 0.5 mm error. (Note that their relative positions were precisely known.) The seed density was about 1.56 seed/cc. Five data sets were collected with the number of seeds varying from 40 to. For each data set, six images within a $20°$ cone around the AP axis were taken using a *Phillips integris V3000* fluoroscope and dewarped using the pin-cushion test. We used four, five and six images to reconstruct the seeds, by using all the combinations of the six available images, i.e. 15 experiments using four images, 6 using five images, and 1 using six images for each data set. The reconstructed seeds were compared with the computed ground truth, and the results were shown in Table 2.

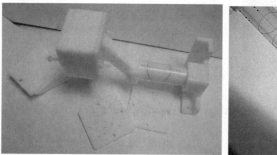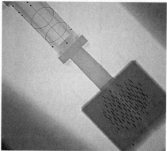

Fig. 4. (Left) An image of the seed phantom attached to the FTRAC fiducial. (Right) A typical X-ray image of the combination (with 100 seeds inserted).

It was shown in [12] that in prostate brachytherapy, 95% of the implanted seeds must be recovered in order to obtain clinically accurate estimation of the dose. Our results showed that (1) from six images more than 98% seeds can be successfully reconstructed, and (2) six images were sufficient for deriving clinically accurate dose estimation. Furthermore, the number of required images depends on the number of seeds implanted. For a smaller number of seeds (40, 55, 70), only four to five images were required. Additionally the performance of our method depends on the ratio between the number of FP seeds and the implanted seeds, which in turn depends on both the number of images used and the number of implanted seeds. Generally the lower is this ratio, the higher is the seed reconstruction ratio we may achieve.

Table 2. Seed reconstruction results on phantom data using different number of images

Number of images used	Number of seeds implanted	Number of candidate seeds before FP removal	Correctly reconstructed seeds after FP removal (%)	Mean reconstruction error (mm)	Reconstruction error STD (mm)
6	40	46	100	1.04	0.56
	55	58	100	0.67	0.39
	70	82	98.6	0.72	0.42
	85	94	100	0.97	0.44
	100	112	98	0.94	0.52
5	40	46.3	99.5	1.02	0.53
	55	68.3	98.8	0.85	0.46
	70	92.3	97.8	0.85	0.46
	85	105.3	97.0	1.00	0.57
	100	121.3	92.5	1.19	0.81
4	40	53.7	96.8	1.24	0.76
	55	82.1	94.7	0.99	0.69
	70	112	94.3	0.91	0.77
	85	135.8	90.1	1.13	0.62
	100	159.7	86.3	1.44	0.91

In summary, we presented a novel method for prostate brachytherapy seed reconstruction using C-arm images. We generate distance maps from the 2D projection images, then a 3D volume is then reconstructed using tomosynthesis using the distance maps, and finally true seeds are extracted from the voxel volume. The attractive feature of our method is that it does not require exact seed segmentation of the X-ray images. As a tradeoff, our method requires slightly higher number of images than the methods that requires elaborate explicit segmentation. Our method yields near 100% correct reconstruction from only six images with an average reconstruction accuracy of 0.86 mm (std=0.46mm). The method was robust to pose error present in radiographic C-arm tracking.

Acknowledgements. This work was funded by NSF grant EEC-9741748, NIH grant 2R44CA099374, and DoD grant PC050170.

References

[1] Zelefsky, M.J., et al.: Five-year outcome of intraoperative conformal permanent I-125 interstitial implantation for patients with clinically localized prostate cancer. Int. J. Radia.t Oncol. Biol. Phy.s 67(1), 65–70 (2007)

[2] Tubic, D., et al.: Automated seed detection and three-dimensional reconstruction II., reconstruction of permanent prostate implants using simulated annealing. Med. Phys 28(11), 2272–2279 (2001)

[3] Narayanan, S., Cho, P., Marks, R.: Fast cross-projection algorithm for reconstruction of seeds in prostate brachytherapy. Med. Phys. 29(7), 1572–1579 (2002)

[4] Todor, D., et al.: Operator-free, film-based 3D seed reconstruction in brachytherapy. Phys. Med. Biol. 47(12), 2031–2048 (2002)
[5] Lam, S.T., et al.: Three-dimensional seed reconstruction for prostate brachytherapy using Hough trajectories. Phys. Med. Biol. 49(4), 557–569 (2004)
[6] Jain, A., et al.: Matching and reconstruction of brachytherapy seeds using the Hungarian algorithm (MARSHAL). Med. Phys. 32(11), 3475–3492 (2005)
[7] Su, Y., et al.: Prostate brachytherapy seed localization by analysis of multiple projections: identifying and addressing the seed overlap problem. Med. Phy. 31(5), 1277–1287 (2004)
[8] Tutar, I.B., et al.: Tomosynthesis-based localization of radioactive seeds in prostate brachytherapy. Med. Phys. 30(12), 3135–3142 (2003)
[9] Grant, D.G.: Tomosynthesis: A three-dimensional radiographic imaging technique. IEEE Trans. Biomed. Eng. 19, 20–28 (1972)
[10] Herman, G.T., Kuba, A.: Discrete tomography in medical imaging. Proceeding of the IEEE 91(10), 1612–1626 (2003)
[11] Marengoni, M., Draper, B., Hanson, A., Sitaraman, R.: A system to place observers on a polyhedral terrain in polynomial time. Image and Vision Computing 18(10), 773–780 (2000)
[12] Su, Y., et al.: Examination of dosimetry accuracy as a function of seed detection rate in permanent prostate brachytherapy. Med. Phys. 32(9), 3049–3056 (2005)
[13] Jain, A., et al.: Robust Fluoroscope Tracking Fiducial. Med. Phys. 32(10), 3185–3198 (2005)

A New and General Method for Blind Shift-Variant Deconvolution of Biomedical Images

Moritz Blume[1], Darko Zikic[1], Wolfgang Wein[1,2], and Nassir Navab[1]

[1] Computer Aided Medical Procedures (CAMP), Technische Universität München, Germany
{blume,zikic,navab}@cs.tum.edu
[2] Siemens Corporate Research, Princeton, USA
wolfgang.wein@siemens.com

Abstract. We present a new method for blind deconvolution of multiple noisy images blurred by a shift-variant point-spread-function (PSF). We focus on a setting in which several images of the same object are available, and a transformation between these images is known. This setting occurs frequently in biomedical imaging, for example in microscopy or in medical ultrasound imaging. By using the information from multiple observations, we are able to improve the quality of images blurred by a shift-variant filter, *without* prior knowledge of this filter. Also, in contrast to other work on blind and shift-variant deconvolution, in our approach no parametrization of the PSF is required. We evaluate the proposed method quantitatively on synthetically degraded data as well as qualitatively on 3D ultrasound images of liver. The algorithm yields good restoration results and proves to be robust even in presence of high noise levels in the images.

1 Introduction

Biomedical imaging techniques suffer - like all measurements - from errors introduced in the acquisition process. Techniques which are able to remove these errors can improve the quality of the images and thus enhance their diagnostic value. Since blur is one of the most common image degradations, deconvolution methods which undo the effects of blurring and thus reveal structures not visible in the uncorrected images are extremely important in biomedical imaging. For medical imaging devices such as ultrasound or microscopy, especially the case in which the blur is not constant in the image - the so-called *shift-variant* blur - is important. The case of constant (*shift-invariant*) blur hardly occurs in biomedical applications.

The problem of deconvolution of shift-variantly blurred images is an extremely challenging task. One part of the difficulty is to determine the point-spread-function (PSF), that is, the function characterizing the blur. Up to now, this is achieved by either theoretical predictions (see e. g. [1] for medical ultrasound) or measurements. Both have to be performed for every single device and are time-consuming, complicated, error-prone, and in some cases even not feasible. Deconvolution methods that build on this previous step can not be considered as general.

As a remedy, most of the existing work assumes a simplified model, the shift-invariant one. This is tempting since it allows for the very attractive option of restoring both the image and the PSF within one method, without the need of measuring or theoretically

N. Ayache, S. Ourselin, A. Maeder (Eds.): MICCAI 2007, Part I, LNCS 4791, pp. 743–750, 2007.
© Springer-Verlag Berlin Heidelberg 2007

predicting the PSF. This class of methods is denoted as *blind* deconvolution methods. Unfortunately, assuming a shift-invariant model very often comes at the price of not adequately describing biomedical reality. Therefore, in many cases such methods do not yield optimal restorations. It would be very attractive to have both: the shift-variant model *and* a blind restoration method able to deal with this model.

In this paper, we present such a *blind* and *shift-variant* method. Our method uses multiple images of the same object together with the information about the transformation between the images. This is a setting readily available in many medical and microscopic applications, and, thanks to advancing image registration techniques (especially deformable registration), will be more and more widespread in the future. Since in this setting the observations are blurred by the same PSF, each additional observation provides information about the present degradation. Our method takes this information into account for the restoration of both the image and the PSF.

To the best of our knowledge, this is the first method capable of performing an *unparameterized*, *blind*, and *shift-variant* deconvolution. These properties make our method extremely general and widely and easily applicable to many applications in the biomedical imaging field.

1.1   Related Work

Single-view deconvolution is a standard post-processing procedure in biomedical applications such as ultrasound [2] or microscopy [3]. Unfortunately, restoration from a single-view is a dramatically ill-posed problem, and in the best case allows for blind shift-invariant deconvolution in a low noise scenario. In photography, several semi-blind shift-variant methods have been proposed [4,5,6,7,8]. However, these methods rely on *a priori* information about the blur, e. g. that the PSF is an instance of motion blur or out-of-focus blur, and thus can not be considered as general. For microscopy, some dedicated methods are known: in [9], the volume subject to restoration is reconstructed block-wise, and shift-invariance is assumed for each block. Preza and Conchello [10] assume to know the PSF at several points in space and restrict shift-variance to the depth direction.

Already in the 1970's researchers found that the multi-view scenario has advantages over single-view restoration, since each additional observation adds information that can be taken into account for the restoration process [11]. Since then, especially dedicated devices for this multi-view setting have been developed for both microscopy and ultrasound [12,13,14,15,16]. Existing restoration methods from the single-view setting have been adapted and new methods especially dedicated to the multi-view setting have been invented. Shaw *et al.* [17] combine several blurred observations by taking the maximum in Fourier space. Their restoration is fast and simple to implement. However it is not optimal, even for synthetic images, and also dramatically amplifies noise. Kikuchi *et al.* calculate synthetic projections from two blurred observations and then use those projections that are less affected by blur for a standard computed tomography reconstruction algorithm [18]. Though being well suited for their specific scenario, this is not quite general since it only works for the shift-invariant case and the direction of the blur has to be known in advance. Often, very simple restoration techniques like linear combination are applied and are reported to lead to a significant improvement of the resolution [14,15]. Soler *et al.* propose a non-blind shift-invariant deconvolution method for ultrasound that relies on a measured PSF [16].

2 Method

2.1 Model

In contrast to other multi-view techniques, we use the shift-variant image formation model

$$z_i = (u \circ \varphi_i) \star h + \eta \ , \tag{1}$$

where $z_i \in F$ is the actual measurement (F denotes the functional space of all images $\Omega \to \mathbb{R}$ where Ω is a bounded domain $\Omega = [0,1]^2 \subset \mathbb{R}^2$), $u \in F$ is the original image, $\varphi_i : \Omega \to \Omega$ is the spatial transformation between measurement and original image, $h : (\Omega \times \Omega) \to \mathbb{R}$ is the shift-variant PSF, "'$\star$'" is the shift-variant convolution operator and $\eta \in F$ represents arbitrary noise. Using this model, we assume that the PSF is equal for each observation, that is, not changing over time. This is a valid assumption for most biomedical applications. Please note that we do not restrict the transformation φ to rigid transformations which implies that also deformations are within our model.

In presence of noise, we can not assume that $z_i = u(\varphi_i) \star h$ holds exactly, so we formulate the cost function which is subject to minimization as

$$\mathcal{D}[u,h] = \frac{1}{2} \sum_{i=1}^{P} \int_{\Omega_i} e_i(\mathbf{x})^2 \, d\mathbf{x} \ , \tag{2}$$

where we suppose to dispose of P measurements. $e_i(\mathbf{x})$ is an error term that measures the difference of the convolved real image to the measurements at position $\mathbf{x}$ by

$$e_i(\mathbf{x}) = ((u \circ \varphi_i) \star h - z_i)(\mathbf{x}) = \int_{\Omega} u(\varphi_i(\xi))h(\mathbf{x}, \xi - \mathbf{x}) \, d\xi - z_i(\mathbf{x}) \ . \tag{3}$$

The set Ω_i denotes the overlapping domain of the original image u and the image transformed by φ_i.

The problem of minimizing the functional from Equation (2) is ill-posed. In order to render the problem well-posed we introduce regularizing terms $\mathcal{U}$ and $\mathcal{H}$. While $\mathcal{U}$ operates on the image u, the term $\mathcal{H}$ imposes restrictions on the point-spread-function h.

So we define the regularized functional $\mathcal{J} : F \times F \to \mathbb{R}$ to be minimized which models the problem as

$$\mathcal{J}[u,h] = \mathcal{D}[u,h] + \alpha \mathcal{U}[u] + \beta \mathcal{H}[h] \ . \tag{4}$$

Here, the positive real coefficients α and β determine the influence of the respective regularization term.

Additionally, since we assume to deal with an intensity PSF, we restrict h to zero and positive values, that is, $h(\mathbf{x}, \mathbf{s}) \geq 0$. We also assume that the imaging system neither emits nor absorbs energy and so the PSF has to be normed to one at every spatial

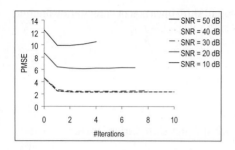 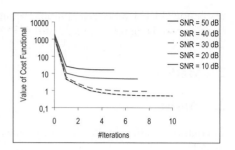

Fig. 1. The percentage mean squared error (PMSE, left plot) and the cost functional from equation (4) (right plot) are plotted over the iterations for the hippocampal rat neurons example - compare Figure (2). For low noise levels, the PMSE is reduced to approximately half of its initial value. Even for extremely noisy images our method provides a significant reduction of the PMSE. The cost function is reduced for each iteration and the algorithm terminates when its reduction is stagnating.

position $\mathbf{x}$ in the image , that is $\int_\Omega h(\mathbf{x},\mathbf{s})\,d\mathbf{s} = 1$. The final goal then is to find functions u and h that minimize $\mathcal{J}$ subject to constraints, that is, compute

$$\underset{u,h}{\operatorname{argmin}}\ J[u,h]\quad \text{subject to}\quad h(\mathbf{x},\mathbf{s})\geq 0\ \text{ and }\ \int_\Omega h(\mathbf{x},\mathbf{s})\,d\mathbf{s} = 1\ \forall \mathbf{x},\mathbf{s}\in\Omega\ . \quad (5)$$

Regularization Term $\mathcal{U}$. Total variation [19] has proven to be a very successful method for image regularization since it discourages noise while edges are preserved

$$\mathcal{U}[u] = \int_\Omega |\nabla_\mathbf{x} u(\mathbf{x})|\,d\mathbf{x}\ . \quad (6)$$

This regularization term penalizes too large gradients in the image to be reconstructed.

Regularization Term $\mathcal{H}$. As mentioned, the lack of information due to the shift-variant PSF is tremendous. In order to account for this lack of information and the resulting ill-posedness of the problem, we introduce a regularization term $\mathcal{H}$ which operates on the PSF:

$$\mathcal{H}[h] = \iint_\Omega |\nabla_\mathbf{x} h(\mathbf{x},\mathbf{s})|^2\,d\mathbf{s}\,d\mathbf{x}\ . \quad (7)$$

A shift-variant PSF can be considered as a set of shift-invariant PSFs for each pixel $\mathbf{x}$. The regularization term $\mathcal{H}$ penalizes the difference between the shift-invariant PSFs at neighboring pixels. It is important to note that this regularization *will not* impose smoothness on the PSF itself but only on their transitions.

2.2 Algorithm

The main difficulty of blind deconvolution in general is that we neither have u nor h. For this type of problem, You and Kaveh identify a scale problem [20] and so justify an algorithmic scheme that is alternating between the calculation of h and u. For the

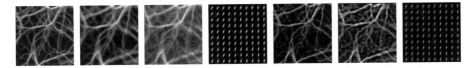

Fig. 2. The original image of hippocampal rat neurons (left) is blurred by a shift-variant PSF (fourth from left) and noise of different strength is added (second and third). Only the first of four observations for each noise case is shown. The restored images and the restored PSF for the 50 dB noise case are shown aside. For 2D images, a shift-variant PSF can be considered as a 2D grid of shift-invariant PSFs for each pixel. For the sake of a clear visualization, the PSF is only imaged for a region of interest of 10×10 image pixels.

calculation of h we assume that u is given, and for the calculation of u we assume h to be given. These two steps are executed alternately until convergence

First step: $h \leftarrow \mathrm{argmin}_h \, \mathcal{J}[u,h]$ subject to constraints on h (8)

Second step: $u \leftarrow \mathrm{argmin}_u \, \mathcal{J}[u,h]$.   (9)

These two optimization problems are treated completely independently. In first step, we assume that u is perfectly known and on this base h is sought. As an initial guess for u we take the first observation z_1. After discretization, any constrained least-squares optimizer can be used. In the second optimization problem we assume that h is perfectly known and on this base u is sought. We derive the Euler-Lagrange first order optimality equation corresponding to this optimization problem by extending the derivation of [8] to the multi-view scenario:

$$\sum_i \int_{\Omega_i} e_i(\xi + \varphi_i^{-1}(\mathbf{x})) h(\xi + \varphi_i^{-1}(\mathbf{x}), \xi) \, d\xi = -\alpha \nabla_{\mathbf{x}}^{\top} \frac{1}{\sqrt{u_{x_1}^2 + u_{x_2}^2 + \varepsilon^2}} \nabla_{\mathbf{x}} u. \quad (10)$$

The image which is subject to reconstruction is found by solving this PDE.

We discretize equation (10) with implicit finite-differences. This leads to a nonlinear system of equations. The nonlinearity can be faced by rearranging it as a fixed-point equation which leads to an iterative solution scheme. Each iteration then involves the solution of a very large linear system of equations that can be solved by any standard method. We use the method of conjugate gradients.

3 Results

3.1 Quantitative Evaluation

We use a simulation of the degradation process with known ground truth. We evaluate our method for several test cases with different noise levels. In each case, four observations are synthetically generated by transforming and degrading an original image. We simulate the image acquisition process by a device suffering from shift-variant blurring and noise. For the simulation, we perform the following steps for each observation:

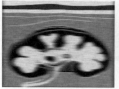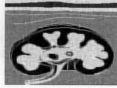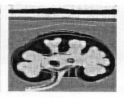

Fig. 3. Comparison of our blind shift-variant method to Soler's non-blind shift-invariant method: Soler *et al.* simulate a multi-view setting by degrading a synthetic image of the kidney with shift-invariant Gaussian blur and noise. Only the first of two generated observations is shown (left). For their restoration in (second from left), they use the known PSF. Our method restores both the image and the PSF (third and fourth from left), without any *a priori* knowledge about the PSF. Even so, our results are comparable.

(i) rotation and translation, (ii) blurring (simulated by shift-variant filtering) and finally (iii) addition of white Gaussian noise. The test cases differ in the amount of added noise. We measure the noise level by the signal to noise ratio $SNR = P_{z_i}/P_{Noise}$, where the signal power P_{z_i} is the power of the observations z_i and P_{Noise} is the noise power. The quality of reconstruction for the image is measured by the percentage mean squared error $PMSE_u = |u - u^{orig}|^2/(|\Omega||u^{orig}|^2)$.

For low noise levels, Figure 2 shows clearly that the obtained restoration of both the image and the PSF comes close to their respective originals. Our restoration leads to better defined structures even for very high noise levels. The reduction of the PMSE as well as the evaluation of the cost functional of equation (4) is presented in Figure 1. We observe fast and robust convergence of the algorithm for all test cases.

3.2 3D Ultrasound Restoration of a Volunteer's Liver

We apply our algorithm to a 3D ultrasound acquisition of a volunteer's liver acquired with the Siemens SONOLINE Antares ©. We acquire two volumes of size of 100^3 voxels each, and the second volume is rotated by an angle of approximately $90°$ about the axial direction. Figure 4 shows selected slices of different orientations of the first observation. The corresponding restoration disposes of better defined structures and reveals some details not quite visible in the observation. Note that the blur extension of the restored PSF varies spatially. Our algorithm performs five iterations until convergence and in our current C++ implementation this takes about six hours.

3.3 Comparison to a Non-blind Shift-Invariant Method

Comparison of our method to other deconvolution methods is a delicate matter, since - to the best of our knowledge - there is no method that performs blind shift-variant deconvolution without assuming an *a priori* blur model. However, we compare our method to the recently proposed non-blind shift-invariant method of Soler *et al.* [16]. There, synthetic images of a kidney are blurred by shift-invariant Gaussian blur and noise is added and the known PSF is used for restoration. Figure 3 shows that though our method does not use the PSF and assumes a shift-variant blur, it produces competitive results. It restores both the image and the PSF. The restored PSF fits to the specifications made in [16].

A New and General Method for Blind Shift-Variant Deconvolution

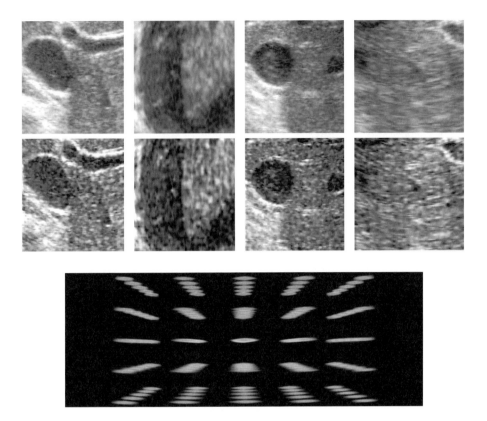

Fig. 4. Multi-view unparameterized blind shift-variant deconvolution of 3D ultrasound acquisitions of a volunteer's liver: two 3D spatially transformed observations are used for restoration. The transformation between the two observations is obtained by deformable registration as described in [21]. The first row shows selected slices of the first observation. The corresponding restored slices are shown in the second row. Last row: restored PSF. For 3D images, a shift-variant PSF can be considered as a 3D grid of shift-invariant PSFs for each voxel (for the sake of a clear visualization we use a coarser grid). It can be clearly seen that the PSF is changing its shape from the lower layers to the upper layers.

4   Conclusion

We present a new method for multi-view blind deconvolution. Existing blind methods assume a stationary blur that is not changing over the image. In contrast, we use a shift-variant blur model that allows the blur to vary with the spatial position in the image. This makes our method better suited for biomedical applications than shift-invariant methods. Due to its blind character, there is no need for previous measurements or theoretical predictions of the PSF. We show experimentally that our method is even competitive to non-blind shift-invariant methods. Our experiments prove robustness, also for extremely high noise levels.

References

1. Ng, J., Prager, R., Kingsbury, N., Treece, G., Gee, A.: Modeling ultrasound imaging as a linear, shift-variant system. Ultrasonics, Ferroelectrics and Frequency Control, IEEE Transactions on 53(3), 549–563 (2006)
2. Jirik, R., Taxt, T.: Two-dimensional blind iterative deconvolution of medical ultrasound images. In: Ultrasonics Symposium, IEEE Computer Society Press, Los Alamitos (2004)
3. Sarder, P., Nehorai, A.: Deconvolution methods for 3-d fluorescence microscopy images. IEEE Signal Processing Magazine 23(3), 32–45 (2006)
4. Sawchuk, A.: Space-variant image motion degradation and restoration. Proceedings of the IEEE 60(7), 854–861 (1972)
5. Tekalp, A.M., Kaufman, H., Woods, J.W.: Model-based segmentation and space-variant restoration of blurred images by decision-directed filtering. Signal Process. 15(3), 259–269 (1988)
6. Lagendijk, R.L., Biemond, J.: Block-adaptive image identification and restoration. In: Acoustics, Speech, and Signal Processing, 1991. ICASSP 1991. 1991 International Conference on, Toronto, Ont. Canada pp. 2497–2500 (1991)
7. Trussell, H., Fogel, S.: Identification and restoration of spatially variant motion blurs in sequential images. IEEE Transactions on Image Processing 1(1), 123–126 (1992)
8. You, Y.L., Kaveh, M.: Blind image restoration by anisotropic regularization. Image Processing, IEEE Transactions on 8(3), 396–407 (1999)
9. Avinash, G.B.: Data-driven, simultaneous blur and image restoration in 3-d fluorescence microscopy. Journal of Microscopy 183(2), 145–157 (1996)
10. Preza, C., Conchello, J.A.: Depth-variant maximum-likelihood restoration for three-dimensional fluorescence microscopy. J. Opt. Soc. Am. A 21, 1593–1601 (2004)
11. Skaer, R., Whytock, S.: Interpretation of the three-dimensional structure of living nuclei by specimen tilt. J. Cell. Sci. 19(1), 1–10 (1975)
12. Kikuchi, S., Sonobe, K., Shinohara, D., Shinro Mashiko, N.O., Hiraoka, Y.: A double-axis microscope and its three-dimensional image position adjustment based on an optical marker method. Optics Communications 129, 237–244 (1996)
13. Kozubek, M., Matula, P., Eipel, H., Hausmann, M.: Automated multi-view 3d image acquisition in human genome research. In: 3D Data Processing Visualization and Transmission. In: Proceedings. First International Symposium on pp. 91–98 (2002)
14. Swoger, J., Huisken, J., Stelzer, E.H.K.: Multiple imaging axis microscopy improves resolution for thick-sample applications. Optics Letters 28, 1654–1656 (2003)
15. Huisken, J., Swoger, J., Bene, F.D., Wittbrodt, J., Stelzer, E.H.K.: Optical sectioning deep inside live embryos by selective plane illumination microscopy. Science 305(5686), 1007–1009 (2004)
16. Soler, P., Villain, N., Bloch, I., Angelini, E.: Volume reconstruction of breast echography from anisotropically degraded scans. In: Proceedings of the IASTED International Conference on Biomedical Engineering, vol. 9, pp. 349–355 (2005)
17. Shaw, P.J., Agard, D.A., Hiroaka, Y., Sedat, J.W.: Tilted view reconstruction in optical microscopy. Biophysical Journal 55, 101–110 (1989)
18. Kikuchi, S., Sonobe, K., Sidharta, L.S., Ohyama, N.: Three-dimensional computed tomography for optical microscopes. Optics Communications 107, 432–444 (1994)
19. Rudin, L.I., Osher, S., Fatemi, E.: Nonlinear total variation based noise removal algorithms. Physica D 60, 259–268 (1992)
20. You, Y.L., Kaveh, M.: A regularization approach to joint blur identification and image restoration. IEEE Transactions on 5(3), 416–428 (1996)
21. Zikic, D., Wein, W., Khamene, A., Clevert, D.A., Navab, N.: Fast deformable registration of 3D-ultrasound using a variational approach. In: Larsen, R., Nielsen, M., Sporring, J. (eds.) MICCAI 2006. LNCS, vol. 4190, Springer, Heidelberg (2006)

Registration of Lung Tissue Between Fluoroscope and CT Images: Determination of Beam Gating Parameters in Radiotherapy

Sukmoon Chang[1,2], Jinghao Zhou[2], Qingshan Liu[2], Dimitris N. Metaxas[2],
Bruce G. Haffty[3], Sung N. Kim[3], Salma J. Jabbour[3], and Ning j. Yue[3]

[1] Computer Science, Capital College, Penn State University, PA, USA
[2] Center for CBIM, Rutgers, The State University of New Jersey, NJ, USA
{sukmoon,qsliu,dnm}@cs.rutgers.edu, jhzhou@eden.rutgers.edu
[3] Dept. of Radiation Oncology, UMDNJ-RWJ Medical School, NJ, USA
{hafftybg,jabbousk,kim18,yuenj}@umdnj.edu

Abstract. Significant research has been conducted in radiation beam gating technology to manage target and organ motions in radiotherapy treatment of cancer patients. As more and more on-board imagers are installed onto linear accelerators, fluoroscopic imaging becomes readily available at the radiation treatment stage. Thus, beam gating parameters, such as beam-on timing and beam-on window can be potentially determined by employing image registration between treatment planning CT images and fluoroscopic images. We propose a new registration method on deformable soft tissue between fluoroscopic images and DRR (Digitally Reconstructed Radiograph) images from planning CT images using active shape models. We present very promising results of our method applied to 30 clinical datasets. These preliminary results show that the method is very robust for the registration of deformable soft tissue. The proposed method can be used to determine beam-on timing and treatment window for radiation beam gating technology, and can potentially greatly improve radiation treatment quality.

1 Introduction

Radiation therapy is an important treatment modality for various cancers. The goals of radiation therapy can be better achieved by delivering conformal radiation dose to target volume while sparing normal or critical structures as much as possible. Various radiation delivery technologies, such as the three dimensional conformal radiation therapy (3DCRT) and the intensity modulated radiation therapy (IMRT), have been adopted and used to serve the purpose. However, the efficacy of these technologies may be compromised because of organ motion during treatment. It has been well known that organs and tumors located in the thorax and upper abdomen may exhibit significant respiratory induced motions [1,2]. These physiologically related motions might well compromise the efficacy of radiation treatment of the tumors since larger margins are needed to provide adequate coverage of the targets, which may subsequently lead to

N. Ayache, S. Ourselin, A. Maeder (Eds.): MICCAI 2007, Part I, LNCS 4791, pp. 751–758, 2007.
© Springer-Verlag Berlin Heidelberg 2007

increased toxicity and prevent dose escalation [3,4]. Many techniques have been proposed and utilized to address the negative impact of respiratory motion during radiation treatment [5,6,7]. Although the method proposed in this paper is potentially applicable to all these techniques, we will limit our discussion only to the beam gating technique for simplicity.

In radiation therapy, treatment planning is usually conducted based on simulation CT images before treatment. At the planning stage, target volume is delineated on the CT image and the plan is designed so that the target volume will be adequately covered with radiation beams. The principle of using beam gating technology is to establish a feedback mechanism between tumor movement and radiation beam-on control during treatment: if the tumor moves outside the designed target volume, the radiation beam is turned off; otherwise, the radiation beam remains on.

In the current beam gating technology, the beam-on timing and treatment window are determined by a target surrogate that is placed outside the patient's body. With this method, to correctly deliver doses to the target, not only is a reliable correlation between the motions of the surrogate and the tumor required, but also this correlation needs to be reproducible from the simulation planning stage to the treatment stage. These two prerequisites, however, are difficult to satisfy. Another alternative is to implant a few markers into the target volume and use the markers as tracers to control the beam gating. The drawback of this approach is that it involves a surgical procedure and it may complicate the radiation treatment process. Furthermore, if the implanted markers migrate away from their original locations in the plan, not only is the tumor missed, but also normal tissue will be unnecessarily damaged.

As more and more on-board imagers are installed onto linear accelerators, fluoroscopic imaging becomes readily available at the radiation treatment stage. Since fluoroscopic imaging is able to detect target or organ motion, in this paper, we propose an automatic and robust registration method for soft tissues registration between fluoroscopic images and planning CT images (e.g., DRR). Then, we can derive temporal and spatial information of target volumes at the treatment stage. This information, instead of the artificial surrogate or implanted markers, can be used to determine beam-on timing and treatment window.

2   Method

Suppose that N fluoroscopic images are acquired during a period of time at the treatment stage. Let $I(\boldsymbol{r}^T(t_i))$ and $I(\boldsymbol{r}^O(t_i))$ denote the representations of the target and the organ, respectively, on a fluoroscopic image I taken at time t_i, $1 \leq i \leq N$. Also let $I(\boldsymbol{r}^T_{\mathrm{CT}})$ and $I(\boldsymbol{r}^O_{\mathrm{CT}})$ denote the representations of the target and the organ, respectively, projected onto the digitally reconstructed radiographs (DRR) from the treatment planning CT or in 3D CT volume. An image registration algorithm will need to search through $I(\boldsymbol{r}^T(t_i))$ and $I(\boldsymbol{r}^O(t_i))$ and determine t_k such that an entropy function

$$H\left[\, I(\boldsymbol{r}^T(t_k)) - I(\boldsymbol{r}^T_{\mathrm{CT}}),\;\; I(\boldsymbol{r}^O(t_k)) - I(\boldsymbol{r}^O_{\mathrm{CT}}) \,\right] \tag{1}$$

reaches at its minimum. This time t_k can be considered as the time at which the target and organ move to the locations that match those on the planning CT images. Therefore, to accurately deliver the radiation dose, the radiation beam needs to be turned on at t_k. However, in reality, if the beam were turned on only at time t_k, the gated radiation treatment would be prolonged to an unacceptable level. A practical approach to avoid the unacceptably prolonged treatment is to allow a beam-on window, during which the movements of the target and the organ are within a pre-specified margin $\boldsymbol{\delta}$. This beam-on window $[t_{k_1}, t_{k_2}]$ can be determined by minimizing the following two entropy functions:

$$H\left[\, I(\boldsymbol{r}^T(t_{k_1})) - I(\boldsymbol{r}^{\boldsymbol{T}}_{\mathrm{CT}} - \boldsymbol{\delta}),\ \ I(\boldsymbol{r}^O(t_{k_1})) - I(\boldsymbol{r}^{\boldsymbol{O}}_{\mathrm{CT}} - \boldsymbol{\delta})\,\right] \tag{2}$$

$$H\left[\, I(\boldsymbol{r}^T(t_{k_2})) - I(\boldsymbol{r}^{\boldsymbol{T}}_{\mathrm{CT}} + \boldsymbol{\delta}),\ \ I(\boldsymbol{r}^O(t_{k_2})) - I(\boldsymbol{r}^{\boldsymbol{O}}_{\mathrm{CT}} + \boldsymbol{\delta})\,\right] \tag{3}$$

Although various registration algorithms between fluoroscopic images and CT images have been proposed, the registration of soft tissue remains a major challenge. For example, [8] discussed a method based on robust similarity measurement, while [9] proposed a method based on both robust similarity measurement and optimization technique. In [10], a 3D volume is reconstructed from fluoroscopic images and compared to 3D CT. Soft tissues are not considered in any of these methods. In [11], deformable soft tissues are considered in the evaluation of the accuracy of similarity measurements; however, the image organ was a phantom spine and only a region of interest defined by user was registered.

In this section, we describe an automatic and robust method for the registration of deformable organs in medical images taken at different times using different modalities. Specifically, we propose a method for the registration of the lungs in fluoroscopic images to those in DRR images from planning CT. The proposed method consists of two steps: (1) accurate delineation of lung areas from both fluoroscopic and DRR images and (2) registration of the delineated lung areas. For the accurate delineation of lung areas, we use the active shape model approach with significant improvements [12,13,14,15].

2.1 Active Shape Models (ASM) and Their Limitations

An active shape model (ASM) represents the features of a shape as the point distribution model (PDM) [12]. Given a set of training images, the feature of interest in each image is manually labeled with n landmark points and represented as a vector in $2n$-dimensional space, i.e., $\boldsymbol{x} = \langle x_0, y_0, x_1, y_1, \cdots, x_{n-1}, y_{n-1} \rangle$. After aligning these vectors into a common coordinate system, a set of orthogonal bases $\boldsymbol{P}$ is computed with the principal component analysis. Then, each aligned shape can be reconstructed as $\boldsymbol{x} = \bar{\boldsymbol{x}} + \boldsymbol{P}\boldsymbol{b}$, where $\bar{\boldsymbol{x}}$ and $\boldsymbol{b}$ are the mean shape and the shape parameter vector, respectively. This equation also allows us to search for a new example of the shape in an unlabeled image by varying $\boldsymbol{b}$ appropriately, often based on low-level image features such as the gradients along normal directions to the boundary of an initial shape toward the strongest edge in the image [12]. Although it has been used successfully in many applications, ASM has two important limitations for the delineation of lung areas from both

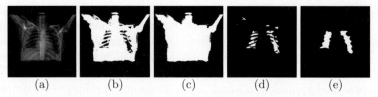

Fig. 1. The coarse segmentation of lung areas from DRR images. (a) Original DRR image, (b) Image after thresholding, (c) Image after morphological filling, (d) Image after XOR operation, and (e) Image after dilation and erosion operations.

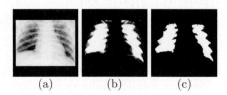

Fig. 2. The coarse segmentation of lung areas of fluoroscopic images. (a) Original fluoroscopic image, (b) Image after thresholding, (c) Image after dilation and erosion operations.

Fig. 3. Lung area segmentation. (a) and (b) DRR and fluoroscopic images by ASM with M-estimator, (c) Fluoroscopic image by ASM without M-estimator.

fluoroscopic and DDR images. In the next two sections, we will address these limitations and propose methods to overcome these drawbacks.

2.2   Automatic Initialization of ASM

The major drawback of ASM for searching for a new example of the shape in an unlabeled image is the initialization of the model. If the model is initialized too far from the feature of interest, the process may fail. To automate the accurate initialization of the model, we first rapidly extract the lung areas from unlabeled images by applying a series of morphological operators. The coarse segmentation process is illustrated in Figs. 1 and 2.

For DRR images (Fig. 1), the given image in (a) is first normalized and thresholded, using the mean intensity value of the normalized image as the threshold value, to generate a binary images shown in (b). Next, we perform the morphological filling on (b) to obtain (c). Then, we combine (b) and (c) with XOR operation to obtain (d). Finally, after applying dilation and erosion operations on (d), we obtain the coarse lung areas as shown in (e). For fluoroscopic images (Fig. 2), the given image in (a) is also normalized and thresholded, using the mean intensity value of the normalized image as the threshold value, to produce a binary image shown in (b). After applying dilation and erosion operations on (b), we obtain the coarse lung areas as shown in (c).

Note that our interest at this step is not to accurately segment the lung areas. The coarse lung areas obtained here are used only to automate the accurate initialization of the shape model on unlabeled images. We achieve the automatic and accurate initialization by aligning the centers of the shape models to the centers of the segmented coarse lung areas.

2.3 Occluded Lung Area Segmentation

Another limitation of ASM in finding an object in unlabeled images is that it heavily relies on the low-level image features to guide the search for the optimal positions of the feature points. For example, the gradient descent search on the image intensity profile has been widely used to move the model points toward the strongest edge in the image [12]. However, this approach is not suitable for the accurate delineation of the lung areas in DDR and fluoroscopic images since the ribs occlude the lungs and appear as the strongest edge as can be seen in Fig 1(a) and 2(a). We overcome this difficulty by introducing a robust error function based on the M-estimator [13,16].

Given an orthogonal basis $\boldsymbol{P}$ obtained in Sec. 2.1, the projection $\boldsymbol{C}$ of a new example shape $\boldsymbol{X}$ is given by $\boldsymbol{C} = \boldsymbol{P}^T d\boldsymbol{X}$, where $\boldsymbol{X} = \bar{\boldsymbol{X}} + d\boldsymbol{X}$ and $\bar{\boldsymbol{X}}$ is the mean shape of the aligned shapes from the training images. Using the projection $\boldsymbol{C}$, we can also find a corresponding shape as $\hat{\boldsymbol{X}} = \bar{\boldsymbol{X}} + \boldsymbol{P}\boldsymbol{C}$, in which $\hat{\boldsymbol{X}}$ and $\boldsymbol{P}\boldsymbol{C}$ approximates $\boldsymbol{X}$ and $d\boldsymbol{X}$, respectively. Therefore, in addition to optimizaing $\boldsymbol{X}$ and $d\boldsymbol{X}$ by the gradient descent search normal to the boundary only, our goal is to also find the optimal $\boldsymbol{C}$ by minimizing the robust energy function, $\boldsymbol{E}(\boldsymbol{C}) = \min_{\boldsymbol{C}} \rho(\|d\boldsymbol{X} - \boldsymbol{P}\boldsymbol{C}\|, \sigma)$, where $\rho(x, \sigma) = x^2/(x^2 + \sigma^2)$ is the Geman-McClure error function and σ is a scale parameter that controls the convexity of the robust function. With an iterative gradient descent search on $\boldsymbol{E}$, we get $\boldsymbol{C}^{(n+1)} = \boldsymbol{C}^{(n)} + \lambda \Delta \boldsymbol{C}$, where λ is a small constant that determines the step size and

$$\Delta \boldsymbol{C} = \frac{\partial \boldsymbol{E}_{rpca}}{\partial \boldsymbol{C}} = -2\boldsymbol{P}(d\boldsymbol{X} - \boldsymbol{P}\boldsymbol{C}) \frac{\sigma^2}{(\|d\boldsymbol{X} - \boldsymbol{P}\boldsymbol{C}\|^2)^2}$$

By continuing the iterative process until $\|\boldsymbol{E}^{(n+1)} - \boldsymbol{E}^{(n)}\| < \epsilon$, where ϵ is a pre-selected tolerance, we obtain the optimal project $\boldsymbol{C}^*$ and a robust shape in the shape space as $\hat{\boldsymbol{X}} = \bar{\boldsymbol{X}} + \boldsymbol{P}\boldsymbol{C}^*$. Fig. 3 shows the typical results of the process applied to 30 clinical datasets, 25 of which were used as a training set. In the figure, (a) and (b) show the results of the ASM with M-estimator, where the lung areas occluded by the ribs are accurately segmented, while (c) shows the inaccruate result of the ASM without M-estimator.

2.4 Registration of the Segmented Lung Areas

Let $\boldsymbol{x}^F$ and $\boldsymbol{x}^D$ be the shape models of the lungs in fluoroscopic and DRR images obtained from the previous section, each containing n landmark points. The registration of $\boldsymbol{x}^F$ onto $\boldsymbol{x}^D$ is achieved by finding the parameters of a 2D transformation that minimizes the weighted least square error:

$$\epsilon = \sum_{i=0}^{n} \left(\boldsymbol{p}_i^D - \boldsymbol{M}(s, \theta, t_x, t_y) \cdot \boldsymbol{p}_i^F \right)^T \boldsymbol{W} \left(\boldsymbol{p}_i^D - \boldsymbol{M}(s, \theta, t_x, t_y) \cdot \boldsymbol{p}_i^F \right)$$

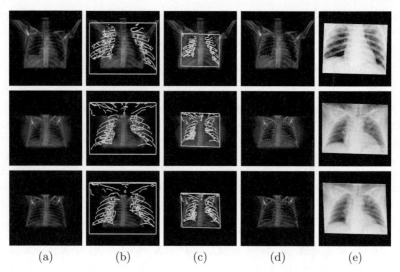

Fig. 4. Registration. (a) DRR image, (b) and (c) Fluoroscopic image before and after registration, superimposed on DRR image (only salient edges of the fluoroscopic image are shown for display purposes), (d) ASM contours on DRR image (red: ASM of DRR; yellow: ASM of registered fluoroscopic image), and (e) Registered fluoroscopic image.

where, $\boldsymbol{p}_i$ is the i-th point of a shape model in homogeneous coordinate system,

$$\boldsymbol{M}(s, \theta, t_x, t_y) = \begin{pmatrix} s\cos\theta & -s\sin\theta & t_x \\ s\sin\theta & s\cos\theta & t_y \\ 0 & 0 & 1 \end{pmatrix}$$

and $\boldsymbol{W}$ is a diagonal matrix of weights for each $\boldsymbol{p}_i$ that can be chosen to give more weights to the stable points [12]. The results of the registration process are shown in Fig. 4 and discussed in the next section.

3   Results

We applied our method to 30 clinical datasets from different patients. Fig. 4 illustrates the results of the proposed method applied to three typical datasets. The given fixed images (DRR images) are shown in Fig. 4(a). Fig. 4(b) shows the original fluoroscopic images superimposed on the corresponding fixed images before registration, while (c) shows the same fluoroscopic images after registration. Note that, in Fig. 4(b) and (c), only the salient edges of the fluoroscopic images are shown for display purposes. As can be seen from Fig. 4(d), the ASM models from the fluoroscopic images are accurately registered onto the corresponding DRR images. Finally, Fig. 4(e) shows the fluoroscopic images transformed and registered to the corresponding fixed images.

The results are also summarized in Table 1. The table shows that, on average, the mean distance and the root-mean-square error (RMSE) of the corresponding model points between the fixed image and the registered moving image are less than 7 pixels. The table also shows the overlap ratios of the lung areas between the DRR images and the registered fluoroscopic images. These overlap ratios can be used to determine the beam-on windows $[t_{k_1}, t_{k_2}]$ that minimize the two entropy functions in Eq. (2) and (3) given in Section 2. For example, in the table, one of the fluoroscopic images registered onto the corresponding DRR image shows that the lung areas in the two images overlap well over 93%. Thus, the time that this particular fluoroscopic image was taken can be interpreted as the t_k that minimizes the entropy function in Eq. (1).

4   Discussion

We proposed an automatic and robust method for the registration of fluoroscopic images and DRR images from planning CT on deformable soft tissue, using an improved active shape model. We also presented various results of our method applied to 30 clinical datasets. With these promising results, the method can be used to determine beam-on timing and treatment window for beam gating technology without requiring a monitor or implanted markers. Since each of the fluoroscopic images is time stamped in segquence, the time that corresponds to the fluoroscopic image that matches the CT image set with the largest overlap ratio is when the radiation beam should be turned on. In this paper, we limited our discussion only to the beam gating techniques for simplicity. However, the proposed method is also applicable to the real-time target tracking as well as the dynamic multileaf collimator tracking.

Though the method is presented for the registration between fluoroscopic images and a 3D CT image set, the principle can also be applied to 4D computed tomography (4DCT) images. 4DCT technology has been introduced and becomes commercially available for clinical applications [17,18]. 4DCT images are usually reconstructed through time-resolved 3D CT data acquisition and contain spatiotemporal patient anatomic information. With the 4DCT technology, it is possible to obtain more information on organ and tumor motions at the simulation and planning stage. Theoretically, a dynamic treatment plan can be designed based on the 4DCT images, but the dynamically designed treatment requires higher degree of motion verification at the treatment stage. With the registration between the fluoroscopic images and 4DCT images, the derived

Table 1. Summary on 30 clinical datasets (MD, RMSE: mean distance and root mean square error of the corresponding points between two models; Overlap(L/R): overlap ratios between two registered left (or, right) lung areas)

Dataset	MD	RMSE	Overlap(L)	Overlap(R)
Best	5.618	6.665	0.930	0.980
Worst	9.515	10.163	0.819	0.821
Average	6.036	6.979	0.880	0.901

temporal and spatial information can be used not only for the determination of
the gating parameters but also for the verification of motion pattern to ensure
a safe dynamic treatment delivery of the highest possible quality.

References

1. Seppenwoolde, Y., et al.: Precise and real-time measurement of 3D tumor motion in lung due to breathing and heartbeat, measured during radiotherapy. Int. J. Padiat. Oncol. Biol. Phys. 53(4), 822–834 (2002)
2. Brandner, E., et al.: Abdominal organ motion measured using 4D CT. Int. J. Padiat. Oncol. Biol. Phys. 65(2), 554–560 (2006)
3. Bos, L., et al.: The sensitivity of dose distributions for organ motion and set-up uncertainties in prostate IMRT. Radiother. Oncol. 76, 18–26 (2005)
4. Hong, T., et al.: The impact of daily setup variations on head-and-neck intensity-modulated radiation therapy. Int. J. Radiat. Oncol. Biol. Phys. 61, 779–788 (2005)
5. Ozhasoglu, C., et al.: Issues in respiratory motion compensation during external-beam radiotherapy. Int. J. Padiat. Oncol. Biol. Phys. 52, 1389–1399 (2002)
6. Wijesooriya, K., et al.: Determination of maximum leaf velocity and acceleration of a dynamic multileaf collimator: Implications for 4D radiotherapy. Med. Phys. 32, 932–941 (2005)
7. Vedam, S., Keall, P., Kini, V., Mohan, R.: Determining parameters for respiration gated radiotherapy. Med. Phys. 28, 2139–2146 (2001)
8. Livyatan, H., Yaniv, Z., Joskowicz, L.: Gradient-based 2-d/3-d rigid registration of fluoroscopic X-ray to CT. IEEE Trans. Med. Imag. 22(11), 1395–1406 (2003)
9. Zollei, L., et al.: 2d-3d rigid registration of X-ray fluoroscopy and CT images using mutual information and sparsely sampled histogram estimators. In: CVPR, pp. 696–703 (2001)
10. Tomazevic, D., Likar, B., Permus, F.: 3-d/2-d registration by integrating 2-d information in 3-d. IEEE Trans. Med. Imag. 25(1), 17–27 (2006)
11. Penney, G., et al.: A comparison of similarity measures for use in 2-d/3-d medical image registration. IEEE Trans. Med. Imag. 17(4), 586–595 (1998)
12. Cootes, T., Taylor, C., Cooper, D., Graham, J.: Active shape models—their training and application. Comp. Vis. Imag. Under. 61(1), 38–59 (1995)
13. Rogers, M., Graham, J.: Robust active shape model search. In: Heyden, A., Sparr, G., Nielsen, M., Johansen, P. (eds.) ECCV 2002. LNCS, vol. 2353, pp. 517–530. Springer, Heidelberg (2002)
14. Beichel, R., Bischof, H., Leberl, F., Sonka, M.: Robust active appearance models and their application to medical image analysis. IEEE Trans. Med. Imag. 24(9), 1151–1169 (2005)
15. van Ginneken, B., Stegmann, M., Loog, M.: Segmentation of anatomical structures in chest radiographs using supervised methods: A comparative study on a public database. Med. Imag. Anal. 10(1), 19–40 (2006)
16. De La Torre, F., Black, M.: A framework for robust subspace learning. Int. J. Comput. Vis. 54(1-3), 117–142 (2003)
17. Keall, P., et al.: Acquiring 4D thoracic CT scans using a multislice helical method. Phys. Med. Biol. 49, 2053–2067 (2004)
18. Rietzel, E., Pan, T., Chen, G.: 4D computed tomography: Image formation and clinical protocol. Med. Phys. 32, 874–889 (2005)

Null Point Imaging: A Joint Acquisition/Analysis Paradigm for MR Classification

Alain Pitiot[1], John Totman[1], and Penny Gowland[2]

[1] Brain & Body Centre
[2] Sir Peter Mansfield Magnetique Resonance Centre
University of Nottingham, UK
{alain.pitiot,john.totman,penny.gowland}@nottingham.ac.uk

Abstract. Automatic classification of neurological tissues is a first step to many structural analysis pipelines. Most computational approaches are designed to extract the best possible classification results out of MR data acquired with standard clinical protocols. We observe that the characteristics of the latter owe more to the historical circumstances under which they were developed and the visual appreciation of the radiographer who acquires the images than to the optimality with which they can be classified with an automatic algorithm.

We submit that better performances could be obtained by considering the acquisition and analysis processes *conjointly* rather than optimising them independently. Here, we propose such a joint approach to MR tissue classification in the form of a fast MR sequence, which nulls the magnitude and changes the sign of the phase at the boundary between tissue types. A simple phase-based thresholding algorithm then suffices to segment the tissues. Preliminary results show promises to simplify and shorten the overall classification process.

1 Introduction

The explosive growth in medical imaging technologies such as Magnetic Resonance Imaging MRI), computer assisted tomography (CT) or positron emission tomography (PET) has fuelled an unprecedented drive to explore the structural and functional organization of the human body. Arguably one of the most complex organs, the human brain has been the primary beneficiary of these fast paced developments. A major objective of neuroscience is to understand both the anatomical characteristics of the various structures of the brain and their inter-relationships. From the structural standpoint (our main focus here), this ambitious goal is often translated into statistical analysis of anatomical variability, within groups, through development, or between normal and diseased populations [1]. A pivotal first step to most MR based structural studies, automatic tissue classification forms the basis for a variety of neuro-informatics applications: quantitative measurement of tissue loss or gain in healthy and diseases populations [2], analysis of cortical thickness and folding [3], automated diagnosis of diseases [4], or morphological analysis such as voxel based morphometry [5] amongst others.

N. Ayache, S. Ourselin, A. Maeder (Eds.): MICCAI 2007, Part I, LNCS 4791, pp. 759–766, 2007.
© Springer-Verlag Berlin Heidelberg 2007

Formally, tissue classification consists in partitioning the input brain MR volume into disjoint regions corresponding to the three main tissue types: white matter (WM), gray matter (GM) and cerebro-spinal fluid (CSF). Non brain tissues such as bone, skin, dura or the meninges are often collected into a fourth category ("other").

A whole menagerie of image analysis techniques are available to classify brain tissues from either monospectral (often T1-weighted MRI) or multisprectral MR images. They rely on a no less varied selection of parametric and non-parametric statistical classifiers, from k-nearest neighbours [6] to neural networks [7]. The necessity to deal with intensity inhomogeneities (bias field) and partial volume effect voxels (those voxels that contain a mixture of several tissue types) called for techniques capable of estimating the relative fraction of each tissue class in each voxel. EM-type algorithms and Hidden Markov Random Field approaches [8,9,10] in particular have proved very popular (see [11] for a thorough review of classification approaches).

1.1   Sub-optimality of Independent Acquisition and Analysis

For a variety of logistics and historical reasons, developments in computational tissue classification have been mostly limited to the processing of clinical MR sequences (i.e. sequences developed specifically for clinical applications) independently of their optimality in distinguishing between tissue types.

As an illustration, the now standard T1/T2/PD multispectral acquisition protocol comes from an era when most brain sequences were based on Spin Echo imaging. Though time consuming, Spin Echo produced good tissue contrast and allowed for the simultaneous acquisition of T2-weighted and proton density (PD) images. The latter provided useful additional information for pathologies. With the development of faster Turbo/Fast Spin Echo sequences, this speed-up trick was not available any longer. However PD had already become part of the standard protocol, causing an effective doubling of the (admittedly now shorter) examination time. Meanwhile, most modern T1 sequences now rely on the even faster 3D Gradient Echo imaging, which also allows for much higher resolution than 2D slice based approaches like Fast Spin Echo.

Incidentally, while the T1/T2/PD combination of contrasts often yields good classification results, other spectral combinations offer markedly better classification performances over acquisition time ratios. For example, the joint use of standard anatomical protocols and contrast-enhanced sequences has proved particularly efficient in cancer and multiple sclerosis research [12].

Regrettably, we note that all too often, analysis only follows acquisition, in that the parameters of the MR sequences are optimized *before* the analysis, following criteria best suited for human operators, not algorithms. For instance, a radiographer or physicist in charge of an MR scanner will often strive to achieve the best visual compromise between contrast and noise whereas, from a computational standpoint, within-class noise matters less than interclass separability.

1.2   A Joint Approach to Classification

We submit that better overall results could be obtained by considering the acquisition and analysis processes *conjointly* rather than optimising them independently. Here we propose such an approach developed specifically for tissue classification in cerebral MR imaging. It consists of a novel MR sequence, which we dubbed Null Point Imaging (NPI), and a very simple phase-based classification algorithm. By imaging half way between the GM and WM null points (see below for detail), the proposed MR sequence introduces *at the acquisition stage* a nulled boundary layer between GM and WM tissues. This layer coincides with the partial volume effects (PVE) voxels resulting from the mix of GM and WM along the gray/white surface. Remarkably, because we image between the two null points, the phase image acquired with this protocol is positive for predominantly gray voxels and negative for predominantly white voxels, which makes it trivial to segment once unwrapped. Using the same principle we also introduce a boundary layer between GM and CSF and segment them in phase space.

We first describe our joint acquisition/analysis approach in Section 2 before presenting the first classification results and some elements of validation in Section 3.

2   Method

2.1   Imaging Brain Tissues with MR

When placed in the strong magnetic field of the scanner (B_0), hydrogen nuclei (protons) align so as to create a net equilibrium magnetization (M_0), parallel to the applied magnetic field, the longitudinal direction. Excitation of the protons by a radio frequency pulse will tip this net magnetization away from the longitudinal direction, and the time taken for the magnetization to recover to its equilibrium value M_0 is characterized by the longitudinal recovery time T1 . In standard T1-weighted imaging, tissue contrast is created by the differences in T1 between different tissues. Figure 1(a) plots the recovery of the longitudinal magnetization for GM, WM and CSF as a function of time, after an RF pulse that had inverted the longitudinal magnetization at $t = 0s$.

In most clinical sequences, imaging is performed at the point in time where the difference between the longitudinal magnetization of WM, GM and CSF is greatest ($960ms$ in Figure 1(a)).

A common technique to increase contrast, inversion recovery uses a preparatory RF pulse to rotate the net magnetization 180° down the B_0 axis. Before the magnetization reaches its equilibrium, another RF pulse is applied at time TI seconds. The preparatory pulse greatly lengthens the duration of the recovery process and consequently increases the contrast between tissues. Remarkably, while the direction of the net magnetization changes sign with this technique, its modulus seems to drop to a null point before recovering. This effect has been exploited in sequence development as a means to selectively remove signal from particular tissue types. In a classical MPRAGE sequence for instance (a fast high-resolution T1-weighted 3D sequence [13]) , TI is chosen to coincide with the time at which contrast is maximum after the initial inversion pulse ($960ms$).

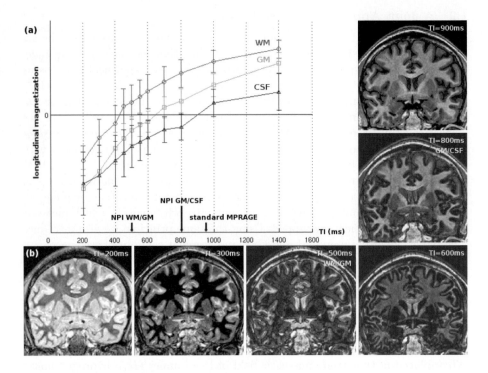

Fig. 1. Imaging characteristics of a standard MPRAGE sequence for various values of TI: (a) longitudinal magnetization (mean and standard deviation) of GM,WM and CSF as a function of the TI parameter; (b) sagittal sections of rigidly registered scans of the same volunteer's brain for different TIs

2.2   Imaging Tissue Boundaries with NPI

Here, we propose to use this nulling effect as a means to classify brain tissues. Our Null Point Imaging sequence is an MPRAGE sequence whose TI value is the barycentre of the GM and WM null points. Since the net magnetization vectors of GM and WM have the same modulus and different signs at that point, the MR signal of those partial volume effect voxels which contain a equal mixture of both GM and WM is nulled. This creates a black line between GM and WM voxels in the modulus image (see middle column of Figure 2). It also makes for a particularly "classification friendly" phase image where GM voxels have negative values and WM voxels positive ones, once the phase has been unwrapped [14]. We then segment the input volume by thresholding the unwrapped phase image at zero. Note that even though tissue contrast between GM and WM is almost null, this does not impact the performance of our classifier since thresholding is done in phase space. Alternatively, by selecting a TI value half way between the GM and CSF null points, our NPI technique outlines in black the pial surface (GM/CSF boundary) and a similar phase-based thresholding approach enables the segmentation of GM and CSF.

Determining the optimal TI value for the NPI sequence is a simple three-stepped approach. First, we acquire a series of structural images of a volunteer's brain by varying the TI parameter of a conventional T1-weighted sequence. All acquisitions were performed on a Philips Achieva, 1.5T with an 8-channel SENSE head coil. Note that we chose MPRAGE as our base sequence even though any inversion recovery sequence could have been employed. We then classify the volume corresponding to the standard clinical choice of TI (TI = 960ms for maximal contrast between WM,GM and CSF) using a standard off-the-shelf tissue classification technique (in our case, the MNI neural network classifier [7]). From these GM, WM and CSF maps, we compute the average intensity value per tissue for each value of TI (see Figure 1(a)). Finally, we determine the optimal value for TI by estimating the zero crossing point for the GM, WM and CSF curves and computing their barycentres. Note that although there is some inter- and intra- individual variation in T1 times for these tissue types it has been shown to be fairly uniform in the absence of pathology. Therefore, this optimization process only needs to be done once per scanner, on a limited number of brains.

From Figure 1(a), we get: $TI = 500ms$ for GM/WM segmentation and $TI = 800ms$ for GM/CSF segmentation. This can be visually confirmed on Figure 1(b) where a black line indeed separates GM from WM at $500ms$ and GM from CSF at $800ms$.

Note that as opposed to susceptibility weighted imaging [15] which uses naturally occurring phase variation to enhance the quality of the acquired magnitude images, our approach imposes a specific phase contrast.

3   Results

Figure 2 illustrates on a volunteer's brain the ability of our NPI approach to distinguish between WM, GM and CSF voxels. We show on the left column a selection of sagittal, coronal and axial slices cut through a standard T1-weighed volume, the corresponding section (after rigid registration) through the NPI magnitude at $TI = 500ms$ (black line between GM and WM) in the middle and the classification maps on the right column (CSF is black, GM is gray and WM is white). Note that we skull-stripped the classification maps in the interest of visual clarity.

3.1   Elements of Validation

Since our joint acquisition/analysis approach is based on a custom MR sequence, we did not have the possibility of using brain simulators (e.g. BrainWeb [16]) to estimate its performances. In the absence of a gold standard, we used as a straw-man standard the classification maps obtained with a standard classification package (the MNI neural network classifier [7]) on the average of 5 rigidly registered standard T1 + T2/PD scans of the same volunteer's brain. The increased signal to noise ratio of the average image yielded an adequate classification against which

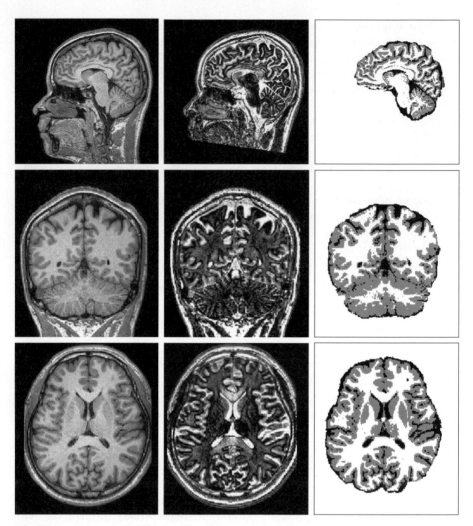

Fig. 2. A selection of corresponding slices cut through the same volunteer's brain: standard T1-weighted sequence (left column); NPI sequence with $TI = 500ms$, a black line follows the GM/WM boundary (center column); binary classification map (right column)

we compared the maps obtained with our approach on two NPI scans of the same volunteer (NPI with $TI = 500ms$ and with $TI = 800ms$).

Following Van Leemput et al. [9], we used the Dice metric [17]. Let Map_T^{mni} denote the classification map for tissue T obtained with the selected standard package, and let Map_T^{npi} be the NPI classification map. The Dice metric is given by: $D_T = 2|Map_T^{mni} \cap Map_T^{npi}|/(|Map_T^{mni}| + |Map_T^{npi}|)$ where $|.|$ is the set size operator.

Overall, our fast, phase-based thresholding approach gave, with only 2 images, results remarkably close to those obtained with the sophisticated MNI classifier on the average images ($D_{WM} = 84\%$, $D_{GM} = 82\%$ and $D_{CSF} = 72\%$). Visual inspection confirmed this finding and showed that discrepancies where for the most part due to isolated voxels (these could be corrected with a morphological filter), overestimation of CSF in the temporal lobes (due to issues with phase unwrapping in the presence of scanner inhomogeneities), and differences in areas where the MNI approach was arguably wrong (in particular around some of the deep gray nuclei -thalamus- for GM).

4   Conclusion

We have presented a joint acquisition/analysis approach to MR tissue classification where information obtained in a preliminary analysis stage (graph of longitudinal magnetization as a function of TI parameter) helped optimize the acquisition sequence. In turn, the acquired images proved much easier to classify than standard T1-weighted or T2/PD multispectral sequences. Indeed, the phase image changed sign at the transition between predominantly gray and predominantly white PVE voxels, which yielded a very simple thresholding algorithm.

Our NPI classification technique is particularly efficient with respect to standard approaches. Typically, on a Philips 1.5T scanner, one or two $15mn$ long scans ($1mm^3$ isotropic T1-weighted sequence for monospectral and/or a $1 \times 1 \times 2mm$ T2/PD sequence for multispectral) followed by sophisticated image processing could be replaced by two fast $6mn$ sequences with a trivial classification algorithm. Note that in a standard computational pipeline, T1-weighted images are often used for other purposes than just classification: for instance they serve to extract the brain from the skull, or to correct for intensity inhomogeneities. Incidentally, even though our approach is not intended for use as a diagnostic tool, its behaviour in the presence of pathological defects such as lesions or tumours would be worth evaluating.

Preliminary results are very encouraging and show performances on par with a standard package even without any pre- or post-processing (inhomogeneity correction or morphological filtering for instance). We are currently working on a thorough validation where comparison against a variety of publicly available classifiers will be performed within the STAPLE framework [18].

Finally, we are also exploring the possibility of using the phase value in each voxel to roughly estimate the mixture of tissues within that voxel, rather than simply thresholding the phase image at zero to obtain a ternary classification map.

References

1. Toga, A., Mazziotta, J.: Brain Mapping: The Methods. Academic Press, London (2002)
2. Thompson, P., Hayashi, K., de Zubicaray, G., Janke, A., Rose, S., Semple, J., Hong, M., Herman, D., Gravano, D., Dittmer, S., Doddrell, D., Toga, A.: Dynamics of Gray Matter Loss in Alzheimer's Disease. Journal of Neuroscience 23, 994–1005 (2003)

3. Fischl, B., Dale, A.: Measuring the Thickness of the Human Cerebral Cortex from Magnetic Resonance Images. Proceedings of the National Academy of Sciences 97, 11044–11049 (2000)
4. Stoeckel, J., Malandain, G., Migneco, O., Koulibaly, P., Robert, P., Ayache, N., Darcourt, J.: Classification of SPECT Images of Normal Subjects versus Images of Alzheimer's Disease Patients. In: Niessen, W.J., Viergever, M.A. (eds.) MICCAI 2001. LNCS, vol. 2208, pp. 666–674. Springer, Heidelberg (2001)
5. Ashburner, J., Friston, K.: Voxel-based morphometry: the methods. NeuroImage 11, 805–821 (2000)
6. Warfield, S.K.: Fast k-NN classification for multichannel image data. Pattern Recognition Letters 17, 713–721 (1996)
7. Collins, D.L., Zijdenbos, A.P., Baaré, W.F.C., Evans, A.C.: ANIMAL+INSECT: Improved Cortical Structure Segmentation. In: Proc. of IPMI 1999, pp. 210–223 (1999)
8. Held, K., Kops, E., Krause, B., Wells, W., Kikinis, R., Müller-Gärtner, H.: Markov random field segmentation of brain MR images. IEEE Transactions on Medical Imaging 16 (1997)
9. Leemput, K.V., Maes, F., Suetens, P.: Automated model-based tissue classification of MR images of the brain. IEEE trans. on medical imaging 18, 897–908 (1999)
10. Zhang, Y., Brady, M., Smith, S.: Segmentation of brain MR images through a hidden markov random field model and the expectation-maximization algorithm. IEEE trans. on medical imaging 20, 45–57 (2001)
11. Pham, D., Xu, C., Prince, J.: Current Methods in Medical Image Segmentation. Annual Reviews 2, 315–337 (1996)
12. Dugas-Phocion, G., Lebrun, C., Chanalet, S., Chatel, M., Ayache, N., Malandain, G.: Automatic segmentation of white matter lesions in multi-sequence MRI of relapsing-remitting multiple sclerosis patients. In: ECTRIMS, Thessaloniki, Greece (2005)
13. Brant-Zawadzki, M., Gillan, G., Nitz, W.: MP RAGE: a three-dimensional, T1-weighted, gradient-echo sequence– initial experience in the brain. Radiology 182, 769–775 (1992)
14. Xu, W., Cumming, I.: A region growing algorithm for insar phase unwrapping. IEEE Trans. Geosci. Remote Sensing 37, 124–134 (1999)
15. Haacke, E., Xu, Y., Cheng, Y., Reichenbach, J.: Susceptibility weighted imaging (SWI). Magnetic Resonance Imaging 52, 612–618 (2004)
16. Collins, D., Zijdenbos, A., Kollokian, V., Sled, J., Kabani, N., Holmes, C., Evans, A.: Design and Construction of a Realistic Digital Brain Phantom. IEEE Transactions on Medical Imaging 26, 463–468 (1998)
17. Dice, L.: Measures of the amount of ecologic association between species. Ecology 26, 297–302 (1945)
18. Warfield, S.K., Zou, K.H., Wells, W.M.: Simultaneous truth and performance level estimation (STAPLE): an algorithm for the validation of image segmentation. IEEE Trans. Med. Imaging 23, 903–921 (2004)

Characterizing Task-Related Temporal Dynamics of Spatial Activation Distributions in fMRI BOLD Signals

Bernard Ng[1], Rafeef Abugharbieh[1], Samantha J. Palmer[2,3], and Martin J. McKeown[3]

[1] Department of Electrical and Computer Engineering
[2] Department of Neuroscience
[3] Department of Medicine (Neurology), Pacific Parkinson's Research Center, University of British Columbia, Vancouver, BC, Canada
bernardn@ece.ubc.ca, rafeef@ece.ubc.ca,
sjpalmer@interchange.ubc.ca, mmckeown@interchange.ubc.ca

Abstract. We present a new functional magnetic resonance imaging (fMRI) analysis method that incorporates both spatial and temporal dynamics of blood-oxygen-level dependent (BOLD) signals within a region of interest (ROI). 3D moment descriptors are used to characterize the spatial changes in BOLD signals over time. The method is tested on fMRI data collected from eight healthy subjects performing a bulb-squeezing motor task with their right-hand at various frequencies. Multiple brain regions including the left cerebellum, both primary motor cortices (M1), both supplementary motor areas (SMA), left prefrontal cortex (PFC), and left anterior cingulate cortex (ACC) demonstrate significant task-related changes. Furthermore, our method is able to discriminate differences in activation patterns at the various task frequencies, whereas using a traditional intensity based method, no significant activation difference is detected. This suggests that temporal dynamics of the spatial distribution of BOLD signal provide additional information regarding task-related activation thus complementing conventional intensity-based approaches.

Keywords: functional imaging, spatio-temporal fMRI analysis, region of interest (ROI), brain activation, 3D moments.

1 Introduction

The most common application of functional magnetic resonance imaging (fMRI) is in mapping neural region(s) to particular function(s) by examining which brain areas activate when a certain task is performed. Most conventional analysis methods, such as statistical parametric mapping (SPM) [1], analyze each voxel's timecourse independently and assign a statistics value to that voxel based on its probability of being activated. To make group inferences under this approach, spatial warping of each subject's brain to a common exemplar shape is often performed to create a correspondence between voxels across subjects [2]. However, spatial normalization, which is typically followed by spatial smoothing, may inappropriately pool responses

N. Ayache, S. Ourselin, A. Maeder (Eds.): MICCAI 2007, Part I, LNCS 4791, pp. 767–774, 2007.
© Springer-Verlag Berlin Heidelberg 2007

from functionally dissimilar regions [3], thus degrading important spatial information. An alternative approach that involves drawing regions of interest (ROIs) individually for each subject, and examining the statistical properties of regional activation across subjects, has been shown to offer finer localization and increased sensitivity to task-related effects [3]. This subject-specific ROI-based approach is thus followed in this study.

To determine whether an ROI is activated or not, a simple approach is to calculate the average intensity over an ROI at every time point, and determine if the resulting average time course significantly correlates with the stimulus [4]. This approach, however, ignores any spatial information of activity within an ROI and assumes that only signal amplitude is modulated by task. However, spatial information might be an important attribute of brain activity. Preliminary evidence supporting this idea of spatial characterization was first shown by Thickbroom et al. [5], where the spatial extent of activation, as opposed to response magnitude, was found to be modulated by different levels of force during a sustained finger flexion task. Their results were based on visual inspection and counting the number of activated voxels within an ROI. Recently, we presented a more elaborate study of the spatial patterns of activity within an ROI where quantitative measures of invariant spatial properties were used to discriminate task-related differences in brain activity [6]. Results demonstrated that, by examining changes in different spatial aspects of an activation distribution, sensitivity in detecting functional changes is enhanced as compared to using intensity means only.

Previous analyses examining spatial patterns of activation, including that in [6], were performed on T-maps where the spatial information is collapsed over time, thus only considered the time-averaged spatial patterns of brain activity. In this paper, we extend our previously proposed spatial characterization approach to the temporal domain to explore whether the spatial distribution of the blood oxygenation level-dependent (BOLD) signal itself is modulated in time by task performance. We note an important difference between our current and previous work [6] is that the generated spatial feature time courses can be used to infer ROI activation, as opposed to only comparing 2 groups of time-averaged activation statistical maps. To characterize the spatial changes, three dimensional (3D) moment descriptors were used as features and were calculated at each time point. The magnitudes of these features, however, are normally not comparable across subjects due to inter-subject variability in brain shapes and sizes, but are comparable for the same subject over time. Thus, any detected modulations of the spatial features over time for a given subject may in fact represent meaningful spatial changes in activation.

In this study, eight healthy subjects were recruited to perform a bulb-squeezing task at various frequencies. The cerebellum, primary motor cortex (M1), supplementary motor area (SMA), prefrontal cortex (PFC), and anterior cingulate cortex (ACC) were chosen as regions of interest. We demonstrate that our method can both detect activation within an ROI, as well as discriminate differences in activation patterns at the various task frequencies. This confirms previous findings of the value in incorporating spatial information into traditional intensity-based fMRI analyses.

2 Data Acquisition and Preprocessing

In this study, after informed consent was obtained, fMRI data were collected from 8 healthy subjects. Each subject was required to perform a right-handed motor task that involved squeezing a bulb with sufficient pressure such that an 'inflatable ring', shown as a black horizontal bar on a screen, was kept within an undulating pathway (Fig. 1-a). The pathway remains straight during rest periods and becomes sinusoidal at time of stimulus. Each run lasted 260 s, consisting of a 20 s rest period at the beginning and end, 6 stimuli of 20 s duration, and 20 s rest periods between the stimuli, as shown in Fig. 1-b. At time of stimulus, the subject was required to squeeze the bulb at 0.25, 0.5 or 0.75 Hz, corresponding to 'Slow', 'Med', and 'Fast' in Fig 1-b. The data were collected as part of a larger experiment exploring the rate of change of force production in older subjects and subjects with Parkinson's disease.

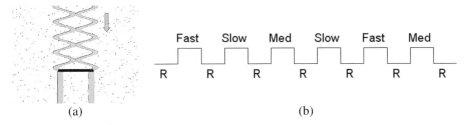

Fig. 1. Experimental task and stimulus timing. (a) Subjects were required to keep the side of the black ring on the gray path (see text). (b) R = rest, Slow, Med, and Fast = stimulus at 0.25, 0.5, and 0.75 Hz, respectively. Each block is 20 s in duration.

2.1 fMRI Data Acquisition

Functional MRI was performed on a Philips Gyroscan Intera 3.0 T scanner (Philips, Best, Netherlands) equipped with a head-coil. We collected echo-planar (EPI) T2*-weighted images with BOLD contrast. Scanning parameters were: repetition time 1985 ms, echo time 3.7 ms, flip angle 90°, field of view (FOV) 216×143×240 mm, in plane resolution 128×128 pixels, pixel size 1.9×1.9 mm. Each functional run lasted 4 minutes where 36 axial slices of 3 mm thickness were collected in each volume, with a gap thickness of 1 mm. We selected slices to cover the dorsal surface of the brain and included the cerebellum ventrally. A high resolution 3D T1-weighted image consisting of 170 axial slices was acquired of the whole brain to facilitate anatomical localization of activation for each subject.

2.2 fMRI PreProcessing

The fMRI data was preprocessed for each subject, using Brain Voyager's (Brain Innovation B.V.) trilinear interpolation for 3D motion correction and sinc interpolation for slice time correction. Further motion correction was performed using motion corrected independent component analysis (MCICA) [7]. To handle temporal autocorrelations, a 'coloring' scheme was used [8], where the time series were high-pass filtered at 0.02 Hz (task-frequency being 0.025 Hz) to remove the majority of the low frequency noise, and temporally smoothened with a Gaussian of width 2.8 s [8]. The first and last 20 s of the time series were truncated to mitigate transient effects. No spatial smoothing was performed.

The Brain Extraction Tool (BET) in MRIcro [9] was used to strip the skull off of the anatomical and first functional image from each run to enable a more accurate alignment of the functional and anatomical scans. Custom scripts to co-register the anatomical and functional images were generated using the Amira software (Mercury Computer Systems, San Diego, USA).

Ten specific ROIs were manually drawn on each unwarped structural scan using Amira. The following ROIs were drawn separately in each hemisphere, based upon anatomical landmarks and guided by a neurological atlas [10]: cerebellum, M1 (Brodman Area 4), SMA (Brodman Area 6), PFC (Brodman Area 9 and 10), and ACC (Brodman Area 28 and 32). The labels on the segmented anatomical scans were resliced at the fMRI resolution. The raw time courses of the voxels within each ROI were then extracted for analysis as described in the next section.

3   Methods

The main goal of the proposed method is to demonstrate that temporal dynamics of the spatial distribution in BOLD signals can be used to infer whether an ROI is activated, as well as to discriminate differences in activation patterns at various task frequencies. Details of feature time course extraction, activation detection, and activation pattern discrimination are discussed below.

3.1   Feature Time Course Extraction

The spatial feature descriptors used in this paper are based on centralized 3D moments, defined as:

$$\mu_{pqr}(t) = \int_{-\infty}^{\infty}\int_{-\infty}^{\infty}\int_{-\infty}^{\infty}(x-\bar{x})^p(y-\bar{y})^q(z-\bar{z})^r\rho(x,y,z,t)dxdydz \ , \tag{1}$$

where $n = p + q + r$ is the order of the moment, (x,y,z) are the coordinates of a voxel, $\rho(x,y,z,t)$ is the intensity of a voxel located at (x,y,z) inside a given ROI at time t, and $\bar{x}$, $\bar{y}$, and $\bar{z}$ are the centroid coordinates of $\rho(x,y,z,t)$. To untangle the effect of amplitude changes, $\rho(x,y,z,t)$ is normalized such that the intensity values of the voxels within the ROI sums up to one at every time point t. This step ensures that the mean ROI intensity does not change with time. Thus, any detected modulations in the spatial feature will be purely due to spatial changes in the BOLD signal. To ease interpretation of the results and since higher order moments are less robust to noise [11], only 2nd and 3rd order 3D moment descriptors characterizing spatial variance [12] and skewness, respectively, were used:

$$J_1(t) = \mu_{200}(t) + \mu_{020}(t) + \mu_{002}(t) \ , \tag{2}$$

$$S(t) = \mu_{300}(t) + \mu_{030}(t) + \mu_{003}(t) \; , \tag{3}$$

To compare with the results obtained using the proposed spatial feature time courses, the traditionally used mean intensity time course, $I(t)$, for each ROI of a given subject is calculated by averaging the intensity over the ROI at every time point.

3.2 Activation Detection

To make group inference as to whether a given ROI is activated, each subject's ROI feature time courses (spatial or mean intensity) are first correlated with a box-car that is time-locked to stimulus with a delay of 4 s [13]. We did not convolve the box-car with a haemodynamic response function since spatial changes, as governed by the different onsets of the active voxels, may exhibit a different temporal profile than that of the haemodynamic response. For each subject, this results in thirty correlation values, one per combination of feature and ROI (e.g. $J_I(t)$, left M1). Each correlation value is then converted into a T-value (4):

$$T = |r|\sqrt{\frac{N-2}{1-r^2}} \; , \tag{4}$$

where r is the correlation value and N is the number of samples used in generating r. The set of T-values of a particular combination of feature and ROI from all subjects is then tested against 1.96 using a T-test to determine the probability (p-value) that the T-values are lower than 1.96 (i.e. the probability that ROI is not activated). The critical p-value was chosen at 0.05.

3.3 Activation Pattern Discrimination

To discriminate the differences in activation pattern at the various task frequencies, each subject's ROI feature time courses (spatial or mean intensity) are first segmented according to Fig. 2. Except for the first and last segments, each segment consists of a

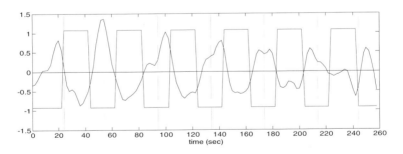

Fig. 2. Feature time course segmentation. The box-car curve corresponds to timing of the stimulus delayed by 4 s. The solid line is a sample feature time course (spatial variance, $J_I(t)$, of the left M1 averaged over subjects with its temporal mean removed and divided by its standard deviation). The dotted lines show how the feature time courses are parsed into 6 segments. Slow, Med, and Fast correspond to the task frequencies of 0.25, 0.5, and 0.75 Hz, respectively.

10 s rest before and after the 20 s stimulus. Segments of the same task frequency are concatenated and correlated with the corresponding segments of the shifted reference signal (see Fig. 2). This results in ninety correlation values per subject, one for each combination of frequency, feature, and ROI (e.g. slow, $J_1(t)$, left M1). Each correlation value is then converted into a T-value using (4).

For each combination of feature and ROI, the set of T-values of a particular frequency from all subjects are tested pair-wise against the other two frequencies (i.e. fast versus slow, fast versus medium, medium versus slow). This is performed using a T-test to determine the probability (p-value) that the sets of T-values from the two task frequencies are the same (i.e. the probability that activation patterns at the two frequencies are the same). The critical p-value was chosen at 0.05.

4   Results and Discussion

Table 1 summarizes the activation detection results generated by extracting the spatial and intensity features from real fMRI data as described in Section 3.2, and correlating the resulting feature time courses with the reference signal.

Table 1. p-values of ROI activation. CER = cerebellum, $J_1(t)$ = spatial variance, $S(t)$ = skewness, $\bar{I}(t)$ = mean intensity, L = left, R = right, * = statically significant at $\alpha = 0.05$

Feature	$J_1(t)$	$S(t)$	$\bar{I}(t)$
LCER	**0.002***	0.077	0.469
RCER	0.220	0.066	**0.042***
LM1	**0.002***	0.051	0.162
RM1	0.157	**0.047***	0.164
LSMA	**0.027***	**0.034***	**0.021***
RSMA	**0.044***	**0.035***	**0.034***
LPFC	**0.036***	**0.020***	**0.034***
RPFC	0.341	0.185	0.058
LACC	**0.001***	0.301	**0.023***
RACC	0.056	0.112	**0.045***

Using spatial variance, $J_1(t)$, the left cerebellum, left M1, both SMAs, left PFC, and left ACC were detected as active. We expected the left M1 to be activated, as typically observed for right-handed motor tasks. It is worth noting that the left M1's BOLD signal distribution shown reduced spatial variance (i.e. focuses) during the time of stimulus (see Fig. 2). Skewness, $S(t)$, additionally detected activation in the right M1. These results demonstrate that the spatial distribution of BOLD signals is, in fact, modulated by stimulus, which supports our hypothesis that spatial changes in BOLD signals are task-related and can be used to infer activation within an ROI.

Using the traditional mean intensity measure, the right cerebellum, both SMAs, left PFC, and both ACCs were detected as active. Comparing to the results generated with the proposed spatial features, some consistencies are shown. In fact, based on the results in Table 1, activation within an ROI appears to modulate both in amplitude and in space.

Segmenting the feature time courses according to task frequencies and using the proposed spatial features, significant frequency-related activation differences were detected in the right cerebellum and right M1 when comparing fast versus slow frequencies (Table 2). These results matched our expectations since the modulation of movement speed is known to involve a complex network of brain areas, including the right cerebellum and right M1 [14]. Also, significant activation differences were found in the right PFC and right ACC using the proposed spatial features. In contrast, no significant activation differences were found using mean intensity. Also, no significant activation differences were detected when comparing fast versus medium frequencies and medium versus slow frequencies for any of the features, thus these results were excluded in Table 2.

Table 2. p-values of activation differences comparing fast versus slow frequencies. CER = cerebellum, $J_l(t)$ = spatial variance, $S(t)$ = skewness, $\overline{I}(t)$ = mean intensity, L = left, R = right, *statically significant at $\alpha = 0.05$.

Feature	$J_1(t)$	$S(t)$	$\overline{I}(t)$
LCER	0.1834	0.1931	0.1528
RCER	0.9993	**0.0096***	0.2757
LM1	0.2932	0.4017	0.4190
RM1	**0.0442***	0.3223	0.1524
LSMA	0.6872	0.2499	0.1836
RSMA	0.7887	0.9066	0.0579
LPFC	0.5981	0.3059	0.2760
RPFC	**0.0398***	0.3668	0.7416
LACC	0.2551	0.4029	0.2126
RACC	**0.0311***	0.1028	0.3248

Examining the results in Table 2, spatial changes appear to provide greater sensitivity in detecting subtle activation differences as compared to intensity.

5 Conclusions

In this paper, we proposed using 3D moment-based spatial descriptors to characterize the temporal dynamics of spatial activation distribution within an ROI for fMRI analysis. We demonstrated with real fMRI data that certain spatial aspects of activation, as opposed to just amplitude, are modulated by stimulus - a result that appeared consistent across subjects. Furthermore, we showed that our method was able to better discriminate frequency-related differences in activation patterns during motor task performance when compared to using mean intensity only. These results suggest that spatial characterization of BOLD signal can complement traditional intensity-based fMRI analysis. A direct extension of the proposed method would be to examine functional connectivity and phase relations between ROIs using spatial feature time courses, an approach currently being pursued.

References

1. Friston, K.J., Toga, A.W., Mazziotta, J.C. (eds.): Statistical parametric mapping and other analyses of functional imaging data. Brain mapping, the methods, pp. 363–396. Academic Press, San Diego (1996)
2. Lancaster, J.L., Rainey, L.H., Summerlin, J.L., Freitas, C.S., Fox, P.T., Evans, A.C., Toga, A.W., Mazziotta, J.C.: Automated labeling of the human brain: a preliminary report on the development and evaluation of a forward-transform method. Hum. Brain Mapp. 5(4), 238–242 (1997)
3. Castanon, A.N., Ghosh, S.S., Tourville, J.A., Guenther, F.H.: Region of interest based analysis of functional imaging data. NeuroImage 19, 1303–1316 (2003)
4. Liu, Y., Gao, J.H., Liotti, M., Pu, Y., Fox, P.T.: Temporal dissociation of parallel processing in the human subcortical outputs. Nature 400(6742), 364–367 (1999)
5. Thickbroom, G.W., Phillips, B.A., Morris, I., Byrnes, M.L., Mastaglia, F.L.: Isometric force-related activity in sensorimotor cortex measured with functional MRI. Exp. Brain Res. 121, 59–64 (1998)
6. Ng, B., Abugharbieh, R., Huang, X., McKeown, M.J.: Characterizing fMRI Activations within Regions of Interest (ROIs) Using 3D Moment Invariants. In: IEEE Worshop on Mathematical Methods in Biomedical Image Analysis, New York (June 17-18, 2006)
7. Liao, R., Krolik, J.L., McKeown, M.J.: An information-theoretic criterion for intrasubject alignment of fMRI time series: Motion corrected independent component analysis. IEEE Trans. Med. Imaging 24, 29–44 (2005)
8. Friston, K.J., Holmes, A.P., Poline, J.B., Grasby, P.J., Williams, S.C.R., Frackowiak, R.S.J., Turner, R.: Analysis of fMRI Time-Series Revisited. NeuroImage 2, 45–53 (1995)
9. Rorden, C., Brett, M.: Stereotaxic display of brain lesions. Behavioural Neurology 12, 191–200 (2000)
10. Talairach, J., Tournoux, P.: Co-Planar Stereotaxic Atlas of the Human Brain: 3-Dimensional Proportional System - an Approach to Cerebral Imaging. Thieme Medical Publishers, New York (1988)
11. Press, W.H., Teukolsky, S.A., Vetterling, W.T., Flannery, B.P.: Nurmerical Recipes in C. Cambridge University Press, Cambridge (1999)
12. Sadjadi, F.A., Hall, E.L.: Three-Dimensional Moment Invariants. IEEE Trans. Pattern. Anal. Machine Intell. PAMI- 2, 127–136 (1980)
13. Svensen, M., Kruggel, F., von Cramon, Y.: Probabilitic modeling of single-trial fMRI data. IEEE Trans. Med. Imaging 19(1), 25–35 (2000)
14. Verstynen, T., Diedrichsen, J., Albert, N., Aparicio, P., Ivry, R.B.: Ipsilateral motor cortex activity during unimanual hand movements relates to task complexity. J. Neurophysiol. 93, 1209–1222 (2005)

Contraction Detection in Small Bowel from an Image Sequence of Wireless Capsule Endoscopy

Hai Vu[1], Tomio Echigo[2], Ryusuke Sagawa[1], Keiko Yagi[3], Masatsugu Shiba[4],
Kazuhide Higuchi[4], Tetsuo Arakawa[4], and Yasushi Yagi[1]

[1] The Institute of Scientific and Industrial Research, Osaka University
[2] Osaka Electro-Communication University
[3] Kobe Pharmaceutical University
[4] Graduate School of Medicine, Osaka City University

Abstract. This paper describes a method for automatic detection of contractions in the small bowel through analyzing Wireless Capsule Endoscopic images. Based on the characteristics of contraction images, a coherent procedure that includes analyzes of the temporal and spatial features is proposed. For temporal features, the image sequence is examined to detect candidate contractions through the changing number of edges and an evaluation of similarities between the frames of each possible contraction to eliminate cases of low probability. For spatial features, descriptions of the directions at the edge pixels are used to determine contractions utilizing a classification method. The experimental results show the effectiveness of our method that can detect a total of 83% of cases. Thus, this is a feasible method for developing tools to assist in diagnostic procedures in the small bowel.

1   Introduction

Information about contractions in the small bowel, in particular the number of contractions, distributions and their visualization along the Gastrointestinal (GI) tract usually reveals clinical pathologies in diagnostic procedures. For example, weak and disorganized contractions are stated as bacterial overgrowth disease; dysfunctions or the absence of contractions in a long duration is present in some patients with functional dyspepsia [1]. The current techniques to measure motility patterns in the small bowel are well tolerated but still invasive tests. Recently, a new clinical device using a system known as Wireless Capsule Endoscopy (WCE) [2,3] has become widely used. It allows examinations in the small bowel to be both more intensive yet comfortable for patients. Using these image data as the source for recognition of contractions presents intuitively opportunities for developing tools to assist in diagnostic procedures.

In a typical examination, the WCE goes through the GI tract in 7-8 hours capturing images at 2 fps, with around 20,000 to 30,000 frames of intestinal images [3]. Visualization of the contractions is rendered in consecutive frames showing shrinkage of intestinal folds. Particularly, at center of the contractions, a wrinkle pattern that presents a state of occlusion of the intestinal lumen has

N. Ayache, S. Ourselin, A. Maeder (Eds.): MICCAI 2007, Part I, LNCS 4791, pp. 775–783, 2007.
© Springer-Verlag Berlin Heidelberg 2007

strong and sharp edges of wrinkles toward to a center point. Thus, contractions are highly recognizable in a WCE image sequence from the combination of the spatial and temporal features.

Addressing the issue of the detection of contractions is still at an initial state. To recognize wrinkle patterns, extracted features from a structured tensor of the intestinal images are mapped into a star-wise pattern in [4]; or in [5] the features of "steerable filters" are coded into radial shape patterns. On the other hand, along a time dimension the contractions are determined by examining 5 wrinkle frames within a window of a ±5 frames neighborhood (in [5]) by an evaluation of intestinal lumen features (solidity, sharpness, deepness) of each image in an interval of 9 continuous frames (in [6]). Accordingly, contractions are generated in the form of a fixed number of frames by using features of separate frames.

Different from these systems, we examine continuous changes of features over time and evaluated the relationship between frames and other frames to detect possible contractions. Then, the spatial features are analyzed by describing the structural pattern to determine contractions utilizing a classification method. Following this strategy, the detection of contractions is more reasonable because the duration of the contractions is not constrained but varies along the small bowel. Implementations are undertaken in a coherent procedure that includes three stages to automatically detect the contractions. The experimental results imply that the method provides a useful way to recognize contractions.

The rest of this paper is organized as follows: Sec. 2 describes the characteristics of the contractions. Sec. 3 explains the techniques for implementation of a three-stage procedure. In Sec. 4, experimental results and discussions are presented. Finally, Sec. 5 concludes the work and suggests further research.

2   Characteristics of Contractions in a WCE Image Sequence

In terms of physiology, contractions are produced by the shrinkage of circular muscle layers. A cycle of contractions begins at the widest state of the intestinal lumen and rapidly occludes the lumen area until reaching the strongest shrinkage state of the inner wall, then these folds relax at an ending state. Fig. 1 marks contractions in an image sequence that is made up of 60 frames.

As showing of the marked frames, the edge features are important cues for detecting contraction events. The number of edge pixels in the images increases rapidly and then decreases, resulting in a strong peak at the contractions. Moreover, because of the movement of the WCE, the changes between successive frames at contraction positions is more discriminative than others.

On the other hand, the center of the contractions presents a muscular structure, as shown in Fig. 2. These patterns include strong edges of the intestinal wrinkles when the inner walls are folded. The muscular tone is toward a center point and produces a state of occlusion of the intestinal lumen. The structure of wrinkle patterns thus can be expressed by directional information.

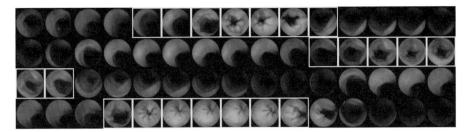

Fig. 1. Some contractions are marked in boxes of 60 continuous frames (from left to right and top to bottom)

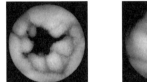 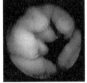 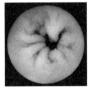

Fig. 2. Some examples of the contractile patterns

For these characteristics, detecting maximal local peaks along the edge signal and evaluating the similarity of successive frames allows for the detection of events, which are considered as possible contractions. These results are highly recognizable for final decisions based on analyzing the directions at the edge pixels. A coherent procedure for implementation is described below.

3   Contractions Detection by Temporal and Spatial Features

3.1   Edges Extractions to Detect Possible Contractions

To detect possible contractions, denote $f(x)$ as a function of the edge number:

$$f(x) = \sum_i \delta \text{ with } \begin{cases} \delta = 1 \text{ if i is an edge pixel} \\ \delta = 0 \text{ otherwise} \end{cases} \text{ (with x is frame number)} \quad (1)$$

The Canny edge detector [7] is used to extract edges from an image. Edge pixels are counted in a region where most of the edges appear. The size of the region (192x192 pixels) is large enough to ensure that no important edges are lost (with image resolution is 256x256 pixels). The signal $f(x)$ is normalized in the range of $[0, 1]$ and smoothed by a Gaussian function to remove noise.

Possible contractions are located where $f(x)$ is in a triangular shape. However, not all signals perfectly present this type of pattern because of the length and the strength during the contractions. Thus, a morphological opening operator is applied to create a simpler graph than the original signal. The opening signal suggests locations of positive peaks that are thinner than a structural element.

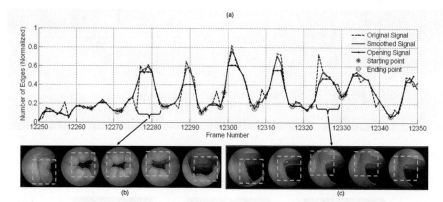

Fig. 3. (a) Possible contractions are marked on an original signal with starting (star points) and ending (circle points) frames. (b) A positive case; (c) a negative case for a contraction. The most edges regions are also marked in rectangles in (b) and (c)

A procedure to look for a number of consecutive frames within an opening signal that exceeds the structuring element duration is implemented. Fig. 3 shows the positions of contractions detected in a sequence of 100 consecutive frames.

3.2 Evaluations of Similarity for Eliminating Non Contractions

Figure 3 shows two cases of possible contractions in which sharp variations between consecutive frames in the positive case (3b) are opposed to the high similarity in the negative case (3c). Shrinkage of the intestinal folds in the positive cases make most regions that have low similarity, whereas the negative cases imply a high similarity of homogeneous regions spanning consecutive frames. These regions can be grouped into clusters by grouping similarity feature space then evaluating similarity to discard redundant cases. Therefore, an unsupervised clustering method that adopted from works in [8] are applied. Based on an observation that a block of image pixels is more likely to belong to a certain cluster if it is located near the cluster centroid. It is reasonable to assume that the similarity of blocks and their positions is represented by a Gaussian distribution, and a set of regions are generated by a mixture of Gaussians.

First, N frames of a possible contraction are divided into $Nblocks$ (Fig. 4a) and an intensity histogram H (with $Nbins$) for each block is calculated. The similarity sim of block t between frames j and $j+1$ are:

$$sim_{j,j+1}^t = \sum_{m \in Nbins} |H_j^t(m) - H_{j+1}^t(m)|$$

$$With\ H(m) = \sum_{x,y \in block} \begin{cases} 1\ if\ IntegerRound(\dfrac{I(x,y)}{Nbins}) = m \\ 0\ Otherwise \end{cases} \qquad (2)$$

A feature vector is notated by: $\chi = \{sim_{0,1}^t, ..., sim_{N-1,N}^t, pos_x, pos_y\}$, including the similarity of blocks and their positions pos_x and pos_y. For a mixture of K Gaussians, the random variable χ presents a probability for a Gaussian component k by:

$$f_k(\chi|\theta) = \alpha_k \frac{1}{\sqrt{(2\pi)^d |\Sigma_k|}} exp\{-\frac{1}{2}(\chi - \mu_k)^T \Sigma_k^{-1}(\chi - \mu_k)\} \qquad (3)$$

where the parameter set $\theta = \{\alpha_i, \mu_k, \Sigma_k\}_{k=1}^{K}$ consists of: $\alpha_k > 0$, $\sum_{k=1}^{K}\alpha_k = 1$ and $\mu_k \in R^d$ and Σ_k is a $[d \times d]$ positive definite matrix (in this case, $d = N-1$).

Given a set of feature vectors $\chi_1, ..., \chi_{Nblocks}$, a Maximum Likelihood (ML) criterion is used to train the data to derive a parameters set θ, yielding:

$$\theta_{ML} = \arg\max_{\theta} f(\chi_1, ..., \chi_{Nblocks}|\theta) \qquad (4)$$

The EM algorithm [9] is an iterative method to obtain θ_{ML}. The parameter set θ_{ML} then provides probabilities following Eq. 3 to assign a feature vector χ to a cluster using a Maximum A Posteriori (MAP) principle. The MIXMOD library [10] is used for this implementation. The results of clustering are then assessed through examining similarity data of the largest clusters. If these regions include high similarity values, it implies a low probability of a true contraction and so is decided as being non contractions. For example, Fig. 4 shows the results for a negative case of contractions in Fig. 3c. With number of clusters $K = 3$, $Nblocks = 144$ and $Nbins = 16$ are preselected in order to obtain a trade-off between number of clusters regions and computational time, two largest clusters 1 and 2 include 60% and 28% total blocks. The average of similarity in these regions are 0.63 and 0.52, respectively. This result show large homogenous regions along the frames that are reasons to assign this case as one of non contractions.

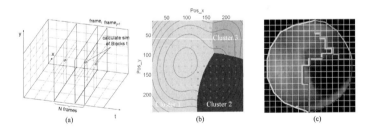

Fig. 4. (a) A configuration to obtain feature vectors. (b) Results of clustering similarity data using GMM for the possible contraction in Fig. 3(c). (c) Borders of the clusters are superimposed on middle frames.

3.3 Detect True Contractions Through Spatial Features

As descriptions of the wrinkle patterns, orientations distribution of edge pixels appears to be a powerful feature for discriminating between contractions and non contractions. For the natural characteristics of contractions, not all of the directions of wrinkles are isotropic and these patterns are not always purely symmetric. Thus, we describe the structure of an image by using an edge direction histogram that seems well able to deal with more general cases of contractile patterns. The frame that has the maximum edge number of each possible contraction is selected for this procedure.

For each edge pixel p, its gradient vector is defined as: $D(p) = \{dx, dy\}$. The amplitude and direction of gradient vectors are:

$$Amp(p) = |dx| + |dy| \text{ and } \theta(p) = \arctan(\frac{dy}{dx}) \tag{5}$$

To express directional features, a polar histogram H is built with the assumption that the directions range from 0 to 360° and are divided into K bins (predefined with K = 256, $\triangle\theta = 360/K = 1.4°$):

$$H(\alpha_i) = \frac{N(\alpha_i)}{SN} \text{ where } N(\alpha_i) = \sum_{p \in \Theta} \log(Amp(p)) \text{ and } SN = \sum_{i=1}^{K} N(\alpha_i) \tag{6}$$

$$\Theta = \{p | \alpha_i - \frac{\triangle\theta}{2} \le \theta(p) < \alpha_i + \frac{\triangle\theta}{2}\}$$

Figure 5 shows the polar histograms H of non contraction (5a) and contraction (5b) cases. The patterns of the polar histogram show the directions are spread every way in the contraction case, whereas in the non contraction case, the polar histogram is distributed in only a dominant direction.

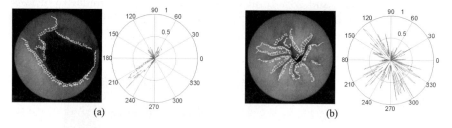

Fig. 5. Direction histogram of a non contraction (a) and contraction (b). Left side shows the original frames with gradient direction at edge pixels, right side is a polar histogram

Based on the signal of H, a simple K-Nearest-Neighbours classifier is used to decide the contraction pattern. The structural similarity between two feature vectors Hx and Hy is estimated by calculating the correlation coefficient $corre(x, y)$, that is:

$$corre(x, y) = \frac{\delta_{xy} + C}{\delta_x \delta_y + C} \tag{7}$$

where δ_x and δ_x are standard deviations of Hx and Hy; δ_{xy} is the covariance of vectors and C is a small constant to avoid the denominator being zero. The K-NN classifier trained with a data set which includes 1000 frames has been labeled manually as non contraction and contraction cases.

4   Experimental Results

The experimental data were supported by the Graduate School of Medicine, Osaka City University, Japan. Six sequences were extracted from different parts of the WCE image sequences in the small bowel. The length of each sequence is 10 minutes. For each sequence, to get ground truth data, manual detections were implemented by medical doctors. The positions at starting and ending frames and the strongest position of each contraction are also marked.

According to the proposed method, the procedures are set up and implemented by C++ programs on a PC Pentium IV 3.2 GHz, 1 GB RAM. Fig. 6 shows the results of the method for an example of 60 continuous frames (from left to right and top to bottom). To evaluate the performance of the proposed method, data as below are calculated for each sequence:

- The number of true contractions detected (True positives – TP)
- The number of wrong contractions detected (False Positives – FP)
- The number of lost contractions (False Negatives – FN)

Using these data, two criteria for the evaluation are:

$$Sensitivity = \frac{TP}{TP + FN} \text{ and } FalseAlarmRate = \frac{FP}{TP + FP} \qquad (8)$$

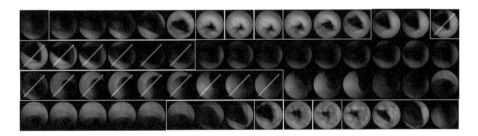

Fig. 6. An illustration the effectiveness of the method. Possible contractions are marked inside rectangle boxes. The redundant cases are removed after evaluating the similarities between frames (marked by slanting). Contractions are recognized as positive cases after utilizing the classification method (marked in square boxes).

The two first stages aim to effectively reduce non contractions with a minimum loss of true positives. The sensitivity of Stage 1 and Stage 2 are 96% and 92%, whereas the false positive rates are 68% and 52%, respectively. For an evaluation of the overall performance of the entire process, Table 1 shows detailed results of each sequence.

Comparisons of the average of the results with those reported in [5] and [6] are 71.5% and 73.5% for sensitivity, and 71% and 44% for false alarm rate, respectively. Obviously, with the proposed method, which combines both spatial and temporal features, the performance is more robust and thus more reliable.

Table 1. Results of the overall process for each sequence

Sequence	Manual Detection	Proposed method	True Pos.	Lost Rate	Sensitivity	FAR
Seq_1	20	56	19	5%	95%	66%
Seq_2	30	44	27	10%	90%	38%
Seq_3	16	25	13	19%	81%	48%
Seq_4	48	50	40	17%	83%	20%
Seq_5	46	60	35	24%	76%	41%
Seq_6	33	41	24	27%	73%	41%
Mean				17%	83%	42%

However, the loss rate is still high in Seq_5 and Seq_6. The reason being that the direction features are less effective for frames at the end of the small bowel because of the weak contractions (Seq_6) or that some contractions have ambiguous patterns (Seq_5). To overcome this issue, more features as changes in the darkness area, or variations of wrinkles patterns (ex., using linear radial patterns in [5]) along the time dimension can be added into the learning paradigm.

5 Conclusion

This paper presented a method to recognize contractions in the small bowel based on analyzing temporal and spatial features. Contractions were successfully detected through a coherent procedure. For temporal features, variations of edge features and evaluations of similarity data between interval frames were implemented to detect possible contractions. To detect a true contraction, the spatial features of the possible contractions were presented through descriptions of an edge direction histogram. From the experimental results, the overall performance implied that the proposed method could detect 83% of the total contractions. Thus, analyzing WCE image sequences by a combination of spatial and temporal features appears a useful way to characterize contractions in the small bowel. However, to ensure more reliable results with different types of data, in future work we need to consider and examine other features to be factored into the classification. In this way, the method proposed here will become a feasible method for developing tools to assist in diagnostic procedures.

References

1. Hansen, M.B.: Small intestinal manometry. Physiological Research 51, 541–556 (2002)
2. Iddan, G., Meron, G., Glukovsky, A., Swain, P.: Wireless capsule endoscope. Nature 405, 417 (2000)
3. Swain, P., Fritscher-Ravens, A.: Role of video endoscopy in managing small bowel disease. GUT 53, 1866–1875 (2004)

4. Spyridonos, P., Vilarino, F., Vitria, J., Azpiroz, F., Radeva, P.: Anisotropic feature extraction from endoluminal images for detection of intestinal contractions. In: Larsen, R., Nielsen, M., Sporring, J. (eds.) MICCAI 2006. LNCS, vol. 4191, pp. 161–168. Springer, Heidelberg (2006)
5. Vilarino, F., Spyridonos, P., Vitria, J., Azpiroz, F., Radeva, P.: Linear radial patterns characterization for automatic detection of tonic intestinal contractions. In: Martínez-Trinidad, J.F., Carrasco Ochoa, J.A., Kittler, J. (eds.) CIARP 2006. LNCS, vol. 4225, pp. 178–187. Springer, Heidelberg (2006)
6. Spyridonos, P., Vilarino, F., Vitria, J., Azpiroz, F., Radeva, P.: Identification of intestinal motility events of capsule endoscopy video analysis. In: Blanc-Talon, J., Philips, W., Popescu, D.C., Scheunders, P. (eds.) ACIVS 2005. LNCS, vol. 3708, Springer, Heidelberg (2005)
7. Canny, J.: A computational approach to edge detection. IEEE T-PAMI 8, 679–698 (1986)
8. Greenspan, H., Goldberger, J., Mayer, A.: A probabilistic framework for spatio-temporal video representation. In: Heyden, A., Sparr, G., Nielsen, M., Johansen, P. (eds.) ECCV 2002. LNCS, vol. 2350, pp. 461–475. Springer, Heidelberg (2002)
9. Dempster, A., Laird, N., Rubin, D.: Maximum likelihood from incomplete data via the em algorithm. Journal Royal Statistical Society B, 39 (1), 1–38 (1997)
10. MIXMOD Ver. 2.0.1: (2007),
    http://www-math.univ-fcomte.fr/mixmod/index.php

Boundary-Specific Cost Functions for Quantitative Airway Analysis

Atilla P. Kiraly[1], Benjamin L. Odry[1], David P. Naidich[2],
and Carol L. Novak[1]

[1]Siemens Corporate Research, Princeton, NJ
{atilla.kiraly,benjamin.odry,carol.novak}@siemens.com
[2]Department of Radiology, NYU Medical University, New York, NY
david.naidich@nyumc.org

Abstract. Computed tomography (CT) images of the lungs provide high resolution views of the airways. Quantitative measurements such as lumen diameter and wall thickness help diagnose and localize airway diseases, assist in surgical planning, and determine progress of treatment. Automated quantitative analysis of such images is needed due to the number of airways per patient. We present an approach involving dynamic programming coupled with boundary-specific cost functions that is capable of differentiating inner and outer borders. The method allows for precise delineation of the inner lumen and outer wall. The results are demonstrated on synthetic data, evaluated on human datasets compared to human operators, and verified on phantom CT scans to sub-voxel accuracy.

1 Introduction

Diseases and abnormalities of the airways can manifest themselves as observable changes in airway lumen diameters and wall thicknesses [1]. These changes can also occur in response to treatment. High-resolution computed tomography (CT) images of the chest offer high resolution views of the airways that potentially allow one to obtain detailed quantitative measurements. However systematic analysis of such images is not feasible without automation due to the sheer number of airways involved. Certain airway abnormalities can affect only localized regions, making analysis of multiple locations throughout the lungs necessary. Automated analysis of such images helps reduce or eliminate reader variability and allows for the entire patient dataset to be analyzed within a reasonable amount of time.

Automated methods for quantitative airway analysis attempt to precisely determine the boundaries of the inner lumen and outer airway wall. These methods face several challenges in providing accurate measurements, especially in smaller airways. Partial volume artifacts result when regions of different densities exist within the volume of a single voxel [2], making it more difficult to find the exact wall location. Additional difficulties arise from the scanner's Point Spread Function (PSF) [3] and CT reconstruction artifacts, which distort the image and create additional noise. Finally, a problem specific to the airways is identifying the outer wall boundary when there is an adjacent artery, which in many situations, obscures the true boundary.

N. Ayache, S. Ourselin, A. Maeder (Eds.): MICCAI 2007, Part I, LNCS 4791, pp. 784–791, 2007.
© Springer-Verlag Berlin Heidelberg 2007

The full-width half-max (FWHM) approach is a popular method that is frequently used as a point of comparison. This method determines the location of the inner and outer boundaries based on the maximum intensity within the wall and the minimum intensities of the air region [4]. The location of the intensity computed from the average of these two is judged as the wall position. This method has been shown to underestimate the inner lumen boundary and overestimate the outer boundary [3]. In [5] the airway segmentation added robustness by defining an initial boundary.

A sub-voxel accurate method for determining airway lumen and wall thickness was presented in [3,6]. These methods estimate the scanner's PSF to help fit a cylindrical model to the data. Although the results show high accuracy, the method depends on an assumed cylindrical shape, which is not always the case for the airways.

In [7], a phase-congruency space is used to recover the borders by predicting intensity crossing points obtained from different reconstruction kernels. The authors suggest it as a "bronze standard" since it shows little variance with different reconstruction kernels and is accurate up to discretization error.

A group of methods depend on an optimal fit based upon gradient computations. In [12], a dual tube model is fit to the inner and outer lumina. Fully automated methods often depend on a definition of the airway centerlines [8-11] to offer a central location as well as a perpendicular direction to perform the measurement. The above methods also have these requirements. An alternate method eliminates the need for direction vectors by using a sphere [13]. Although subvoxel accuracy is achieved, only the average diameter is computed. A promising method [14] finds the borders directly from the airway segmentation, allowing for an inner lumen definition without a dependence on airway centerlines. However, the method's accuracy is not yet established.

Minimum-path based methods operate by defining a minimum cost path through a cost function image via dynamic programming. This concept was originally applied to vessels [15,16], but was adapted for airways [11,17]. In these applications, the data is resampled into a polar space and two balanced edge filters are used to obtain an accurate inner lumen boundary. The results show excellent accuracy and robustness, but the defined cost function limits its potential for obtaining the outer boundary and can make it vulnerable to other strong edge artifacts.

We propose a dynamic programming approach allowing for accurate inner and outer wall measurements. Our paper introduces cost functions targeted specifically for the inner and outer boundaries of airway walls. The functions can also be individually tuned to particular sizes, and increase robustness by limiting artifacts from non-boundary edges. Additionally, the determined inner border is used to influence the computation of the outer border to prevent intersection.

2 Method

The method computes cost functions locally at each site perpendicular to the direction of the airway. The airway centerlines are used to obtain these sites and directions. The cost functions are based on an airway model of a very low density lumen, a high density airway wall, and an intermediate density parenchyma outside the wall.

2.1   Airway Centerline Extraction

The airway centerlines are the prerequisite for fully automated analysis. They describe airway tree hierarchy as a series of branches where each branch contains a series of sites giving the lumen center location as well as a direction heading. This location and the perpendicular plane defined by the heading give the two necessary components to define an isotropic 2D cross-sectional image of the site, allowing measurements to be computed at that point. Fig 1a shows a 2D image obtained from a given location and direction. We used a two step process of skeletonization of the segmented airways followed by refinement to obtain smooth centerlines. Complete details and validation are found in [10,5]. Other centerline methods can be used for this step [8-13]. Sites can also be manually specified if a single airway location is to be measured.

2.2   Boundary Determination

Given the 2D cross-sectional image of the site to be measured, it is first radially resampled into a polar form, as shown in Fig. 1b. The vertical direction corresponds to the distance from the airway center, while the horizontal direction corresponds to different angles around the airway axis. We used 360 different angles to form the images. Note that in Figs. 1b through 1e the images are horizontally compressed for space and are sampled to a sub-pixel level.

This polar image C_{polar} is used to create two cost function images, C_{inner} and C_{outer}, (Figs. 1d and 1e) corresponding to the inner and outer boundaries. These cost functions assign a cost to each pixel in the radial image. The goal is to find a path with minimum cost spanning the horizontal length of the cost function image. A dynamic programming method is applied with the constraint that the vertical level of the starting position corresponds to that of the ending position [18]. Additionally, the path must be piece-wise congruent.

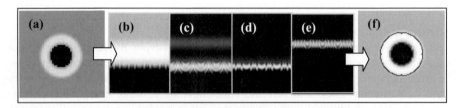

Fig. 1. Outline of the proposed method on synthetic airway data. The perpendicular cross section of the airway (a) is radially resampled (b). Cost functions are then determined from resampled image. (Brighter response = lower cost) (c) is a previously proposed cost function [11]. The proposed cost functions (d) and (e) are targeted towards the inner and outer boundaries. Horizontal paths through the cost functions then determine the boundaries as shown in (f).

Since two boundaries are determined, two minimum paths are computed. In the proposed method, first the inner boundary is determined. This boundary is then used to assign very high cost to the inner portions of the outer boundary cost function to prevent the two boundaries from crossing. The computed outer boundary then never intersects the inner boundary. The radially transformed image creates an almost linear structure from the airway wall along with a dark-light-dark pattern in the vertical direction, as illustrated in Fig. 2 (top). A straighter airway wall can also be induced by incrementally offsetting the image with regards to the segmentation of the airway lumen [11]. We make use of the unique placement of the wall within the polar image to accurately determine both boundaries, as shown in Fig. 2.

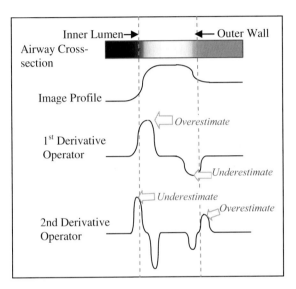

Fig. 2. An illustration of two directional filters that are combined to accurately detect inner and outer airway boundaries. A cross-section of an airway along a radial line is shown on top. The result of the 1st and 2nd order derivative operators are shown below. Examining the extremum, the 1st derivative operator overestimates the inner lumen while underestimating the outer diameter. The opposite is true for the positive extremum in the 2nd derivative operator. Hence, combining variations of each of these operators can allow for accurate localization of the inner lumen or outer wall.

We propose the following cost functions to allow for accurate inner and outer boundary characterization:

$$C_{inner} = w_i \cdot H\big(D'_y(C_{polar})\big) \cdot D'_y(C_{polar}) + (1 - w_i) \cdot D''_y(C_{polar}) \text{, and} \qquad (1)$$

$$C_{outer} = w_o \cdot \big(1 - H(D'_y(C_{polar}))\big) \cdot D'_y(C_{polar}) + (1 - w_o) \cdot D''_y(C_{polar}) \text{,} \qquad (2)$$

where H() is the Heaviside step function, returning 1 for positive values and 0 for negative values. These functions are composed of linear combinations of small scale directional 1st and 2nd order derivatives of the image C_{polar}. The terms w_i and w_o have a possible range of [0,1] and determine the weightings applied to each directional derivative to balance the under and over estimations. The inner boundary filter (1) is composed of a linear combination of the positive portions of the 1st derivative and the 2nd order derivative. As shown in Fig. 2, the 1st derivative operator overestimates while the 2nd derivative operator underestimates. The outer border filter consists of a linear combination of the inverted negative portion of the 1st derivative and the 2nd order derivative. In this case, the 1st order derivative underestimates while the 2nd order derivative overestimates.

The results of these filters on synthetic data are shown in Fig. 1d and 1e. The outer boundary produces a weaker response relative to the inner boundary as predicted by Fig. 2. Note that this weaker response has no impact on the proposed method since the boundaries are computed separately. Also note that in each case the particular boundary not targeted has virtually no response.

The cost function of a previously proposed method [11] does not differentiate between inner and outer walls. Both boundaries appear in the cost function, as shown in Fig. 1c. This effect can distract the inner boundary computation. Further distractions can result in an emphasis of non-linear edges. This latter effect was compensated for by giving emphasis to specific edges depending upon gradient direction. This step can also be applied to the proposed method, but the focus is on developing specialized filters.

Fig. 3 shows an example of derived cost functions from a real airway along with the resultant boundaries. The adjacent artery creates an error in the outer boundary when using the standard minimum path algorithm, as shown in the left image. On the right, using the exact same cost functions, the minimum path is computed by assigning an additional cost for deviating from the predicted straight border. Note that imposing this additional cost does not significantly impact the inner boundary determined. Additionally possibilities are discussed in the conclusion.

Since a linear combination of underestimates and overestimates is involved, their weighting must be calibrated to produce accurate border estimates across different size ranges. These calibration parameters are obtained from materials of similar density to airways to account for the PSF and partial volume effects at different scales. During measurement, the airway segmentation is used to determine an inner size estimate and a linear interpolation between calibrated parameters of the nearest scale is applied for both parameters. It is possible to incorporate an outer size estimate to determine w_o separately.

4 Results

Two different evaluations were performed. The method was first calibrated and evaluated on a scanned phantom airway. The phantom consists of 5 tubes of known dimensions, varying in inner diameter from 2mm to 10mm with wall thicknesses from 1mm to 3mm. It is constructed of PVC pipe and nylon tubing and scanned at a voxel resolution of $0.35\times0.35\times0.5$ mm^3. We determined values of w_i =[0.17, 0.22, 0.15, 0.30, 0.27] and w_o =[0.49, 0.17, 0.32, 0.20, 0.21] for the range of sizes to provide optimal measurements and then applied them along multiple locations of the same tube. Again, linear interpolation is used based upon the size estimate from the segmentation. The method accurately measured the tube dimensions, demonstrating the validity of the cost function in determining the true boundaries to sub-voxel accuracy. Table 1 lists the errors and standard deviations.

The second experiment compared the measurements against two operators on a human airway CT dataset with $0.58 \times 0.58 \times 0.79$ mm^3 voxel resolution. A total of 34 airways with lumen diameters ranging from 1.2 to 3.6mm and outer diameters ranging from 3.2 to 6.1mm were randomly selected. Each operator independently performed inner and outer diameter measurements twice using digital calipers. Some locations included nearby arteries. The results show that the method produces measurement results within the error of the human operators. In the smallest airway, the method produced the largest variation (0.5mm), although still achieving sub-voxel accuracy.

The average running time for each site was 1.1s. The path computation occupied the majority of the time (70%) at 390ms per path on average.

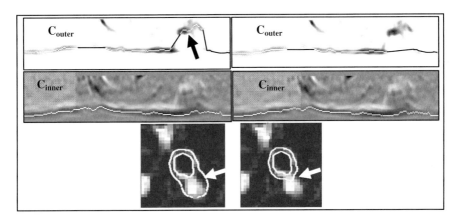

Fig. 3. The left and right sides show a comparison of two different minimum path computation methods. In both cases the results for the outer wall filter (*top*) and the inner wall filter (*middle*) are shown along with the minimum cost path. In each case the cost functions are the same with lower gray levels indicating lower cost. The subsequent boundary results are shown at the bottom. In the left case, a standard minimum path was computed, resulting in an error with the outer boundary due to the artery, (*white arrow*). In the right case, the path cost was increased when not heading straight. The outer boundary is correctly captured. Note that the inner boundary has not changed with this additional requirement.

Table 1. Absolute errors and standard deviations for the computed inner and outer diameters obtained from phantom data of hollow cylinders of known radii and wall thickness.

	Mean Absolute Error of Inner Diameter (mm)	Mean Absolute Error of Outer Diameter (mm)	Std. Dev. Inner Diameter (mm)	Std. Dev Outer Diameter (mm)
Tube 1	0.02	0.03	0.0215	0.0259
Tube 2	0.05	0.06	0.0417	0.0661
Tube 3	0.11	0.07	0.0766	0.0772
Tube 4	0.06	0.30	0.0551	0.0408
Tube 5	0.15	0.10	0.1014	0.0549

5 Conclusions

We have presented a method based on boundary-specific cost functions for quantitative airway measurements. Previous airway cost function methods use generalized cost functions not geared toward specific boundaries and produce extraneous responses. The proposed functions accurately target specific boundaries while producing little or no response to other boundaries. The computed inner path was also used to influence the outer cost function. This feature prevented the outer boundary from intersecting the inner boundary.

The method demonstrated robustness in cases of image noise and adjacent arteries when enforcing a straight path. Further experiments in the cost function definition and minimum path computation can be done to determine still more robust methods. Additional possibilities include allowing both paths to influence each other during computation as opposed to sequential computation. Modifications to the cost functions seem promising. Applying the Heaviside function to the second derivative operator eliminates negative responses, which may increase robustness. We find that assigning higher cost to regions above the high intensity areas occupied by arteries eliminates the need for enforcing a straighter path in cases such as Fig. 3. This change defines the cost functions with elements taken directly from the polar image in addition to the operators. Calibration based upon wall thickness also seems promising.

The method demonstrated accurate inner lumen and outer wall boundary determination for airway walls within phantom and human airway data. Further tests on multiple phantoms and reconstruction kernels are the subject of future work. Currently, it appears that the method needs re-calibration for different reconstruction kernels and CT-scanner machines. Finally, measurement tests with more human operators and locations will help further establish the method's robustness.

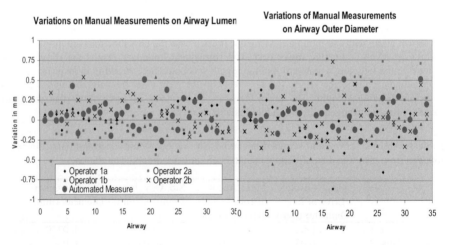

Fig. 4. A comparison of the proposed method against two human operators on a total of 34 airways. Operator 1a and 1b refer to the measurements of the first operator at times 1 and 2. Similarly 2a and 2b correspond to operator 2's measurements at times 1 and 2. The results show that the obtained measurements are within the range of the inter- and intra- operator measurement variation. No airway size dependent variation was noticed.

References

1. Matsuoka, S., Kurihara, Y., Nakajima, Y., Niimi, H., Ashida, H., Kaneoya, K.: Serial Change in Airway Lumen and Wall Thickness at Thin-Section CT in Asymptomatic Subjects. Radiology (December 2004)
2. Santago, P., Gage, H.D.: Statistical Models of Partial Volume Effect. IEEE Trans. Img. Proc. pp. 1531–1540 (November 1995)
3. Reinhardt, J.M., D'Souza, N.D., Hoffman, E.A.: Accurate measurement of intra-thoracic airways. IEEE Trans Med. Imag. 16(6), 820–827 (1997)
4. Nakano, Y., Muro, S., Sakai, H., Iría, T., Chin, K., Tsukino, M., Nishimura, K., Itoh, H., Pare, P.D., Hogg, J.C., Mishima, M.: Computed Tomographic Measurements of Airway Dimensions and Emphysema in Smokers. J. Respiratory Crit. Care Med. 161, 574–580 (2000)
5. Kiraly, A.P., Reinhardt, J.M., Hoffman, E.A., et al.: Virtual bronchoscopy for quantitative airway analysis. SPIE Medical Imaging 2005 5746 (2005)
6. Saba, O., Hoffmann, E.A., Reinhardt, J.M.: Maximizing quantitative accuracy of the lung airway lumen and wall measures obtained from X-ray CT imaging. J. Applied Physiology 95, 1063–1095 (2003)
7. Estépar, R.S.J., Washko, G.G., Silverman, E.K., Reilly, J.J., Kikinis, R., Westin, C.F.: Accurate Airway Wall Estimation Using Phase Congruency. In: Larsen, R., Nielsen, M., Sporring, J. (eds.) MICCAI 2006. LNCS, vol. 4191, Springer, Heidelberg (2006)
8. Preteux, F., Fetita, C.I., Grenier, P., Capderou, A.: Modeling, segmentation, and caliber estimation of bronchi in high-resolution computerized tomography. J. Electron. Imag. 8(1), 36–45 (1999)
9. Mori, K., Suenaga, Y., Toriwaki, J.: Automated anatomical labeling of the bronchial branch and its applications to the virtual bronchoscopy. Med. Imag. 19(2), 103–114 (2000)
10. Kiraly, A.P., Helferty, J.P, Hoffman, E.A., McLennan, G., Higgins, W.E.: 3D Path Planning for Virtual Bronchoscopy. IEEE Trans. Med. Imag. 23(11) (2004)
11. Tschirren, J., Hoffman, E.A., McLennan, G., Sonka, M.: Intrathoracic Airway Trees: Segmentation and Airway Morphology Analysis From Low-Dose CT Scans. IEEE Trans. Med. Imag. 24(12) (2005)
12. Odry, B.L., Kiraly, A.P., Novak, C.L., et al.: Automated airway evaluation system for multi-slice computed tomography using airway lumen diameter, airway wall thickness and broncho-arterial ratio. In: Proc. SPIE Medical Imaging 2006, vol. 6143 (2006)
13. Wiemker, R., Blaffert, T., Bülow, T., Renisch, S., Lorenz, C.: Automated assessment of bronchial lumen, wall thickness and bronchoarterial diameter ratio of the tracheobronchial tree using high-resolution CT. I.C.S. 1268 CARS (2004), pp. 973–977 (2004)
14. Saragalia, A., Fetita, C.I., Preteux, F.J.: Airway wall thickness assessment: a new functionality in virtual bronchoscopy investigation. SPIE Medical Imaging (2007)
15. Fleagle, S.R., Johnson, M.R., Wilbricht, C.J., Skorton, D.J., Wilson, R.F., White, C.W., Marcus, M.L., Collins, S.M.: Automated Analysis of Coronary Arterial Morphology in Cineangiograms: Geometric and Physiologic Validation in Humans. IEEE Trans. Med. Imag.8(4) (1989)
16. Sonka, M., Reddy, G.K., Winniford, M.D., Collins, S.M.: Adaptive Approach to Accurate Analysis of Small-Diameter Vessels in Cineangiograms. IEEE Trans. Med. Imag. 16(1) (1997)
17. Li, K., Wu, X., Chen, D.Z., Sonka, M.: Efficient Optimal Surface Detection: Theory, Implementation and Experimental Validation. SPIE Medical Imaging (2004)
18. Moon, T.K., Stirling, W.C.: Mathematical Methods and Algorithms for Signal Processing. Prentice Hall, Inc, Englewood Cliffs (2000)

Automatic Dry Eye Detection

Tamir Yedidya[1], Richard Hartley[1], Jean-Pierre Guillon[2],
and Yogesan Kanagasingam[2]

[1] The Australian National University, and National ICT Australia*
{tamir,hartley}@rsise.anu.edu.au
[2] Faculty of Medicine and Health Sciences, Lions Eye Institute, Australia
jp@eye5.com.au,yoge@lei.org.au

Abstract. Dry Eye Syndrome is a common disease in the western world, with effects from uncomfortable itchiness to permanent damage to the ocular surface. Nevertheless, there is still no objective test that provides reliable results. We have developed a new method for the automated detection of dry areas in videos taken after instilling fluorescein in the tear film. The method consists of a multi-step algorithm to first locate the iris in each image, then align the images and finally analyze the aligned sequence in order to find the regions of interest. Since the fluorescein spreads on the ocular surface of the eye the edges of the iris are fuzzy making the detection of the iris challenging. We use RANSAC to first detect the upper and lower eyelids and then the iris. Then we align the images by finding differences in intensities at different scales and using a least squares optimization method (Levenberg-Marquardt), to overcome the movement of the iris and the camera. The method has been tested on videos taken from different patients. It is demonstrated to find the dry areas accurately and to provide a measure of the extent of the disease.

1   Introduction

One of the roles of the tear film is the maintenance of corneal epithelial integrity and transparency which is achieved by keeping the ocular surface continuously moist. The pre-ocular tear film in humans does not remain stable for long periods of time [3]. When blinking is prevented, the tear film ruptures and dry spots appear over the cornea [5].

The Fluorescein Break Up Time (FBUT) test was designed by Norn [8] and called corneal wetting time. A moistened fluorescein strip is applied to the bulbar conjunctiva and after a few blinks to spread the fluorescein evenly, the tear film is viewed with the help of a yellow filter in front of a slit-lamp biomicroscope. When a dark area appears, it represents the rupture of the tear film and the time elapsed since the last blink is recorded as break-up time (BUT). The shorter the BUT, the more likely the diagnosis of dry eye [9]. The degree of blackness is related to the depth of the breakup. The deeper the break, the greater the

---

* National ICT Australia is funded by the Australian Government's Backing Australia's Ability initiative, in part through the Australia Research Council.

N. Ayache, S. Ourselin, A. Maeder (Eds.): MICCAI 2007, Part I, LNCS 4791, pp. 792–799, 2007.
© Springer-Verlag Berlin Heidelberg 2007

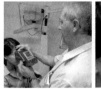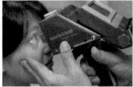

Fig. 1. EyeScan portable imaging system for Fluorescein tear film recording

chances of ocular surface damage. If the eyes are kept open, the area of the break will increase in size and breaks may appear in new areas over the cornea.

This is the test of tear film stability most commonly used by clinicians and a few improvements have been presented over the years [4]. A BUT inferior to 10 seconds usually reveals an anomaly of the pre-ocular tear film. If the film ruptures repeatedly in the same spot a superficial epithelial abnormality must be suspected. If the break up occurs over the center of the cornea, a decrease in visual acuity will be induced.

The location, shape, progression and depth of the original and successive breaks give clinical indications as to the cause of the break and what treatment to choose and are incorporated into our method. This is not possible with our current subjective observation and grading clinical routines. With the development of the EyeScan system, as seen in Fig. 1, an affordable and easy to operate system of video recording of anterior ocular structures is available.

To our knowledge, automatic methods towards finding the dry eye areas are sparse in the current literature. However, there are some existing approaches for locating the iris as part of another applications. Usually assuming its shape is a perfect circle, the methods mostly use circle fitting algorithms. Daugman [1] focused on iris recognition, but he first finds the pupil-iris and iris-sclera borders by searching over all circles in different radii for the ones that gives the maximum contour integral derivative. Ma and el [7] also locate the iris as part of their iris recognition procedure. They first locate the darker pupil and then the iris using Canny edge detector and Hough transform to estimate the iris location. However, in our videos the pupil is not visible at all as shown in Fig. 2, and the boundaries

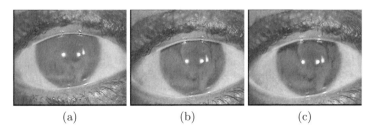

(a)   (b)   (c)

Fig. 2. Samples of eye images after instilling fluorescein. (a) Immediately after a blink (b) half way between blinks (c) just before a blink. The darker areas are the dry eye areas which evolve through the sequence. In (c) the upper eyelid opened.

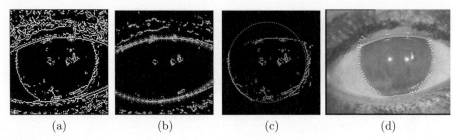

(a)   (b)   (c)   (d)

Fig. 3. Steps for locating the iris (a) cropped edge map (b) cropped edge map for locating the eyelids and their detection (c) cropped image after removing outliers and the fitted iris (d) selected pixels used for LM on the original image

between the iris and the sclera are much fuzzier due to the fluorescein spreading. The Hough transform is a commonly used method for circle detection, however it is very slow and needs a few iterations to find the correct radius. The Fast Radial Symmetry [6] algorithm is equivalent to circular Hough, but also takes gradient direction into account. The method is robust to patrial occlusion, but had difficulties finding the exact radius in our images.

2 Algorithm

The dry areas always appear as darker areas in the fluorescent image, as seen in Fig. 2(c). Trying to apply a single threshold to the grey values does not work, since the spreading of the fluorescein and the lighting conditions change from patient to patient. Therefore, the intensity of the fluorescein cannot be predicted. Moreover, dry areas might become visible only at parts of the sequence, for example, as the eyelids open or close. Finally, the camera is hand held, therefore there is a considerable movement of the iris. To address these problems, we present our algorithm that is based on aligning the video.

2.1 Fitting a Circular Model

The images of interest in the video are those between blinks. To that end, we first find all the blinks and half-blinks and treat each sequence individually. Blinks are detected when consecutive images have big difference in intensity. An edge map of the image immediately after a blink is created using the sobel operator and non-maximal edges are suppressed. We use RANSAC [2] with three parameters, (x, y, r), on the edge map to locate the iris. At each iteration a set of three points is used for fitting a circle and the number of pixels passing through it is counted. In order for RANSAC to perform well the outliers need to occupy a small percentage of the total pixels as demonstrated in [2]. However, the edges of the iris are usually not strong and are hindered by the eyelashes and strong illumination changes around the iris's borders. In some cases, the ratio between the inliers (the iris) and the outliers is 1 to 10 as seen in Fig. 3(a).

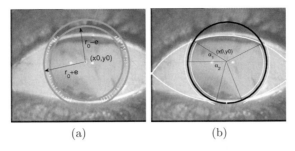

Fig. 4. Explanation of the LM (a) the area between the two circles is used as the search area for the iris. The white pixels are those found by LM to best fit the iris (b) the detected eyelids and the iris are segmented, the white arcs are those corresponding to the circles from part (a). Only the area between the two arcs is used for searching.

Therefore, we initially segment the upper and lower eyelids and then remove all pixels above and below them respectively. The eyelids are detected by creating another edge map with a higher threshold and then running RANSAC with three parameters and assuming the eyelids are circles with a very big radius, see Fig. 3(b). The method proves to be a reliable way to detect the eyelids. However, sometimes the lower eyelids might not be visible, so extra care is taken to ensure parts of the iris are not removed. Then it is possible for RANSAC to find the iris as seen in Fig. 3(c). At each iteration three points are randomly picked up and a few rules are imposed regarding the points distribution and limiting the search for the expected range of iris's radii existing in patients.

After the iris has been detected we use Levenberg-Marquardt(LM) [2] to do the fine-tuning by iteratively minimizing a non-linear function for fitting a circle. The initial estimation (x_0, y_0, r_0) is the one found for the iris in the RANSAC step. We define the maximum error e to be a few pixels, usually around four, and then compute the gradient's magnitude for all pixels in the annulus formed by the circles of radii $r_0 - e$ and $r_0 + e$ and the center (x_0, y_0), as depicted in Fig. 4(a). However, since the iris is usually only partly visible, we find the angles α_1 and α_2 between the estimated iris and the upper and lower eyelids respectively, see Fig. 4(b). Only the pixels that are on the arc between the eyelids are taken. If the whole iris is visible all pixels are taken. These pixels are sorted according to their magnitude and the strongest 150 are considered for the LM minimization. The parameter to the function to be minimized is the vector (x, y, r) and at each iteration the set of pixels found are used to compute the sum of squares of the Huber distance $D_h(x_k, y_k)$ of each pixel (x_k, y_k) to the estimated iris:

$$\text{define} \quad d = \sqrt{(x_0 - x_k)^2 + (y_0 - y_k)^2} - r$$

$$D_h(x_k, y_k) = \begin{cases} d & \text{when } |d| \leq \epsilon \\ \text{sign}(d) \sqrt{(2|d| - \epsilon)\epsilon} & \text{when } |d| > \epsilon \end{cases} \quad (1)$$

The use of the Huber distance makes the penalty linear above the threshold ϵ, avoiding quadratic penalties to faraway outliers. Results of the LM with the

chosen pixels are depicted in Fig. 3(d). The detection of the iris in the rest of
the sequence is done in a similar way, each time using the previous estimation as
the initial guess. Since, we do not expect drastic movements of the iris, the LM
converges quickly. It is worth mentioning that the time-consuming RANSAC is
computed only once, for the first image.

2.2   Computing Image Translation

After locating the iris in each of the images, it is possible to align the images
over the iris area. The need for such alignment is demonstrated in Fig. 5. Since,
the iris is represented as a circle, we first simply align by scaling and translating
one circle to another circle. Then a second alignment is done by using the grey
levels of the iris area to find the best homography between the images. Every
few images are treated as a block. The first image in the block is aligned to an
image in the previous block and the other images are aligned to the first image
in the block to avoid accumulating error. The alignment procedure is as follows:

1. Initialize the homography matrix H_0 to be the identity matrix. Since, we are interested only in translation and scaling the matrix has three unknowns. Define
   the initial region of interest(ROI) as the area that includes the iris and the eyelids, since they differ in grey level from the iris and help the alignment process.
2. The homography H_0 is used as our initial guess. A pyramid of scaled images
   for both images is built. For each scale the best homography is found starting from the smallest scale. Going up the pyramid is done by rescaling the
   transformation and the ROI.
3. Compute the homography by minimizing:

$$C(H) = \sum_{x \in ROI} (I_x^{(j)} - I_{Hx}^{(k)})^2 \tag{2}$$

   where Hx is the transformed pixel in I_k, and j and k are indices for the two
   images being aligned.
4. The process is repeated for every image in the sequence.

It is difficult to show the results of an alignment unless in a video. However,
Fig. 5 shows the averaged images over a sequence. The non-aligned image is
completely blurred and cannot provide information regarding the dry areas. It
is expected since the camera is hand held and the patient's gaze can move.

2.3   Segmentation of the Dry Area

Based on the two previous steps, the task of segmenting correctly the dry areas
becomes possible. In section 2.1 we found the circle equations of the iris and the
upper and lower eyelids. Since, the dry areas appear only on the iris, the area to
be searched for dryness can be extracted. The pixels of interest will be those that
become darker during the sequence. However, the intensities of the dry areas can

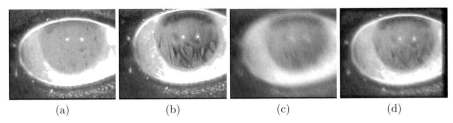

| (a) | (b) | (c) | (d) |

Fig. 5. Since the camera is hand held and the iris can move, it is necessary to align the video: (a) image after a blink (b) last image before the next blink. The averaged image of all the images in the (c) non-aligned video (d) aligned video. The non-aligned result is blurred showing that the dry areas cannot be detected without aligning the images or by just taking the difference between images (a) and (b).

change a lot from patient to patient as the fluorescein spreading varies and light conditions are not the same. To that end, we calculate a difference image:

$$D(x,y) = \sum_{k=i_0}^{i_0+\Delta} I_k(x,y) - \sum_{k=n-\Delta}^{n-1} I_k(x,y) < T_1 \tag{3}$$

assuming the number of images in the sequence is n, Δ is a small number of images and i_0 is chosen to be close to zero.

Ideally each pixel will have a monotonically decreasing intensity function through the sequence. However, it is not always the case. It is often that the dark areas are revealed only in parts of the sequence, for example, if the eyelids open or if a few pixels are aligned incorrectly especially near the borders of the iris with the eyelids. To overcome this, for each frame k we compute an average value $V_k(x,y)$ for the pixels in the frame over a small neighborhood about a pixel (x,y). A smoothing is done by convolving with a gaussian to minimize the effects of erratic movement. Then we compute the following downs-ups ratio:

$$R(x,y) = \frac{\#downs}{\#ups} = \frac{\sum_{k=0}^{n-1}[V_{k+1}(x,y) < V_k(x,y) - d]}{\sum_{k=0}^{n-1}[V_{k+1}(x,y) > V_k(x,y) + d]} \tag{4}$$

where d is a small number around 0.5. The ratio $R(x,y)$ provides information how the pixel changes through the sequence and is dependent on the sequence length. Unlike Eq. 3, $R(x,y)$ detects pixels that only mildly become dry and also dry pixels near the iris's borders that their intensity fluctuates through the sequence. These pixels usually have low or unpredicted $D(x,y)$ value. A weighted average of equations (3) and (4) and the intensity in the last frame serve as the criterion for a dry pixel. Finally, isolated pixels are deleted, since they have a high chance of being erroneous. The result is a confidence map of the dry areas, computed as follows:

$$\tilde{I}(x,y) = \lambda_1 D(x,y) + \lambda_2 R(x,y) + \lambda_3 I_{n-1}(x,y) \tag{5}$$

where the parameters are at present chosen according to our empirical observations. In ongoing work, we are determining ways to choose them through learning

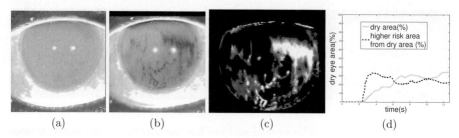

(a)   (b)   (c)   (d)

Fig. 6. Dry eye area segmentation results (a) image after a blink (b) last image before the next blink (c) Confidence map of the dry area. Brighter shades represent drier areas (d) graph of the evolution of the dry area in the sequence. About 35 percent of the eye became dry, but from that only 22 percent is severely dry.

techniques. However, λ_3 should be relatively small, since low intensity at the final frame does not always mean that the pixel became dry. The brighter the pixel is in $\tilde{I}(x, y)$, the drier it is likely to be. Darker pixels still exhibit some dryness, but might not be so substantial. The area of the dryness is calculated and we separate between higher risk and lower risk areas as seen in Fig. 6.

3   Results

We used 8 videos of different patients to evaluate our results. The videos are of size 355 x 282 pixels in RGB format. Each video usually had 3 to 5 good sequences that could be checked for the dry areas. The patients varied from having a very dry eye to an eye with no visible dryness. The videos were taken at different times with different illumination conditions.

Evaluating the robustness of our detection algorithm is a difficult task, since the area of dryness is subjective and cannot be exactly defined. This is the advantage of building the confidence map. In order to measure our performance, an optometrist was given the videos and hand segmented the dry areas over the last image (for reasons of convenience) in 12 sequences taken from 3 different patients with different degree of dryness (see Fig. 7(a) and (c)). We chose a fixed threshold for our confidence maps and used the following figure of merit:

$$S(\tilde{I}_x^t, I_x^h) = \frac{\sum_{x \in ROI} \tilde{I}_x^t == I_x^h}{|ROI|} \qquad (6)$$

where $\tilde{I}_x^t$ results from thresholding the confidence map, I_x^h is the hand segmented image and $|ROI|$ is the number of pixels in the iris. On average our method had 91% of accuracy, ranging from 84% to 96% and a standard deviation of 4%. Our algorithm found 61 out of the total 68 areas that were hand segmented for dryness, and in two images segmented an extra area. The main differences between the segmentations were in the exact boundaries of the dry areas and the difficulty of our method to find thin areas next to the eyelids that were revealed only partly through the sequence. By choosing different thresholds for

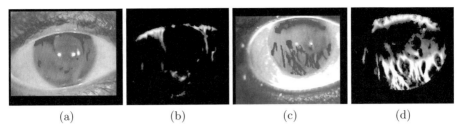

(a)   (b)   (c)   (d)

Fig. 7. Comparison of the dry eye area segmentation results. (a) & (c) Hand segmented areas for Fig. 2 and Fig. 5. (b) & (d) Our confidence maps for Fig. 2 and Fig. 5.

the confidence maps and changing the parameters in Eq. 5 the results can be adjusted to match better to specific hand segmentations.

4 Conclusion and Future Research

In this paper, a new method for automatic detection of the tear film breakup area was developed. We demonstrated that the method can find the relevant area and size and build a confidence map.

This method will be tested on larger data sets and provide a comprehensive evaluation including the BUT value and confidence level for that value and a new standard to distinguish between the thinning of the tear film and the break based on the progression through the sequence. This should prove this method clinically useful by the optometrists. Our long term goal is to implement a non-invasive method to automatically detect the stability of the tear film.

References

1. Daugman, J.: The importance of being random: statistical principles of iris recognition. Pattern Recognition 36(2), 279–291 (2003)
2. Hartley, R.I., Zisserman, A.: Multiple View Geometry in Computer Vision, 2nd edn. Cambridge University Press, Cambridge (2004)
3. Holly, F.J.: Formation and rupture of the tear film. Exp. Eye. Res. 15, 515–525 (1973)
4. Korb, D., Greiner, J., Herman, J.: Comparison of fluorescein break-up time measurement reproducibility using standard fluorescein strips versus the dry eye test (det) method. Cornea 20(8), 811–815 (2001)
5. Lemp, M.A., Hamill, J.R.: Factors affecting tear film break up in normal eyes. Arch. Ophthalmol. 89(2), 103–105 (1973)
6. Loy, G., Zelinsky, A.: A fast radial symmetry transform for detecting points of interest. In: Heyden, A., Sparr, G., Nielsen, M., Johansen, P. (eds.) ECCV 2002. LNCS, vol. 2350, pp. 358–368. Springer, Heidelberg (2002)
7. Ma, L., Tan, T., Wang, Y., Zhang, D.: Efficient iris recognition by characterizing key local variations. IEEE Transactions on Image Processing 13(6), 739–750 (2004)
8. Norn, M.S.: Desiccation of the pre corneal film. Acta Ophthalmol 47(4), 865–880 (1969)
9. Tsubota, K.: Tear dynamics and dry eye. Progress in Retinal and Eye Research 17, 556–596 (1998)

Ultrasound Myocardial Elastography and Registered 3D Tagged MRI: Quantitative Strain Comparison

Zhen Qian[1], Wei-Ning Lee[2], Elisa E. Konofagou[2], Dimitris N. Metaxas[1], and Leon Axel[3]

[1] Center for Computational Biomedicine Imaging and Modeling (CBIM), Rutgers University, New Brunswick, NJ, USA
[2] Department of Biomedical Engineering, Columbia University, New York, NY, USA
[3] Department of Radiology, New York University, New York, NY, USA

Abstract. Ultrasound Myocardial Elastography (UME) and Tagged Magnetic Resonance Imaging (tMRI) are two imaging modalities that were developed in the recent years to quantitatively estimate the myocardial deformations. Tagged MRI is currently considered as the gold standard for myocardial strain mapping in vivo. However, despite the low SNR nature of ultrasound signals, echocardiography enjoys the widespread availability in the clinic, as well as its low cost and high temporal resolution. Comparing the strain estimation performances of the two techniques has been of great interests to the community. In order to assess the cardiac deformation across different imaging modalities, in this paper, we developed a semi-automatic intensity and gradient based registration framework that rigidly registers the 3D tagged MRIs with the 2D ultrasound images. Based on the two registered modalities, we conducted spatially and temporally more detailed quantitative strain comparison of the RF-based UME technique and tagged MRI. From the experimental results, we conclude that qualitatively the two modalities share similar overall trends. But error and variations in UME accumulate over time. Quantitatively tMRI is more robust and accurate than UME.

1 Introduction

Many cardiovascular diseases, such as ischemia and infarction, are associated with the alteration of the global or local contractility of the myocardium. Accurately assessing the detailed myocardial deformation, such as the estimation of the local strain values, could be critical for the early diagnosis of cardiac diseases and dysfunctions. Tagged Magnetic Resonance Imaging (tMRI) and Ultrasound Myocardial Elastography (UME) are two imaging modalities that have been developed in the recent years to quantitatively estimate the myocardial deformations in vivo. The technique of tMRI generates sets of equally spaced parallel tagging planes within the myocardium as temporary material markers at end-diastole through spatial modulation of the magnetization. We have 2 sets of

N. Ayache, S. Ourselin, A. Maeder (Eds.): MICCAI 2007, Part I, LNCS 4791, pp. 800–808, 2007.
© Springer-Verlag Berlin Heidelberg 2007

orthogonal tagging planes for strain assessment. Imaging planes are perpendicular to the tagging planes, so that the tags appear as dark grids and deform with the underlying myocardium during a cardiac cycle. This can yield detailed motion information on the myocardium.

Ultrasound Myocardial Elastography is a radio-frequency (RF) based speckle tracking technique [1]. Despite the low SNR nature of ultrasound signals, echocardiography enjoys widespread availability in the clinic, as well as its relatively low cost and high temporal resolution. In UME, the two in-plane orthogonal displacement components (lateral and axial) are estimated using 1D cross-correlation and recorrelation of RF signals in a 2D search [2]. Then, the incremental displacements are integrated to obtain a cumulative motion estimation.

Tagged MRI is currently considered the most accurate noninvasive myocardial motion and strain estimator. Several studies have compared the estimates from ultrasound with those from tMRI. Notomi et al. [3], Helle-Valle et al. [4] and Cho et al. [5] have demonstrated that left-ventricular torsion measured from B-mode-based speckle tracking methods is consistent with that from tMRI in short-axis (SA) views. In [6] 2D motion and strain estimates from UME are shown to be highly comparable with those from tMRI. However due to the different characteristics of ultrasonic imaging and tMRI, a main limitation of these comparisons is that the two modalities are not registered in 3D. Thus, the ultrasound and tMR images may not be acquired at the same SA slice with the same orientation. To address this potential discrepancy, in this paper we have developed a semi-automatic intensity and gradient based mutual information registration framework that rigidly registers the 3D corresponding tagged MRIs with the 2D ultrasonic images. Based on the two registered modalities, we are able to conduct more detailed quantitative strain comparison of the RF-based UME technique and tagged MRI.

2 Methods

2.1 Ultrasound and Tagged MRI Data Acquisition

Both RF ultrasound and 3D tMRI images were acquired in 2D short-axis (SA) views from two healthy subjects with breath-holding and ECG gating. A clinical echocardiography ultrasound scanner (GE Vivid FiVe, GE Vingmed Ultrasound, Horten, Norway) with a phased array probe (FPA 2.5MHz 1C) was used to acquire cardiac ultrasound in-phase and quadrature (I/Q) data at the papillary muscle level at a frame rate of 136 fps. The I/Q data were upsampled to retrieve the RF signals.

Tagged MR images were obtained from a Siemens Trio 3T MR scanner with 2D grid tagging. The 3D tagged MR images consists of a stack of 6 equally spaced SA image sets from near the left ventricle (LV) base to the LV apex. The SA orientation of the ultrasound was approximately consistent with that of the tMRI, but was not guaranteed to be the same. Both modalities utilized full ECG gating during the scans so that they can be registered temporally in a heart beat cycle.

2.2   Rigid-Body Registration of 2D Elastography with 3D Tagged MRI

For the purpose of inter-modal comparison, we assume that the overall pattern of the heart shape, size and function of the same subject did not change between acquisition by the different imaging modalities. Previous work on inter-modal registration of cardiac ultrasound (US) with MR images has been very limited [7]. It has two main difficulties. First, the cardiac left ventricle (LV) in SA view has a circular shape that lacks reliable anatomical landmarks. Second, the US images have very different appearances compared to MR images. In [8], an approach combining intensity and gradient information was proposed to address the registration of brain US with MR images. In [9] a dynamic cardiac US and MR image registration is achieved by optical tracking of the US probe and fine-tuned by a mutual information registration method.

In our system, since the US probe is not tracked during the imaging process, the semi-automatic registration has to rely on user interactions as well as the image information from the myocardium and the neighboring anatomical structures. The main idea of our registration framework is that we allow the user to freely translate and rotate the US imaging plane w.r.t. the 3D tMRI data and manually find a proper initial registration. Then, a 2D pseudo US image is reconstructed from tMRI, which has an appearance comparable with the 2D US image, so that a mutual information based method can automatically fine-tune the initial manual registration by optimizing the translation (t_x, t_y, t_z) and rotation $(\theta_x, \theta_y, \theta_z)$ of the imaging plane.

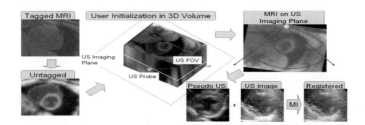

Fig. 1. The flowchart of the rigid-body registration framework. The stack of the untagged images is interpolated using splines to achieve a 3D isotropic volume. The user can freely tune the translation and rotation parameters of the US imaging plane. After manual initialization, a pseudo US image is constructed from the untagged MRI. The position of the simulated US probe gives the US beam direction. Finally an MI based registration procedure is performed to fine-tune the manual initialization.

Both modalities are ECG gated, which easily makes them temporally aligned. First, the tagged MR images at a mid-systolic phase undergo a Gabor filter bank-based tag removal process [10], which essentially enhances the tag-patterned regions. The tag patterns in the blood are flushed out very quickly after the initial tagging modulation, as shown in Fig. 1, this tag removal method enhances the areas of the chest wall, the myocardium and the other surrounding organs, and suppresses the areas of the blood pools and lungs. This de-tagging process increases the image's readability. It is helpful for both the user initialization and the following mutual information based registration algorithm.

The characteristic appearance of cardiac US images comes from two main sources. First, the speckle intensity levels vary in different tissues. For instance, we observe that the blood pool area is darker than the myocardium. Second, because of the impedance mismatch effect, US images usually enhance the interfaces between successive tissue layers [8]. We further observe that the angles between the interfaces with the incoming US beam affect the enhancement magnitude. Here we denote vector $\mathbf{b}$ as the direction of the incoming US beam. Therefore we model the transformation T from the tag removed tMRI, I_u, to the reconstructed image by:

$$T(I_u(x,y)) = \alpha I_u(x,y) + \beta \nabla I_u(x,y) \cdot \mathbf{b}(x,y) + \gamma I_v(x,y) \qquad (1)$$

The right hand side of the equation is a linear combination of three terms, where the relative weighting parameters α, β and γ are experimentally determined. The first term is the tag removed image. The second term is an edge detector, which is sensitive to orientation . In order to detect the dark strips between the myocardium and the neighboring liver, the third term I_v acts as a valley detector. Suppose $\mathbf{H}(x,y)$ is the Hessian matrix at $I_u(x,y)$, and λ_1 and λ_2 are the eigenvalues of $\mathbf{H}$. If $\lambda_1 < -|\lambda_2|$, then at pixel (x,y) an intensity valley exists, whose width is proportional to $|\lambda_1|$, and its orientation is determined by the eigenvector $\mathbf{v}_1$. Hence we model the valley detector as:

$$I_v(x,y) = \begin{cases} \lambda_1^2 \mathbf{v}_1(x,y) \cdot \mathbf{b}(x,y), & if\ \lambda_1 < -|\lambda_2| \\ 0, & otherwise \end{cases} \qquad (2)$$

The mutual information based optimization of the translation and rotation parameters is found by using gradient decent. Since the tag removed image I_u is heavily blurred, the algorithm tends to get stuck in local maxima. Thus a proper manual initialization is necessary. Multiple initializations are also helpful to find the global maximum.

2.3   Strain Estimation

Ultrasound Myocardial Elastography. In the UME technique, the two in-plane orthogonal displacement components (lateral and axial) were estimated using one-dimensional (1D) cross-correlation and recorrelation of RF signals in a 2D search [2]. The cross-correlation technique employed a 1D matching kernel of 7.7 mm and 80% overlap. The reference and comparison frames respectively contained the RF signals before and after deformation. An 8 : 1 linear interpolation scheme between two adjacent original RF signal segments of the comparison frame within the 1D kernel was employed to improve the lateral resolution [2]. The maximal cross-correlated value yielded from the RF signal segment in the comparison frame was considered the best match with the RF signal segment in the reference frame. Cosine interpolation was then applied around this maximum of the cross-correlation function for a more refined peak search.

The correction (or, recorrelation) in axial displacement estimation [2], was performed to reduce the decorrelation resulting from axial motion. In UME, recorrelation was implemented by shifting RF signal segments according to the estimated axial displacement in the comparison frame, prior to the second lateral displacement estimation.

The incremental displacements were integrated to obtain the cumulative displacement that occurred from ED to ES. Appropriate registration for each pixel on two consecutive displacement images was performed to further ensure that the cumulative displacement depicted the motion of the same tissue region.

Strain is defined in terms of the gradient of the displacement. A displacement vector $\mathbf{u}$, is written as $\mathbf{u} = u_x\mathbf{e}_x + u_y\mathbf{e}_y$, where u_x and u_y are lateral and axial displacement components, respectively, and $\mathbf{e}_x$ and $\mathbf{e}_y$ are the unit vectors in the lateral and axial directions, respectively. The displacement gradient tensor $\mathbf{G}$ in Cartesian coordinates (x, y) is thus defined as $\mathbf{G} = \nabla\mathbf{u}$.

The in-plane Lagrangian finite strain tensor, $\mathbf{E}$, is formulated as in [11]:

$$\mathbf{E} = \frac{1}{2}(\mathbf{G} + \mathbf{G}^T + \mathbf{G}^T\mathbf{G}) \tag{3}$$

Lateral and axial strains are the diagonal components of $\mathbf{E}$, i.e., $\mathbf{E}_{xx}$ and $\mathbf{E}_{yy}$, respectively. In UME, a least-squares strain estimator (LSQSE) [12] with a kernel of $13.4mm$ in both the lateral and axial directions was used in order to improve the signal-to-noise ratio (SNR) in the strain image (i.e., elastogram) and simultaneously have similar image resolutions between tMRI and UME in order to better facilitate subsequent comparison.

The above mentioned 2D (or, lateral and axial) Lagrangian finite strains are dependent on the orientation of the ultrasound transducer relative to the ventricle. This angle-dependence may complicate the interpretation of the myocardial deformation in the left ventricle. Therefore, radial and circumferential strains are obtained by defining an angle, θ, about the centroid of the left ventricle and by transforming the finite strain tensor $\mathbf{E}$ into a radial-circumferential strain tensor $\dot{\mathbf{E}}$ with a rotation matrix $\mathbf{Q}$: $\dot{\mathbf{E}} = \mathbf{Q}\mathbf{E}\mathbf{Q}^T$ [11].

Positive and negative radial strains indicate myocardial thickening and thinning, respectively, while myocardial stretching and shortening are represented by positive and negative circumferential strains, respectively.

Tagged MRI. The registered imaging plane may not be the same as one of the tMRI SA slices. Simply interpolating in between the slices might blur the tagging grids and result in inaccurate strain calculations. We observe that the 2D tagging grids are actually the intersections of two sets of orthogonal tagging sheets and the tMRI imaging planes. If we recover the geometry of the tagging sheets, then by finding their intersections with the registered US imaging plane, we are able to calculate the strain values in the registered imaging plane. Therefore we chose to track the tagging sheets over time [13].

First we decompose the grid tagged images into two sets of horizontal and vertical line tagged images by suppressing the component of one direction of the tagging grids via band-stop filtering in the images' Fourier domain. Then the two sets of 3D tagged MR images are filtered with a tunable 3D Gabor filter bank so that the tagging sheets can be enhanced, where the parameters of the 3D Gabor are adaptive to the spacing and orientation of the local tagging sheets. In the tracking step, we impose a set of deformable meshes onto the initial tagging sheets and let them deform according to the enhanced tagging sheets over time. The tracking process is controlled by a dynamic model, and the deformable mesh is smoothed with an internal spring force as well as an inter-mesh spring force.

During tracking, the displacements $\mathbf{u}$ of the intersection points of the two sets of perpendicular tagging sheets and the registered imaging plane are recorded. Then for all the other pixels in the myocardial area, their displacements $\mathbf{u}$ are interpolated by a spline interpolation method.

The strain calculations is the same as that employed in the previous UME section. Lateral, axial, radial and circumferential strains are calculated.

3   Experimental Results

In our experiments, active contraction (i.e., systole) was only considered for the assessment of the contractility of cardiac muscle. The strain estimates of these two imaging modalities have qualitatively good agreement. A visual comparison of the strain patterns can be found in Fig. 2. For a normal subject (top panel in Fig. 2), the lateral and axial strains of this clinical data show similar patterns to those of the theoretical framework proposed by Lee et al. [2] . Furthermore, polar strains (bottom panel in Fig. 2) show radial thickening and circumferential shortening except for the anterior and septal walls in the ultrasound images due to the low signal-to-noise (SNR) ratio, which results from the rib and the lung.

As shown in Fig. 4(a), for more spatially localized quantitative analysis, we divide the LV into 6 sectors: the septum 1, the septum 2, the posterior wall, the lateral wall 1, the lateral wall 2, and the anterior wall. According to the quantitative results shown in Fig. 3, both modalities show that the total radial and circumferential strains, from ED to ES, in six different myocardial regions show similar trend of strain value accumulation. In tMRI results, we observe that for intra-subject case, the mean strain values in each sector have similar shapes and slopes, which means the myocardial strain grows evenly and stably over time. Even for inter-subject case, the strain patterns of the two subjects look similar, which shows tMRI strain estimation is quite robust. In addition, the relatively small and stable standard deviations of tMRI strains also show the robustness of tMRI. In UME results, for the case of subject 1, the mean strain values of sectors posterior, lateral 1 and lateral 2, which are opposite to the US probe, are higher than those of the tMRI, while the other 3 sectors, which are near the chest wall and closer to the US probe, have smaller strains. This suggests that UME may be affected by the US beam direction. On the other hand, in general, ultrasound elastographic strain estimates exhibit higher spatial resolution but larger

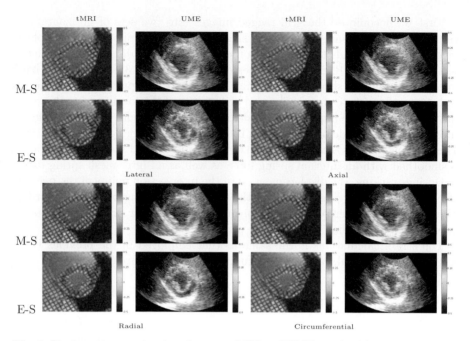

Fig. 2. Strain pattern comparison between tMRI and UME on a healthy subject. Clockwisely starting from the top-left 4 images, lateral, axial, circumferential and radial strains of the left ventricle are displayed. For each strain component, the first row is taken at a mid-systole (M-S) phase, and the second row is taken at end-systole (ES). The pseudo color is displayed on a scale of the strain value from −0.5 to 0.5.

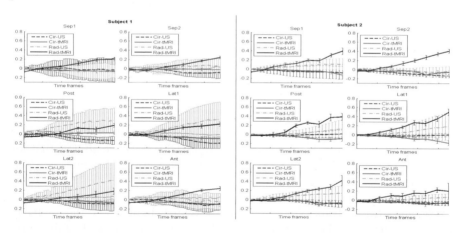

Fig. 3. In each sector of the LV, the mean and standard deviation of the radial and circumferential strain values are calculated from end-diastole to end-systole. We find that the UME results have an overall trend which is similar with that of the tMRI. However the standard deviation of the US results tends to keep growing quickly, while that of the tMRI remains stable.

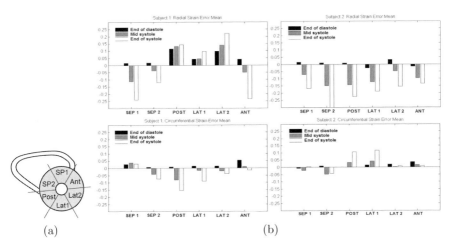

Fig. 4. (a) illustrates the division of the 6 sectors. (b) is the strain error mean of the UME technique compared with tMRI. We find in UME modality, from ED to ES, the error are also accumulative.

noise. Even though the original pixel resolution in both tagged MR and ultrasonic images is adjusted to the same scale, the overestimation from ultrasound elastography for subject 1 may also owes to its high resolution of estimation. As shown in Fig. 4, the mean strain discrepancies between UME and tMRI increase over from ED to ES. In addition, the ultrasound elastographic estimation errors accumulate during systole can also be depicted from the increasing standard deviations. The circumferential strain estimates depicts the strongest agreement between the two modalities.

4   Conclusion

Ultrasound Myocardial Elastography is qualitatively able to assess myocardial motion and deformation with values well comparable to those obtained with tagged MRI in normal subjects. However, for quantitative strain measurement, tMRI will provide much more accurate and robust estimates. Future work will focus on the assessment of the role of the sonographic SNR on the myocardial elastographic strain estimates and study of the tradeoff between spatial resolution and strain accuracy for precise quantification in both normal and acute infarction patients. We will also carry out more UME and tMRI comparisons.

References

1. Konofagou, E.E., Dhhooge, J., Ophir, J.: Myocardial elastography-a feasibility study in vivo. Ultrasound in Med. & Bio. 28(4), 475–482 (2002)
2. Lee, W.N., Konofagou, E.E.: Analysis of 3D motion effects in 2D myocardial elastography. In: IEEE-UFFC Symp. Proc. pp. 1217–1220 (2006)

3. Notomi, Y., et al.: Measurement of ventricular torsion by two-dimensional ultrasound speckle tracking imaging. J. Am. Coll. Cardiol. 45, 2034–2041 (2005)
4. Helle-Valle, T., et al.: New noninvasive method for assessment of left ventricular rotation - speckle tracking echocardiography. Circulation 112, 3149–3156 (2005)
5. Cho, G., et al.: Comparison of two-dimensional speckle and tissue velocity based strain and validation with harmonic phase magnetic resonance imaging. The American Journal of Cardiology 97, 1661–1666 (2006)
6. Lee, W., et al.: Validation of ultrasound myocardial elastography using MR tagging in normal human hearts in vivo. In: ISBI (2007)
7. Makela, T., et al.: A review of cardiac image registration methods. IEEE Trans. Med. Imaging 21(9), 1011–1021 (2002)
8. Roche, A., Pennec, X., Malandain, G., Ayache, N.: Rigid registration of 3D ultrasound with MR images: a new approach combining intensity and gradient information. IEEE Trans. Med. Imaging 20(10), 1038–1049 (2001)
9. Huang, X., et al.: Dynamic 3D ultrasound and MR image registration of the beating heart. In: Duncan, J.S., Gerig, G. (eds.) MICCAI 2005. LNCS, vol. 3750, pp. 171–178. Springer, Heidelberg (2005)
10. Manglik, T., et al.: Use of bandpass Gabor filters for enhancing blood-myocardium contrast and filling-in tags in tagged MR images. In: Proc of ISMRM p. 1793 (2004)
11. Lai, W.M.: Introduction to Continuum Mechanics, 3rd edn. Butterworth-Heinemann (1993)
12. Kallel, F., Ophir, J.: A least-squares strain estimator for elastography. Ultrasound Imaging 19, 195–208 (1997)
13. Qian, Z., Metaxas, D., Axel, L.: Extraction and tracking of MRI tagging sheets using a 3D Gabor filter bank. In: Proc. of Int'l. Conf. of the Engineering in Medicine and Biology Society (2006)

Robust Kernel Methods for Sparse MR Image Reconstruction

Joshua Trzasko[1], Armando Manduca[1], and Eric Borisch[2]

[1] Department of Physiology and Biomedical Engineering
[2] Magnetic Resonance Research Lab
Mayo Clinic College of Medicine, Rochester, MN, USA
{trzasko.joshua,manduca,borisch.eric}@mayo.edu

Abstract. A major challenge in contemporary magnetic resonance imaging (MRI) lies in providing the highest resolution exam possible in the shortest acquisition period. Recently, several authors have proposed the use of L_1-norm minimization for the reconstruction of sparse MR images from highly-undersampled k-space data. Despite promising results demonstrating the ability to accurately reconstruct images sampled at rates significantly below the Nyquist criterion, the extensive computational complexity associated with the existing framework limits its clinical practicality. In this work, we propose an alternative recovery framework based on homotopic approximation of the L_0-norm and extend the reconstruction problem to a multiscale formulation. In addition to several interesting theoretical properties, practical implementation of this technique effectively resorts to a simple iterative alternation between bilteral filtering and projection of the measured k-space sample set that can be computed in a matter of seconds on a standard PC.

1 Introduction

One of the fundamental limitations of MRI is the linear relation between scan time and the number of measured data samples. With the recent drive towards dynamic imaging as well as high-resolution scans and those covering an extended field-of-view (FOV), the need for shorter examination times to improve patient comfort and improve clinical throughput is substantial. Barring the introduction of additional hardware such as is used in parallel imaging techniques, conventional undersampled MRI reconstruction techniques such as homodyne detection [1] and projections onto convex sets (POCS) [2] are often inherently limited by the Nyquist criterion to a maximum theoretical sampling reduction of 50%. In practice, even less undersampling is typically employed when using these approaches.

Recently, there has been great interest in "compressed sensing" methods for reconstructing MR images from only a small fraction of the complete k-space sample set [3,4,5]. For naturally sparse scenarios such as MR angiography, high-quality recovery has been demonstrated even at up to 80% undersampling,

N. Ayache, S. Ourselin, A. Maeder (Eds.): MICCAI 2007, Part I, LNCS 4791, pp. 809–816, 2007.
© Springer-Verlag Berlin Heidelberg 2007

offering the potential for dramatically reducing clinical scan times. The main limitation of the existing compressed sensing framework lies in the extensive computation that is required to generate a solution, e.g. the reconstruction of a single 256x256 image can take on the order of several hours [6] using standard descent methods and even several minutes using state- of-the-art matrix-based solvers [7]. The considerable computational burden of these techniques precludes their use in clinical practice, especially when considering the extension to 3D data.

In this paper, we consider an alternative formulation of the sparse reconstruction problem that is both theoretically alluring and computationally practical. While compressed sensing methods typically deal with L_1-norm minimization as they are the closest convex approximation to the ideal L_0-minimization problem, we attack the L_0 problem directly using a quasiconvex homotopy scheme. This approximation is closely related to work on robust anisotropic diffusion [8] and, when considering image gradients across multiple scales, kernel regression methods such as the bilateral filter [9,10]. Following these developments, we address the handling of complex MR image data and discuss practical and simple numerical implementation of the technique.

2   Methods

For many MR images, the underlying image structure is piecewise smooth and thus the signal is sparse in the gradient domain. Let Φ represent a k-space measurement matrix such as that defined by the trajectory of a projection reconstruction or spiral-type acquisition after gridding. The goal of the sparse MRI reconstruction problem is to recover an image, f, from only a small subset of Fourier transform samples, $\Phi\hat{f}$. The ideal approach to recovering a signal with limited support involves solving the following combinatorial optimization problem:

$$\min_u \|\nabla u\|_0 \quad s.t. \quad \Phi\hat{u} = \Phi\hat{f}, \tag{1}$$

where $\hat{f}$ denotes the Fourier transform of f and u is the recovered image; however, as (1) is NP-complete, it is computationally intractable except for very small problems. In the recent work by Candès et al. [11] and Donoho [12], it has been shown that, given sufficient gradient sparsity, f can be almost exactly recovered with overwhelming probability by solving the L_1 analog of (1),

$$\min_u \|\nabla u\|_1 \quad s.t. \quad \Phi\hat{u} = \Phi\hat{f}. \tag{2}$$

While few signals are truly sparse in practice, most are compressible within some transform domain, e.g. the spatial gradient of a piecewise-smooth image exhibits exponential decay upon enumeration. In this scenario, the "compressed sensing" paradigm offers reconstruction whose error is comparable to the best possible K-term approximation within the sparsity basis [13].

Although (2) is a convex optimization problem closely related to basis pursuit [14] that can be solved using standard Interior Point methods [14,11,7], many of these modern numerical solvers rely heavily on matrix-based operators that are not only computationally expensive but also require extensive parameterization. For example, Kim et al. [7] have recently proposed a method for solving (2) based on preconditioned conjugate gradients (PCG) which, while converging in only around 100 iterations, requires several minutes to reconstruct a single 256x256 image. In effect, this class of approaches is neither readily implimentable nor computationally practical and this may preclude their widespread usage in clinical application.

2.1   Robust Error Norms and L_0-Continuation

Although (1) is generally impossible to solve directly, it is the ideal formulation to address for the sparse reconstruction problem whether for MRI or any other application. Begin by realizing that the zero semi-norm can be defined as

$$\|\nabla u\|_0 = \sum_{\Omega} \mathbf{1}\left(|\nabla u| > 0\right), \tag{3}$$

where Ω is the image domain and $\mathbf{1}$ is the indicator function. Consequently,

$$\{\mathbf{1}\left(|\nabla u| > 0\right) = 1\} \Longleftrightarrow \{\exists n \in [1, N] \,|\, |u_{x_n}| > 0\}, \tag{4}$$

where $N = \dim\{\Omega\}$ and u_{x_n} is the partial derivative of u along the n-th dimension. Given (4),

$$\mathbf{1}\left(|\nabla u| > 0\right) \leq \sum_{n=1}^{N} \mathbf{1}\left(|u_{x_n}| > 0\right) \tag{5}$$

follows trivially and a new sparsity semi-norm can be defined as

$$\|\nabla u\|_{0^*} = \sum_{\Omega} \sum_{n=1}^{N} \mathbf{1}\left(|u_{x_n}| > 0\right); \tag{6}$$

note that this is essentially just a migration of u to Markovian form.

At this point, (6) is still combinatorial much like $\|\nabla u\|_0$ and thus of little practical use. Suppose a continuous function, ρ, can be defined such that it is homotopic with $\mathbf{1}$ through the limit function, i.e.

$$\lim_{\sigma \to 0} \rho\left(x, \sigma\right) = \mathbf{1}\left(|x| > 0\right). \tag{7}$$

Consequently, (6) can be redefined as

$$\|\nabla u\|_{0^*} = \lim_{\sigma \to 0} \sum_{\Omega} \sum_{n=1}^{N} \rho\left(u_{x_n}, \sigma\right) \tag{8}$$

yielding the new reconstruction problem,

$$\min_{u} \|\nabla u\|_{0^*} \quad s.t. \quad \Phi\hat{u} = \Phi\hat{f}. \tag{9}$$

Although there is no guarantee of achieving a global minima when using non-convex priors, standard continuation schemes simliar to those developed to numerically handle the discontinuity of the total variation (TV) semi-norm at the origin [15] yield local minima which are more than acceptable in practice.

While one approach to defining ρ includes using a $p < 1$ semi-norm as utilized in [6], the non-differentiability of these functionals requisites need for additional continuation, limiting their practicality within our approach. Alternatively, consider the class of robust error functions known as redescending M-estimators [16]. Two of the more common examples, the Gaussian and Tukey Biweight error functions, are respectively described by

$$\rho(x,\sigma) = 1 - e^{-\frac{x^2}{2\sigma^2}} \qquad \rho(x,\sigma) = \begin{cases} \frac{3x^2}{\sigma^2} - \frac{3x^4}{\sigma^4} + \frac{x^6}{\sigma^6}, & |x| \leq \sigma \\ 1, & \text{else} \end{cases}. \qquad (10)$$

For both measures in (10), σ is a scale parameter that controls the dilation of the error functions. Unlike traditional error norms such as the various p-norms, the influence of outlier values beyond a threshold determined by σ is reduced. More interestingly, as $\sigma \to 0$, these redescending functions naturally approach the indicator function, and they remain continuous until that limit is reached. We note that the use of such non-convex estimators have been previously employed in the imaging community for denoising [17,8] and deconvolution [18]; however, to our knowledge, this approach has not been utilized for the highly-undersampled reconstruction problem.

2.2   Multiscale Image Sparsity

One approach to discretizing the partial derivatives of u in (9) involves computing the finite differences between u at a point x and its immediate neighbors. If the set of all immediate neighbors is denoted as η, then (8) can be approximated by

$$\|\nabla u\|_{0^*} = \lim_{\sigma \to 0} \sum_{x \in \Omega} \sum_{n \in \eta} \rho\left(u\left(x + \xi_n\right) - u\left(x\right), \sigma\right), \qquad (11)$$

where the vector $\xi_n = n - x$.

Enforcement of image sparsity can subsequently be generalized to address multiple scales of image gradients by simply extending the neighborhood over which finite differences are computed. Spatial proximity can easily be incorporated into (11) through the addition of an auxiliary influence function, namely

$$\|\nabla u\|_{0^*} = \lim_{\sigma \to 0} \sum_{x \in \Omega} \sum_{n \in \eta} \rho\left(u\left(x + \xi_n\right) - u\left(x\right), \sigma\right) \phi\left(|\xi_n|, \kappa\right), \qquad (12)$$

where ϕ is commonly defined by a Gaussian function with scale κ.

2.3   Practical Implementation and Numerical Considerations

For a fixed value of σ, a minima of (12) is given when,

$$\sum_{n \in \eta} \psi\left(u\left(x + \xi_n\right) - u\left(x\right), \sigma\right) \phi\left(|\xi_n|, \kappa\right) = 0, \qquad \forall x \in \Omega \qquad (13)$$

where the influence function $\psi = \rho'$. Letting $g(x) = \psi(x)/x$, (13) can be written in operator form as

$$\left[\sum_{n\in\eta} g\left(u\left(x+\xi_n\right)-u\left(x\right),\sigma\right)\phi\left(\left|\xi_n\right|,\kappa\right)\left(\delta\left(x+\xi_n\right)-\delta\left(x\right)\right)\otimes\right]u = 0, \quad (14)$$

where δ is the Kronecker delta function and $\otimes$ is the convolution operator. When considering (14) in the homogeneous form $A(u)u = 0$, and noting that $A(u)$ is non-expansive and strongly connected, (14) can be solved for iteratively using a nonlinear Jacobi or Fixed-Point iteration, resulting in

$$u^{t+1}(x) = \frac{\sum_{n\in\eta} g\left(u^t\left(x+\xi_n\right)-u^t\left(x\right),\sigma\right)\phi\left(\left|\xi_n\right|,\kappa\right)u^t\left(x+\xi_n\right)}{\sum_{n\in\eta} g\left(u^t\left(x+\xi_n\right)-u^t\left(x\right),\sigma\right)\phi\left(\left|\xi_n\right|,\kappa\right)}. \quad (15)$$

(15) can be interpreted as an iterative zero-order or Nadaraya-Watson type kernel regression estimator, or more familiarly as a bilateral filter [9]. Recently, kernel regression estimators [10] (including higher-order) have been applied to the related problems of super-resolution and deconvolution and shown excellent results. In effect, the derived form in (15) is very promising as there has been extensive work on developing fast implementations and approximations of the bilateral filter. In particular, it has been shown that a separable version of (15) [19], where 1D bilateral filtering is performed sequentially along each data dimension, can provide a dramatic computational speed-up with no substantial degradation of the result.

When dealing with complex image data such as in MRI, addressing $|\nabla u|$ is not as straighforward as for the strictly real case. For our application, we choose to assess sparsity in the real and imaginary data channels separately as mentioned in [4] and is commonly used for MR image denoising. Given (15), the complex multiscale extension of (9) can be solved using the following iterated projection procedure with continuation:

```
Let û⁰ = Φf̂ , σ >> 0
1. ℜ{v^{t+1}} = BilateralFilter[ℜ{u^t}, σ]
2. ℑ{v^{t+1}} = BilateralFilter[ℑ{u^t}, σ]
3. Φv^{t+1} = Φf̂
4. if ‖v^{t+1} − u^t‖ < tol , σ = σ * β
   else u^{t+1} = v^{t+1} , go to Step 1.
```

In the above algorithm, $\Re$ and $\Im$ denote the real and imaginary operators, respectively, *tol* is a threshold indicating when filtering at a given σ-level has numerically reached steady-state, and $\beta \in (0,1)$ controls the reduction rate of σ in the continuation procedure. The number of iterations can either be specified *a priori* or an intelligent termination scheme can be incorporated when some target level for σ has been achieved.

Note that the presented algorithm is significantly less intimidating than its matrix-based counterparts for the sparse reconstruction problem as it requires little more than a simple filtering and Fourier tranform operation. Consequently, we hope the inherent simplicity and resultant speed of this method will promote its use in practical application.

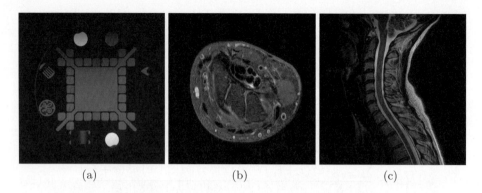

(a)   (b)   (c)

Fig. 1. Example MR images: standard phantom (a), wrist (b), and spine (c)

3   Results

Examples of the presented reconstruction algorithm are given for the three images in Fig. 1. For each case, image intensities were normalized to unity and the following parameterizations were used: $tol = 1e-4$, $\beta = 0.5$, $\sigma_0 = 1$, and $iter = 80$. Additionally, bilateral filters were implemented in separable form as described in [19]. On a 3.4 GHz Pentium IV machine with 4GB RAM, a C++ implementation of the reconstruction algorithm using the FFTW library runs at roughly 80ms/iteration for a 256x256 image, yielding a total reconstruction time of around 7s.

The k-space patterns in Fig. 2 imposed 82% (2a), 77% (2b), and 75% (2c) undersampling, respectively. Additionally, the difference between the fully-sampled and reconstructed images, shown in Figs. 2j-l, was quantified using a standard root-mean-square (RMS) measure to yield a per-pixel average intensity error of only 1.687e-5, 2.256e-5, and 1.989e-5, respectively. While some expected textural loss is present in the anatomical image examples, notice that all of the main structural components of the images are accurately recovered as are many of the smaller objects. Some prominent areas of focus showcasing this capability include the comb object inside the physical resolution phantom (Fig. 2j), the carpal tunnel region of the wrist (Fig. 2k), and the walls of the spinal column (Fig. 2l). We note that these results are similar in quality to those obtained by L_1 methods but we do not show a comparison here for sake of brevity.

4   Summary

In this work, we have developed a novel approach to the sparse image reconstruction problem and shown the application of our methods to phantom and clinical MR images. As detailed in Section 2, we offer a new approach at directly handling the L_0-minimization problem and extend the formulation to incorporate multiscale information. Numerically, solving the proposed formulation of the sparse reconstruction problem resorts to a simple iterative scheme based on

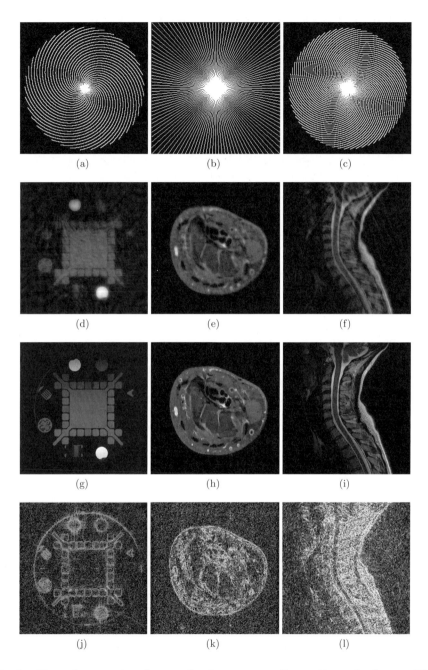

Fig. 2. Example reconstruction results: k-space sampling patterns (a-c), zero-filled reconstructions (d-f), proposed reconstructions (g-i), and reconstruction errors (j-l). Note that images (a-i) are scaled uniformly; images (j-l) have been amplified by 10x. For more details, see Section 3.

alternating between bilateral filtering in image space and reinforcement of the measured Fourier samples in frequency space, two operations which are very computationally efficient and relatively trivial to implement. Consequently, we are able to achieve reconstruction results which are comparable to those of L_1-based methods in a clinically practical amount of time and with relatively little effort spent in the development of the numerical sovler.

References

1. Noll, D., Nishimura, D., Macovski, A.: Homodyne detection in magnetic resonance imaging. IEEE Trans. Med. Imag. 10(2), 154–163 (1991)
2. Haacke, E., Lindskog, E., Lin, W.: A fast, iterative, partial-fourier technique capable of local phase recovery. J. Mag. Res. 92, 125–146 (1991)
3. Lustig, M., Donoho, D., Pauly, J.: Sparse MRI: the application of compressed sensing for rapid MR imaging. Manuscript (2007)
4. He, L., Chang, T., Osher, S., Fang, T., Speier, P.: MR image reconstruction by using the iterative refinement method and nonlinear inverse scale space methods. UCLA CAM Reports 06-35 (2006)
5. Boubertakh, R., Giovanelli, J., Cesare, A.D., Herment, A.: Non-quadratic convex regularized reconstruction of MR images from spiral acquisitions. Sig. Proc. 86, 2479–2494 (2006)
6. Chartrand, R.: Exact reconstruction of sparse signal via nonconvex minimization. Manuscript (2007)
7. Kim, S., Koh, K., Lustig, M., Boyd, S., Gorinevsky, D.: A method for large-scale l1-regularized least squares problems with applications in signal processing and statistics. Manuscript (2007)
8. Black, M., Sapiro, G., Marimon, D., Heeger, D.: Robust anisotropic diffusion. IEEE Trans. Imag. Proc. 7(3), 421–432 (1998)
9. Tomasi, C., Manduchi, R.: Bilateral filtering for gray and color images. In: Proc. IEEE ICIP (1998)
10. Takeda, H., Farsiu, S., Milanfar, P.: Kernel regression for image processing and reconstruction. IEEE Trans. Imag. Proc. 16(2), 349–366 (2007)
11. Candés, E., Romberg, J., Tao, T.: Robust uncertainty principles: exact signal reconstruction from highly incomplete frequency information. IEEE Trans. Info. Theory 52(2), 489–509 (2006)
12. Donoho, D.: Compressed sensing. IEEE Trans. Info. Theory 52(4), 1289–1306 (2006)
13. Candés, E., Romberg, J., Tao, T.: Stable signal recovery from incomplete and inaccurate measurements. Comm. Pure Appl. Math. 59, 1207–1223 (2006)
14. Chen, S., Donoho, D., Saunders, M.: Atomic decomposition by basis pursuit. SIAM J.Sci. Comp. 20(1), 33–61 (1998)
15. Chan, T., Zhou, H., Chan, R.: Continuation method for total variation denoising. UCLA CAM Reports 95-28 (1995)
16. Huber, P.: Robust Statistics. Wiley, New York (1981)
17. Perona, P., Malik, J.: Scale-space and edge detection using anisotropic diffusion. IEEE Trans. Patt. Anal. Mach. Intel. 12(7), 629–639 (1990)
18. Geman, D., Reynolds, G.: Constrained restoration and the recovery of discontinuities. IEEE Trans. Patt. Anal. Mach. Intel. 14(3), 367–383 (1990)
19. Pham, T., van Vliet, L.: Separable bilateral filtering for fast video preprocessing. In: Proc. IEEE ICME (2005)

How Do Registration Parameters Affect Quantitation of Lung Kinematics?

Tessa Sundaram Cook[1], Nicholas Tustison[1], Jürgen Biederer[2,3], Ralf Tetzlaff[3], and James Gee[1]

[1] Dept. of Radiology, University of Pennsylvania, Philadelphia, PA, USA
[2] Dept. of Diag. Radiology, Univ. Hosp. Schleswig-Holstein, Campus Kiel, Germany
[3] Dept. of Radiology, German Cancer Research Center, Heidelberg, Germany

Abstract. Assessing the quality of motion estimation in the lung remains challenging. We approach the problem by imaging isolated porcine lungs within an artificial thorax with four-dimensional computed tomography (4DCT). Respiratory kinematics are estimated via pairwise non-rigid registration using different metrics and image resolutions. Landmarks are manually identified on the images and used to assess accuracy by comparing known displacements to the registration-derived displacements. We find that motion quantitation becomes less precise as the inflation interval between images increases. In addition, its sensitivity to image resolution varies anatomically. Mutual information and cross-correlation perform similarly, while mean squares is significantly poorer. However, none of the metrics compensate for the difficulty of registering over a large inflation interval. We intend to use the results of these experiments to more effectively and efficiently quantify pulmonary kinematics in future, and to explore additional parameter combinations.

1 Introduction

The ability to quantify pulmonary deformation is useful in early detection of disease, evaluation of treatment efficacy and improved assessment of disease staging and prognosis. Structural imaging modalities can be used to capture *in vivo* deformation of the lung between sequential images by harnessing the power of non-rigid registration algorithms. Dougherty and Li have applied optical flow to computed tomography (CT) images of the lung to construct an atlas of normal pulmonary anatomy [1,2], while Hatabu et al. have developed magnetic resonance protocols for imaging the lung, [3]. In addition, Sarrut et al. have proposed an interpolation scheme for upsampling 4DCT image sequences, [4].

We have shown that non-rigid registration of serial MR images can be used to quantify lung kinematics, [5]. But validating the accuracy of these motion estimates is difficult; ground-truth motion cannot be determined without disruptive methods (such as implantation of tissue fiducials). Less invasive validation approaches for non-rigid registration in general include tracking landmarks on images, [6], comparison with known synthetic deformations, [7], tracking known

N. Ayache, S. Ourselin, A. Maeder (Eds.): MICCAI 2007, Part I, LNCS 4791, pp. 817–824, 2007.
© Springer-Verlag Berlin Heidelberg 2007

818   T.S. Cook et al.

displacements of a phantom, [8], assessment of anatomic overlap, [9], and comparison to other modalities, [10]. However, these methods are often sub-optimal when validating motion quantitation of *in vivo* dynamic organs.

We have previously used landmark-based validation: identifying and tracking structures which are visible within the lungs, such as airway and vessel bifurcations, [11]. The challenges we encountered include the inability to consistently identify points in successive images as well as a limit on the total number of landmarks that can be identified. Here, we image porcine lung explants ventilated using an artificial thorax, [12]. Nearly 350 landmarks are identified within the lungs, along the artificial diaphragm, and (as controls) on the hull of the artificial thorax. The "ground-truth" motion of these points is compared with the registration-derived motion estimate to assess the accuracy of the parenchymal dynamics computation with respect to image resolution and similarity metric. We also seek to quantify the optimal inflation interval for motion analysis.

Table 1. Summary of 36 experiments performed. "Iterations" indicates the # of iterations at each of the four levels (from $\frac{1}{8}$ of full resolution to full resolution).

Iterations		Metric		Intervals
100/1/1/1		MI		sequential (0%-25%, 25%-50%, etc.)
100/100/1/1	×	MSQ	×	alternating (0%-50%, 50%-100%)
100/100/100/1		CC		phase (0%-100%)
100/100/100/100				

2   Materials and Methods

2.1   Data Acquisition

Porcine lung explants from a healthy animal are placed inside a dedicated chest phantom designed by Biederer and colleagues, [12]. The phantom is sealed and evacuated to make the lung expand passively. A water-filled elastic diaphragm is used to simulate tidal respiration by cyclic variation of the filling volume at a frequency of 8 cycles/min. 4DCT images are acquired in dynamic mode with a pitch of 0.1 (Siemens Somatom, slice collimation 24 × 1.2 mm, rotation time 1 sec, slice thickness 1.5 mm, increment 0.8 mm, 120 kV, 400 mAs, Kernel B50s). Images are reconstructed retrospectively at 0, 25, 50, 75 and 100% inspiration. The data are acquired with a matrix of 512 × 512. To accommodate technical limitations, image volumes are resampled to dimensions of 256 × 256 × 243 with 1.17-mm isotropic voxels.

2.2   Symmetric, Diffeomorphic Non-rigid Registration

We use an intrinsically symmetric image registration for the experiments in this paper, [13]. The method is able to capture large, diffeomorphic transformations between two images I and J, and may be guided by a variety of similarity metrics to give a dense space-time mapping. Normally, the metric derivative is taken with respect to either I or J (whichever is the transforming image), creating a dependence on the gradients of that image. This symmetric approach resolves this bias in a fundamental way, using the transformation model, and optimizes the registration with respect to both ϕ_1 and ϕ_2 (the forward and inverse transformations). The forward and backward registrations both contribute via $I(\phi_1(\mathbf{x}, t))$ and $J(\phi_2(\mathbf{z}, 1 - t))$, respectively, where t is the path between I and J, $\mathbf{x}$ is the coordinate system of I, $\mathbf{z}$ is the coordinate system of J, ϕ_1 is the forward mapping that warps J into the space of I, and ϕ_2 is the inverse mapping that warps I into the space of J.

Performance of the algorithm has previously been evaluated for brain registration, [13]. Here, we test its effectiveness specifically for lung motion quantitation. We compare the effect of three different similarity metrics on our motion estimates: mean squares (MSQ), a $5 \times 5 \times 5$-neighborhood cross-correlation (CC) based on the implementation in [14], and mutual information (MI). All three are adapted to the symmetric formulation of the registration. We also explore the dependence of the motion quantitation process on the resolution of the image.

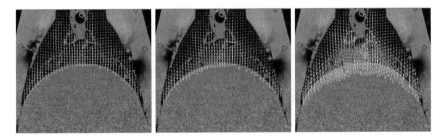

Fig. 1. Sample mid-coronal vector fields (extracted from the 3-D displacements) representing expansion from (left) 0% to 25%, (middle) 0% to 50% and (right) 0% to 100%. Vector magnitudes increase nonlinearly as the degree of expansion increases; there is greater motion at the lung bases than the apices.

2.3 Estimation of Pulmonary Motion

Our image sequence is processed multiple times to study the effect of image resolution and image similarity on the accuracy of motion quantitation over progressively larger inflation intervals. First, we study the sensitivity of our motion estimates to the number of resolution levels processed. We run registrations at four increasing levels of resolution (from $\frac{1}{8}$ to 1) using MI as the similarity in all cases. Next, we examine the effect of metric choice on our motion estimates by running registrations at all four resolution levels with each of the three metrics under investigation. In both cases, three types of inflation interval are used: sequential, alternating, and phase (see table 1); the latter covers the entire inspiratory phase of respiration. Each level of the multi-resolution pyramid is used for no more than 100 iterations.

We anticipate that registration accuracy will decrease as the inflation interval increases, and that mutual information and cross-correlation will perform better than mean squares because of their regional coverage and statistical sampling, respectively. Furthermore, we expect that most of the global motion of the lung will be captured by registration at the lowest resolution level, and that endpoint errors will generally be higher at the diaphragm than within the lung.

2.4 Assessment of Motion Quantitation Accuracy

A specially trained physician manually selects point landmarks on the 0% inspiration image and then identifies them on subsequent images (figure 2). Branching structures (both airway and vascular) are chosen on each image because of their reproducibility and distribution throughout the lungs. In addition, landmarks are placed on the diaphragm—site of greatest pulmonary deformation—and on the phantom itself. 125 landmarks identify airway and vessel bifurcations, while 142 points are selected on the diaphragm and 76 points on the hull of the phantom. This distribution of the landmarks throughout the lungs is useful because it allows us to quantify the uncertainty of our registration measurements in different anatomic regions.

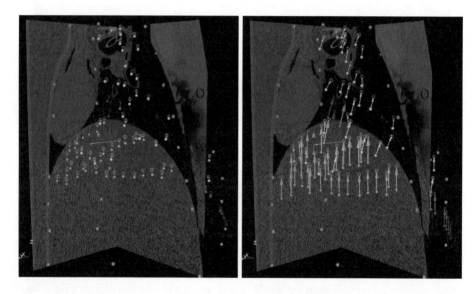

Fig. 2. 3-D renderings of the landmark displacements between (left) 0% and 25% inflation and (right) 0% and 100% inflation. Vectors are rendered in 3-D space, while orthogonal cross-sections of the image volume are provided for reference. Note that the points on the phantom's hull serve as controls and therefore lack displacement vectors.

The error between the known landmark displacement dx_l and the registration-derived displacement dx_r at each landmark location is computed as the distance between the endpoints of the two displacement vectors ($|dx_l - dx_r|$). In the discussion that follows, we report the mean of this endpoint error over the landmarks within the indicated anatomic region (diaphragmatic or parenchymal).

3 Results

The runtime of the 36 experiments described above depends on the number of resolutions at which an upper limit of 100 iterations is prescribed. Registration at the lower resolutions is achieved in 10-20 minutes, while registration at all four levels requires 2-3 hours for MI and 6-10 hours for CC. All registrations utilize up to 2.5 gigabytes of RAM. Figure 1 provides examples of the displacement fields generated via registration of the 0% inflation image to subsequent images in the sequence. Figure 3 summarizes the errors observed in our experiments.

3.1 Effect of Image Resolution

When estimating lung motion sequentially, the final result is almost completely achieved at the lowest image resolution, while the error within the lung drops by 0.5-2 mm with processing at higher levels. Errors tend to be 1-2 mm higher at the diaphragm than within the lung, likely because the diaphragm and lung bases move more than the apical parenchyma. Upon visualization of the registration-derived displacements at the landmarks, it appears that the error at the diaphragm is angular (vectors are of appropriate magnitude but point in a different direction), while within the parenchyma it is scalar (the vectors point in an appropriate direction but are not of the correct magnitude).

Using the alternating inflation intervals, we again observe a 1 mm gain in accuracy within the lung by registering at higher levels; errors at the diaphragm remain almost constant. This is likely because the soft tissue-air interface at the diaphragm is not compromised by downsampling and remains a strong contributor to the gradient of the similarity at low image resolutions.

When registering the entire inspiratory phase, we again observe an increase in accuracy intraparenchymally with higher levels of processing. However, it is important to note that the mean endpoint error throughout the lung and diaphragm is 11 mm as a result of the large degree of inflation. By acquiring one additional image (and using alternating intervals), we are able to cut our error in half. By further doubling our sampling frequency, we gain another 25-50%.

Overall, errors are at least 1 mm higher along the diaphragm than within the lung parenchyma. In most cases, the magnitude of the resulting endpoint errors is less than 40% of the actual motion in the region. There does not appear to be much improvement between the 128^3 level and the 256^3 level. This suggests that processing at the highest data resolution does not significantly alter the final result, and is encouraging because this level is the most time-consuming.

3.2 Effect of Image Similarity Metrics

Regardless of inflation interval, mean squares is consistently the least accurate of the three metrics studied. It results in a diaphragmatic error of 0.5-4.5 mm for sequential registrations, 1.9-4 mm for alternating registrations and 1.8-6.3 mm for the inspiratory phase registrations. Within the lung however, the MSQ

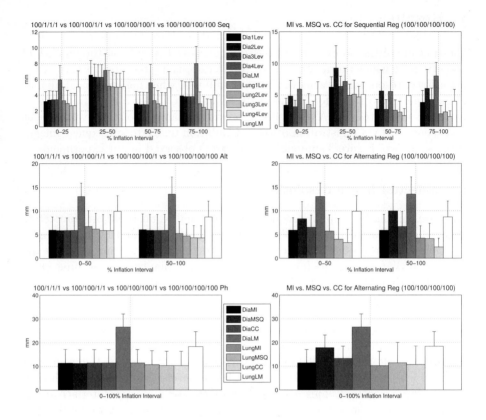

Fig. 3. Mean±SD endpoint errors for the resolution (left—top legend) and similarity (right—bottom legend) experiments at each of the three intervals (rows). The middle and last bars in each group indicate (for reference) the average motion at each landmark along the diaphragm and within the lung, respectively. #Lev = # of resolution levels used, Dia = diaphragm.

error is within 0.5-1 mm of the MI and CC errors, and occasionally less than the former.

Comparison of the performance of MI and CC yields some interesting observations. For the sequential registrations, the accuracy of the two metrics is within 0.5 mm of one another. As the inflation interval increases, MI outperforms CC (by an average of 1.8 mm in the phase registrations). However, within the lung CC is 1.4-1.9 mm better in the alternating registrations (the two metrics are within 0.4 mm of one another in the other experiments). This motivates the anatomic customization of similarity computations. Matching at the diaphragm may be easier because of the clear tissue interface between air and muscle, while matching in the parenchyma may require additional regional information (such as that provided the neighborhood integration of CC).

Again, it is important to note that the phase registrations with MI and CC are only accurate to within 11-13 mm at the diaphragm and 10-11 mm within the lung. Adding just one additional image reduces the mean error to 6-7 mm at the diaphragm and only 3-6 mm within the lung.

4 Discussion

We present a quantitative evaluation of the sensitivity of pulmonary motion estimation to image resolution, similarity metric and inflation interval. As expected, accuracy drops as the inflation interval increases. It is conceivable that registering for additional iterations may reduce this error; however, the sequential and alternating registrations rarely reached the limit of 100 iterations per level.

With only one set of landmarks, it is difficult to quantify the accuracy of the points themselves. It is realistic to assume that there is an inherent error associated with identifying the same anatomic point in different images. However, this can only be quantified by performing a multi-observer experiment in which two or more physicians independently identify the same landmarks, enabling the computation of inter-observer vs. registration-observer errors.

Ideally, we would be able to analyze data at the acquired resolution, instead of halving the resolution due to memory limitations. However, it is important to note that the results at the top two resolution levels are very similar. This suggests that slightly augmenting system memory may allow us to register data at the original resolution ($0.5{\times}0.5{\times}0.8$ mm in this case), and result in even better accuracy. Furthermore, we can reduce the number of iterations at the highest level and drastically reduce the runtime required to process an image pair without sacrificing the quality of our motion estimates.

Though we process only one image sequence in this experiment, the importance of small inflation intervals is clear. Attempting to quantify lung motion over an entire phase (i.e., end-inspiration to end-expiration), whether we use tidal limits or respiratory extremes, is inaccurate. If a 1-cm error is acceptable, then it is appropriate to acquire only two images, reducing scan time and radiation exposure. However, most clinical applications of this work would not tolerate such a large inaccuracy. Hence, this work motivates the need for finer sampling of the respiratory cycle.

In the future, we hope to further explore the issues in this paper with additional image sequences and multi-observer validation. Evaluation of different registration algorithms would also be interesting to determine if our current motion quantitation approach can be improved. Another avenue of exploration is the sensitivity of our methods to different degrees of image noise. It would also be interesting to investigate the sampling frequency problem in greater detail, as well as to compare motion quantitation in CT and MR. The ultimate goal of our work is to develop robust methods for motion quantitation that allow the development of a thorough spatio-temporal analysis of pulmonary motion and the subsequent construction of dynamic atlases of human lung motion.

References

1. Dougherty, L., Asmuth, J.C., Gefter, W.B.: Alignment of CT lung volumes with an optical flow method. Acad. Rad. 10(3), 249–254 (2003)
2. Li, B., Christensen, G.E., Hoffman, E.A., McLennan, G., Reinhardt, J.M.: Establishing a normative atlas of the human lung: intersubject warping and registration of volumetric CT images. Acad. Rad. 10, 255–265 (2003)
3. Hatabu, H., Ohno, Y., Uematsu, H., Oshio, K., Gefter, W.B., Gee, J.C.: Lung biomechanics via non-rigid reg. of serial MR images. Rad. 221P, 630 (2001)
4. Sarrut, D., Boldea, V., Miguet, S., Ginestet, C.: Simulation of four-dimensional CT images from deformable registration between inhale and exhale breath-hold CT scans. Med. Phys. 33(3), 605–617 (2006)
5. Sundaram, T., Gee, J.: Towards a model of lung biomechanics: pulmonary kinematics via registration of serial lung images. Med. Img. Anal. 9, 524–537 (2005)
6. Betke, M., Hong, H., Thoams, D., Prince, C., Ko, J.: Landmark detection in the chest and registration of lung surfaces with an application to nodule registration. Med. Image Anal. 7, 265–281 (2003)
7. Schnabel, J.A., Tanner, C., Castellano-Smith, A.D., Degenhard, A., Leach, M.O., Hose, D.R., Hill, D.L.G., Hawkes, D.J.: Validation of nonrigid image registration using finite-element methods: application to breast MR images. IEEE TMI 22(2), 238–247 (2003)
8. Dougherty, L., Asmuth, J., Blom, A., Axel, L., Kumar, R.: Validation of an optical flow method for tag displacement estimation. IEEE TMI 18(4), 359–363 (1999)
9. Woods, R.P., Grafton, S.T., Holmes, C.J., Cherry, S.R., Mazziotta, J.: Automated Image Registration: I General methods and intra-subject intra-modality validation. J. Comp. Asst. Tomo. 22, 141–154 (1998)
10. Ledesma-Carbayo, M.J., Mahia-Casado, P., Santos, A., Perez-David, E., Garcia-Fernandez, M.A., Desco, M.: Cardiac motion analysis from ultrasound sequences using nonrigid registration: validation against doppler tissue velocity. Ultrasound in Med. and Biol. 32(4), 483–490 (2006)
11. Sundaram, T.A., Gee, J.C.: Quantitative comparison of registration-based lung motion estimates from whole-lung MR images and corresponding two-dimensional slices. In: Proc. ISMRM 15th Mtg, p. 3039 (2007)
12. Biederer, J., Plathow, C., Schoebinger, M., Tetzlaff, R., Puderbach, M., Bolte, H., Zaporozhan, J., Meinzer, H.P., Heller, M., Kauczor, H.U.: Reproducible simulation of respiratory motion in porcine lung explants. Röontgenstr 178(11), 1067–1072 (2006)
13. Avants, B.B., Grossman, M., Gee, J.C.: Symmetric diffeomorphic image registration: Evaluating automated labeling of elderly and neurodegenerative cortex and frontal lobe. In: Pluim, J.P.W., Likar, B., Gerritsen, F.A. (eds.) WBIR 2006. LNCS, vol. 4057, pp. 50–57. Springer, Heidelberg (2006)
14. Hermosillo, G., Chefd'Hotel, C., Faugeras, O.: A variational approach to multimodal image matching. Intl. J. Comp. Vis. 50(3), 329–343 (2002)

Diffuse Parenchymal Lung Diseases: 3D Automated Detection in MDCT

Catalin Fetita[1], Kuang-Che Chang-Chien[1,4], Pierre-Yves Brillet[1,2],
Françoise Prêteux[1], and Philippe Grenier[3]

[1] Dept. ARTEMIS, INT, Groupe des Ecoles des Télécommunications, Evry, France
[2] AP-HP, Avicenne Hospital, Bobigny, France
[3] Université Paris 6 and AP-HP, Pitié-Salpêtrière Hospital, Paris, France
[4] National Chung Cheng University, Chia-yi, Taiwan, R.O.C

Abstract. Characterization and quantification of diffuse parenchymal lung disease (DPLD) severity using MDCT, mainly in interstitial lung diseases and emphysema, is an important issue in clinical research for the evaluation of new therapies. This paper develops a 3D automated approach for detection and diagnosis of DPLDs (emphysema, fibrosis, honeycombing, ground glass).The proposed methodology combines multi-resolution image decomposition based on 3D morphological filtering, and graph-based classification for a full characterization of the parenchymal tissue. The very promising results obtained on a small patient database are good premises for a near implementation and validation of the proposed approach in clinical routine.

1 Introduction

Diffuse parenchymal lung diseases (DPLDs) include chronic obstructive lung disease which is defined by lung destruction (emphysema), and idiopathic interstitial pneumonias which are characterized by lung infiltrates (ground glass) and fibrosis.

High-resolution computed tomography (HRCT) with 1-mm-thick sections obtained at 10-mm intervals has been widely accepted as the imaging reference standard for assessing DPLDs. Based on HRCT images, the diagnosis is done by analysing the different patterns of lung texture, and the severity of the disease can be evaluated by quotation of the extent of lesions. Nowadays, multidetector row CT (MDCT) generates isotropic volumetric high-resolution data and allows contiguous visualization of the lung parenchyma. MDCT tends to replace HRCT examinations since it allows creating three-dimensional reformatted images of excellent quality and significance.

Unfortunately, pathology features on the MDCT images sometimes would be subtle, especially in the early stage, and cause inter-observer variability even among the experienced radiologists. Hence, computer-aided diagnosis (CAD) is required for objective quantitative assessment of alterations in the lung [1]. Several studies in the medical and technical literature have addressed the classification problem of the lung parenchyma. Without claiming an exhaustive analysis, these studies can be roughly divided into two categories, density-based and

N. Ayache, S. Ourselin, A. Maeder (Eds.): MICCAI 2007, Part I, LNCS 4791, pp. 825–833, 2007.
© Springer-Verlag Berlin Heidelberg 2007

texture-based. The principle of the density-based analysis is to investigate the relationship between a defined threshold value and the ratio of the lung tissue area/volume below this threshold [2]. However, these methods cannot discriminate between several pathologies of the lung parenchyma occurring at the same time. In order to solve this problem, Blechschmidt et al. [3] defined an additional Bulae index which combines density measures with some texture-based approaches to quantify emphysema with concomitant fibrosis. The texture-based methods compute several measures in order to describe the CT attenuation characteristics. Then, a classifier (Bayesian, support vector machines, ...), performs an automated discrimination of the experimented samples. Malone et al. [4] proposed a texture-based approach to evaluate the pulmonary parenchyma from CT images. They split each image into grids with three block sizes, 4, 8, and 16 pixels, and computed 18 textural features for each block. Xu et al. [5] extended a run-length encoding method to three-dimensional (3D) data for volumetric texture analysis. Chabat et al. [6] adopted 13 features for extracting texture information from CT images. These features can be divided into three categories: n^{th} order statistical moments, spatial dependence of gray-scale distribution, and acquisition-length parameters. Recently, Xu et al. [7,8] used 3D texture features to enhance a previous two-dimensional (2D) classification system, the adaptive multiple feature method. The new system would be able to consider co-existing pathologies and to provide a simultaneous classification for differentiating between emphysema-like tissues found in normal smokers versus non-smokers.

In this paper we develop an original, fully-3D approach for automated detection of DPLDs in MDCT, based on the analysis of low-density patterns of the lung parenchyma. The proposed approach performs a multiresolution image data decomposition according to a specific morphological filtering. The result of the decomposition is synthesized into a hierarchic tree graph which nodes are analyzed in terms of textural and spatial relationship. Such analysis provides a classification of the decomposition patterns in normal and DPLD types.

The paper is organized as follows. Section 2 presents the image multiresolution decomposition scheme, and recalls the 3D morphological filter there considered. Section 3 describes and illustrates the generation of the descriptive tree graph and the performed classification analysis. The results are presented and discussed in Section 4.

2   Multiresolution Decomposition of Image Lung Parenchyma

Lung parenchyma tissue can be roughly described as a collection of vascularized structures of tree-like topology and of various calibers decreasing with the subdivision order and crossing each other, namely the arterial, venous and tracheobronchial trees. From an image analysis point of view, such a multiple crossing, coupled with the influence of the MDCT acquisition protocol, results in a complex parenchymal texture which can be described and characterized by the distribution and the size of the low-density patterns delimited by the vascularized structures.

Within normal tissue, the low-density patterns have a small size and are uniformly distributed (Fig. 1(a)). Such patterns change in the case of DPLDs due to tissue damages. Emphysema is characterized by larger, round-shape patterns of nearly-constant low gray value, surrounded by normal tissue (Fig. 1(b)). The appearance of emphysema/fibrosis patterns is similar, but their border is of a higher density than normal tissue. Honeycombing is characterized by agglomerations of several low-density patterns of similar size and dense thin or thick borders (Fig. 1(c)). Finally, ground glass tissue "infiltrates" the normal zones with medium-high opacities (Fig. 1(d)).

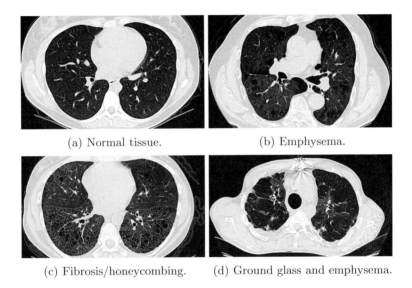

(a) Normal tissue.   (b) Emphysema.

(c) Fibrosis/honeycombing.   (d) Ground glass and emphysema.

Fig. 1. Some examples of MDCT axial images showing the patterns specific of different lung diseases

The idea exploited in this paper is the possibility to discriminate between normal and pathologic lung tissues by analyzing the size and distribution of, and the relationship between the low-density patterns. A one-dimensionnal schematic representation of the lung tissue, according to the previous remarks, is given in Fig. 2. Such "relief" representation will be exploited in the following in order to illustrate the principle of the developed approach.

In order to detect and analyze the different low-density patterns of the lung texture (local valleys on the lung "relief", Fig. 2) we have developed an image multiresolution decomposition scheme based on a 3D morphological filter, the *sup-constrained connection cost* introduced in [9]. Such a filter, denoted by $\mathcal{RC}_f^n$, will affect a function "relief" $f : \Re^n \to \Re$ by "filling in", at constant level, all local "basins" of f, of spatial extent smaller than n and disconnected from larger "basins". Note that the considered filter do not modify the "basins" shape. They can be at most flooded if enclosed in larger "basins" of higher "walls". The *increasing* property of $\mathcal{RC}_f^n$ allows to apply such filter recursively, with increasing size, in order to progressively select all "basins" of a f "relief".

The multiresolution decomposition scheme, illustrated in Fig. 3 for 4 levels of decomposition, exploits the $\mathcal{RC}_f^n$ properties and builds-up a hierarchic relief of the lung parenchyma, $g : \Re^3 \rightarrow \Re$, as follows.

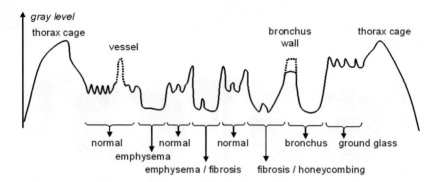

Fig. 2. 1-D schematic representation of normal and pathologic lung tissues. The dashed line symbolizes that a connectivity is possible at that level between the left and the right sides.

If L denotes the maximum image value of the 3D thorax CT data, n_i the filter size at level i, $n_j > n_i \ \forall \ j > i$, and N_{max} the maximum filter size, the decomposition procedure is given by:

$g = 0; \quad i = 0;$
while $(n_i \leq N_{max})$ **do**

- **extract** $i-$**level patterns** $l_i = \begin{cases} L - n_i, if \ \mathcal{RC}_f^{n_i} - f > 0 \\ 0, \qquad otherwise \end{cases}$ (1)

- **update** $\mathbf{g}$ $g = max(g, \ l_i)$
- **reiterate** $f = \mathcal{RC}_f^{n_i}; \quad i = i + 1$

end while

Finally, the eventual ground glass zones, which cannot be selected with the above procedure, are included as the lowest level of g. Their segmentation is based on a gray-scale reconstruction [10] of $\mathcal{RC}_f^{N_{max}}$ with respect to its largest plateaux and suppression of the high-density thorax cage (Fig. 3).

Fig. 4 shows the corresponding axial cross-section images of the 3D hierarchic decomposition obtained with 10 resolution levels for the patients in Fig. 1 (histogram-equalized). Note that the descriptive information is free of high-density tissues (vessels, thorax cage) and concerns only the lung parenchyma and the airway structure. A level of such decomposition informs on the size of the lung patterns at this level and also on a possible pathologic status (isolated larger patterns could point to disorders like emphysema/fibrosis/honeycombing). Conversely, patterns extracted at a decomposition level are independent of the native data values (for example, in Fig. 3, the 0-level patterns come from both normal and pathologic tissues).

By combining the information of the lung image decomposition (patterns size, 3D spatial and inter-level relationships) and the corresponding native image density values, a classification of the lung texture can be more confidently achieved. For an effective analysis, all this information is gathered in a 3D hierarchic descriptive graph built-up from the multi-level decomposition and presented in the following section.

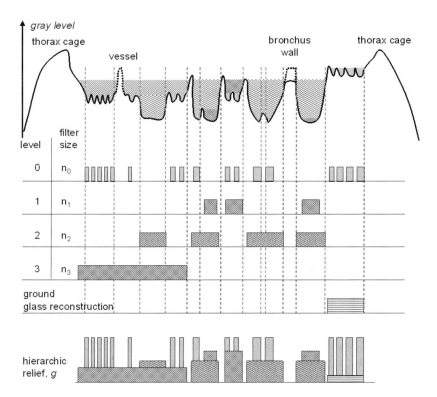

Fig. 3. Multiresolution decomposition of the schematic lung relief of Fig. 2

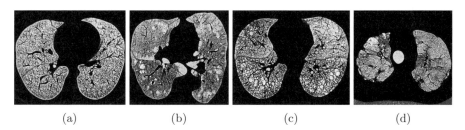

(a)   (b)   (c)   (d)

Fig. 4. Example of multiresolution hierarchic decomposition of data from Fig. 1

3   Hierarchic Classification of the Lung Tissue

The objective is to obtain a compact, multi-valued description of the lung parenchyma based on the previous image decomposition and original data information. We shall show in the following that an information node can be associated with each pattern extracted at each resolution level of the decomposition and that a connectivity relationship can be established between such nodes, providing a descriptive tree graph.

Starting from the hierarchic relief g (Fig. 3), the patterns of a level i can be reconstructed by means of morphological operations, as follows. Using the notations of eq. 1:

$$
\begin{aligned}
&i = 0; \\
&\textbf{while } (n_i \leq N_{max} + 1) \textbf{ do} \\
&\quad \bullet \textbf{ extract pattern subset of level i} \qquad l_i' = T_{L-n_i}^{L-n_i}(g) \subseteq l_i \\
&\quad \bullet \textbf{ reconstruct connected patterns} \qquad p_i = T_{L-n_i}^{L-n_i}\left(R_g^\delta(l_i')\right) \\
&\quad \bullet \forall \, p_i, \textbf{ create a node in the tree graph } t_i \leftrightarrow p_i \qquad\qquad (2) \\
&\quad \bullet \textbf{ update nodes connectivity} \qquad C\left\{t_i, t_j\right\}_{j<i} \\
&\quad \bullet \textbf{ reiterate} \qquad i = i+1 \\
&\textbf{end while,}
\end{aligned}
$$

where T_a^b denotes the thresholding operator between a and b, $R_g^\delta(f)$ the grayscale reconstruction by geodesic dilation of f inside g [10], and l_i the initial patterns extracted at resolution level i (eq. 1). Note that a reconstructed pattern p_i at resolution level i will always include initial patterns l_j of levels $j < i$, $p_i \supseteq l_j$, if l_i and l_j are either (partially) overlapping or 3D connected. In this situation, the associated nodes, t_i, t_j have a *parent-child* relationship and a tree graph results (Fig. 5, see also [12] for a step-by-step 3D illustration).

Each node t_i of the descriptive graph carries out information related to 3D spatial location, resolution level, connected patterns, first order statistics (mean μ and standard deviation σ) of the native density values within p_i pattern, p_i volume (number of voxels), p_i fractal dimension computed using box counting [11], p_i relative volume with respect to its "children".

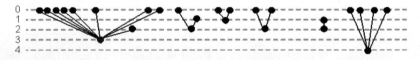

Fig. 5. Descriptive tree graph of the hierarchic relief g of Fig. 3

The lung parenchyma descriptive tree graph $\{t_i\}_i$ is investigated and each node classified into normal or DPLD tissue according to a set of intuitive rules established with respect to intrinsic node properties and to those of its hierarchy [12]. Three significant density classes have been defined for MDCT native data: low-density (LD) values within [-1000, -950] Hounsfield Units (HU), medium-density (MD) values within (-950, -765] HU and medium-high density (MHD) values within (-765, -450] HU. The main structural properties of DPLDs as described in §2 are reflected in the following parameter evaluation: (1) categorize $\mu(t_i)$ as LD, MD or MHD; (2) categorize the t_i children mean $\mu\left(\{t_j\}_j\right)$ as LD, MD, MHD; (3) categorize the mean of the disjoint pattern $\mu\left(t_i \setminus \{t_j\}_j\right)$ as LD, MD or MHD; (4) evaluate the density dispersion within the pattern: $\mu(t_i)/\sigma(t_i) \geq 3.0$ denotes a narrow dispersion, otherwise we consider a spread dispersion; (5) categorize the tissue density in the pattern (close) neighborhood; (6) estimate the pattern compactness according to the fractal dimension: $d_f(t_i) < 2.0$ denotes a compact, otherwise "porous", pattern; (7) evaluate the pattern relative volume with respect to its "children" $\frac{V(t_i)-V(\{t_j\}_j)}{V(\{t_j\}_j)}$. After classification, each node is assigned one of the following labels: EM (emphysema), FHC (fibrosis/honeycombing), GDG (ground glass), N (normal), and the corresponding image pattern is labeled with a comprehensive color code [12].

4   Results and Discussion

The developed classification approach was tested on a MDCT database including 10 patients suspected of DPLD, of which 4 representative cases are illustrated Fig. 1. Their corresponding classification is illustrated Figs. 6 and 7 both locally, in axial cross-sections, and globally, by using a volume rendering approach. Here, the proximal airways are labeled distinctly by means of a region-growing procedure initiated at the top of the trachea. The pathology detection sensitivity/specificity were estimated by one experienced radiologist: EM: 94%/80.5%, FHC: 81.2%/90%, GDG: 97%/95%. Missclassification of EM *vs.* FHC occured sometimes (13% EM classed as FHC, 22% FHC classed as EM) which also explains the low specificity value. This is due to the fact that some high-density tissues surrounding FHC patterns do not subsist in the hierarchic decomposition (Fig. 4) and, consequently, they are not considered in classification. Our future work will take into account such information together with additional features [8] for a more confident discrimination between various types of DPLDs.

To conclude, the main advances of the proposed approach with respect to the recent literature [6,7,8] consists in an automatic partitioning of the lung regions based on multiresolution decomposition and graph description, a fully-3D

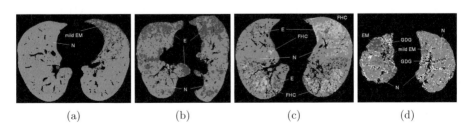

| (a) | (b) | (c) | (d) |

Fig. 6. Example of lung tissue classification of data from Fig. 1 (color plates in [12])

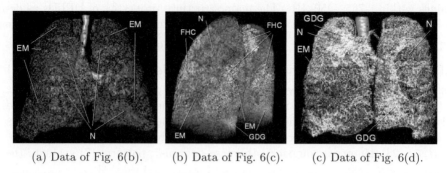

(a) Data of Fig. 6(b).   (b) Data of Fig. 6(c).   (c) Data of Fig. 6(d).

Fig. 7. Volume rendering of the lung tissue 3D classification (color plates in [12])

classification of the whole lung and the absence of training/interaction. Further improvement of the DLPD discrimination rules will be evaluated on a larger database. Note also that the rule-based pattern classification can be replaced by a Bayesian, neural network or support vector machines (SVM) approach.

References

1. Doi, K., Macmahon', H., Katsuragawa, S., Nishikawa, M.R., Jiang, Y.: Computer-aided diagnosis in radiology: potential and pitfalls. Eur. J. Radiol. 31(2), 97–109 (1999)
2. Coxson, H.O., Rogers, R.M., Whittall, K.P., D'yachkova, Y., Pare, P.D., Sciurba, F.C., Hogg, J.C.: A quantification of the lung surface area in emphysema using computed tomography. Am. J. Respir. Crit. Care Med. 163(6), 1500–1501 (2001)
3. Blechschmidt, R.A., Werthschutzky, R., Lorcher, U.: Automated CT image evaluation of the lung: a morphology-based concept. IEEE Trans. Med. Imag. 20(5), 434–442 (2001)
4. Malone, J., Rossiter, J.M., Prabhu, S., Goddard, P.: Identification of disease in CT of the lung using texture-based image analysis. Proc. IEEE Conf. Signals, Systems and Computers 2, 1620–1624 (2004)
5. Xu, D.H., Kurani, A.S., Furst, J.D., Raicu, D.S.: Run-length encoding for volumetric texture. In: Proc. Visualization, Imaging and Image Processing (2004)
6. Chabat, F., Yang, G.Z., Hansell, D.M.: Obstructive lung diseases: texture classification for differentiation at CT. Radiology 228(3), 871–877 (2003)
7. Xu, Y., Sonka, M., McLennan, G., Junfeng, G., Hoffman, E.A.: MDCT-based 3D texture classification of emphysema and early smoking related lung pathologies. IEEE Trans. Med. Imag. 25(4), 463–475 (2006)
8. Xu, Y., Vanbeek, E.J.R., Yu, H., McLennan, G., Guo, J., Hoffman, E.A.: Computer-aided Classification of Interstitial Lung Disease via MDCT: 3D Adaptive Multiple Feature Method (3D AMFM). Acad. Radiol. 13(8), 969–978 (2006)
9. Fetita, C., Lucidarme, O., Preteux, F.: Automated 3D vascular segmentation in CT hepatic venography. In: Proc. SPIE Conference on Mathematical Methods in Pattern and Image Analysis, San Diego, CA, vol. 5916, pp. 114–125 (2005)

10. Vincent, L.: Morphological gray scale reconstruction in image analysis: applications and efficient algorithms. IEEE Trans. on Imag. Proc. 2(2), 176–201 (1993)
11. Liebovitch, L.S., Toth, T.: A fast algorithm to determine fractal dimensions by box counting. Physics Letters A 141(11), 386–390 (1989)
12. Fetita, C.: Classification of lung parenchyma ROIs resulting from hierarchic decomposition. in Internal report (2007),
    http://www-artemis.int-evry.fr/~fetita/classif.html

Unsupervised Reconstruction of a Patient-Specific Surface Model of a Proximal Femur from Calibrated Fluoroscopic Images

Guoyan Zheng, Xiao Dong, and Miguel A. Gonzalez Ballester

MEM Research Center - ISTB, University of Bern, Stauffacherstrasse 78,
CH-3014, Bern, Switzerland
guoyan.zheng@ieee.org

Abstract. In this paper, we present an unsupervised 2D/3D reconstruction scheme combining a parameterized multiple-component geometrical model and a point distribution model, and show its application to automatically reconstruct a surface model of a proximal femur from a limited number of calibrated fluoroscopic images with no user intervention at all. The parameterized multiple-component geometrical model is regarded as a simplified description capturing the geometrical features of a proximal femur. Its parameters are optimally and automatically estimated from the input images using a particle filter based inference method. The estimated geometrical parameters are then used to initialize a point distribution model based 2D/3D reconstruction scheme for an accurate reconstruction of a surface model of the proximal femur. We designed and conducted *in vitro* and *in vivo* experiments to compare the present unsupervised reconstruction scheme to a supervised one. An average mean error of 1.2 mm was found when the supervised reconstruction scheme was used. It increased to 1.3 mm when the unsupervised one was used. However, the unsupervised reconstruction scheme has the advantage of elimination of user intervention, which holds the potential to facilitate the application of the 2D/3D reconstruction in surgical navigation.

Keywords: proximal femur, fluoroscopy, surface reconstruction, particle filter, multiple-component geometrical model, point distribution model.

1 Introduction

A patient-specific surface model of a proximal femur plays an important role in planning and supporting various computer-assisted surgical procedures including total hip replacement, hip resurfacing, and proximal femur osteotomy. Accordingly, various reconstruction methods have been developed.

One of these methods is to extract a three-dimensional (3D) surface model from volume data pre-operatively acquired from Computed Tomography (CT) or Magnetic Resonance Imaging (MRI) and then intra-operatively to register the extracted surface model to the patient anatomy. However, the high logistic effort and cost, the extra radiation involved with the CT imaging, and the

N. Ayache, S. Ourselin, A. Maeder (Eds.): MICCAI 2007, Part I, LNCS 4791, pp. 834–841, 2007.
© Springer-Verlag Berlin Heidelberg 2007

large quantity of data to be acquired and processed make them less functional. The alternative is to reconstruct a patient-specific surface model from a limited number of intra-operatively acquired two-dimensional (2D) fluoroscopic images using a statistical model.

Several research groups have explored the methods for reconstructing a patient specific model from a statistical model and a limited number of calibrated X-ray images [1][2][3][4]. Except the method presented in Yao and Taylor [1], which depends on a deformable 2D/3D registration between an appearance based statistical model and a limited number of X-ray images, all other methods have their reliance on a point distribution model (PDM) in common. The common disadvantage of all these PDM based reconstruction methods lies in the fact that they require either knowledge about anatomical landmarks [4], which are normally obtained by interactive reconstruction from the input images, or an interactive alignment of the model with the input images [2][3]. Such a supervised initialization is not appreciated in a surgical navigation application, largely due to the strict sterilization requirement.

To eliminate the user intervention constraint, we propose in this paper an unsupervised 2D/3D reconstruction scheme combining a parameterized multiple-component geometrical model and a point distribution model, and show its application to automatically reconstruct a surface model of the proximal femur with no user intervention at all. The parameterized multiple-component geometrical model is regarded as a simplified description capturing the geometrical features of a proximal femur. The constraints between different components are described by a causal Bayesian network. A particle filter based inference algorithm [5] is applied to automatically estimate their parameters from the input X-ray images. The estimated geometrical parameters of the proximal femur are then used to initialize a point distribution model based 2D/3D reconstruction scheme for an accurate reconstruction of a surface model of the proximal femur.

This paper is organized as follows. Section 2 briefly recalls the supervised 2D/3D reconstruction scheme. Section 3 describes the approach for unsupervised initialization. Section 4 reports the experimental results, followed by conclusions in Section 5.

2   Supervised 2D/3D Reconstruction Scheme

2.1   Image Acquisition

We use calibrated fluoroscopic images. Due to the limited imaging volume of a fluoroscope, we ask for four images for the proximal femur from different view direction, of which two images focus on the proximal femoral head and the other two focus on the femoral shaft. The calibrated fluoroscopic image set is represented by **I**. Although all four images are used to estimate the parameters of the multiple-component geometrical model, only those two images that focus on the proximal femur are used for surface reconstruction.

2.2   Statistical Model of the Proximal Femur

The PDM used in this paper was constructed from a training database consisted of proximal femoral surfaces from above the less trochanter. Let $\mathbf{x}_i, i = 0, 1, ..., m-1$, be $m = 30$ members of the aligned training surfaces. Each member is described by a vectors $\mathbf{x}_i$ with $N = 4098$ vertices:

$$\mathbf{x}_i = \{x_0, y_0, z_0, x_1, y_1, z_1, ..., x_{N-1}, y_{N-1}, z_{N-1}\} \qquad (1)$$

The PDM is obtained by applying principal component analysis.

$$\mathbf{D} = \frac{1}{(m-1)} \cdot \sum_{i=0}^{m-1} (\mathbf{x}_i - \bar{\mathbf{x}}) \cdot (\mathbf{x}_i - \bar{\mathbf{x}})^T$$
$$\sigma_0 \geq \sigma_1 \geq \cdots \geq \sigma_{m_1-1} > 0; \ m_1 \leq m - 1 \qquad (2)$$
$$\mathbf{D} \cdot \mathbf{p}_i = \sigma_i^2 \cdot \mathbf{p}_i; \ i = 0, \cdots, m_1 - 1$$

where $\bar{\mathbf{x}}$ and $\mathbf{D}$ are the mean vector and the covariance matrix, respectively. $\{\sigma_i^2\}$ are non-zero eigenvalues of the covariance matrix $\mathbf{D}$, and $\{\mathbf{p}_i\}$ are the corresponding eigenvectors. The sorted eigenvalues σ_i^2 and the corresponding eigenvectors $\mathbf{p}_i$ are the principal directions spanning a shape space with $\bar{\mathbf{x}}$ representing its origin.

Then, an instance $\mathcal{M}$ generated from the statistical model with parameter set $\mathbf{Q} = \{s, \alpha_0, \alpha_1, \cdots, \alpha_{m_1-1}\}$ can be described as:

$$\mathcal{M} : \mathbf{x}(\mathbf{Q}) = s \cdot (\bar{\mathbf{x}} + \sum_{i=0}^{m_1-1} (\alpha_i \cdot \mathbf{p}_i)) \qquad (3)$$

where s is the scaling factor; $\{\alpha_i\}$ are the weights calculated by projecting vector $(\mathbf{x}/s - \bar{\mathbf{x}})$ into the shape space. The mean surface model $\bar{\mathbf{x}}$ is shown in Fig. 1, left.

2.3   2D/3D Reconstruction Scheme

Our 2D-3D reconstruction scheme is a further improvement of the approach we introduced in [4], which combines statistical instantiation and regularized shape deformation with an iterative image-to-model correspondence establishing algorithm. The image-to-model correspondence is established using a non-rigid 2D point matching process, which iteratively uses a symmetric injective nearest-neighbor mapping operator and 2D thin-plate splines based deformation to find a fraction of best matched 2D point pairs between features detected from the fluoroscopic images and those extracted from the 3D model. The image contours of the proximal femur are extracted from the input images by a graphical model based Bayesian inference [6] whereas the apparent contours of the 3D model are extracted using an approach described in [7]. The obtained 2D point pairs are then used to set up a set of 3D point pairs such that we turn a 2D-3D reconstruction problem to a 3D-3D one. The 3D/3D reconstruction problem is then solved optimally in three sequential stages. For details, we refer to our previous works [4] and [6].

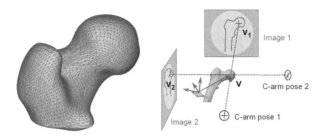

Fig. 1. The mean surface model of our point distribution model (left) and a schematic view of landmark reconstruction (right)

2.4   Supervised Initialization

The convergence of the 2D/3D reconstruction scheme introduced in [4] relies on a proper initialization of scale and pose of the mean surface model of the PDM. In our previous work [4], three anatomical landmarks, i.e., the center of the femoral head, a point on the axis of the femoral neck, and the apex of the greater trochanter were reconstructed interactively from the input fluoroscopic images, as shown in Fig. 1, right, and were used to compute the initial scale s_0 and the initial rigid transformation T_0 of the mean surface model of the PDM in relative to the input images.

3   Approach for Unsupervised Initialization

3.1   Proximal Femur Model

The proximal femur is approximated by a simplified geometrical model consisting of 3 components: head, neck and shaft, which are described by a sphere, a trunked cone and a cylinder with parameter set $\mathbf{X}_{Femur} = \{\mathbf{X}_{Head}, \mathbf{X}_{Neck}, \mathbf{X}_{Shaft}\}$ respectively as shown in Fig. 2, left. These three components are constrained by the anatomical structure of the proximal femur. The advantage of using such a model is apparent. On the one hand, this simplified 3D model has the capability to catch the global structure of the anatomy from the fluoroscopic images and is not dependent on the view directions of the input images. On the other hand, using such a model to estimate the geometrical parameters of the proximal femur is much less computational expensive than using a point distribution model, largely due to the simple and parameterized geometrical shape of its components.

The constraints among components are represented by a causal Bayesian network as shown in Fig. 2, right, where all $\pi(\cdot)$'s are prior distributions and all $p(\cdot)$'s are conditional distributions. The prior distributions are designed according to the information estimated from the two images that focus on the proximal femur and the prior information about the geometrical features of each component, e.g., the centroids of three components are assumed uniformly distributed in the common view volume of the fluoroscopic images, which can be obtained by calculating the intersection of their projection frustums; the radii and the lengths (for neck and shaft) of different components are assumed to be uniformly distributed in their associated anatomical ranges. The structural constraints among components are set so that the component configuration that fulfills these constraints will show a higher probability of being assembled to represent a proper proximal femur. These constraints are regarded as the conditional distributions of those components when the configuration of their parent components is given. The reason why the network starts from shaft component is that the shaft component is much easier to be detected from the images than other two components, which will accelerate the convergence of the model fitting algorithm as described below.

3.2   Geometrical Model Fitting by Particle Filter

Particle filter, also known as the Condensation algorithm [8] is a robust filtering technique, based on the Bayesian framework. This technique provides a suitable basic framework for estimating paramerers of a multiple-component geometrical model from images: particle filter estimates the states by recursively updating sample approximations of posterior distribution. In this work, we implement a particle filter based inference algorithm as follows.

1. Initialization: Generate the first generation of particle set with M particles $\{P_i^0 = \mathbf{X}_{Femur,i}^0\}_{i=0,\ldots,M-1}$ from the proposal distributions

$$q^0(\mathbf{X}_{Shaft}) = \pi(\mathbf{X}_{Shaft})$$
$$q^0(\mathbf{X}_{Neck}) = \pi(\mathbf{X}_{Neck})q^0(\mathbf{X}_{Shaft})p(\mathbf{X}_{Neck}|\mathbf{X}_{Shaft})$$
$$q^0(\mathbf{X}_{Head}) = \pi(\mathbf{X}_{Head})q^0(\mathbf{X}_{Neck})p(\mathbf{X}_{Head}|\mathbf{X}_{Neck})$$

2. Observation: Given the current generation of particle set, calculate the weight of each particle as $w_i^n \propto Prob(\mathbf{I}|\mathbf{X}_{Femur,i}^n)$, where $Prob(\mathbf{I}|\mathbf{X}_{Femur,i}^n)$ is called observation model and is defined by the product of two items:

$$p(\mathbf{I}|\mathbf{X}_{Femur,i}^n) = \prod_{(I \in \mathbf{I})} p_E(I|\mathbf{X}_{Femur,i}^n) \cdot p_G(I|\mathbf{X}_{Femur,i}^n) \qquad (4)$$

The first item $p_E(I|\mathbf{X}_{Femur,i}^n)$ measures discrepancies between extremal contours of the model obtained by simulating X-ray projection to the Ith image and the edges $E(I)$ extracted from the Ith image by applying a Canny edge detector. For details about this similarity measure, we refer to chapter 6 of [10].

The second item $p_G(I|\mathbf{X}_{Femur,i}^n)$ measures differences between the intensity distribution of the projected silhouettes of the model and that of the fluoroscopic image along the profile normal to the projected extremal contours of the model. For details about this similarity measure, we refer to chapter 7 of [10].

3. Update: Update the proposal distributions as

$$q^{n+1}(\mathbf{X}_{Shaft}) = NPDE(w_i^n, \mathbf{X}_{Shaft,i}^n)$$
$$q^{n+1}(\mathbf{X}_{Neck}) = \pi(\mathbf{X}_{Neck})q^{n+1}(\mathbf{X}_{Shaft})p(\mathbf{X}_{Neck}|\mathbf{X}_{Shaft})$$

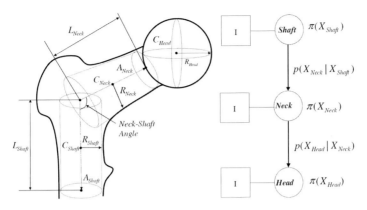

Fig. 2. The parameterized multiple-component geometrical model (left) and a causal Bayesian network for encoding the conditional distribution among components (right)

$$q^{n+1}(\mathbf{X}_{Head}) = \pi(\mathbf{X}_{Head})q^{n+1}(\mathbf{X}_{Neck})p(\mathbf{X}_{Head}|\mathbf{X}_{Neck})$$

where $NPDE(w_i^n, \mathbf{X}_{Shaft,i}^n)$ is a *nonparametric density estimation* [9] . Generate the next generation of particle set from the updated proposal distributions.

4. Go to 2 until the particle set converges.

3.3 Unsupervised Initialization of the PDM

From the mean surface model $\bar{\mathbf{x}}$ of the PDM, the model vertices can be classified into three regions, femoral head, neck and shaft. The femoral head center and radius, axes of femoral neck and shaft can be determined in the mean surface model coordinate space by a 3D sphere fitting to the femoral head region and cylinder fittings to the femoral neck and shaft regions. The initial rigid transformation and scale can then be computed to fit the PDM (the scaled mean surface model) to the estimated geometrical model of the proximal femur.

4 Experimental Results

We designed and conducted two experiments to validate the present approach. The first experiment was conducted on 3 clinical dataset. Due to the lack of ground truth, we used the clinical dataset to verify the robustness of the particle filter based inference algorithm. We run the algorithm for 10 trials on each dataset with particle number $M = 200$. In each trial the proximal femur was correctly identified in about 4 minutes on a 3.0 GHz Pentium IV computer with 1 GB RAM, when the algorithm was implemented with GCC 4.0 on a Fedora 4.0 Linux system. The statistical results are shown in Table 1. An example of the unsupervised initialization using the inference results is shown in Fig. 3.

The second experiment was performed on 10 dry cadaveric femurs with different sizes and shapes. The purpose was to evaluate the accuracy of the unsupervised 2D/3D reconstruction. For each bone, two studies were performed.

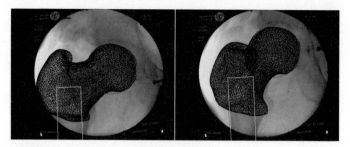

Fig. 3. An example of unsupervised initialization of the PDM. The color lines show the projected extremal contours of different components.

Table 1. Satistical results of the particel filter based inference algorithm, all results are relative to the mean values of the 10 trials

Parameter	Data Set 1	Data Set 2	Data Set 3
Head Center (mm)	1.4±1.1	0.1±0.1	0.1±0.2
Head Radius (mm)	0.3±0.4	0.6±0.2	1.0±0.8
Neck Length (mm)	1.0±1.4	1.3±1.8	1.2±1.7
Neck Axis (degree)	0.8±0.7	2.3±1.0	1.8±1.1
Shaft Radius(mm)	0.2±0.3	0.1±0.2	0.2±0.2
Neck/Shaft Angle(degree)	0.8±1.0	2.0±2.5	1.8±2.6

Table 2. The reconstruction errors when different initialization methods were used

Bone Index	No. 1	No. 2	No. 3	No. 4	No. 5	No. 6	No. 7	No. 8	No. 9	No. 10
Errors of supervised reconstruction										
Median (mm)	1.7	1.3	0.8	0.9	1.3	1.0	0.9	0.8	0.8	1.1
Mean (mm)	1.7	1.4	0.9	1.3	1.4	1.1	1.1	1.0	1.0	1.2
Errors of unsupervised reconstruction										
Median (mm)	1.8	1.4	0.9	1.6	1.3	1.2	1.0	1.2	1.5	0.8
Mean (mm)	1.9	1.6	0.9	1.5	1.2	1.2	1.2	1.1	1.5	1.1

In the first study, the 2D/3D reconstruction scheme was initialized using the interactionvely reconstructed landmarks as described in Section 2, whereas in the second study, the present unspervised initialization was used to initialize the 2D/3D reconstruction scheme. It took about 1 minute to interatctively reconstruct the landmarks for a supervised initilization for each case in the first study. To evaluate the reconstruction accuracy, 200 points were digitized from each bone surface. The distance between these points to the reconstructed surface of the associated bone were calculated and used to evaluate the reconstruction accuracy. The median and mean reconstruction errors for each study when using different initialization methods were recorded. The results are presented in Table 2. It was found that the unsupervised reconstruction was a little bit less accurate when compared to the supervised one. An average mean reconstruction error of

1.3 mm was found for the unsupervised reconstruction. It decreased to 1.2 mm when the supervised one was used.

5 Conclusions

In this paper, an unsupervised 2D/3D reconstruction scheme combining a parameterized multiple-component geometrical model with a point distribution model was presented. We solved the supervised initialization problem by using a particle filter based inference algorithm to automatically determine the geometrical parameters of a proximal femur from the calibrated fluoroscopic images. No user intervention is required any more. The qualitative and quantitative evaluation results on 3 clinical dataset and on dataset of 10 dry cadaveric bones indicate the validity of the present approach. Although the unsupervised reconstruction is a little bit less accurate and needs longer time than the supervised one, it has the advantage of elimination of user intervention, which holds the potential to facilitate the application of the 2D/3D reconstruction in surgical navigation.

References

1. Yao, J., Taylor, R.H.: Assessing accuracy factors in deformable 2D/3D medical image registration using a statistical pelvis model. In: ICCV 2003, vol. 2 pp. 1329–1334 (2003)
2. Fleute, M., Lavallée, S.: Nonrigid 3D/2D registration of images using a statistical model. In: Taylor, C., Colchester, A. (eds.) MICCAI'99. LNCS, vol. 1679, pp. 138–147. Springer, Heidelberg (1999)
3. Benameur, S., Mignotte, M., Parent, S., et al.: A hierarchical statistical modeling approach for the unsupervised 3D biplanar reconstruction of the scoliotic spine. IEEE Trans. Biomed. Eng. 52, 2041–2057 (2005)
4. Zheng, G., Gonzalez Ballester, M.A., Styner, M., Nolte, L.-P.: Reconstruction of patient-specific 3D bone surface from 2D calibrated fluoroscopic images and point distribution model. In: Larsen, R., Nielsen, M., Sporring, J. (eds.) MICCAI 2006. LNCS, vol. 4190, pp. 25–32. Springer, Heidelberg (2006)
5. Dong, X., Zheng, G.: A computational framework for automatic determination of morphological parameters of proximal femur from intraoperative fluoroscopic images. In: ICPR 2006, Part I pp. 1008–1013 (2006)
6. Dong, X., Gonzalez Ballester, M.A., Zheng, G.: Automatic extraction of femur contours from calibrated fluoroscopic images. WACV 2007, p. 55 (2007)
7. Hertzmann, A., Zorin, D.: Illustrating smooth surface. In: SIGGRAPH 2000, pp. 517–526 (2000)
8. Isard, M., Blake, A.: Contour tracking by stochastic propagation of conditional density. In: Buxton, B.F., Cipolla, R. (eds.) ECCV 1996. LNCS, vol. 1064, pp. 343–356. Springer, Heidelberg (1996)
9. Scott, D.W.: Multivariate Density Estimation. Wiley, Chichester (1992)
10. Cootes, T., Taylor, C.: Statistical models of appearance for computer vision. Technical report, University of Manschester, United Kingdom, ch. 6 & 7, pp. 34–42 (2004)

A New Method for Spherical Object Detection and Its Application to Computer Aided Detection of Pulmonary Nodules in CT Images

Xiangwei Zhang[1], Jonathan Stockel[2], Matthias Wolf[2], Pascal Cathier[2], Geoffrey McLennan[1], Eric A. Hoffman[1], and Milan Sonka[1]

[1] University of Iowa, Iowa City, IA, 52242, USA
[2] Siemens Medical Solutions, Malvern, PA, 19355, USA

Abstract. A novel method called local shape controlled voting has been developed for spherical object detection in 3D voxel images. By introducing local shape properties into the voting procedure of normal overlap, the proposed method improves the capability of differentiating spherical objects from other structures, as the normal overlap technique only measures the 'density' of normal overlapping, while how the normals are distributed in 3D is not discovered. The proposed method was applied to computer aided detection of pulmonary nodules based on helical CT images. Experiments showed that this method attained a better performance compared to the original normal overlap technique.

1   Introduction

Lung cancer is one of the most lethal kinds of cancer worldwide. Its cure depends critically on disease detection in the early stages. Computed tomography (CT) is an important tool for early detection of nodules, but interpreting the large amount of thoracic CT images is a very challenging task for radiologists. Computer-aided detection (CAD) is considered as a promising tool to aid the radiologist in lung nodule CT interpretation.

Many techniques of nodule detection have been developed based on thoracic CT images. Giger [1] proposed multiple gray-level thresholding and a rule based method. Armato [2] introduced some 3D geometric features and a linear discriminant analysis (LDA) classifier. Kanazawa [3] used fuzzy clustering method and a rule-based method. Lee [4] used pherical/half-circle templates to detect in-field/pleural nodules respectively. Surface normal overlap method [5] was proposed to capture the concentration of surface normals. Surface curvature/local shape feature was also utilized for detecting lung nodules [6], [7].

In this work, we developed a new method called local shape controlled voting for spherical object detection in 3D voxel images. This new scheme integrates surface curvature feature into the voting procedure of normal overlap [5]. Specifically, we applied the proposed method to lung nodule CAD. The overall scheme of the CAD system is described in Sect. 2; the method is described in Sect. 3; then the experimental results are presented in Sect. 4; and the conclusion is given in Sect. 5.

N. Ayache, S. Ourselin, A. Maeder (Eds.): MICCAI 2007, Part I, LNCS 4791, pp. 842–849, 2007.
© Springer-Verlag Berlin Heidelberg 2007

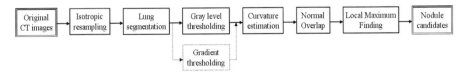

Fig. 1. Schematic view of the CAD for nodule detection

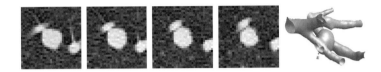

Fig. 2. A nodule attached to vessels. The left four images are neighboring slices in axial view, the most right one is an iso-surface rendering image.

2   Overall Scheme

The proposed method for pulmonary nodule detection is outlined in Fig. 1. First, the original CT data are resampled to isotropic using tri-linear interpolation. Then the lung is extracted. Next, thresholding gives us high intensity regions. For each voxel near the boundary, shape index/curvedness features can be calculated using iso-surface curvatures. These features are used to control the voting procedure of normal overlap. For each voxel, the resulted value is a confidence score indicating the possibility of being the center of a nodule. The nodule candidate positions are obtained using local maximum criteria and thresholding.

3   Methods

3.1   Basic Shape of Pulmonary Nodules

In automated detection of nodules, dealing with non-isolated nodules (attaching to other structures) are major difficulties. Most methods first obtain suspected nodule areas (SNAs) based on intensity, then these SNAs are classified using associated features. Problem arises if a non-isolated nodule is segmented as part of normal structures, so it is difficult to be located afterwards.

Basic observations show that a nodule usually takes a sphere-like shape (or partly), while vessels have tubular structures. See, for example, Fig. 2. Usually this shape property was used as a feature of a segmented object, i.e., a SNA. In order to prevent from treating a non-isolated nodule as a part of attached structures, we need some local shape feature to distinguish between a non-isolated nodule and the contact normal anatomical structures.

3.2   Surface Normal Overlap

In order to detect sphere-like structures, a Hough transform type method, called surface normal overlap method [5] is developed to capture the concentration of

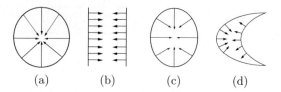

Fig. 3. Illustration of 2D boundary normal overlap

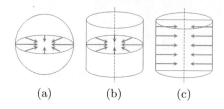

Fig. 4. Illustration of 3D boundary normal overlap

normals, illustrated in Fig. 3. The normals on the object boundary is assumed going inside. For a circle, all normals will meet at the center; for a strap like shape, a normal vector will only meet one normal from the other side; for an ellipse, the normals are less concentrated than a circle; for a complicated shape, the normals on the convex part will concentrate, while the normals on the concave part will diversify. 3D case is shown in Fig. 4. A sphere has the most concentrated normals at the center; any great circle will have a distribution same as a circle in 2D. For a cylinder, the cross section perpendicular to the axis is a circle; the cross section passing the axis is a strap like shape.

Assuming unit line/surface density on the boundary, then for a circle with radius r, the corresponding 'density' at the center is the circumference $2\pi r$; for a strap-type object, the 'density' will be no more than two. For a sphere with radius r, the 'density' at the center will be the surface area of sphere $4\pi r^2$; for a cylinder with directrix being a circle with radius r, the 'density' at the center line will be $2\pi r$.

Thus, gradient directions can be used to detect circular/spherical structures in digital images. For pixels satisfying some boundary conditions, a tracking operation is performed in the gradient direction. This can be considered as a voting: every object pixel is a candidate; every boundary pixel is an individual voter who selects the favorite candidates (any object pixel on the gradient direction). The positions around the center of circular/spherical structures may have a high value after the voting procedure.

In a specific application, usually the maximum size of the object of interest is known in advance, thus the maximum voting distance can be set. Another idea is that the voting does not always need to reach the maximum distance, as the nodule candidate position should be inside the high intensity objects.

3.3   Air/Non-air Segmentation Using Optimal Thresholding

Optimal thresholding [8] is used to automatically determine a threshold for segmentation between the background (parenchyma) and objects (nodules, vessels, and so on). Let T^t be the threshold at iteration step t, and μ_b^t and μ_o^t be the mean intensity of background and objects. μ_b^t and μ_o^t are obtained by applying T^t to the image. Then for the next step $t + 1$, the threshold is updated by $T^{t+1} = (\mu_b^t + \mu_o^t)/2$. This updating is iterated until the threshold does not change. The initial threshold T^0 is chosen as the mean value of the whole image.

3.4   Local Maximum Finding

After the voting, the pixels around the center of a circle/sphere will possibly have a higher value not only than their neighbors, but also higher than other non-circle or non-sphere structures. So the positions of nodule candidates can be generated by a combination of thresholding and local maximum criterion. In this work, the neighborhood used to check the local maximum criterion for a pixel is chosen as $3 \times 3 \times 3$. The rule to decide a local maximum is that a pixel is not less than any neighbor.

3.5   Local Shape Features

According to Sect. 3.2, the ratio of maximum 'density' of normals between a sphere with radius r_1 and a cylinder with radius r_2 is $4\pi r_1^2$ to $2\pi r_2$. With same radius r (assuming that $r \geq 1$ for our applications), the sphere will have a higher density than the cylinder. But if r_2 is much larger than r_1, the cylinder will possibly give a higher response. This shows that the normal overlap method fails to distinguish between a small size sphere and a much larger size cylinder.

Practically, a nodule is usually not perfectly spherical; and vessels may have distortions resulting more concentrated normals; in addition, non-isolated nodules may only show spherical-like structure partly. All these factors can destroy the possible difference between nodules and non-nodules. To deal with these problems, we introduces local shape information to improve the original normal overlap technique [5].

A local surface shape can be completely described by its two principal curvatures, i.e., the maximal and the minimal curvatures k_1, k_2, or equivalently by the Gaussian curvature K and the mean curvature H, see the HK segmentation [9]. Neither the HK curvatures pair nor the two principal curvatures pair capture the intuitive notion of "local shape" very well. In both schemes, two parameters are needed to "tell" the local shape. Koenderink [10] proposed two measures – "shape index" S and "curvedness" C. The shape index is scale-invariant and captures the intuitive notion of "local shape", whereas the curvedness specifies the amount of curvature.

$$S = \frac{2}{\pi} \cdot arctan\frac{k_1 + k_2}{k_1 - k_2}, \quad C = \sqrt{\frac{k_1^2 + k_2^2}{2}}, \quad \text{for } k_1 \geq k_2 \tag{1}$$

The S and C decouple the shape and the magnitude of the curvatures. This is done by transforming a k_1, k_2 Cartesian coordinate description of a local shape into a polar coordinate system description. Every distinct shape, except for the plane, corresponds to a unique value of S. $S = 1$ indicates a cap, $S = -1$ describes a cup; $S = 0.5$ (ridge) and $S = -0.5$ (rut) correspond to parabolic points (cylindrical shapes). For $0 < S < 0.5$, the local shape is a saddle (hyperbolic) ridge. For $-0.5 < S < 0$, saddle ruts are obtained. And symmetrical saddles have $S = 0$. The range $-1 < S < -0.5$ represents the concavities, and the range $0.5 < S < 1$ represents the convexities. A plane has a zero value C and indeterminate S.

By assuming the surface of interest to be a level surface (iso-intensity surface) locally, curvatures can be computed from up to the second order partial derivatives (Gaussian smoothing with window size $7 \times 7 \times 7$ is used in the partial derivatives estimation in this work) of the image function [11]:

$$
\begin{aligned}
K = \frac{1}{(f_x^2 + f_y^2 + f_z^2)^2} \{ & f_x^2 (f_{yy} f_{zz} - f_{yz}^2) + 2 f_y f_z (f_{xy} f_{xz} - f_{xx} f_{yz}) \\
& + f_y^2 (f_{xx} f_{zz} - f_{xz}^2) + 2 f_x f_z (f_{xy} f_{yz} - f_{xz} f_{yy}) \\
& + f_z^2 (f_{xx} f_{yy} - f_{xy}^2) + 2 f_x f_y (f_{xz} f_{yz} - f_{xy} f_{zz}) \}
\end{aligned}
\tag{2}
$$

$$
\begin{aligned}
H = \frac{-1}{2(f_x^2 + f_y^2 + f_z^2)^{3/2}} \{ & (f_y^2 + f_z^2) f_{xx} + (f_x^2 + f_z^2) f_{yy} + (f_x^2 + f_y^2) f_{zz} \\
& - 2 f_x f_y f_{xy} - 2 f_x f_z f_{xz} - 2 f_y f_z f_{yz} \}
\end{aligned}
\tag{3}
$$

The shape index of each voxel on the boundary of nodules tends to be around 1 due to the sphere-like local shape. And tubular vessels have the shape index value of 0.5. For the airway walls, the voxels near the outer surface show the shape index value of 0.5, while the voxels near the inner surface take the value -0.5. This analysis shows that the shape index value can be used to differentiate the boundaries between of a nodule and vessels/airway walls. But this differentiation tends to be not very reliable due to noise, as it only depends on operation in a small neighborhood. What is needed is to synthesize these local information in a global way to give a more robust shape feature. Normal overlap technique will serve as the global level information processing tool in this work.

3.6   Local Shape Controlled Voting

In the original normal overlap scheme, every boundary point stimulates a tracking procedure. Such a system treats all voter equally. This rule is modified in the proposed local shape controlled voting: only boundary points satisfying some local shape conditions are allowed to vote, and the voting weights also depend on the local shape feature.

To exclude tubular structures (vessels, airways), a threshold S_t can be set so that boundary points with $S \le S_t$ are prohibited from the voting. Experiments

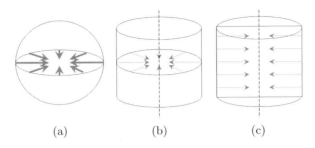

(a)   (b)   (c)

Fig. 5. Illustration of 3D local shape controlled voting.

show that $S_t \in [0.5, 0.6]$ is a good choice for nodule detection. For boundary points with $S > S_t$, a voting procedure is started along the gradient direction, with the voting weight being $b(S - S_t)$, in order to enhance sphere-like local structures. Here b is a positive coefficient. This local shape controlled voting is illustrated in Fig. 5: the thicker arrows represent larger weights; the thinner arrows indicate smaller weights.

It is also possible to use curvedness C to drive the voting. If a boundary point has a very small curvedness, it is probably located at the slowly changing pleural surface, rather than on the boundary of a nodule with very limited size. So an upper bound threshold C_u can be set to prohibit the voting. It is also possible to set a lower bound threshold C_l in order to reduce the response from too tiny structures or noise.

Compared to the normal overlap method, it seems that we always pay extra cost for calculating local shape, but this is not true, because there are many boundary points not allowed to vote due to non-qualification. In the applications of nodule detection in CT images, most of the anatomical structures will either be tubular, such as vessels and airways, or be a slowly changing surface, such as pleural surface and lobe fissure. This situation is very suitable for the proposed method, as boundary points on these objects will not stimulate a voting. And experiments also showed the efficiency of the scheme, see Sect. 4.

4   Experimental Methods and Results

4.1   Database

The database consisted of 42 clinical high resolution helical thoracic CT cases. In this work, the independent standard is the nodule center positions created by human experts, i.e., the x, y, z coordinates. Furthermore, the maximum 2D diameters of these nodules were measured manually.

4.2   Validation

A nodule is said to be detected by the CAD system if there is a position given by the CAD that is located closer than the size (the 2D maximum diameter

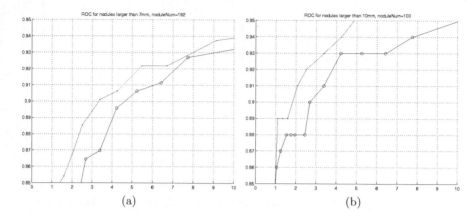

Fig. 6. Comparison of FROCs for the proposed method (.) and the original normal overlap method (o). The horizontal axis indicates the false positive number per case, and the vertical axis indicates the nodule detection sensitivity. (a) FROCs for nodule as small as $7\,mm$; (b) FROCs for nodule larger than $10\,mm$.

created manually, as described above) of the nodule. If there are more than one such positions for a single true nodule, only the position nearest to the true nodule is treated as the detected true nodule position, all the other positions are considered as FPs.

The value of the local maximum positions obtained from local shape controlled voting can be considered as the confidence score of being the center of nodules. FROC curves can be obtained accordingly, shown in Fig 6. It showed that the proposed local shape controlled voting method attained a better overall performance than the original surface normal overlap method. Here only nodules larger than $7mm$ are evaluated, as these nodules are of significant clinical importance.

The efficiency of the proposed method is also investigated. The average processing time of local shape controlled voting (excluding isotropic resampling, lung segmentation) for each case is around 24.2 seconds, compared to the average time 30.1 seconds for surface normal overlap. The reason for this is that the average number of qualified voter decreased dramatically, only 12.9% of the boundary points in the direct normal overlap procedure was allowed to stimulate a tracking under the local shape standards.

5   Conclusions

A novel method called local shape controlled voting was proposed for spherical object detection in 3D voxel images. This scheme improved surface normal overlap method proposed for detection of spherical objects by integrating differential characteristics into the global tracking procedure of normal overlap. The proposed method has been applied to computer aided detection of pulmonary nodules based on helical CT images. Validation on 42 high resolution clinical cases showed that this method attains a better performance compared to the original normal overlap technique. Additionally, the time efficiency is also improved.

References

1. Giger, M.L., Bae, K.T., MacMahon, H.: Computerized detection of pulmonary nodules in computed tomography images. Investigate. Radiol. 29, 459–465 (1994)
2. Armato, S.G., Giger, M.L., Moran, C.J., Blackburn, J.T., Doi, K., MacMahon, H.: Computerized detection of pulmonary nodules on CT scans. Radiographics 19, 1303–1311 (1999)
3. Kanazawa, K., Kawata, Y., Niki, N., Satoh, H., Ohmatsu, H., Kakinuma, R., Kaneko, M., Moriyama, N., Eguchi, K.: Computer-aided diagnostic system for pulmonary nodules based on helical CT images. In: Doi, K., MacMahon, H., Giger, M.L., Hoffmann, K. (eds.) Computer-Aided Diagnosis Medical Imaging, pp. 131–136. Elsevier, Amesterdam, The Netherlands (1999)
4. Lee, Y., Hara, T., Fujita, H., Itoh, S., Ishigaki, T.: Automated detection of pulmonary nodules in helical CT images based on an improved template-matching technique. IEEE Transactions on Medical Imaging 20, 595–604 (2001)
5. Paik, D.S., Beaulieu, C.F., Rubin, G.D., Acar, B., Jeffrey, R.B., Yee Jr., J., Dey, J., Napel, S.: Surface normal overlap: a computer-aided detection algorithm with application to colonic polyps and lung nodules in helical CT. IEEE Transactions on Medical Imaging 23, 661–675 (2004)
6. Zhang, X., McLennan, G., Hoffman, E.A.: Automated detection of small-size pulmonary nodules based on helical CT images. In: Christensen, G.E., Sonka, M. (eds.) IPMI 2005. LNCS, vol. 3565, pp. 664–676. Springer, Heidelberg (2005)
7. Mendoca, P.R.S., Bhotika, R., Sirohey, S.A., Turner, W.D., Miller, J.V.: Model-based analysis of local shape for lesion detection in CT scans. In: Duncan, J.S., Gerig, G. (eds.) MICCAI 2005. LNCS, vol. 3749, pp. 688–695. Springer, Heidelberg (2005)
8. Ridler, T.W., Calvard, S.: Picture thresholding using an iterative selection method. Man and Cybernetics 8, 630–632 (1978)
9. Besl, P.J., Jain, R.C.: Segmentation through variable-order surface fitting. IEEE Trans. Patt. Anal. Machine Intell. 10, 167–192 (1988)
10. Koenderink, J.J., van Doorn, A.J.: Surface shape and curvature scales. Image and Vision Computing 10, 557–565 (1992)
11. Thirion, J.P., Gourdon, A.: Computing the differential characteristics of isointensity surfaces. Computer Vision and Image Understanding 61, 190–202 (1995)

Global Medical Shape Analysis Using the Laplace-Beltrami Spectrum

Marc Niethammer[1,2,5], Martin Reuter[3,4], Franz-Erich Wolter[3,4],
Sylvain Bouix[1,2,5], Niklas Peinecke[3], Min-Seong Koo[6],
and Martha E. Shenton[1,5]

[1] Psychiatry Neuroimaging Laboratory
[2] Laboratory of Mathematics in Imaging,
Brigham and Women's Hospital, Harvard Medical School, Boston MA, USA
[3] Welfenlab, Leibniz University of Hannover, Germany
[4] Deslab, Massachusetts Institute of Technology, Boston MA, USA
[5] Laboratory of Neuroscience, VA Boston Healthcare System, Brockton MA, USA
[6] Dept. of Psychiatry, Kwandong University College of Medicine, Kangnung, Korea

Abstract. This paper proposes to use the Laplace-Beltrami spectrum (LBS) as a global shape descriptor for medical shape analysis, allowing for shape comparisons using minimal shape preprocessing: no registration, mapping, or remeshing is necessary. The discriminatory power of the method is tested on a population of female caudate shapes of normal control subjects and of subjects with schizotypal personality disorder.

1 Motivation and Background

Morphometric studies of brain structures have classically been based on volume measurements. More recently, shape studies of gray matter brain structures have become popular. Methodologies for shape comparison may be divided into global and local shape analysis approaches. While local shape comparisons [1,2] yield powerful, spatially localized results that are relatively straightforward to interpret, they usually rely on a number of preprocessing steps: one-to-one correspondences between surfaces need to be established, shapes need to be registered and resampled, possibly influencing shape comparisons. While global shape comparison methods cannot spatially localize shape changes they may be used to indicate the existence of shape differences between populations. Global approaches may be formulated with a significantly reduced number of assumptions and preprocessing steps in comparison to local approaches, staying as true as possible to the original data.

This paper describes a methodology for global shape comparison based on the Laplace-Beltrami spectrum (LBS) [3,4] of a Riemannian manifold (of closed surfaces in space). Previous approaches for global shape analysis in medical imaging include the use of invariant moments [5], the shape index [6], and global shape descriptors based on spherical harmonics [7]. The proposed methodology based on the LBS differs in the following ways from these previous approaches:

N. Ayache, S. Ourselin, A. Maeder (Eds.): MICCAI 2007, Part I, LNCS 4791, pp. 850–857, 2007.
© Springer-Verlag Berlin Heidelberg 2007

- It works for any Riemannian manifold, whereas spherical harmonics based methods are restricted to surfaces with spherical topology, and invariant moments do not easily generalize to arbitrary Riemannian manifolds. It may thus be used to analyze surfaces, solids, non-spherical objects, etc.
- The only preprocessing required is the extraction of a surface approximation from a manually segmented binary volume. No registration, remeshing, or additional mappings are necessary. Further the description is invariant to isometries and remeshing.

2 Shape-DNA: The Laplace-Beltrami Spectrum

In this section we introduce the necessary background for the computation of the LBS beginning sequence (also called "Shape-DNA"). The "Shape-DNA" is a signature computed only from the intrinsic geometry of an object. It is the beginning sequence of the spectrum of the LB operator defined for real valued functions on Riemannian manifolds and can be used to identify and compare objects like surfaces and solids independent of their representation, position and, if desired, independent of their size. This methodology was first introduced in [8] with a first description of basic ideas given in [9]. The LBS can be regarded as the set of squared frequencies (the so called natural or resonant frequencies) that are associated to the eigenmodes of an oscillating membrane defined on the manifold. (E.g., the eigenmodes of a sphere are the spherical harmonics.) Let us review the basic theory in the general case (see [3,4] for details).

Let f be a real-valued function, with $f \in C^2$, defined on a Riemannian manifold M. The **Laplace-Beltrami Operator** Δ is: $\Delta f := \operatorname{div}(\operatorname{grad} f)$ with grad f the **gradient** of f and div the **divergence** on the manifold. The LB operator is a linear differential operator. It can be calculated in local coordinates. Given a local parametrization $\psi : \mathbb{R}^n \to \mathbb{R}^{n+k}$ of a submanifold M of $\mathbb{R}^{n+k}$ with

$$g_{ij} := \langle \partial_i \psi, \ \partial_j \psi \rangle, \ \ G := (g_{ij}), \ \ W := \sqrt{\det G}, \ \ (g^{ij}) := G^{-1} \qquad (1)$$

(where $i, j = 1(1)n$, det is the determinant) we get: $\Delta f = \frac{1}{W} \sum_{i,j} \partial_i(g^{ij} W \partial_j f)$. If M is a domain in the Euclidean plane $M \subset \mathbb{R}^2$ the LB operator is the well known Laplacian $\Delta f = \frac{\partial^2 f}{(\partial x)^2} + \frac{\partial^2 f}{(\partial y)^2}$. The **Laplacian eigenvalue problem** is

$$\Delta f = -\lambda f, \qquad (2)$$

its solutions represent the spatial part of the solutions of the wave eq. (with an infinite number of eigenvalue λ and eigenfunction f pairs). In the case where the Riemannian manifold M is a planar region, $f(u, v)$ in eq. (2) can be understood as the natural vibration form (also **eigenfunction**) of a homogeneous membrane with **eigenvalue** λ. Any properties of the material are ignored. The standard boundary condition of a fixed membrane is $f \equiv 0$ on the boundary of the surface domain (Dirichlet boundary condition).

The **spectrum** is defined to be the family of eigenvalues of eq. 2, consisting of a diverging sequence $0 \le \lambda_1 \le \lambda_2 \le \cdots \uparrow +\infty$, with each eigenvalue repeated according to its multiplicity and with each associated finite dimensional eigenspace. In the case of a closed manifold without a boundary the first eigen-value λ_1 is always equal to zero, because in this case the constant functions are non-trivial solutions of the Laplacian eigenvalue problem.

The spectrum is an **isometric invariant** as it only depends on the gradient and divergence which in turn are defined to be dependent only on the Riemannian structure of the manifold, i.e., the intrinsic geometry. Furthermore, **scaling** an n-dimensional manifold by a factor a results in eigenvalues scaled by a factor $\frac{1}{a^2}$. Thus, by normalizing the eigenvalues, shape can be compared regardless of the object's scale and position. The spectrum **depends continuously** on the shape of the manifold [10]. We use cubic triangular finite elements for the computation of the spectra [3,4].

Normalization: The LBS is a diverging sequence. Analytic solutions for the spectrum are only known for a limited number of shapes. For the unit 2-sphere the eigenvalues are $\lambda_i = i(i+1)$, $i \in \mathbb{N}_0$ with multiplicity $2i + 1$. In general the eigenvalues asymptotically tend to a line with a slope dependent on the surface area of the 2D manifold M: $\lambda_n \sim \frac{4\pi n}{\text{area}(M)}$, as $n \uparrow \infty$. Therefore, a difference in surface area manifests itself in different slopes of the eigenvalue asymptotes. Fig. 1 shows the behavior of the spectra of a population of spheres

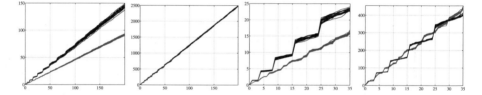

Fig. 1. Spectral behavior from left to right: (a) unnormalized, (b) Area normalized, (c) unnormalized (zoom), (d) Area normalized (zoom). Eigenvalue (ordinate) versus eigenvalue number (abscissa).

and a population of ellipsoids respectively. The sphere population is based on a unit sphere where Gaussian noise is added in the direction normal to the surface of the noise-free sphere. Gaussian noise is added in the same way to the ellipsoid population. Since the two basic shapes (sphere and ellipsoid) differ in surface area, their unnormalized spectra diverge (Fig. 1 a). Area normalization greatly improves the spectral alignment (Fig. 1 b). Figs 1 c) and d) show zoom-ins of the spectra for small eigenvalues. For the unnormalized as well as for the surface area normalized case, the spectra of the two populations clearly differ, demonstrating that the LBS can detect shape- as well as size-differences.

Statistical testing results depend on the chosen normalization. When unnormalized spectra of populations with widely different surface areas are compared, larger eigenvalues lead to better discrimination of the groups (Fig. 1 a), however, this mainly reflects the surface area differences. A surface area normalization shows if *additional* shape differences exist. Having identical noise levels for the populations under investigation is essential, since different noise levels will affect surface areas differently, with increased surface areas for increased noise levels (see Fig. 2 for an illustration). Violating this assumption may yield to the detection of noise level differences as opposed to shape differences, as demonstrated in Fig. 2. For the analysis of identically acquired and processed shapes – e.g., obtained through manual segmentations – identical noise levels are a reasonable assumption; also, the expected accuracy of the spectra calculations is expected to be independent of population.

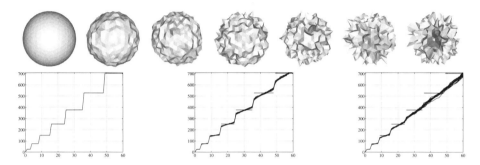

Fig. 2. Spectra of a sphere with different noise levels. The noise-free case on the left demonstrates the accuracy of the numerical eigenvalue computations. Spectra were normalized to unit surface area. Black horizontal lines: analytic spectrum of the noise-free sphere. Increasing levels of noise from left to right. Eigenvalue (ordinate) versus eigenvalue number (abscissa).

3   Statistical Analysis of Groups of LB Spectra

Given the (possibly normalized) LB spectra we use permutation tests to compare group features to each other (200,000 permutations were used for all tests). We use three different kinds of statistical analyses[1] (see [11] for details on permutation testing): **(i)** A two-sided, nonparametric, permutation test to analyze the scalar quantities: volume and surface area; **(ii)** a two-sided, nonparametric, multivariate permutation test based on the maximum t-statistic to analyze the high-dimensional spectral feature vectors (Shape-DNA); and **(iii)** independent permutation tests of the spectral feature vector components across groups (as in (ii)), followed by a false discovery rate (FDR) approach to correct for multiple comparisons, to analyze the significance of individual vector components.

To test scalar values the absolute mean difference is used as the test statistic $s = |\mu_a - \mu_b|$, where the μ_i indicates the group means. Due to the small number of samples compared to the dimensionality of the feature vectors (preventing the use of the Hotelling T^2 statistic), the maximum t-statistic

$$t_{max} = \max_{1 \leq j \leq N} \frac{|\overline{e}_{a,j} - \overline{e}_{b,j}|}{SE_j} \qquad (3)$$

---

[1] All shapes are initially corrected for brain volume differences.

is chosen as the test statistic for the spectral feature vectors. Here, N is the vector dimension, $\bar{e}_{a,j}$ indicates the mean of the j-th vector component of group a, and SE_j is the pooled standard error estimate of the j-th vector component, defined as

$$SE_j = \frac{\sqrt{(n_a - 1)\sigma_{a,j}^2 + (n_b - 1)\sigma_{b,j}^2}}{\sqrt{\frac{1}{n_a} + \frac{1}{n_b}}}, \tag{4}$$

where n_i is the number of subjects in group i and $\sigma_{i,j}$ is the standard deviation of vector component j of group i. To account for the multiple comparison problem when testing individual vector components, the significance levels are corrected based on an FDR of 5% [12].

4   Results

Volume measurements are the simplest means of morphometric analysis. While volume analysis results are easy to interpret, they only characterize one morphometric aspect of a structure. The following Sections introduce the LBS as a method for a more complete global structural description using the analysis of a caudate as an exemplary brain structure. For brevity all results are presented for the right caudate only.

Populations: Magnetic Resonance (MR) images of the brains of 32 neuroleptic-naïve female subjects diagnosed with Schizotypal Personality Disorder (SPD) and of 29 female normal control subjects were acquired on a 1.5-T General Electric MR scanner. Spoiled-gradient recalled acquisition images (voxel dimensions, 0.9375 x 0.9375 x 1.5 mm) were obtained coronally. The images were used to delineate the caudate nucleus and to estimate the intracranial content [13].

Preprocessing: The caudate nucleus was delineated manually by an expert. Interrater reliability (based on intraclass correlation coefficients) among three raters for the right caudate volume were high (r=.94). Interrater reliabilities were computed by three raters on the brain scans of five randomly selected subjects from the pool of subjects [13]. The isosurfaces separating the binary label maps of the caudate shapes from the background were extracted using marching cubes (assuring spherical topology). Analysis was performed on the resulting triangulated surfaces directly (referred to as unsmoothed surfaces) as well as on the same set of surfaces smoothed and resampled using spherical harmonics[2] (referred to as smoothed surfaces). The unsmoothed surfaces are used as a benchmark dataset subject to only minimal preprocessing, whereas the smoothed surfaces are used to demonstrate the influence of additional preprocessing. See Fig. 3 for an example of a smoothed and an unsmoothed caudate.

Volume and Area Analysis: For comparison, results for a volume and a surface area analysis are shown in Fig. 3. As has been previously reported for this

---

[2] We used the spherical harmonics surfaces as generated by the UNC shape analysis package [1].

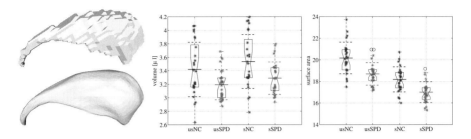

Fig. 3. Exemplary caudate shape unsmoothed and with spherical harmonics smoothing (left). Group comparisons for volume differences (middle) and surface area differences (right). Smoothed results prefix 's', unsmoothed results prefix 'us'. Volume and surface area reductions are observed for the SPD population in comparison to the normal control population.

dataset [13], subjects with schizotypal personality disorder exhibit a statistically significant volume reduction compared to the normal control subjects. While smoothing plays a negligible role for the volume results (smoothed: $p = 0.008$, volume loss 7.0%, i.e., there is a chance of $p = 0.008$ that the volume loss is a random effect; unsmoothed: $p = 0.013$, volume loss 6.7%), the absolute values of the surface area are affected more, since smoothing impacts surface area more than volume. While surface smoothing is desirable to reduce noise effects, the result for the female caudates shows the same trend for the surface areas (but not for magnitude) in the smoothed and the unsmoothed cases (smoothed: $p = 0.00019$; unsmoothed: $p = 0.000085$).

Laplace-Beltrami Spectrum Analysis: The LB spectrum was computed for the female caudate population using surface area normalization. A maximum t-statistic permutation test on a 100-dimensional spectral shape descriptor shows significant shape differences (see Tab. 1) for surface area normalization for the unsmoothed surfaces, but not for the smoothed ones. Surface area normalization is the strictest normalization in terms of spectral alignment. Testing for surface area independently yields statistically significant results.

Fig. 4 indicates that using too many eigenvalues has a slightly detrimental effect on the observed statistical significance. This is sensible, since higher order modes correspond to higher frequencies and are thus more likely noise, which can overwhelm the statistical testing. In this particular example, a few small eigenvalues distinguish the shapes (explaining the sharp initial drop in Fig. 4), while the upward slope is explained by adding an increasing number of eigenvalues that no longer contribute to the shape discrimination of the two populations. It is thus sensible to restrict oneself only to a subset of the spectrum (e.g., the first 20). However, this subset needs to be agreed upon before the testing and cannot be selected after the fact. Note, that the LBS results of Tab. 1 show statistically significant shape differences even when the strong influence of surface area is removed, which suggests that the LBS indeed picks up shape differences that complement area and volume findings. The LBS can detect surface area differences (since the surface areas may be extracted from the spectrum) and can distinguish objects with identical surface area or volume based on their shape. Future work, computing the LBS of solids, will try to disentangle the influence of volume and area differences further. Our shape difference findings are consistent with results previously reported in [6,13] for a population of male caudates and the same population of female caudates used in this paper.

Table 1. Shape comparison results for the maximum t-statistic permutation test for the unsmoothed and smoothed dataset. Volume and area results for comparison.

	normalization	p-value (unsmoothed)	p-value (smoothed)
LBS (N=20)	unit brain volume	0.0026	0.0013
	unit caudate surface area	0.0050	0.63
LBS (N=100)	unit brain volume	0.00032	0.00092
	unit caudate surface area	0.026	0.84
Volume	unit brain volume	0.013	0.0078
	unit caudate surface area	0.0011	0.011
Area	unit brain volume	0.000045	0.00022
	unit caudate volume	0.001	0.011

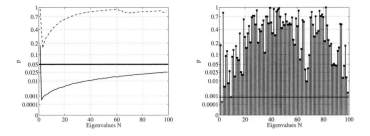

Fig. 4. Maximum t-statistic results of area normalized case (**left**) for the first n eigenvalues (solid line: unsmoothed, dashed line: smoothed) and (**right**) for individual eigenvalues (unsmoothed case) with FDR multiple comparison correction. The black horizontal lines correspond to the 5% significance level and the 5% FDR corrected significance level respectively. The left plot shows statistical results for the analysis of shape-DNAs of different lengths. The right plot shows statistical results for individual spectral components. Since the statistically most significant eigenvalue cannot be selected after the statistical analysis, a shape-DNA-based analysis with prespecified length is useful.

5   Conclusion

This paper showed the applicability and utility of the LBS for shape analysis in medical imaging. The maximum t-statistic was used for a group analysis of LB spectra. In particular, the paper demonstrates that the LBS can reliably be computed on (iso)surfaces without preprocessing, e.g., surface smoothing, and that the normalizations of the spectra greatly influence the outcome of the statistical procedure. In particular, the surface area normalized results indicate that there are true shape differences. Future work will focus on the computation of volume spectra.

Acknowledgements

This work was supported in part by a Dept. of Veteran Affairs Merit Award (SB,MS), a Research Enhancement Award Program (MS), NIH grants R01 MH50747 (SB,MS), K05 MH070047 (MS), U54 EB005149 (MN,SB,MS), and a Humboldt Foundation postdoctoral fellowship (MR).

References

1. Styner, M., Oguz, I., Xu, S., Brechbühler, C., Pantazis, D., Levitt, J.J., Shenton, M.E., Gerig, G.: Framework for the statistical shape analysis of brain structures using SPHARM-PDM. In: Open Science Workshop at MICCAI (2006)
2. Nain, D., Styner, M., Niethammer, M., Levitt, J.J., Shenton, M.E., Gerig, G., Bobick, A., Tannenbaum, A.: Statistical shape analysis of brain structures using spherical wavelets. In: ISBI (2007)
3. Reuter, M., Wolter, F.E., Peinecke, N.: Laplace-Beltrami spectra as "Shape-DNA" of surfaces and solids. Computer-Aided Design 38(4), 342–366 (2006)
4. Reuter, M.: Laplace Spectra for Shape Recognition. Books on Demand (2006)
5. Mangin, J.F., Poupon, F., Duchesnay, E., Riviere, D., Cachia, A., Collins, D.L., Evans, A.C., Regis, J.: Brain morphometry using 3D moment invariants. Medical Image Analysis 8, 187–196 (2004)
6. Levitt, J.J., Westin, C.-F., Nestor, P.G., Estepar, R.S.J., Dickey, C.C., Voglmaier, M.M., Seidman, L.J., Kikinis, R., Jolesz, F.A., McCarley, R.W., Shenton, M.E.: Shape of the caudate nucleus and its cognitive correlates in neuroleptic-naive schizotypal personality disorder. Biological Psychiatry 55, 177–184 (2004)
7. Gerig, G., Styner, M., Jones, D., Weinberger, D., Lieberman, J.: Shape analysis of brain ventricles using SPHARM. In: MMBIA Workshop, pp. 171–178 (2001)
8. Reuter, M., Wolter, F.-E., Peinecke, N.: Laplace-spectra as fingerprints for shape matching. In: SPM 2005: ACM Symposium on Solid and Physical Modeling, pp. 101–106. ACM Press, New York (2005)
9. Wolter, F.E., Friese, K.: Local and global geometric methods for analysis, interrogation, reconstruction, modification and design of shape. In: CGI 2000, pp. 137–151 (2000)
10. Courant, R., Hilbert, D.: Methods of Mathematical Physics. Interscience (1953)
11. Good, P.: Permutation, Parametric, and Bootstrap Tests of Hypotheses, 3rd edn. Springer, Heidelberg (2005)
12. Genovese, C.R., Lazar, N.A., Nichols, T.: Thresholding of statistical maps in functional neuroimaging using the false discovery rate. Neuroimage 15, 870–878 (2002)
13. Min-Seong, K., Levitt, J., McCarley, R.W., Seidman, L.J., Dickey, C.C., Niznikiewicz, M.A., Voglmaier, M.M., Zamani, P., Long, K.R., Kim, S.S., Shenton, M.E.: Reduction of caudate nucleus volumes in neuroleptic-naive female subjects with schizotypal personality disorder. Biological Psychiatry 60, 40–48 (2006)

Real-Time Tracking of the Left Ventricle in 3D Echocardiography Using a State Estimation Approach

Fredrik Orderud[1], Jøger Hansgård[2], and Stein I. Rabben[3]

[1] Norwegian University of Science and Technology, Norway
fredrik.orderud@idi.ntnu.no
[2] University of Oslo, Norway
jogerh@ifi.uio.no
[3] GE Vingmed Ultrasound, Norway
stein.rabben@med.ge.com

Abstract. In this paper we present a framework for real-time tracking of deformable contours in volumetric datasets. The framework supports composite deformation models, controlled by parameters for contour shape in addition to global pose. Tracking is performed in a sequential state estimation fashion, using an extended Kalman filter, with measurement processing in information space to effectively predict and update contour deformations in real-time. A deformable B-spline surface coupled with a global pose transform is used to model shape changes of the left ventricle of the heart.

Successful tracking of global motion and local shape changes without user intervention is demonstrated on a dataset consisting of 21 3D echocardiography recordings. Real-time tracking using the proposed approach requires a modest CPU load of 13% on a modern computer. The segmented volumes compare to a semi-automatic segmentation tool with 95% limits of agreement in the interval 4.1 ± 24.6 ml ($r = 0.92$).

1 Introduction

The emergence of volumetric image acquisition within the field of medical imaging has attracted a lot of scientific interest over the last years. In a recent survey, Noble *et al.* [1] presented a review of the most significant attempts for automatic segmentation within the field of ultrasonics. However, all of these attempts are limited to being used as postprocessing tools, due to extensive processing requirements, even though volumetric acquisition may be performed in real-time with the latest generation of 3D ultrasound technology. Availability of technology for real-time tracking and segmentation in volumetric datasets would open up possibilities for instant feedback and diagnosis during data acquisition. Automatic tracking of the main chamber of the heart, the left ventricle (LV), would here serve as an excellent application.

Orderud [2] recently presented a tracking approach that allows for real-time tracking of rigid bodies in volumetric datasets. The approach treats the tracking

N. Ayache, S. Ourselin, A. Maeder (Eds.): MICCAI 2007, Part I, LNCS 4791, pp. 858–865, 2007.
© Springer-Verlag Berlin Heidelberg 2007

problem as a state estimation problem, and uses an extended Kalman filter to recursively track global pose parameters using a combination of state predictions and measurement updates. Experimental validation of LV tracking in 3D echocardiography, using a simple truncated ellipsoid model, was performed to demonstrate the feasibility of the approach.

This state estimation approach is based on prior work by Blake *et al.* [3,4], who used a Kalman filter to track B-spline contours deformed by linear transforms within a model subspace referred to as *shape space*. Later, the same approach was applied to real-time LV tracking in 2D echocardiography by Jacob *et al.* [5,6,7]. All these papers did, however, lack a separation between global pose and local shape. They were also restricted to linear deformations, such as principal component analysis deformation models, and to tracking in 2D datasets.

This paper extends [2] to support contours with composite deformation models, consisting of both local shape changes and global pose. We also propose to use a 3D B-spline surface model to circumvent the limitations of rigid ellipsoidal models for LV tracking. This model is coupled with a global pose transform, and successful LV tracking in 3D echocardiography is demonstrated.

This model somewhat resembles the deformable superquadrics model [8], and a 3D active shape model [9], but is spline-based, and allows for free-form shape deformations [10] by letting the control points move independently perpendicular to the surface.

2   Deformable Contour

The tracking framework is based upon a contour deformation model $\mathbf{T}$, which is decomposed into local deformations and global transformations. Local shape deformations are used to alter contour shape, by deforming points on a shape template $\mathbf{p}_0$ into intermediate contour shape points $\mathbf{p}_l$, using a local shape deformation model $\mathbf{T}_l$ with local state vector $\mathbf{x}_l$ as parameters:

$$\mathbf{p}_l = \mathbf{T}_l(\mathbf{p}_0, \mathbf{x}_l) \ . \tag{1}$$

The intermediate contour shape points $\mathbf{p}_l$ are subsequently transformed into final contour points $\mathbf{p}$, using a global pose transformation model $\mathbf{T}_g$ with global state vector $\mathbf{x}_g$ as parameters:

$$\mathbf{p} = \mathbf{T}_g(\mathbf{p}_l, \mathbf{x}_g) \ . \tag{2}$$

A composite deformation model $\mathbf{T}$ is then constructed by combining local and global deformations of shape template points into a joint model, as shown in Fig. 1. This yields a composite state vector $\mathbf{x} \equiv \left[\mathbf{x}_g^T, \mathbf{x}_l^T\right]^T$ consisting of N_g global and N_l local deformation parameters. Calculation and propagation of associated contour normals $\mathbf{n}$ through $\mathbf{T}$ must also be performed, since they are required to specify the search direction for the later edge-detection.

This separation between local and global deformations is intended to ease modeling, since changes in shape are often parameterized differently compared

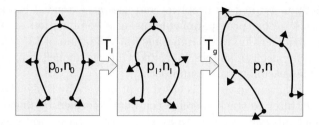

Fig. 1. Overview over the contour deformation and transformation process: The shape template $\mathbf{p}_0,\mathbf{n}_0$ is first deformed locally into $\mathbf{p}_l,\mathbf{n}_l$, followed by a global transformation into the final contour $\mathbf{p},\mathbf{n}$

to deformations associated with global position, size and orientation. It also puts very few restrictions on the allowable deformations, so a wide range of parameterized deformation models can be used, including nonlinear models, as opposed to previous *shape space* models that are limited to linear deformations.

3   Tracking Framework

The proposed tracking framework follows the processing chain of the Kalman filter, starting by predicting contour state using a motion model (section 3.1). The shape template is subsequently deformed to form a predicted contour, and associated normal vectors and state-space Jacobi matrices are computed (section 3.2). Edge detection is then performed locally along the normal vectors. Finally, all measurement information is assimilated in information space [11], and combined with the predicted contour to compute an updated contour state estimate (section 3.3). Figure 2 shows an overview over these steps.

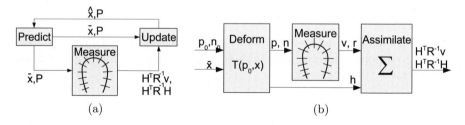

Fig. 2. (a) Overview of the tracking scheme. (b) Illustration of how points on the shape template $\mathbf{p}_0$, $\mathbf{n}_0$ are first deformed using a predicted state $\bar{\mathbf{x}}$, yielding a deformed contour $\mathbf{p}$, $\mathbf{n}$ and measurement vector $\mathbf{h}$. Edges are then measured relative to the predicted contour, resulting in normal displacements v with associated measurement error variances r. The edge measurements are finally assimilated into an information vector and matrix for efficient processing.

3.1   Motion Model

Modeling of motion, in addition to position, is accomplished in the prediction stage of Kalman filter by augmenting the state vector to contain the last two successive state estimates. A *motion model* which predicts the state $\bar{\mathbf{x}}$ at timestep $k + 1$, is then expressed as:

$$\bar{\mathbf{x}}_{k+1} - \mathbf{x}_0 = \mathbf{A}_1(\hat{\mathbf{x}}_k - \mathbf{x}_0) + \mathbf{A}_2(\hat{\mathbf{x}}_{k-1} - \mathbf{x}_0) \ , \tag{3}$$

where $\hat{\mathbf{x}}_k$ is the estimated state from timestep k. Tuning of properties like damping and regularization towards the mean state $\mathbf{x}_0$ for all deformation parameters can then be accomplished by adjusting the coefficients in matrices $\mathbf{A}_1$ and $\mathbf{A}_2$. Prediction uncertainty can similarly be adjusted by manipulating the process noise covariance matrix $\mathbf{B}_0$ used in the associated covariance update equation. The latter will then restrict the change rate of parameter values.

3.2   Edge Measurements

Processing of edge measurements using an extended Kalman filter [12] requires *state-space* Jacobi matrices to relate changes in contour point positions to changes in contour state. Separate Jacobi matrices for each contour point must therefore be calculated. The choice of composite deformations leads to state-space Jacobi matrices consisting of two separate parts, namely of global and local derivatives:

$$\frac{\partial \mathbf{T}(\mathbf{p}_0, \mathbf{x})_i}{\partial \mathbf{x}} \equiv \left[\frac{\partial \mathbf{T}_g(\mathbf{p}_l, \mathbf{x}_g)_i}{\partial \mathbf{x}_g}, \quad \sum_{n \in x,y,z} \frac{\partial \mathbf{T}_g(\mathbf{p}_l, \mathbf{x}_g)_i}{\partial \mathbf{p}_{l,n}} \frac{\partial \mathbf{T}_l(\mathbf{p}_0, \mathbf{x}_l)_n}{\partial \mathbf{x}_l} \right] \ . \tag{4}$$

The global Jacobian becomes a $3 \times N_g$ matrix, while the Jacobian for the local shape deformations becomes the product of a 3×3 matrix by a $3 \times N_l$ matrix using the chain rule for multivariate calculus.

Edge detection is performed by measuring the distance between points $\mathbf{p}_i$ on a predicted contour inferred from the motion model, and edges $\mathbf{p}_{obs,i}$ detected by searching in normal direction $\mathbf{n}_i$ of the contour surface. This type of edge detection is referred to as *normal displacement* [4], and is calculated as follows:

$$v_i = \mathbf{n}_i^T (\mathbf{p}_{obs,i} - \mathbf{p}_i) \ . \tag{5}$$

Each normal displacement measurement is coupled with a measurement noise value r_i that specifies the uncertainty associated with the edge, which may either be constant for all edges, or dependent on edge strength, or other measure of uncertainty.

Linearized measurement models [12], which are required in the Kalman filter for each edge measurement, are constructed by transforming the state-space Jacobi matrices the same way as the edge measurements, namely by projecting them onto the normal vector:

$$\mathbf{h}_i^T = \mathbf{n}_i^T \frac{\partial \mathbf{T}(\mathbf{p}_0, \mathbf{x})_i}{\partial \mathbf{x}} \ . \tag{6}$$

This yields a separate *measurement vector* $\mathbf{h}_i$ for each normal displacement measurement, to relate normal displacements to changes in contour state.

3.3   Measurement Assimilation and State Update

Contour tracking forms a special problem structure, since the number of measurements far exceeds the number of state dimensions. Ordinary Kalman gain calculations then becomes intractable, since they involve inverting matrices of dimensions equal to the number of measurements. An alternative approach is to assimilate measurements in *information space* prior to the state update step. This enables very efficient processing if we assume that measurements are independent. All measurement information can then be summed into an information vector and matrix of dimensions invariant to the number of measurements:

$$\mathbf{H}^T\mathbf{R}^{-1}\mathbf{v} = \sum_i \mathbf{h}_i r_i^{-1} v_i \tag{7}$$

$$\mathbf{H}^T\mathbf{R}^{-1}\mathbf{H} = \sum_i \mathbf{h}_i r_i^{-1} \mathbf{h}_i^T \ . \tag{8}$$

Measurements in information filter form require some alterations to the state update step in the Kalman filter. This can be accomplished by using the information filter formula [11] for the updated state estimate $\hat{\mathbf{x}}$ at timestep k:

$$\hat{\mathbf{x}}_k = \bar{\mathbf{x}}_k + \hat{\mathbf{P}}_k\mathbf{H}^T\mathbf{R}^{-1}\mathbf{v}_k \ . \tag{9}$$

The updated error covariance matrix $\hat{\mathbf{P}}$ can similarly be calculated in information space to avoid inverting matrices with dimensions larger than the state dimension:

$$\hat{\mathbf{P}}_k^{-1} = \bar{\mathbf{P}}_k^{-1} + \mathbf{H}^T\mathbf{R}^{-1}\mathbf{H} \ . \tag{10}$$

4   Experiments

We used a quadratic B-spline surface consisting of 24 control points arranged in a prolate spheroid grid as a LV model. Shape deformations were enabled by allowing the control points to move perpendicularly to the surface. This was combined with a global model for translation and scaling in three dimensions, as well as rotation around two of the axes. In total, this resulted in a deformation model consisting of 32 parameters. Edge detection was performed in the normal direction of approximately 450 contour points distributed evenly over the surface, using 30 samples spaced 1 mm apart. A simple edge detector based upon the transition criterion with variable height [13] is used to determine the position of the strongest edge along each normal. This detector assumes edges to form a transition in image intensity, from a dark cavity to a bright myocardium, and calculates the edge position that minimizes the sum of squared errors between a transition model and the data. Weak and outlier edges were automatically rejected to improve robustness.

4.1   Results

A collection of 21 apical 3D echocardiography recordings of adult patients, of which half were diagnosed with heart diseases, were used to validate the method.

The recordings were acquired with a Vivid 7 scanner (GE Vingmed Ultrasound, Norway), using sub-volume stitching to form a contiguous wide-angle recording of the LV. The exact same tracking configuration was used for all recordings, with an initial LV contour placed at a predefined position in the first frame. The tracking were then run for a couple of heartbeats to give the contour enough time to lock on to the LV. Tracking accuracy was evaluated by comparing the segmentations with the results from a custom-made semiautomatic segmentation tool (GE Vingmed Ultrasound), that facilitates manual editing. The reference segmentations were validated and, if needed, edited by an expert operator.

Figure 3 shows the overall volume correspondence throughout the cardiac cycle, for all frames in all of the 21 recordings. Bland-Altman analysis of the volume points in Fig. 3(a) yields a 4.1 ml bias, with 95% limits of agreement in the interval 4.1 ± 24.6 ml, and a strong correlation ($r = 0.92$). The average point to surface distance between the contour and the reference surfaces was 2.7 mm.

The volume curves were usually very similar in shape compared to the reference method. However, some per-recording bias was seen. This is illustrated in Fig. 3(b), where each volume curve is more or less parallel to the identity line, but have different offset. If we subtract the 'per-recording' bias from each volume curve, the limits of agreement is improved to ± 11.0 ml, indicating that much of the disagreement stems from the varying bias from recording to recording.

Figure 4 shows the intersection between the segmented contour and several slices throughout the volume in one of the recordings, as well as a plot of the volume of the segmented contour throughout the cardiac cycle.

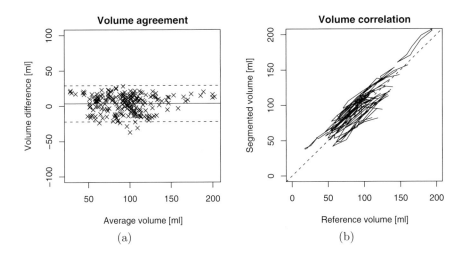

Fig. 3. Bland-Altman plot for the overall correspondence between automatically real-time segmented volumes and the reference (a), along with the mean volume difference (solid) and 95% limits of agreement (dashed). Associated volume correlation plot (b), where segmented volume curves from each recording is compared to the reference and shown as separate lines, along with the identity line (dashed).

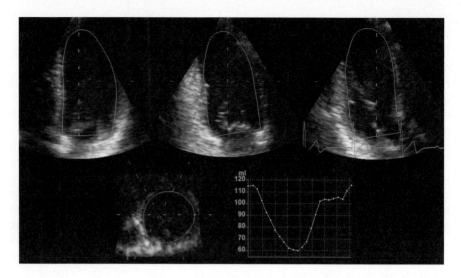

Fig. 4. Example of successful real-time tracking, showing intersections between the segmented contour and several slices through the volume, as well as a plot of the volume of the segmented contour for one cardiac cycle

The CPU load required to maintain real-time segmentation at 25 frames per second (fps) was approximately 13% when visualization was disabled[1].

5   Discussion and Conclusion

A novel framework for real-time tracking of deformable contours in volumetric datasets using a state estimation approach has been proposed. It extends prior work [2] by enabling tracking of contours with both local and global modes of deformation, both of which may be nonlinear. Compared to traditional deformable model based segmentation methods, the non-iterative Kalman filter algorithm leads to outstanding computational performance.

The feasibility of real-time LV tracking in 3D echocardiography has been demonstrated by successful tracking and segmentation in 21 recordings using a quadratic B-spline model coupled to a global pose transform. This represents a significant improvement over [2], that solely tracked chamber position, orientation and size, using an ellipsoid model, and were thus inherently unable of segmenting shape changes of the LV. The framework is well suited for rapid analysis of LV volumes and global function, since it operates without user interaction. Other applications, like patient monitoring, and automatic initialization of other methods are also possible.

Tracking accuracy is primarily limited by the difficulty of edge detection in echocardiography recordings, which suffers from inherently poor image quality.

---

[1] The experiments were performed using a C++ implementation on a 2.16 GHz Intel Core 2 duo processor.

It is in fact difficult, even for experts, to accurately determine the endocardial border in such recordings. Replacement of the simplistic transition criterion with a more advanced edge-detector, specifically designed for the ultrasound modality, is therefore believed to give better tracking accuracy.

Acknowledgment. The authors would like to thank Brage Amundsen at the Norwegian University of Science and Technology for providing the 3D echocardiography datasets.

References

1. Noble, J.A., Boukerroui, D.: Ultrasound image segmentation: A survey. Medical Imaging, IEEE Transactions on 25(8), 987–1010 (2006)
2. Orderud, F.: A framework for real-time left ventricular tracking in 3D+T echocardiography, using nonlinear deformable contours and kalman filter based tracking. In: Computers in Cardiology (2006)
3. Blake, A., Curwen, R., Zisserman, A.: A framework for spatiotemporal control in the tracking of visual contours. International Journal of Computer Vision 11(2), 127–145 (1993)
4. Blake, A., Isard, M.: Active Contours: The Application of Techniques from Graphics, Vision, Control Theory and Statistics to Visual Tracking of Shapes in Motion. Springer-Verlag, New York, Inc. Secaucus, NJ, USA (1998)
5. Jacob, G., Noble, J.A., Mulet-Parada, M., Blake, A.: Evaluating a robust contour tracker on echocardiographic sequences. Medical Image Analysis 3(1), 63–75 (1999)
6. Jacob, G., Noble, J.A., Kelion, A.D., Banning, A.P.: Quantitative regional analysis of myocardial wall motion. Ultrasound in Medicine & Biology 27(6), 773–784 (2001)
7. Jacob, G., Noble, J.A., Behrenbruch, C., Kelion, A.D., Banning, A.P.: A shape-space-based approach to tracking myocardial borders and quantifying regional left-ventricular function applied in echocardiography. Medical Imaging, IEEE Transactions on 21(3), 226–238 (2002)
8. Park, J., Metaxas, D., Young, A.A., Axel, L.: Deformable models with parameter functions for cardiac motion analysis from tagged MRI data. Medical Imaging, IEEE Transactions on 15(3), 278–289 (1996)
9. Cootes, T.F., Taylor, C.J., Cooper, D.H., Graham, J.: Active shape models - Their training and application. Computer Vision and Image Understanding 61(1), 38–59 (1995)
10. Rueckert, D., Sonoda, L.I., Hayes, C., Hill, D.L.G., Leach, M.O., Hawkes, D.J.: Nonrigid registration using free-form deformations: application to breast MR images. Medical Imaging, IEEE Transactions on 18(8), 712–721 (1999)
11. Comaniciu, D., Zhou, X.S., Krishnan, S.: Robust real-time myocardial border tracking for echocardiography: An information fusion approach. Medical Imaging, IEEE Transactions on 23(7), 849–860 (2004)
12. Bar-Shalom, Y., Li, X.R., Kirubarajan, T.: Estimation with Applications to Tracking and Navigation. Wiley-Interscience, Chichester (2001)
13. Rabben, S.I., Torp, A.H., Støylen, A., Slørdahl, S., Bjørnstad, K., Haugen, B.O., Angelsen, B.: Semiautomatic contour detection in ultrasound M-mode images. Ultrasound in Med. & Biol. 26(2), 287–296 (2000)

Vessel and Intracranial Aneurysm Segmentation Using Multi-range Filters and Local Variances

Max W.K. Law and Albert C.S. Chung

Lo Kwee-Seong Medical Image Analysis Laboratory,
Department of Computer Science and Engineering,
The Hong Kong University of Science and Technology, Hong Kong
{maxlawwk,achung}@cse.ust.hk

Abstract. Segmentation of vessels and brain aneurysms on non-invasive and flow-sensitive phase contrast magnetic resonance angiographic (PCMRA) images is essential in the detection of vascular diseases, in particular, intracranial aneurysms. In this paper, we devise a novel method based on multi-range filters and local variances to perform segmentation of vessels and intracranial aneurysms on PCMRA images. The proposed method is validated and compared using a synthetic and numerical image volume and four clinical cases. It is experimentally shown that the proposed method is capable of segmenting vessels and aneurysms with various sizes on PCMRA images.

1 Introduction

Brain aneurysms are vascular diseases caused by abnormal dilation of the cerebral arteries. The presence of brain aneurysms is potentially fatal as the burst of aneurysms can lead to severe internal bleeding. In the past decade, there has been a growing interest in the detection of brain vessels and aneurysms by performing analysis on angiography. Hernandez *et al.* proposed two training based geodesic active region methods in [1,2], and a technique using the Hessian matrix [3] and a Gaussian mixture model in [4] to segment aneurysms in computed tomography (CT) angiography. Kawata *et al.* made use of a template that a sphere was attached on a tube to discover aneurysms based on cone-beam CT images. In [5], Bruijne *et al.* described how to perform segmentation of aneurysms in multi-spectral magnetic resonance images with the help of user interaction when training data was limited.

As a non-invasive and flow-sensitive acquisition technique, phase contrast magnetic resonance angiographic (PCMRA) images are useful to assess patient conditions. One of the limitations of the PCMRA images is the low image contrast of vasculature, especially the regions inside aneurysms. Furthermore, due to slow blood flow inside aneurysms, the intensity values of aneurysms are significantly lower than those of the vessels in PCMRA. The intensity drops between vessels and the attached aneurysms create large intensity changes which are easy to be misinterpreted as vessel boundaries and cause incorrect segmentation of aneurysms by the traditional vascular segmentation approaches such as [6,7].

In this paper, a novel method is proposed for the segmentation of intracranial aneurysms in PCMRA images. The proposed method requires neither training,

N. Ayache, S. Ourselin, A. Maeder (Eds.): MICCAI 2007, Part I, LNCS 4791, pp. 866–874, 2007.
© Springer-Verlag Berlin Heidelberg 2007

which causes the segmentation results depending on the training data; nor shape assumption, which is possibly inflexible to handle variation of aneurysm shapes. To cope with the aforementioned limitations of PCMRA images, the proposed method makes use of a new detection filter and local variances. This detection filter aims at recognizing the intensity changes of the aneurysm boundaries. This filter complements with local variances to reduce the effect of noise and suppress the responses induced from high intensity vessels to avoid the missing of low intensity aneurysms. Furthermore, a multi-range scheme is employed to provide a detection response to handle the size variations of aneurysms. The proposed method is validated and compared using a synthetic and numeric image volume, and four PCMRA images acquired from a collaborating hospital. It is experimentally shown that the proposed method is capable of segmenting low contrast aneurysms with various sizes on PCMRA images.

2   Methodology

A New Detection Filter

To determine whether a local voxel is inside an aneurysm, it is necessary to detect the intensity changes induced by the aneurysm boundaries. Along a line from a voxel inside an aneurysm to any position of the image background, an intensity drop can be observed at the aneurysm boundary. The first part of this work is to devise a filter to detect such intensity changes. Due to the variations of sizes and shapes of aneurysms, this filter is required to be sensitive to the intensity changes that occur in different directions and distances relative to a local voxel in an aneurysm.

To design such a detection filter, a set of translated and rotated first derivative of Gaussian filters are added up as a single detection filter. To illustrate this idea, we firstly consider the filter in a 1D case, i.e. $f_{l,\sigma}^{1D}(x) = \frac{1}{2}(G_x^\sigma(x+l)+G_{-x}^\sigma(-x-l))$, where G_x^σ is the first derivative of a Gaussian function with the scale parameter σ along x. $f_{l,\sigma}^{1D}$ includes translating and differentiating the Gaussian function in both the x and $-x$ directions to detect intensity changes that occur in any direction in 1D (including the positive and negative directions) and distance l away from a local pixel (see Fig. 1a and Fig. 1c is in the case of 2D). In 3D cases, the filter is given by,

$$f_{l,\sigma}(x,y,z) = \frac{1}{K}\sum_k^K G_{\hat{n}_k}^\sigma(x+l\hat{n}_k\cdot(1,0,0)^T, y+l\hat{n}_k\cdot(0,1,0)^T, z+l\hat{n}_k\cdot(0,0,1)^T),$$

(1)

where $\hat{n}_k$ is the k-th orientation sample and K is the total number of the orientation samples which sweep across the surface of a sphere (see an example in Fig. 1d). In our implementation, the total number of orientation samples K guarantees that there is at least one orientation sample for each unit area on the surface of a sphere having radius l. This isotropic filter is capable of detecting intensity changes that take place in any direction with distance l away from a local voxel. As such, for a local voxel located in l voxels away from the aneurysm boundary, the filtering response of this local voxel is negative if it is inside an aneurysm, or positive if it is outside an aneurysm.

Multi-Range Detection and Local Variances

Using the above detection filter, a multi-range scheme is employed to recognize intensity changes that occur in various distances away from a local voxel. The multi-range scheme is based on obtaining responses using a group of $f_{l,\sigma}$ with various values of l and a small constant value σ. The main purpose of utilizing various values of l instead of σ is that the enlargement of σ intends to anni-hilate low contrast structures. Based on the multi-range scheme, there are as many filtering responses as the number of ranges being utilized. However, for a range that does not match the distance between a local voxel and the aneurysm boundary, the corresponding filtering response is possibly driven by noise and becomes unreliable. It is essential to have another measurement to appropriately suppress the responses associated with undesired ranges prior to the employment of a multi-range scheme.

To suppress the responses of undesired ranges, local variances are utilized,

$$V_{l,\sigma}(x,y,z) = \int B_{l,\sigma}(u,v,w)\{I(x+u,y+v,z+w) - \mu_{l,\sigma}(x,y,z)\}^2 dudvdw, \quad (2)$$

where μ is the averaged intensity of the local region covered by $B_{l,\sigma}(x,y,z)$, $\mu_{l,\sigma}(x,y,z) = \int B_{l,\sigma}(u,v,w)I(x+u,y+v,z+w)dudvdw$, and $B_{l,\sigma}$ is a filter of smoothed spherical step function with radius $l+\sigma$, defined as,

$$B_{l,\sigma} = G^\sigma * b_{l+\sigma} \text{ where } b_r(x,y,z) = \begin{cases} 1/4\pi r^3 & \text{if } \sqrt{x^2+y^2+z^2} \le r \\ 0 & \text{otherwise.} \end{cases} \quad (3)$$

An 1D example of the above filter, denoted as $B_{l,\sigma}^{1D}$, is shown in Fig. 1b. This filter $B_{l,\sigma}$ is designed to cover a region that $f_{l,\sigma}$ is close to or equal to zero. The local variance $V_{l,\sigma}(x,y,z)$ based on this filter quantifies the local intensity similarity within the coverage of $B_{l,\sigma}$. It returns a large value if the intensity values inside the filter coverage are fluctuating. Such fluctuation implies that an object boundary passes though the filter coverage and thus, this local region possibly belongs to different objects. Therefore, the filtering response of $f_{l,\sigma} * I$ is unreliable for deciding whether a local voxel is inside an aneurysm. Hence, we weight the response $f_{l,\sigma} * I$ by the local variance $V_{l,\sigma}$ to acquire a reliable measure, which reflects how likely a local voxel is inside an aneurysm,

$$R_{l,\sigma}(x,y,z) = \frac{f_{l,\sigma} * I(x,y,z)}{\sqrt{V_{l,\sigma}(x,y,z)} + \rho}, \quad (4)$$

where ρ is a parameter which should be assigned with the consideration of the intensity values of the dimmest part of the target aneurysm. Since the coverage of the spherical filter $B_{l,\sigma}$ (Eq. 3) used by $V_{l,\sigma}$ includes the coverage of $f_{l,\sigma}$ (see Figs. 1a and b), the intensity changes which can be detected by $f_{l,\sigma}$ also affect the local variance $V_{l,\sigma}$. For a high contrast boundary, such as boundaries of vessels connected with aneurysms, it can result in a local variance value which

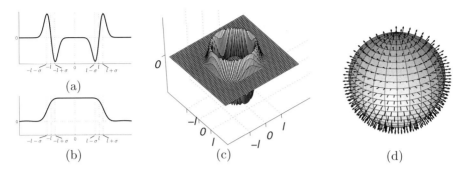

Fig. 1. (a) $f_{l,\sigma}^{1D}(x)$. (b) $B_{l,\sigma}^{1D}(x)$. (c) $f_{l,\sigma}^{2D}(x,y)$. (d) An example of orientation samples taken for computation of $f_{l,\sigma}^{3D}(x,y,z)$.

is large relative to ρ (i.e. $\sqrt{V_{l,\sigma}} \gg \rho$). Weighting the filtering responses $f_{l,\sigma}$ by $\sqrt{V_{l,\sigma}} + \rho$ not only suppresses the responses obtained in undesired ranges, but also restrains the value of $R_{l,\sigma}$ from being too large with the presence of high contrast boundaries where both the values of $f_{l,\sigma} * I$ and $V_{l,\sigma}$ increase. It is beneficial to avoid the high contrast vessel boundaries dominating the detection results and causing missing of low intensity aneurysms in segmentation results.

Grounded on the detection response in Eq. 4, a set of detection ranges l, denoted as $L = \{l_1, l_2, ..., l_P\}, l_1 < l_2 < .... < l_P$, is used for multi-range detection,

$$S_{L,\sigma}(x,y,z) = \max\{R_{l_1,\sigma}(x,y,z), 0\} + \min\{\min_q(R_{l_q,\sigma}(x,y,z)), 0\}. \quad (5)$$

The minimum range, l_1 should be assigned with the consideration of the narrowest part of the aneurysm. The rest of the ranges in L are suggested to ensure that the voxels inside the aneurysm can reach the aneurysm boundary by a distance included in L. $S_{L,\sigma}$ in Eq. 5 embodies two components, the former part is positive valued, which determines if a local voxel is outside an aneurysm away from the boundary of the aneurysm with distance l_1. It is zero if $R_{l_1,\sigma}(x,y,z)$ is negative which indicates that in the range l_1, the voxel is located inside an aneurysm. For the later component, it is negative valued and judges how likely a local voxel is inside an aneurysm. It searches all ranges for the highest negative detection response which indicates that the local voxel is inside an aneurysm.

Active Surface Model

The multi-range detection response described above is able to indicate how likely a voxel belongs to an aneurysm (negative responses) or outside an aneurysm (non-negative responses). Based on this detection response, a level set framework [8] is utilized to find a region which maximizes the negative multi-range detection response. As such, a level set function ψ is evolved as $\frac{d\psi}{dt} = S|\nabla\psi| + \kappa\left(\nabla\frac{\nabla\psi}{|\nabla\psi|}\right)$, where κ is a length regularization term which is 0.05 in our implementation to maintain surface smoothness. The other parameters to solve the differential equation follow the description in [9] and the implementation is based on [10].

The evolution of the level set function is stopped when the accumulated per-voxel update of the level set function was less than 10^{-5} for 10 iterations.

3   Experimental Results

A synthetic and numerical volume and four clinical PCMRA images were utilized in the experiments. Two gradient based active surface segmentation methods (Geodesic Active Contour, **GAC** [6]; Flux Maximizing Geometric Flows, **FLUX** [7]) were implemented and compared with the proposed method (**MRFLV**). In **FLUX** and **GAC**, all the images involved were pre-smoothed by a Gaussian with the scale parameter 1. In **GAC**, an edge detector $1/(1 + |m\nabla I_\sigma|^n)$ was employed, where I_σ was the smoothed image, $n = 4$ and $n = 2$ for the synthetic and clinical volumes respectively; $m = 32$ and $m = 1$ for synthetic and clinical volumes respectively to enlarge the intensity changes of edges for the edge detector so that the object boundaries can be located correctly. The above parameters were set carefully to provide the best segmentation results for **GAC** in the experiments. For **MRFLV**, σ was 1 (Eq. 4) in all the experiments. Other parameters such as the radii associated with the multiscale scheme of **FLUX**, the range set L (Eq.5) and ρ (Eq.4) of **MRFLV** were assigned according to the conditions of images based on the description presented in Section 2. The values of those parameters are indicated individually in the figure captions for different cases, Figs. 3, 4, 5.

A synthetic and numerical image volume
In the first experiment, a synthetic and numerical image volume was used (Fig. 2). In this volume, a tube was attached with eight spheres with various combinations of sizes and intensities (Figs. 2a and b). This volume was smoothed

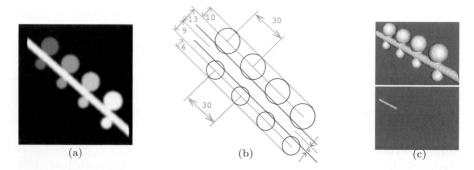

(a)   (b)   (c)

Fig. 2. The $128 \times 128 \times 128$ voxel synthetic and numerical image volume. (a) A maximum intensity projection of the image volume. From the upper left corner to the lower right corner, the intensity values for each pair of spheres with radii 10 and 6 voxels are 0.4, 0.6, 0.8 and 1.0 respectively. (b) The description of the settings of the image volume, the numbers are in unit voxel. (c) Top: The isosurface of the image volume. Bottom: The initial level set function utilized in the experiments.

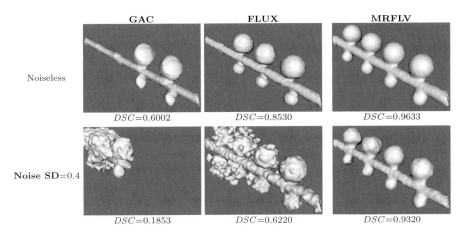

Fig. 3. The segmentation results of **GAC**; **FLUX**, radii=$\{2,3...6\}$; and **MRFLV**, $\rho = 4, L = \{2,3...6\}$

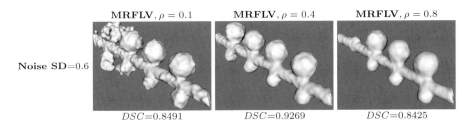

Fig. 4. Segmentation results of **MRFLV**, $L = \{2,3...6\}$ various values of ρ

with a Gaussian filter ($\sigma = 1$) to mimic the smooth intensity transition between different structures. In addition, Rayleigh noise with different noise levels (specified by standard deviation and mentioned as **Noise SD** hereafter) was utilized to corrupt the image. The noise levels, **Noise SD**s, were assigned according to the fact that the image background intensity standard deviation is similar to the intensity of aneurysms in the clinical cases. There are two challenges to segment all spheres attached on the tube without leakage. First, the high intensity changes occurred at the connection between the tube and the low intensity spheres prohibit the active surface to propagate into the low intensity spheres. Second, the low contrast boundaries of the low intensity spheres result in inadequate intensity changes to stop the evolution of surface and lead to leakages.

    MRFLV, **FLUX** and **GAC** were applied on the noiseless and **Noise SD**=0.4 cases with the initial level set function shown in the bottom of Fig. 2c. In Fig. 3, the segmentation results and Dice Similarity Coefficient (DSC) [11] are shown. In the noiseless case (first row of Fig. 3), both **GAC** and **FLUX** were not able to pick all the spheres as the surfaces were halted by the high intensity changes of the connections between the low intensity spheres and the tube. For the noisy case (second row of Fig. 3), **GAC** and **FLUX** had leakages. It is worth to mention that leakages or unfaithful halts of surfaces lead to unsatisfactory performance of aneurysm segmentation. On the contrary, **MRFLV** (Fig. 3) that was able to pick all the spheres without leakage in the both cases is suitable to discover low intensity aneurysms attached to high intensity vessels.

For **Noise SD**=0.6, only **MRFLV** was examined as other methods were failed when **Noise SD**=0.4. This case demonstrated the results of **MRFLV** using various values of ρ (Eq. 4). As stated previously, the value of ρ should be assigned with the intensity value of the dimmest part of the target aneurysm. An undersized ρ resulted in high sensitivity of low contrast voxels which leads to leakage (left of Fig. 4). On the other hand, a large value of ρ causes missing of low contrast structures (right of Fig. 4). With properly assigned values of ρ, $\rho = 0.4$, **MRFLV** provided the best results (middle of Fig. 4). Furthermore, the slight drop of DSC values of **MRFLV** between different noisy cases and the noiseless case (the third column of Fig. 3 and middle of Fig. 4) implies that **MRFLV** is robust to handle noisy cases. Such robustness is essential to prevent leakages when performing segmentation of low intensity aneurysms.

Clinical cases

In the clinical cases, to demonstrate the results of **MRFLV**, the slices of the aneurysmal regions and the resultant contours of **MRFLV** are shown in Fig. 5. Since the voxel intensity inside aneurysms are significantly lower than the vessels which the aneurysms attached on, to display the aneurysms along with the vessels, the pixels having intensity larger than 350 are displayed as having intensity value 350. Due to the space limitation, the result comparison is focused on the regions containing aneurysms. The cases that no observable result was obtained due to severe leakages at the position of aneurysms are indicated as "Failed". The initial seeds for these four cases were obtained by thresholding the 0.2% of the total number of voxels with the highest intensity values.

The segmentation results of these clinical cases are presented in Fig. 5. It is observed that **GAC** has leakages and cannot segment the aneurysms in these cases (Figs. 5b, c, f, g, j and l). Also, **FLUX** has leakage in the first case (Figs. 5b and c). The main cause of leakages is that the evolving surfaces followed the noise attached on the aneurysm boundaries. Although **FLUX** had no leakage in the second, third and forth cases (Figs. 5f, g, j and l), **FLUX** could not discover the low intensity parts of the aneurysms (Figs. 5f, g, j and l). In contrast, **MRFLV** demonstrated a promising performance to cope with the aneurysms in different shapes (irregular shape in the first and second cases, Figs 5a-h; and blob shapes in the rest of the cases, Figs 5i-m) and various sizes (see the differences of the detection ranges utilized in the first, second cases in Figs. 5b, c, f, g and the third, forth cases in Figs. 5j and l). Furthermore, since the initial seeds were obtained by intensity thresholding and they were located in the high intensity major vessels, the active surfaces of **MRFLV** were able to evolve from the high intensity vessels to the low intensity aneurysms. As such, the proposed method is shown to be able to handle the intensity drops in the connection of the vessels and the aneurysms (see the contours in Figs 5d, h, k and m, and the vessel

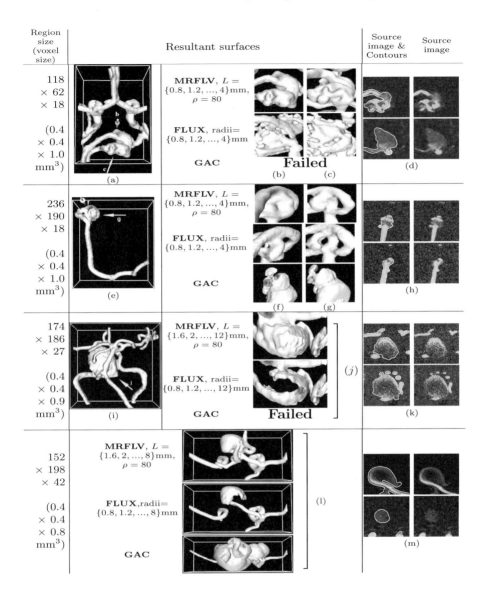

Fig. 5. The segmentation results of clinical cases corresponding to four regions of interest extracted from four distinct PCMRA images. (a-d) The first case; (e-h) the second case; (i-k) the third case; (l, m) the forth case. (a, e, i, l(top)) The resultant surfaces of **MRFLV** in the regions of interest. (a, e, i) The white arrows show the positions of the aneurysms and the view angles to obtain the zoomed-views shown in (b, c, f, g, j). (l(middle, bottom)) The resultant surfaces of different methods in the regions of interest. (b, c, f, g, j) The zoomed-views of the segmentation results of different methods at the aneurysm regions. (d, h, k, m) Slices of the aneurysmal regions and the corresponding contours of **MRFLV**, the pixels having intensity larger than 350 are shown as having intensity value 350 for the purpose of illustration.

intensities are higher than those appeared in these figures as the intensity above 350 were cropped for better visualization only).

4 Conclusion

We have presented a new method to segment vessels and intracranial aneurysms in PCMRA image volumes. The proposed method, called **MRFLV**, is validated using a synthetic and numerical image volume and four clinical cases. In the experiments, **MRFLV** is capable of selecting the low intensity aneurysms having various sizes and shapes without leakages of active surfaces, as well as coping with the intensity changes occurred in the connection between vessels and aneurysms. Two gradient based vascular segmentation approaches are utilized to compare with **MRFLV**. It is experimentally demonstrated that **MRFLV** can provide promising segmentation results of aneurysms on PCMRA images.

References

1. Hernandez, M., Frangi, A.: Geodesic active regions using non-parametric satistical regional description and their application to aneurysm segmentation from cta. In: MIAR, pp. 94–102 (2004)
2. Hernandez, M., Frangi, A., Sapiro, G.: Three-dimensional segmentation of brain aneurysms in cta using non-parametric region-based information and implicit deformable models: method and evaluation. In: Ellis, R.E., Peters, T.M. (eds.) MICCAI 2003. LNCS, vol. 2879, pp. 594–602. Springer, Heidelberg (2003)
3. Sato, Y., Nakajima, S., et al.: Three-dimensional multi-scale line filter for segmentation and visualization of curvilinear structures in medical images. MedIA. 2(2), 143–168 (1998)
4. Hernandez, M., Barrena, R., et al.: Pre-clincial evaluation of implicit deformable models for three-dimensional segmentation of brain aneurysms in cta. In: SPIE MI pp. 1264–1274 (2003)
5. Bruijne, M., Ginneken, B., et al.: Automated segmentation of abdominal aortic aneurysms in multi-spectral mr images. In: Ellis, R.E., Peters, T.M. (eds.) MICCAI 2003. LNCS, vol. 2879, pp. 538–545. Springer, Heidelberg (2003)
6. Caselles, V., Kimmel, R., Sapiro, G.: Geodesic Active Contours. ICCV 22, 61–79 (1997)
7. Vasilevskiy, A., Siddiqi, K.: Flux Maximizing Geometric Flows. T. PAMI. 24(12), 1565–1578 (2002)
8. Malladi, R., Sethian, J., Vemuri, B.: Shape Modeling with Front Propagation: A Level Set Approach. T. PAMI 17(2), 158–175 (1995)
9. Whitaker, R.: A Level-Set Approach to 3D Reconstruction from Range Data. IJCV 29(33), 203–231 (1998)
10. Ibanez, L., Schroeder, W., Ng, L., Cates, J. (The ITK Software ToolKit)
11. Zijdenbos, A., Dawant, B., et al.: Morphometric analysis of white matter lesions in mr images: Method and validation. IEEE. TMI 13(4), 716–724 (1994)

Fully Automatic Segmentation of the Hippocampus and the Amygdala from MRI Using Hybrid Prior Knowledge

Marie Chupin[1,2], Alexander Hammers[3], Eric Bardinet[2], Olivier Colliot[2], Rebecca S.N. Liu[4], John S. Duncan[1], Line Garnero[2], and Louis Lemieux[1]

[1] Department of Clinical and Experimental Epilepsy, IoN, UCL, London, UK
m.chupin@ion.ucl.ac.uk, l.lemieux@ion.ucl.ac.uk[*]
[2] Cognitive Neuroscience and Brain Imaging, CNRS UPR640, UPMC, Paris, France
[3] Faculty of Medicine, ICL, London, UK
[4] National Hospital for Neurology and Neurosurgery, UCLH, London, UK

Abstract. The segmentation of macroscopically ill-defined and highly variable structures, such as the hippocampus Hc and the amygdala Am, from MRI requires specific constraints. Here, we describe and evaluate a hybrid segmentation method that uses knowledge derived from a probabilistic atlas and from anatomical landmarks based on stable anatomical characteristics of the structures. Combined in a previously published semi-automatic segmentation method, they lead to a fast, robust and accurate fully automatic segmentation of Hc and Am. The probabilistic atlas was built from 16 young controls and registered with the "unified segmentation" of SPM5. The algorithm was quantitatively evaluated with respect to manual segmentation on two MRI datasets: the 16 young controls, with a leave-one-out strategy, and a mixed cohort of 8 controls and 15 subjects with epilepsy with variable hippocampal sclerosis. The segmentation driven by hybrid knowledge leads to greatly improved results compared to that obtained by registration of the thresholded atlas alone: mean overlap for Hc on the 16 young controls increased from 78% to 87% ($p < 0.001$) and on the mixed cohort from 73% to 82% ($p < 0.001$) while the error on volumes decreased from 10% to 7% ($p < 0.005$) and from 18% to 8% ($p < 0.001$), respectively. Automatic results were better than the semi-automatic results: for the 16 young controls, average overlap increased from 84% to 87% ($p < 0.001$) for Hc and from 81% to 84% ($p < 0.002$) for Am, with equivalent improvements in volume error.

1 Introduction

Volumetric analyzes of brain structures can inform on mechanisms underlying disease progression. The hippocampus Hc and the amygdala Am are of major interest, due to their implication in epilepsy and Alzheimer's disease. Manual volume measurement still remains the norm, making large cohort studies difficult. Poor boundary definition makes segmentation of these two grey matter

---

[*] MC was funded by a European post doctoral Marie Curie fellowship.

N. Ayache, S. Ourselin, A. Maeder (Eds.): MICCAI 2007, Part I, LNCS 4791, pp. 875–882, 2007.
© Springer-Verlag Berlin Heidelberg 2007

structures from Magnetic Resonance Imaging (MRI) scans challenging. Prior knowledge from anatomical atlases is necessary to their coherent manual delineation. For automation, this knowledge can come from statistical information on shape [1][2] or deformations [3][4], which may not be suitable for diseased structures. Registering an atlas template derived from a single subject [5][6] has been shown to be influenced by the choice of the atlas [7], even if combined registration-segmentation methods [8] may prove less sensitive. Registration and segmentation using probabilistic information [9][10][11] offer more thorough global spatial knowledge. It is complementary to anatomical knowledge [12] [13], which formalizes stable global and local anatomical relationships.

Fully automatic, fast and robust segmentation of healthy and pathological hippocampi and amygdale suitable for routine use has yet to be demonstrated. On the one hand, segmentation methods based on probabilistic information require high dimensional deformations [10], in order to achieve precise extraction. On the other hand, methods based mainly on image intensity can be fast, but need a good initialisation to be accurate. We describe a new fully automatic hybrid segmentation algorithm that combines the two methods by using global spatial knowledge from a probabilistic atlases within a previously published semi-automatic algorithm driven by anatomical knowledge [13]. The new algorithm's performance is evaluated on data from healthy controls and a mixed cohort including subjects with hippocampal sclerosis associated with chronic epilepsy.

2 Method

The method is based on iterative two-object competitive deformation [13]. Two regions deform following local topology-preserving transformations from two initial objects, within an extracted bounding box embedding Hc and Am. Bounding box and initial objects are automatically retrieved from probabilistic atlases. Here, the deformation process is constrained by hybrid prior knowledge derived from probabilistic atlases and neuroanatomical landmarks automatically detected during the deformation. The process is driven by minimizing a global energy functional in a Markovian framework. A competitive scheme allows the identification of the partly visible Hc-Am interface. At each iteration, the energy functional is modified according to probabilistic and anatomical likelihood.

2.1 Construction of the Am and Hc Probabilistic Atlases

MRI data from 16 young controls (S1-S16) were manually segmented by an expert following a 3D protocol [13], ensuring 3D-coherent structures. This results in a set of 32 binary labeled datasets, 16 with both Hc $\{Hc_i, i = 1...16\}$ and 16 with both Am $\{Am_i, i = 1...16\}$. The transformation from native to MNI standard space, $\{T_i, i = 1...16\}$, is computed with the unified segmentation module of SPM5 [14], which allows to iteratively optimize registration parameters (linear combination of cosine transformation bases), tissue classification, and intensity

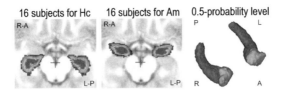

Fig. 1. Axial section showing probabilistic atlases for Hc and Am and 3D renderings of the 0.5-level of the probability maps (Hc in red, Am in green)

non-uniformity correction. The SPM5 default parameters are used. The probabilistic atlases PA_{Hc} and PA_{Am} (Fig 1) are created as follows:

$$\forall v \in \Omega, PA_{Hc}(v) = \frac{1}{16}\sum_{i=1}^{16} T_i(Hc_i)(v) \ and \ PA_{Am}(v) = \frac{1}{16}\sum_{i=1}^{16} T_i(Am_i)(v) \quad (1)$$

where v is a voxel in the MRI set Ω. $PA_{Hc}(v)$, resp. $PA_{Am}(v)$, is the probability that v belongs to Hc, resp. Am, according to the probabilistic atlas prior.

2.2 Initialization of the Deformation

For a given subject, individual atlases IPA_{Hc} and IPA_{Am} are created by back registering the atlases PA_{Hc} and PA_{Am} to the subject's space, using the inverse deformation $\{(T_i,)^{-1}, i = 1...16\}$ computed by the SPM5 unified segmentation.

Bounding box: The bounding box BB_{HcAm} must fully embed Hc and Am but is not used as a geometrical constraint. It is defined as the smallest parallelepiped subvolume in Ω around the non-null probability object $HcAm^{min} = [v \in \Omega, \ IPA_{Hc}(v) > 0 \ or \ IPA_{Am}(v) > 0]$ (Fig 2).

Initial objects: The initial object Hc^{init}, resp. Am^{init}, is created from the maximum probability object Hc^{max}, resp. Am^{max}. Hc^{max} is defined as the 1-level of the probability map IPA_{Hc}. It is built by keeping the voxels for which the probability equals one, while regularising to prevent holes ($IPA_{Hc}(v) < 1$ but v is "inside" Hc^{max}) and wires ($IPA_{Hc}(v) = 1$ but v "spikes" from Hc^{max})

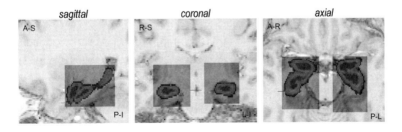

Fig. 2. Bounding box extraction, illustrated on sagittal, coronal and axial slices

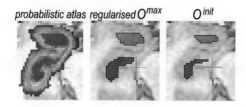

Fig. 3. Atlas, regularised object and initial object, for Hc and Am (axial slice)

to appear. Let $N^{6N}_{Hc^{max}}$ be the number of 6-neighbours of v labelled in Hc^{max}. If $N^{6N}_{Hc^{max}}$ is larger than 3, rejecting v from Hc^{max} will result in a hole in Hc^{max}; if $N^{6N}_{Hc^{max}}$ is smaller than 1, including v in Hc^{max} will result in a wire. Combining regularity rule and probability threshold iteratively, we get:

$$\begin{cases} [Hc^{max}]^0 = [v \in BB_{HcAm}, IPA_{Hc}(v) > 0] \\ [Hc^{max}]^i = \begin{bmatrix} IPA_{Hc}(v) = 1 \ and \ N^{6N}_{[Hc^{max}]^{i-1}}(v) \geq 1 \\ or \ IPA_{Hc}(v) \neq 1 \ and \ N^{6N}_{[Hc^{max}]^{i-1}}(v) \geq 3 \end{bmatrix} \end{cases}. \quad (2)$$

The iterations proceed until Hc^{max} (resp. Am^{max}) remains unchanged. Hc^{max} (resp. Am^{max}) is then eroded with a 1mm-structuring element, and the largest connected component is kept to create the initial object Hc^{init} (resp. Am^{init}) (Fig 3). The erosion step is introduced to increase robustness in case of atrophy.

2.3 Introduction of Hybrid Prior Knowledge

The regularisation term of the energy functional in [13] is modified to take into account the probability of the voxel v to belong to the deforming object O (Hc or Am), derived from IPA_{Hc} and IPA_{Am}. This term is locally expressed as the comparison of the number of O-labelled neighbours of v, $N_O(v)$, and a standard number of neighbours $\tilde{N}$, with σ^I a standard deviation around $\tilde{N}$:

$$E^I_O = \left(\frac{\tilde{N} - \gamma^{PZ}_O(v)\gamma^{AZ}_O(v)N_O(v)}{\sigma^I} \right)^5. \quad (3)$$

The γ parameters influence the classification according to prior probabilities for v to belong to O; for γ superior to 1, $N_O(v)$ is artificially increased, decreasing the energy, and vice versa for γ inferior to 1. γ^{AZ}_O models anatomical zones AZ defined by the anatomical landmarks ($\gamma^{AZ}_O(v) = 2$ if v is likely for O and 0.5 if v is unlikely for O). γ^{PZ}_O models probability zones PZ given by IPA_O: $\gamma^{PZ}_O(v) = 0.75$ if $IPA_O(v) = 0$, $\gamma^{PZ}_O(v) = 1.5$ if $0.75 \leq IPA_O(v) < 1$ and $\gamma^{PZ}_O(v) = 2$ if $IPA_O(v) = 1$; otherwise, $\gamma^{PZ}_O = 1$. Values are chosen empirically.

2.4 Atlas Mismatch: Automatic Detection and Correction Strategies

Atlas-based segmentation methods face a common problem: a possible initial mismatch of the atlas. An automatic strategy is used to detect such occurrences,

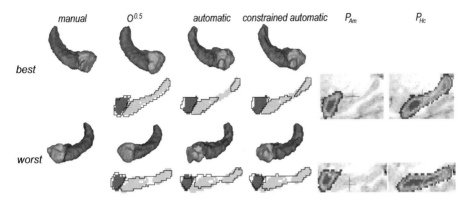

Fig. 4. 3D-renderings of automatic and manual segmentations, and overlap between segmentations (manual segmentations in shades of grey) and probabilistic atlases

based on two successive tests comparing intensity distributions for the grey matter (GM) and for the 0.5-level object for Hc: $Hc^{0.5} = [v \in \Omega, \; IPA_{Hc}(v) \geq 0.5]$. The first test detects cases when the deformed atlas fails to match the Hc sclerosis. It compares the average intensity on $Hc^{0.5}$ to that of GM; the assumption is that an overestimated $Hc^{0.5}$ when Hc is sclerotic will include cerebrospinal fluid dark voxels. The second test detects atlas misalignment in the region of interest. It compares the standard deviation on $Hc^{0.5}$ to that on an eroded version of $Hc^{0.5}$. The assumption is that a misaligned $Hc^{0.5}$ will include voxels of several tissues; for large misplacements, erosion will not reduce the standard deviation. An automatic correction strategy was introduced: if the atlas IPA_{Hc} is misaligned, the correction relies on decreasing the probabilistic constraint; if IPA_{Hc} is overestimated, the correction relies on shrinking IPA_{Hc} by erosion.

3   Performance Evaluation

The impact of the new automatic initialisation process and probabilistic atlas constraint on segmentation performance was evaluated with qualitative and quantitative comparisons between automatic (without and with atlas constraint), semi-automatic (with manual initialisation [13]) and manual segmentations [13] together with comparisons to the 0.5-level object derived from the registered atlas in subject's space ($Hc^{0.5}$ and $Am^{0.5}$), as a simple atlas-based segmentation.

3.1   Validation Data

The atlas is created using the 16 controls data (S1-S16 included in [13]), acquired in the axial plane; a leave-one-out procedure is followed, the atlas being derived from the remaining 15 subjects for each subject. Data from 23 subjects (mixed cohort), acquired in the coronal plane [15] were split into 3 groups: 8 healthy controls (C1-C8, Hc volume: $2.9 \pm 0.5 cm^3 (1.8 - 3.6)$), 8 subjects with epilepsy

Table 1. Segmentation performance index values in data from 16 healthy controls (top) and from the 23 subjects in the mixed cohort (bottom)

		semi-auto	$0^{0.5}$	automatic	constrained	corrected
			16 young controls			
Hc	RV	7 ± 4(0-14)	10 ± 6(1-26)	9 ± 6(0-25)	7 ± 4(0-15)	7 ± 4(0-15)
	K	84 ± 3(78-89)	78 ± 4(64-84)	82 ± 4(74-89)	87 ± 2(80-90)	87 ± 2(80-90)
	MIV	1.1 ± 1(0-4)	0.8 ± 1(0-5)	1.6 ± 2.3(0-9)	0.8 ± 0.8(0-4)	0.8 ± 0.8(0-4)
	DM	4.5 ± 1.5(3-9)	4 ± 1.3(3-9)	5.1 ± 2.4(2-15)	3.5 ± 1.2(2-8)	3.5 ± 1.2(2-8)
Am	RV	12 ± 7(1-27)	10 ± 8(0-33)	14 ± 9(1-35)	10 ± 6(0-26)	10 ± 6(0-26)
	K	81 ± 4(69-88)	82 ± 4(70-89)	77 ± 6(62-86)	84 ± 4(76-91)	84 ± 4(76-91)
	MIV	1.5 ± 1(0-4)	1.9 ± 2.2(0-9)	1.1 ± 0.7(0-2)	1.1 ± 1(0-5)	1.1 ± 1(0-5)
	DM	3.9 ± 0.9(3-6)	2.8 ± 0.5(2-4)	4.5 ± 1.1(3-7)	3.3 ± 0.7(2-7)	3.3 ± 0.7(2-7)
			mixed cohort			
Hc	RV			18 ± 15(0-74)	25 ± 39(0-200)	10 ± 11(0-64)	9 ± 7(0-33)
	K		73 ± 11(41-86)	70 ± 18(0-87)	81 ± 8(59-89)	82 ± 6(64-89)
	MIV		2.3 ± 4.7(0-28)	11 ± 14(0-68)	3.5 ± 8(0-48)	3.0 ± 5.6(0-33)
	DM		4.5 ± 2.9(2-20)	10 ± 5.5(3-27)	5.3 ± 2.9(3-14)	5.1 ± 2.6(3-14)
Am	RV		15 ± 10(0-44)	32 ± 42(0-200)	20 ± 14(1-58)	20 ± 13(1-54)
	K		75 ± 8(35-86)	63 ± 18(0-85)	77 ± 9(34-88)	77 ± 7(50-88)
	MIV		2.9 ± 3.4(0-13)	1.2 ± 0.9(0-10)	1.8 ± 2.3(0-10)	1.8 ± 2.3(0-10)
	DM		2.8 ± 3.6(2-7)	6.2 ± 2.7(3-16)	3.7 ± 0.9(2-6)	3.7 ± 0.9(2-6)

and known Hc sclerosis (HS1-HS8, $2.0 \pm 0.8 cm^3 (0.7 - 3.5)$), 7 subjects with temporal lobe epilepsy and normal Hc volumes (TL1-TL7, $2.6 \pm 0.5 cm^3 (1.6 - 3.4)$)). All datasets were manually segmented according to the same protocol as that used to create the atlas, by the same investigator. All processing apart from registration is run within the Anatomist software environment [16]. The whole segmentation procedure for both Hc and Am requires around 15min. Four indices are used to compare the segmentation S with the reference R [13]: $RV(S, R) = 2.|V_S - V_R|/(V_S + V_R)$, the error on volumes; $K(S, R) = 2.V_{S \cap R}/(V_S + V_R)$, the Dice overlap; $MIV(S_1, R_1, R_2) = 2.V_{S_1 \cap R_2}/(V_{S_1} + V_{R_1})$, the missclassified interface voxels and $DM(S, R) = \max[\max_{v \in \hat{S}}(d(v, \hat{R})), \max_{v \in \hat{R}}(d(v, \hat{S}))]$, the symmetric maximal distance, with $\hat{S}$ the 6-connectivity border of S. Significance for the variation of these values was tested using a two-tailed Student's t-test.

3.2   Validation Results in Young Healthy Controls

The segmentation results were found to be qualitatively correct. The two cases chosen for illustration (Fig 4) are those with the best and worst results in [13]. Table 1, top rows, summarizes the quantitative results. The automatic initialisation gives better results than the registered 0.5-level object, but inferior to the semi-automatic results [13]; the automatic results with atlas constraint are better than those from all other methods. No need for correction was detected.

3.3   Evaluation on Data from Mixed Cohort

Quantitative comparisons between automatic and manual segmentations (Table 1, bottom rows), show the importance of the atlas constraint on the results, even if the automatic results for Am were not significantly better than $Am^{0.5}$. Occasional initial atlas misalignments were observed; most were not detected as atlas mismatch but were nonetheless successfully corrected in the course of the automatic segmentation. Atlas mismatch was detected in 3 Hc out of 78, as illustrated in Fig. 5: atlas overestimation for two highly sclerotic Hc and atlas misalignment in another one. Segmentation failures were prevented with the correction strategy, as shown in the right column of Table 1. Note that the worst value for RV (33%) in our method was obtained for the smallest Hc in the group studied according to the manually estimated volume. $0.7cm^3$.

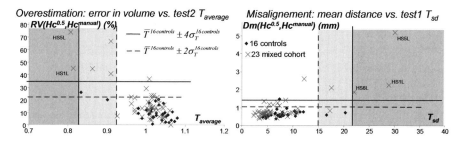

Fig. 5. Qualitative indices vs. detection test characterizing atlas mismatch (defined vs. the test value average on the 16 young controls with a range of 4 standard deviations).

4   Discussion and Conclusion

The combination of probabilistic knowledge and anatomical prior knowledge within the competitive deformation algorithm [13] allows accurate fully automatic segmentation of Hc and Am on healthy controls. The automatic detection and correction of initial atlas mismatch resulted in highly encouraging Hc segmentation on data from a representative group of subjects with epilepsy, including cases with high degrees of hippocampal sclerosis.

The fully automatic method performed better than both semi-automatic segmentation and 0.5-level probability object. For controls, the segmentation results (a K value of 87% for Hc and 84% for Am) compare favourably with the literature. In fact, K values are 83% for Hc [5] after manual placement of 28 landmarks, or 80% for Hc and 65% for Am [9], with similar errors on volumes. Using a method that requires the placement of 50 manual landmarks, a K of 88% for Hc was obtained [2]. The results for an entirely probabilistic method were 82% for Hc and 81% for Am [10]. Moreover, our results on patient data compare favourably with published results in subjects with epilepsy. Values for the 9 sclerotic Hc in HS1-8 (average volume: $1.4cm^3$ (0.7-2)) are K=76% (64-83) and RV=16% (4-33) for Hc, while in [5], they were, for 5 sclerotic Hc (average volume: $1.3cm^3$ (1.2-1.4), $K=67\%$ (57-75) and $RV=16\%$ (6-19). A recent study in sclerotic Hc ($1.2cm^3$ (1.1-1.6)) achieved similar overlap ($K=76\%$ (71-83)) but at the expense of about 2 weeks of CPU time [17].

References

1. Kelemen, A., et al.: Elastic model-based segmentation of 3-D neuroradiological data sets. IEEE TMI 18, 828–839 (1999)
2. Shen, D., et al.: Measuring size and shape of the hippocampus in MR images using a deformable shape model. Neuroimage 15, 422–434 (2002)
3. Duchesne, S., et al.: Appearance-based segmentation of medial temporal lobe structures. Neuroimage 17, 515–531 (2002)
4. Klemenčič, J., et al.: Non-rigid registration based active appearance models for 3D medical image segmentation. J. Imag. Sci. and Tech. 48(2), 166–171 (2004)
5. Hogan, R., et al.: Mesial temporal sclerosis and temporal lobe epilepsy: MR imaging deformation-based segmentation of the hippocampus in five patients. Radiology 216, 291–297 (2000)
6. Dawant, B., et al.: Automatic 3-D segmentation of internal structures of the head in MR images using a combination of similarity and free-form transformation. IEEE TMI 18, 909–916 (1999)
7. Carmichael, O., et al.: Atlas-based hippocampus segmentation in Alzheimer's disease and mild cognitive impairment. Neuroimage 27(4), 979–990 (2005)
8. Wang, F., et al.: Joint registration and segmentation of neuroanatomic structures from brain MRI. Academic Radiology 13, 1104–1111 (2006)
9. Fischl, B., et al.: Whole brain segmentation: Automated labelling of neuroanatomical structures in the human brain. Neuron. 33, 341–355 (2002)
10. Heckemann, R., et al.: Automatic anatomical brain MRI segmentation combining label propagation and decision fusion. Neuroimage 33, 115–126 (2006)
11. Pitiot, A., et al.: Expert knowledge-guided segmentation system for brain MRI. Neuroimage 23, S85–S96 (2004)
12. Bloch, I., et al.: Fusion of spatial relationships for guiding recognition, example of brain structure recognition in 3D MRI. Pattern Recogn. Let. 26, 449–457 (2005)
13. Chupin, M., et al.: Automated segmentation of the hippocampus and the amygdala driven by competition and anatomical priors: Method and validation on healthy subjects and patients with Alzheimer's disease. Neuroimage 34, 996–1019 (2007)
14. Ashburner, J., Friston, K.: Unified segmentation. Neuroimage 26, 839–851 (2005)
15. Liu, R., et al.: A longitudinal quantitative MRI study of community-based patients with chronic epilepsy and newly diagnosed seizures: Methodology and preliminary findings. Neuroimage 14, 231–243 (2001)
16. Rivière, D., et al.: A structural browser for human brain mapping. In: Human Brain Mapping p. 912 (2000)
17. Hammers, A., et al.: Automatic detection and quantification of hippocampal atrophy on MRI in temporal lobe epilepsy: A proof-of-principle study. Neuroimage 36, 38–47 (2007)

Clinical Neonatal Brain MRI Segmentation Using Adaptive Nonparametric Data Models and Intensity-Based Markov Priors

Zhuang Song[1], Suyash P. Awate[1], Daniel J. Licht[2], and James C. Gee[1]

[1] Departments of Radiology, University of Pennsylvania
[2] Division of Neurology, The Children's Hospital of Philadelphia
Philadelphia, PA, USA 19104
songz@seas.upenn.edu

Abstract. This paper presents a Bayesian framework for neonatal brain-tissue segmentation in *clinical* magnetic resonance (MR) images. This is a challenging task because of the low contrast-to-noise ratio and large variance in both tissue intensities and brain structures, as well as imaging artifacts and partial-volume effects in clinical neonatal scanning. We propose to incorporate a spatially adaptive likelihood model using a data-driven nonparametric statistical technique. The method initially learns an *intensity-based prior*, relying on the empirical Markov statistics from training data, using fuzzy nonlinear support vector machines (SVM). In an iterative scheme, the models adapt to spatial variations of image intensities via nonparametric density estimation. The method is effective even in the absence of anatomical atlas priors. The implementation, however, can naturally incorporate probabilistic atlas priors and Markov-smoothness priors to impose additional regularity on segmentation. The maximum-a-posteriori (MAP) segmentation is obtained within a graph-cut framework. Cross validation on clinical neonatal brain-MR images demonstrates the efficacy of the proposed method, both qualitatively and quantitatively.

1 Introduction

Magnetic resonance imaging (MRI) has become an important tool for the clinical study of neonatal brain development and neurodevelopmental disorders [1,2,3]. In neonatal brain MRIs, biological tissue properties, such as ongoing white-matter myelination and large water content, inherently limit inter-tissue intensity contrast-to-noise ratio (CNR), which is much lower than that of adult brain MRIs [1,2,4]. Compared to adult brains, neonatal brains have larger variation in size, shape, and cortical-folding patterns. Furthermore, time constraints and subject motion may introduce significant imaging artifacts, noise, and field inhomogeneities. These problems are exacerbated in *clinical* neonatal brain imaging, which is typically optimized for visual inspection with low inter-slice resolution causing significant partial-volume effects.

N. Ayache, S. Ourselin, A. Maeder (Eds.): MICCAI 2007, Part I, LNCS 4791, pp. 883–890, 2007.
© Springer-Verlag Berlin Heidelberg 2007

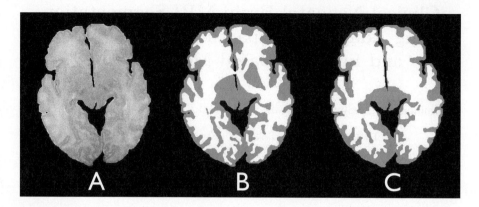

Fig. 1. An example slice of a neonatal brain T2-weighted axial MR image (A) and two manual segmentations of the same slice (B and C), showing significant disagreement

Several recent segmentation approaches [4,5] rely on probabilistic atlas priors that capture the spatial variability in the tissue structure of neonates. High quality atlases, however, are difficult to obtain, as there is often significant variability (especially near tissue boundaries and regions of myelination) in ground-truth manual segmentations from which the priors are derived (Figure 1). Because of low CNR and large variation in brain size and structures, incorporation of atlas priors also entails image registration which introduces another methodological challenge. These factors undermine the efficacy of the atlas-based approaches.

Another common element in segmentation approaches is the use of Gaussian probability density functions (PDFs) to model the tissue intensities. Such approaches have faced problems in adult brain MR tissue segmentation for producing anomalous behavior at low noise levels [6,7]. In tissue intensity histograms of neonatal brain MR images based on manual segmentations, the distributions are significantly different from Gaussians, which is consistent with the previously reported observation [4]. Awate et al. modeled the Markov statistics of each tissue nonparametrically and have shown improvements over the Gaussian scheme in adult brain MR tissue segmentation [8,9].

We propose a Bayesian framework for neonatal brain tissue segmentation in clinical magnetic resonance (MR) images. It incorporates adaptive models using data-driven nonparametric statistical estimation schemes. Furthermore, the models adapt to spatial variations in image statistics that arise from variations in brain structure and tissue composition, in addition to imaging inhomogeneity. We present an effective strategy for constructing intensity-based Markov priors using fuzzy nonlinear support vector machines (SVMs) [10]. The proposed method can naturally incorporate atlas priors for additional regularity on the segmentation, although it is shown to be reasonably effective even without atlas priors. In this way, our method reduces the dependence on atlas priors, which helps to address the challenges in neonatal atlas construction. We compute the maximum-a-posteriori segmentation using graph cuts. Graph-cut techniques efficiently find global, or near global, optima for MRF-based energy function [11].

2   Bayesian Segmentation with Markov Random Fields

Consider an image I defined on a set of voxels $\mathcal{T}$, the associated Markov neighborhood system $\mathcal{N}$, and an image of segmentation labels L. For voxel t, we denote the intensity by I_t, the segmentation label by L_t, the voxels in its Markov neighborhood by $\mathcal{N}_t$, and the intensities in the Markov neighborhood by $I_{\mathcal{N}_t}$. We consider the segmentation task as a Bayesian inference problem in a Markov-random-field (MRF) framework. The optimal label assignment minimizes the Gibbs energy:

$$E(L) = \sum_{t \in \mathcal{T}} V_1(L_t) + \sum_{t \in \mathcal{T}} \sum_{s \in \mathcal{N}_t} V_2(L_t, L_s), \qquad (1)$$

where $V_1(\cdot)$ and $V_2(\cdot)$ are the clique potentials associated with cliques of sizes 1 and 2, respectively, in a homogeneous MRF. We define

$$V_1(L_t) \propto -\lambda_1 \log P_{\mathrm{np}}(L_t|I_t) - \lambda_2 \log P_{\mathrm{svm}}(L_t|I_{\mathcal{N}_t}) - \lambda_3 \log P_{\mathrm{atlas}}(L_t), \qquad (2)$$

where $P_{\mathrm{np}}(\cdot)$ is the likelihood term obtained from a data-driven spatially-varying nonparametric model (described in Section 3), $P_{\mathrm{svm}}(\cdot)$ is the intensity-based prior learned using a fuzzy nonlinear SVM (described in Section 4), $P_{\mathrm{atlas}}(\cdot)$ is the probabilistic atlas prior, and $\lambda_1, \lambda_2, \lambda_3 \geq 0$ are the weight parameters, which are set empirically. Setting $\lambda_3 = 0$ ignores the atlas prior. The second term on the right side of the Gibbs energy function in (1) is defined as: $V_2(L_t, L_s) = 1$ when $L_t \neq L_s$, otherwise $V_2(L_t, L_s) = 0$. V_2 penalizes the differing label values in neighboring voxels, regularizing the segmentation. We minimize the energy in (1) using an efficient max-flow/min-cut algorithm [11], similar to that in [5].

3   Adaptive, Nonparametric Tissue-Intensity Models

Parametric modeling of tissue-intensity PDFs assumes that the forms of the PDFs are known. In many practical situations, especially those concerning neonatal MR images, simple parametric models may not accurately model the underlying data [4]. The proposed method employs the *Parzen-window nonparametric density estimation* technique, which does not make strong assumptions about the forms of the PDFs, but rather infers the PDF structure from the input data. The Parzen-window probability estimate for each tissue-intensity PDF $P(I_t)$, at voxel t, is:

$$P_{np}(I_t|L_t) = \frac{1}{|\mathcal{S}'_t|} \sum_{i' \in \mathcal{S}'_t} G(I_t; i', \sigma), \qquad (3)$$

where $\mathcal{S}'_t$ is a random sample drawn from the tissue-intensity histogram for class L_t, and $G(I_t; i', \sigma)$ is a Gaussian kernel with mean i' and variance σ^2. This allows us to compute the first term in (2), using Bayes rule,

$$P_{np}(L_t|I_t) \propto P_{np}(I_t|L_t)/P_{np}(I_t). \qquad (4)$$

We have found that tissue-intensity statistics in virtually all MR images depict significant variability in different regions of the brain—this results from both biological properties and imaging artifacts. To adapt the model to such spatial variations, we use a *local-sampling* strategy. In this local-sampling framework, for each voxel t, we draw a unique random sample S'_t from an isotropic Gaussian PDF, defined on the image-coordinate space, with mean at the voxel t and variance $\sigma^2_{\text{spatial}}$. Thus, the sample S'_t is spatially biased and contains more voxels near the voxel t being processed. Our experiments show that the method performs well for reasonable choices of σ_{spatial} and encompasses more than a few hundred voxels. We choose $\sigma_{\text{spatial}} = 6cm$ and $|S'_t| = 500$. Fixing σ_{spatial} and $|S'|$, we chose a value for the kernel bandwidth σ based on a standard penalized-maximum-likelihood scheme [12].

4   Probabilistic Markov Intensity Priors Using SVMs

This section describes the proposed strategy of learning intensity-based Markov priors using fuzzy nonlinear SVMs. The key idea underlying SVMs is to implicitly transform the data into a high-dimensional feature space and, subsequently, learn a linear classifier (hyperplane) in the transformed space [10]. In this way, SVMs effectively learn complex nonlinear classifiers in the original feature space. Furthermore, finding linear classifiers reduces the optimization to a quadratic programming problem (involving inner product of feature vectors) that yields fast algorithms for finding the global optimum. SVMs avoid overfitting by computing an optimal classifier that maximizes the margin of separation between the classes. The classifier that separates the classes is described by only a fraction of training points in the feature space—namely, the *support vectors*, leading to efficient data representation and computation.

SVMs employ kernel functions $K(\cdot, \cdot)$ to implicitly transform the feature vectors (say z_i, z_j) to a higher-dimensional space $\mathcal{F}$ and evaluate their inner product, i.e. $\mathcal{F}(z_i) \cdot \mathcal{F}(z_j) = K(z_i, z_j)$. The proposed method effectively uses Gaussian kernels $K(z_i, z_j) = \exp(-\parallel z_i - z_j \parallel^2 / \sigma^2_{\text{SVM}})$. We chose σ^2_{SVM} to be 10% of the image intensity range—the SVM output is fairly robust to small changes in this value.

Fuzziness is often required in segmentations to deal with uncertainty in decision making. This becomes more important for neonatal brain MR images because the myelination process makes it more difficult to differentiate between white matter and gray matter based on intensity alone. Fuzzy learning with SVMs, which allows misclassification on some training data, decreases the sensitivity to manual segmentation errors in a principled manner, and reduces chances of overfitting. As with typical fuzzy classifiers, the degree of fuzziness is specified by a free parameter, namely C [13]. We chose $C = 0.01$ to enforce a reasonable degree of fuzziness in the learned classifier. Figure 2(C) shows an example slice of the output of a fuzzy SVM.

The SVM outputs numbers that indicate the distance of the test data point from the learned boundary that separates the classes. To *calibrate* the SVM outputs into probabilities, researchers have proposed, and rigorously analyzed, schemes akin to regularized maximum-likelihood approaches in statistics [14]. We employ a standard technique which fits a sigmoid function to the SVM outputs and converts them into prior probabilities [14].

5   Experiments and Validation

The difficulty of accurate manual segmentations on clinical neonatal brain MRI makes validation a challenging task. Figure 1 demonstrates the degree of disagreement between different human raters. In the light of these limitations, we propose to validate the segmentation of the proposed method, not only by quantitative comparison to the manual segmentations, but also by qualitative visual inspection. The challenges in automatic neonatal brain MRI segmentation often require multi-spectral image data [4,15]. Due to the poor image quality of the T1 weighted MRIs in our current dataset (based on the opinion of pediatric neurologists), we used only T2 weighted MRIs in the validation of our method. The proposed framework can handle multi-spectral images in a straightforward manner.

We performed cross validation (leave-one-out strategy) on clinical axial T2-weighted images ($512 \times 384 \times 28$ with voxel size $0.35 \times 0.35 \times 3$ mm) scanned using a spin-echo pulse sequence on ten neonates—all term newborn infants with ages less than ten days. The proposed method considers myelinated and non-myelinated white matter as a single tissue class—a postprocessing stage can help further differentiate the white matter, as in [4]. Gray and white matter of all ten T2-weighted MR images were manually segmented by two experts. The skull and other brain tissues were removed using manual delineation. Probabilistic atlas priors were constructed by registering pre-segmented MRIs to a canonical atlas space. For this purpose, we used diffeomorphic flow-based registration and unbiased population-atlas construction [16]. We preprocessed the scanned MR images using standard techniques: (a) edge-preserving anisotropic smoothing, followed by (b) inhomogeneity correction using an information minimization method [17], and (c) adaptive histogram equalization to enhance local contrast [18]. For effective SVM training, we ensured a reasonable match of the histograms of the preprocessed images. Because of the low inter-slice resolution typically found in clinical neonatal MR images, we chose the neighborhood $N(t)$, for each voxel t, as the 3×3 voxel neighborhood in the corresponding axial slice. We rescaled all images so that the intensities lie in the range of $[0, 100]$. SVM training, using nine of the ten images, takes about two hours using SVMTorch [13].

Qualitatively, Figure 2 shows that the proposed method obtained an improved segmentation, in the marked areas, as compared to that using a Gaussian model based method. Note that the quantitative comparisons should be interpreted conservatively because of the challenges in ground-truth construction, as discussed previously. Figure 3(A) shows the Dice overlap metric for the ten neonates, for

888   Z. Song et al.

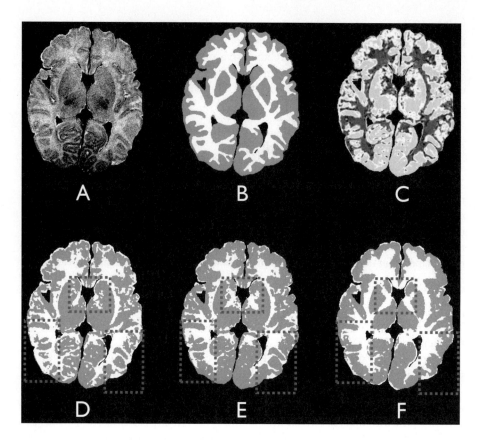

Fig. 2. Qualitative comparison of segmentation results. (A) original neonatal T2-weighted MR image with only white matter and gray matter.(B) Manual segmentation by rater A. (C) Output of a fuzzy SVM for this image. Segmentations using: (D) conventional Gaussian tissue-intensity models, (E) adaptive nonparametric modeling using Markov-intensity-based priors learned by the fuzzy SVM $(\lambda_1 = 1, \lambda_2 = 1, \lambda_3 = 0)$, and (F) adaptive nonparametric modeling coupled with atlas priors$(\lambda_1 = 1, \lambda_2 = 1, \lambda_3 = 0.2)$.

both gray and white matter, to compare the automatic segmentations with the manual segmentations by rater A. As a reference, it also shows the performance of rater B based on the segmentations of rater A as the ground truth. In comparison to the results of the Gaussian model based method, the proposed method has higher Dice overlap values for gray matter. For the proposed method, using the atlas prior produces segmentations with slightly higher Dice overlap values. Figure 3(B) shows that the average brain-tissue volumes calculated from the segmentations of the proposed method lie between the volumes calculated from the two manual segmentations (with similar variances in all three cases). This indicates that the tissue-volume estimation by the proposed method can be as accurate as that provided by human experts.

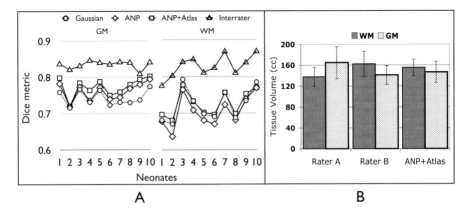

Fig. 3. Quantitative comparison of cross validation results: (A) Dice overlap metric of gray and white matters between the manual segmentation by rater A and four different segmentations based on: (i) the manual segmentation by rater B, (ii) Gaussian model with adaptive inhomogeneity correction, (iii) the proposed adaptive nonparametric (ANP) method, (iv) the proposed ANP method including the atlas prior (ANP+Atlas). (B) Volume of brain tissues given by the segmentations by rater A, rater B, and the proposed automatic method (ANP+Atlas).

6   Conclusion

We present a neonatal brain-MR segmentation method that produces a MAP segmentation using nonparametric likelihood models and intensity-based priors learnt by fuzzy nonlinear SVMs. The proposed nonparametric modeling adapts to the spatial variability in the intensity statistics that arises from variations in brain structure and image inhomogeneity. The proposed method produces reasonable segmentations even in the absence of atlas prior. Moreover, we find that intensity-based priors relying on empirical Markov statistics are more effective, than atlas-based priors, given high variability in manual segmentations and the challenges for registering neonatal images. Fuzzy learning with SVMs decreases the sensitivity to manual segmentation errors in a principled manner. Cross validation using ten neonatal brain-MR images demonstrates the efficacy of the proposed segmentation method. Although it is hard to quantify the advantage of the proposed method over other methods without accurate ground-truth manual segmentations, the utility of the proposed method could be more evident in studies involving cortical-thickness measurements and folding-pattern analysis.

Acknowledgments

This work was funded in part by the USPHS under grants DA-015886, MZ-402069, NS-045839, MH-072576, NINDS K23, and NS052380-03.

References

1. van der Knaap, M., Valik, J.: MR imaging of the various stages of normal myelination during the first year of life. Neuroradiology 31(6), 459–470 (1990)
2. Dietrich, R.: Maturation, Myelination, and Dysmyelination. In: Magnetic Resonance Imaging. Mosby pp. 1425–1447 (1999)
3. Barkovich, A.: Magnetic resonance techniques in the assessment of myelin and myelination. J Inherit Metab Dis. 28(3), 311–343 (2005)
4. Prastawa, M., Gilmore, J., Lin, W., Gerig, G.: Automatic segmentation of MR images of the developing newborn brain. Med Image Anal. 9(5), 457–466 (2005)
5. Song, Z., Tustison, N., Avants, B., Gee, J.: Integrated graph cuts for brain mri segmentation. In: Larsen, R., Nielsen, M., Sporring, J. (eds.) MICCAI 2006. LNCS, vol. 4191, pp. 831–838. Springer, Heidelberg (2006)
6. Leemput, K.V., Maes, F., Vandermeulen, D., Seutens, P.: Automated model-based tissue classification of MR images of the brain. IEEE Tr. Med. Imaging 18, 897–908 (1999)
7. Greenspan, H., Ruf, A., Goldberger, J.: Constrained gaussian mixture model framework for automatic segmentation of MR brain images. IEEE Trans. Medical Imaging 25(9), 1233–1245 (2006)
8. Awate, S., Tasdizen, T., Foster, N., Whitaker, R.: Adaptive, nonparametric markov modeling for unsupervised, MRI brain-tissue classification. Medical Image Analysis 10(5), 726–739 (2006)
9. Awate, S.P., Gee, J.C.: A fuzzy, nonparametric segmentation framework for DTI and MRI analysis. In: Proc. Info. Proc. in Med. Imag (IPMI), (to appear, 2007)
10. Burges, C.: A tutorial on support vector machines for pattern recognition. Data Mining and Knowledge Discovery 2, 121–167 (1998)
11. Boykov, Y., Veksler, O., Zabih, R.: Fast approximate energy minimization via graph cuts. IEEE Trans. Pattern Anal. Machine Intell. 23(11), 1222–1239 (2001)
12. Chow, Y., Geman, S., Wu, L.: Consistent cross-validated density estimation. Annals of Statistics 11(1), 25–38 (1983)
13. Collobert, R., Bengio, S.: Svmtorch: Support vector machines for large-scale regression problems. Journal of machine learning research 1, 143–160 (2001)
14. Platt, J.: Probabilistic outputs for support vector machines and comparison to regularized likelihood methods. In: Advances in Large Margin Classifiers, MIT Press, Cambridge (1999)
15. Weisenfeld, N., Mewes, A., Warfield, S.: Highly accurate segmentation of brain tissue and subcortical gray matter from newborn mri. In: Larsen, R., Nielsen, M., Sporring, J. (eds.) MICCAI 2006. LNCS, vol. 4190, pp. 199–206. Springer, Heidelberg (2006)
16. Avants, B., Gee, J.: Geodesic estimation for large deformation anatomical shape and intensity averaging. Neuroimage Suppl. 1, S139–150 (2004)
17. Likar, B., Viergever, M.A., Pernus, F.: Retrospective correction of MR intensity inhomogeneity by information minimization. IEEE Trans. Med. Imaging 20(12), 1398–1410 (2001)
18. Stark, J.: Adaptive image contrast enhancement using generalizations of histogram equalization. IEEE Trans. Image Processing 9(5), 889–896 (2000)

Active-Contour-Based Image Segmentation Using Machine Learning Techniques

Patrick Etyngier, Florent Ségonne, and Renaud Keriven

Odyssée Team / Certis - Ecole des Ponts - France
etyngier@certis.enpc.fr

Abstract. We introduce a non-linear shape prior for the deformable model framework that we learn from a set of shape samples using recent manifold learning techniques. We model a category of shapes as a finite dimensional manifold which we approximate using Diffusion maps. Our method computes a Delaunay triangulation of the reduced space, considered as Euclidean, and uses the resulting space partition to identify the closest neighbors of any given shape based on its Nyström extension. We derive a non-linear shape prior term designed to attract a shape towards the shape prior manifold at given constant embedding. Results on shapes of ventricle nuclei demonstrate the potential of our method for segmentation tasks.

1 Introduction

1.1 Motivation

Accurate segmentation of anatomical structures from medical images is a fundamental but difficult task that often dictates the outcome of the entire clinical or research analysis (e.g. visualization, neuro-surgical planning, surface-based processing of functional data, inter-subject registration, among others). The challenge is that images are usually corrupted by several artifacts, such as image noise, missing or occluded parts, image intensity inhomogeneity or non-uniformity, and partial volume averaging effect. When dealing with complex images, some prior shape knowledge may be necessary to disambiguate the segmentation process.

In medical imaging, excluding uncommon pathological cases, the overall shape of most macroscopic anatomical structures is prescribed by medical knowledge: it is usually known a priori, does not vary much between individuals, and its observed geometric variability seems to be governed by a small set of unknown parameters. In this paper, we assume that the set of shapes of a specific anatomical structure (e.g. left or right ventricle, hippocampus nucleus) evolves in a low-dimensional, but not necessarily linear, space that we term the *shape prior manifold*. This is clearly exemplified in Fig. 1 which displays some shapes corresponding to the right ventricle nucleus for different subjects at different time points in their life. Even shapes extracted from subjects with Alzheimer's Disease, a relatively slowly evolving pathology, exhibits some shape similarity with normal controls.

Knowledge of the underlying structure encoding the geometric variability of anatomy provides shape constraints for image segmentation. We propose to discover the structure of the *shape prior manifold* using recent manifold learning techniques, and to exploit it

N. Ayache, S. Ourselin, A. Maeder (Eds.): MICCAI 2007, Part I, LNCS 4791, pp. 891–899, 2007.
© Springer-Verlag Berlin Heidelberg 2007

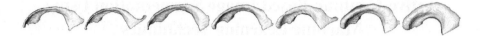

Fig. 1. Aligned shape samples of the right ventricle nucleus from different subjects corresponding, from left to right, to 2 young, 2 mid-age, and 2 old subjects; the last shape sample originates
from a subject with Alzheimer's Disease. While shapes appear quite similar, they usually cannot
be considered as small deformations around a mean shape.

to carefully design a non-linear shape prior integrated into the deformable model framework for the purpose of image segmentation.

1.2   Previous Work

The use of shape prior information in the deformable model framework has long been
limited to a smoothness assumption or to simple parametric families of shapes. But a
recent and important trend in this domain is the development of deformable models
integrating more elaborate shape information.

An important work in this direction is the *active shape model* of Cootes et al. [1]. A
principal component analysis (PCA) on the position of some landmark points placed in
a coherent way on all the training contours is used to reduce the number of degrees of
freedom to the principal modes of variation. Although successfully applied to various
types of shapes (hands, faces, organs), the reliance on a parameterized representation
and the manual positioning of the landmarks, particularly tedious in 3D images, seri-
ously limits it applicability.

Leventon, Grimson and Faugeras [2] circumvent these limitations by computing
parameterization-independent shape statistics within the level set representation [3]. Basically, they perform a PCA on the signed distance functions of the training shapes, and
the resulting statistical model is integrated into a geodesic active contour framework.
The evolution equation contains a term which attracts the model towards an optimal
prior shape as a combination of the mean shape and of the principal modes of variation. Several improvements to this approach have been proposed [4,5], and in particular
an elegant integration of the statistical shape model into a unique MAP Bayesian optimization. Let us also mention another neat Bayesian prior shape formulation, based on
a B-spline representation, proposed by Cremers, Kohlberger and Schnörr in [6].

Performing PCA on distance functions might be problematic since they do not define
a vector space. To cope with this, Charpiat, Faugeras and Keriven [7] proposed shape
statistics based on differentiable approximations of the Hausdorff distance. However,
their work is limited to a linearized shape space with small deformation modes around
a mean shape. Such an approach is relevant only when the learning set is composed of
very similar shapes. Finally, let's also mention the elegant M-reps approach [8], that is
restricted to a specific type of deformable models.

1.3   Novelty of Our Approach

In this paper, we depart from the small deformation assumption and introduce a new
deformable model framework that integrates more general non-linear shape priors. We

model a category of shapes as a smooth finite-dimensional sub-manifold of the infinite-dimensional shape space, termed the *shape prior manifold*. This manifold which cannot be represented explicitly is approximated from a collection of shape samples using a recent manifold learning technique called Diffusion maps [9,10]. Manifold learning, which is already an established tool in object recognition and image classification, has been recently applied to shape analysis [11]. Yet, to our knowledge, such techniques have not been used in the context of image segmentation with shape priors.

Diffusion maps generate a mapping, called an embedding, from the original shape space into a low-dimensional space, which can *advantageously* be considered as Euclidean [9]. We design a shape prior term based on the Nyström extension [12] which provides a sound and efficient framework for extending embedding coordinates to the full infinite dimensional shape space. Motivated by its Euclidean nature, a Delaunay partitioning of the reduced space is used to identify the closest neighbors (in the training set) of any shape in the original infinite dimensional shape space. The neighboring shapes are then integrated into a variational functional designed to attract any given shape towards the *shape prior manifold*.

The remainder of this paper is organized as follows. Section 2 introduces the necessary background in manifold learning: it is dedicated to learning the *shape prior manifold* from a finite set of shape samples using Diffusion maps. Section 3 presents our deformable model framework using non-linear shape priors. Section 4 reports some preliminary numerical experiments which yield promising results with real shapes.

2   Learning the Shape Prior Manifold

In the sequel, we define a *shape* as a simple compact (i.e. closed and non-intersecting) surface, and we denote by $\mathbb{S}$ the (infinite-dimensional) space of such shapes[1]. We make the assumption that a category of shapes, i.e. the set of shapes that can be identified with a common anatomical structure, e.g. left or right ventricle, hippocampus nucleus, can be modeled as a finite-dimensional manifold, termed the *shape prior manifold*.

Dimensionality reduction, i.e. the process of recovering the underlying low dimensional structure of a manifold $\mathcal{M}$ embedded into a higher-dimensional space, has enjoyed renewed interest over the past years. Among the most recent and popular techniques are the Locally Linear Embedding (LLE) [13], Laplacian eigenmaps [14], Diffusion maps [9,15].

In this work, we learn the *shape prior manifold* using Diffusion maps. For the sake of clarity, we present the mathematical formulation for data living in $\mathbb{R}^n$. An extension to infinite-dimensional shape manifolds is straightforward (We refer the reader to [9,10,15] for more detail).

2.1   Manifold Learning and Diffusion Maps

Let $\mathcal{M}$ be a manifold of dimension m lying in $\mathbb{R}^n$ ($m << n$). Diffusion maps rely on discrete approximations of the Laplace-Beltrami operator $\Delta_{\mathcal{M}}$ defined on the manifold

---

[1] Note that, although this paper only deals with 2-dimensional surfaces embedded in the 3-dimensional Euclidean space, all ideas and results seamlessly extend to higher dimensions.

$\mathcal{M}$ to generate a mapping (called an embedding) $f : \mathcal{M} \longrightarrow \mathbb{R}^m$ such that if two points x and z are *close* in $\mathcal{M}$, so are $f(x)$ and $f(z)$. The optimal mapping is given by the eigen-functions of the Laplace-Beltrami operator corresponding to the m smallest non-zero eigenvalues, where m is the target dimension. Note that the latter dimension can either be known *a priori* or be inferred from the profile of the eigen spectrum [9]. In practice, a discrete counterpart to this continuous formulation must be used since we only have access to a discrete and finite set, denoted Γ, of example shapes in this category.

2.1.a   Distance in the Shape Space

The approximation of the Laplace-Beltrami operator requires the choice of a distance between shapes. Many different definitions of the distance between two shapes have been proposed in the computer vision literature but there is no agreement on the correct way of measuring shape similarity. The definition used in the experiments presented in Sect. 4 are based on the representation of a surface S in the Euclidean embedding space $\mathbb{R}^3$ by its signed distance function. In this context, we define the distance between two shapes to be the Sobolev $W^{1,2}$-norm of the difference between their signed distance functions [7]:

$$d_{W^{1,2}}(S_1, S_2)^2 = ||\bar{D}_{S_1} - \bar{D}_{S_2}||^2_{L^2(\Omega, \mathbb{R})} + ||\nabla\bar{D}_{S_1} - \nabla\bar{D}_{S_2}||^2_{L^2(\Omega, \mathbb{R}^n)} ,$$

where $\bar{D}_{S_i}$ denotes the signed distance function of shape S_i ($i = 1, 2$), and $\nabla\bar{D}_{S_i}$ its gradient. Note that to define a distance between shapes that is invariant to rigid displacements (rotations and translations), we first align the shapes using their principal moments before computing distances. Note also that the proposed method is obviously not limited to a specific choice of distance [7].

2.1.b   Approximation to the Laplace-Beltrami Operator

Once a distance has been chosen, classical manifold learning techniques can be applied by building an adjacency graph of the learning set of shape examples. Let $\Gamma = \{x_1 \cdots x_p \in \mathbb{R}^n\}$ be p sample points of the m dimensional manifold $\mathcal{M}$ sampled under an unknown density $q_{\mathcal{M}}$. An adjacency matrix $(W_{i,j})_{i,j \in 1,...,p}$ is then constructed, the coefficients of which measure the strength of the different edges in the adjacency graph. Typically, $W_{i,j}$, also denoted $w(x_i, x_j)$, is a decreasing function of the distance between x_i and x_j. In this work, $w(x_i, x_j) = \exp\left(-d^2(x_i, x_j)/2\sigma^2\right)$, with σ estimated as the median of all the distances between all shapes.

Classical manifold learning methods provide an embedding that combines the information of both the density $q_{\mathcal{M}}$ and the geometry [10,15]. In order to construct an approximation of the Laplace-Beltrami operator that is independent of the unknown density $q_{\mathcal{M}}$, we renormalize the adjacency matrix $(W_{i,j})$. Briefly, we form the new adjacency matrix $\left(\tilde{W}_{i,j}\right)$ by $\tilde{w}(x_i, x_j) = \frac{w(x_i, x_j)}{q(x_i)q(x_j)}$, with $q(x) = \sum_{y \in \Gamma} w(x, y)$. We then define the anisotropic transition kernel $(P_{i,j})_{i,j \in 1,...,p}$ such that $p(x_i, x_j) = \frac{\tilde{w}(x_i, x_j)}{\tilde{q}(x_i)\tilde{q}(x_j)}$ with $\tilde{q}(x) = \sum_{y \in \Gamma} \tilde{w}(x, y)$. The kernel $(P_{i,j})$ is a density-independent approximation of the operator $\mathbb{1} - \Delta_{\mathcal{M}}$ [9]. From the definition of the adjacency matrix, we find that:

$$p(x_i, x_j) = \frac{w(x_i, x_j)}{\sum_b K_{jb} w(x_i, x_b)} \text{ with } K_{jb} = \frac{q(x_j)}{q(x_b)} = \frac{\sum_{y \in \Gamma} w(x_j, y)}{\sum_{y \in \Gamma} w(x_b, y)}. \quad (1)$$

2.1.c   Generating the Embedding Using Diffusion Maps

Let's denote $\{\lambda_i\}_{i,j \in 1,\ldots,p}$ (with $|\lambda_0| \geq |\lambda_1| \geq \ldots$) and Ψ_i the associated eigenvalues and eigenvectors of $(P_{i,j})$. Coifman and coworkers have shown in [9] that the eigenvectors of $(P_{i,j})$ converge to those of the Laplace-Beltrami operator on $\mathcal{M}$ and that a mapping Φ_t that embeds the data into the *Euclidean* space $\mathbb{R}^m$ *isometrically* with respect to a Diffusion distance in the original shape space $\mathbb{S}$ can be constructed:

$$\Phi_t : \Gamma \subset \mathcal{M} \to \mathbb{R}^m, \; x_i \mapsto \left(\lambda_1^t \Psi_1(x_i), \ldots, \lambda_m^t \Psi_m(x_i) \right). \quad (2)$$

Diffusion distance reflects the intrinsic geometry of the data set defined via the adjacency graph in a diffusion process. It was shown to be more robust to outliers than geodesic distances [9], thereby motivating its use to estimate the embedding (Fig. 2-c). In this formulation, t is a time parameter controlling the diffusivity of the adjacency graph and can be chosen arbitrarily. We used $t = 1$ for our experiments (Sect. 4).

2.2   Extending the Embedding Based on Nyström Extension

The mapping Φ_t is only defined on the training samples. The Nyström extension method is a popular technique employed for the extension of empirical functions from the training set Γ to new samples. Noticing that every training sample verifies:

$$\forall x \in \Gamma \quad \forall k \in 1, \ldots, p \quad \sum_{y \in \Gamma} p(x, y) \Psi_k(y) = \lambda_k \Psi_k(x),$$

the embedding of new data points located outside the set Γ can similarly be computed by extension (Lafon and coworkers define another elegant extension in [15]):

$$\tilde{\Phi}_t : \mathbb{R}^n \to \mathbb{R}^m, \; x \mapsto \left(\lambda_1^{t-1} \sum_{y \in \Gamma} p(x, y) \Psi_1(y), \ldots, \lambda_m^{t-1} \sum_{y \in \Gamma} p(x, y) \Psi_m(y) \right) \quad (3)$$

3   Image Segmentation Using the Shape Prior Manifold

In this section, we propose to use the embedding to carefully design a shape prior term integrated into a deformable model framework for the purpose of image segmentation.

3.1   Image Segmentation as a Variational Problem

Without loss of generality, we cast the segmentation problem as a variational one, where the objective is to find a surface S minimizing a global energy functional E^{ac}. Depending on the segmentation task and the available information, the energy functional E^{ac} can take on different, more or less complex, forms, but, generally , E^{ac} can be written as a combination of image terms, designed to drive the surface towards the searched contour, and regularization terms, enforcing smoothness constraints. Directly finding the global minimum of E^{ac} is usually impossible and one often has to resort to a sub-optimal gradient-descent strategy starting from a guess S_0. That is we assume that the image segmentation problem amounts to solving the following evolution problem: find the active contour $S : \tau \in \mathbb{R}^+ \mapsto S(\tau) \in \mathbb{S}$ such that $S(0) = S_0$, $\frac{dS}{d\tau} = -\nabla E^{ac}$.

3.2 Designing and Integrating the Shape Prior Term

We define a shape prior functional E^{sp} designed to attract any given shape S towards the shape prior manifold. Unfortunately, Diffusion maps do not give access to an explicit projection operator onto the reduced manifold. To alleviate this problem, we exploit the Euclidean nature of the reduced space by computing a Delaunay triangulation in $\mathbb{R}^m$ of the training data. The space partition is then used to identify the $m+1$ closest neighbors (in the training set Γ) of the shape S in the $\mathbb{S}$ by computing its embedding coordinates $\tilde{\Phi}(S)$ and finding the corresponding Delaunay triangle formed by $m+1$-vertices in $\mathbb{R}^m$. By doing so, we identify the $m+1$ closest neighbors $\mathcal{N} = (S_0, ..., S_m)$ of S in $\mathbb{S}$ for the Diffusion metric [9]. This neighborhood $\mathcal{N}$ will then be used to attract S towards the manifold.

To this end, we compute the barycentric coordinates $\Theta = (\theta_0, \cdots, \theta_m)$ of the shape S in the reduced space $\mathbb{R}^m$ and define the shape prior functional in $\mathbb{S}$:

$$E^{sp}_{\mathcal{N},\Theta}(S) = \sum_{i=0}^{m} \theta_i d^2 \left(S_i, S \right) \text{ with } \tilde{\Phi}(S) = \sum \theta_i \tilde{\Phi}(S_i), \ \theta_i \geq 0, \ \sum \theta_i = 1$$

designed to attract the shape S towards a *weighted mean shape* that interpolates between the $m+1$ samples $S_i \in \mathcal{N}$.

Minimization of the energy $E^{sp}_{\mathcal{N},\Theta}(S)$ by gradient descent might change the embedding coordinates $\tilde{\Phi}_t(S)$ of the evolving shape S. Therefore, denoting by $\mathbb{S}_x = \tilde{\Phi}_t^{-1}(x)$ the x-level set in $\mathbb{S}$ of the embedding $\tilde{\Phi}_t$ (note that $\mathbb{S}_x$ has codimension m), we define the shape prior term $\overrightarrow{v}_{sp}$ as the projection of the velocity field $\overrightarrow{v} = -\nabla E^{sp}_{\mathcal{N},\Theta}$ onto the tangent space $\mathbb{T}_{\tilde{\Phi}_t(S)}$ of $\mathbb{S}_{\tilde{\Phi}_t(S)}$ at S. Using Eq. 1 and Eq. 3, $\mathbb{T}_{\tilde{\Phi}_t(S)}$ can be expressed by m simple orthogonality conditions in the tangent space $\mathbb{T}_{\mathbb{S}}(S)$ of $\mathbb{S}$ at S:

$$\mathbb{T}_{\tilde{\Phi}_t(S)} = \left\{ \overrightarrow{v} \in \mathbb{T}_{\mathbb{S}}(S) \text{ s.t. } \forall k = 1, \ldots, m \sum_{S_j \in \Gamma} \langle \nabla sp(S, S_j) | \overrightarrow{v} \rangle_{\mathbb{L}^2} \Psi_k(S_j) = 0 \right\},$$

where $\langle . | . \rangle_{\mathbb{L}^2}$ corresponds to the $\mathbb{L}^2$-dot product in the tangent shape space $\mathbb{T}_{\mathbb{S}}(S)$. Projection of the velocity field $-\nabla E^{sp}_{\mathcal{N},\Theta}$ onto $\mathbb{T}_{\tilde{\Phi}_t(S)}$ can then be achieved using the orthogonalization Gram-Schmidt process.

Finally, the general deformable model framework corresponds to solving the following evolution problem:

$$S(0) = S_0, \ \frac{dS}{d\tau} = -\nabla E^{ac} + \alpha \overrightarrow{v}_{sp},$$

where α is a weighting parameter. Note that at each step of the evolution, we have to align the shape with the training samples using the principal moments before computing its embedding and dering the shape prior term $\overrightarrow{v}_{sp}$.

4   Results and Discussion

We illustrate the potential benefits of our approach on a simple segmentation task, the segmentation of the ventricle nucleus from Magnetic Resonance Image (MRI). Training shape samples were obtained from 39 manually segmented images of 10 young, 10 mid-age, and 9 old normal controls and of 11 demented adults (Fig. 1). 39 data points form an insufficiently small data set and more shape samples are desirable to recover a satisfactory embedding. Note also that the artificial nature of the proposed segmentation task is only dedicated to reveal the influence of the shape prior term.

4.1   Estimating the Dimension of the Shape Prior Manifold

The dimension m is usually estimated from the profile of the eigenspectrum (Fig. 2-a). Yet, there is not always an obvious choice (especially when the number of data points is insufficient). In our case, $m = 2$, $m = 3$, or $m = 4$ appear to be a realistic guess. However, in the case of labeled data, one can disambiguate this choice by also requiring the embedding $\tilde{\Phi}_t$ to separate/cluster "well" the different groups. We simply define the degree of separability $d_{i,j}$ between two groups i and j by the distance $d_{i,j} = \frac{\|\mu_i - \mu_j\|}{\sqrt{\sigma_i^2 + \sigma_j^2}}$, where μ_i and σ_i^2 are the mean and variance in $\mathbb{R}^m$ of data points corresponding to group #i. The degree of separability of the mapping $\tilde{\Phi}_t$ is then $\sum_{i,j} d_{i,j}$. Note that this method can also be used to determine an optimal value for the parameter t. Finally, on this unsatisfactory small data set, we find that the optimal mapping requires $m = 2$ (Fig. 2-a,b).

4.2   Closest Neighbors

Diffusion maps embed *advantageously* the data set in the Euclidean space R^m *isometrically* with respect to a Diffusion distance in $\mathbb{S}$. This distance was shown to be more robust to outliers than geodesic distances [9]. To illustrate this point, we show in Fig. 2-c a manually corrupted shape with its two closest neighbors in $\mathbb{S}$ and $\mathbb{R}^m$. At least visually, the identified shapes in $\mathbb{R}^m$ appear more similar to the corrupted shape than the ones in $\mathbb{S}$.

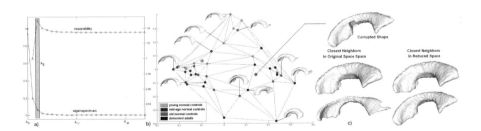

Fig. 2. a) Eigenspectrum profile and degree of separability: on this restricted data set with 39 shapes only, $m = 2$ appears to be the optimal dimension. b) The two-dimensional embedding partitioned by a Delaunay triangulation. c) A manually corrupted shape and its two closest neighbors in $\mathbb{S}$ and in the reduced space: visually, the ones in the reduced space appear more similar.

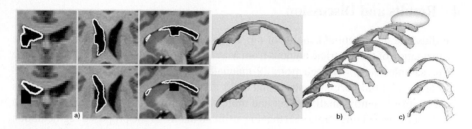

Fig. 3. a) Coronal, horizontal, and sagital slices of the MRI volume with the final segmentations without (top) and with (bottom) the shape prior. b) Some snapshots of the shape evolution - the shape prior term was not used during the first steps. c) The closest neighbors of the final surface.

4.3   Ventricle Nucleus Segmentation from MRI with Occlusion

we consider a simple segmentation task which consists of segmenting the ventricle nucleus from an MRI that was corrupted by white noise and degraded with an artificial occlusion (clearly visible in Fig. 3-a). Motivated by our choice of representing a shape S by its signed distance function $\bar{D}_S$, our surface deformation is implemented in the level set framework. The level set evolution is guided by a *simple* intensity-based velocity term, a curvature term, and the non-linear shape prior term:

$$\partial_\tau \bar{D}_S(x, \tau) = [\beta(I(x) - T(x)) - \kappa] \, |\nabla_x \bar{D}_S(x, \tau)| - \alpha \vec{v}_{sp} \cdot \nabla_x \bar{D}_S(x, \tau)$$

where $I(x)$ and κ represents the image intensity and mean curvature respectively at location x, T is a threshold computed locally from image intensities, β and α two weighting coefficients equal to $\beta = 0.1$ and $\alpha = 0.1$. Figure 3 displays our segmentation results. Despite the artificial occlusion, the shape prior term was able to recover the correct shape by attracting the shape onto the *shape prior manifold*. Yet, the final surface is geometrically-accurate because the active contour can evolve freely inside the manifold $\mathcal{M}$ subject to the image term. The red-cross in Fig. 2 locates the final segmented shape in the embedding. Finally, note that, in practice, the shape prior term is not used during the first steps of the evolution (a robust alignment being impossible).

5   Conclusion and Future Work

We have proposed a new deformable model framework for image segmentation that incorporates non-linear shape priors by learning a shape prior manifold using recent manifold learning techniques. Our approach exploits carefully the properties of Diffusion maps to derive an innovative shape prior term designed to attract an active contour towards the shape manifold. While preliminary, our segmentation results on shapes of ventricle nucleus demonstrate the potential of our approach.

The proposed method is quite general and is not necessarily restricted to specific 3-dimensional segmentation tasks. In particular, the only requirement is a differentiable kernel. We plan to apply our approach to more general data sets, such as diffusion weighted imaging as well as combined anatomical and functional MRI, in future work.

References

1. Cootes, T., Taylor, C., Cooper, D., Graham, J.: Active shape models-their training and application. Computer Vision and Image Understanding 61(1), 38–59 (1995)
2. Leventon, M., Grimson, E., Faugeras, O.: Statistical shape influence in geodesic active contours. In: IEEE Conference on Computer Vision and Pattern Recognition, pp. 316–323. IEEE Computer Society Press, Los Alamitos (2000)
3. Osher, S., Sethian, J.: Fronts propagating with curvature-dependent speed: Algorithms based on Hamilton–Jacobi formulations. Journal of Computational Physics 79(1), 12–49 (1988)
4. Rousson, M., Paragios, N.: Shape priors for level set representations. In: European Conference on Computer Vision. vol 2, pp. 78–92 (2002)
5. Tsai, A., Yezzi, A., Wells, W., Tempany, C., Tucker, D., Fan, A., Grimson, W., Willsky, A.: A shape-based approach to the segmentation of medical imagery using level sets. IEEE Transactions on Medical Imaging 22(2), 137–154 (2003)
6. Cremers, D., Kohlberger, T., Schnörr, C.: Nonlinear shape statistics in mumford shah based segmentation. In: European Conference on Computer Vision, pp. 93–108 (2002)
7. Charpiat, G., Faugeras, O., Keriven, R.: Approximations of shape metrics and application to shape warping and empirical shape statistics. Foundations of Computational Mathematics 5(1), 1–58 (2005)
8. Pizer, S.M., et al.: Deformable M-Reps for 3D medical image segmentation. International Journal of Computer Vision 55(2–3), 85–106 (2003)
9. Coifman, R., Lafon, S., et al.: Geometric diffusions as a tool for harmonic analysis and structure definition of data: Diffusion maps. PNAS 102(21), 7426–7431 (2005)
10. Lafon, S., Lee, A.B.: Diffusion maps and coarse-graining: a unified framework for dimensionality reduction, graph partitioning, and data set parameterization. IEEE Transactions on 28(9), 1393–1403 (2006)
11. Charpiat, G., Faugeras, O., Keriven, R., Maurel, P.: Distance-based shape statistics. IEEE International Conference on Acoustics, Speech and Signal Processing 5, 925–928 (2006)
12. Bengio, Y., Vincent, P., et al.: Spectral clustering and kernel pca are learning eigenfunctions. Technical Report 1239, Département d'informatique et recherche opérationnelle, Université de Montréal (2003)
13. Roweis, S., Saul, L.: Nonlinear dimensionality reduction by locally linear embedding. Science 290, 2323–2326 (2000)
14. Belkin, M., Niyogi, P.: Laplacian eigenmaps for dimensionality reduction and data representation. Neural Computation 15(6), 1373–1396 (2003)
15. Lafon, S., Keller, Y., Coifman, R.R.: Data fusion and multicue data matching by diffusion maps. IEEE Transactions on Pattern Analysis and Machine Intelligence 28(11), 1784–1797 (2006)

Methods for Inverting Dense Displacement Fields: Evaluation in Brain Image Registration*

William R. Crum[1], Oscar Camara[1], and David J. Hawkes[1]

Centre for Medical Image Computing, University College London, UK
b.crum@ucl.ac.uk

Abstract. In medical image analysis there is frequently a need to invert dense displacement fields which map one image space to another. In this paper we describe inversion techniques and determine their accuracy in the context of 18 inter-subject brain image registrations. Scattered data interpolation (SDI) is used to initialise locally and globally consistent iterative techniques. The inverse-consistency error, E_{IC} is computed over the whole image and over 10 specific brain regions. SDI produced good results with mean (max) $E_{IC} \sim 0.02$mm (2.0mm). Both iterative method produced mean errors of ~ 0.005mm but the globally consistent method resulted in a smaller maximum error (1.9mm compared with 1.4mm). The largest errors were in the cerebral cortex with large outlier errors in the ventricles. Simple iterative techniques are, on this evidence, able to produce reasonable estimates of inverse displacement fields provided there is good initialisation.

1 Introduction

In most pair-wise non-rigid registration applications, either by design or because of the available registration software, there is an implied direction i.e. one image is designated the target (reference) and the other is the source (floating image). The transformation, T, is defined at points t in the target space and specifies the point in source space $s = t + T(t)$ corresponding to each target voxel. The transformation may be parameterised at a coarser level but voxel-wise displacements can always be obtained by interpolation. Often the choice of target and source is application-specific e.g. to propagate a mesh from one image to another requires the mesh to be defined in the target space but to propagate a set of dense labels requires the labels to be defined in the source space. Similarly, to create a group average template requires the template space to be the target, but to subsequently transform labels from the template space to individual scans requires the template to be the source. The inverse transformation (from source to target) cannot be trivially deduced from the forward transformation. A registration algorithm can be run in reverse (i.e. with target

---

* This work is supported by the EPSRC Integrated Brain Image Modelling, Medical Image and Signals IRC and Modelling and Understanding and Predicting Structural Brain Change projects We are thankful to David Kennedy, Centre for Morphometric Analysis, MGH, Boston for the brain images used in this work.

N. Ayache, S. Ourselin, A. Maeder (Eds.): MICCAI 2007, Part I, LNCS 4791, pp. 900–907, 2007.
© Springer-Verlag Berlin Heidelberg 2007

and source exchanged) but the reverse transformation is not generally consistent with the forward transformation.

Some registration algorithms are designed to be inverse-consistent [1][2] and compute consistent forward and backward transformations. The related symmetric approaches [3] are conceptually similar but improve robustness without computing explicit inverses. In theory, inverse-consistent algorithms should remove the need to worry about the reverse transformation. In practice, these algorithms are not all that mature or widely available and the effect of enforcing strict inverse-consistency on the registration optimisation can be computationally expensive and has not been studied in any detail. In addition, it is clear that for many applications strict inverse-consistency is not appropriate. For instance, registering scans of a single patient anatomy subject to some mechanical deformation is a case where inverse-consistency is appropriate. However registering inter-subject brain scans is a case where strict inverse consistency has little biological foundation [4].

Some study of the computation of inverse transformations has been made in the registration literature, most notably in [1] and [5]. In [6] methods for making a discrete transformation topology-preserving, and therefore invertible, are described which could be embedded in a registration algorithm. However, to date there has not been a systematic evaluation of numerical methods for inversion of non-rigid registration transformations. Therefore, in this paper we evaluate different methods for computing the inverse of a dense, non-parametric, displacement field. We make no assumptions beyond assuming that the Jacobian determinant remains positive and comment on exceptions later. We focus on two classes of techniques (i) scattered data interpolation (SDI) and (ii) inverse-consistent iterative approaches. We evaluate the acuracy of these techniques globally and over specific neuroanatomical regions for transformations obtained from inter-subject MR brain registration.

2   Method

2.1   Inversion Problem

The inversion problem is sketched in figure 1. We assume the forward transformation is known at the target voxel centres, t, where solid arrows point to corresponding points in the source space. To invert this transformation the magnitude and direction of the dashed arrows must be deduced at voxel-centres, s, in the source space.

Inversion Using Direct Interpolation. The simplest interpolated inversion is a nearest-neighbour (NN) approach where the inverse transformation is defined as the negative nearest forward transformation vector. We adopted an extended NN method (NNe) as the simplest initialiser for the iterative methods described below. Where the nearest forward transformed point did not lie within the current source voxel because of local divergence, an average of forward transformed points in surrounding voxels was used. This was computed hierachically so that

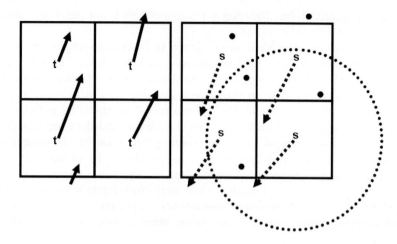

Fig. 1. Left: The forward transformation is defined in the target space at t. Right: The inverse transformation must be deduced in the source space at s. Filled dots indicate where the inverse transformation is defined by the forward transformation. The dashed circle indicates a possible search space for a scattered data interpolation approach.

averages with the highest number of nearest-neighbours were computed before averages with a smaller number of neighbours.

Inversion can also be cast as a simple scattered data interpolation (SDI) problem. In figure 1, the inverse transformation is known by definition at the points in the source image pointed to by the forward transformation and can be deduced at the voxel centres s by interpolation [7]. A distance weighting function, $w()$ sets the relative contribution of each scattered point to the interpolated inverse displacement; we chose an inverse-square (Shepard) weighting function (equation 1) where d_i is the distance from the interpolated point to the ith data point.

$$ I(s) = \frac{\sum_i w(d_i) * I(t_i + T_i)}{\sum_i w(d_i)} \tag{1} $$

As only local points contribute significantly, we use a modified weighting function incorporating a search radius, R, given by $w(d_i; R) = \left(\frac{1}{d_i} - \frac{1}{R}\right)^2$ when $d_i \leq R$ and $w(d_i; R) = 0$ otherwise. R is initially chosen to be twice the maximum voxel dimension but if no points are found it is arbitrarily increased until at least 4 scattered points are included.

Inversion Using Iterative Techniques. We compared two iterative techniques, one inverting point-by-point iteratively in target space (the **local** method) and one inverting the entire field iteratively in source space (the **global** method).

The **local** method is implemented as described in [1] and searches for the position in target-space, t where the trilinearly interpolated forward transformation,

```
FOREACH VOXEL, t
    i = 0
    DO
        R_L = t + T(t) − s
        t^{i+1} = t^i − R_L/2
        i = i + 1
    UNTIL (R_L ≤ tol) OR (i > 200)
    I(t) = −T(t^{i−1})
NEXT VOXEL
```

Fig. 2. Pseudo-code for **local** iterative inversion

$t + T(t)$ points to the current source voxel centre, s. A residual error R_L is used to update the current estimate of t at each voxel. Figure 2 shows pseudo-code for the **local** method.

The **global** method uses the current estimate of the inverse transformation I to interpolate (trilinearly) the forward transformation T to each source voxel-centre, s. Then the residual difference between the estimated inverse and the interpolated forward transformation is used to update the inverse as before. The magnitude of the update is capped for stability and each iteration is computed over the whole field before the next iteration. Figure 3 shows pseudo-code for the **global** method.

Both methods have a maximum number of iterations (200) specified and a stopping criterion based on residual size. The stopping criterion (residual < 0.01mm) for the **local** method is inherently stricter than for the **global** method as it is computed on a point-by-point basis rather than averaged over the volume. For this reason the **global** method has an additional stopping criterion based on the maximum inverse-consistency error being ≤ 0.1mm.

```
i = 0
DO
    max = av = 0
    INTERPOLATE T(s) FROM T(t) USING I()
    FOREACH VOXEL, t
        R_G(s) = I(s) + T(s)
        I^{i+1}(s) = I^i(s) − αR_G(s)
        av = av + |R_G|
        max = MAX(|R_G|, max)
        i = i + 1
    NEXT VOXEL
    av = av/nvox
UNTIL ((av ≤ tol) AND (max ≤ tolmax)) OR (i > 200)
```

Fig. 3. Pseudo-code for **global** iterative inversion

2.2   Image Registration Experiment

Image-data and structural labels from 18 subjects were supplied by the Centre for Morphometric Analysis, Boston. The scans were MRI T1-weighted coronal volume acquisitions of dimensions 256x256x128 and voxel sizes 1.0x1.0x1.5mm. All subjects were of normal appearance (i.e. had no obvious pathology or re-section). A standard (i.e. not inverse-consistent) non-rigid (fluid) registration algorithm [8] was used with two multi-resolution steps with a maximum of 200 iterations per step, driven by intensity cross-correlation. The 18 images were grouped randomly into 9 pairs and registered in both directions giving 18 registrations, i.e 9 forward and 9 reverse, so that the inherent inverse-consistency error of the registration algorithm could also be computed. Then the inverse of each registration transformation was computed using (a) SDI (b) NNe+**local** (c) SDI+**local** (d) NNe+**global** (e) SDI+**global**.

$$E_{IC} = |t' - t| \text{ where } t' = t + T(t) + I(t + T(t)) \tag{2}$$

We evaluated the different inversion methods by computing the inverse-consistency error (equation 2) at each point and compared this with the inherent registration inverse-consistency in corresponding forward and reverse registrations. We also computed the inversion error over ten specific brain structures (amygdala, caudate, cerebellum, cortex, hippocampus, lateral ventricles, pallidum, putamen, thalamus, white-matter). To assess how the error scaled with transformation magnitude a single transformation from the test set was (a) composed with global rotational components between 2.5° and 25.0° (b) globally scaled by factors in the range 1.25 to 5.00, and inverted as above.

3   Results

Figure 4 shows the mean and maximum global inverse-consistency error for the five inversion techniques. SDI produces sub-voxel inverse-consistency on average

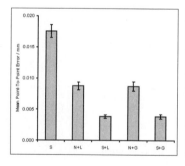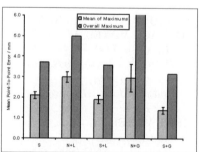

Fig. 4. The mean (left) and maximum (right) inverse-consistency error over 18 inter-subject brain registrations. S=Scattered Data Interpolation, N = Nearest-Neighbour-extended, L = Local Iterative and G = Global Iterative.

and using SDI to initialise either iterative method reduces the mean error further by $\sim 75\%$. In this experiment the SDI+**local** and SDI+**global** iterative methods are virtually indistinguishable as regards mean error but there is some regional variation apparent from maps of E_{IC} (figure 5). The SDI+**global** method had a lower maximum error averaged over all the registrations but the SDI+**local** method had a lower worst-case maximum error. By comparison, the inverse-consistency error determined directly from the forward and reverse non-rigid registration was much larger (0.7mm compared with 0.02mm for the SDI case).

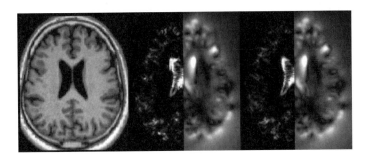

Fig. 5. Example of an inverse consistency error map for a single subject. Left Panel = subject anatomy. The left-hand-side of the middle and right panels shows the error distribution for S+L and S+G inversion methods respectively ranging from 0.0mm=black $\geq$ 0.6mm=white. For comparison the error distribution for fwd-rev registration is shown on the right-hand-side scaled from 0.0mm = black $\geq$ 6.0mm = white.

Figure 6 shows that the mean inversion error for all brain structures was $\ll 0.1$mm and that with the exception of the cerebral cortex (where the **global** error had signifcantly smaller mean error), the performance of **local** and **global** techniques is virtually identical. These errors should be considered in the context of the mean (maximum) displacements computed over all registrations for all structures of 4.2 (20.7)mm. We expect most inversion problems in the cortex region as inter-subject variation results in particularly tortuous non-rigid transformations. Figure 6 also shows the maximum inversion error over all registrations associated with each label. Overall the **global** inverses have lower maxima than the **local** with the most notable exception being in the hippocampus. Most structures have maximum errors $\leq$ 1mm, but the cortex, lateral ventricles and white matter structures have maximum errors $\sim$ 3mm. The ventricle results are dominated by two outlier cases with mean errors 10 times the rest of the cohort. Excluding these outliers gives a mean (maximum) error of 0.03 (0.08)mm for ventricles for both **local** and **global** methods. More detailed analysis is required to understand these cases which do not exhibit significantly larger deformation magnitudes than the rest of the cohort or have ventricle errors correlated with errors in the cortex. Figure 7 shows how the inversion error increases with the maximum rotational or scaled displacement. Note that the rotational displacement, which preserves local volume change, has a shallow linear error relationship

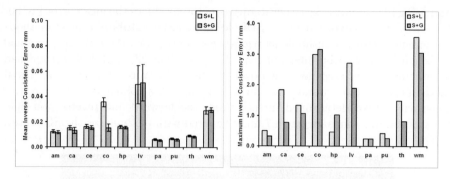

Fig. 6. The mean (left) and maximum (right) inverse-consistency error over 18 inter-subject brain registrations. am=amygdala, ca=caudate, ce=cerebellum, co=cortex, hp=hippocampus, lv = lateral ventricles, pa=pallidum, pu=putamen, th=thalamus, wm=white-matter.

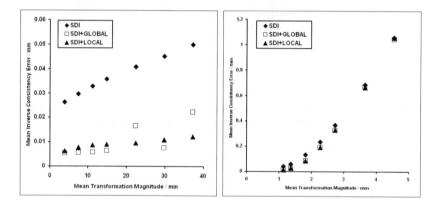

Fig. 7. The scaling of the mean inverse-consistency error with applied (left) rotation and (right) scaling

but the scaled displacement, which results in negative Jacobian determinants, has a polynomial error relationship.

4   Discussion

We have evaluated simple techniques for inversion of dense displacement fields in the context of inter-subject non-rigid registration algorithms and quantified the inversion error over a range of neuroanatomical structures. Both locally and globally consistent techniques initialised with a scattered data interpolation approach proved generally reliable and accurate in this study. We confirmed that inverting transformations matching convoluted structures such as the cortex is prone to relatively higher errors. While this is not unexpected it suggests that inverse-consistent registration approaches which rely on an explicit inverse calculation to enforce inverse-consistency will also perform less well in these regions.

All the original registration transformations were diffeomorphic i.e. the Jacobian determinant $|J| > 0$ everywhere and the transformation inverse was therefore well-defined throughout the domain. Many non-rigid algorithms do not guarantee a positive Jacobian determinant and therefore some transformation regularisation or transformation model-based constraints may be necessary.

The methods described here are completely generic and make no assumptions about the classes of permitted displacements. However these methods should be considered the "lowest common denominator" of inversion techniques and more sophisticated approaches will improve robustness. In future work we will analyze regions of displacement fields with high E_{IC} and investigate the use of regularising techniques in the spirit of [6] for regions with $|J| < 0$. These findings will be used to improve the performance of inverse-consistent registration algorithms.

References

1. Christensen, G.E, Johnson, H.J: Consistent image registration. IEEE Transactions on Medical Imaging 20(7), 568–582 (2001)
2. Cachier, P., Rey, D.: Symmetrization of the non-rigid registration problem using invertion-invariant energies: application to multiple sclerosis. In: Medical Image Computing and Computer-Assisted Intervention, pp. 472–481 (2000)
3. Rogelj, P., Kovačič, S.R.: Symmetric image registration. Medical Image Analysis 10(3), 484–493 (2006)
4. Crum, W.R, Griffin, L.D., Hill, D.L., Hawkes, D.J: Zen and the art of medical image registration: Correspondence, homology and quality. NeuroImage 20, 1425–1437 (2003)
5. Rao, A., Chandrashekara, R., Sanchez-Ortiz, G.I., Mohiaddin, R., Aljabar, P., Hajnal, J.V., Puri, B.K., Rueckert, D.: Spatial transformation of motion and deformation fields using nonrigid registration. IEEE Transactions on Medical Imaging 23(9), 1065–1076 (2004)
6. Karacali, B., Davatzikos, C.: Estimating topology preserving and smooth displacement fields. Journal of Electronic Imaging 23(7), 868–880 (2004)
7. Amidror, I.: Scattered data interpolation methods for electronic imaging systems: a survey. Journal of Electronic Imaging 11(2), 157–176 (2002)
8. Crum, W.R, Tanner, C., Hawkes, D.J: Multiresolution, anisotropic fluid registration: Evaluation in magnetic resonance breast imaging. Physics in Medicine and Biology 50, 5153–5174 (2005)

Registration of High Angular Resolution Diffusion MRI Images Using 4th Order Tensors*

Angelos Barmpoutis, Baba C. Vemuri, and John R. Forder

University of Florida, Gainesville FL 32611, USA
{abarmpou,vemuri}@cise.ufl.edu, jforder@mbi.ufl.edu

Abstract. Registration of Diffusion Weighted (DW)-MRI datasets has been commonly achieved to date in literature by using either scalar or 2nd-order tensorial information. However, scalar or 2nd-order tensors fail to capture complex local tissue structures, such as fiber crossings, and therefore, datasets containing fiber-crossings cannot be registered accurately by using these techniques. In this paper we present a novel method for non-rigidly registering DW-MRI datasets that are represented by a field of 4th-order tensors. We use the Hellinger distance between the normalized 4th-order tensors represented as distributions, in order to achieve this registration. Hellinger distance is easy to compute, is scale and rotation invariant and hence allows for comparison of the true shape of distributions. Furthermore, we propose a novel 4th-order tensor re-transformation operator, which plays an essential role in the registration procedure and shows significantly better performance compared to the re-orientation operator used in literature for DTI registration. We validate and compare our technique with other existing scalar image and DTI registration methods using simulated diffusion MR data and real HARDI datasets.

1   Introduction

In medical imaging, during the last decade, it has become possible to collect magnetic resonance image (MRI) data that measures the apparent diffusivity of water in tissue *in vivo*. A 2nd order tensor has commonly been used to approximate the diffusivity profile at each image lattice point in a DW-MRI [4]. The approximated diffusivity function is given by

$$d(\mathbf{g}) = \mathbf{g}^T \mathbf{D} \mathbf{g} \tag{1}$$

where $\mathbf{g} = [g_1 \ g_2 \ g_3]^T$ is the magnetic field gradient direction and $\mathbf{D}$ is the estimated 2nd-order tensor.

Registration of DW-MRI datasets by using 2nd-order tensors has been proposed by Alexander et al. [2]. In this work a tensor re-orientation operation was

* This research was in part supported by RO1 EB007082 and NS42075 to BCV and the data collection was in part supported by the grants R01 NS36992 and P41 RR16105. We thank Dr. Stephen Blackband for supporting the data collection and Dr. Shepherd for collecting the data.

N. Ayache, S. Ourselin, A. Maeder (Eds.): MICCAI 2007, Part I, LNCS 4791, pp. 908–915, 2007.
© Springer-Verlag Berlin Heidelberg 2007

proposed as a significant part of the diffusion tensor field transformation procedure. A framework for non-rigid registration of multi-modal medical images was proposed in [12]. This technique performs registration based on extraction of highly structured features from the datasets and it was applied to tensor fields. Registration of DTI using quantities which are invariant to rigid transformations and computed from the diffusion tensors was proposed in [7]. By registering the rigid-tranformation invariant maps, one avoids the re-orientation step and thus can reduce the time complexity. The locally affine multi-resolution scalar image registration proposed in [8] was extended to DTI images in [17]. In this method the image domain of the image being registered is subdivided (using a multi-resolution framework) into smaller regions, and each region is registered using affine transformation. The affine transformation is parametrized using a transformation vector, a rotation, and an SPD matrix. By using this parametrization one can avoid the polar decomposition step which is required in order to extract the rotation component for re-orientation purposes.

All the above methods perform registration of DW-MRI datasets based on scalar images or 2nd-order tensorial approximations of the local diffusivity. This approximation fails to represent complex local tissue structures, such as fiber crossings, and therefore DTI registration of dataset containing such crossings leads to inaccurate transformations of the local tissue structures.

In this paper we present a novel registration method for DW-MRI datasets represented by a field of 4th-order tensors. We propose to use the Hellinger distance measure between 4th-order tensors represented by angular distributions (corresponding to the normalized coefficients of these tensors), and employ it in the registration procedure. Hellinger distance is very commonly used in communication networks and also in density estimation techniques as it is quite robust and has attractive asymptotics [5]. From our point of view, this distance is easy to compute and is scale and rotation invariant, thus allowing for true shape comparison [9]. Another key contribution of our work is the higher-order tensor re-transformation operation, which is applied in our registration algorithm. We validate our framework and compare it with existing techniques using simulated MR and real datasets.

2   Registration of 4th-Order Tensor Fields

This section is organized as follows: First, in 2.1 we briefly review the formulation of 4th-order tensors in DW-MRI. Then, in section 2.2 we define the Hellinger distance between 4th-order tensors represented by angular distributions, which will be employed in section 2.3 for registration of 4th-order tensor fields.

2.1 4th-Order Symmetric Positive Tensors from DW-MRI

The diffusivity function can be modeled by Eq. 1 using a 2nd-order tensor. Studies have shown that this approximation fails to model complex local diffusivity profiles in real tissues [14,10,11,1] and a higher-order approximation must be employed instead. Several higher-order approximations have been proposed in literature and among them, spherical harmonics [14,6], cartesian tensors [10] etc. have been popular. A 4th-order tensor can be employed in the following diffusivity function

$$d(\mathbf{g}) = \sum_{i+j+k=4} D_{i,j,k} g_1^i g_2^j g_3^k \tag{2}$$

where $\mathbf{g} = [g_1\ g_2\ g_3]^T$ is the magnetic field gradient direction. It should be noted that in the case of 4th-order symmetric tensors there are 15 unique coefficients $D_{i,j,k}$, while in the case of 2nd-order tensors we only have 6.

A positive definite 4th-order tensor field can be estimated from a DW-MRI dataset using the parametrization proposed in [3]. In this parametrization, a 4th-order symmetric positive definite tensor is expressed as a sum of squares of three quadratic forms as $d(\mathbf{g}) = (\mathbf{v}^T\mathbf{q}_1)^2 + (\mathbf{v}^T\mathbf{q}_2)^2 + (\mathbf{v}^T\mathbf{q}_3)^2 = \mathbf{v}^T\mathbf{Q}\mathbf{Q}^T\mathbf{v} = \mathbf{v}^T\mathbf{G}\mathbf{v}$ where $\mathbf{v}$ is a properly chosen vector of monomials, (e.g. $[g_1^2\ g_2^2\ g_3^2\ g_1g_2\ g_1g_3\ g_2g_3]^T$), $\mathbf{Q} = [\mathbf{q}_1|\mathbf{q}_2|\mathbf{q}_3]$ is a 6×3 matrix obtained by stacking the 6 coefficient vectors $\mathbf{q}_i$ and $\mathbf{G} = \mathbf{Q}\mathbf{Q}^T$ is the so called *Gram matrix*. Gram matrix $\mathbf{G}$ is symmetric positive semi-definite and has rank=3. By using this parametrization and following the algorithm presented in [3], a Gram matrix $\mathbf{G}$ is estimated at each voxel of a DW-MRI dataset. Then, one can uniquely compute the tensor coefficients $D_{i,j,k}$ from the coefficients of $\mathbf{G}$.

Given two different DW-MRI datasets depicting the same or different subjects, one can register them by using the information provided by the coefficients $D_{i,j,k}$ of the corresponding 4th-order tensor fields. For this purpose, we need to define the appropriate metric between higher-order tensors, which will be later employed by the registration algorithm.

2.2   Distance Measure

In this section we define a distance measure between symmetric positive definite 4th-order tensors using their corresponding normalized representations which are angular distributions. A family of angular distributions for modeling antipodal symmetric directional data is the angular central Gaussian distribution family, which has a simple formula and a number of properties discussed in [16].

The family of angular central Gaussian distributions on the q-dimensional sphere S_q with radius one is given by $p(\mathbf{g}) = \frac{1}{Z_q(\mathbf{T})}(\mathbf{g}^T\mathbf{T}^{-1}\mathbf{g})^{-\frac{q+1}{2}}$ where $\mathbf{g}$ is a $(q+1)$-dimensional unit vector, $\mathbf{T}$ is a symmetric positive-definite matrix and $Z_q(\mathbf{T})$ is a normalizing factor. In the S_2 case, $\mathbf{g}$ is a 3 dimensional unit vector, $Z_2(\mathbf{T}) = 4\pi\sqrt{|\mathbf{T}|}$, and $\mathbf{T}$ is a 3×3 symmetric positive-definite matrix similar to the 2nd-order tensor used in DTI. A generalization of this distribution family for the case of higher-order tensors should involve an appropriate generalized normalizing factor as a function of higher-order tensors and a generalization of the tensor inversion operation, which may not lead to a closed-form expression. In order to get closed-form expressions we define a new higher-order angular distribution as

$$p(\mathbf{g}) = \frac{1}{\int_{S_2} d(\mathbf{g})^2} d(\mathbf{g})^2 \tag{3}$$

where in the case of 4th-order tensors $d(\mathbf{g})$ is given by Eq. (2) and the integral is over S_2 (i.e. over all unit vectors $\mathbf{g}$). The integral in Eq. (3) can be analytically computed and it can be written in a sum-of-squares form [3].

Given two angular distributions we need to define a scale and rotation invariant metric in order to make true shape (obtained after removing scale and orientation) comparison between them. This can be efficiently done by the Hellinger distance between 4th-order tensors $\mathbf{D}_1$ and $\mathbf{D}_2$:

$$dist^2(\mathbf{D}_1, \mathbf{D}_2) = \int_{S_2} (\sqrt{p_1(\mathbf{g})} - \sqrt{p_2(\mathbf{g})})^2 = \int_{S_2} (\frac{d_1(\mathbf{g})}{\sqrt{\int_{S_2}(d_1(\mathbf{g}))^2}} - \frac{d_2(\mathbf{g})}{\sqrt{\int_{S_2}(d_2(\mathbf{g}))^2}})^2 \tag{4}$$

Here we use the notation $\mathbf{D}$ to denote the 15-dimensional vector consisting of the unique coefficients $D_{i,j,k}$ of a 4th-order tensor. Eq. 4 can also be analytically expressed in a sum-of-squares form and it is invariant to scale and rotations of the 3D space, i.e. the distance between $p_1(\mathbf{g})$ and $p_2(\mathbf{g})$ is equal to the distance between $p_1(s\mathbf{Rg})$ and $p_2(s\mathbf{Rg})$, where $\mathbf{R}$ is a 3×3 rotation matrix and s is a scale parameter.

In the following section we use the above distance measure for registering a pair of misaligned 4th-order tensor fields.

2.3   Registration

In this section we present an algorithm for 4th-order tensor field registration. Given two 4th-order tensor fields $I_1(\mathbf{x})$ and $I_2(\mathbf{x})$, where $\mathbf{x}$ is the 3D lattice index, we need to estimate the unknown transformation $F(\mathbf{x})$, which transforms the dataset $I_1(F(\mathbf{x}))$ in order to better match $I_2(\mathbf{x})$. In the case of an affine transformation we have $F(\mathbf{x}) = \mathbf{Ax} + \mathbf{T}$, where $\mathbf{A}$ is a 3×3 transformation matrix and $\mathbf{T}$ is the translational component of the transformation.

The estimation of the unknown transformation parameters can be done by minimizing the following energy function

$$E(\mathbf{A}, \mathbf{T}) = \int_{\Re^3} dist^2(I_1(\mathbf{Ax} + \mathbf{T}), \mathbf{A}^{-1} \times I_2(\mathbf{x}))d\mathbf{x} \tag{5}$$

where $dist(.,.)$ is the distance measuere between 4th-order tensors defined in section 2.2, and the integral is over the 3D image domain. $\mathbf{A}^{-1} \times I_2(\mathbf{x})$ denotes some higher-order tensor re-transformation operation. This operation applies the inverse transformation to the tensors of the dataset I_2 in order to compare them with the corresponding tensors of the transformed image I_1.

In the case of registering 2nd-order tensor fields, it has been shown that the unknown transformation parameters can be successfully estimated by applying only the rotation component of the transformation to the dataset I_2 [2]. This happens because of the fact that 2nd-order tensors can approximate only single fiber distributions, whose principal direction transformation can be adequately performed by applying rotations only to the tensors.

In the case of 4th-order tensors, multiple fiber distributions can be resolved by a single tensor, whose relative orientations can also be affected by the deformation part of the applied transformation. Therefore, tensor re-orientation is not meaningful for higher-order tensors and in this case a tensor re-transformation operation must be performed instead, using the full affine matrix $\mathbf{A}$, which is defined in section 2.4. Affine transformation has been also used in DTI; for more details and justification of the scheme, the reader is referred to [15].

Equation (5) can be extended for non-rigid registration of 4th-order tensor fields by dividing the domain of image I_1 into N smaller regions and then registering each smaller region by using affine transformations. Similar method has been used for scalar image registration [8] and DTI registration [17]. The unknown transformation parameters can be estimated by minimizing

$$E(\mathbf{A}_1, \mathbf{T}_1, \ldots, \mathbf{A}_N, \mathbf{T}_N) = \sum_{r=1}^{N} \int_{\Re^3} dist^2(I_{1,r}(\mathbf{A}_r\mathbf{x} + \mathbf{T_r}), \mathbf{A}_r^{-1} \times I_2(\mathbf{x}))d\mathbf{x} \quad (6)$$

Eq. 6 can be efficiently minimized by a conjugate gradient algorithm used in a multi-resolution framework, similar to that used in [8] and [17].

2.4   3D Affine Transformation of 4th-Order Tensors

Assume that we have vectorized the coefficients $D_{i,j,k}$ into a 1×15 vector $\mathbf{D}$ in some specific order $D_n = D_{i_n,j_n,k_n}$, (e.g. $D_1 = D_{4,0,0}$, $D_2 = D_{2,2,0}$, etc.). By using this vector, Eq. 2 can be written as $\sum_{n=1}^{15} D_n g_1^{i_n} g_2^{j_n} g_3^{k_n}$. If we apply an affine transformation defined by the 3×3 matrix $\mathbf{A}$ to the 3D space, the previous equation becomes $\sum_{n=1}^{15} D_n (\mathbf{a}_1\mathbf{g})^{i_n} (\mathbf{a}_2\mathbf{g})^{j_n} (\mathbf{a}_3\mathbf{g})^{k_n}$, where $(\mathbf{a}_1\mathbf{g})^{i_n} (\mathbf{a}_2\mathbf{g})^{j_n} (\mathbf{a}_3\mathbf{g})^{k_n}$ is a polynomial of order 4 in 3 variables g_1, g_2, g_3, and a_i is the ith raw of $\mathbf{A}$. In this summation there are 15 such polynomials and each of them can be expanded as $\sum_{m=1}^{15} C_{m,n} g_1^{i_m} g_2^{j_m} g_3^{k_m}$, by computing the corresponding coefficients $C_{m,n}$ as functions of matrix $\mathbf{A}$. For example if we use the same vectorization as we did in the previous example, we have $C_{1,1} = (A_{1,1})^4$, $C_{1,2} = (A_{1,1})^2(A_{2,1})^2$, etc. Therefore, we can construct the 15×15 matrix $\mathbf{C}$, whose elements $C_{m,n}$ are simple functions of $\mathbf{A}$, and use it to define the operation of transforming a 4th-order tensor $\mathbf{D}$ by a 3D affine transformation $\mathbf{A}$ as

$$\mathbf{A} \times \mathbf{D} = \mathbf{C}(A) \cdot D \quad (7)$$

3   Experimental Results

In the experiments presented in this section, we tested the performance of our method using simulated diffusion-weighted MR data and real HARDI data sets. The figures in this section are depicting probability profiles estimated from the 4th-order tensors [11]. The synthetic data were generated by simulating the MR signal from single fibers and fiber crossings using the simulation model in [13]. A

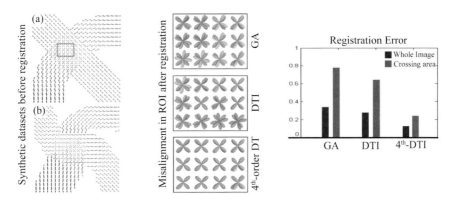

Fig. 1. Left: a) Synthetically generated dataset by simulating the MR signal [13]. b) Dataset generated by applying a non-rigid transformation to (a). Center: Crossing misalignment in ROI after registering datasets (a) and (b) using various methods. Right: Quantitative comparison of the registration errors. The errors were measured by Eq. 4 for the whole field.

dataset of size 128×128 was generated by simulating two fiber bundles crossing each other (Fig. 1a). Then, a non-rigid deformation was randomly generated as a b-spline displacement field and then applied to the original dataset. The obtained dataset is shown in Fig. 1b.

In order to compare the accuracy of our 4th-order tensor field registration method with other methods that perform DTI regitration or registration of scalar quantities computed from tensors (e.g. GA), we registered the dataset of Fig. 1a with that of Fig. 1b by performing: a) General Anisotropy (GA) map registration using the method in [8], b) DTI registration using the algorithm in [17] and c) 4th-order tensor registration using our proposed method. Fig. 1 (center) shows a comparison of the registration results in the region of interest (ROI) shown in the box of Fig. 1a. Each plate in this column shows the misalignment of the fiber crossing profiles after registering using the above methods. By observing the results, our proposed method performs significantly better than the other methods, and motivates the use of 4th-order tensors for registering DW-MRI datasets. Figure 1 (right) shows a quantitative comparison of the above results by measuring the distance between the corresponding misaligned tensors by using the measure defined in section 2.2. The results conclusively validate the accuracy of our method and demonstrate its superior performance compared to the other existing methods.

Furthermore, another dataset (shown in Fig. 2 left) was simulated using [13], by stretching the fibers of Fig.1a along the x-axis by a factor s. In this simulation the fiber orientations were taken to form an angle $\phi' = atan(tan(\phi)/s)$ with x-axis, where ϕ is the original angle between the fiber orientation and x-axis, which was used in the simulation of dataset in Fig. 1a.

In order to demonstrate the need of the tensor re-transformation operation defined in section 2.4, we registered the dataset in Fig. 1a with that in Fig. 2(left)

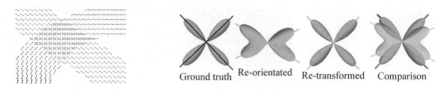

Ground truth   Re-orientated   Re-transformed   Comparison

Fig. 2. Left: Simulated dataset generated by stretching the fibers of Fig 1a. Rest of the plates: Comparison of results after registering dataset in Fig.2(left) to that of Fig.1a using tensor re-orientation only and our proposed tensor re-transformation.

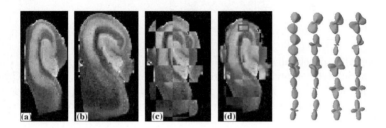

Fig. 3. a and b) S_0 images from two HARDI volumes of human hippocampi. c,d) datasets before and after registration. Tensors from the ROI in (d) showing crossings.

by using: a) re-orientation only in Eq. (5), and b) our proposed re-transformation operation. Fig. 2 depict: a single tensor from the crossing region of the dataset in Fig. 2(left) after registering the datasets using the two methods. By observing the results, we conclude that by re-orienting only the tensors, the fiber orientations were inaccurately estimated, and this motivates the use of our proposed re-transformation.

In the data acquisition first an image without diffusion-weighting was collected, and then 21 diffusion-weighted images were collected with a 415 mT/m diffusion gradient (T_d =17 ms, δ = 2.4ms, b = 1250 s/mm^2). Figure 3 shows two S_0 images from the two 3D volumes (a,b), and two "checkers" images showing the datasets before (c) and after registration (d). A "checkers" image is a way to display two images at the same time, presenting one image in the half boxes, and the other in the rest of the boxes. Based on knowledge of hippocampal anatomy, fiber crossings are observed in several hippocampal regions such as CA3 stratum pyramidale and stratum lucidum. Therefore, one should employ our 4th-order tensor method instead of DTI registration. By observing Fig.3d all the hippocampal regions were successfully alligned by our method, transforming appropriately the fiber crossings Fig. 3(right).

4   Conclusions

Registration of DW-MRI datasets has been commonly performed by using either scalar or DTI information [17]. However scalar or 2nd-order tensorial approximation fails to represent complex local tissue structures, such as fiber crossings, resulting in inaccurate transformations in regions where such complex structures are present. In this paper we presented a method for registering diffusion weighted MRI represented by 4th-order tensor fields. This method employs a novel scale and rotation invariant distance measure between 4th-order tensors. We also proposed a 4th-order tensor re-transformation operation and showed that it plays essential role in the registration procedure. We applied our method to both synthetically generated datasets from simulated MR signal, and real high angular resolution diffusion weighted MR datasets. We compared and validated our method, showing superior performance over other existing methods.

References

1. Alexander, D.C.: Maximum entropy spherical deconvolution for diffusion MRI. In: IPMI, pp. 76–87 (2005)
2. Alexander, D.C., Pierpaoli, C., Basser, P.J., Gee, J.C.: Spatial transformations of diffusion tensor magnetic resonance images. TMI 20(11), 1131–1139 (2001)
3. Barmpoutis, A., et al.: Symmetric positive 4th order tensor and their estimation from diffusion weighted MRI. In: Karssemeijer, N., Lelieveldt, B. (eds.) IPMI 2007. LNCS, vol. 4584, pp. 308–319. Springer, Heidelberg (2007)
4. Basser, P.J., Mattiello, J., Lebihan, D.: Estimation of the Effective Self-Diffusion Tensor from the NMR Spin Echo. J. Magn. Reson. B 103, 247–254 (1994)
5. Beran, R.: Minimum hellinger distance estimates for parametric models. The Annals of Statistics 5(3), 445–463 (1977)
6. Frank, L.R.: Characterization of anisotropy in high angular resolution diffusion-weighted MRI. Magn. Reson. Med. 47(6), 1083–1099 (2002)
7. Guimond, A., et al.: Deformable registration of DT-MRI data based on transformation invariant tensor characteristics. ISBI (2002)
8. Ju, S.X., Black, M.J., Jepson, A.D.: Skin and bones: Multi-layer, locally affine, optical flow regularization with transparency. In: CVPR, pp. 307–314 (1996)
9. Kendall, D.G.: Shape manifolds, procrustean metrics, and complex projective spaces. Bulletin of the London Mathematical Society 16(2), 81–121 (1984)
10. Ozarslan, E., Mareci, T.H.: Generalized diffusion tensor imaging and analytical relationships between DTI and HARDI. MRM 50(5), 955–965 (2003)
11. Özarslan, E., et al.: Resolution of complex tissue microarchitecture using the diffusion orientation transform (DOT). NeuroImage 31, 1086–1103 (2006)
12. Ruiz-Azola, J., Westin, C.F., Warfield, S.K., Alberola, C., Maier, S., Kikinis, R.: Non rigid registration of 3d tonsor medical data. Med. Im. Anal. 6, 143–161 (2002)
13. Söderman, O., Jönsson, B.: Restricted diffusion in cylindrical geometry. J. Magn. Reson. A(117), 94–97 (1995)
14. Tuch, D.: Q-ball imaging. Magn. Reson. Med. 52, 1358–1372 (2004)
15. Wang, Z., Vemuri, B.C.: DTI segmentation using an information theoretic tensor dissimilarity measure. IEEE TMI 24(10), 1267–1277 (2005)
16. Watson, G.S.: Statistics on Spheres. Wiley, New York (1983)
17. Zhang, H., Yushkevich, P.A., Gee, J.C.: Registration of Diffusion Tensor Images. CVPR 1, 842–847 (2004)

Non-rigid Image Registration Using Graph-cuts

Tommy W.H. Tang and Albert C.S. Chung

Lo Kwee-Seong Medical Image Analysis Laboratory,
Department of Computer Science and Engineering, The Hong Kong University of
Science and Technology, Hong Kong
{cstommy,achung}@cse.ust.hk

Abstract. Non-rigid image registration is an ill-posed yet challenging problem due to its supernormal high degree of freedoms and inherent requirement of smoothness. Graph-cuts method is a powerful combinatorial optimization tool which has been successfully applied into image segmentation and stereo matching. Under some specific constraints, graph-cuts method yields either a global minimum or a local minimum in a strong sense. Thus, it is interesting to see the effects of using graph-cuts in non-rigid image registration. In this paper, we formulate non-rigid image registration as a discrete labeling problem. Each pixel in the source image is assigned a displacement label (which is a vector) indicating which position in the floating image it is spatially corresponding to. A smoothness constraint based on first derivative is used to penalize sharp changes in displacement labels across pixels. The whole system can be optimized by using the graph-cuts method via alpha-expansions. We compare 2D and 3D registration results of our method with two state-of-the-art approaches. It is found that our method is more robust to different challenging non-rigid registration cases with higher registration accuracy.

1 Introduction

Image registration is actively applied in the field of medical image analysis. Unlike rigid registration, non-rigid registration is an ill-posed problem due to its supernormal high degree of freedoms and inherent requirement of smoothness. Yet, there are a wide range of applications for non-rigid image registration [1].

The task of image registration is to find a transformation T such that I and $T(J)$ are spatially matched, according to an image-to-image dissimilarity measure, $C(I, T(J))$. I and J are referred as the source image and the floating image respectively and $T(J)$ refers to the resultant image after applying T to J. Mathematically, the registration problem can be defined as finding the optimal transformation T^* such that

$$T^* = \arg\min_T C(I, T(J)). \tag{1}$$

Unlike rigid image registration in which T is restricted to a rigid transformation, for non-rigid image registration, there is still no common consensus in the literature regarding how the transformation T should be modeled. Some models restrict T to be of low degree of freedoms, such as affine, polyaffine [2] or

N. Ayache, S. Ourselin, A. Maeder (Eds.): MICCAI 2007, Part I, LNCS 4791, pp. 916–924, 2007.
© Springer-Verlag Berlin Heidelberg 2007

control-points interpolated deformation [3] models. These models intrinsically constrain T to be smooth or elastic and they are usually capable of representing an intra-patient deformation across time since there is a real physical underlying deformation between the images. However, in the case of inter-patient image registration, anatomical structures can vary significantly across patients both geometrically and topologically, a transformation of low degree of freedoms may not have the flexibility to represent these complex changes. Therefore, in principal, any hard constraints on the domain of T should not be imposed. However, in Eqn. 1, we are optimizing $C(I, T(J))$ without posing any restrictions on T and T can map any points in J to any points in I without correlation across neighborhood pixels. Thus, T needs regularization by adding a penalizing function $S(T)$ to penalize those T, which are not smooth. By modifying Eqn. 1, we get

$$T^* = \arg\min_{T} \quad C(I, T(J)) + \lambda S(T), \tag{2}$$

where λ is a positive constant that controls the level of penalty for non-smooth T. If we consider T as a displacement vector field, integrated magnitude of different derivatives is usually used as a criterion of smoothness in practice.

Two pioneer works of formulating non-rigid image registration, namely, Free-Form Deformations Based Method (denoted as **FFD** later) and Demons Based Method (denoted as **DEMONS** later), are widely used in the medical image analysis field and can be considered state-of-the-art. Rueckert *et al.* [3] proposed a method which modeled the local deformation by free-form deformation based on B-splines. In this method, only a regular grid of control points on the image are allowed to displace freely. The displacement of any other point is obtained from the displacements of its neighborhood control points, via B-spline interpolation functions. If a sparse set of control points is used, the transformation may not allow flexible movements of pixels to represent complicated deformation. We will show the effects in the experimental results section. Thirion [4] proposed a diffusion-based approach to non-rigid image registration. No hard constraints were imposed on the transformation T so that each pixel can have its own displacement. In each iteration, the movement of any pixel in the floating image is based on its local intensity gradient and its intensity difference with the source image at the same position. It will naturally guarantee a decrease in (sum squared differences) SSD or (sum absolute differences) SAD by each iteration if the movement steps are sufficiently small. Since all pixels can move freely, a Gaussian smoothing step is applied at the end of each iteration in order to regularize the transformation. However, since the regularization is done after each iteration but not incorporated into the cost function, large displacements of pixels or sharp changes in the displacement field may not be penalized. Moreover, since the motions of pixels are highly depending on local intensity gradient, this method is highly sensitive to local artifacts. The effect will be demonstrated in the experimental results section.

In this paper, we formulate a new non-rigid image registration framework as a discrete labeling problem. Each pixel in the source image has a displacement label (which is a vector) indicating its corresponding position in the floating image, according to a similarity measure. A smoothness constraint based on first derivative is used to penalize sharp changes in displacement labels across pixels. The whole system can be optimized by using the graph-cuts method via alpha-expansions [5]. Through graph-cuts, the optimization process is not easily trapped in local minima and the solution is guaranteed to be within a known factor of the exact minimum. This makes the registration robustness and accuracy of our approach significantly better than other methods. To the best of our knowledge, our work is the first time where 3D labels are used in graph-cuts method, though using 2D labels in graph-cuts has been successfully applied in motion detection [5,6].

2   Theory and Methodology

2.1   Formulation of the Energy Function

Let I and J respectively be the source image and the floating image of dimension d and $\mathbf{X}$ be the continuous spatial domain of both images. For any spatial point $\mathbf{x} = (x_1, x_2, ..., x_d) \in \mathbf{X}$, $I(\mathbf{x})$ and $J(\mathbf{x})$ are the intensity values (or feature vectors in general) at $\mathbf{x}$ of both images. In our formulation, a transformation T is represented by a displacement vector field $\mathbf{D}$ that displaces every point $\mathbf{x}$ in J away from its original position by the vector $\mathbf{D}(\mathbf{x}) \in \mathbb{R}^d$ to the new point $\mathbf{x} + \mathbf{D}(\mathbf{x})$. By modifying Eqn. 2, we can get

$$\mathbf{D}^* = \arg\min_{\mathbf{D}} \ C(I(\mathbf{X}), J(\mathbf{X} + \mathbf{D})) + \lambda S(\mathbf{D}). \tag{3}$$

We use integrated absolute difference as the dissimilarity function C, and magnitide of first derivative terms as the smoothness function S. It yields

$$\mathbf{D}^* = \arg\min_{\mathbf{D}} \ \int_{\mathbf{X}} \|I(\mathbf{x}) - J(\mathbf{x} + \mathbf{D}(\mathbf{x}))\| \, d\mathbf{X} + \lambda \sum_{i=1}^{d} \int_{\mathbf{X}} \|\mathbf{D}_{(x_i)}\| \, d\mathbf{X}, \tag{4}$$

where $\mathbf{D}_{(x_i)}$ is the first derivative of $\mathbf{D}$ along direction x_i and the differential element $d\mathbf{X} = dx_1 dx_2 ... dx_d$. Since everything is in the continuous domain, $\mathbf{D}$ can have infinite degree of freedoms theoretically. Here, we introduce the first discretization step, by discretizing $\mathbf{X}$ into pixels. This is a natural discretizing step as images are usually acquired in a discretized form. By replacing all integrals by summations and derivatives by finite differences, Eqn. 4 becomes

$$\mathbf{D}^* = \arg\min_{\mathbf{D}} \ \sum_{\mathbf{x} \in \mathbf{X}} \|I(\mathbf{x}) - J(\mathbf{x} + \mathbf{D}(\mathbf{x}))\| + \lambda \sum_{(\mathbf{x},\mathbf{y}) \in \mathcal{N}} \|\mathbf{D}(\mathbf{x}) - \mathbf{D}(\mathbf{y})\|, \tag{5}$$

where $(\mathbf{x}, \mathbf{y}) \in \mathcal{N}$ iff x and y are adjacent pixels. Note that at this stage, $\mathbf{D}(\mathbf{x}) \in \mathbb{R}^d$ is still not discretized. Therefore, $\mathbf{x} + \mathbf{D}(\mathbf{x})$ in Eqn. 5 can be any non-integer valued vector, and $J(\mathbf{x} + \mathbf{D}(\mathbf{x}))$ needs to be computed using an interpolation function. Also, when $\mathbf{x} + \mathbf{D}(\mathbf{x})$ is outside the image domain, a pre-assigned background intensity value can be used.

In principle, Eqn. 5 can be optimized by any iterative optimization tools instead of using the graph-cuts method. However, in practice, the degree of freedoms of $\mathbf{D}$ can be as high as a billion. First, it may cost huge amount of time for the optimization process. Second, since $\mathbf{D}$ has value in each pixel position, it is a requirement that the step size of updating $\mathbf{D}$ is sufficiently small in each iteration in order to ensure a smooth field. Not only adding an extra time cost, this makes the optimization process highly sensitive to local minima. Yet, Eqn. 5 is still not solvable by the graph-cuts method without modifications. It will be addressed shortly in the next subsection.

2.2 Optimization Via Graph-cuts

Unlike other general purpose techniques such as simulated annealing, which can be extremely slow in practice to find good optima of an energy function, the graph-cuts method yields either a global minimum or a strong local minimum in polynomial time, under some specific conditions. In general, the graph-cuts method is used to solve labeling problems by minimizing energy function E_f in the following form [5,7],

$$E_f = \sum_{p \in \mathcal{P}} D_p(f_p) + \sum_{(p,q) \in \mathcal{N}} V_{p,q}(f_p, f_q). \tag{6}$$

In Eqn. 6, $\mathcal{P}$ is the set of pixels, $\mathcal{N} \subset \mathcal{P} \times \mathcal{P}$ is a neighborhood system defined on $\mathcal{P}$, $f : \mathcal{P} \to L$ is a labeling function where L is a set of labels, $f_i \in L$ is the label of pixel i in f. The term $D_p(f_p)$ measures the penalty of assigning label f_p to pixel p and the term $V_{p,q}(f_p, f_q)$ measures the penalty of assigning labels f_p, f_q to the neighborhood pixels p, q respectively. The two summations are usually referred as the data term and the smoothness term.

Comparing with the form of function solvable by the graph-cuts method in Eqn. 6, it is not difficult to observe that our current energy function in Eqn. 5 is already in that form if we consider a 4-connected neighborhood system $\mathcal{N}$, i.e., $(\mathbf{x}, \mathbf{y}) \in \mathcal{N}$ iff $\mathbf{x}, \mathbf{y}$ are adjacent pixels.

To convert our optimization to a labeling problem, $\mathbf{D}(\mathbf{x}) \in \mathbb{R}^d$ should be limited into a finite set. Here, we perform the second discretization step. Also acting as a restriction of how far a pixel can be displaced, a discretized window $W = \{0, \pm s, \pm 2s, ..., \pm ws\}^d$ of dimension d is chosen such that $\mathbf{D}(\mathbf{x}) \in W$. Note that W is the discretization of the continuous dimension-d region $[-ws, ws]^d$ with sampling period s along all directions. Also, if $s < 1$, displacements with sub-pixel units can be considered. Now, by using W as the set of labels that every $\mathbf{D}(\mathbf{x})$ can be assigned, the optimization in Eqn. 5 can readily be solved by using graph-cuts via a sequence of alpha-expansion (α-expansion) [5] moves.

Given the current labeling f for the set of pixels $\mathcal{P}$ and a new label α, an α-expansion move means: For any pixel $p \in \mathcal{P}$, it is considered either keeping its current label f_p or changing its label to α in the next labeling f'. Obviously, an α-expansion move is a two-label problem, with label 0 meaning $f'_p = f_p$ and label 1 meaning $f'_p = \alpha$. Kolmogorov & Zabih [7] showed that the graph-cuts method can find the exact minimum of a two-label problem if every $V_{p,q}$ term in Eqn. 6 satisfies the following inequality.

$$V_{p,q}(0,0) + V_{p,q}(1,1) \leq V_{p,q}(0,1) + V_{p,q}(1,0). \tag{7}$$

We now show that any expansion move of our formulation satisfies Eqn. 7. Given a current labeling f and two adjacent pixels $\mathbf{x}, \mathbf{y}$ with $f_{\mathbf{x}} = \beta$ and $f_{\mathbf{y}} = \gamma$, where $\beta, \gamma \in \mathcal{W}$, an expansion move of new label $\alpha \in \mathcal{W}$ is considered.

- $V_{\mathbf{x},\mathbf{y}}(0,0) = \|\beta - \gamma\|$ is the cost when both $\mathbf{x}, \mathbf{y}$ choose their old labels β, γ.
- $V_{\mathbf{x},\mathbf{y}}(1,1) = \|\alpha - \alpha\| = \mathbf{0}$ is the cost when both $\mathbf{x}, \mathbf{y}$ choose new label α.
- $V_{\mathbf{x},\mathbf{y}}(0,1) = \|\beta - \alpha\|$ is the cost when $\mathbf{x}$ retains β but $\mathbf{y}$ chooses new label α.
- $V_{\mathbf{x},\mathbf{y}}(1,0) = \|\alpha - \gamma\|$ is the cost when $\mathbf{x}$ chooses new label α but $\mathbf{y}$ retains γ.

Since $\alpha, \beta, \gamma \in \mathcal{W} \subset \mathbb{R}^d$ and $\| \cdot \|$ is the L2-norm operator, by the triangle inequality, we have $\|\beta - \gamma\| \leq \|\beta - \alpha\| + \|\alpha - \gamma\|$ for any vectors α, β, γ. Thus, the inequality in Eqn. 7 is satisfied for any adjacent pixels $\mathbf{x}, \mathbf{y}$ and each of our α-expansion move is globally optimal. Boykov et al. [5] have further proved that, in such a case, the α-expansion algorithm can finally converge to a local minimum, which is within a guaranteed factor of the exact minimum.

3   Experimental Results

In all experiments, it is assumed that all pairs of images are affinely pre-registered and the intensities of the images are normalized to be within 0 and 255. For **FFD** and **DEMONS**, we used the implementations obtained from ITK [8]. In **FFD**, we used a 15×15 control point grid. In our method, we used $\lambda = 0.05 \times 255$ and $\mathcal{W} = \{0, \pm 1, \pm 2, ..., \pm 15\}^2$ ($\{0, \pm 1, \pm 2, ..., \pm 12\}^3$ for 3D) so that displacement label of a pixel was chosen from a 31×31 window ($25 \times 25 \times 25$ for 3D) centered at that pixel. For the graph-cuts algorithm, we used the source codes provided by Kolmogorov & Zabih [7]. All MR and segmented data used in our experiments were obtained from BrainWeb [9]. Some slices are shown in Fig. 1.

Registration Robustness. The left of Fig. 1 shows an axial slice from an MR dataset which was used as the source image and four different artificial deformations (Case A-D) were applied to generate four floating images shown in the left column of Fig. 2. These artificial deformations can resemble different intra-subject and inter-subject mapping behaviors. The registration outputs of **DEMONS**, **FFD** and our method are shown in the last three columns in Fig. 2. From the registration output, it is obvious that **FFD** failed in Cases B and D and **DEMONS** failed in Cases C and D. All other cases were successful.

The failures of **FFD** in Cases B and D were situations where a transformation with low degree of freedoms cannot model a complicated or high-frequency deformation. **FFD** only allows control points to freely displace but restricts other pixels' displacements to be an interpolation of the displacements of neighborhood control points. As predicted, both **DEMONS** and our method are capable of

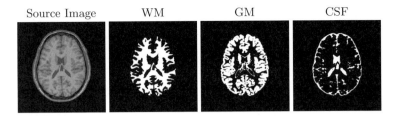

Fig. 1. Some original and segmented slices from BrainWeb used in our experiments

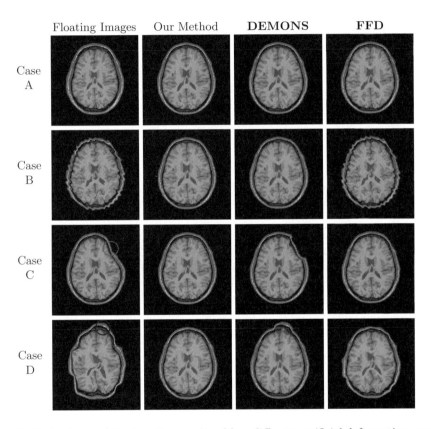

Fig. 2. *(Color Images)* Registration results of four different artificial deformation cases

restoring the images in such cases since no hard constraints are posed in the deformation models. The failures of **DEMONS** in Cases C and D were caused by local minima in the optimization process. The deformations in Cases C and D were considered large as some points are displaced more than 10 pixel-units. In Case C|D, before registration, some portions of the skull (circled red|blue in Fig. 2) in the floating image had its whole thickness being overlapping with the interior|background of the brain in the source image. Since **DEMONS** uses local intensity gradient to drive the movement of pixels, these initial overlapping

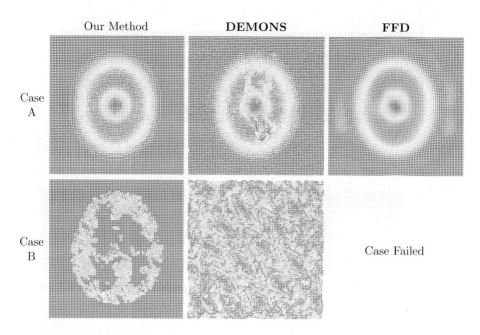

Fig. 3. *(Color Images)* Recovered deformation fields in Case A and Case B. Red color represents large displacements while blue color represents small displacements.

caused some pixels move towards the wrong directions and finally got trapped in local minima. Although our transformation model also has high degree of freedoms, our method still survive in this situation. It is because the graph-cuts method considers the labels of all pixels in a global manner in an α-expansion move. Once the energy barrier is overcome, a group of pixels will together pursuit a large displacement in an α-expansion step, without moving gradually through a series of small displacements.

Smoothness of the Recovered Deformation Fields. To compare the smoothness of the recovered deformation fields from different registration methods, we plot the fields for Cases A and B in Fig. 3. Case A corresponds to a squeeze-in deformation. As predicted, the fields recovered by **FFD** is the smoothest since **FFD** internally constrains the field to be a B-Spline interpolated transform. Comparing **DEMONS** and our method in both Cases A and B, it can be clearly seen that the field recovered by our method is much smoother than that recovered by **DEMONS**. It is because the smoothness constraint is kept globally in the cost function during the whole optimization process in our method.

Registration Accuracy. To evaluate for registration accuracy, we performed 10 (4 full and 6 downsampled) sets of 3D inter-patient registration by using **FFD**, **DEMONS** and our method. Fig. 4 shows the images and results of one of the sets using our method. Table 1 lists the distributions of pre/post-registration

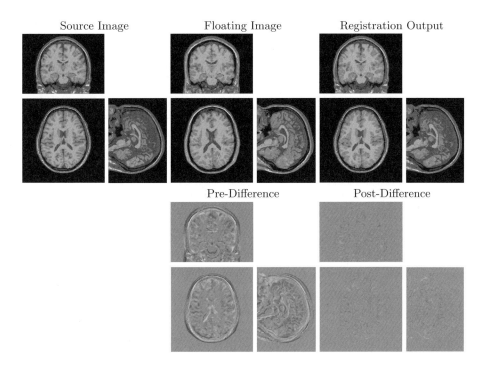

Source Image   Floating Image   Registration Output

Pre-Difference   Post-Difference

Fig. 4. 3D Registration results across two MR volumes. For each sub-figure, the middle slice across each axis of the volume is shown.

Table 1. Pre- and post-registration absolute intensity difference and tissue overlap measures of **FFD**, **DEMONS** and our method. Each number gives the mean value over all 3D registration tests.

Tissue Class	Pre-Registration	**FFD**	**DEMONS**	Our Method
	Absolute Intensity Difference (Mean $\pm$ SD)			
Whole Image	9.66 ± 22.15	7.31 ± 17.17	4.84 ± 12.01	2.65 ± 6.30
	Tissue Overlap Measure			
WM	0.4479	0.5041	0.6123	0.6754
GM	0.4575	0.5175	0.6282	0.7109
CSF	0.2395	0.3605	0.4721	0.5844

absolute intensity difference and the pre/post-registration overlap measures of three tissue classes, grey matter (GM), white matter (WM) and cerebrospinal fluid (CSF). We adopted the overlap measure $\frac{\#(A \cap B)}{\#(A \cup B)}$, used by Crum *et al.* [10], where A and B denote the regions of the two images that belong to a specific tissue class. From the table, it is found that our method can consistently achieve higher registration accuracy than **FFD** and **DEMONS**.

4   Conclusion

We have proposed a new formulation to non-rigid image registration problem. First, we adopt a flexible deformation model, which allows every pixel to displace freely. This is essential for our method to recover any complicated deformation fields. Next, we present an energy function associated with the parameters of the deformation model, which are the displacement vector field **D**. This function considers the dissimilarity measure of the images together with the smoothness requirement of the deformation field. Despite the supernormal high degree of freedoms in **D** as well as its smoothness requirement, we have successfully proved that our energy function can be globally optimized by using the graphcuts method. The graph-cuts method also provides a solution with some degree of guarantee. Experimental results have demonstrated that our proposed method shows robustness to different challenging registration cases, e.g. large deformation, ripple distortion. It can be explained by the flexibility of our deformation model, as well as the power of the graph-cuts method to perform optimization in a global manner. Moreover, our method can achieve high registration accuracy.

References

1. Rueckert, D.: Non-rigid registration: techniques and applications. In: Medical Image Registration, CRC Press (2001)
2. Arsigny, V., Pennec, X., Ayache, N.: Polyrigid and polyaffine transformations: a novel geometrical tool to deal with non-rigid deformations - application to the registration of histological slices. Medical Image Analysis 9(6), 507–523 (2005)
3. Rueckert, D., Sonoda, L.I., et al.: Non-rigid registration using free-form deformations: Application to breast MR images. TMI 18(8), 712–721 (1999)
4. Thirion, J.P.: Image matching as a diffusion process: an analogy with maxwell's demons. Medical Image Analysis 2(3), 243–260 (1998)
5. Boykov, Y., Veksler, O., Zabih, R.: Fast approximate energy minimization via graph cuts. PAMI 23(11), 1222–1239 (2001)
6. Winn, J., Jojic, N.: Locus: Learning object classes with unsupervised segmentation. In: ICCV, pp. 756–763 (2005)
7. Kolmogorov, V., Zabih, R.: What energy functions can be minimized via graph cuts? PAMI 26(2), 147–159 (2004)
8. Ibanez, L., Schroeder, W., et al.: The ITK Software Guide, 1st edn. Kitware, Inc (2003)
9. Aubert-Broche, B., Evans, A., Collins, L.: A new improved version of the realistic digital brain phantom. NeuroImage 32(1), 138–145 (2006)
10. Crum, W.R., Rueckert, D., et al.: A framework for detailed objective comparison of non-rigid registration algorithms in neuroimaging. In: Barillot, C., Haynor, D.R., Hellier, P. (eds.) MICCAI 2004. LNCS, vol. 3216, pp. 679–686. Springer, Heidelberg (2004)

Probabilistic Speckle Decorrelation for 3D Ultrasound

Catherine Laporte and Tal Arbel

Centre for Intelligent Machines, McGill University, Montréal, Canada
{cathy,arbel}@cim.mcgill.ca

Abstract. Recent developments in freehand 3D ultrasound (US) have shown how image registration and speckle decorrelation methods can be used for 3D reconstruction instead of relying on a tracking device. Estimating elevational separation between untracked US images using speckle decorrelation is error prone due to the uncertainty that plagues the correlation measurements. In this paper, using maximum entropy estimation methods, the uncertainty is directly modeled from the calibration data normally used to estimate an average decorrelation curve. Multiple correlation measurements can then be fused within a maximum likelihood estimation framework in order to reduce the drift in elevational pose estimation over large image sequences. The approach is shown to be effective through empirical results on simulated and phantom US data.

1   Introduction

Freehand 3D ultrasound (US) involves integrating the information contained in 2D US images into a 3D model. For this difficult task, the positions of the 2D images relative to each other must be known. A typical implementation involves attaching a tracking device to the US probe. Unfortunately, the position tracking device is often cumbersome to the clinician. Furthermore, the accuracy of the pose measurements depends on temporal and spatial calibration procedures [9] which are technically non trivial and often time consuming. This has led to the development of a position tracking methodology based entirely on image content. In-plane probe motion can be estimated through standard image registration techniques. This paper focuses on the estimation of out-of-plane motion from the elevational decorrelation of US speckle between image frames [4,13,10,3,6].

A typical framework for estimating the elevational separation between US images involves a calibration phase where a speckle phantom is scanned at regular intervals, allowing the construction of a decorrelation curve, depicting the measured average correlation coefficient between pairs of images separated by known elevational distances. The shape of this curve is more or less Gaussian, with width dependent on the elevational beam width of the transducer and the axial depth at which correlations were measured [13]. To estimate the distance between two US image patches, their correlation coefficient is subsequently measured and the corresponding elevational distance estimate is read off the curve. This process is subject to error, especially in the nonlinear portions of the curve

N. Ayache, S. Ourselin, A. Maeder (Eds.): MICCAI 2007, Part I, LNCS 4791, pp. 925–932, 2007.
© Springer-Verlag Berlin Heidelberg 2007

(very high and very low correlations) [12]. This results in significant large scale drift error when attempting to estimate the relative positions of a large number of frames. Large scale accuracy is of paramount importance when measuring the dimensions of organs from 3D reconstructions of the US data, for instance.

Each pair of frames (not necessarily subsequent) in an US scan provides correlation measurements which can be used for estimating their positions. Recent work [6] has attempted to reduce the impact of measurement errors by averaging independent interleaved reconstructions using only correlation measurements lying on the "well-behaved" (i.e. linear) portion of the decorrelation curve. This paper presents an alternative approach which allows for more measurements to be exploited simultaneously, with the goal of further reducing drift error. Measurement uncertainty is represented by a probabilistic speckle decorrelation (PSD) model which captures statistical information available at calibration time but not represented by the average decorrelation curve. The model is used within a maximum likelihood estimation framework to fuse multiple correlation measurements of arbitrary quality in order to reduce residual uncertainty for the benefit of additional processing steps such as 3D interpolation. Preliminary results obtained with parallel frames of simulated and phantom US data show the approach to be effective at limiting drift error over long image sequences.

The remainder of this paper is structured as follows. Section 2 describes the PSD model. The maximum likelihood data fusion method is presented in section 3. Finally, the experimental results on simulated and phantom US data are discussed in section 4.

2   Probabilistic Speckle Decorrelation Model

Inspired by the approach taken in [10], the approach proposed here begins with the subdivision of the US image into a number of small patches, each having its own speckle decorrelation model (see figure 1). This accounts for the variation of correlation length with axial depth. Moreover, such a subdivision yields as many correlation measurements per frame pair as there are patches: enough to estimate yaw and tilt as well as elevational translation.

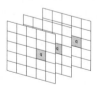

Fig. 1. The images are divided into non-overlapping patches. Corresponding patches (*e.g.* the highlighted patches labeled q) in different images are used to build local decorrelation models and are treated as mini-frames when estimating elevational positions.

Given two correlated random signals X and Y with correlation coefficient ρ_0, the sample correlation coefficient of realisations x and y of X and Y, respectively, of length N is given by

$$\rho(x, y) = \frac{N \sum x_i y_i - \sum x_i \sum y_i}{\sqrt{[N \sum x_i^2 - (\sum x_i)^2][N \sum y_i^2 - (\sum y_i)^2]}}. \tag{1}$$

For multiple realisations of X and Y, the average sample correlation coefficient should tend towards the nominal value ρ_0. However, the individual sample correlation coefficients will exhibit some variability due to the finite length of the realisations x and y. This is true of any kind of random signal, including US image patches. In this case, the length N corresponds to the number of pixels.

The uncertainty intrinsic to correlation measurements can be modeled explicitly by a probability density function $p(\rho|\delta, q)$ relating the sample correlation coefficient ρ to elevational separation δ in patch q. Assuming that the relationship between elevational separation and the nominal correlation coefficient ρ_0 is one-to-one, as depicted by the decorrelation curves used in [4,13,6], $p(\rho|\delta, q) = p(\rho|\rho_0, q)$. The statistical variability of the sample correlation coefficient depends on ρ_0, and on the statistical distributions of X and Y.

$p(\rho|\delta, q)$ can be estimated from data samples acquired by scanning a speckle phantom at regular distance intervals at calibration time. These are the same data required to construct decorrelation curves used in related work. While the decorrelation curve represents the *average* ρ as a function of distance, the probability density function $p(\rho|\delta, q)$ also captures higher order statistics of ρ, such as variance. Since no theoretical results are available concerning the form of $p(\rho|\delta, q)$, it is estimated using a empirical maximum entropy method by Baker [2].

From a set of correlation measurements $\{\rho_i\}, i = 1, ...N$, acquired between frames separated by a distance δ in patch q, Baker's method computes a number of probability densities from the exponential family given by

$$p_K(\rho|\delta, q; \mu) = p_0(\rho) \exp \left(\lambda_0(\mu) + \sum_{k=1}^{K} \lambda_k(\mu) \rho^k \right), \tag{2}$$

where p_0 is a uniform probability density function over the range D of the data (here, $D = [-1, 1]$) and μ is a vector of the sample moments of the data of order 1 to K. The normalisation constant $\lambda_0(\mu)$ is given by

$$\lambda_0(\mu) = -\ln \left\{ \int_D p_0(\rho) \exp \left(\sum_{j=1}^{K} \lambda_j(\mu) \rho^j \right) d\rho \right\}, \tag{3}$$

and the parameters $\lambda(\mu)$ are obtained from the first K sample moments by solving the system of nonlinear equations

$$\frac{\int_D \rho^k p_0(\rho) \exp \left(\sum_{j=1}^{K} \lambda_j(\mu) \rho^j \right) d\rho}{\int_D p_0(\rho) \exp \left(\sum_{j=1}^{K} \lambda_j(\mu) \rho^j \right) d\rho} = \mu_k, k = 1, ..., K. \tag{4}$$

K is then selected such that the Akaike information criterion (AIC) [1],

$$AIC = 2K - 2 \sum_{j=1}^{N} \ln p_K(\rho_j|\delta, q; \mu), \tag{5}$$

is minimised. This application of the AIC encourages model goodness of fit while discouraging model complexity [2]. Using this method, conditional probability density functions $p(\rho|\delta_j, q)$ are obtained from sample correlation coefficients measured between frames of elevational separation $\delta_j = j\delta_0$ at patch q, where δ_0 is the elevational distance between consecutive frames in the calibration scan. The PSD model is illustrated by an example in figure 2.

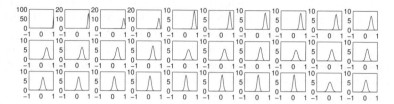

Fig. 2. The PSD model for an US image patch q obtained from speckle phantom data. Each plot is the estimated probability density function $p(\rho|\delta, q)$ (vertical axis) of the correlation coefficient ρ (horizontal axis) corresponding to elevational separation δ, with δ starting at 0.05 mm and increasing at a rate of 0.05 mm per plot from left to right and top to bottom.

Given correlation measurement ρ, the likelihood $p(\rho|\delta, q)$ for the unknown elevational separation δ can be estimated from the PSD model. The model provides samples of the likelihood at discrete values of δ corresponding to the regular intervals used for calibration. Interpolation is used to estimate the log-likelihood $L(\rho|\delta, q) = \ln p(\rho|\delta, q)$ at arbitrary δ.

3   Estimation of Elevational Separations

Consider a set of US images whose relative positions must be estimated. In this paper, it is assumed that: (1) there is no in-plane probe motion or the images have been correctly aligned by some registration procedure; (2) the frames do not intersect; (3) the motion of the probe in the elevational direction is monotonic; (4) the images are made of fully developed speckle. These assumptions may be relaxed through the use of complementary algorithms [5,6] as an add-on to the proposed drift-reduction scheme. They are adopted here for simplicity, and in the experimental protocol to minimise the influence of sources of error outside the control of the proposed method in the analysis of results.

Subdividing the frames in the data set into M patches corresponding to those used to define the speckle decorrelation model yields M individual US data sets consisting of "mini-frames" the size of the individual image patches (see figure 1). The first problem considered is that of estimating the maximum likelihood positions Z_i, $i = 1, ..., n$ along the elevational direction of n mini-frames corresponding to patch q, with respect to a reference mini-frame with position $Z_0 = 0$. A correlation measurement ρ_{ij} between mini-frames i and j provides an uncertain measurement of the elevational separation $\delta_{ij} = |Z_i - Z_j|$ between them through the log-likelihood $L(\rho_{ij}|\delta_{ij}, q)$. Enforcing the assumption of motion monotonicity, the absolute value is dropped and $\delta_{ij} = Z_i - Z_j, i > j$. Assuming mutual independence of measurements given the the configuration of the frames, the maximum likelihood position vector $\mathbf{Z}$ is given by

$$\mathbf{Z}^* = \underset{\mathbf{Z}}{\operatorname{argmax}} \sum_{i>j} L(\rho_{ij}|Z_i - Z_j, q). \tag{6}$$

This is a difficult non-linear optimisation problem for arbitrary L. However, it was observed the log-likelihood terms in (6) are generally unimodal, suggesting that a Gaussian approximation of L is both possible and useful. This amounts to assuming that $\delta_{ij} = Z_i - Z_j$ is Gaussian with mean $\bar{\delta}_{ij} = \underset{\delta_{ij}}{\operatorname{argmax}} L(\rho_{ij}|\delta_{ij}, q)$, and variance $\sigma_{ij}^2 = -1 / \left(\frac{d^2}{d\delta_{ij}^2} L(\rho_{ij}|\bar{\delta}_{ij}, q) \right)$. The approximate solution $\tilde{\mathbf{Z}}^*$ is

$$\tilde{\mathbf{Z}}^* = \underset{\mathbf{Z}}{\operatorname{argmin}} \sum_{i>j} \frac{(Z_i - Z_j - \bar{\delta}_{ij})^2}{\sigma_{ij}^2}. \tag{7}$$

This simpler optimisation problem was addressed for the context of robot localisation and can be solved analytically [8]. Re-expressing (7) in matrix form,

$$\tilde{\mathbf{Z}}^* = \underset{\mathbf{Z}}{\operatorname{argmin}} (\bar{\delta} - \mathbf{HZ})^T \mathbf{C}^{-1} (\bar{\delta} - \mathbf{HZ}), \tag{8}$$

where $\bar{\delta}$ is the vector of all distance measurements, $\mathbf{H}$ is a matrix consisting exclusively of 0, 1 and -1 entries expressing the linear relationships between distances and absolute positions, and $\mathbf{C}$ is a diagonal covariance matrix made of all the σ_{ij}. The solution to the problem of (8) is [8]

$$\tilde{\mathbf{Z}}^* = (\mathbf{H}^T \mathbf{C}^{-1} \mathbf{H})^{-1} \mathbf{H}^T \mathbf{C}^{-1} \bar{\delta}, \tag{9}$$

whose computation is simplified by $\mathbf{C}$ being diagonal due to the assumed independence of measurement errors. The approach also allows for the computation of the residual uncertainty in $\mathbf{Z}$, which could eventually be used to embed uncertainty in tasks such as volume interpolation or re-slicing.

Having obtained an elevational position estimate for each mini-frame, knowing that all image patches belonging to the same frame of the original data set lie on a plane provides an additional constraint. This is enforced by calculating the final position of each full frame as the least squares rigid transformation mapping the positions of the patch centers from every frame to the first.

4   Experiments

In order to demonstrate the feasibility of the proposed approach with data from a clinical US scanner, experiments were carried out on both simulated US imagery and real US data of a speckle phantom. The simulations were run on a parallel processing cluster using Field II [7], with a 3.5 MHz linear transducer scanning a moving speckle phantom at a depth of 6 cm, and the resulting RF data were scan converted and log compressed to emulate the action of a clinical US scanner. The real imagery was acquired through a video frame grabber connected to an Acuson Cypress ultrasound system using a 5 MHz sector probe at a depth setting of 2.7 cm. The probe was moved using a sub-millimeter positioning device which approximately restricted motion to the elevational direction. Calibration scans were obtained for both imaging devices, at intervals of 0.1 mm for the simulations and 0.05 mm for the phantom data. The simulated images were divided into 64 patches of 60x60 pixels and the real images were divided into 19 patches of 50x50 pixels. The log compression was reversed using the technique presented in [11].

The PSD method for computing out-of-plane probe motion was applied to 16 different parallel image sequences. A minimum correlation threshold was defined for each patch such that the lowest 20% of the range of correlation values observed during calibration was cut off. A maximum number of measurements per frame was determined as the average number of consecutive frames needed to reach this threshold. This rougly amounts to assuming that variations in probe velocity are small, and reduces the sensitivity of the method to local variations in speckle decorrelation rates.

The PSD approach was compared to two base-line methods, both of which rely only on the average decorrelation curve. The first, nearest neighbour (NN), consists in positioning each frame relative to its immediate predecessor using only the correlations between subsequent frames. The second, shifting reference (SR), consists in positioning each frame using its correlation to a reference frame until the correlation falls below the minimum value or the maximum number of frames is exceeded, at which point the last frame positioned becomes the reference. The thresholds involved are the same as for the PSD method.

The accuracy of the recovered frame positions (which include elevational translation from a global reference, frame yaw and frame tilt) was measured in terms of the average RMS error between the inferred 3D positions of the centers of the image patches and the ground truth. Results are summarised in table 1.

Predictably, the NN strategy exhibits poor performance on long sequences due to the accumulation of large relative error at every frame. The PSD and SR approaches both did much better, with PSD generally outperforming SR and relative improvement varying from -4.5% (Sequence 6) to $+62.6\%$ (Sequence 11). Detailed results for these two extreme cases are shown in figure 3. Qualitatively, the PSD method yields more stable error in elevation, yaw and tilt over time, implying that in addition to reducing large scale drift error, the proposed method improves local accuracy. In the context of 3D volume interpolation, this should lead to more accurate large scale measurements (within the limitations imposed by the sensorless framework) and better rendition of local tissue structure.

Table 1. Average RMS error (mm) for different test image sequences reconstructed with the proposed PSD approach, the NN approach and the SR approach. The best result for each sequence is in bold font. The frame positions in the random simulated sequences were sampled at exponentially distributed intervals with mean 0.15 mm.

Sequence	Type	Description	RMS error (mm)		
			PSD	NN	SR
1	Simulated	178 frame calibration scan	**0.038**	0.667	0.051
2	Simulated	67 frames 0.3 mm apart	**0.087**	0.152	0.133
3	Simulated	150 frames 0.15 mm apart	**0.059**	0.564	0.074
4	Simulated	150 frames 0.15 mm apart	**0.066**	0.560	0.074
5	Simulated	134 frames 0.05 mm apart	**0.036**	1.400	0.048
6	Simulated	128 frames, random	0.114	0.606	**0.109**
7	Simulated	130 frames, random	**0.078**	0.641	0.099
8	Simulated	123 frames, random	**0.105**	0.541	0.188
9	Simulated	149 frames, random	**0.095**	0.757	0.113
10	Simulated	149 frames, random	**0.097**	0.752	0.113
11	Simulated	134 frames, random	**0.104**	0.609	0.278
12	Real	101 frame calibration scan	**0.036**	0.124	0.071
13	Real	111 frames, 0.05 mm apart	0.171	0.196	**0.168**
14	Real	101 frames, 0.03 mm apart	**0.086**	0.145	0.100
15	Real	126 frames, 0.04 mm apart	**0.165**	0.253	0.180
16	Real	201 frames, 0.05 mm apart	**0.221**	0.515	0.352

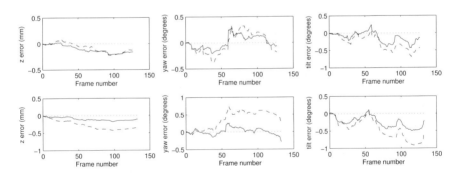

Fig. 3. Error in frame elevational translation, yaw and tilt as a function of frame number for image sequences 6 (top) and 11 (bottom). The solid line plots the results for the PSD approach, and the dashed line represents the SR approach.

5   Conclusions

This paper presented a probabilistic model for elevational speckle decorrelation in US imagery which embeds measurement uncertainty into the recovery of positional information. The model was applied to the task of fusing multiple correlation measurements obtained from long US image sequences in an attempt to recover their relative out-of-plane separations. According to the experimental results presented in this paper, the approach is promising as it leads to a reduction of drift compared to methods which only use one correlation measurement per frame. Future work will investigate the inclusion of tissue models in the proposed probabilistic formulation in order to robustly account for local variations in scatterer organisation and density in the scanned subject, as well as global variations which occur outside the context of fully developed speckle [5].

Acknowledgments. Catherine Laporte is funded by a NSERC scholarship.

References

1. Akaike, H.: A new look at the statistical model identification. IEEE T. Automat. Contr. 19(6), 716–723 (1974)
2. Baker, R.: Probability estimation and information principles. Struct. Saf. 9, 97–116 (1990)
3. Chang, R.-F., Wu, W.-J., Chen, D.-R., Chen, W.-M., Shu, W., Lee, J.-H., Jeng, L.-B.: 3-D US frame positioning using speckle decorrelation and image registration. Ultrasound Med. Biol. 29(6), 801–812 (2003)
4. Chen, J.-F., Fowlkes, J.B., Carson, P.L., Rubin, J.M.: Determination of scan-plane motion using speckle decorrelation: theoretical considerations and initial test. Int. J. Imag. Syst. Tech. 8(1), 38–44 (1997)
5. Gee, A.H., Housden, R.J., Hassenpflug, P., Treece, G.M., Prager, R.W.: Sensorless freehand 3D ultrasound in real tissue: speckle decorrelation without fully developped speckle. Med. Image Anal. 10(2), 137–149 (2006)
6. Housden, R.J., Gee, A.H., Treece, G.M., Prager, R.W.: Sensorless reconstruction of unconstrained freehand 3D ultrasound data. Ultrasound Med. Biol. 33(3), 408–419 (2007)
7. Jensen, J.A.: Field: a program for simulating ultrasound systems. Med. Biol. Eng. Comput. 34, 351–353 (1996)
8. Lu, F., Milios, E.: Globally consistent range scan alignment for environment mapping. Auton. Robots 4(4), 333–349 (1997)
9. Mercier, L., Langø, T., Lindseth, F., Collins, D.L.: A review of calibration techniques for freehand 3-D ultrasound systems. Ultrasound Med. Biol. 31(4), 449–471 (2005)
10. Prager, R.W., Gee, A.H., Treece, G., Cash, C.J.C., Berman, L.H.: Sensorless freehand 3-D ultrasound using regression of the echo intensity. Ultrasound Med. Biol. 29(3), 437–446 (2003)
11. Prager, R.W., Gee, A.H., Treece, G.M., Berman, L.H.: Decompression and speckle detection for ultrasound images using the homodyned k-distribution. Pattern Recogn. Lett. 24, 705–713 (2003)
12. Smith, W., Fenster, A.: Statistical analysis of decorrelation-based transducer tracking for three-dimensional ultrasound. Med. Phys. 30(7), 1580–1591 (2003)
13. Tuthill, T.A., Krücker, J.F., Fowlkes, J.B., Carson, P.L.: Automated three-dimensional US frame positioning computed from elevational speckle decorrelation. Radiology 209(2), 575–582 (1998)

De-enhancing the Dynamic Contrast-Enhanced Breast MRI for Robust Registration

Yuanjie Zheng[1,2], Jingyi Yu[2], Chandra Kambhamettu[2], Sarah Englander[1],
Mitchell D. Schnall[1], and Dinggang Shen[1]

[1] Department of Radiology, University of Pennsylvania, Philadelphia, PA 19104, USA
[2] Department of Computer and Information Sciences, University of Delaware,
Newark, DE 19716, USA

Abstract. Dynamic enhancement causes serious problems for registration of contrast enhanced breast MRI, due to variable uptakes of agent on different tissues or even same tissues in the breast. We present an iterative optimization algorithm to de-enhance the dynamic contrast-enhanced breast MRI and then register them for avoiding the effects of enhancement on image registration. In particular, the spatially varying enhancements are modeled by a Markov Random Field, and estimated by a locally smooth function with boundaries using a graph cut algorithm. The de-enhanced images are then registered by conventional B-spline based registration algorithm. These two steps benefit from each other and are repeated until the results converge. Experimental results show that our two-step registration algorithm performs much better than conventional mutual information based registration algorithm. Also, the effects of tumor shrinking in the conventional registration algorithms can be effectively avoided by our registration algorithm.

1 Introduction

Image registration is a fundamental problem in medical imaging. Classical image registration techniques assume corresponding pixels in two images have consistent intensities or at least are strongly correlated [1]. For instance, it is commonly assumed that if two pixels have the same intensity in one image, they will have the same intensity in the other image [2]. However, this assumption is not always valid in many applications. For example, in dynamic contrast enhanced (DCE) magnetic resonance (MR) images, tumor and non-tumor tissues may have similar intensities at a pre-contrast image, but then appear very dissimilar at post-contrast images due to variable signal enhancements [3,2]. Moreover, even same tissue (such as tumor tissue) [4] can appear different at various contrast enhancement stages, due to different uptakes of the contrast agent. These spatially varying enhancements lead to serious problems for the conventional registration algorithms which assume consistent intensities or strongly correlated intensities in the two images under registration [5]. One typical problem is that a tumor region can be significantly deformed during registration of DCE-MR images in order to maximize the mutual information as reported in [6].

N. Ayache, S. Ourselin, A. Maeder (Eds.): MICCAI 2007, Part I, LNCS 4791, pp. 933–941, 2007.
© Springer-Verlag Berlin Heidelberg 2007

Many research efforts have been proposed to design good correlation metrics in order to cancel out intensity inconsistencies across the images. Normalized mutual information (NMI) [7,3] has been used to account for the change of image intensity and contrast in registering DCE-MR images. However, NMI only works well in the regions with similar enhancement characteristics [8] and poorly handles the images with spatially varying enhancement like the DCE-MR breast images [4]. Model-based approaches, such as the pharmacokinetic (PK) model [2], have also been used to characterize pixel-wise enhancement-time signal. In theory, one can combine the PK model with conventional registration algorithms to get better performance, provided that the temporal enhanced signals comply well with the PK model. In practice, the PK model alone is often insufficient to model the intensity variations. Although the PK model with addition of a noise term can potentially better represent temporal enhanced signals [9], the noise term alone is insufficient to model inconsistency of intensity enhancements between the two images.

In this paper, we present a different approach to solve the intensity inconsistency of DCE-MR images. Instead of finding the physical model that represent this inconsistency, we set out to find the intensity transformation between the images, i.e., estimating enhancements. Specifically, we calculate the ratio of the intensity for each tissue point over the two images. The resulting ratio image is called the enhancement map. For perfectly registered images, the enhancement map is simply the ratio between the reference and the target images. For time-lapse DCE-MR images, computing the enhancement map requires registration between the target and the reference image due to possible patient motion.

We model the enhancement map by a Markov Random Field, and estimate it by a locally smooth function with boundaries using a graph cut algorithm [10]. Then, we use the estimated enhancement map to eliminate the enhancements between two images under registration, and further use a B-spline based registration method to register those de-enhanced images. These two steps are incorporated into an iterative optimization algorithm, and are repeated iteratively until convergence, similar to [11]. Experimental results show that the elimination of spatially variable enhancements in the DCE-MR images can significantly improve the registration accuracy, compared to the conventional mutual information based registration algorithms [7].

2   Methods

2.1   Problem Definition

Given two images I and J, our goal is to find the correspondence mapping T that warps every pixel from I to J. We use notion $T(I)$ to represent the resulting image after applying T on I. An ideal registration should perfectly align $T(I)$ with J. However, $T(I)$ and J can be different due to intensity changes η between I and J, e.g., enhancement variations in DCE-MR breast images. In addition, both I and J can be corrupted by noise ε. Therefore, registration methods that directly measure similarity of pixels intensities between the images might fail.

Notice, if we know η in prior, we can simply cancel out the enhancement between I and J and then apply existing registration algorithms to recover T. Similarly, if we know T in prior, we can then solve η using $T(I)$ and J. However, neither η nor T is known to us. Therefore, our goal is to simultaneously find the optimal T and η by maximizing a posteriori (MAP) given I and J:

$$T, \eta = \arg\max_{T,\eta} \mathcal{P}(T, \eta | I, J) \tag{1}$$

We propose an iterative optimization algorithm to approximate the MAP of T and η. We start with a rough registration using existing algorithms. At each iteration, we first estimate the optimal η given the current estimation of T. We then re-compute the registration by cancelling out η in J. The iteration continues until the results converge.

2.2 Enhancement Map

Assume we have estimated the registration T from I to J, our goal is to compute the enhancement map η between I' and J, where $I' = T(I)$. The enhancement is defined as

$$C'(s) = \frac{J(s) - I'(s)}{I'(s)}, \quad s \in \Omega \tag{2}$$

where s represent the pixels inside image region Ω.

Enhancement map has been widely used to analyze DCE-MR images in breast cancer diagnosis [12,4]. We assume the enhancements change spatially in a smooth way, with discontinuities appeared between different kinds of enhancements, e.g., tumor boundaries.

2.3 Estimating Enhancement Map

If the registration T is exact, then η can be directly computed using equation (2). In practice, T can be inaccurate and both images are corrupted by noise ϵ. Notice, the spatial smoothness and tumor boundary discontinuity of the enhancement map are very similar to those seen in disparity maps in computer vision. Recent research [10] have shown that fields satisfying such properties can be modeled as a Markov Random Field. Methods such as belief propagation or graph-cut are very efficient to solve the MAP of Markov Random Fields.

We start with an initial estimation of the enhancement map by computing C' using equation (2). We then discretize the range of the enhancements into a finite number (e.g., 15) of levels, which are initially obtained by clustering with k-means algorithm. Our goal is to assign every pixel in C' with an enhancement label and find the MAP of the enhancement MRF η. In our implementation, we modify the graph cut algorithm [10] to compute η that maximizes the labeling consistency and overall smoothness. The energy function we choose to minimize is defined as

$$E = \sum_{s \in \Omega} E_1(\eta'(s)) + \lambda_1 \sum_{<s,t> \in \mathcal{N}} E_2(\eta'(s), \eta'(t)) + \lambda_2 \sum_{<s,t> \in \mathcal{N}} E_3(\eta'(s), \eta'(t)) \tag{3}$$

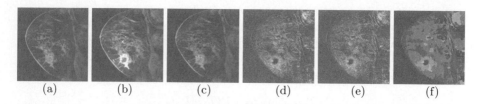

|(a)|(b)|(c)|(d)|(e)|(f)|

Fig. 1. Demonstration of enhancement estimation result by our method. (a) Pre-contrast image. (b) Post-contrast image. (c) De-enhanced post-contrast image. (d) Initial enhancement map calculated from (a) to (b). (e) Enhancement map clustered by a k-means algorithm. (f) Enhancement map segmented by a graph cut algorithm.

E_1 computes the difference between the assigned level value and enhancement computed by equation (2) for all pixels, which is defined as:

$$E_1(\eta'(s)) = \mathcal{G}(|\eta'(s) - C'(s)|) \tag{4}$$

where $\mathcal{G}(x) = \frac{x}{x+1}$.

E_2 corresponds to the smoothness term in standard graph cut algorithms. It measures the consistency of the enhancement levels between the neighboring pixels in $\mathcal{N}$:

$$E_2(\eta'(s), \eta'(t)) = 1 - \delta(\eta'(s) - \eta'(t)) \tag{5}$$

where δ is a Kronecker delta function.

Finally, we introduce a new term E_3 that further constrains the enhancement variations between pixels, where

$$E_3(\eta'(s), \eta'(t)) = \mathcal{G}(|\eta'(s) - \eta'(t)|). \tag{6}$$

The use of E_3 guarantees that even if the neighboring pixels have different enhancement levels, their differences should be constrained within a small range. In our experiments, we find the use of E_3 is critical to maintain spatial smoothness of the recovered enhancement map.

In equation (3), λ_1 and λ_2 are used for adjusting the relative importance of the three energy terms. They are both set to 1 in our experiments. We also find 15 levels clustered by k-means are sufficient to accurately approximate an enhancement map for a typical pair of DCE-MR breast images. This can be shown from the results of enhancement map estimated by our graph cut on a pair of typical enhanced images in Fig. 1.

Once we recover the enhancement map η between I' and J, we can then "de-enhance" J to the same level of I' using η. Notice $J_{de-enhanced}$ should be approximately the same as I'. Therefore, we can reuse equation (2) to compute $J_{de-enhanced}$ as

$$J_{de-enhanced} \approx I' = \frac{J}{\eta + 1} \quad s \in \Omega. \tag{7}$$

In Fig. 1, we use the estimated η to de-enhance the post-contrast MR breast image. The resulting image maintains similar spatial characteristics as the un-enhanced one while preserving important features such as tumor boundaries.

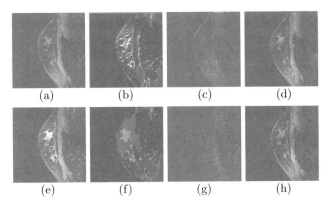

(a)   (b)   (c)   (d)

(e)   (f)   (g)   (h)

Fig. 2. Demonstration on the process of iterative enhancement estimation, elimination, and image registration. (a) and (e) are pre-contrast and post-contrast images, respectively. The results from the 1st and 2nd iterations are respectively shown in upper panels of (b), (c), and (d), and in lower panels of (f), (g), and (h). For each set of results, from left to right, they are the estimated enhancement map (b,f), the difference between the warped pre-contrast image and the de-enhanced post-contrast image (c,g), and the de-enhanced post-contrast image (d,h), respectively. These results show the progressive improvement of registration with iterations, reflected as smaller differences in (g), compared to those in (c).

2.4   Iterative Optimization

We have developed a two-step iterative optimization algorithm to simultaneously recover the MAP registration T^* and enhancement map η^*. We start with an initial registration using the conventional B-spline based non-rigid registration on the pre-contrast and the post-contrast MR images [7]. We then:

1. Find the initial estimate η' for η based on methods explained in section 2.3.
2. Repeat below steps until convergence:
   (a) Compute $T' = \arg\max_T \mathcal{P}(T|\eta', I, J)$
   (b) Compute $\eta' = \arg\max_\eta \mathcal{P}(\eta|T', I, J)$

In step (a) of each iteration, we de-enhance the target image using equation (7), to obtain $J_{de-enhanced}$. We then estimate T' by finding the optimal $T' = \arg\max_T \mathcal{P}(T|I, J_{de-enhanced})$. This optimization can be easily computed using many existing registration algorithm. We use the B-spline based registration algorithm [7]. In step (b), we use the estimated T' to register I with J. We then use the graph-cut algorithm to find the optimal enhancement map η'.

Fig. 2 illustrates the intermediate results using our method on MR breast images for registration and enhancement map estimation. From the results, we can see the steps of enhancement estimation and registration help each other for achieving better results.

3   Experimental Results

The performance of our enhancement estimation and image registration algorithm is extensively evaluated on both simulated data and real data as described by separate sections next.

3.1   Experiments on Simulated Data

For generating the simulated dataset, we first select a pre-contrast image of a real patient, such as the one shown in Fig. 1 (a). Second, we use the enhancements computed between this pre-contrast image and one post-contrast image of the same patient by equation (2) as a simulated enhancement map, to enhance our selected pre-contrast image and obtain a simulated post-contrast image. Third, we further use simulated motions, represented by B-Splines, to deform this simulated post-contrast image. Finally, we add Gaussian noise (with zero mean and standard deviation of 20) to this simulated post-contrast image.

The pre-contrast image and its final simulated post-contrast image are shown in Fig. 3 (a) and (b), respectively. To be clear, we only show the region around tumor. Notice that both simulated enhancement map and motions are pre-known.

We have compared our algorithm with the NMI-based method on this simulated dataset. Notice that both algorithms use the B-spline-based deformation representation [7] with 1 degree and 13 control points for each axis. To compensate for the intensity inconsistencies between the pre- and post-contrast images, the NMI-based approach estimates different intensity distributions in the two images while our algorithm first computes and removes the enhancement map and then directly uses the intensity difference metric. The results are shown in Fig. 3.

These results demonstrate at least three pieces of better performance of our algorithm. First, after removing the estimated enhancements (Fig. 3(c)), the simulated post-contrast image looks very similar to the original pre-contrast image (Fig. 3(a)). This shows the effectiveness of our graph cut algorithm in estimating enhancements. Second, the conventional registration algorithm produced errors especially at tumor as reflected by an enlarged tumor (Fig. 3(d)), while our algorithm still worked very well (Fig. 3(e)). Finally, the better registration result by our algorithm can also be observed as more similarity between the estimated (Fig. 3(h)) and the simulated enhancement maps (Fig. 3(f)), compared to that produced by the conventional registration algorithm (Fig. 3(g)). This is further demonstrated by the difference maps between the simulated and the estimated enhancements for our registration algorithm (Fig. 3(j)) and conventional registration algorithm (Fig. 3(i)), respectively.

Quantitatively, our registration algorithm is also better than the conventional registration algorithm. For example, by comparing the simulated motions with the estimated motions, our registration algorithm produced mean error of 0.44 pixel, standard deviation of 0.38 pixel, and maximum error of 2.4 pixels.

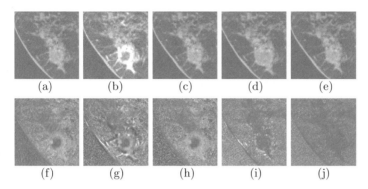

Fig. 3. Results on simulated data. (a) A pre-contrast image with tumor, selected from Fig. 1 (a). (b) A simulated post-contrast image, using simulated enhancement in (f). (c) An de-enhanced post-contrast image by our algorithm. (d) Warped pre-contrast image using a conventional registration algorithm to transform (a) to (b). (e) Warped pre-contrast image using our algorithm to transform (a) to (c). (f) Simulated enhancement map. (g) Estimated enhancement map from (d) to (b) by conventional registration algorithm. (h) Estimated enhancement map from (e) to (b) by our method. (i) Difference map between (f) and (g). (j) Difference map between (f) and (h).

In contrast, the conventional registration algorithm produced mean error of 0.82 pixel, standard deviation of 0.57 pixel, and maximum error of 10.8 pixels.

3.2 Experiments on Real Data

Data acquired from eight patients are also used to further compare the performances of our method and conventional registration algorithm. For each DCE-MR image sequence, the pre-contrast and the last post-contrast images are selected for evaluation of both registration algorithms. Typical results on three subjects are shown in Fig. 4. Each row corresponds to one individual subject. The first column shows the pre-contrast images, while the second column shows the post-contrast images. The de-enhanced images by our method are shown in the third column. It can be observed that the de-enhanced images are very similar to the pre-contrast images in the first column, which indicates the effectiveness of our enhancement estimation method.

The difference maps between the warped pre-contrast images and the de-enhanced images are shown in the fourth and the fifth columns for conventional registration method and our registration method, respectively. It can be observed that our method generally produces smaller difference maps, indicating better registration results.

Our algorithm completes the registration within 15 seconds on a PC of 1.2 GHz Intel Pentium M CPU and 2GB memory for images of a resolution 512×512 while the conventional algorithm takes about 3 seconds. For all the experiments demonstrated in this paper, our two-step optimization converges after 3 iterations.

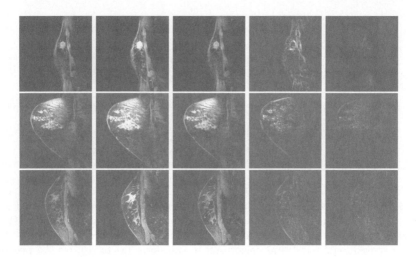

Fig. 4. Comparisons of our registration algorithm with conventional registration algorithm on real data. Each row corresponds to one individual subject. See text for details.

4   Conclusion

We have presented an iterative two-step optimization algorithm to simultaneously estimate dynamic enhancements in DCE-MR images and eliminate them for robust registration. The estimation of dynamic enhancement map is particularly formulated by a MRF model, and completed by a graph cut algorithm. The experimental results on both real and simulated datasets show the relative accuracy of registration after de-enhancing the DCE-MR images by our method. Also, by comparing with conventional registration methods using NMI, our registration algorithm can effectively register the tumor regions across different images, thus potentially avoiding the effects of tumor shrinking or enlarging that commonly happen in conventional registration methods. In the future, we will test our algorithm on more datasets available in our institute, adapt it to 3D case, and re-formulate it for group-wise registration of multiple contrast-enhanced breast images.

References

1. Maintz, J., Viergever, M.: A Survey of Medical Image Registration. Medical Image Analysis 2, 1–36 (1998)
2. Hayton, P., et al.: Analysis of dynamic MR breast images using a model of contrast enhancement. Medical Image Analysis 1, 207–224 (1997)
3. Tanner, C., et al.: Volume and shape preservation of enhancing lesions when applying non-rigid registration to a time series of contrast enhancing MR breast images. In: Delp, S.L., DiGoia, A.M., Jaramaz, B. (eds.) MICCAI 2000. LNCS, vol. 1935, pp. 327–337. Springer, Heidelberg (2000)

4. Schnall, M.D., Ikeda, D.M.: Lesions diagnosis working group report. Journal of Magnetic Resonance Imaging 10, 982–990 (1999)
5. Papademetris, X.: Integrated intensity and point-feature nonrigid registration. In: Barillot, C., Haynor, D.R., Hellier, P. (eds.) MICCAI 2004. LNCS, vol. 3216, Springer, Heidelberg (2004)
6. Rohlfing, R., et al.: Volume-preserving nonrigid registration of mr breast images using free-form deformation with an incompressibility constraint. IEEE Trans. Med. Imaging 22, 730–741 (2003)
7. Rueckert, D., et al.: Nonrigid registration using free-form deformations: application to breast MR images. IEEE Trans. Med. Imag. 18, 712–721 (1999)
8. Pluim, J.P.W., et al.: Mutual information based registration of medical images: survey. IEEE Trans. Med. Imaging 22, 986–1004 (2003)
9. Chen, X., et al.: Simultanous segmentation and registration of contrast-enhanced breast MRI. In: Christensen, G.E., Sonka, M. (eds.) IPMI 2005. LNCS, vol. 3565, Springer, Heidelberg (2005)
10. Boykov, Y., et al.: Fast approximate energy minimization via graph cuts. IEEE Trans. PAMI 23, 1222–1239 (2001)
11. Wells, W.M., et al.: Adaptive segmentation of MRI data. IEEE Trans. Med. Imaging 20, 1398–1410 (2001)
12. Chen, X., et al.: Simultanous segmentation and registration for medical image. In: Barillot, C., Haynor, D.R., Hellier, P. (eds.) MICCAI 2004. LNCS, vol. 3216, Springer, Heidelberg (2004)

Deformable Density Matching for 3D Non-rigid Registration of Shapes

Arunabha S. Roy[1], Ajay Gopinath[1], and Anand Rangarajan[2],[*]

[1] Imaging Technologies Laboratory, GE Global Research Center, Bangalore, India
[2] Department of CISE, University of Florida, Gainesville, FL, USA

Abstract. There exists a large body of literature on shape matching and registration in medical image analysis. However, most of the previous work is focused on matching particular sets of features—point-sets, lines, curves and surfaces. In this work, we forsake specific geometric shape representations and instead seek probabilistic representations—specifically Gaussian mixture models—of shapes. We evaluate a closed-form distance between two probabilistic shape representations for the general case where the mixture models differ in variance and the number of components. We then cast non-rigid registration as a deformable density matching problem. In our approach, we take one mixture density onto another by deforming the component centroids via a thin-plate spline (TPS) and also minimizing the distance with respect to the variance parameters. We validate our approach on synthetic and 3D arterial tree data and evaluate it on 3D hippocampal shapes.

1   Introduction

The need for shape matching occurs in diverse sub-domains of medical image analysis. Whenever a biomedical image is segmented or parsed into a set of shapes, the need for shape analysis and comparison usually arises [1]. In brain mapping for example [2], we frequently require the comparison of cortical and subcortical structures such as the thalamus, putamen etc. extracted from subject neuroanatomical MRI images. Image databases often use shape features and here the need is to index and query the shape database. In MR angiography, the complex network of blood vessels in the brain can be represented as trees or graphs and need to be compared across subjects. And in cardiac applications, if heart chamber information is available and extracted as a set of shapes, the wall tracking problem requires us to solve for shape correspondences in the cardiac cycle [3].

The need for shape matching is followed by a need for good shape representations. When shape features are extracted from medical images, they can be represented using an entire gamut of representations—points, line segments, curves, surfaces, trees, graphs and hybrid representations. What should be noted here is that an inferential stage is present in any shape representation. That is,

---

[*] A.R. was partially supported by NSF IIS 0307712 and NIH RO1 NS046812.

N. Ayache, S. Ourselin, A. Maeder (Eds.): MICCAI 2007, Part I, LNCS 4791, pp. 942–949, 2007.
© Springer-Verlag Berlin Heidelberg 2007

the raw features extracted from the underlying images are then converted into one of the above mentioned shape representations. Consequently, once a shape representation is adopted, we are immediately faced with the problem of *robustness* when we seek to compare two shapes. Some of the raw features present in (or extracted from) one image may not be present in the other. A second problem we face is that there may be no or poor *correspondences* between the features. It is for this reason that most methods seek to fit curves or surfaces to the data. Once such representations are fitted, there is no need to seek for correspondences at the point feature level. However, methods that rely on fitting curves and surfaces to the data face a more difficult robustness problem. How do you match one shape consisting of 10 curves to another shape consisting of 15 curves?

For these reasons, we elect to go the probabilistic route. Beginning with raw point features, we fit probability density functions to the feature vectors [4]. Each feature set is converted into a probability density function. The advantage here is that we can now compare probability density functions rather than the original images or other feature representations extracted from the images. The robustness problem is alleviated since the density functions are compared at all locations in $\mathbb{R}^3$ and we are not faced with the problem of matching incommensurate entities such as one curve in one shape to two curves in the other. There is no correspondence problem since we are not conducting comparisons at the point feature level. Shape comparison by matching the density functions between shapes also has the advantage that the point feature counts (in the two feature sets) can differ considerably.

We summarize our new method as follows: i) We fit Gaussian mixture models to point features extracted from the two images. A standard maximum likelihood expectation-maximization (EM) approach is used for this step. ii) We derive a *closed-form distance* between the two Gaussian mixture models by comparing the probability density functions at each point in $\mathbb{R}^3$. iii) Since the problem of minimizing this distance w.r.t. non-rigid deformations is ill-posed, we add a thin-plate spline regularization term to the cost. iv) We use a standard conjugate-gradient (CG) optimization strategy to minimize the above objective function. It should be stressed that we minimize the objective function w.r.t. both the deformation parameters and the variance parameters of the Gaussian mixture model. The result is a deformable density matching (DDM) method which seeks to register two shapes by moving the density function parameters of one shape until the first density closely approximates the other.

2   Previous Work

There exists an enormous literature on feature matching. We restrict our focus to methods that seek to fit and/or match probabilistic representations of shape features. The joint clustering and matching (JCM) approach [5] begins as we do with fitting Gaussian mixture models to feature point-sets. However, instead of minimizing a distance between the two density functions, they seek to augment the mixture model objective by linking a diffeomorphism between the centroid parameters of the mixture model. Consequently, they are forced to keep two sets of cluster centers in correspondence which we do not require. The methods in [6] and in [7] seek to convert a point matching problem into an image matching problem which is somewhat similar to density matching. However, the methods make no attempt to fit a probabilistic shape representation via maximum likelihood (or equivalent) to the features. Essentially, both methods convert the sparse feature set into dense images and then employ an image matching strategy. Furthermore, the method in [6] uses a deformation field parametrization which has to be applied at each point in $\mathbb{R}^3$ and this is computationally expensive compared to our approach. The method in [7] does not use a deformation field parametrization but the main differences are that they restrict their approach to point matching and make no attempt to fit a density function to the data via maximum likelihood or minimize their distance w.r.t. the centroid and variance parameters. Instead, they apply a thin-plate spline (TPS) on the original, noisy data. Perhaps the method that is closest in spirit to our approach is the recent work in [4]. They minimize the Jensen-Shannon divergence between the feature point-sets w.r.t. a non-rigid deformation. The Jensen-Shannon divergence cannot be computed in closed form for a mixture model and is estimated from the data using a law of large numbers approach. In sharp contrast, our distance between the two densities is in closed form and we apply the deformation parametrization to the centroidal parameters of the Gaussian mixture model.

3   Theory

3.1   Maximum-Likelihood Model for Shape Representation

As mentioned in the Introduction, the first step in our overall method is probabilistic shape representation based on the raw shape features.

The notation used in this paper is as follows. The two sets of input shape features are denoted by $\{X_i^{(1)} \in \mathbb{R}^d, i \in \{1, \ldots, N_1\}\}$ and $\{X_j^{(2)} \in \mathbb{R}^d, j \in \{1, \ldots, N_2\}\}$. The maximum likelihood approach assumes that the shape features $\{X_i^{(1)}\}$ and $\{X_j^{(2)}\}$ are independent and identically distributed (i.i.d.). The features of shape $X^{(1)}$ are represented by a Gaussian mixture model [8]

$$p(\mathbf{x}|\theta^{(1)}) = \sum_{a=1}^{K_1} \Omega_a^{(1)} \frac{1}{(2\pi)^{\frac{d}{2}}|\Sigma_a|^{\frac{1}{2}}} \exp\{-\frac{1}{2}(\mathbf{x} - \mu_a)^T \Sigma_a^{-1}(\mathbf{x} - \mu_a)\} \qquad (1)$$

(where $\mathbf{x} \in \mathbb{R}^3$) and that of shape $X^{(2)}$ is represented by a second Gaussian mixture model with parameter set $\theta^{(2)} = \{\Omega_\alpha^{(2)}, \nu_\alpha, \Xi_\alpha\}$. Constraints on $\Omega^{(\cdot)}$ are $\{\Omega_a^{(\cdot)} > 0, \sum_{a=1}^{K_1} \Omega_a^{(\cdot)} = 1\}$ where the superscript index can be either 1 or 2 corresponding to the two shapes respectively. Both probability density functions define measures on location with $\mathbf{x} \in \mathbb{R}^3$. We see that the set of model parameters for shape $X^{(1)}$ is $\theta^{(1)} = \{\Omega_a^{(1)}, \mu_a, \Sigma_a, a \in \{1, \ldots, K_1\}\}$ and

$\theta^{(2)} = \{\Omega_\alpha^{(2)}, \nu_\alpha, \Xi_\alpha, \alpha \in \{1,\ldots,K_2\}\}$ for shape $X^{(2)}$. Since $\{X_i^{(1)}\}$ and $\{X_j^{(2)}\}$ are assumed to be i.i.d., the likelihood of the set of features of $X^{(1)}$ is

$$p(\{X_i^{(1)}\}|\theta^{(1)}) = \prod_{i=1}^{N_1}\sum_{a=1}^{K_1}\Omega_a^{(1)}\frac{1}{(2\pi)^{\frac{d}{2}}|\Sigma_a|^{\frac{1}{2}}}\exp\{-\frac{1}{2}(X_i^{(1)} - \mu_a)^T\Sigma_a^{-1}(X_i^{(1)} - \mu_a)\}$$

(2)

where $\{X_i^{(1)}\}$ is the set of instances of $X^{(1)}$. For both shapes, we fit the model parameters by minimizing the negative log-likelihood objective function of the above mixture model w.r.t. the model parameters. In the experiments, we specialize to the case where the occupancy probabilities are uniform $(\Omega_a^{(1)} = \frac{1}{K_1})$ and where we have one isotropic covariance matrix $(\Sigma^2 = \sigma^2 I_3)$, for the entire shape. This is done for reasons of computational efficiency. The objective function for this reduced version is minimized over its parameter set $(\{\mu_a\}, \sigma)$ to obtain the model representation of the feature set.

We use the well known expectation-maximization (EM) algorithm [8] for the above minimization. While fitting mixture models is computationally difficult in the general case, in our special case of uniform occupancy probabilities and isotropic covariances it is not as difficult. Also, this computation is done offline for all the shapes once we fix the number of centroids (K_1 and K_2). Model selection for mixture models needs to be performed to fix the number of centroids.

3.2   A Closed-Form Distance Measure Between Two Gaussian Mixtures

We now derive the distance measure between the two probabilistic shape representations. Since this distance measure can be derived in closed form for the most general Gaussian mixture model case, we present this below. (Other distance measures like Kullback-Leibler cannot be derived in closed form for the Gaussian mixture model.) We hasten to add that the general mixture model can be quite unwieldy in practice and that specializations of the sort considered in the paper—like isotropic covariances and uniform occupancy probabilities—are very useful. Below we derive the distance measure as the squared pointwise difference between the two Gaussian mixture models with parameter sets ($\theta^{(1)}$ and $\theta^{(2)}$) integrated over $\mathbb{R}^d$ (where $d = 3$). [We have dropped terms that do not depend on $\theta^{(2)}$ since it is only $\theta^{(2)}$ that is deformed during the optimization.]

$$D[p(\mathbf{x}|\theta^{(1)}), p(\mathbf{x}|\theta^{(2)})] = \int_{\mathbb{R}^d}[p(\mathbf{x}|\theta^{(1)}) - p(\mathbf{x}|\theta^{(2)})]^2 dx \propto$$

$$-\sum_{a=1}^{K_1}\sum_{\alpha=1}^{K_2}\frac{2\exp\{-\frac{1}{2(\sigma^2+\xi^2)}||\mu_a - \nu_\alpha||^2\}}{K_1K_2(\sigma^2 + \xi^2)^{\frac{3}{2}}} + \sum_{\alpha=1}^{K_2}\sum_{\beta=1}^{K_2}\frac{\exp\{-\frac{1}{4\xi^2}||\nu_\alpha - \nu_\beta||^2\}}{2^{\frac{3}{2}}K_2^2\xi^3}. \quad (3)$$

This is the final expression for the distance function used in this paper. The number of centroids and the variances of the two models can be different.

3.3   Deformable Density Matching

We now turn to the description of the deformation model. We assume that the parameters $\theta^{(1)}$ of shape 1 are held fixed and that the parameters $\theta^{(2)} = (\{\nu_\alpha\}, \xi)$ (comprising the centroids and variance) of shape 2 are deformed so that $p(\mathbf{x}|\theta^{(2)})$ approaches $p(\mathbf{x}|\theta^{(1)})$.

We use the familiar thin-plate spline (TPS) deformation model [9] for the centroids. That is, the action of the deformation takes the centroids $\{\nu_\alpha\}$ to new locations $\{\tilde{\nu}_\alpha \overset{\text{def}}{=} A\nu_a + \sum_{\beta=1}^{K_2} K(v_\alpha, \nu_\beta) Q_2 \gamma_\beta\}$ where A is the unknown (4×3) affine matrix, the TPS kernel $K(\nu_\alpha, \nu_\beta) = -||\nu_\alpha - \nu_\beta||$ in 3D, Q_2 is the $K_2 \times (K_2 - 4)$ part of the QR decomposition of ν (in homogeneous coordinates) and γ is the unknown $(K_2 - 4) \times 3$ matrix of deformation parameters. To avoid degenerate solutions which include all permutations of ν when $K_1 = K_2$, we add a deformation regularization term $\lambda \operatorname{trace}(\gamma^T Q_2^T K Q_2 \gamma)$ to the objective function in (3) with λ being a regularization parameter. In addition a regularization term $\lambda_A \operatorname{trace}[(A - I)^T (A - I)]$ is added to prevent reflections and unphysical affine transformations. We use a standard nonlinear conjugate-gradient (CG) algorithm (with line search) on the affine and deformation parameters (A, γ) and a 1-D search on the variance ξ^2. The variance parameter is updated separately from the remaining parameters and is not allowed to abruptly change.

4   Results

4.1   Synthetic Example: Sphere to Ellipsoid Density Matching

To showcase our approach of density matching, we begin with a synthetic example. We generate a sphere and an ellipsoid with 600 points each. We run a mixture model EM algorithm on the ellipsoid and sphere representing them with 120 and 60 centroids respectively. We then warp the ellipsoid using a Gaussian radial basis function (GRBF) using the 120 centroids as the centers for the GRBF. Subsequently, we run the deformable density matching (DDM) on the two synthetic datasets. The goal is to deform the sphere so that it matches the warped ellipsoid. Here the fixed variance σ^2 was set to the mean of the cluster variances resulting from the EM algorithm ($\sigma = 0.04$) and a 1-D search was performed over the parameter ξ, obtaining $\xi = 0.06$ as the optimum. The initial overlay of the sphere and the warped ellipsoid, the overlay of the centroids after matching and the final overlay of the warped sphere (using the recovered deformation parameters) are shown in Figure 1. Our results clearly demonstrate that the lack of correspondences at the point level as seen in the final shape overlay in Figure 1 is no deterrent to recovering the shape of the deformed ellipsoid.

4.2   Validation of Recovered Deformation: Bending and Stretching

Our approach to validation is based on comparing the recovered deformation vectors against the true (synthetically generated) deformation vectors generated at

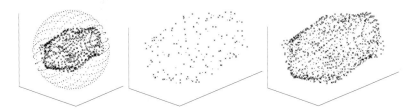

Fig. 1. Left: Initial overlay of sphere and warped ellipsoid, Middle: Cluster centers of the two shapes after density matching and Right: Overlay after registration

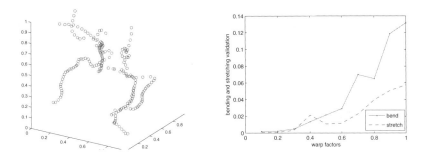

Fig. 2. Left: Vessel tree structure; Right: Validation over 30 noise trials, 10 warps

a set of vessel tree structure feature points [Figure 2]. Since we are not performing point matching, we cannot validate our results by using prior correspondence information. We begin with a point-set X consisting of about 200 points. A deformation field is applied to the point-set X to obtain a deformed point-set Y. We remove 50% of the points in Y to get a reduced set and this is done so that the two mixture densities have a large discrepancy in the number of centroids. Then we match X to the reduced Y using deformable density matching using 60 and 30 centroids for the two sets respectively. The recovered TPS parameters are used to compute the estimated displacement vector at each point in X. We compare the estimated displacement to the true displacement by separately plotting the stretching and bending components of the mean-squared displacement error: $\frac{1}{N_2}\sum_i \|\hat{u}_i - u_i\|^2 = \frac{1}{N_2}\sum(\|\hat{u}_i\| - \|u_i\|)^2 + \frac{1}{N_2}\sum_i 2\|\hat{u}_i\|\|u_i\|(1 - \frac{\hat{u}_i^T u_i}{\|\hat{u}_i\|\|u_i\|})$ where $\hat{u}_i$ is the estimated deformation, u_i is the true deformation and we have separated the total error into stretching (first term) and bending (second term) components. We executed 30 noise trials at different TPS warp factors w ranging from 0.1 to 1 in steps of 0.1. The TPS warp factor specifies that the TPS coefficients be uniformly generated from the interval $[-w, w]$. Higher the warp factor, greater the degree of deformation. The medians of the two error measures are shown in Figure 2, illustrating the difference between bending and stretching. The bending errors are more sensitive and increase more rapidly with w.

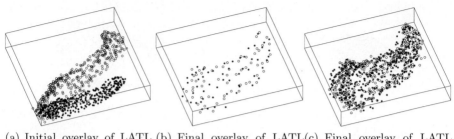

(a) Initial overlay of LATL (b) Final overlay of LATL(c) Final overlay of LATL
hippocampal datasets   hippocampal clusters   hippocampal datasets

Fig. 3.

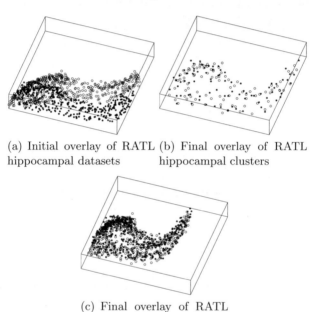

(a) Initial overlay of RATL (b) Final overlay of RATL
hippocampal datasets   hippocampal clusters

(c) Final overlay of RATL
hippocampal datasets

Fig. 4.

4.3   Evaluation on 3D Hippocampal Datasets

The general problem of building a hippocampal atlas is a clinical application
requiring multiple registrations of shapes from different patients. Here we use
deformable density matching to register 3D hippocampal point-set pairs from a
database of 60 cases. We showcase results on two pairs of patients scheduled for
left and right anterior temporal lobectomy (LATL and RATL) respectively. The
point-sets consisting of a few hundred points each are clustered into about 80
centroids, and we set $\lambda = 0.01$. After matching, we overlay the two point-sets by
warping one set onto the other using the recovered TPS parameters. The initial
overlay of the data, the final overlay of the centroids and the final overlay of the

warped datasets are shown in Figures 3 and 4 for LATL and RATL respectively. In both cases, the final overlay shows that we have achieved good registration. We are currently looking at entropic registration measures for more objective evaluation of all pairwise registrations across our database.

5 Discussion

In summary: i) We used a maximum likelihood EM approach to fit centroids and variances to raw feature data. ii) We determined a closed-form distance between two Gaussian mixture models. iii) We recovered a TPS deformation of the centroids of one shape while also allowing the shape variance parameter to change in order to best match the two shape representations. iv) Finally, we applied the recovered TPS deformation to the original data and showed that shape matching was possible even though there were few correspondences at the point feature level.

Our goal was to obtain a robust shape distance with very few free parameters and with the deformation parameters only affecting the model parameters and not specified over $\mathbb{R}^3$. The TPS model only warps the centroids and the variance parameters are allowed to move until the best fit is achieved. There are four free parameters in our model: K_1, K_2 and the regularization parameters λ, λ_A. Since the process of fitting probabilistic representations is offline, we can take recourse to model selection in order to fit K_1 and K_2. The regularization parameters can be learned via a Bayesian MAP procedure. There also do not appear to be any technical barriers to generalizing the TPS deformation parametrization to a diffeomorphism and optimizing over the occupancy probabilities as well.

References

1. Davies, R.H., Twining, C., Cootes, T.F., Taylor, C.J.: A minimum description length approach to statistical shape modelling. IEEE Trans. Med. Imag. 21, 525–537 (2002)
2. Toga, A., Mazziotta, J.: Brain Mapping: The Methods. Academic Press, London (1996)
3. Tagare, H.: Shape-based nonrigid correspondence with application to heart motion analysis. IEEE Transactions on Medical Imaging 18(7), 570–579 (1999)
4. Wang, F., Vemuri, B.C., Rangarajan, A., Schmalfuss, I.M., Eisenschenck, S.J.: Simultaneous registration of multiple point-sets and atlas construction. In: Leonardis, A., Bischof, H., Pinz, A. (eds.) ECCV 2006. LNCS, vol. 3953, pp. 551–563. Springer, Heidelberg (2006)
5. Guo, H., Rangarajan, A., Joshi, S.C.: 3-D diffeomorphic shape registration on hippocampal data sets. In: Duncan, J.S., Gerig, G. (eds.) MICCAI 2005. LNCS, vol. 3750, pp. 984–991. Springer, Heidelberg (2005)
6. Glaunes, J., Trouve, A., Younes, L.: Diffeomorphic matching of distributions: A new approach for unlabelled point-sets and sub-manifolds matching. In: IEEE Conf. on Computer Vision and Pattern Recognition, vol. 2, pp. 712–718 (2004)
7. Jian, B., Vemuri, B.C.: A robust algorithm for point set registration using mixture of Gaussians. In: Intl. Conf. on Computer Vision (ICCV), pp. 1246–1251 (2006)
8. McLachlan, G.J., Basford, K.E.: Mixture models: inference and applications to clustering. Marcel Dekker, New York (1988)
9. Wahba, G.: Spline models for observational data. SIAM, Philadelphia, PA (1990)

Robust Computation of Mutual Information Using Spatially Adaptive Meshes

Hari Sundar[1,2], Dinggang Shen[1], George Biros[1], Chenyang Xu[2], and Christos Davatzikos[1]

[1] Section for Biomedical Image Analysis, Department of Radiology, University of Pennsylvania
[2] Imaging and Visualization Department, Siemens Corporate Research, Princeton, NJ

Abstract. We present a new method for the fast and robust computation of information theoretic similarity measures for alignment of multi-modality medical images. The proposed method defines a non-uniform, adaptive sampling scheme for estimating the entropies of the images, which is less vulnerable to local maxima as compared to uniform and random sampling. The sampling is defined using an octree partition of the template image, and is preferable over other proposed methods of non-uniform sampling since it respects the underlying data distribution. It also extends naturally to a multi-resolution registration approach, which is commonly employed in the alignment of medical images. The effectiveness of the proposed method is demonstrated using both simulated MR images obtained from the BrainWeb database and clinical CT and SPECT images.

1 Introduction

Inter-modality image alignment is a fundamental step in medical image analysis. It is required to bring image data from different modalities to a common coordinate frame in order to accumulate information. It is usually presented as an optimization problem requiring the minimization of a certain objective function. Objective functions, or similarity measures based on information theoretic principles have been successful in aligning images from differing modalities. Mutual Information (MI) was proposed as an image similarity measure by Collignon [1], Viola [2] and Wells [3] and is widely used for rigid inter-modality registration. Several modifications have been proposed to make MI more robust and increase its capture range, including Normalized Mutual Information [4]. However, MI-based methods are very sensitive to the way the probability distributions are estimated and the accuracy of the estimated probability distributions have a great influence in the accuracy and robustness of the registration results [5].

A common assumption made in estimating the probability distribution is that each voxel is an i.i.d. realization of a random variable. Therefore, the probability distributions (including the joint distribution) can be computed by using all voxels in the reference image and the corresponding voxels in the transformed subject image. In general this can be quite expensive to compute and several multi-resolution and sampling techniques have been proposed for faster estimation of the probability distribution. Downsampling, both uniform and random, have been used quite commonly to speed up the estimation of the distributions [5]. Nonlinear sampling techniques where the local sampling rate is proportional to the gradient magnitude have also been proposed [6].

N. Ayache, S. Ourselin, A. Maeder (Eds.): MICCAI 2007, Part I, LNCS 4791, pp. 950–958, 2007.
© Springer-Verlag Berlin Heidelberg 2007

In general, although these methods have performed quite well for registering different structural modalities (like CT and MR), they have been less successful in being able to register structural modalities to functional modalities,which is important for diagnosis and treatment planning applications. Functional modalities do not image all tissues and are therefore more sensitive to errors in the estimation of probability distributions. We shall use the example of registering Single Photon Emission Computed Tomography (SPECT) with CT images of the same patient to demonstrate this problem.

In this paper we present a new method for rigid alignment of multi-modality images using an octree based partitioning of the reference image. Octrees allow us to partition the image into spatially adaptive regions (octants) such that homogeneous regions produce large octants. The octree allows us to define a non-linear sampling of the image that is proportional to the underlying image complexity. The samples thus obtained are closer to the usual i.i.d. assumption in that they tend to be less statistically interdependent, which in turn help us obtain more accurate estimates of entropy. The MI is the sum of the entropy of the subject image and the entropy of subject conditional on the target. Consequently, improved entropy estimates provide better estimates of MI.

The rest of the paper is organized as follows. In Section 2 we present a brief introduction to estimating entropy in images, and lay the foundation for our arguments in favor of the octree-based estimation of distributions, which is described in Section 3. Section 4 discusses the incorporation of the octree-based mutual information metric into a registration framework for inter-modality alignment of images, within a multi-resolution framework. Experimental results and comparisons with other methods are provided in Section 5.

2 Estimating the Entropy of Images

Shannon's entropy [7] for a discrete random variable X with a probability distribution $\mathbf{p}(X) = (p_1, \cdots, p_n)$, is defined as,

$$H(X) \overset{\Delta}{=} - \sum_{i=0}^{n} p_i \log p_i. \tag{1}$$

The definition can be extended to images by assuming the image intensities to be samples from a high dimensional signal. A common assumption made while defining entropy for images is that each voxel is an i.i.d. realization and that the underlying probability of pixel intensities can be estimated via the normalized histogram. The probability of a pixel having an intensity y_i, $p(y_i) = \text{hist}_Y(y_i)/d$, where $\text{hist}_Y(y_i)$ is the number of voxels in image Y with intensity y_i and d is the total number of voxels. Equation 1 can be then used to estimate the entropy of the image. This however does not capture the spatial complexity of the underlying image. For example, if we shuffle the pixels within the image, we will lose structure and be left with an image which is spatially random. However since the histogram is unchanged, the entropy is the same. This is demonstrated in Figure 1, where Figure 1(a) is highly structured and the red and blue blocks are placed at regular intervals. It can be seen that although the image in Figure 1(b) is produced from that in Figure 1(a) by adding random noise to the position of the

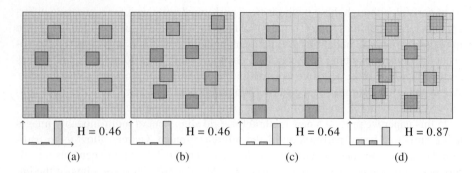

Fig. 1. The difficulty in estimating the entropy of images. **(a)** An image with the corresponding histogram and entropy estimate, **(b)** An image with objects moved within the image to make it appear more *random* than (a). The standard estimate for the entropy does not change, since the histogram is still the same. **(c)** Octree-based entropy estimation for the image shown in (a), and **(d)** octree-based entropy estimation for the image shown in (b). Note that in this case the increase in entropy was captured by the octree.

objects in the scene, the entropy is unaffected. This happens because of our assumption that each voxel intensity is an independent sample. This is not true since voxel intensities depend on the underlying objects, and samples from the same object cannot be assumed to be independent. Also observe that the gradient based approaches will not be able to capture this difference either, because it is not affected by the spatial variation between the two configurations shown in Figures 1(a) and (b).

It is widely accepted that images can be successfully modeled as Markov random fields [8,9]. Now, assuming that instead of an i.i.d. assumption, the samples form a Markov random field, then the error in the estimation of the entropy is lowered if the samples are largely independent of each other. Sabuncu et al. [6] suggest two non-linear sampling strategies based on the magnitude of the image gradient, in order to make the samples more independent. These suggested sampling methods, however, are for 2D images, expensive to compute and not easily extensible for 3D images. Algorithms have been proposed to make mutual information more robust by incorporating geometric information using gradients [10] and image salience [11]. However, the gradient captures only the local image complexity and it is not straightforward to extend this within a scale independent framework. This suggests using an adaptive sampling strategy, and adaptive image representations have been commonly used in non-linear image registration for representing the transformation [12] and for estimating local image similarities. However, to the best of our knowledge, it has not been used to estimate the global similarity of images.

3   Octrees Based Estimation of MI

If we can define a partitioning on the image that is spatially adaptive, and creates largely independent regions, we will be able to use the partition to define a better sampling strategy. Binary space partitions (BSP) [13] allow us to generate such spatially adaptive

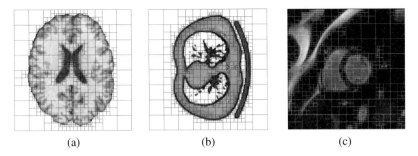

(a)   (b)   (c)

Fig. 2. (a) An example of a quadtree generated from a 2D slice of a MR brain image demonstrating how the quadtree adapts to the underlying data, **(b)** an example of a quadtree generated from a 2D slice of a thoracic CT image, and **(c)** the quadtree generated from a cardiac short axis MR image

partitions of data by recursively subdividing a space into convex sets by hyperplanes. BSP trees can be used in spaces with any number of dimensions, but *quadtrees* [14] and *octrees* [15] are most useful in partitioning 2D and 3D domains, respectively. Quadtrees and octrees use axis aligned lines and planes, respectively, instead of arbitrary hyperplanes and are efficient for the specific domains they are intended to work on.

The octree structure introduces non-stationarity in space [16]. This is important since the resulting octree is not shift-invariant and can create block artifacts. Such artifacts have been reported before [17,18]. Approaches like generating octrees with overlapping leaves [19] could possibly be applied for estimating shift-invariant octrees. Making the samples shift-invariant is left for future work.

We use a standard top-down approach to construct the octree for a given image. Starting with the entire domain, we test each block to see if it meets some criterion of homogeneity. If a block meets the criterion, it is not divided any further. If it does not meet the criterion, it is subdivided and the test criterion is applied to those blocks. This process is repeated iteratively until each block meets the criterion. In the experiments reported in this paper, we used a simple intensity based test criterion of homogeneity, wherein a block is split if all the voxels within it are not within a specified threshold, which was based on the number of bins of the histogram used to estimate the probability distribution. An example of a quadtree constructed from a 2D slice of a MR image of the human brain, a 2D slice of a Cardiac CT image, and a cardiac short axis MR image are shown in Figure 2.

In our sampling method, the same number of samples are used per octant. In other words the density of octants specifies the sampling frequency. The octree-based entropy can be computed by using the following estimate of the probability distribution in (1),

$$p_i = \frac{\sum_x (T(x) \in \text{bin}(i))}{\sum_x 1}, \quad \forall x \in \text{Oct}(T), \qquad (2)$$

where $\text{bin}(\cdot)$ defines the histogram binning operator and $\text{Oct}(T)$ is the octree computed for the template image T. In order to understand why an octree-based sampling appears to be better than uniform or gradient based sampling, consider the example discussed earlier, shown in Figure 1. We showed earlier that traditional sampling methods (both uniform and gradient based) estimate the same entropy for the images shown in Figures 1(a) and (b). However, the octree-based sampling is able to capture this difference, as seen in Figures 1(c) and (d). This is because the spatial complexity of the octree increases as a result of the change in the randomness of the scene. The octree captures the spatial complexity of the scene and consequently the entropy of a complex scene is higher as it has a denser octree. It is important to point out that the octree is not necessarily the best estimate of spatial complexity, since it is partial towards objects that are axis aligned and will not be able to capture such variations. A better estimate of the scene complexity would be a connectivity graph of segmented objects. This however would increase the complexity of both computing such a graph and also in using it during the registration. It would be difficult and computationally expensive to define transformations and interpolation functions on a connectivity graph of segmented tissues. The octree is a compromise that provides a sufficiently accurate and robust estimate of the entropy (see Section 5) and is also easy to compute and manipulate. Interpolation and transformations (linear and non-linear) can be easily defined on the octree. Importantly, octree-representations are amenable to parallel computing, which can dramatically expedite the performance of algorithms that use it. In all the experiments reported in this paper, the octree was computed only for the template image and each octant was sampled at the center of each octant in the template image. Although, it would be better to average over the entire octant instead of sampling at the center, we opted for the latter to improve the computational efficiency of the method.

4   Rigid Inter-modality Registration Using Adaptive MI

Given a template image, $T : \Omega \rightarrow \mathbb{R}^n$ and a subject image $S : \Omega \rightarrow \mathbb{R}^n$, where $\Omega \in \mathbb{R}^d$, the goal is to determine a rigid transformation χ that aligns the two images. The similarity measure is the metric that quantifies the degree of alignment and allows us to present the alignment problem as an optimization problem. We use the octree-based similarity measures as described in Section 3. We formulate the determination of the optimal transformation, $\hat{\chi}$, as an optimization problem:

$$\hat{\chi} = \arg \max_{\chi} I(T(x), S(\chi(x))), \quad \forall x \in \mathrm{Oct}(T), \tag{3}$$

where, $I(.;.)$ is the Mutual Information. Powell's multidimensional set method [20] is used to iteratively search for the maxima along each parameter using Brent's method [20]. In order to increase the robustness and to improve speed, we use a multi-resolution framework defined on the octree. The octree at lower (coarser) resolutions are generated by skipping all octants at the finer levels.

5   Results

In this section we describe experiments that were carried out to test the effectiveness of octree-based MI in the rigid registration of inter-modality images. We first describe

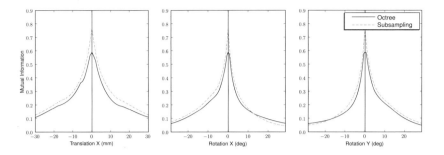

Fig. 3. Comparison of the mutual information computed via uniform sampling (dotted lines) and using the proposed octree-based sampling (solid lines), on BrainWeb datasets. The plots shown are for a comparison between a T1-weighted (T1) image and a proton density (PD) image with 9% noise and 40% intensity non-uniformity.

the similarity profiles when an artificial transformation is introduced between two registered images. We compared the octree-based method with uniform sampling based estimation of mutual information. The first experiment was performed using simulated MR datasets obtained from the BrainWeb database [21]. The second experiment was performed with 13 CT datasets with corresponding SPECT images. These images were all acquired using a Siemens Symbia™ T, a TruePoint SPECT-CT system and are assumed self registered. We analyzed the mutual information profiles while varying the transformation. The transformation parameters were varied one at a time, and the similarity profiles were plotted. The plots for translation along the x-axis, and for rotation about the x and y axes are shown in Figures 3 and 4, for T1-PD MR images and CT-SPECT images, respectively[1]. The profiles for translation and rotation along the other axes were similar. In all cases we compare the octree-based sampling with uniform sampling, where the total number of samples are similar. The octree reduced the number of samples by a factor of 8 on an average, therefore we subsampled by a factor of 2, along each direction, for the uniform sampling strategy, to have the same number of samples in both cases. As can be seen from Figure 3, both methods perform equally well on the BrainWeb datasets. Both sampling techniques have smooth curves with sharp peaks and very good capture ranges. However, when we look at the results from the CT-SPECT comparison, shown in Figure 4, we observe that the octree-based sampling performs much better. Although, both approaches have good profiles subject to translation, for the profiles subject to rotation, the uniform sampling approach exhibits a weak maxima at the optimal value with a very small capture range. In contrast the octree-based approach exhibits a strong maximum at the optimal value and also has a much larger capture range. The fact that the neighboring maxima in the vicinity of the optimum are lower further implies that it is likely that a multi-resolution approach can potentially be used to increase the capture range. The uniform sampling approach will in most cases converge to the wrong result since the neighboring maxima are much larger in that case.

---

[1] The profiles generated from using all the voxels in the image were almost identical to those obtained by uniform subsampling, and are not presented here for clarity.

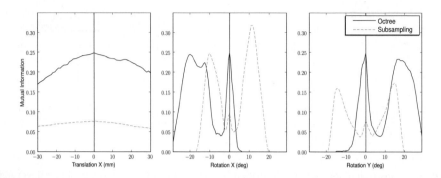

Fig. 4. Comparison of the mutual information computed via uniform sampling (dotted lines) and using the proposed octree-based sampling (solid lines), with CT-SPECT datasets. The plots shown are for a comparison between a CT cardiac image ($512 \times 512 \times 25$) and a SPECT image ($128 \times 128 \times 128$).

Table 1. Means and standard deviations of the registration errors for the different test cases

Dataset	Uniform sampling			Octree-based		
	Success	Trans. error (mm)	Rot. error (deg)	Success	Trans. error (mm)	Rot. error (deg)
T1 - T2	82.4%	0.48 ± 0.63	0.17 ± 0.24	86.1%	0.53 ± 0.59	0.21 ± 0.19
T1 - PD	79.7%	0.57 ± 0.66	0.2 ± 0.33	81.3%	0.59 ± 0.62	0.22 ± 0.23
CT - SPECT	31.1%	0.73 ± 0.69	0.23 ± 0.28	68.5%	0.64 ± 0.57	0.21 ± 0.31

Registration was performed on a number of datasets to quantitatively assess the performance of the octree-based mutual information within the registration framework. We selected a T1-weighted image with no noise and uniform intensity as the template image. T2-weighted and Proton Density (PD) images with varying levels of noise ($0-9\%$) and intensity non-uniformity ($0 - 40\%$) were registered to the template image, with a pseudo-random initial transform applied. The random transform was selected such that the initial translation was at most half the size of the image (to ensure overlap) and the rotational components were less than $60°$. The same set of pseudo-random transformations were used for both methods. The registration was considered successful if the final error was less than 2mm for the translational parameters and less than $2°$ for the rotational parameters. Similar experiments were performed for the CT-SPECT dataset and are summarized in Table 1. The error in the estimation of the translation and rotation parameters is calculated using only the cases in which a successful registration was performed. We can see from Table 1, that the octree-based sampling performs slightly better than uniform sampling in case of T1-T2 and T1-PD registration. We would like to emphasize that the success rate for the CT-SPECT registration is much better using the octree-based sampling as compared to uniform sampling, owing mainly to the broader capture range of the octree-based method. The average time to perform the registration was 13 seconds using the octree-based approach, 14 seconds for uniformly sampled approach and 85 seconds when using all voxels. All experiments were performed on an Intel Xeon 2.8GHz with 2GB of RAM. The time for the octree-based method includes the time to compute the octree.

6   Conclusion

We have presented a spatially adaptive sampling method for the estimation of image entropies and mutual information. We also demonstrate the improvements in the rigid registration of CT and SPECT images using the new sampling method. The proposed sampling offers flexibility between robustness and speed. When used at full resolution, octree-based sampling provides better estimates of image entropy and mutual information between images. In addition, it is better to use octree-based sampling in order to speed up the estimation of the similarity measure as opposed to using uniform sampling approaches. When compared with uniform sampling approaches, the octree-based sampling was more accurate for comparable computational speeds, and appears to be a better method for speeding up the estimation of MI.

Acknowledgments

The authors would like to thank Dr. Parmeshwar Khurd for useful discussions. This research was partially funded by a research grant from Siemens Corporate Research, Princeton, NJ.

References

1. Collignon, A., et al.: Automated multimodality medical image registration using information theory. Proc. Information Processing in Medical Imaging 3, 263–274 (1995)
2. Viola, P.: Alignment by Maximization of Mutual Information. PhD thesis, Massachusetts Institute of Technology (MIT), Cambridge, Massachusetts (1995)
3. Wells, W., Viola, P., Atsumi, H., Nakajima, S., Kikinis, R.: Multi-modal volume registration by maximization of mutual information. Medical Image Analysis 1(1), 35–51 (1996)
4. Studholme, C., Hill, D., Hawkes, D.: An overlap invariant entropy measure of 3D medical image alignment. Pattern Recognition 32(1), 71–86 (1999)
5. Pluim, J., Maintz, J., Viergever, M.: Mutual-information-based registration of medical images: a survey. IEEE Trans. on Medical Imaging 22(8), 986–1004 (2003)
6. Sabuncu, M.R., Ramadge, P.J.: Gradient based nonuniform sampling for information theoretic alignment methods. In: Proc. Int. Conf. of the IEEE EMBS, San Francisco, CA, IEEE Computer Society Press, Los Alamitos (2004)
7. Shannon, C.E.: A mathematical theory of communication. The Bell System Technical Journal 27 (1948)
8. Li, S.Z.: Markov random field modeling in computer vision. Springer, Heidelberg (1995)
9. Prez, P.: Markov random fields and images. CWI Quarterly 11(4), 413–437 (1998)
10. Pluim, J.P.W., Maintz, J.B.A., Viergever, M.A.: Image registration by maximization of combined mutual information and gradient information. IEEE Trans. on Medical Imaging 19(8), 809–814 (2000)
11. Luan, H., Qi, F., Shen, D.: Multi-modal image registration by quantitative-qualitative measure of mutual information Q-MI. In: Proc. CVBIA, pp. 378–387 (2005)
12. Timoner, S.: Compact Representations for Fast Nonrigid Registration of Medical Images. PhD thesis, Massachusetts Institute of Technology (MIT), Cambridge, Massachusetts (2003)
13. Fuchs, H., Kedem, Z.M., Naylor, B.F.: On visible surface generation by a priori tree structures. In: Proc. SIGGRAPH, pp. 124–133 (1980)

14. Finkel, R.A., Bentley, J.L.: Quad trees: A data structure for retrieval on composite keys. Acta. Inf. 4, 1–9 (1974)
15. Meagher, D.: Geometric modeling using octree encoding. Computer Graphics and Image Processing 19, 129–147 (1982)
16. Laferté, J., Perez, P., Heitz, F.: Discrete Markov image modeling and inference on the quadtree. IEEE Trans. on Image Processing 9(3), 390–404 (2000)
17. Bouman, C.A., Shapiro, M.: A multiscale random field model for Bayesian image segmentation. IEEE Trans. on Image Processing 3(2), 162–177 (1994)
18. Luettgen, M.R., Karl, W.C., Willsky, A.S.: Efficient multiscale regularization with applications to the computation of optical flow. IEEE Trans. on Image Processing 3(1), 41–64 (1994)
19. Irving, W.W., et al.: An overlapping tree approach to multiscale stochastic modeling and estimation. IEEE Trans. on Image Processing 6(11), 1517–1529 (1997)
20. Press, W.H., Teukolsky, S.A., Vetterling, W.T., Flannery, B.P.: Numerical Recipes in C: The Art of Scientific Computing. Cambridge University Press, New York (1992)
21. Collins, D.L., et al.: Design and construction of a realistic digital brain phantom. IEEE Trans. on Medical Imaging 17(3), 463–468 (1998)

Shape Analysis
Using a Point-Based Statistical Shape Model
Built on Correspondence Probabilities

Heike Hufnagel[1,2], Xavier Pennec[1], Jan Ehrhardt[2], Heinz Handels[2],
and Nicholas Ayache[1]

[1] Asclepios Project, INRIA, Sophia Antipolis, France
heike.hufnagel@sophia.inria.fr
[2] Medical Informatics, Universitätsklinikum Hamburg-Eppendorf, Germany

Abstract. A fundamental problem when computing statistical shape
models is the determination of correspondences between the instances of
the associated data set. Often, homologies between points that represent
the surfaces are assumed which might lead to imprecise mean shape and
variability results. We propose an approach where exact correspondences
are replaced by evolving correspondence probabilities. These are the basis for a novel algorithm that computes a generative statistical shape
model. We developed an unified MAP framework to compute the model
parameters ('mean shape' and 'modes of variation') and the nuisance
parameters which leads to an optimal adaption of the model to the set
of observations. The registration of the model on the instances is solved
using the Expectation Maximization - Iterative Closest Point algorithm
which is based on probabilistic correspondences and proved to be robust
and fast. The alternated optimization of the MAP explanation with respect to the observation and the generative model parameters leads to
very efficient and closed-form solutions for (almost) all parameters. Experimental results on brain structure data sets demonstrate the efficiency
and well-posedness of the approach. The algorithm is then extended to
an automatic classification method using the k-means clustering and applied to synthetic data as well as brain structure classification problems.

1 Introduction

One of the central difficulties of analyzing different organ shapes in a statistical manner is the identification of correspondences between the shapes. As
the manual identification of landmarks is not a feasible option in 3D, several
preprocessing techniques were developed to automatically find exact one-to-one
correspondences [1,2] between surfaces. Some approaches solve this with a search
for the registration transformation using an atlas [3] or the ICP algorithm [4].
Other methods directly combine the search of correspondences and of the statistical shape model (SSM) [5,6,7]. However, exact correspondences can only be
determined between continuous surfaces, not between point cloud representations of surfaces. Thus, using imprecise homologies leads to variability modes

N. Ayache, S. Ourselin, A. Maeder (Eds.): MICCAI 2007, Part I, LNCS 4791, pp. 959–967, 2007.
© Springer-Verlag Berlin Heidelberg 2007

that not only represent the organ shape variations but also artificial variations whose importance is linked to the local sampling. The SoftAssign algorithm tries to solve this problem with some kind of probabilistic formulation [8]. Another recent approach proposes an entropy based criterion to find shape correspondences, but requires implicit surface representations [9]. Other recent methods combine the shape analysis with the search for correspondences, however, these methods are not easily adaptable to multiple observations of unstructured point sets [10,11,12] or focus only on the mean shape [13]. In order to build an SSM based on inexact correspondences between point clouds, we pursue a probabilistic concept and base our work on a EM-ICP registration algorithm which proved to be robust, precise, and fast [14]. In section 2, we realize a Maximum a Posteriori (MAP) estimation of the model and observation parameters which lead to a unique criterion. We then compute the mean shape and eigenmodes which best fit the given data set by optimizing the global criterion iteratively with respect to all model and observation parameters. A key part of our method is that we can find a closed-form solution for almost each of the parameters. In particular, the approach solves for the mean shape and the eigenmodes *without* the need of one-to-one correspondences as is usually required by the PCA. Experiments in section 3 demonstrate that the resulting deformation coefficients can be used as an efficient measure to classify each observation.

2   Construction of the Statistical Shape Model

2.1   Model and Observation Parameters

In the process of computing the SSM, we distinguish strictly between **model parameters** and **observation parameters**. The generative SSM is explicitly defined by 4 **model parameters**:

- mean shape $\bar{M} \in \mathbb{R}^{3N_m}$ parametrized by N_m points $m_j \in \mathbb{R}^3$,
- eigenmodes v_p consisting of N_m 3D vectors v_{pj},
- associated standard deviations λ_p which describe - similar to the classical eigenvalues in the PCA - the impact of the eigenmodes,
- number n of eigenmodes.

Using the generative model $\Theta = \{\bar{M}, v_p, \lambda_p, n\}$ of a given structure, the shape variations of that structure can be generated by $M_k = \bar{M} + \sum_{p=1}^{n} \omega_{kp} v_p$ with $\omega_{kp} \in \mathbb{R}$ being the deformation coefficients. The shape variations along the modes follow a Gaussian probability with variance λ_p:

$$p(M_k|\Theta) = p(\Omega_k|\Theta) = \prod_{p=1}^{n} p(\omega_{kp}|\Theta) = \frac{1}{(2\pi)^{n/2} \prod_{p=1}^{n} \lambda_p} \exp\left(-\sum_{p=1}^{n} \frac{\omega_{kp}^2}{2\lambda_p^2}\right). \quad (1)$$

In order to account for the unknown position and orientation of the model in space, we introduce the random (uniform) rigid or affine transformation T_k. A model point m_j can then be deformed and placed by $T_k \star m_{kj} = T_k \star (\bar{m}_j +$

$\sum_p \omega_{kp} v_p$). Finally, we specify the sampling of the model surface: Each sampling (e.g. observation) point s_{ki} is modeled as a Gaussian measurement of a (transformed) model point m_{kj}. The probability of the observation $p(s_{ki}|m_{kj}, T_k)$ knowing the originating model point m_{kj} is given by $p(s_{ki}|m_{kj}, T_k) = (2\pi)^{-3/2}$ $\sigma^{-1} \exp(-\frac{1}{2\sigma^2}(s_{ki} - T_k \star m_{kj})^T.(s_{ki} - T_k \star m_{kj})$. As we do not know the originating model point for each s_{ki}, the probability of a given observation point s_{ki} is described by a Mixture of Gaussians and the probability for the whole scene S_k becomes:

$$p(S_k|M, T_k) = \prod_{i=1}^{N_k} \frac{1}{N_m} \sum_{j=1}^{N_m} p(s_{ki}|m_{kj}, T_k). \tag{2}$$

We summarize the **observation parameters** as $Q_k = \{\Omega_k, T_k\}$. Notice that the correspondences are hidden parameters that do not belong to the observation parameters of interest.

2.2 Derivation of the Global Criterion Using a MAP Approach

When building the SSM, we deal with the inverse problem of the approach in section 2.1: We have N observations $S_k \in \mathbb{R}^{3N_k}$, and we are interested in the parameters linked to the observations $Q = \{Q_k\}$ as well as the unknown model parameters Θ. In order to determine all parameters of interest, we optimize a MAP on Q and Θ rather than an ML to take into account that Q and Θ are not independent.

$$\text{MAP} = -\sum_{k=1}^{N} \log(p(Q_k, \Theta|S_k)) = -\sum_{k=1}^{N} \log\left(\frac{p(S_k|Q_k, \Theta)p(Q_k|\Theta)p(\Theta)}{p(S_k)}\right). \tag{3}$$

As $p(S_k)$ does not depend on Θ and $p(\Theta)$ is assumed to be uniform, the global criterion integrating our unified framework is the following:

$$C(Q, \Theta) = -\sum_{k=1}^{N} \left(\log(p(S_k|Q_k, \Theta)) + \log(p(Q_k|\Theta))\right). \tag{4}$$

The first term describes the ML criterion (2) whereas the second term is the prior on the deformation coefficients ω_{kp} as described in (1). Dropping the constants, our criterion simplifies to $C(Q, \Theta) \sim \sum_{k=1}^{N} C_k(Q_k, \Theta)$ with

$$C_k(Q_k, \Theta) = \sum_{p=1}^{n} \left(\log(\lambda_p) + \frac{\omega_{kp}^2}{2\lambda_p^2}\right) - \sum_{i=1}^{N_k} \log\left(\sum_{j=1}^{N_m} \exp\left(-\frac{\|s_{ki} - T_k \star m_{kj}\|^2}{2\sigma^2}\right)\right). \tag{5}$$

This equation is the heart of the unified framework for the model computation and its fitting to observations. By optimizing it alternately with respect to the operands in $\{Q, \Theta\}$, we are able to determine all parameters we are interested in. Starting from the initial model parameters Θ, we fit the model to each of the observations (section 2.3). Next, we fix the observation parameters Q_k and update the model parameters (section 2.4). Some terms will recur in the different optimizations, so we introduce the following notation for the derivation of the second term $\xi_{kij}(T_k, \Omega_k, \bar{M}, v_p, \lambda_p) = \log \sum_{j=1}^{N_m} \exp\left(\frac{-\|s_{ki} - T_k \star m_{kj}\|^2}{2\sigma^2}\right)$ with respect to one of the function's parameters (let's say x):

$$\frac{\partial \xi}{\partial x} = \sum_{j=1}^{N_m} \gamma_{kij} \frac{(s_{ki} - T_k \star m_{kj})^T}{\sigma^2} \frac{\partial(s_{ki} - T_k \star m_{kj})}{\partial x} \tag{6}$$

where the weights $\gamma_{ijk} = \exp\left(-\frac{\|s_{ki} - T_k \star m_{kj}\|^2}{2\sigma^2}\right) \left[\sum_{l=1}^{N_m} \exp\left(-\frac{\|s_{ki} - T_k \star m_{kl}\|^2}{2\sigma^2}\right)\right]^{-1}$ are sometimes interpreted as soft labels/correspondences.

2.3   Mapping the Model to the Observations

Optimization with respect to the Transformations. As no closed form solution exists for the optimization of criterion (2), we employ an EM algorithm where the correspondence probabilities between S_k and M are modeled as the hidden variable $H_k \in \mathbb{R}^{N_k \times N_m}$. An instance point s_{ki} corresponds to a model point m_j with probability $E(H_{k_{ij}})$. By computing the expectation of the log-likelihood of the complete data distribution with T_k fixed, we find in the *expectation step* $E(H_{k_{ij}}) = \gamma_{kij}$. As defined above, the γ_{kij} represent the weights of each pair (s_{ki}, m_j) in the criterion. Next, $T_k = \{A_k, t_k\}$ is computed in the *maximization step* by maximizing the global criterion in (5) with all γ_{kij} fixed in a closed-form solution. The implementation of the EM-ICP algorithm is realized in a multi-scaling frame regarding the variance [14]. $\sigma_{initial}$ and its decrease rate have to be carefully adapted to the data at hand (σ_{final} should be in the order of the average point distance).

Optimization with respect to the Deformation Coefficients. The observation parameter T_k and Θ are fixed, and we compute the ω_{kp} which solve $\partial C_k(Q_k, \Theta)/\partial \omega_{kp} = 0$. This leads to a matrix equation of the form $\Omega_k = (B_k - \sigma^2 \Lambda_{nn})^{-1} d_k$ with $d_{kp} = \sum_{i=1}^{N_k} \sum_{j=1}^{N_m} \gamma_{kij}(s_{ki} - t_k - A_k \bar{m}_j)^T A_k v_{pj}$, $d_{kp} \in \mathbb{R}$ and $b_{kqp} = \sum_{i=1}^{N_k} \sum_{j=1}^{N_m} \gamma_{kij} v_{qj}^T A_k^T A_k v_{pj}$, $b_{kqp} \in \mathbb{R}$ $b_{kqp} = b_{kpq}$.

2.4   Learning the Model from the Observations

Optimization with respect to the Standard Deviations. The computation of the optimal standard deviation λ_p with parameters $\bar{M}, v_p$ and Q_k fixed is simply:

$$\frac{\partial C(Q, \Theta)}{\partial \lambda_p} = \sum_{k=1}^{N} \left(\frac{1}{\lambda_p} - \frac{\omega_{kp}^2}{\lambda_p^3}\right) = 0 \quad \Leftrightarrow \quad \lambda_p^2 = \frac{1}{N} \sum_{k=1}^{N} \omega_{kp}^2. \tag{7}$$

Optimization with respect to the Mean Shape. Setting $\partial C(Q, \Theta)/\partial \bar{m}_j$ to 0 and using the general derivation presented in (6), we find

$$\bar{m}_j = \left(\sum_{k=1}^{N} \sum_{i=1}^{N_k} \gamma_{kij} A_k^T A_k \right)^{-1} \sum_{k=1}^{N} \sum_{i=1}^{N_k} \gamma_{kij} A_k^T \left(s_{ki} - t_k - A_k \sum_{p=1}^{n} \omega_{kp} v_{pj} \right) \quad (8)$$

Optimization with respect to the Eigenmodes. (The parameters $\lambda_p, \bar{M}$ and Q_k are fixed.) Let us first define the matrix $V \in \mathbb{R}^{3N_m \times n}$ containing the eigenmodes $v_p \in \mathbb{R}^{3N_m}$ in its columns. The $v_{pj} \in \mathbb{R}^3$ referred to in the equations are the eigenmode information associated to point $\bar{m}_j$. As we want the eigenmodes to be orthonormal, we add a Lagrange multiplier by introducing the symmetric matrix $Z \in \mathbb{R}^{n \times n}$ to our global criterion in the form: $\Lambda = C + \frac{1}{2} tr \left(Z(V^T V - I_{n \times n}) \right)$. Deriving the Lagrangian with respect to v_{pj} gives in the rigid case

$$\frac{\partial \Lambda}{\partial v_{pj}} = \sum_{q=1}^{n} z_{qp} v_{qj} - \sum_{q=1}^{n} b_{pq} v_{qj} + q_{pj}$$

where $q_{pj} = \frac{1}{\sigma^2} \sum_{k=1}^{N} \sum_{i=1}^{N_k} \gamma_{kij} (s_{ki} - t_k - A_k \bar{m}_j)^T \omega_{kp} A_k$, $q_{pj} \in \mathbb{R}^3$ and $b_{pqj} = \frac{1}{\sigma^2} \sum_{k=1}^{N} \sum_{i=1}^{N_k} \gamma_{kij} \omega_{kq} \omega_{kp} I_{3 \times 3}$ $b_{pqj} \in \mathbb{R}^{3 \times 3}$.

Hence we find $\sum_{q=1}^{n} v_{jq}(z_{qp} + b_{pqj}) = q_{jp}$. We approach the problem regarding each of the N_m bands $[V]_{\{j\}} \in \mathbb{R}^{3 \times n}$ of matrix $V \in \mathbb{R}^{3N_m \times n}$ separately with $[V]_{\{j\}} = [v_{j1}, ..., v_{jq}, ..., v_{jn}]$ and $[V]_{\{j\}} (B_j + Z) = [Q]_{\{j\}}$. We iterate the following two steps until $\|V^{t+1} - V^t\|^2 \leq \epsilon$.

1. For Z known, we compute V: $[V]_{\{j\}} = [Q]_{\{j\}} (B_j + Z)^{-1}$ for all model point indices j. To enforce V to be orthonormal, we apply first a singular value decomposition $V = USR^T$ and then replace V by UR^T.
2. For all $[V]_{\{j\}}$ known, we determine Z: $Z = V^T \tilde{Q}$ with $[\tilde{Q}]_{\{j\}} = [Q]_{\{j\}} - [V]_{\{j\}} B_j$. As Z has to be symmetric, we set $Z \leftarrow \frac{1}{2}(Z + Z^T)$.

3   Experiments and Results

3.1   Validation of Algorithm on Synthetic Data

We generated a data set consisting of ellipsoids with and without bump. Each ellipsoid was transformed using a random affine transformation, and then an uniform noise was added, see Fig. 1a) for some observation examples.

Building the SSM on Ellipsoids. The data set contained 18 ellipsoids, half with bump, half without. An initial mean shape was randomly chosen from the data set, Fig. 1d). The results of the alignment as seen in Fig. 1b) were obtained with the EM-ICP registration. The final mean shape and the deformations according to the first eigenmode are depicted in Fig. 1d). As can be seen in Fig. 1c),

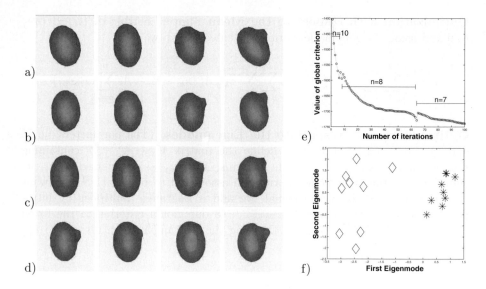

Fig. 1. SSM on synthetic data set. Row a) shows 4 observation examples. Row b) shows the same observation after being aligned to the mean shape. Row c) shows the shapes generated by using the SSM and the deformation coefficients associated with the observations. Row d) shows (from left to right) the initial mean shape (a randomly chosen observation), the final mean shape, and the mean shape deformed with respect to the first eigenmode ($\bar{M} - 3\lambda_1 v_1$ and $\bar{M} + 3\lambda_1 v_1$). e): Values of global criterion after each iteration. f): 2D deformation coefficient feature vectors (ω_{k1}, ω_{k2}) for the first two eigenmodes, 'with bump' observations (diamonds) and 'without bump' (stars).

all observation shapes can be generated using the resulting SSM and the deformation coefficients as $S_k = \bar{M} + \sum_{kp} \omega_{kp} v_p$. Figure 1e) shows the converging values of the global criterion (5) during the iterations of the SSM computation. Since we discard eigenvectors whose standard deviation falls below a certain threshold, n diminishes from 10 to 7 during computation. The results show that the algorithm computes a representative SSM for a given data set.

Classification of Ellipsoids. The deformation coefficients Ω computed during the optimization of (5) serve as a classification measure regarding the shape of the observations S_k. We formed feature vectors $\omega_k = (\omega_{k1}, \omega_{k2}, ..., \omega_{kn})$ and used them as input for a k-means clustering. The resulting two classes coincide with the 'bump' and 'without bump' classes with an average Rand index [15] of 0.95. See Fig. 1f) for the values of the 2D feature vectors (ω_{k1}, ω_{k2}).

3.2 Shape Analysis of Brain Structure

Here, we focus on the putamen. The data set consists of $N = 21$ right and left segmented instances (approximately $20mm \times 20mm \times 40mm$) which are represented by min 994 and max 1673 points, see Fig. 2a),b) for some shape examples. The MR images ($255 \times 255 \times 105$ voxels of size $0.94mm \times 0.94mm \times$

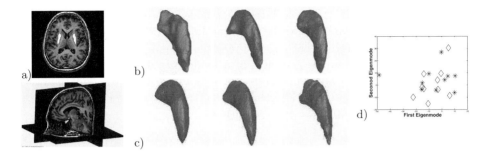

Fig. 2. Shape analysis of the putamen. a) CT-images with segmented left putamen. b) Observation examples of the data set. c) Mean shape (middle) and its deformations according to the first eigenmode ($\bar{M} - 3\lambda_1 \boldsymbol{v}_1$ and $\bar{M} + 3\lambda_1 \boldsymbol{v}_1$). d) 2D deformation coefficient feature vectors (ω_{k1}, ω_{k2}) for the first two eigenmodes, 'control' observations are represented as diamonds and 'patient' as stars.

$1.50mm$) as well as the segmentations were kindly provided by the Hôpital La Pitié-Salpêtrière, Paris, France. The data was collected in the framework of a study on hand dystonia. We chose the following parameters as input: Number of eigenmodes $n = 20$, initial sigma in the EM-ICP $\sigma = 4mm$, EM-ICP iterations 4, variance multi-scaling factor of the EM-ICP 0.7. The computation of the SSM converges after 30 iterations. The resulting smooth mean shape and the deformations according to the first two eigenmodes are shown Fig. 2c). In order to analyse the shapes, again we formed feature vectors $\omega_k = (\omega_{k1}, \omega_{k2}, ..., \omega_{kn})$ and used them as input for a k-means clustering. In this case, no two distinct shape classes were found (Fig.2d)).

3.3 Practical Aspects

Initial Model Parameters. As the computation of the observation parameters is based on known model parameters $\Theta = \{\bar{M}, v_p, \lambda_p\}$, we initialize $\bar{M}$ with one of the observations S_k in the given data set, preferably with a typical shape. Next, by applying the EM-ICP registration, we evaluate the resulting correspondence probabilities between $\bar{M}$ and each S_k and determine "virtual" one-to-one correspondences. These are then used as input for the Principal Components Analysis to compute the initial eigenvectors v_p and the initial eigenvalues λ_p. In order to test for the sensibility of our SSM computation with respect to the initialization, we compared the mean shape results which are obtained when using dissimilar initial mean shapes M_1 and M_2 (e.g.the first two shapes in Fig. 2b)). We established that M_1 can be generated based on the SSM found with M_2 with statistically very small deformation coefficients ω_{1p}: $M_1 = M_2 + \sum_p \omega_{1p} v_p$ with e.g. $\omega_{11} = 3.8 << \lambda_{21} = 15.7$.

Model Selection. As we want to find a good balance between complexity and simplicity of the model, we reduce the dimension of the eigenvector space during the iterated computation of the parameters. If the standard deviation

λ_p becomes "too small", the associated eigenmodes v_p are no longer taken into account. Finally, we want to add the Bayesian Information Criterion [16] to our global criterion with $BIC(n, N, N_k) = C(Q, \Theta) + \frac{n}{2} \log \sum_{k=1}^{N} N_k$. The Bayesian selection approach rates the goodness of a model based on the probability it assigns to the observed data while preferring a more constrained model than the Akaike Information Criterion. This suits our needs as we assume that several of the eigenmodes only represent noise variations.

4   Discussion

We developed a novel algorithm to generate statistical shape models (SSMs) which does not need one-to-one point correspondences but relies solely on point correspondence probabilities for the computation of mean shape and eigenmodes. Therefore, elaborate preprocessing of the observations in the data set to establish correspondences becomes obsolete, no questionable correspondences between point clouds representing surfaces are assumed, and the number of points in the observation may vary. The approach can be used for non-spherical surfaces and can be adapted to applications on data sets with different topologies as the connectivity between points does not play a role. We developed a mathematically sound and unified framework for the computation of model parameters and observation parameters and succeeded in determining a closed form solution for optimizing the associated criterion alternately for all parameters. Experiments showed that our algorithm works well and leads to plausible results. It proved to be robust to different initial mean shape choices and is stable even for a small number of observations. The explicit computation of all parameters involved allows a in-depth analysis of the data set. By evaluating the standard deviation and associated deformation coefficients for each eigenmode and each observation, a direct automatic classification of the data set is possible as we showed for the synthetic data set. We then performed a shape analysis on a putamen data set and found no statistically significant shape differences between dystonia patients and control group after affine normalizations (which confirms the presumption of the concerned physicians). From a theoretical point of view, a very powerful feature of our method is that we are optimizing a unique criterion. Thus, the convergence is ensured. However, the practical convergence rate has to be investigated more carefully. For instance, a fast decrease of the multi-scale variance σ^2 easily freezes the model in local minima. For further validation, we intend to study other kinds of data (e.g. hippocampus or ganglion) whose shapes are less convex than the putamen. In order to ensure robustness, we will extend the distance measure in the EM-ICP to include the normals.

References

1. Lorenz, C., Krahnstoever, N.: Generation of point-based 3D statistical shape models for anatomical objects. CVIU 77(2), 175–191 (2000)
2. Styner, M., Gerig, G., Lieberman, J., Jones, D., Weinberger, D.: Statistical shape analysis of neuroanatomical structures based on medial models. MedIA (03)

3. Shelton, C.R.: Morphable surface models. IJCV 38(1), 75–91 (2000)
4. Besl, P.J., McKay, N.D.: A method for registration of 3D shapes. IEEE Trans. PAMI, 239–256 (1992)
5. Davies, R., Twining, C., Cootes, T.: A minimum description length approach to statistical shape modeling. IEEE Trans. Med. Imag. 21(5) (2002)
6. Heimann, T., Wolf, I., Williams, T., Meinzer, H.: 3D active shape models using gradient descent optimization of description length. In: Christensen, G.E., Sonka, M. (eds.) IPMI 2005. LNCS, vol. 3565, Springer, Heidelberg (2005)
7. Zhao, Z., Theo, E.K.: A novel framework for automated 3D PDM construction using deformable models. In: Medical Imaging 2005, SPIE Proc. (2005)
8. Rangarajan, A., Chui, H., Bookstein, F.L.: The softassign procrustes matching algorithm. In: Duncan, J.S., Gindi, G. (eds.) IPMI 1997. LNCS, vol. 1230, pp. 29–42. Springer, Heidelberg (1997)
9. Cates, J., Meyer, M., Fletcher, P., Whitaker, R.: Entropy-based particle systems for shape correspondences. In: MICCAI 2006 (2006)
10. Tsai, A., Wells, W.M., Warfield, S.K., Willsky, A.S.: An EM algorithm for shape classification based on level sets. MedIA 9, 491–502 (2005)
11. Peter, A., Rangarajan, A.: Shape analysis using the Fisher-Rao Riemannian metric: Unifying shape representation and deformation. In: IEEE ISBI (2006)
12. Kodipaka, S., Vemuri, B., Rangarajan, A., Leonard, C., Schmallfuss, I., Eisenschenk, S.: Kernel fisher discriminant for shape-based classification in epilepsy. Medical Image Analysis 11 (2007)
13. Rangarajan, H.C.A., Zhang, J., Leonard, C.: Unsupervised learning of an atlas from unlabeld point-sets. IEEE Transactions on PAMI 26(2) (2004)
14. Granger, S., Pennec, X.: Multi-scale EM-ICP: A fast and robust approach for surface registration. In: Heyden, A., Sparr, G., Nielsen, M., Johansen, P. (eds.) ECCV 2002. LNCS, vol. 2353, pp. 418–432. Springer, Heidelberg (2002)
15. Rand, W.M.: Objective criteria for the evaluation of clustering methods. American Statistical. Association 66 (1971)
16. Schwarz, G.: Estimating the dimension of a model. Ann. of Stat. 6(2) (1978)

Robust Autonomous Model Learning
from 2D and 3D Data Sets[*]

Georg Langs[1,2], René Donner[2,4], Philipp Peloschek[3], and Horst Bischof[2]

[1] GALEN Group, Laboratoire de Mathématiques Appliquées aux Systèmes,
Ecole Centrale de Paris, France
[2] Institute for Computer Graphics and Vision, Graz University of Technology, Austria
[3] Department of Radiology, Medical University of Vienna, Austria
[4] Pattern Recognition and Image Processing Group, Vienna University of Technology, Austria
georg.langs@ecp.fr, donner@prip.tuwien.ac.at,
philipp.peloschek@meduniwien.ac.at, bischof@icg.tugraz.at

Abstract. In this paper we propose a weakly supervised learning algorithm for appearance models based on the minimum description length (MDL) principle. From a set of training images or volumes depicting examples of an anatomical structure, correspondences for a set of landmarks are established by group-wise registration. The approach does not require any annotation. In contrast to existing methods no assumptions about the topology of the data are made, and the topology can change throughout the data set. Instead of a continuous representation of the volumes or images, only sparse finite sets of interest points are used to represent the examples during optimization. This enables the algorithm to efficiently use distinctive points, and to handle texture variations robustly. In contrast to standard elasticity based deformation constraints the MDL criterion accounts for systematic deformations typical for training sets stemming from medical image data. Experimental results are reported for five different 2D and 3D data sets.

1   Introduction

Model based approaches like active shape models (ASMs) or active appearance models (AAMs) [1] capture shape and texture variation of a specific structure or object. They utilize this a priori knowledge to provide robust segmentation while allowing for repeatable identification of specific landmarks in the data. They are employed in various medical imaging tasks, like the segmentation of the diaphragm in CT data [2], vertebral morphometry in dual x-ray absorptiometry data [3], and registration in functional heart imaging [4]. The necessity for a large number of manually annotated training examples in order to obtain a sufficiently representative power of the model poses a major drawback for model based approaches, since the annotation is time consuming and the results are often sub-optimal. The problem of automatic model building or equivalently that of establishing correspondences over landmark positions in a set of images has been tackled from different directions: in [5] temporal continuity of image sequences is

---

[*] This research has been supported by the Austrian Science Fund (FWF) under the grant P17083-N04 (AAMIR). It has been partially supported from the Region Île-de-France.

N. Ayache, S. Ourselin, A. Maeder (Eds.): MICCAI 2007, Part I, LNCS 4791, pp. 968–976, 2007.
© Springer-Verlag Berlin Heidelberg 2007

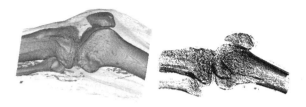

Fig. 1. Left: volume rendering of knee CT data. right: interest points on the bone structure.

used to determine correspondences. Given a set of manual continuous contour annotations in [6,7,8] landmarks are placed automatically along contours or surfaces that are mapped to a circle or a sphere using minimum description length (MDL). The reference manifold limits the approach to a topological class. Even-though these purely shape based approaches provide good landmark positions for constructing a compact shape model, in [9] the authors conclude that the lack of texture information poses a limitation hampering the capturing of *true* correspondences, like anatomical landmarks. In a line of work correspondences are established by one-to-many [10] or by group-wise registration of the entire images or volumes [11,12]. Non of these approaches can handle partially missing data. They are either dependent on a prior segmentation of objects, or deform the entire image continuously. In Fig. 1 on the left a surface rendering of the bones in knee CT data is shown. Such structures cannot be handled with a single reference manifold, and manual prior segmentation is tedious. A continuous deformation of the whole volume would not account for the compound structure, and would include large parts of soft tissue that deforms only loosely correlated with the bone surfaces. On the right the interest points, to which we restrict the calculation in this work, are depicted. Only local texture information is utilized giving sufficient information about the bone structure to perform model building.

Contribution. In this paper we propose a method to autonomously build appearance models based on group-wise registration of sparse representations of the training data. Instead of deforming dense texture maps we formulate the task as a search for correspondences between finite lists of interest points and local features in the training examples. This has several advantages: (1) the use of specific local features enables the algorithm to omit texture variations that yield no relevant information for the model, and to handle overlaps present in projective modalities, like x-ray. (2) The approach does not rely on a mapping to a reference manifold, therefore it is not constrained to an a priori topological class. (3) Occlusions and partially missing data sets are dealt with by outlier detection and robust model estimation. In contrast to purely shape based approaches local features add more specific information with regard to the correspondences of anatomical structures. These properties are relevant for complex anatomical structures that pose an obstacle to supervised model learning strategies, which would demand for an a priori definition of the topology, the structure or the connectivity constraints of the entity and a complete training set, i.e. no missing data. The approach is aimed at overcoming the necessity for the time consuming manual annotation prone to errors and variations in expert opinions.

2   Model Building

From a set of n training images or volumes $\mathbf{I}_i$, $i = 1, 2, \ldots, n$ depicting examples of a structure or an object, n sets of m_i interest points each is extracted. Initial correspondences for a random subset of k of these points are established by pairwise matching of a single reference image $\mathbf{I}_1$ to the remaining $n - 1$ images. This results in correspondences for the k landmarks $\{l_1, \ldots, l_k\}$, which are encoded in a $k \times n$ matrix $\mathbf{G}$. Each column represents an image, and the entry $\mathbf{G}_{ji} \in \{1, \ldots, m_i\}$ with $j \in \{1, \ldots, k\}$ is the index of the interest point in image $\mathbf{I}_i$, at which the landmark l_j is positioned. Starting from these correspondences groupwise registration is performed by minimizing a criterion function that captures the compactness of the appearance model comprising the variation of landmark positions and local texture variation at the landmark positions in the different training images. The interest points in the images or volumes are treated as landmark candidates. Each point (i, q) with $q \in \{1, \ldots, m_i\}$ is assigned its coordinate information $\mathbf{p}(i, q)$ and local features $\mathbf{f}(i, q)$ (e.g. SIFT, steerable filters). By assigning $\mathbf{G}_{ji} = q$ the landmark l_j in image $\mathbf{I}_i$ has position $\mathbf{p}_{ij} = \mathbf{p}(i, q)$ and feature vector $\mathbf{f}_{ij} = \mathbf{f}(i, q)$. During model building the matrix $\mathbf{G}$ is modified to minimize the criterion function, resulting in *optimal* positions for each landmark in each image.

2.1   Criterion Based on Minimum Description Length

The criterion function that is minimized during model building comprises the compactness of the model that describes shape and local texture variation, and an elasticity regularization that is used during the initial phase of the optimization.

Compactness of the shape model. We use a standard linear multivariate Gaussian model for the shape representation [1]. The shape model compactness criterion is based on minimum description length, see [6] for an extensive derivation. An optimal shape model should minimize the cost L of communicating the model $\mathcal{M}$ itself and the data D (i.e. the landmark positions) encoded with the model: $L(D, \mathcal{M}) = L(\mathcal{M}) + L(D|\mathcal{M})$. Since we do not represent the entire image content but only a sparse set of landmarks and their variation a normalization term has to be introduced, that prohibits the landmarks from collapsing to a single position. The shape term is normalized by the entropy of the landmark positions in the individual examples $L_{ref} = \sum_{i=1,\ldots,N} entropy_{j=1,\ldots,k}(\mathbf{p}_{ij})$ and captures the gain of compactness achieved by the model in contrast to the complexity of the original data without exploiting its structure. The normalization is not essential to the quality of the model, but fosters the more even covering of the training images by the model landmarks. The final shape model criterion is $\mathcal{C}_S = L(\mathcal{M}_S) + L(D_S|\mathcal{M}_S) + \mathcal{R}_S - Lref$, where $L(\mathcal{M}_S)$ is the cost of communicating the shape model, $L(D_S|\mathcal{M}_S)$ is the cost of the shape data encoded with help if the model, and $\mathcal{R}_S$ is a penalty for the residual error not captured by the model.

Local texture. The image content is captured by local descriptors that extract features at the landmark candidate positions in the training images (e.g. SIFT features). For a landmark l_j the component-wise median of the individual entries in the feature vectors $\mathbf{f}_{ij}$ for $i = 1, \ldots, n$ from the landmark positions in all training images is calculated resulting in the center $\hat{\mathbf{f}}_j$. The local appearance is then modeled by a Gaussian centered at $\hat{\mathbf{f}}_j$, and the description length is utilized as criterion for the compactness of the feature model $\mathcal{M}_T$ analogously to the shape model. Hence the criterion is $\mathcal{C}_T = L(\mathcal{M}_T) + L(D_T|\mathcal{M}_T) + \mathcal{R}_T$, where $L(\mathcal{M}_T)$ is the cost for the model, $L(D_T|\mathcal{M}_T)$ the cost of the local features encoded with the model, and $\mathcal{R}_T$ a penalty for the residual error.

Elasticity regularization. Since at the beginning of the model building the model has poor generalization behavior an elasticity cost term is introduced to regularize the deformations during the early phase of the optimization. A standard elasticity term $C_E = |\nabla \mathbf{d}(\mathbf{x})|^2$, where d is the displacement of the landmark x throughout the training set, helps avoiding a degenerate model.

Criterion function The final criterion function encompasses the compactness of models for shape and local texture information and the elasticity regularization: $\mathcal{C} = \mathcal{C}_S + \mathcal{C}_T + \alpha(t)\mathcal{C}_E$. The weight $\alpha(t)$ controls the influence of the elasticity, and is gradually decreased to 0 during optimization, to ensure a final result depending on the model costs only. During model building the criterion function is minimized by altering the matrix $\mathbf{G}$ that holds the correspondences between the landmarks and the interest points in the training images. A change of a single entry in $\mathbf{G}$ corresponds to a change of the position of a landmark in one image.

2.2   Dealing with Incomplete Data

Due to occlusions, irregular contrast or pose changes certain landmarks may not be present in all of the images. In order to still be able to build a model if parts of the data are missing the values are imputed based on previous estimates of the shape model $\mathcal{M}_S$, which is then re-estimated from the completed data vectors. The algorithm starts with estimates of the positions of the landmarks in all images i.e. no landmark is reported as missing. For a missing landmark l_j in image $\mathbf{I}_i$ the corresponding value in a matrix $\mathbf{R} \in [0,1]^{k \times n}$ is set to $\mathbf{R}_{ji} = 0$ and $\mathbf{R}_{ji} = 1$ if the landmark is present. During model building the algorithm decides at each iteration for each landmark in an image whether it is to be considered an outlier or not. The underlying idea is to perform an expectation maximization (EM) algorithm on the incomplete data set, by iteratively re-estimating mean and covariance matrix of the data [13]. Each of the shape vectors $\mathbf{x}_i$ is partitioned into $\mathbf{x}_i^a \in \mathbb{R}^{p_a}$, the vector of p_a values that are available for this particular image and $\mathbf{x}_i^m \in \mathbb{R}^{p_m}$ the vector of p_m values that are missing. Accordingly the mean is partitioned into $\bar{\mathbf{x}}_a$ and $\bar{\mathbf{x}}_m$. The relationship between available and missing records is modeled by a linear regression model $\mathbf{x}_m = \bar{\mathbf{x}}_m + (\mathbf{x}_a - \bar{\mathbf{x}}_a)\mathbf{B} + \mathbf{e}$, where $\mathbf{e}$ is the residual error. The regression matrix $\mathbf{B}$ is based on estimates of the mean $\hat{\mathbf{x}}$ and covariance matrix $\hat{\Sigma}$ of the entire data set from the preceding model building iteration. The missing values of all shape vectors are imputed, and based on the completed data the mean $\hat{\bar{x}}$ and the covariance matrix $\hat{\Sigma}$ are re-estimated. See [14] for a concise explanation of imputation.

2.3   Optimization

Initialization For each image interest points and corresponding local features are extracted. The group-wise registration is initialized by a one-to-many registration of one

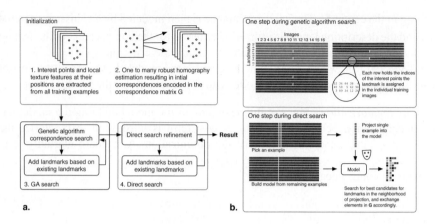

Fig. 2. a.: Scheme of the algorithm; b.: For the two ways of optimizing landmark correspondences, one step is shown: top: genetic algorithm, the correspondence matrix **G** serves as genome, two parent genomes and the resulting child are depicted. Below: direct search scheme, a model is build from all but one example, and the remaining example is changed to better fit the model.

of the images $\mathbf{I}_1$ to the remaining $n-1$ training images $\{\mathbf{I}_2, \ldots, \mathbf{I}_n\}$. In order to provide for a reliable initialization the feature vectors $\mathbf{f}_{1q}$ are matched to the feature vectors in each of the remaining images, and a transformation $\mathcal{H}_i$ (e.g. similarity transform) with a low number of parameters is estimated robustly by RANSAC. The correspondence matrix **G** is then initialized by choosing a small random set of k landmarks in $\mathbf{I}_1$ and propagating them across the images. In each image the interest points closest to the positions calculated by $\mathcal{H}_i$ are chosen as initial landmark positions, resulting in the initial correspondence matrix $\mathbf{G}_{init}$.

Optimizing the Criterion function. The algorithm is outlined in Fig. 2. After the coarse initialization of the correspondences the criterion function is minimized by updating the correspondence matrix **G**. For an efficient optimization a neighborhood concept in the space of possible landmark positions has to be used. In [6] and [7] contours or surfaces of objects are mapped onto a circle or sphere. In contrast to this parameterization we employ k-D trees to efficiently search for candidates close to the current landmark position, while being independent from a parameterization reference. This enables the algorithm to adapt to complex and even changing topological configurations not defined a priori, like in three dimensional medical data where the behavior of anatomical structures needs to be modeled.

The optimization starts with a small number of landmarks (e.g. 10). After the learning process converges, additional landmarks are added to the model. This leads to an increasingly fine definition of the object. The new landmarks can either be chosen automatically by enforcing an even distribution, or they can be placed manually in a single reference frame. Their positions in the training set are estimated by interpolating the deformation field established by already existing landmark correspondences. Subsequently the entire larger set of landmarks is refined. The coarse deformations are learned by relatively few landmarks, and only after a good fit is achieved, fine local details are modeled by a larger landmark set. Thereby a considerable speedup is achieved. We optimize the criterion function with two algorithms:

Genetic algorithm search. First the criterion is optimized by a genetic algorithm [15], with a set of correspondence matrices **G** serving as genomes of intermediate solutions (*individuals*), making a straight-forward implementation of mutations and cross-over functions possible (Fig. 2(b)).

Fine search. After the genetic algorithm converges a fine direct search is performed. It exploits two properties of the criterion to increase speed, and provide for robustness (Fig. 2(b)). During an iterative process a single example is chosen, a model is build from the remaining examples and the landmarks of the examples are projected into this model. The criterion function is calculated for interest points in the vicinity of the landmark position suggested by the model, and the landmark is moved to the position with lowest cost. This is similar to [11] but no parameterization of the landmark space is used. A search by evaluating the criterion function for small displacements of the current landmark positions is possible but results in far slower convergence. Landmark outliers are detected by comparing the current estimate for an image to the model built from the remaining images. If the cost for including the closest interest point to the landmark position estimate generated by the model is high, either due to its position or to its texture features, it is considered missing in this image. If the landmark is considered to be missing $\mathbf{R}_{ji}$ is set to 0 and its position is estimated from the model instead from an interest point candidate, as described in Sec. 2.2.

3   Experiments

Setup Evaluation results are reported for five data sets: **1.** 20 hand radiographs with a resolution of 0.34 mm / pixel, and semi-manual expert standard of reference annotations of 256 landmarks each on metacarpals and proximal phalanges. **2.** 20 randomly picked frames from a sequence of face images [16] with 576×720 pixel resolution and semi-manual ground truth annotation. The temporal coherence of the frames was not utilized. **3.** The same data as in 2. but with random occlusions covering up to 10% of the face. **4.** A synthetic data set of two 3D surfaces with an approximate diameter of 60 voxels consisting of a deformed torus and a sphere was generated using a single mode of deformation. To assess the capability of the algorithm to deal with 3D data independent of its topology, the topology of the setup changes throughout the data set. The model building was performed on dense sets of points on the surfaces. No texture information was used in this experiment, and correspondences were initialized with nearest neighbors, after the examples were centered and normalized w.r.t. to their standard deviation. **5.** 10 computed tomography data sets of the knee region (Fig. 1). For this data set no standard of reference was available and the model quality is assessed by means of the model compactness. For data sets 1.-4. the accuracy with regard to a semi-manual standard of reference annotation was assessed: the landmark correspondences define a deformation field between examples. One example was selected and the corresponding annotation was propagated to the other examples by piece wise affine interpolation according to the deformation field. The mean and median distance between propagated and standard of

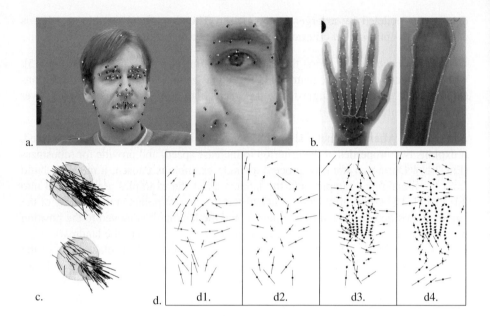

Fig. 3. a. Face data, and b. hand data: ground truth landmarks (green) and propagated landmarks, after autonomous model building (red circles), white crosses are the landmarks learned by the algorithm. c. 1st shape mode for artificial 3D data, before and after optimization. d. 1st and 2nd shape model for hand data, d1. and d2. during early optimization, d3. and d4 after fine search. The positions of the bones correspond to b.

Table 1. Landmark deviation between propagated and standard of reference landmarks

Data	Hand	Hand cont.	3D	Face	F. occl.
Mean	5.84	2.27	2.14	10.10	13.08
Median	4.91	1.03	1.25	5.34	7.80

reference landmarks on the remaining images were recorded. It provides for a measure of how the model building captures the structure of the data.

Results In Fig. 3(a) and (b) the standard of reference (green) and the landmarks propagated according to the learned model (red) are depicted for face and hand data. White crosses show the positions of the landmarks learned automatically, used as control points for the landmark propagation. The accuracy of the resulting landmark correspondences is given in Tab. 1. The median error for the hand data is 4.91 pixels. Larger errors occur predominantly in regions where only few interest points are available because of low contrast. The error to the continuous standard of reference bone contours are reported, too, since salient features like the contours are modeled with high accuracy (mean error is 2.27 pixel). In this case a splitting of the model according to the separate bones can be expected to improve the landmark accuracy, since the variation in hand posture superposes the shape variation of individual bones [17]. For the face data the landmark error increases if the images exhibit occlusions, however the moderate increase of the error indicates that the method can deal with incomplete data without resulting in a degenerate model. The percentage of landmarks reported missing was in the range of $8-10\%$. In Fig. 3(c) and (d) the modes of shape variation before and after optimization for sets (1) and (4) are depicted. The single mode that generates the data (4) is adequately captured by the resulting landmarks. For the hands the modes properly capture the aspect ratio change and the variation of finger positions. The results indicate that the approach is capable of generating reliable landmark correspondences which can replace semi-manual annotations, and that the resulting statistical model reflects the properties of the data. The criterion terms corresponding to shape and texture can be weighted according to the reliability of the image structure. This is subject of ongoing research. In [18] a similar evaluation was performed for registration of labeled magnetic resonance images, and the surface to surface distance after registration was in the range of 1.5 to 3.3 voxels. For the knee data (5) the compactness of the shape model increases significantly during optimization. After initialization 5 modes are necessary to represent 85% of the data variation, while after optimization 2 modes are sufficient.

4   Conclusion

In this paper we propose a method to autonomously learn appearance models. The algorithm does not need manual annotations, and establishes correspondences of landmarks by group-wise robust registration of a sparse set of interest points. No mapping onto a reference shape is used, and thereby a restriction to an a priori topological class is avoided. Instead of deforming the entire image local features are used to capture image content in an efficient way. In contrast to elasticity based registration techniques, the evolving shape model allows to deal with partially missing data in a natural way, by using the statistical properties of the training population. The results indicate that the resulting correspondences are good, that the approach produces compact models capturing the relevant information in the data, and that it has the potential to overcome the need for manual annotation. Future research will focus on the evaluation and the improvement of the method on a wider range of medical data, to model complex structures with minimal training effort and with the accuracy necessary for clinical application.

References

1. Cootes, T., Edwards, G.J., Taylor, C.J.: Active appearance models. IEEE TPAMI 23(6), 681–685 (2001)
2. Beichel, R., Gotschuli, G., Sorantin, E., Leberl, F., Sonka, M.: Diaphragm dome surface segmentation in CT data sets: A 3D active appearance model approach. In: Sonka, M., Fitzpatrick, J. (eds.) SPIE: Medical Imaging, vol. 4684, pp. 475–484 (2002)
3. Roberts, M., Cootes, T., Adams, J.: Vertebral shape: Automatic measurement with dynamically sequenced active appearance models. In: Proc. of MICCAI 2005 pp. 733–740 (2005)
4. Stegmann, M.B., Ólafsdóttir, H., Larsson, H.B.W.: Unsupervised motion-compensation of multi-slice cardiac perfusion MRI. Medical Image Analysis 9(4), 394–410 (2005)
5. Walker, K., Cootes, T., Taylor, C.: Automatically building appearance models from image sequences using salient features. IVC 20(5), 435–440 (2002)

6. Davies, R.H., Twining, C., Cootes, T.F., Waterton, J.C., Taylor, C.J.: A minimum description length approach to statistical shape modeling. IEEE TMI 21(5), 525–537 (2002)
7. Davies, R.H., Twining, C.J., Cootes, T.F., Waterton, J.C., Taylor, C.J.: 3D statistical shape models using direct optimisation of description length. In: Heyden, A., Sparr, G., Nielsen, M., Johansen, P. (eds.) ECCV 2002. LNCS, vol. 2352, pp. 3–20. Springer, Heidelberg (2002)
8. Thodberg, H.H., Olafsdottir, H.: Adding curvature to minimum description length shape models. In: Proc. of BMVC 2003, vol. 2, pp. 251–260 (2003)
9. Ericsson, A., Karlsson, J.: Benchmarking of algorithms for automatic correspondence localisation. In: Proc. of BMVC 2006. vol. 2, pp. 759–768 (2006)
10. Rueckert, D., Frangi, A., Schnabel, J.: Automatic construction of 3-D statistical deformation models of the brain using nonrigid registration. IEEE TMI 22(8), 1014–1025 (2003)
11. Cootes, T., Twining, C., Petrović, V., Taylor, C.: Groupwise construction of appearance models using piece-wise affine deformations. In: Proc. of BMVC 2005 (2005)
12. Twining, C.J., Cootes, T., Marsland, S., Petrovic, V., Schestowitz, R., Taylor, C.J.: A unified information-theoretic approach to groupwise non-rigid registration and model building. In: Proc. of Information Processing in Medical Imaging IPMI, pp. 1–14 (2005)
13. Little, R., Rubin, D.: Statistical Analysis with Missing Data. Wiley and Sons, Chichester (1987)
14. Schneider, T.: Analysis of incomplete climate data: Estimation of mean values and covariance matrices and imputation of missing values. Journal of Climate 14, 853–871 (2001)
15. Mitchell, M.: An Introduction to Genetic Algorithms. MIT Press, Cambridge, MA (1996)
16. (FGnet - IST-, -26434, Face and Gesture Recognition Working Group) (2000)
17. Langs, G., Peloschek, P., Donner, R., Bischof, H.: Multiple appearance models. Pattern Recognition 40(9), 2485–2495 (2007)
18. Babalola, K.O., Cootes, T.F.: Groupwise registration of richly labelled images. Proc. Medical Image Understanding and Analysis 2, 226–230 (2006)

On Simulating Subjective Evaluation Using Combined Objective Metrics for Validation of 3D Tumor Segmentation

Xiang Deng[1], Lei Zhu[1], Yiyong Sun[2], Chenyang Xu[2], Lan Song[5],
Jiuhong Chen[3], Reto D. Merges[3], Marie-Pierre Jolly[2], Michael Suehling[4],
and Xiaodong Xu[1]

[1] Corporate Technology, Siemens Ltd., China
xiang.deng@siemens.com
[2] Siemens Corporate Research, USA
[3] Medical Solutions, Siemens Ltd., China
[4] Siemens Medical Solutions, Germany
[5] Peking Union Medical College Hospital, China[*]

Abstract. In this paper, we present a new segmentation evaluation method that can simulate radiologist's subjective assessment of 3D tumor segmentation in CT images. The method uses a new metric defined as a linear combination of a set of commonly used objective metrics. The weighing parameters of the linear combination are determined by maximizing the rank correlation between radiologist's subjective rating and objective measurements. Experimental results on 93 lesions demonstrate that the new composite metric shows better performance in segmentation evaluation than each individual objective metric. Also, segmentation rating using the composite metric compares well with radiologist's subjective evaluation. Our method has the potential to facilitate the development of new tumor segmentation algorithms and assist large scale segmentation evaluation studies.

1 Introduction

Tumor volume measured from CT images has been shown to provide more accurate estimate of lesion size than 1D and 2D measurements [1,2] in cancer diagnosis and evaluation of treatment response [3]. Quantitative validation of image segmentation techniques for computing lesion volume is essential for routine clinical use of tumor volumetry.

The quality of the lesion segmentation is traditionally evaluated using either subjective or objective methods [4]. While the subjective evaluation by radiologists, such as five-level rating [5], is considered as gold standard in clinical

---

[*] We would like to thank Guangwei Du and Haibin Huang at Corporate Technology, Siemens Ltd., China, Dr. Zhengyu Jin at Peking Union Medical College Hospital, China, and Daniel Rinck at Siemens Medical Solutions, Germany for their support on this work.

N. Ayache, S. Ourselin, A. Maeder (Eds.): MICCAI 2007, Part I, LNCS 4791, pp. 977–984, 2007.
© Springer-Verlag Berlin Heidelberg 2007

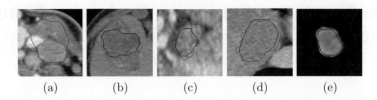

(a)   (b)   (c)   (d)   (e)

Fig. 1. Tumor segmentations with scores 1 to 5 ((a)-(e)) rated by a radiologist. The red contours are the ground truth defined by the radiologist. The blue contours are the results from the semi-automatic segmentation technique.

setting, it is costly and time consuming, especially for large scale validation studies. Also, the intra-rater and inter-rater variability might result in inconsistent ratings. Compared to the subjective evaluation, the objective metrics are easy to compute, but may not provide an overall assessment of the segmentation quality because each metric only captures certain aspect of the difference between the segmentation and the ground truth. Recently, several methods based on combined objective metrics have been proposed to provide evaluation more relevant to subjective assessment of generic object segmentation [6,7,8,9]. The weights in these combined measures, however, are determined rather empirically, and may not be applicable for tumor segmentation evaluation due to the medical expertise required in the assessment. To date, little work has been done to study radiologist's qualitative evaluation of 3D tumor segmentation.

In this paper, we present a new method for evaluating 3D tumor segmentation. By quantitatively studying the relation between the subjective and objective measures, we propose a new composite metric that can simulate radiologist's subjective rating. The composite metric is defined as a linear combination of a set of objective metrics. Compared to the previously published empirically defined combined metrics, the weighing parameters of the linear combination in our method are determined by maximizing the Spearman rank correlation coefficient between the composite metric and radiologist's subjective rating. Five cluster centers defined by the composite metric are derived from training data to simulate the five-level scale. A segmentation is rated using the corresponding composite metric value according to the distance to the five cluster centers.

The composite metric in our method shows better performance in rating segmentation than each individual objective metric, and compare well with radiologist's subjective rating. Our method has the potential to facilitate the development of new tumor segmentation algorithms and assist large scale segmentation evaluation studies when radiologist's rating is not available.

2   Method

2.1   Subjective Evaluation and Objective Metrics

The radiologist's subjective evaluation for the 3D tumor segmentation was obtained in three steps. First, the ground truth for all lesions was defined by an experienced radiologist on the CT images. Second, all lesions were segmented using an in-house developed technique based on algorithm described in [10]. Third, the quality of the 3D tumor segmentation was evaluated by the same radiologist using a five-point scale, as shown in Fig. 1, where 1 = segmentation is highly inaccurate, 2 = segmentation is moderately inaccurate, 3 = segmentation is marginally accurate, 4 = segmentation is moderately accurate, and 5 = segmentation is highly accurate.

We investigated a total of ten commonly used volume related objective metrics[1]. These metrics reflect different aspects of discrepancy in segmented and ground truth volumes, such as relative position and volume difference. Three of the ten metrics with highest correlation with radiologist's subjective rating were selected as candidates to construct a composite metric, which is described in the next section. The three objective metrics are defined as follows

a) Volume overlap (m_1)

$$m_1 = (\mathrm{Vol_{seg}} \cap \mathrm{Vol_{gt}})/(\mathrm{Vol_{seg}} \cup \mathrm{Vol_{gt}}) \tag{1}$$

where $\mathrm{Vol_{seg}}$ denotes segmented volume. $\mathrm{Vol_{gt}}$ denotes ground truth volume.

b) Absolute value of normalized volume difference (m_2)

$$m_2 = |\mathrm{Vol_{seg}} - \mathrm{Vol_{gt}}|/\mathrm{Vol_{gt}} \tag{2}$$

c) RMS surface distance (m_3)

$$m_3 = \sqrt{\frac{\sum_{a \in A} [\min_{b \in B}\{\mathrm{dist}(a,b)\}]^2 + \sum_{b \in B} [\min_{a \in A}\{\mathrm{dist}(a,b)\}]^2}{N_A + N_B}} \tag{3}$$

where A and B denote the surfaces of segmented and ground truth volumes. a and b are mesh point on A and B respectively. $\mathrm{dist}(a,b)$ denotes the distance between a and b. N_A and N_B are the number of points on A and B.

2.2 New Composite Metric

Motivated by the work in [11], we propose a new metric that can simulate the radiologist's subjective rating in segmentation evaluation. It is defined as a linear combination of a set of objective metrics described in previous section,

$$u = \sum_{i=1}^{n} c_i \cdot m_i \tag{4}$$

where u is the composite metric, c_i is the weighing parameter, m_i is the objective metric, n is the number of objective metrics.

---

[1] The ten volume related objective metrics are volume overlap, over-segmentation ratio, under-segmentation ratio, volume difference, absolute value of volume difference, normalized volume difference, absolute value of normalized volume difference, RMS surface distance, maximum of surface distance, and 75 percentile of surface distance.

Let Q denote the number of lesions used in this study, we can stack the objective measurements obtained from segmentation of all these lesions into the matrix equation

$$\mathbf{u} = \mathbf{Mc}. \tag{5}$$

where $\mathbf{u}$ is a $Q \times 1$ vector of the measurements from the composite metric. $\mathbf{M}$ is a $Q \times n$ matrix of the measurements from the objective metrics. $\mathbf{c}$ is a $n \times 1$ vector of weighing parameters.

To simulate the radiologist's five-level ratings of 3D tumor segmentation using the composite metrics, we first quantify the relation between these two measures. Because the radiologist's rating is based on ranking of the quality of the segmentation, the relation can be described using the correlation of the order of the same set of segmentation defined by radiologist's rating and the composite metric.

One method to quantitatively compute the strength of such correlation is to use Spearman rank correlation coefficient. See [12] for details on Spearman rank correlation coefficient.

To avoid negative value in the computed rank correlation, all objective metrics used in this study except volume overlap are linearly mapped into the interval [0,1], in which higher value is associated with better segmentation quality. From (5), the composite measure computed using normalized objective metrics on all lesions can be expressed as

$$\bar{\mathbf{u}} = \bar{\mathbf{M}}\mathbf{c} \tag{6}$$

where $\bar{\mathbf{u}}$ is a $Q \times 1$ vector of the measurements from the composite metric, $\bar{\mathbf{M}}$ is a $Q \times n$ matrix of normalized objective measurements.

Let $\mathbf{w}$, a $Q \times 1$ vector, denote the radiologist's five-level ratings for segmentation of all the Q lesions. The Spearman rank correlation coefficient between the subjective and composite measures is computed as

$$r_s(\mathbf{w}, \bar{\mathbf{u}}) = 1 - \frac{6\sum_{i=1}^{Q}[\mathcal{R}_i(\mathbf{w}) - \mathcal{R}_i(\bar{\mathbf{u}})]^2}{Q(Q^2 - 1)}, \tag{7}$$

where r_s is the Spearman rank correlation coefficient, $\mathcal{R}_i(\cdot)$ denotes the rank of the i-th element in the vector.

For tied ranks in either subjective or composite group, ranks are computed using the mean value of the ranks those segmentations would have had, if they had been distinguishable [12].

We can make the two sets of rankings as similar as possible by maximizing the Spearman rank correlation coefficient in (7). For a fixed set of objective metrics, i.e., n and $m_i, i = 1, \ldots, n$ are fixed, the optimal weighing parameters are determined by

$$\mathbf{c}^* = \arg\max_{\mathbf{c}} \{r_s(\mathbf{w}, \bar{\mathbf{u}})\}, \tag{8}$$

Using the results from (5) and (7), the optimization problem in (8) is equivalent to

$$\mathbf{c}^* = \arg\min_{\mathbf{c}} \{\sum_{i=1}^{Q}[\mathcal{R}_i(\mathbf{w}) - \mathcal{R}_i(\bar{\mathbf{M}}\mathbf{c})]^2\}. \tag{9}$$

We use "lsqnonlin", a non-linear least square optimization function in MAT-LAB[2], to compute the optimal weighing parameters in (9). Once the weighing parameters are determined, the value of the composite metric for segmentation of all lesions can be obtained from the objective measurements using Eq. (6).

2.3 Evaluation of Segmentation

The composite metric computed from all training data is used to determine five cluster centers for segmentation evaluation. Each cluster center is computed using the mean value of the composite metric from lesions in each of the five categories defined by the radiologist. All five centers are sorted in ascending order and assigned labels of 1 to 5 to simulate the radiologist's five-level scale.

To rate segmentation of a testing lesion, the value of the composite metric for this lesion is first computed using the method described in previous section. A list of five possible scores is generated in such a way that the label of the nearest cluster center is on the top, and the label of the farthest center at the bottom. Note that the top two scores in the list are always adjacent scores, e.g., 1 and 2, 4 and 3, due to the monotonically increased composite metric value for the five cluster centers. This property is desirable in simulating radiologist's rating because it is common in clinical practice for a radiologist to adjust the rating by one level, as the result of fuzzily defined adjacent classes in the 5-point scale.

3 Results

3.1 Accuracy of Segmentation Evaluation

We tested our segmentation evaluation method using a set of 93 tumors from patients with a variety of cancer, including liver, lymphoma, lung, and so on. All the image datasets were acquired on a 64-slice Siemens SOMATOM Sensation CT scanner. The results of the radiologist's subjective evaluation for all 93 lesions using the five-level scale are briefly described as follows. The number of lesions with rating from 1 to 5 are 7, 10, 19, 39 and 18 respectively.

We evaluated our technique using leave-one-out cross validation [13]. The performance was measured using average correct rank and frequency of correct score in the top ranks of the rating list [14]. The average correct rank is computed as the rank of the correct score, i.e., the radiologist's rating, in the generated rating list averaged over all 93 trials. Smaller value of average correct rank indicates better performance of evaluation. For comparison purpose, Spearman rank correlation coefficient between radiologist's rating and quantitative measures averaged over all 93 trials was computed as well.

To select the best set of objective metrics for the composite metric, the leave-one-out procedure was repeated on all combinations of the candidate objective metrics. This is feasible because of the relatively small number of objective metrics used in this study. Rating segmentation using single objective metric was

---

[2] MATLAB is a product of The Mathworks, Natick, MA.

implemented in a way similar to that for composite metric described in Section 2.3.

The segmentation evaluation results are shown in Table 1 and Fig. 2. For the sake of brevity, Fig. 2 only shows results from three combinations with smallest average rank of correct scores. These three combinations also showed the highest percentage of correct score in the top ranks of rating list among all combinations using either single or multiple objective metrics. Compared to other combinations, the composite metric computed using all three objective metrics showed the best value for each performance measure. The average correct rank is 1.44, and the average Spearman correlation coefficient is 0.83. The percentage of correct rating in the first place of the list is 66.7%, and increases to 90.8% for top two choices. This result suggests that there is $\sim 90\%$ of chance that one of the two ratings in the top two positions in the list will match radiologist's score.

Table 1. Rank of correct label in the rating list and Spearman rank correlation coefficient (r_s) between radiologist's qualitative rating and quantitative measures for all combinations of objective metrics averaged over all 93 leave-one-out trials. A p value less than 0.05 is considered significant. u denotes composite measure from objective metrics m_1, m_2 and m_3.

Metric	Average rank	r_s	p
m_1	1.70	0.80	< 0.0001
m_2	1.60	0.75	< 0.0001
m_3	1.98	0.70	< 0.0001
u_{m_1,m_2}	1.48	0.83	< 0.0001
u_{m_1,m_3}	1.62	0.80	< 0.0001
u_{m_2,m_3}	1.55	0.77	< 0.0001
u_{m_1,m_2,m_3}	1.44	0.83	< 0.0001

The performance of composite metric from objective metrics m_1, m_2 and m_3 was slightly better than that from m_1 and m_2. This is probably because the RMS surface distance (m_3) and volume overlap (m_1) both reflect the relative position of two segmentations, although m_3 may be more sensitive than m_1. Using more similar metrics in the composite metric provides only limited help for improving the performance.

From the experimental results above, we chose all the three objective metrics as the optimal combination, and used this combination for the remaining experiments. The composite metric determined from all the 93 lesions is given by

$$u_{m_1,m_2,m_3} = 0.39m_1 + 0.15m_2 + 0.42m_3. \tag{10}$$

3.2   Parameter Sensitivity

We studied the variation of the optimal weighing parameters of the composite metric and the five cluster centers for rating segmentation in the leave-one-out cross validation. The variation is measured by coefficient of variation, which is defined as ratio of standard variation to the mean of data. Table 2 shows the

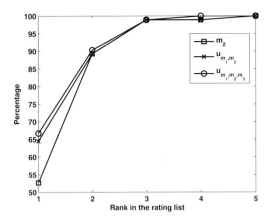

Fig. 2. Frequency of the correct score in the top ranks of the rating list for three representative combinations of objective metrics

Table 2. Coefficient of variation of weighing parameters in the composite metric and five cluster centers for rating segmentation in the 93 leave-one-out trials

Weight			Cluster Center				
c_1	c_2	c_3	ctr_1	ctr_2	ctr_3	ctr_4	ctr_5
7.6%	8.7%	17.4%	8.8%	9.1%	8.9%	8.8%	8.8%

coefficient of variation for the weighing parameters and cluster centers. Results from 4 of the 93 trials showed significantly different values than others, and were removed as outliers. The weighing parameter for RMS surface distance showed larger variation than those for volume overlap and absolute value of normalized volume difference. This is mainly because RMS surface distance is more sensitive to lesion size. The value of all the five cluster centers showed relatively small change.

4   Discussion and Conclusion

We presented a method for evaluating 3D tumor segmentation using a new composite metric. The composite metric is defined as a linear combination of a set of objective metrics. The segmentation is rated using the composite metric on a five-point scale to simulate the radiologist's criterion routinely used in clinical setting.

Experimental results on 93 lesions demonstrated that the new composite metric showed better performance in rating segmentation than each individual objective metric. Our method is also relatively robust to the selection of training data. These results suggest that our method can provide a more adequate and reproducible evaluation of the quality of tumor segmentation.

The combined objective metrics for segmentation evaluation in [6,7,8,9] were determined empirically. In comparison, the weighing parameters of the new composite metric were computed by quantitatively correlating the objective and subjective measures. Consequently, our method can be applied to evaluate different segmentation algorithms and segmentation results on images from other imaging modalities, such as MRI.

Results on 93 lesions showed that segmentation rating from the new composite metric compared well with radiologist's score using top two selection in the rating list. This result suggests that our method can facilitate segmentation evaluation on large scale clinical study by predicting radiologist's five-level rating, especially when such scores are not available for all the data.

Future work includes deriving a composite metric that can simulate subjective evaluation from multiple radiologists, and investigating the reproducibility of radiologist's rating and the optimal sample size in the training stage.

References

1. Therasse, P., et al.: New guideline to evaluate the response to treatment in solid tumors. Journal of National Cancer Institute 92(3), 205–216 (2000)
2. World Health Organization: WHO Handbook for Reporting Results of Cancer Treatment. World Health Organization (1979)
3. Van Hoe, L., et al.: Size quantification of liver metastases in patients undergoing cancer treatment: reproducibility of one-, two-, and three-dimensional measurements determined with spiral CT. Radiology 202(3), 671–675 (1997)
4. Zhang, Y.J.: A survey on evaluation methods for image segmentation. Pattern Recognition 29(8), 1335–1346 (1996)
5. Armato, S.G., Griger, M.L., MacMahon, H.: Automated lung segmentation in digitized posteroanterior chest radiographs. Academic Radiology 5(4), 245–255 (1998)
6. Correia, P.L., Pereira, F.: Objective evaluation of video segmentation quality. IEEE Transactions on Image Processing 12(2), 186–200 (2003)
7. Villegas, P., Marichal, X.: Perceptually-weighted evaluation criteria for segmentation masks in video sequences. IEEE Transactions on Image Processing 13(8), 1092–1103 (2004)
8. Cavallaro, A., Gelasca, E.D., Ebrahimi, T.: Objective evaluation of segmentation quality. In: Proceedings of IEEE ICIP, pp. 301–304. IEEE Computer Society Press, Los Alamitos (2002)
9. Gelasca, E.D., et al.: A framework for evaluating video object segmentation algorithms. In: Proceedings of IEEE CVPRW, pp. 191–198. IEEE Computer Society Press, Los Alamitos (2006)
10. Grady, L.: Random walks for image segmentation. IEEE Transactions on Pattern Analysis and Machine Intelligence 28(11), 1768–1783 (2006)
11. Delgorge, C., et al.: Towards a new tool for the evaluation of the quality of ultrasound compressed images. IEEE Transactions on Medical Imaging 25(11), 1502–1509 (2006)
12. Sheskin, D.I.: Handbook of Parametric and Nonparametric Statistical Procedures. CRC Press (1997)
13. Duda, R.O., Hart, P.E., Stork, D.G.: Pattern Classification, 2nd edn. John Wiley and Sons, Chichester (2001)
14. Yoon, S., et al.: Automatic skin pixel selection and skin color classification. In: Proceedings of IEEE ICIP, pp. 941–944. IEEE Computer Society Press, Los Alamitos (2006)

Detection and Segmentation of Pathological Structures by the Extended Graph-Shifts Algorithm

Jason J. Corso[1], Alan Yuille[2], Nancy L. Sicotte[3], and Arthur Toga[1]

[1] Center for Computational Biology, Laboratory of Neuro Imaging
[2] Department of Statistics
[3] Department of Neurology, Division of Brain Mapping
University of California, Los Angeles, USA
jcorso@ucla.edu

Abstract. We propose an extended graph-shifts algorithm for image segmentation and labeling. This algorithm performs energy minimization by manipulating a dynamic hierarchical representation of the image. It consists of a set of moves occurring at different levels of the hierarchy where the types of move, and the level of the hierarchy, are chosen automatically so as to maximally decrease the energy. Extended graph-shifts can be applied to a broad range of problems in medical imaging. In this paper, we apply extended graph-shifts to the detection of pathological brain structures: (i) segmentation of brain tumors, and (ii) detection of multiple sclerosis lesions. The energy terms in these tasks are learned from training data by statistical learning algorithms. We demonstrate accurate results, precision and recall in the order of 93%, and also show that the algorithm is computationally efficient, segmenting a full 3D volume in about one minute.

1 Introduction

Automatic detection of pathological brain structures is a problem of great practical clinical importance. From the computer vision perspective, the task is to label regions of an image into pathological and non-pathological components. This is a special case of the well-known image segmentation problem which has a large literature in computer vision [1,2,3] and medical imaging [4,5,6,7,8,9,10]

In previous work [11], we developed a hierarchical algorithm called graph-shifts which we applied to the task of segmenting sub-cortical structures formulated as energy function minimization. The algorithm does energy minimization by iteratively transforming the hierarchical graph representation. A big advantage of graph-shifts is that each iteration can exploit the hierarchical structure and cause a large change in the segmentation, thereby giving rapid convergence while avoiding local minima in the energy function. The algorithm was limited, however, because it required the number of model labels to be fixed and the number of model instances to be known. For example, every brain has a single ventricular system. Nevertheless it was effective for segmenting sub-cortical structures in terms of accuracy and speed. However, such an assumption is not practical in the case of pathological structures, i.e., the number of multiple sclerosis lesions is never known a priori.

In this paper, we present a generalization which we call the *extended graph-shifts algorithm*. This is able to dynamically create new model instances and hence deal with

N. Ayache, S. Ourselin, A. Maeder (Eds.): MICCAI 2007, Part I, LNCS 4791, pp. 985–993, 2007.
© Springer-Verlag Berlin Heidelberg 2007

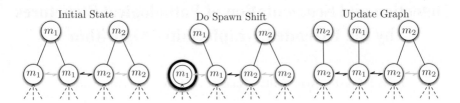

Fig. 1. An intuitive example of the extended graph-shifts algorithm. It shows a spawn shift being selected (middle panel, double-circle) and then the process of updating the graph hierarchy with the new root-level model node (right panel).

situations where the number of structures in the image is unknown. Hence we can apply extended graph-shifts to the detection of pathological structures. We formulate these tasks as energy function minimization where statistical learning techniques [12,13] are used to learn the components of the energy functions. As we will show, extended graph-shifts is also a computationally efficient algorithm and yields good results on the detection of brain tumors and multiple sclerosis lesions.

The hierarchy is structured as a set of nodes on a series of layers. The nodes at the bottom layer form the image lattice. Each node is constrained to have a single parent. All nodes are assigned a model label which is required to be the same as its parent's label. There is a neighborhood structure defined at all layers of the graph. A *graph shift* is a transformation of the hierarchical structure and thus, the model labeling on the image lattice. There are two types of graph-shifts: (1) changing the parent of a node to the parent of a neighbor with a different model label thus altering the model label of the node and its descendants, and (2) spawning a new sub-graph from a node to the root-level that creates a new model instance. We refer the reader to [11] for a discussion of the first type of shift and restrict the discussion in this paper to the new spawn shift. The spawn shift is illustrated in figure 1, which shows a node being selected to spawn a new instance of model m_2 and then the creation of the new root-level model node. Figure 2 shows a synthetic example comparing the original graph-shifts with the extended algorithm to demonstrate the importance of the spawn-shift to detect small, detached structures. In this case, without spawning, only one of four small structures is detected properly. The extended graph-shifts algorithm minimizes a global energy function and at each iteration selects the shift that maximally decreases the energy.

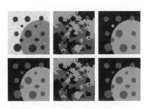

Fig. 2. Extended graph-shifts can detect small structures. Left-col.: image and labels. Middle-col.: initialization. Top-right: no spawning (graph-shifts), bottom-right: with spawning.

We apply this algorithm to brain tumor (*glioblastoma multiforme*, GBM) and multiple sclerosis detection and segmentation. Due to the clinical importance of automatic detection for both diagnosis and treatment, each of these applications has received much attention. Clark et al. [4] integrate knowledge-based techniques and multi-spectral histogram analysis to segment GBM tumors in a multi-channel feature space. Corso et al. [5] extend the Segmentation by Weighted Aggregation (SWA) algorithm [3] to integrate Bayesian model classification into the bottom-up aggregation process to rapidly detect GBM tumors. Fletcher-Heath et al. [6] take a fuzzy clustering approach to the segmentation followed by 3D connected components to build the tumor shape. Prastawa et al. [7] present a detection/segmentation algorithm based on learning voxel-intensity distributions for normal brain matter and detecting outlier voxels, which are considered tumor.

Akselrod-Ballin et al. [8] present a sequential approach to segmentation and classification by using the aggregates from the SWA algorithm as features in a decision tree-based classification for multiple sclerosis. Van Leemput et al. [9] and Dugas-Phocion et al. [10] each use a probabilistic model outlier detection algorithm using a generative i.i.d. model of the normal brain for multiple sclerosis analysis. We next describe the extended graph shifts algorithm, and then we report the experimental results in section (3).

2 Extended Graph-Shifts

First, we discuss the hierarchical graph structure in section (2.1). Then in section (2.2), we review the recursive energy formulation that makes it possible to evaluate graph shifts at any level in the hierarchy. Finally, we present the extended graph-shifts algorithm in section (2.3), the pseudo-code for which is in figure 4.

2.1 The Hierarchical Graph Structure

We define a graph G to be a set of nodes $\mu \in \mathcal{U}$ and a set of edges. The graph is hierarchical and composed of multiple layers. The nodes at the lowest layer are the elements of the lattice D and the edges are defined to link neighbors on the lattice. The coarser layers are computed recursively, as will be described in section (2.3). Two nodes at a coarse layer are joined by an edge if any of their children are joined by an edge.

The nodes are constrained to have a single parent (except for the nodes at the top layer) and every node has at least one child (except for nodes at the bottom layer). We use the notation $C(\mu)$ for the children of μ, and $A(\mu)$ for the parent. A node μ on the bottom layer (i.e. on the lattice) has no children, and hence $C(\mu) = \emptyset$. We use the notation $N(\mu, \nu) = 1$ to indicate that nodes μ, ν on the same layer (or lattice D) are neighbors, with $N(\mu, \nu) = 0$ otherwise.

At the top of the hierarchy, we define a special *root* layer of nodes comprised of a single node for each of the K model labels. We write $\overline{\mu}_k$ for these root nodes and use the notation m_k to denote the model variable associated with it. Each node is assigned a label that is constrained to be the label of its parent. Since, by construction, all non-root nodes can trace their ancestry back to a single root node, an instance of the graph G is equivalent to a labeled segmentation $\{m_\mu : \mu \in D\}$ of the image. Finally, we add a

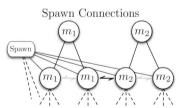

Fig. 3. Example of graph-structure including the connections to the spawn node

spawning node which is the neighbor of all nodes in the forest except the root layer nodes. The spawning node can take any model label. It is used to enable a node to switch to any model, and does not make a direct contribution to the energy function.

Such a construct is used to simplify the representation of potential shifts: both types of shifts are now simply edges in the graph.

2.2 The Energy Models

The input image $\mathbf{I}$ is defined on a lattice D of pixels/voxels. For the medical image applications being studied this is a three-dimensional lattice. The lattice has the standard 6-neighborhood structure. The task is to assign each voxel $\mu \in D$ to one of a fixed set of K models $m_\mu \in \{1, ..., K\}$. This assignment corresponds to a segmentation of the image into K, or more, connected regions.

We want the segmentation to minimize an energy function criterion:

$$E[\{m_\omega : \omega \in D\}] = \sum_{\nu \in D} E_1(\phi(\mathbf{I})(\nu), m_\nu) + \frac{1}{2} \sum_{\substack{\nu \in D, \mu \in D: \\ N(\nu,\mu)=1}} E_2(\mathbf{I}(\nu), \mathbf{I}(\mu), m_\nu, m_\mu).$$

(1)

This energy represents is a hybrid discriminative-generative model and is related to the popular conditional random fields models [14]. The first term E_1 is a *unary term* which gives local evidence that the pixel μ takes model m_μ, where $\phi(\mathbf{I})(\mu)$ denotes a nonlinear filter of the image evaluated at μ. In this paper, we set $E_1(\mu, m_\mu) = -\log P(m_\mu|\phi(\mathbf{I})(\mu))$ where $P(m_\mu|\phi(\mathbf{I})(\mu))$ is the probability distribution for the label m_μ at voxel $\mu \in D$ conditioned on the response of a nonlinear filter $\phi(\mathbf{I})(\mu)$. This filter $\phi(\mathbf{I})(\mu)$ depends on voxels within a local neighborhood of μ, and hence takes local image context into account. $\phi(\mathbf{I})$ is learned from training data from a set of features using boosting techniques [12,13,15]. We discuss the feature-set and learning in more detail in section 3. The second term E_2 is a *pairwise term* which penalizes the length of the segmentation boundaries. It is written as, where δ is the standard delta function: $E_2(\mathbf{I}(\nu), \mathbf{I}(\mu), m_\nu, m_\mu) = 1 - \delta_{m_\nu, m_\mu}$. We don't use the intensities $\mathbf{I}(\cdot)$ in the binary term in this formulation but suggest potential variations in [11].

We now recursively assign an energy to all nodes, and neighboring node pairs in the hierarchy. This enables us to rapidly compute the changes in energy caused by extended graph-shifts at any level of the hierarchy, and will be used in the definition of the extended graph-shifts algorithm.

The unary term for assigning a model m_μ to a node μ is defined recursively by:

$$E_1(\mu, m_\mu) = \begin{cases} E_1(\phi(\mathbf{I})(\mu), m_\mu) & \text{if } C(\mu) = \emptyset \\ \sum_{\nu \in C(\mu)} E_1(\nu, m_\mu) & \text{otherwise .} \end{cases}$$

(2)

The pairwise energy term E_2 between nodes μ_1 and μ_2, with models m_{μ_1} and m_{μ_2} is defined recursively by:

$$E_2(\mu_1, \mu_2, m_{\mu_1}, m_{\mu_2}) =$$
$$\begin{cases} E_2(\mathbf{I}(\mu_1), \mathbf{I}(\mu_2), m_{\mu_1}, m_{\mu_2}) & \text{if } C(\mu_1) = C(\mu_2) = \emptyset \\ \sum_{\substack{\nu_1 \in C(\mu_1), \nu_2 \in C(\mu_2): \\ N(\nu_1,\nu_2)=1}} E_2(\nu_1, \nu_2, m_{\mu_1}, m_{\mu_2}) & \text{otherwise} \end{cases}$$

(3)

where $E_2(\mathbf{I}(\mu_1), \mathbf{I}(\mu_2), m_{\mu_1}, m_{\mu_2})$ is the edge energy for pixels/voxels in equation (1).

2.3   Extended Graph-Shifts

We first initialize the graph hierarchy using a stochastic algorithm which recursively coarsens the graph. The coarsening proceeds in three stages. First, we sample a binary edge activation variable $e_{\mu\nu} \sim \gamma \mathcal{U}(\{0, 1\}) + (1 - \gamma) \exp\left[-\alpha \left|\mathbf{I}(\mu) - \mathbf{I}(\nu)\right|\right]$, for all neighbors μ, ν s.t. $N(\mu, \nu) = 1$ in the current graph layer G^t. ($\mathcal{U}$ is the uniform distribution and γ is a fixed weight). Second, we compute connected components to form node-groups. The size of a connected component is constrained by a threshold τ, which governs the relative degree of coarsening between two graph layers. Third, we create a node at the next graph layer for each component. Nodes in this new layer are connected if any two of their children are connected. The algorithm executes this coarsening procedure until the number of node in the layer G^T falls below a threshold β (related to the number of models). Finally we add a model layer G^M directly above layer G^T so that each node in G^T is the child of its best fit node in G^M (using the recursive unary energy $E_1(\mu, m_\mu)$ from (2)). We do not need to enforce the constraint that each node in G^M has at least one child in G^T because the new spawn shift makes it possible to create new (connected) nodes on G^M for any model type.

The extended graph-shifts algorithm enables a node μ to change its label to any model. This is an extension of the graph-shifts algorithm [11], which allowed a node to change its model only to the model of one of its neighboring nodes (the children of the node must also change to the same model). This original type of shift is straightforward in the hierarchical structure since it corresponds to allowing node μ to change its parent to the parent $A(\nu)$ of a neighboring node ν. In the original graph-shifts algorithm, a list of potential shifts (between nodes having different models only) is maintained. After each shift is taken, this list is quickly updated (the number of updates is logarithmic in the size of the voxel lattice). Thus, graph-shifts can rapidly do the minimization.

In this extension, we permit a node to switch to any other model while maintaining this ability to rapidly and deterministically manage the potential shifts by modifying the graph structure. We create a new *spawning node* to which all nodes in the graph are connected (see figure 3). This spawning node can take the label of any model in the set, and when evaluating the shift on the edge connecting a node to the spawning node, all possible models are evaluated. But, the spawn node contributes nothing to the energy function. A node μ taking a spawning graph shift causes a new sub-graph to be dynamically created. The new sub-graph is a chain of nodes from μ to the top of the hierarchy, i.e., a new ancestry chain $A(\mu)$ is created that terminates at a new model level node on G^M.

Each change of node model will correspond to a change of energy (because the descendant nodes, including the lattice nodes, are also required to make the same change). We need to efficiently compute the change of energy for all nodes and for all changes of models in order to select the best shift to make in the hierarchy. Fortunately, these *shift-gradients* can be computed efficiently using the recursive formulae given above in equations (2) and (3). For example, the change in energy due to node μ changing from model m_μ to model $\hat{m}_\mu$ is given by:

$$\Delta E(m_\mu \to \hat{m}_\mu) = E_1(\mu, \hat{m}_\mu) - E_1(\mu, m_\mu) +$$
$$\sum_{\eta: N(\mu, \eta) = 1} \left[E_2(\mu, \eta, \hat{m}_\mu, m_\eta) - E_2(\mu, \eta, m_\mu, m_\eta)\right] . \qquad (4)$$

We maintain both the original and the spawning shifts in a single list. Computing the shift gradient is equivalent for both types, but effecting a spawn shift, while still logarithmic in order, has a higher computational cost in creating the new sub-graph. When computing a potential graph-shift, we first evaluate the shift-gradient for all of the node's neighbors. Next, we evaluate the shift-gradient to the spawn node, only considering those models for which there was no neighbor. We store those shifts which have negative gradients in an unsorted list (only the best potential shift is stored per node). The size of this list is generally small (empirically about 2% of those possible), very few neighbors in the graph have different models and a spawn shift more often increases the energy than decreases due to the additional boundary energy cost.

Extended graph-shifts proceeds by selecting the steepest shift-gradient in the list and makes the corresponding shift in the hierarchy. This changes the labels in the part of the hierarchy where the shift occurs, but leaves the remainder of the hierarchy unchanged. If the shift is a spawn, then a new sub-graph is dynamically generated. Neighbor connectivity for a newly generated node up the graph is inherited from the node that initiated the spawn. The algorithm recomputes the shift-gradients in the changed part of the hierarchy and updates the weight list. We repeat the process until convergence, when the shift-gradient list is empty (i.e. all shift-gradients are positive or zero). The algorithm tends to initially prefer shifts at coarse levels since those typically alter the labels of many nodes on the lattice and cause large changes in energy. As the algorithm converges, it tends to select shifts at finer levels, but this trend is not monotonic, see examples in [11].

EXTENDED GRAPH-SHIFTS

Input: Volume $\mathbf{I}$ on lattice D.
Output: Label volume $\mathbf{L}$ on lattice D.
0   Initialize graph hierarchy.
1   Compute exhaustive set of potential shifts S.
2   **while** S is not empty
3        $s \leftarrow$ the shift in S that best reduces the energy.
4   Apply shift s to the graph.
5   **if** (s is a spawn)
6   Build new subgraph and create model.
7   Recompute affected shifts and update S.
8   Compute label volume $\mathbf{L}$ from final hierarchy.

Fig. 4. Extended graph-shifts pseudo-code

---

3 Detection of Pathological Brain Structures

We apply extended graph-shifts to detecting and segmenting brain tumors and multiple sclerosis lesions. For the task of modeling the different pathologies, we build a cascade of boosted discriminative classifiers [12,13,15]. Each classifier in the cascade is trained using a set of about 3000 features including the standard location and Harr-based filters but also some novel features including inter-channel box-filters and gradients, local intensity curve-fitting, and morphology filters. The filters are combined to define the unary term in equation (1). As we demonstrate below, the combination of the boosting-based discriminative modeling and the extended graph-shifts algorithm provides a powerful, general approach to pathology detection and segmentation.

3.1 Segmenting Tumors

We work with a set of 20 expert annotated GBM scans. Each scan is comprised of T1 (with and without contrast), Flair and T2 weighted low-resolution MR scans (about $1 \times 1 \times 10$ on average); this is a common instance for diagnostic brain tumor imaging. All sequences from each patient are co-registered (to the T1 with contrast sequence), skull-stripped, and intensity standardized using the standard FSL tools [16]. We learn models of three separate classes: brain-and-background, tumor (including enhancing and necrotic regions), and edema; half of the dataset was arbitrarily selected for training and the other half for testing.

In table 1(a), we give quantified volume scores for the segmentation accuracy on the dataset. Let T be the true positive, F_p be the false positive, and F_n be the false negative. The Jaccard score is $T/(T + F_p + F_n)$, the precision is $T/(T + F_n)$, and the recall is $T/(T + F_p)$. To the best of our knowledge, these scores are superior to the current state-of-the-art in tumor and edema segmentation. However, we note that a direct comparison is difficult due to different data, manual raters, and others. The Jaccard scores for Clark et al. [4] are about 70%, for Prastawa et al. [7] are 80% (both on very limited datasets with seven and three patients respectively), and Corso et al. [5] is 85% (on training data with of five cases) The extended graph-shifts algorithm is also the fastest among these taking about a minute to perform the segmentation on each of these scans (pre-processing takes about five minutes). We show some examples in figure 5.

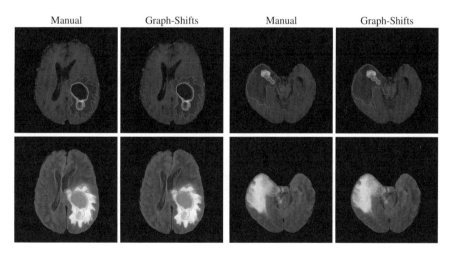

Fig. 5. An example of the brain tumor segmentation. Left case is from the training set and right case is from the testing set. Edema is outlined in red and tumor in green. Top row is the contrast-enhanced T1 weighted sequence, and bottom row is the flair sequence. The results are obtained automatically. Please view in color.

3.2 Detecting MS Lesions

We work with a set of 12 high-lesion-load multi-sequence MR scans. The voxel resolution of these scans is $1 \times 1 \times 3$. In this case, we train a two-class discriminative

992   J.J. Corso et al.

probability model for lesion/not-lesion using the manually annotated dataset. Again, the dataset was split in half for training and testing. Table 1(b) gives the detection rate for the lesion. The detection rate (recall) stresses the importance of picking up most of the lesion mass. Due to its diffuse nature, there is high-variability in expert raters, and detecting each lesion "kernel" is most important. These scores are comparable to the state-of-the-art in automatic lesion detection (#Hit is 80%-85% in [8] and [9] give graphs with varying thresholds showing scores in the 70%s through 90%s). In figure 6 we show some qualitative results

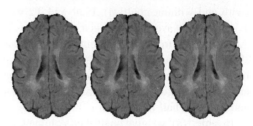

Fig. 6. Extended graph-shifts detects small lesions. Left: manual, middle: no spawning, right: with spawning. Please view in color.

comparing the original graph-shifts to the extended algorithm; the benefit of the spawning functionality is clear from these images. Many smaller lesions are missed by the original algorithm.

Table 1. Quantified accuracy of the extended graph-shifts algorithm on two pathologies

(a) Brain Tumor

	Training Set			Testing Set		
	Jaccard	Precision	Recall	Jaccard	Precision	Recall
Tumor	87%	93%	92%	86%	95%	90%
Edema	87%	90%	96%	88%	89%	98%

(b) Multiple Sclerosis

	Lesion Detection Rate
Training Set	86%
Testing Set	81%

4 Conclusion

In this paper, we define the extended graph-shifts algorithm for segmenting and labeling image data. Extended graph-shifts is a hierarchical energy minimization algorithm. It has potential application in a broad range of problems where the components of the energy functions can be learned from labeled training data using techniques from statistical learning. This extension generalizes our recent graph-shifts algorithm so that it can now deal with an unknown number of model instances. Hence, the algorithm can be applied to the task of detecting pathological structures, where the number of regions is unknown in advance. Extended graph-shifts retains the advantages in speed and robustness to local minima which were demonstrated for the graph-shifts algorithm. We applied extended graph-shifts to the tasks of detecting brain tumors and multiple sclerosis lesions. Our results were accurate (precision and recall on the order of 93%) and fast (segmenting an entire 3D volume, $256 \times 256 \times 50$, in about a minute).

Acknowledgement. This work was funded by the National Institutes of Health through the NIH Roadmap for Medical Research, Grant U54 RR021813 entitled Center for Computational Biology (CCB).

References

1. Geman, S., Geman, D.: Stochastic Relaxation, Gibbs Distributions, and Bayesian Restoration of Images. IEEE Trans. on Pattern Analysis and Machine Intelligence 6, 721–741 (1984)
2. Zhu, S.C., Yuille, A.: Region Competition. IEEE Trans. on Pattern Analysis and Machine Intelligence 18(9), 884–900 (1996)
3. Sharon, E., Brandt, A., Basri, R.: Fast Multiscale Image Segmentation. Proc. of IEEE Conf. on Computer Vision and Pattern Recognition I, 70–77 (2000)
4. Clark, M.C., Hall, L.O., Goldgof, D.B., Velthuizen, R., Murtagh, R., Silbiger, M.S.: Automatic tumor segmentation using knowledge-based techniques. IEEE Trans. on Medical Imaging 17(2), 187–201 (1998)
5. Corso, J.J., Sharon, E., Yuille, A.: Multilevel Segmentation and Integrated Bayesian Model Classification with an Application to Brain Tumor Segmentation. Medical Image Computing and Computer Assisted Intervention 2, 790–798 (2006)
6. Fletcher-Heath, L.M., Hall, L.O., Goldgof, D.B., Reed Murtagh, F.: Automatic segmentation of non-enhancing brain tumors in magnetic resonance images. Artificial Intelligence in Medicine 21, 43–63 (2001)
7. Prastawa, M., Bullitt, E., Ho, S., Gerig, G.: A brain tumor segmentation framework based on outlier detection. Medical Image Analysis Journal 8(3), 275–283 (2004)
8. Akselrod-Ballin, A., Galun, M., Gomori, M.J., Filippi, M., Valsasina, P., Basri, R., Brandt, A.: Integrated Segmentation and Classification Approach Applied to Multiple Sclerosis Analysis. In: Proc. of IEEE Conf. on Computer Vision and Pattern Recognition (2006)
9. Leemput, K.V., Maes, F., Vandermeulen, D., Colchester, A., Suetens, P.: Automated Segmentation of Multiple Sclerosis Lesions by Model Outlier Detection. IEEE Trans. on Medical Imaging 20(8), 677–688 (2001)
10. Dugas-Phocion, G.M.A., Lebrun, C., Channalet, S., Bensa, C., Malandain, G., Ayache, N.: Hierarchical Segmentation of Multiple Sclerosis Lesions in Multi-Sequence MRI. In: Proc. of the IEEE Intl. Symposium on Biomedical Imaging (2004)
11. Corso, J.J., Tu, Z., Yuille, A., Toga, A.W.: Segmentation of Sub-Cortical Structures by the Graph-Shifts Algorithm. In: Proc. of Information Processing in Medical Imaging, pp. 183–197 (2007)
12. Freund, Y., Schapire, R.E.: A Decision-Theoretic Generalization of On-line Learning and an Application to Boosting. Journal of Computer and System Science 55(1), 119–139 (1997)
13. Tu, Z.: Probabilistic Boosting-Tree: Learning Discriminative Models for Classification, Recognition, and Clustering. In: Proc. of International Conference on Computer Vision (2005)
14. Lafferty, J., McCallum, A., Pereira, F.: Conditional Random Fields: Probabilistic Models for Segmenting and Labeling Sequence Data. In: Proc. of International Conference on Machine Learning (2001)
15. Viola, P., Jones, M.: Rapid object detection using a boosted cascade of simple features. In: Proc. of IEEE Conference on Computer Vision and Pattern Recognition (2001)
16. Smith, S.M., Jenkinson, M., Woolrich, M.W., Beckmann, C.F., Behrens, T.E.J., Johansen-Berg, H., Bannister, P.R., Luca, M.D., Drobnjak, I., Flitney, D.E., Niazy, R., Saunders, J., Vickers, J., Zhang, Y., Stefano, N.D., Brady, J.M., Matthews, P.M.: Advances in Functional and Structural MR Image Analysis and Implementation as FSL. NeuroImage 23(S1), 208–219 (2004)

Cutting Tool System to Minimize Soft Tissue Damage for Robot-Assisted Minimally Invasive Orthopedic Surgery

Naohiko Sugita[1], Yoshikazu Nakajima[1], Mamoru Mitsuishi[1], Shosaku Kawata[2], Kazuo Fujiwara[3], Nobuhiro Abe[3], Toshifumi Ozaki[3], and Masahiko Suzuki[4]

[1] School of Engineering, The University of Tokyo, Japan
{sugi,mamoru}@nml.t.u-tokyo.ac.jp
[2] NAKANISHI INC, Japan
[3] Graduate School of Medicine and Density, Okayama University, Japan
[4] Graduate School of Medicine, Chiba University, Japan*

Abstract. Minimally invasive surgery in orthopedic field is considered to be a challenging problem with a milling robot. One objective of this study is to minimize collision of the cutting tool with soft tissue. The authors have developed a robot with redundant axis to avoid the collision so far. Some important components are modeled based on physical requirements, and a geometric optimization approach based on the model has been also proposed to improve performance. In this paper, a protective mechanism to cover the non-working part of the cutting edge is proposed to avoid soft tissue damage. Hardware and software have been developed for this application and the effectiveness of this technique was evaluated with urethane bone.

1 Introduction

The number of surgical procedures with minimally invasive techniques has increased in orthopedics. Minimally invasive surgical approaches utilize small incisions and offer several advantages over traditional open surgery, such as reduced pain and trauma to the body, faster recovery and shorter hospital stays. New ways to open the knee are becoming important in reducing length of the incision. However, difficulty of the procedure increases with smaller incisions, and results of such operations depend on the skill of the surgeon. Mechanical or robot-assisted surgical systems are thus hoped to prove useful for this procedure, and many robots have been developed.

ROBODOC has been developed as a robotic orthopedic surgery system [1] and is the most famous in the orthopedic field. The system has been used in numerous clinical operations. Recent orthopedic robots display unique features. Some work passively to support the surgeon, and others are downsized and mounted directly on bone. For example, "ACROBOT", developed by Davies

---

* We are thankful to Nakashima Propeller Co. Ltd., CORETEC INC and HalleyValley Co.,Ltd.

N. Ayache, S. Ourselin, A. Maeder (Eds.): MICCAI 2007, Part I, LNCS 4791, pp. 994–1001, 2007.
© Springer-Verlag Berlin Heidelberg 2007

et al. passively supports the surgeon, and is used clinically [2]. Dombre et al. developed "BRIGHT", which has a guide jig for a bone saw implemented on the tip of a robot arm [3]. "ARTHROBOT" by Kwon et al. is intended for minimally invasive joint replacement [4], and the robot by Plaskos can be set on bone directly [5]. The recent tendency has been to focus on minimal invasiveness of the surgical procedure in addition to high accuracy.

Many of the robots developed to date, including our multi-axis bone-cutting robot[6], use an end mill as the cutting tool, and some problems must be solved to allow application to minimally invasive orthopedic surgery. Minimally invasive surgery (MIS) makes incisions smaller, reduces pain and trauma to the body, and enables faster recovery. Smaller incisions mean small and narrow opening areas. This means that robot attitude for bone resection becomes restricted, and this can result in collision of the tool with surrounding soft tissue, the existence of untouched areas and the degradation of joint position accuracy. Any approach to minimize soft tissue damage in bone cutting is expected to resolve these issues.

Collision of the cutting edge with soft tissue should be taken into account as a problem of invasiveness. The end mill is a rotational tool, and all angles around the shaft function as a cutter. Therefore, damage to the surrounding soft tissues, vessels and nerves becomes more likely. A protection mechanism to cover the non-working part of the cutting edge is required to avoid this damage. Necrosis of bone cells caused by cutting heat or tool friction heat should also be prevented by cooling the cutting edge.

In this paper, a toolpath generation method and a tool mechanism for the protection of soft tissue are proposed to minimize damage to the surrounding tissues in robotic-assisted minimally invasive orthopedic surgery. With these methods, the cutting tool can approach the resection area through a narrow-opening area, proceed with machining of bone without any damage.

2   Milling System for Minimally Invasive Surgery

2.1   Milling Robot

Fig.1 shows the developed milling robot with 7 degrees of freedom and the kinematics. The problems in the minimally invasive surgical procedure are to approach and resect the target bone through a narrow, visible area. To solve these problems, the machine tool is equipped with a redundant axis (A-axis in Fig. 1) so the cutting tool can avoid interference, such as with soft tissue, under a minimum change of robot attitude.

Figure 2 shows a redundant axis and spindle with the cutting tool. The tool tip does not move during the rotation, and the cutting tool approaches inside the joint and resects the target bone by suitably controlling tool attitude.

Serial kinematics is realized in the order of $Z \to B \to C \to U \to W \to V \to A \to$ from the base part. The attitude matrix and position of the cutting tool are expressed as follows.

Attitude matrix

$$\mathbf{E} = \mathbf{E}^{j\theta_1} \cdot \mathbf{E}^{k\theta_2} \cdot \mathbf{E}^{i\theta_3} \tag{1}$$

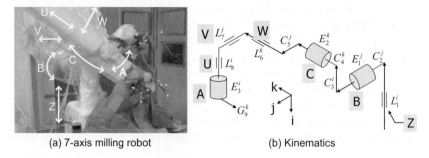

(a) 7-axis milling robot   (b) Kinematics

Fig. 1. Overview and kinematics of milling robot

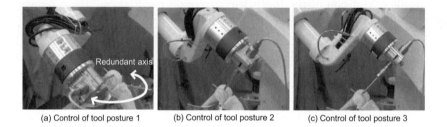

(a) Control of tool posture 1   (b) Control of tool posture 2   (c) Control of tool posture 3

Fig. 2. Redundant axis for minimally invasive surgery

Tool position

$$\mathbf{P} = \mathbf{L}_1^i + \mathbf{C}_2^j + \mathbf{E}^{j\theta_1} \cdot (\mathbf{C}_3^i + \mathbf{C}_4^k + \mathbf{E}^{k\theta_2} \cdot (\mathbf{C}_5^j + \mathbf{L}_6^k + \mathbf{L}_7^j + \mathbf{L}_8^i + \mathbf{E}^{i\theta_3} \cdot \mathbf{G}_9)) \quad (2)$$

where the position of the cutting tool $\mathbf{P}$ is composed of a rotational matrix $\mathbf{E}$, variable matrix $\mathbf{L}$, fixed vector $\mathbf{C}$ and $\mathbf{G}$. Subscripts i, j, k mean the operation is in the U-axis, V-axis and W-axis, respectively.

2.2   Toolpath Generator[7]

Concept. In minimally invasive orthopedic surgery, the cutting tool needs to approach the target through a small hole and resect the large area inside the joint. The opening area, positions and attitudes of the femur and tibia are measured by an infrared positioning sensor, and the workspace for the operation is precisely defined. A toolpath generator has been developed to avoid collisions with surrounding soft tissue (Fig.3).

Measurement of incision area. The opening area is measured using a 3-dimensional optical position sensor. The border of the area is measured as points for the opening plane. Based on the stored data, regression analysis is used.

Calculation of initial cutting tool posture. Utilizing cross detection of the cutting tool vector and target plane, machinable area is calculated at a given

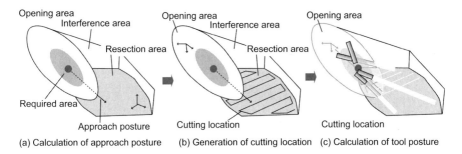

Fig. 3. Strategy for toolpath generation in MIS

cutting tool attitude, and a posture to maximize this area without collision is selected. A local coordinate system is set on the opening area measured with the 3-dimensional sensor. The normal direction is along the Z-axis and is defined. The resection plane is divided into triangular patches, and vertex vectors are set $\mathbf{q_i}$. Tool vector with a attitude vector $\mathbf{l}$ and an offset vector from the origin $\mathbf{p}$ comes to $\mathbf{p} + t\mathbf{l}$.

When it is machinable, collision with the interferences is checked next. The offset vector $\mathbf{p}$ is varied on the opening plane with the parameter of the tool attitude $\mathbf{l}$, and the machinable area is calculated on the triangle patch. Likewise, the machinable area is computed on other triangle patches. Attitude $\mathbf{l}$ to maximize the evaluation function is selected as the initial tool posture.

3   Tool Mechanism to Protect Soft Tissue

3.1   Overview of Design

Damage to soft tissue should be avoided when the bone is machined. Damage will occur for the following reasons: (1) collision of cutting tool and soft tissue; (2) thermal damage caused by cutting temperature; and (3) long cutting time and mechanical stress to the patient. When the opening area is large relatively, the toolpath generator for MIS is sufficient for the operation. However, in the minimally invasive surgery this study targets, completing resection without any collision of cutting tool and soft tissue is difficult, as the opening area is small and interferences surround the target area. A protective mechanism to cover the non-working part of the cutting edge is thus required, and we developed a spindle equipped with a tool cover as shown in Fig.4.

The tool system comprises the cutting tool, tool attachment, tool cover, decelerator and motor, and the tool cover can be controlled in shaft and circumferential directions. From the perspective of requirements for the tool system, the main specifications are as follows: tool diameter, $\phi 8$; rotational speed, 5000 rpm; and shaft length, 70 mm. In addition, the safety of the patient and the surgeon must be ensured and adequate irrigation and sterilization capabilities are provided in a machine tool for medical use. A positive pressure structure is

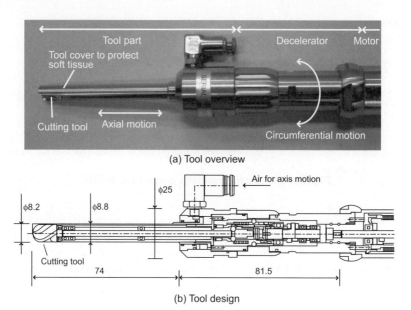

(a) Tool overview

(b) Tool design

Fig. 4. Overview of tool part

adopted in the tool attachment to evacuate the comtaminant, and it is possible to sterilize.

3.2   Mechanism

Axial motion. Motion of the tool cover in shaft direction is realized by air pressure. As shown in Fig.5, when air fills the chamber and pushes a spring to sustain the cover, the tool cover moves to the right side in the figure ((b) in Fig.5). This mode is adopted when the end of the cutting edge needs to be used. The upper side of the cutting tool is covered, and the safety is kept on even when soft tissue comes into contact with the cutting tool. When air is removed from the chamber, the tool cover returns the start position, and the end part is also covered ((c) in Fig.5). This mode is used for cutting with the side edge. All of the upper half is covered, and soft tissue can be further protected.

Circumferential motion. Motion in a circumferential direction is realized by the stepping motor, and the spindle itself rotates(Fig.6). The motion enables control of the position between resection area and the tool cover. The parts of the decelerator and motor are unclean, while the cutting tool and tool attachment are clean. The clean part adopts a pressing system and avoids suction of contaminated objects.

3.3   Control Mode

The tool cover needs to be controlled, as the part of the cutting edge used in machining depends on tool posture. The "End/Side mode" in Fig.7 is general

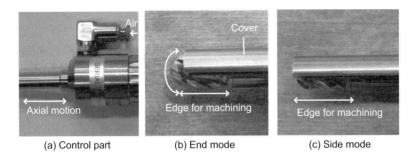

(a) Control part   (b) End mode   (c) Side mode

Fig. 5. Axial motion

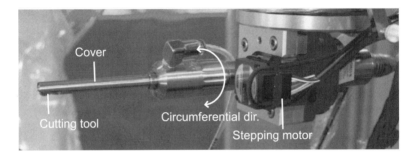

Fig. 6. Circumferential motion

and uses the whole of the cutting edge for the process. "End mode" and "Side mode" represent special cases. To control the area for covering the tool, the mechanism for motion of the tool covering a shaft direction is used. In "Side mode", half of the cutting tool is non-working, and the tool cover is controlled as in Fig.5(c). In "End mode" and "End/Side mode", the ball part of the tool is also used for machining, and half of the side edge is covered to protect soft tissue as in Fig.5(b).

Circumferential motion controls the relationship between the tool cover and resection area. The basic concept is to minimize the non-working area and un-covered cutting edge. To meet the condition, vector in the j-direction of cover coordinates and the normal vector at the cutting location are orthogonal in (a) of Fig.8, and the vector in i-direction of cover coordinates and the normal vector at the cutting location are in reverse. A matrix to express the attitude of the cutting tool $\mathbf{A}$ is represented in the robot coordinates as Eq.3. In the equation, θ_1 to θ_3 means the rotational angles to determine robot posture, and the attitude of the tool cover is finalized by θ_4.

$$\mathbf{A} = \mathbf{E}^{j\theta_1} \cdot \mathbf{E}^{k\theta_2} \cdot \mathbf{E}^{i\theta_3} \cdot \mathbf{E}^{k\theta_4} \tag{3}$$

With the tool cover matrix $\mathbf{A}$, the vector in j-direction $\mathbf{p}$ and the vector in i-direction $\mathbf{q}$ are translated to the robot coordinates in Eq.4.

$$\mathbf{p} = \mathbf{A}(0\ 1\ 0)^T, \quad \mathbf{q} = \mathbf{A}(1\ 0\ 0)^T \tag{4}$$

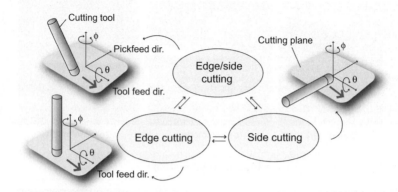

Fig. 7. Machine state

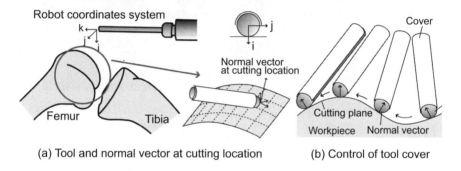

(a) Tool and normal vector at cutting location   (b) Control of tool cover

Fig. 8. Control of tool cover

Tool cover angle θ_4 is determined to meet the following equation with the inner products of the normal vector $\mathbf{n}$ and the vectors $\mathbf{p}$ and $\mathbf{q}$.

$$\mathbf{p} \cdot \mathbf{n} = 0, \quad \mathbf{q} \cdot \mathbf{n} < 0 \tag{5}$$

4   Experimental Results

As shown in Fig.9, an evaluation is conducted with the plastic bone to confirm the effect of toolpath for MIS and the tool cover. Length of the incision is about 80 mm, and the toolpath generated by the proposed method is applied to avoid mechanical conflict. As a result, most of the area can be cut without collision, but the cutting tool touched the soft tissue at the end of stroke in (b) and (c) of Fig.9. However, with adequate control of the tool cover, damage to soft tissues did not occur, showing that the tool cover could protect soft tissue even when contact with the cutting tool was encountered.

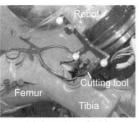 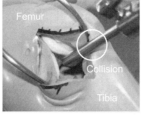 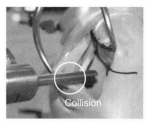

(a) Overview of MIS   (b) Collision at lateral side   (c) Collision at medial side

Fig. 9. Collision check with urethane bone

5 Conclusions

In this paper, a redundant axis is used to avoid interferences by way of a minimal attitude change in a multi-axis bone-cutting robot for a minimally invasive joint replacement. A strategy of toolpath generation and a tool cover were proposed to accomplish the procedure; with this strategy based on an approach through a narrow opening area and machining without damage to soft tissue. Some techniques were described for realizing this strategy. Finally, an experiment was conducted using am incision length of 80 mm, and the toolpath and tool cover were evaluated in minimally invasive procedures.

References

1. Taylor, R., Mittelstadt, B., Paul, H., Hanson, W., Kazanzides, P., Zuhars, J., Williamson, B., Musits, B., Glassman, E., Bargar, W.: An image-directed robotic system for precise orthopaedic surgery. IEEE Trans. on Robotics and Automation 10(3), 261–275 (1994)
2. Rodriguez, F., Harris, S., Jakopec, M., Barrett, A., Gomes, P., Henckel, J., Cobb, J., Davies, B.: Robotic clinical trials of uni-condylar arthroplasty. Int. J. Medical Robotics and Computer Assisted Surgery 1(4), 20–28 (2005)
3. Maillet, P., Nahum, B., Blondel, L., Poignet, P., Dombre, E.: Bright, a robotized tool guide for orthopaedic surgery. In: Proceedings of IEEE Conference on Robotics and Automation (ICRA 2005), pp. 212–217 (2005)
4. Chung, J., Ko, S., Kwon, D., Lee, J., Yoon, Y., Won, C.: Robot-assisted femoral stem implantation using an intramedulla gauge. IEEE Transaction on Robotics and Automation 19(5), 885–892 (2003)
5. Plaskos, C., Cinquin, P.: Praxiteles: a miniature bone-mounted robot for minimal access total knee arthroplasty. Int. J. of Medical Robotics and Computer Assisted Surgery 1(4), 67–79 (2005)
6. Mitsuishi, M., Warisawa, S., Tajima, F., et al.: Development of a 9 axes machine tool for bone cutting. Annals of the CIRP 52(1), 323–328 (2003)
7. Sugita, N., Genma, F., Nakajima, Y., Mitsuishi, M.: Toolpath optimization for a milling robot for minimally invasive orthopedic surgery. In: ICRA 2007, pp. 2273–2278. IEEE Computer Society Press, Los Alamitos (2007)
8. Möoller, T., Trumbore, T.: First,minimum storage ray-triangle intersection. Journal of Graphics Tools 2(1), 21–28 (1997)

Author Index

Printing: Mercedes-Druck, Berlin
Binding: Stein+Lehmann, Berlin

Lecture Notes in Computer Science

Sublibrary 6: Image Processing, Computer Vision, Pattern Recognition, and Graphics

Vol. 4191: R. Larsen, M. Nielsen, J. Sporring (Eds.), Medical Image Computing and Computer-Assisted Intervention – MICCAI 2006, Part II. XXXVIII, 981 pages. 2006.

Vol. 4190: R. Larsen, M. Nielsen, J. Sporring (Eds.), Medical Image Computing and Computer-Assisted Intervention – MICCAI 2006, Part I. XXXVVIII, 949 pages. 2006.

Vol. 4179: J. Blanc-Talon, W. Philips, D. Popescu, P. Scheunders (Eds.), Advanced Concepts for Intelligent Vision Systems. XXIV, 1224 pages. 2006.

Vol. 4174: K. Franke, K.-R. Müller, B. Nickolay, R. Schäfer (Eds.), Pattern Recognition. XX, 773 pages. 2006.

Vol. 4170: J. Ponce, M. Hebert, C. Schmid, A. Zisserman (Eds.), Toward Category-Level Object Recognition. XI, 618 pages. 2006.

Vol. 4153: N. Zheng, X. Jiang, X. Lan (Eds.), Advances in Machine Vision, Image Processing, and Pattern Analysis. XIII, 506 pages. 2006.

Vol. 4142: A. Campilho, M. Kamel (Eds.), Image Analysis and Recognition, Part II. XXVII, 923 pages. 2006.

Vol. 4141: A. Campilho, M. Kamel (Eds.), Image Analysis and Recognition, Part I. XXVIII, 939 pages. 2006.

Vol. 4122: R. Stiefelhagen, J.S. Garofolo (Eds.), Multimodal Technologies for Perception of Humans. XII, 360 pages. 2007.

Vol. 4109: D.-Y. Yeung, J.T. Kwok, A. Fred, F. Roli, D. de Ridder (Eds.), Structural, Syntactic, and Statistical Pattern Recognition. XXI, 939 pages. 2006.

Vol. 4091: G.-Z. Yang, T. Jiang, D. Shen, L. Gu, J. Yang (Eds.), Medical Imaging and Augmented Reality. XIII, 399 pages. 2006.

Vol. 4073: A. Butz, B. Fisher, A. Krüger, P. Olivier (Eds.), Smart Graphics. XI, 263 pages. 2006.

Vol. 4069: F.J. Perales, R.B. Fisher (Eds.), Articulated Motion and Deformable Objects. XV, 526 pages. 2006.

Vol. 4057: J.P.W. Pluim, B. Likar, F.A. Gerritsen (Eds.), Biomedical Image Registration. XII, 324 pages. 2006.

Vol. 4046: S.M. Astley, M. Brady, C. Rose, R. Zwiggelaar (Eds.), Digital Mammography. XVI, 654 pages. 2006.

Vol. 4040: R. Reulke, U. Eckardt, B. Flach, U. Knauer, K. Polthier (Eds.), Combinatorial Image Analysis. XII, 482 pages. 2006.

Vol. 4035: T. Nishita, Q. Peng, H.-P. Seidel (Eds.), Advances in Computer Graphics. XX, 771 pages. 2006.

Vol. 3979: T.S. Huang, N. Sebe, M.S. Lew, V. Pavlović, M. Kölsch, A. Galata, B. Kisačanin (Eds.), Computer Vision in Human-Computer Interaction. XII, 121 pages. 2006.

Vol. 3954: A. Leonardis, H. Bischof, A. Pinz (Eds.), Computer Vision – ECCV 2006, Part IV. XVII, 613 pages. 2006.

Vol. 3953: A. Leonardis, H. Bischof, A. Pinz (Eds.), Computer Vision – ECCV 2006, Part III. XVII, 649 pages. 2006.

Vol. 3952: A. Leonardis, H. Bischof, A. Pinz (Eds.), Computer Vision – ECCV 2006, Part II. XVII, 661 pages. 2006.

Vol. 3951: A. Leonardis, H. Bischof, A. Pinz (Eds.), Computer Vision – ECCV 2006, Part I. XXXV, 639 pages. 2006.

Vol. 3948: H.I. Christensen, H.-H. Nagel (Eds.), Cognitive Vision Systems. VIII, 367 pages. 2006.

Vol. 3926: W. Liu, J. Lladós (Eds.), Graphics Recognition. XII, 428 pages. 2006.

Vol. 3872: H. Bunke, A.L. Spitz (Eds.), Document Analysis Systems VII. XIII, 630 pages. 2006.

Vol. 3852: P.J. Narayanan, S.K. Nayar, H.-Y. Shum (Eds.), Computer Vision – ACCV 2006, Part II. XXXI, 977 pages. 2006.

Vol. 3851: P.J. Narayanan, S.K. Nayar, H.-Y. Shum (Eds.), Computer Vision – ACCV 2006, Part I. XXXI, 973 pages. 2006.

Vol. 3832: D. Zhang, A.K. Jain (Eds.), Advances in Biometrics. XX, 796 pages. 2005.

Vol. 3736: S. Bres, R. Laurini (Eds.), Visual Information and Information Systems. XI, 291 pages. 2006.

Vol. 3667: W.J. MacLean (Ed.), Spatial Coherence for Visual Motion Analysis. IX, 141 pages. 2006.

Vol. 3417: B. Jähne, R. Mester, E. Barth, H. Scharr (Eds.), Complex Motion. X, 235 pages. 2007.

Vol. 2396: T.M. Caelli, A. Amin, R.P.W. Duin, M.S. Kamel, D. de Ridder (Eds.), Structural, Syntactic, and Statistical Pattern Recognition. XVI, 863 pages. 2002.

Vol. 1679: C. Taylor, A. Colchester (Eds.), Medical Image Computing and Computer-Assisted Intervention – MICCAI'99. XXI, 1240 pages. 1999.